Questions, Approaches, and Dialogues in Eastern Mediterranean Archaeology

Studies in Honor of Marie-Henriette and Charles Gates

Edited by
Ekin Kozal, Murat Akar, Yağmur Heffron,
Çiler Çilingiroğlu, Tevfik Emre Şerifoğlu, Canan Çakırlar,
Sinan Ünlüsoy, and Eric Jean

Alter Orient und Altes Testament

Veröffentlichungen zur Kultur und Geschichte des Alten Orients
und des Alten Testaments

Band 445

Ugarit Verlag

Questions, Approaches, and Dialogues in Eastern Mediterranean Archaeology

Studies in Honor of Marie-Henriette and Charles Gates

Edited by
Ekin Kozal, Murat Akar, Yağmur Heffron,
Çiler Çilingiroğlu, Tevfik Emre Şerifoğlu, Canan Çakırlar,
Sinan Ünlüsoy, and Eric Jean

2017
Ugarit-Verlag
Münster

Book design: Sinan Kılıç, Alef Editorial Design

Ekin Kozal, Murat Akar, Yağmur Heffron, Çiler Çilingiroğlu, Tevfik Emre Şerifoğlu, Canan Çakırlar, Sinan Ünlüsoy, and Eric Jean (Eds.):

Questions, Approaches, and Dialogues in Eastern Mediterranean Archaeology. Studies in Honor of Marie-Henriette and Charles Gates

Alter Orient und Altes Testament 445

Printed in Germany

ISBN 978-3-86835-251-1

ISSN 0931-4296

Printed on acid-free paper

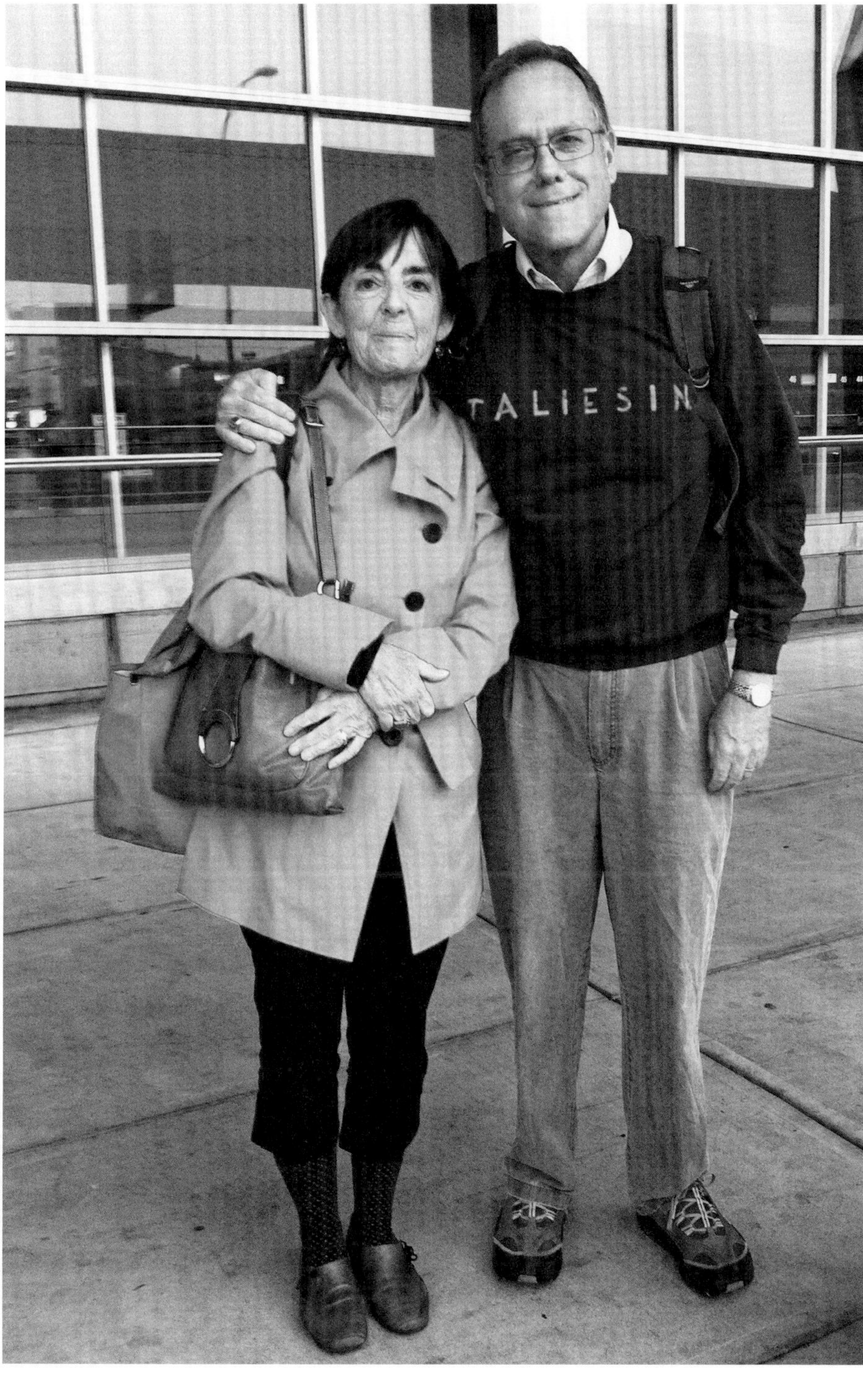

PHOTO BY CAROLINE GATES

Marie-Henriette and Charles Gates at Dulles airport in Washington, DC, 2013

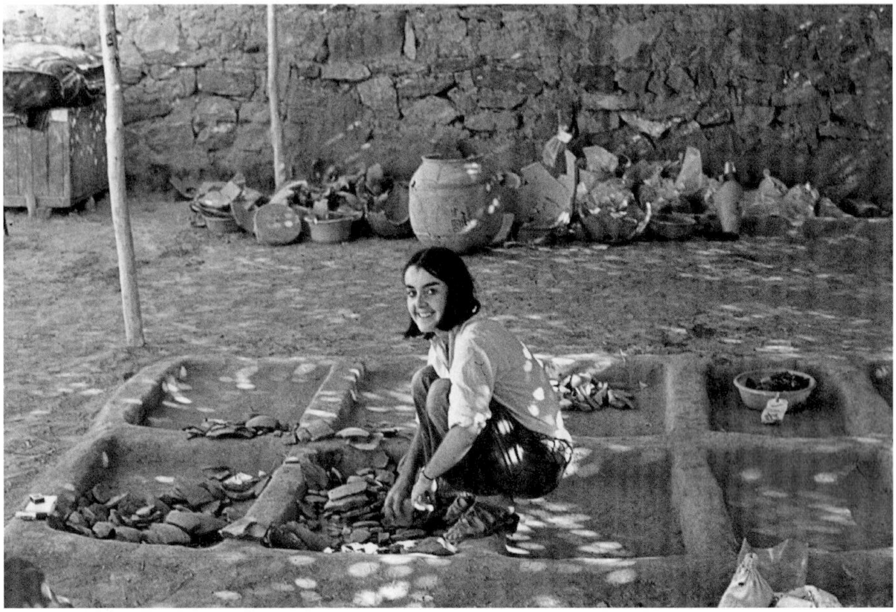

PHOTO BY A. VAN AS

Marie-Henriette Gates sorting pottery at Godin Tepe, 1973

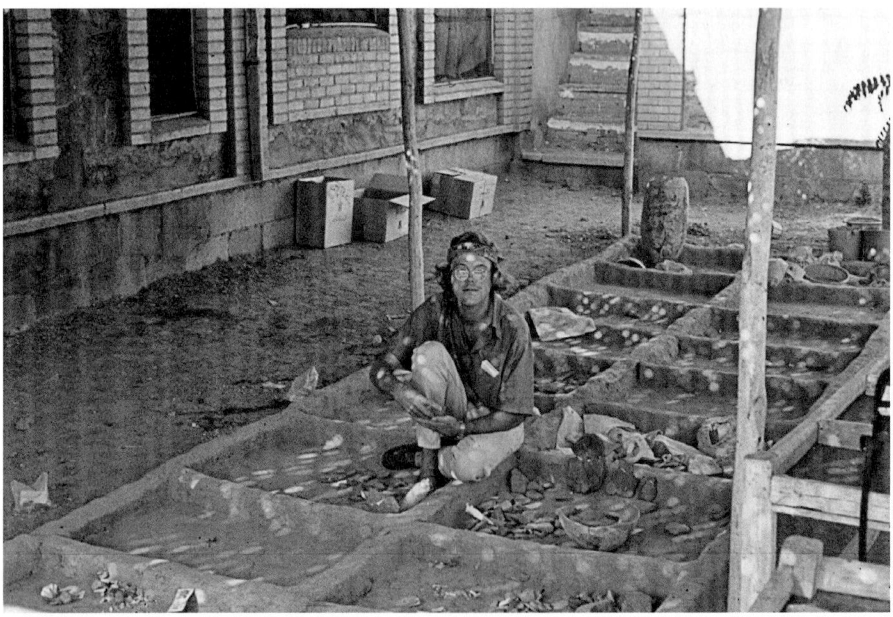

PHOTO BY A. VAN AS

Charles Gates sorting pottery at Godin Tepe, 1973

Contents

Editors' Foreword

It is a privilege to be presenting this book of essays in honor of Marie-Henriette and Charles Gates, two outstanding scholars of Eastern Mediterranean Archaeology, who have made immense contributions to the field. This collection of essays is but an inadequate token of our enormous respect, gratitude, and affection for these two remarkable scholars and their work, which they have always conducted with care and with a generosity of heart. Their dedication to archaeology, and the kindness, patience, and wisdom with which they have inspired students, colleagues and friends, have been truly extraordinary. It is difficult to find the words to express the overwhelming sense of happiness we feel to have 'sprouted' from the seeds planted by such exceptional teachers.

Since 1990, Marie-Henriette and Charles Gates have been teaching at the Department of Archaeology (formerly Department of Archaeology and History of Art) at Bilkent University in Ankara. Both were nominated by their students for Bilkent University's Distinguished Teaching Award in 2008 and 2009 respectively, which Marie-Henriette Gates received in 2008.

Marie-Henriette Gates received her B.A. in Latin and Archaeology from Bryn Mawr College in 1970, following which she entered the graduate program in Near Eastern Languages and Literatures at Yale University. She was awarded her M.Phil. there in 1974 and her Ph.D. in 1976, with a Thesis entitled, *Alalakh-Tell Atchana, Levels VI and V: A Re-examination of a Mid-Second Millennium B.C. Syrian City*, completed under the supervision of Richard S. Ellis. Following her doctorate, Marie-Henriette Gates was awarded a three-year post-doctoral fellowship at the American Research Institute in Turkey (ARIT) in Ankara. During her Fellowship, she also served as Director of ARIT-Ankara between 1977 and 1978.

She returned to the United States in 1979, joining the Classics Department at the University of North Carolina at Chapel Hill, as visiting part-time Assistant Professor. She then became fulltime Assistant Professor, and finally Associate Professor at the same department.

Marie-Henriette Gates first came to Turkey as an undergraduate to participate in the 1969–1971 seasons of the Bryn Mawr excavations at Karataş-Semayük in Elmalı, Antalya, conducted by Machteld Mellink. During 1981–1984, Marie-Henriette Gates was field director of the Gritille salvage excavations near Adıyaman, run by Richard S. Ellis. Also at Gritille were Charles Gates, Christine Eslick, Scott

Redford, and Ann Gunter, who would later form the core team at Kinet Höyük. Marie-Henriette Gates has also excavated at Gordion and Aphrodisias in Turkey, Tell Leilan in Syria, and Godin Tepe in Iran.

In 1990, she joined Bilkent University's then Department of Archaeology and History of Art, for which she served as Chair from 2000 to 2006. Since 1993, she has also been a board member of BLIS, Bilkent Laboratory and International School (formerly BUPS, Bilkent University Preparatory School).

During her time at Bilkent, Marie-Henriette Gates spent the academic year 1997–1998 as Research Associate at the McDonald Institute for Archaeological Research at the University of Cambridge, along with Charles Gates. In 2008 she held a Fellowship at the Institute for Advanced Studies of the Hebrew University of Jerusalem in Israel. She was selected as one of the two American Institute of Archaeology (AIA) Joukowsky Lecturers for 2013–2014, during which period she delivered lectures to AIA societies in Montréal, Toronto, Omaha, Oregon, California, New Mexico, Nevada, Oklahoma, Massachussets, New York, and Ontario.

Marie-Henriette Gates has produced the annual "Archaeology in Turkey" reports for the *American Journal of Archaelogy* during the 1990s and is also on the editorial board of the journal *Anatolia Antiqua*, published by L'Institut Français d'Études Anatoliennes in İstanbul.

Charles Gates received his B.A. in Archaeology at Yale University in 1971, and his Ph.D. in Classical Archaeology from the University of Pennsylvania in 1979 with his Thesis on *Burials at Ialysos and Kameiros (Rhodes) in the Mid-Archaic Period, ca. 625–525 B.C.,* supervised by Donald White.

During 1976–1978 he also held a Fellowship at ARIT-Ankara, and served as Director from 1976 to 1977. Between 1979 and 1990, he taught at the Department of Classics and the Evening College, as Adjunct Professor and Lecturer in Classical Archaeology at the University of North Carolina at Chapel Hill. Prior to joining Bilkent in 1990, Charles Gates was Visiting Assistant Professor in Classics and Director of the Foreign Study Program at Dartmouth College in 1989. In 1997–1998, he was Visiting Fellow at the McDonald Institute for Archaeological Research, and Visiting Scholar at the Faculty of Classics at the University of Cambridge.

Charles Gates is the author of *Ancient Cities: The Archaeology of Urban Life in the Ancient Near East and Egypt, Greece, and Rome* (2003; 2011), recently translated into Turkish as *Antik Kentler: Antik Yakındoğu, Mısır, Yunan ve Roma'da Kentsel Yaşamın Arkeolojisi* (2015). He has co-edited *Sacred Landscapes in Anatolia and Neighboring Regions* (2009) with Jacques Morin and Thomas Zimmermann; and *Anatolian Images* (2013), a collection of short articles by Toni Cross for the newsletter, *Ankara Scene*, with Patricia Ülkü. In 2013 Charles Gates also published *Escape from Smyrna*, a historical mystery for which the author gave his first reading at Kinet Höyük dig-house in 2012.

Prior to Kinet Höyük, Charles Gates excavated at Gordion, Gritille, and Aphrodisias in Turkey, Godin Tepe in Iran, and Oronsay in Scotland.

From 1992 to 2012, Marie-Henriette and Charles Gates have devoted twenty-one years of archaeological work at the multi-period harbor site of Kinet Höyük (Hatay-Dörtyol). The final season of the project was celebrated with a surprise party at the dig-house – affectionately known as Camp Kinet – attended by past and present Kinetters and friends and colleagues from sister excavations.

Kinet Höyük has trained countless students in field archaeology, many of whom are now training students of their own. As is evident from the dedications from many of this volume's contributors, Kinet has made an enormous impact on everyone who has been connected to it in some way. Out of the pitiless humidity of Dörtyol, the spirit of Kinet Höyük – namely, a tireless work ethic, endless generosity, and good-humored appreciation for the hilarity in which archaeology often unfolds – has reached far and wide.

Work towards the final publication of Kinet Höyük Excavations is currently under progress at Bilkent University, where the Kinet study collections are temporarily housed.

Tabula Gratulatoria

Ahmet Şevket Çağan
Ali Umut Türkcan
Ann E. Killebrew
Ann Gunter
Anna Lucia d'Agata
Asa Eger
Aslı Özyar
Asuman Coşkun Abuagla
Aylin Değirmencioğlu
Ayşe Batman
Ayşe Tuğcu
Bahadır Yıldırım
Ben C. Coockson
Bettina Fischer
Brandon R. Olson
Burak Yener
C. Brian Rose
Canan Çakırlar
Carl Knappett
Cécile Michel
Cédric Bodet
Chris Roosevelt
Christine Eslick
Çağatay Karabulut
Çiler Çilingiroğlu
David I. Owen
Delwen Samuel
Derya Yalçıklı
Dominique Collon
Dominique Kassab Tezgör
Ekin Kozal
Elif Denel
Elif Koparal
Elif Ünlü
Eren Koyunoğlu
Eric C. and Roseann M. Schneider
Eric H. Cline
Eric Jean
Erica Hughes
Erkan Akbulut
Esen Öğüş
Fahri Dikkaya
Filiz Tütüncü-Çağlar
Franca L. Cole
Füsun Tülek
Geoffrey D. Summers
Giovanni Salmeri
Glenn Schwartz
Gonca Dardeniz
Gül Pulhan
Gülin Özgönül van Kempen
Günder Varinlioğlu
Gunnar Lehmann
Hatice Pamir
Hayriye Akıl
Hermann Genz
İlknur Taş
Jacques Morin
Jak Yakar
James Osborne
Jan Bouzek
Jason de Block
Jeroen Poblome
Jonathan M. Flood

Julian Bennett
Jürgen Seeher
K. Aslıhan Yener
Karin Kopetzky
Kutalmış Görkay
Lorenzo d'Alfonso
Mara T. Horowitz
Mark Nesbitt
Mary M. Voigt
Mirko Novák
Müge Bulu
Müge Durusu-Tanrıöver
Murat Akar
Mustafa Kaya
Neslihan Yılmaz
N. İlgi Gerçek
Nicholas Postgate
Nicholas Rauh
Onur Ertürk
Özlem Girginer
Philip Bes
Remzi Yağcı
Salima Ikram
Scott Redford
Selim F. Adalı
Serdar Girginer
Sevil Baltalı-Tırpan
Sevil Conka
Sheryl Luzzadder-Beach
Sıla Votruba
Sinan Kılıç
Sinan Ünlüsoy
Stefania Mazzoni
Suna Güven
Tamar Hodos
Tevfik Emre Şerifoğlu
Thomas Zimmermann
Tim Harrison
Timothy Beach
Tuba Ökse
Tuğba Tanyeri-Erdemir
Tuna Şare
Vasıf Şahoğlu
Yağmur Heffron

Marie-Henriette Gates: Publications

Book

1976 *Alalakh-Tell Atchana, Levels VI and V: A Re-examination of a Mid-Second Millennium B.C. Syrian City.* Ann Arbor: University Microfilms International.

Articles

2017 "Gods, Temples, and Cult at the Service of the Hittite State." Pp. 189-210 in Y. Heffron, A. Stone, and M. Worthington (eds.), At the Dawn of History: Ancient Near Eastern Studies in Honour of J. Nicholas Postgate. Winona Lake, IN: Eisenbrauns.

2014 (with C. Çakırlar and S. Ikram) "New Evidence for Fish Processing in the Ancient Near Eastern Mediterranean: Formalized Epinephelus Butcher y in 5th Centur y B.C. Kinet Höyük, Turkey." *International Journal of Osteoarchaeology.*

2014 (with C. Gates, S. Redford and A.A. Eger) "Excavations at Kinet Höyük and Hisn al-Tinat." Pp. 157–171 in *Hatay Arkeolojik Kazı ve Araştırmaları*, ed. by A. Özfırat and Ç. Uygun. Mustafa Kemal Üniversitesi Yayın No: 50. Antakya: Mustafa Kemal Üniversitesi.

2013 "The Hittite Seaport Izziya at Late Bronze Kinet Höyük (Cilicia)." *Near Eastern Archaeology* 76/4: 223–234.

2013 "From Late Bronze to Iron Age on Syria's Northwest Frontier: Cilicia and the Amuq." Pp. 95–116 in S. Mazzoni and S. Soldi (eds.), *Syrian Archaeology in Perspective: Celebrating 20 Years of Excavations at Tell Afis.* Pisa: Edizioni ETS.

2013 "Early Iron Age Newcomers at Kinet Höyük, Eastern Cilicia." Pp. 485–508 in A. E. Killebrew and G. Lehmann (eds.), *The Philistines and Other "Sea Peoples" in Text and Archaeology.* Atlanta: Society of Biblical Literature.

2013 "Southern and Southeastern Anatolia in the Late Bronze Age." Pp. 393–412 in S. R. Steadman and G. McMahon (eds.), *The Oxford Handbook of Ancient Anatolia (8000 – 323 BCE).* Oxford: Oxford University Press.

2011 "Maritime Business in the Bronze Age Eastern Mediterranean: The View from its Ports." Pp. 387–400 in K. Duistermaat and I. Regulski (eds.), *Intercultural Contacts in the Ancient Mediterranean.* Orientalia Lovaniensia Analecta 202. Leuven: Peeters.

2010 "Potters and Consumers in Cilicia and the Amuq during the 'Age of Transformations' (13th–10th Centuries B.C.)." Pp. 65–81 in F. Venturi (ed.), *Societies in Transition: Evolutionary Processes in the Northern Levant between the Late Bronze Age II and the Early Iron Age*. Bologna: Clueb.

2010 (with C. Gates) "Kuzeydoğu Akdeniz'de Bir Kent: Kinet Höyük." *Arkeo-atlas* 7/1:32–35.

2008 (with P. Grave, L. Kealhofer, and B. Marsh) "Using NAA to Identify Scales of Interaction at Kinet Höyük, Turkey." *Journal of Archaeological Science* 35/7:1974–1992.

2007 (with B. Yıldırım) "Archaeology in Turkey, 2004–2005." *American Journal of Archaeology* 111:275–356.

2006 "Dating the Hittite Levels at Kinet Höyük: A Revised Chronology." Pp. 293–309 in D. P. Mielke, U.-D. Schoop, and J. Seeher (eds.), *Strukturierung und Datierung in der hethitischen Archäologie*. Byzas 4. Istanbul: Ege Yayınları.

2005 "Archaeology and the Ancient Near East: Methods and Limits." Pp. 65–78 in D. C. Snell (ed.), *A Companion to the Ancient Near East.* Blackwell Companions to the Ancient World. Oxford: Blackwell.

2003 "Anadolu'nun Güneyinde Bir Yabancı Kazı: Kinet Höyük." *ICOM Türkiye* 3:11–12.

2003 "Kinet Höyük 2002." *Anadolu Akdenizin Arkeoloji Haberleri* 2003/1:17–19.

2001 "Potmarks at Kinet Höyük and the Hittite Ceramic Industry." *Varia Anatolica* 13:137–157.

2000 "Kinet Höyük Hatay, Turkey and MB Levantine Chronology." *Akkadica* 119–120:77–101.

1999 "Kinet Höyük in Eastern Cilicia: A Case Study for Acculturation in Ancient Harbors." *Olba* 2/2:303–312.

1997 "Archaeology in Turkey." *American Journal of Archaeology* 101:241–305.

1996 "Archaeology in Turkey." *American Journal of Archaeology* 100:277–335.

1995 "Archaeology in Turkey." *American Journal of Archaeology* 99:207–255.

1994 "Archaeology in Turkey." *American Journal of Archaeology* 98:249–278.

1992 "Nomadic Pastoralists and the Chalcolithic Hoard from Nahal Mishmar." *Levant* 24:131–139.

1992 "Mycenaean Art for a Levantine Market? The Ivory Lid from Minet el Beidha/Ugarit." *Aegaeum* 8:77–84.

1989 "Artisans and Art in Old Babylonian Mari." Pp. 29–37 in A. C. Gunter (ed.), *Investigating Artistic Environments in the Ancient Near East.* Washington: Smithsonian Institution.

1988 "Dialogues between Ancient Near Eastern Texts and the Archaeological Record: Test Cases from Bronze Age Syria." *Bulletin of the American Schools of Oriental Research* 270:63–91.

1987 "Alalakh and Chronology Again." Pp. 60–86 in P. Åström (ed.), *High, Middle or Low?* Part 2. Göteborg: Paul Åströms.

1986 "The Mitanni." *Biblical Archaeologist* 49:49.

1986 "Casting Tiamat into Another Sphere." *Levant* 1818:75–81.

1986 "From Ebla to Damascus: The Archaeology of Ancient Syria." *Biblical Archaeology Review* 12/3:62–67.

1984 "Zimri-Lim's Palace at Mari." *Biblical Archaeologist* 47:70–87.

1984 "Dura-Europos: A Fortress of Syro-Mesopotamian Art." *Biblical Archaeologist* 47:166–181.

1981 "Alalakh Levels VI and V: A Chronological Reassessment." *Syro-Mesopotamian Studies* 4/2:11–50.

1981 "Report on Idrimi" in J.M. Sasson, "Idrimi and Šarruwa, the Scribe." Pp.318–320 in *Studies in the Civilization and Culture of Nuzi and the Hurrians in Honor of Ernest R. Lacheman*, ed. by M.A. Morrison and D.I. Owen. Winona Lake, IN: Eisenbrauns.

Site Reports

2013 (with A. Eger) "2011 Season at Kinet Höyük (Yeşil-Dörtyol, Hatay)." *Kazı Sonuçları Toplantısı* 34.

2012 "Kinet Höyük (Yeşil-Dörtyol, Hatay) 2010 Sezonu." *Kazı Sonuçları Toplantısı* 33/1:409–417.

2011 "2009 Season at Kinet Höyük (Yeşil-Dörtyol, Hatay)." *Kazı Sonuçları Toplantısı* 32/3:182–195.

2010 "2008 Season at Kinet Höyük (Yeşil-Dörtyol, Hatay)." *Kazı Sonuçları Toplantısı* 31/3:303–320.

2009 "2007 Season at Kinet Höyük (Yeşil-Dörtyol, Hatay)." *Kazı Sonuçları Toplantısı* 30/2:351–368.

2008 "2006 Season at Kinet Höyük (Yeşil-Dörtyol, Hatay)." *Kazı Sonuçları Toplantısı* 29/2:281–298.

2007 "2005 Season at Kinet Höyük (Yeşil-Dörtyol, Hatay)." *Kazı Sonuçları Toplantısı* 28/2:685–700.

2005 "2003 Season at Kinet Höyük (Yeşil-Dörtyol, Hatay)." *Kazı Sonuçları Toplantısı* 26/1:163–174.

2004 "2002 Season at Kinet Höyük (Yeşil-Dörtyol, Hatay)." *Kazı Sonuçları Toplantısı* 25/1:405–416.

2003 "2001 Season at Kinet Höyük (Yeşil-Dörtyol, Hatay)." *Kazı Sonuçları Toplantısı* 24/1:283–298.

2002 "Kinet Höyük 2000 (Yeşil-Dörtyol, Hatay)." *Kazı Sonuçları Toplan-tısı* 23/2:55–62.

2001 "1999 Excavations at Kinet Höyük Hatay: Yeşil-Dörtyol." *Kazı Sonuçları Toplantısı* 22/1:203–222.

2000 "1998 Excavations at Kinet Höyük Hatay: Yeşil-Dörtyol." *Kazı Sonuçları Toplantısı* 21/1:193– 208.

1997 "Archaeological Excavations at Kinet Höyük Hatay: Yeşil-Dörtyol." *Kazı Sonuçları Toplantısı* 20/1:259–281.

1994 "1992 Excavations at Kinet Höyük Hatay: Dörtyol." *Kazı Sonuçları Toplantısı* 15:193–200.

1993 (with I. Özgen) "Report on the Bilkent University Archaeological Survey in Cilicia and the Northern Hatay (1991)." *Araştırma Sonuçları Toplantısı* 10:387–394.

1993 (with S. Ozaner and I. Özgen) "Dating the Coastal Dunes of Karabasamak District, Iskenderun Bay by Geomorphological and Archaeological Methods." *Arkeometri Sonuçları Toplantısı* 8:357–368.

Selected Reviews

1991 Review of *The Early History of the Ancient Near East 9000–2000 B.C.* by Hans J. Nissen, Elizabeth Lutzeier, Kenneth J. Northcott. *The Classical World* 84/5:405–406.

1988 Review of *I tesori di Ebla* by Paolo Matthiae. *Journal of the American Oriental Society* 108/3:518–519.

1982 Review of *The Archaeology of Mesopotamia from the Old Stone Age to the Persian Conquest* by Seton Lloyd; *Babylon* by Joan Oates. *Journal of the American Oriental Society* 102/1:170–171.

1981 Review of *Korucutepe 2: Final Report on the Excavations of the Universities of Chiago, California (Los Angeles) and Amsterdam in the Keban Reservoir, Eastern Anatolia, 1968–1970* by Maurits N. van Loon. *American Journal of Archaeology* 85/4:497–498.

Others

1993 *Mesopotamian Archaeology Slide Set.* 140 slides, 53 pp. caption book. Washington, D.C.: Biblical Archaeology Society.

Charles Gates: Publications

Books

2015 *Antik Kentler. Antik Yakındoğu, Mısır, Yunan ve Roma'da Kentsel Yaşamın Arkeolojisi* [Turkish translation of Ancient Cities, 2nd edn., 2011]. Translated by B. Cezar. Istanbul: Koç Üniversitesi Yayınları.

2013 *Escape from Smyrna*. New Alresford: Top Hat Books.

2011 *Ancient Cities: The Archaeology of Urban Life in the Ancient Near East, Egypt, Greece, and Rome* (2nd ed.). London and New York: Routledge.

2003 *Ancient Cities: The Archaeology of Urban Life in the Ancient Near East, Egypt, Greece, and Rome*. London and New York: Routledge.

2002 *Turkish-English/English-Turkish Dictionary and Phrasebook*. New York: Hippocrene Books.

1983 *From Cremation to Inhumation: Burial Practices at Ialysos and Kameiros During the Mid-Archaic Period, ca. 625–525 B.C.* Occasional Paper **11**, Institute of Archaeology, UCLA. Los Angeles: Institute of Archaeology, University of California, Los Angeles.

Edited books

2013 (with Patricia W. Ülkü) *Anatolian Images*. Toni M. Cross. Istanbul: Libra Books.

2009 (with Jacques Morin and Thomas Zimmermann) *Sacred Landscapes in Anatolia and Neighboring Regions*. BAR International Series 2034. Oxford: Archaeopress.

Articles

2015 "Kinet Höyük (Classical Issos): A Harbor Town in Southeast Cilicia during the Persian and Hellenistic Periods." *Journal of Eastern Mediterranean Archaeological and Heritage Studies* 3/2:81–104.

2014 "Kinet Höyüğün Akamenid Pers ve Helenistic Dönemleri: 1998–2012 Yılları Kazı Sonuçları" [The Achaemenid Persian and Hellenistic Periods at Kinet Höyük: Results from the Excavations of 1998–2012]. Pp. 85–99 in A. Özfırat and Ç. Uygun (eds), *Uluslararası Çağlar Boyunca Hatay ve Çevresi Arkeolojisi Sempozyumu Bildirileri. / Proceedings of the International Symposium on the Archaeology of Hatay and its Vicinity Through the Ages*. Antakya: Mustafa Kemal Üniversitesi Yayınları.

2014 "Ruins and the Archaeologist." Pp. 387–399 in M. Pultar (ed.), *Kültürötesi Bir Gezgin: Gönül Pultar'a Armağan Kitabı / A Transcultural Wanderer: A Festschrift for Gönül Pultar.* Istanbul: Tetragon.

2014 (with M.-H. Gates, S. Redford and A.A. Eger) "Excavations at Kinet Höyük and Hisn al-Tinat." Pp. 157–171 in *Hatay Arkeolojik Kazı ve Araştırmaları*, ed. by A. Özfırat and Ç. Uygun. Mustafa Kemal Üniversitesi Yayın No: 50. Antakya: Mustafa Kemal Üniversitesi.

2013 "Issos: The City and the Battle." *Aktüel Arkeoloji* no. 5/2:88–97.

2012 "Issos – Şehir ve Savaş." *Aktüel Arkeoloji* 5/1:132–139.

2010 "Greeks in the East: A View from Cilicia." Pp. 41–45 in S. Solovyov (ed.), *Archaic Greek Culture: History, Archaeology, Art and Museology. Proceedings of the International Round-Table Conference, June 2005, St-Petersburg, Russia.* BAR International Series 2061. Oxford: Archaeopress.

2010 (with M.-H. Gates) "Kinet Höyük: Kuzeydoğu Akdeniz'de Bir Liman Kenti" ["Kinet Höyük: A Harbor Town in the Northeast Mediterranean"]. *Arkeoatlas* 7/1:32–35.

2006 "Orientalizing and Archaic East Greek Pottery Types from Kinet Höyük (Cilicia)." Pp. 368–372, in B. Avunç (ed.), *Hayat Erkanal'a Armağan: Kültürlerin Yansıması / Studies in Honor of Hayat Erkanal: Cultural Reflections.* Istanbul: Homer Kitabevi.

2005 "The Place of the Achaemenid Persian Period in Archaeological Research in Cilicia and Hatay (Turkey)." Pp. 49–69 in P. Briant and R. Boucharlat (eds.), *L'archéologie de l'empire achéménide: nouvelles recherches.* Paris: De Boccard.

2004 "The Adoption of Pictorial Imagery in Minoan Wall Painting: A Comparativist Perspective." Pp. 27–46 in Anne Chapin (ed.), *Charis. Studies in Honor of Sara A. Immerwahr.* Hesperia Supplement 33. Princeton, NJ: American School of Classical Studies at Athens.

1999 "Research in Late Bronze Age and Iron Age Cilicia: Whence and Whither?" Pp. 265–268, in É. Jean, A. M. Dinçol, and S. Durugönül (eds.), *La Cilicie: espaces et pouvoirs locaux (2e millénaire av. J.-C. – 4e siècle ap. J.-C). Actes de la Table ronde internationale d'Istanbul, 2–5 novembre.* Paris: de Boccard.

1999 "Why Are There No Scenes of Warfare in Minoan Art?" in R. Laffineur (ed.), *POLEMOS. Le contexte guerrier en Egée à l'Âge du bronze. Aegaeum* 19:277–283.

1999 "Kinet Höyük 1992–1997: The Achaemenid Persian and Hellenistic Periods." *Olba* 2:323–332.

1996 "American Archaeologists in Turkey: Intellectual and Social Dimensions." *Journal of the American Studies Association of Turkey* 4:47–68.

1995 "Defining Boundaries of a State: The Mycenaeans and their Anatolian Frontier" in R. Laffineur and W.-D. Niemeier (eds), *POLITEIA. Society and State in the Aegean Bronze Age. Aegaeum* **12**:289–297.

1994 "Priene, Miletus, and Didyma." *Ankara Scene* 21/2:1–8.

1993 "Cappadocia." *Ankara Scene* 20/6:1–7; Reprinted *Ankara Scene* 1998 25/ 31–8.

1992 "Art for Children in Mycenaean Greece" in R. Laffineur and J. L. Crowley (eds.), *EIKON. Aegean Bronze Age Iconography: Shaping a Methodology. Aegaeum* 8:161–171.

1989 "Iconography at the Crossroads: The Aegina Treasure" in R. Laffineur, (ed.), *Transition: Le monde égéen du Bronze moyen au Bronze récent. Aegaeum* 3:215–225.

1985 "Rethinking the Building History of Grave Circle A at Mycenae," *American Journal of Archaeology* 89:263–274.

Encyclopedia Entries

2010 "Acropolis." Pp. 1–2 in R. Hutchison (ed.), *Encyclopedia of Urban Studies*. Thousand Oaks, CA: Sage Publications.

2010 "Agora." Pp. 7–10 in R. Hutchison (ed.), *Encyclopedia of Urban Studies. Thousand* Oaks, CA: Sage Publications.

2010 "City: Historical Overview and Theoretical Issues." Pp. 151–161 in M. Gagarin (ed.), *The Oxford Encyclopedia of Ancient Greece and Rome*, vol. 2. New York: Oxford University Press.

2008 "Cities, Ancient, and Daily Life." Pp. 996–1002, in D. M. Pearsall (ed.), *Encyclopedia of Archaeology*. San Diego, CA: Elsevier/Academic Press.

Reviews

2015 Review of Adam M. Kemezis (ed.), *Urban Dreams and Realities in Antiquity. Remains and Representations of the Ancient City*. (Leiden: Brill, 2015). *Ancient History Bulletin Online Reviews* 5:101–103.

2015 Review of Hadrien Bru and Guy Labarre (eds.), L'Anatolie des peuples, des cités et des cultures. (IIe millénaire av. J.-C. - Ve siècle ap. J.-C.). Colloque international de Besançon - 26–27 novembre 2010. 2 vols. (Besançon: Presses universitaires de Franche-Comté, 2014). Bryn Mawr Classical Review 2015.06.06. http://bmcr.brynmawr.edu/2015/2015–06–06.html.

2014 Review of Scott Redford and Nina Ergin (eds.), *Cities and Citadels in Turkey: from the Iron Age to the Seljuks* (Leuven: Peeters, 2013). *Antiquity* 88, no. 340:674–676.

2014 Review of Zainab Bahrani, Zeynep Çelik and Edhem Eldem (eds.), *Scramble for the Past. A Story of Archaeology in the Ottoman Empire, 1753–1914* (Istanbul: SALT, 2011); Renata Holod and Robert Ousterhout (eds.), *Osman Hamdi Bey and the Americans: Archaeology, Diplomacy, Art* (Istanbul: Pera Museum, 2011); and Robert Ousterhout, John Henry Haynes, *A Photographer and Ar-*

chaeologist in the Ottoman Empire 1881–1900 (Istanbul: Cornucopia Books, 2011). Journal of American Studies of Turkey 39:163–169.

2008 Review of Stephanie Moser, *Wondrous Curiosities: Ancient Egypt at the British Museum* (Chicago: The University of Chicago Press, 2006). *Museum History Journal* 1:288–289.

2007 Review of John E. Curtis and Nigel Tallis (eds.), *Forgotten Empire: The World of Ancient Persia* (Berkeley: University of California Press, 2005). *American Journal of Archaeology* 111:583–584.

2005 Review article. "Tracking the Achaemenid Persians in Anatolia." *American Journal of Archaeology* 109:789–792.

2000 Review of Roger Matthews (ed.), *Ancient Anatolia. Fifty Years' Work by the British Institute of Archaeology at Ankara* (London: British Institute of Archaeology at Ankara, 1998). *American Journal of Archaeology* 104:800–801.

1997 Review of Irene Bald Romano, Gordion Special Studies 2. *The Terracotta Figurines and Related Vessels.* University Museum Monograph 86 (Philadelphia: The University Museum, 1995). *Journal of Hellenic Studies* 117:258–259.

1996 Review of Ian Morris, *Death-Ritual and Social Structure in Classical Antiquity* (Cambridge: Cambridge University Press, 1992) and Ian Morris (ed.), *Classical Greece: Ancient Histories and Modern Archaeologies* (Cambridge: Cambridge University Press, 1994). *Bulletin, Society for the Anthropology of Europe* 10/2:9–10.

1993 Review of Howard Colvin, *Architecture and the After-Life* (New Haven: Yale University Press, n.d.). *Bulletin, Society for the Anthropology of Europe* 7/3:10.

1988 Review of R. Laffineur (ed.), *Thanatos. Les coutumes funéraires en Egée à l'âge du bronze* (Liège: Université de Liège, 1987). *American Journal of Archaeology* 92:605–606.

Blog

Ankara Scribbler www.ankarascribbler.blogspot.com

Life at Kinet Höyük

Roz Schneider — Salima Ikram[1]

The list of attributes that a successful director of a years-long archaeological project needs to combine in order for the project to succeed is legion. As a basis, impeccable scholarship, diplomatic skills, and fund-raising prowess are crucial, supported by a fluency in local languages and social practices, and Dr. Marie-Henriette Gates possesses all these abilities in abundance. Additionally, after coming to Kinet over many years, it seems that successfully combining ever-changing groups of people of extremely varied ages, backgrounds and experiences into a functioning team in often challenging circumstances takes skills that might often go unnoticed - unless they were missing! Running an archaeological excavation can be described as directing a military campaign while running a summer camp for teen-agers mixed in with the periodic addition of government officials, curious neighbors, and willful 2 year olds. But whatever the challenges of running either a military campaign or a summer camp, they cannot have been more wildly varied than those faced by Marie-Henriette during the many years of excavations at Kinet.

As director of the campaign, her work started long before the season, plotting the plan of excavation and survey, and managing to raise the necessary funds to do it all. She had to orchestrate, down to the minutest detail, the arrival and departure of her many and varied team members, organize their accommodation, and cheerfully meet and greet them regardless of the time of day or night they arrived, or on what manner of transport (ranging from chic, sporty cars, to Dr. Scott Redfords's beloved and venerable land rover, to motor-cycles, public buses, *dolmuş*, and once even a gendarme rescue vehicle). Every morning M-H would sit alone on her campstool in the sherd yard contemplating the day's campaign as the rest of us munched our breakfast. Like a good general, she dealt with her fears, worries, and bureaucratic issues in private, always showing the team an untroubled visage.

Throughout the summer, Bayan Gates's personnel management skills were very much at the fore. Most fundamental was the care and respect she showed for all of us whether she had known us only a few days or for many years, and regard-

1 Department of Sociology, Anthropology, Psychology and Egyptology, The American University of Cairo, AUC Avenue, New Cairo 11835, Egypt.

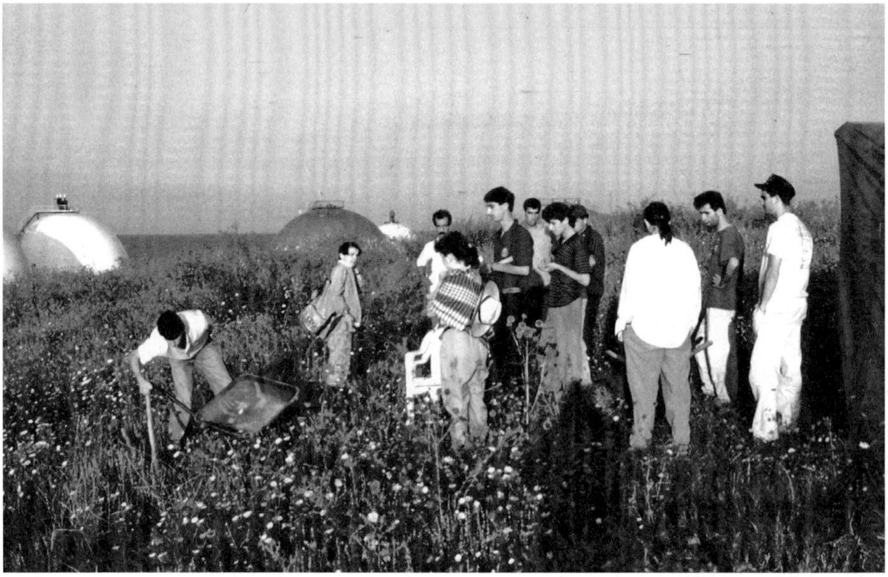

FIG. 1 First excavation day at Kinet Höyük, 1992.

less of our status in the world of academia. This was illustrated by Marie-Henriette's early morning bread runs: in the hot and humid pre-dawn, M-H would drive off to the town bakery in her pumpkin colored Mercedes. She would return a short time later with hot, fresh bread for our breakfast just as the sky lightened to what looked like a photo of dawn on the Serengeti, and the baby swallows above our outdoor tables reached the peak of their noisy pleas for breakfast (with the backdrop of the giant golf-balls of the petrol tanks). That image of open baby bird beaks quickly became the visual symbol of the care M-H showed for our wellbeing.

Years later we were able to have bread delivered in the mornings, so she did not have to go fetch the bread, at least most of the time. But even if no one else was up at 4:15 to prepare and lay out breakfast, she always was there to slice the cheese finely and neatly, cut up the tomatoes and cucumbers, put out the olives, and dish out the jam. And for the rest of us, knowing that whatever else might have happened over night, there would be hot tea or coffee and fresh hot bread, providing a reassuring constant toward which even the most groggy could orient themselves. It made all of us, no matter our age, feel as if someone was really thinking about our comfort and welfare.

Just finding adequate housing for the team was a big challenge for the first few years. In the early years, we often had several houses in a season. One year we began at the grade school in the little town of Yeşilköy, but after a few days, just as we finished the first day of excavation, we were compelled to leave for po-

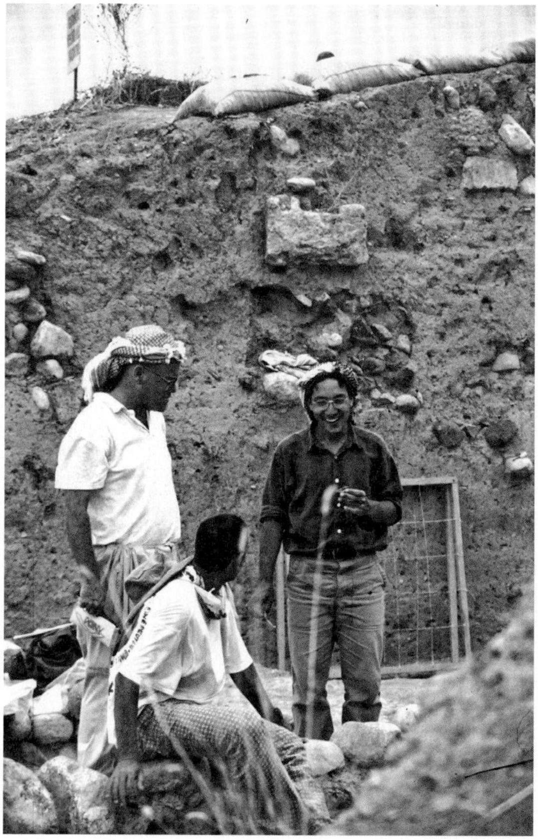

FIG. 2 Charles Gates with the assistants of Emre Tevfik Şerifoğlu and Çağatay Karabulut in Trench E, 1997.

litical/military reasons. This was not entirely unpopular among some of us, since that very day we discovered there were leeches in the squat toilet. No doubt our departure was a terrific disappointment to the neighborhood, since our attempts to organize ourselves had been the source of intense amusement to neighborhood children and adults alike. Somehow, using her extraordinary powers of persuasion, Marie-Henriette managed to convince Delta Petrol that their offices, which were conveniently adjacent to the mound and were empty for the summer, were really quite suitable for the excavation team, so we moved there. The following year began in a spectacular location – the caravanserai at Payaş. The distance to the excavation site was a bit of a drawback, as were the tour groups arriving periodically to see this site of architectural and historical significance, but sadly, the humidity in this vast stone building, which proved sufficient to melt our conservator's humidity test strips, made the idea of working there or conserving any artifact at all utterly laughable. Those who had been met by strange creatures crawling out of one of the open drains in the showers or had mold growing out of their clothes were none too sorry to retreat once more to the relative safety of Delta's offices.

The next year found us at the Yeşilköy middle school, where there was space enough for sleeping, but often no water during the day for washing sherds or bones. Sometimes though, there was an excess of liquid, like when the septic tank, full after a year's school use, overflowed in a flood that caused a mass exodus of staff and artifacts into the relative safety of the schoolyard. Meanwhile, M-H was hard at work getting us a purpose-built dig house. At last, despite various irregularities in the behavior of the architect and builders, the next year the Kinet project had a home. This dear two-story yellow and white building, with its spacious courtyard and small gardens planted by Mustafa Kaya with roses, jasmine and fruit trees, provided a wonderfully stable home for the project for the rest of the time we were there.

Of course, having our own home did not solve all problems; some, like plumbing, were perennial. The famous electrical showers of Ercan Trans were already the stuff of legend, thanks to Dr. Toni Cross' vivid descriptions, as was Dr. Norbert Karg's liquefaction of some plastic plumbing at the grade school by his application of hydrochloric acid in an attempt to clear the drains. Once installed in our own house, most of our plumbing problems were less exotic but no less time and attention consuming: leaks, drips, occasional floods, and an exposed hot water pipe resulted in singed archaeologists. Sometimes there would be no water at all, and M-H would have to order a tank to be delivered by the municipality. Finally, in a brave attempt to secure a more predictable water supply, M-H had a well dug and pumps installed at the dig house. As a result, in these later years our plumbing crises were almost always combined with the failure of the electrical supply. And that, we soon learned, was best met by lying down quietly on one's mattress and attempting not to sweat too much.

Although M-H made sure every season that our food needs were catered for, breakfast, as mentioned above, required a refrigerator. Not surprisingly with so many people, its use was open to a variety of interpretations. Researching the contents of the anonymous, opaque plastic bags which materialized overnight required bravery and daring, and spurred on by M-H (or led by her), the sometimes bizarre and slightly rancid, or occasionally delicious, contents would be unearthed and disposed of – either orally or into the maw of the bin. Occasionally, what seemed like normal food that was stored in the fridge would start behaving in unusual and terrifying ways, like the yogurt that Norbert used to purchase from the Yeşilköy corner store. This occasionally got so enthusiastic that it would bubble out of Norbert's specially bought yogurt container and effervesce joyfully over the shelves of the fridge, baptizing all and sundry in its vicinity.

Wearing her camp director's cap, M-H always made sure that some civilizing influences were available to lighten and enlighten our weeks. Many times on our days off, Dr. Charles Gates or Dr. Scott Redford would generously organize tours

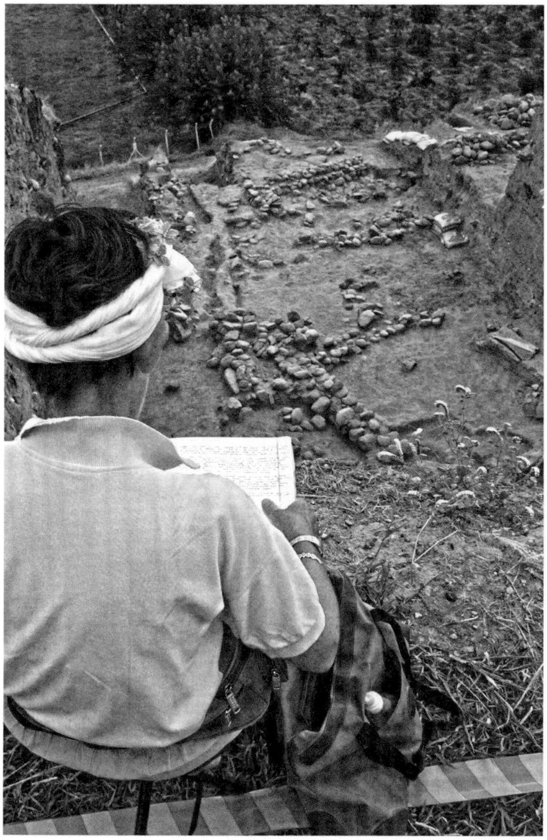

FIG. 3 Marie-Henriette Gates taking daily notes over the deep trench E/H, 2005

of nearby sites. And the bureaucratic requirements of our trips to Antakya almost always left time for lunch at Harbiye or a museum visit, if not both.

One tradition which encouraged a return, however brief, to our shiny clean, non-trench selves was Friday dinners out. During the first years, with the help of Dr. Toni Cross and her husband İhsan, we were allowed access to the Botaş social service facilities just north of Kinet. These Friday dinners took place at the Portofino – a charming restaurant just slightly off shore. The Portofino had marvelous little wooden balconies where you could sit with a drink and contemplate the passage of millennia on the site, or speculate on the life adventures of the various exotic animals, most memorably the llamas, who strolled about the grounds just opposite the bridge to the restaurant.

For several years we were also granted access to the Botaş swimming pool where, as Marie-Henriette's mother, Mimi Hanım, pointed out, even "deep" shade was available to complete the cooling process provided by the pool, the soft drinks, and the ice cream available there. In fact, Mimi Hanım was a major civilizing force herself. Her conversations, whether about French literature and philosophy, university life or her childhood in Algeria, curious flowering plants, or the variety of feline characters she had known, were always reminders of the world outside our immediate field of view and therefore most welcome. Often all that was needed to free us from our tunnel vision was for her to walk past trailing one of her lovely perfumes. Her solutions to problems of daily living were often surprising and innovative, and generally successful. Her personal campaign against squeaky door hinges was of great help to those of us who needed every shred of sleep we could get. Her weapon of choice was any kind of skin or face cream which she applied to the hinge until it stopped misbehaving, ignoring the WD-40 that had proven unsuccessful to the task. She taught us the quick and effective way of cleaning silver jewelry that blackened quite dramatically at Kinet: apply toothpaste and brush!

In subsequent years, the charms of Botaş were succeeded by on-the-premises beer coolers (thanks to Dr. Redford), the discovery of Magnum ice creams at the disco near the *tatil sitesi* (which provided additional joys and entertainment to team members), and walks down the beach to our favorite fish restaurant, the Yakamoz Balık Lokantası, to view the sunset, chat, and unwind after a long week in the trenches. This commanded a marvelous view of sunset at sea, and supplied us with delicious meze and varying beverages of choice, all of which made for very merry evenings, some that ended back at the dig house with Charlie (and others) gyrating madly to various songs, old and new.

The Doctors Gates provided other welcome reminders of a world beyond the intensity of the excavation. For several years, gentle tones from Marie-Henriette's afternoon *ud* practice gracefully drifted through our nap times. And some years Charlie would practice memorizing poetry, which he would declaim on request. Charlie was also most generous with the condiments he procured to enliven the canteen cuisine, particularly the pomegranate molasses and his hot peppers, and we are forever grateful to him and Scott Redford for the fans they provided for the workroom.

Of course, over the years, we came up with some civilizing influences of our own. Among these were a variety of exercise routines, which usually made the practitioners feel less lump-like, and at least amused the onlookers. We had early morning tai chi on weekends and Charlie's pre-dinner yoga group on weekdays, which, like Rado Kabaharova's weightlifting, lasted for years. We also had very sportive years with volleyball or soccer "teams". Most exotic of all however, was Murat Akar's climbing walls where, if you were lucky, you could see him hang by a finger as you checked your email nearby. Some nights while we waited for our bodies to cool down to normal body temperature before attempting to sleep, we would play games like Pictionary or the not too dissimilar, "fictionary-dictionary" or our favorite "happy families". The latter two were often particularly hilarious if we could enlist people with different native languages or cultural backgrounds; there was always more than enough creativity to make for many memorable evenings.

Over the years, non-human animals posed frequent challenges to the dig-house, the artefacts, and the team. There were the scary, dangerous ones: the snakes, the scorpions, the centipedes, and the mysterious creature that bit Fran Cole one night as she and Salima took a cool evening stroll through Yeşilköy. These encounters often resulted in M-H ferrying the afflicted to the *yılancı* (the "snake-man"who would luckily, and often mysteriously, affect a cure. The scourge of the rats, who invaded the house when all the snakes that kept them under control had been killed by the over-zealousness of Mustafa Kaya, meant that many of the bags containing artefacts were eaten away, and huge amounts of rat fecal matter deposited in the crates. Abby Isaac and Müge Bulu (Akar) heroically spent much of two seasons clearing up the mess, while others dealt with the rats themselves.

There were also the mostly harmless but annoying animals: the baby chickens Roz used as a means of ridding herself of unwanted watermelon but who were easily distracted into playing among Salima's carefully sorted bones, much to her irritation. Their rather thuggish, juvenile delinquent-type older siblings strutted right into the middle school where we were staying that year and menaced Dr. Norbert Karg in his room so he had to resort to standing on a chair, and then tried to intimidate Fran Cole in her lab. There were the begging animals, mostly dogs, in varying degrees of desperation. The unlucky adoption of a puppy in the early years turned out very badly when its attraction to the neighbors' chickens proved fatal (to the chickens) and it was relocated only with the greatest difficulty. This disturbing incident resulted in a firm "no (local) pets" policy, was broken only once, by a kitten named Squeak, or isqueak, as the Turkish students called him. He and Fran developed a very close relationship, but alas, since no one present could provide him with a home when the season ended, he did not become a permanent team member. On a few occasions, some of us brought our own cats when there was nowhere else for them to stay. And when Marie- Henriette inherited her mother's cat, Bellisima, despite her luxurious fur coat, she too came to stay the season. Later Charlie and Marie-Henriette's new kitten, Momtaz, replaced Bellisima as our (generally invisible) feline overseer. The wild creatures (other than snakes – the darlings of the bone team, and a very select few others) also were a source of entertainment, fascination, and sometimes repulsion. Roz's regular rescue of doomed baby birds, the tracking of the hedgehogs across the courtyard, the thumping of mating turtles, and the racing of rats across the grape vines were all part of the natural history experience at Camp Kinet.

Work was hard, but a delight. Whether on the mound or at the house, M-H would come by to check on progress, advice on field problems, and discuss ideas, insane or otherwise. Images of her climbing on ladders to photograph trenches, or flying above us trying to photograph Kinet aerially (we laid out sherd baskets in a giant k-h to mark the house) are vivid in our minds – especially as she was caught half in flight in one of the group photos out on the mound.

Respect for the team's diversity was matched by a pervasive sense of common purpose not only of a shared passion for excavating our Höyük, but also, in part resulting from the variety of challenges in our environment. This, together with Bayan Gates's inclusivity, may have also prevented each year's group from splitting into cliques, whether that of field or house, age, background or anything else. Rather, there was a sense of shared excitement which was fed by the weekly mound tours that allowed field and house staff to unify and share their knowledge, shedding light on diverse aspects of ancient Kinet.

This inclusivity extended even to aspects of the project that were a frequent source of annoyance to M-H, like the ever increasing, and invariably deteriorating, bags of heavy residue which stubbornly accumulated under the stairs. These were the result of the (temporarily) orphaned botanical sampling procedure. Thanks to volunteers and staff, the samples continued to be collected and cleaned, and forms filled out according to the protocol established by the original archaeobotanist, but sorting through the dried rocky matrix left behind once the botanical remains were removed was a time-consuming and tedious process. And although a few of the rest of us sometimes enjoyed the two-dimensional excavation of fish bones and tiny sherds, not to mention the occasional flashy bead, it was Marie-Henriette who took the orphan in hand and made sure the whole heap of bags was finally sorted and the results recorded.

In retrospect it's hard to say which of her many "hats" were most important, but we are glad she was willing and able to wear all of them.

Marie-Henriette's many students and colleagues have their own reasons to be grateful to her, but those of us at Kinet who benefitted from her many skills and years of care want to say thank you too.

PART 1

Neolithic and Chalcolithic

Temples as Sacred Houses: A Case Study from Tepe Gawra

Sevil Baltalı Tırpan[1]

Abstract

In this article, I explore the symbolic relationship between 'house' and 'temple' architecture at the northern Mesopotamian site of Tepe Gawra during the Late Chalcolithic period. Through a diachronic and comparative study of house and temple architecture and use of space, I illustrate how standardized temple architecture appropriated and further developed the symbolism already present in the structure of the houses. I argue that temples symbolically represent houses as microcosms of the larger cosmological principles and the social order. The analysis of ritual-architectural elements within the houses suggests that access to ritual knowledge, ancestor veneration, and possession of inalienable items played an important role as the basis for social differences at Tepe Gawra.

The idea that there is a symbolic relationship between Mesopotamian temples and houses is mostly based on textual data such as lexical temple lists.[2] The textual readings suggest that temples were the houses of gods. The archaeological analysis of temples shows that the main tripartite layout of the temples was also used for houses. In this article, I explore the symbolic relationship between temples and houses in northern Mesopotamia by re-visiting the site of Tepe Gawra during the Late Chalcolithic period (*ca.* 4300–3000 BC). This is an important period of political centralization and formation of hierarchical social systems in Mesopotamian history. These changes are revealed through regional centers, long-distance exchange, uses of bureaucratic devices, monumental architecture and institutionalized religion manifested through standardized temple architecture.[3] It is clear that these temples were a direct manifestation of the interrelationship between religion and political social control. I think a nuanced understanding of the relationship between houses and temples is extremely important to be able

1 İnsan ve Toplum Bilimleri Bölümü, Fen-Edebiyat Fakültesi, İstanbul Teknik Üniversitesi, Maslak, 34469, İstanbul, Turkey.

2 George 1993.

3 Frangipane 2002; 2009; Rothman 2002.

to comprehend the underlying socio-political implications and dynamics in this pivotal era of political centralization.

This article consists of two parts. The first part discusses various anthropological theories of architecture and houses that inform my analysis. In the second part, I discuss ritual-architectural elements of selected houses from Tepe Gawra Levels XII and XIA. This part traces the ritual significance of houses through the analyses of organization and use of space within houses. I suggest that the standardized religious architecture appropriated and further developed the cosmological symbolisms already present in the structure of the houses. I also argue that access to ritual knowledge and performance played an important role as the basis of social differences.

The Anthropology of House and Architecture

A detailed understanding of the relationship between temples and houses has been hindered in Mesopotamian archaeology in general due to a lack of contextual data from houses, and the classification of built spaces into the dichotomous functional categories of public/private, temple/house and religious/secular architecture. Western notions of public and private do not necessarily work cross-culturally. In traditional archaeological analysis, houses are usually defined through a room function analysis as well as the size and number of rooms. If the material content of the building reveals 'domestic' and/or craft activities, such as household ceramics, cooking facilities, such as ovens, and storage facilities, then the building is often accepted as a house/domicile. Therefore, houses are perceived merely as dwellings or residential buildings with activity and storage areas mostly secular in character.

The vast array of ethnographic and theoretical work on houses problematizes the categorization of houses only as secular and domestic structures.[4] According to these studies, houses are not merely dwellings, they are the microcosm of larger structures revealing both the material/visible and the immaterial/invisible aspects of society, and can give access to an understanding of social organization.[5] The house is a place of residence, a ritual site and a social unit. In other words, houses can be embodiments of social groups within a society.[6] They can be a place for domestic activity, a residential unit, a burial place and a place for ritual.[7] Houses

4 Carsten and Hugh-Jones 1995; Joyce and Gillespie 2000; Levi-Strauss 1991, 1987; Waterson 1995, 1997.

5 Gillespie 2000, 139.

6 Levi-Strauss 1991.

7 Joyce and Gillespie 2000; McKinnon 2000; Waterson 1990.

can be status symbols, and their variation can enclose hierarchical social order.[8] The rituals practiced within the house can enhance the family's social prestige and rank. The houses' history, long-time occupation, renovation by several generations and generations, family items such as heirlooms that form part of the dwellers' social memory and in-house burials of ancestors can be used in the construction and authentication of social groups.[9] Sources of social power that serve to mark some groups as eminent may include access to cosmological knowledge, religious-ritual, beliefs about the special origins of certain families and exotic knowledge expressed through possession of objects from distant places.[10]

The architectural dimension of houses can provide a starting point for examining larger socio-cosmological principles and symbolic construction of social differentiations within societies. Cosmology can be defined as ideas and theories about the origins and the structure of the universe that determine the perception of time, space and causality.[11] Socio-cosmic refers to the cosmological ideas that cause people within a given culture to perceive things from a particular view and organize their social life according to those ideas.[12] The cosmology of a society affects religion by creating a world view that is used to explain the supernatural, the divine and the ideal life.[13] In many cultures, people conceptualize the universe in the architectonic form of a house.[14]

Through architecture, societies' socio-cultural categories gain material existence. At the same time, these built spaces become lived/experienced spaces which are used and changed by people in the performance of everyday life. Therefore, architecture can be examined simultaneously as "architecture as constituted" and "architecture as lived".[15] "Architecture as constituted" refers to larger socio-cosmological principles that can be described as "the symbolic relations of cultural order"[16] according to which the people design their built spaces. These principles start operating at the level of design in the minds of the builders, and subsequently the imagined design is realized as a result of the performance of construction. The choice of materials that are used and the technology and style of building are

8 Pearson and Richards 1994, 9.

9 McKinnon 2000.

10 Helms 1988, 1998; Joyce and Gillespie 2000; Carsten and Hugh-Jones 1995; Weiner 1992.

11 Flannery and Marcus 1998, 37–38.

12 Bell 1992, 1997; Insoll 2004.

13 Flannery and Marcus 1998, 39.

14 Jones 2000, 113.

15 Baltalı Tırpan 2013, 472.

16 Sahlins 1985; Baltalı Tırpan 2013, 472.

dictated by larger cosmological principles. Therefore, built spaces have a "dual existence", "structure in convention" and "structure in action".[17] Architecture not only reflects society but is also actively manipulated to construct society, illustrating social action and thus agency.[18] An investigation of architecture, therefore, has the potential to provide information about social structure and action.

Ethnographic studies suggest that from the construction of the houses –such as the ritual dedication of the house– through their life-cycle, rituals take place.[19] Ethnographic data reveal that houses are considered to be living beings often believed to have a soul or resident spirit. During the life-cycle of each house, rituals are performed to nourish the house and cleanse it.[20] The thick layer of white plastering of the rooms and the floors can be part of the house life-cycle rituals. In a Swahili example, white plastering is used to cleanse the house from possible evil forces and thus can be associated with ritual purity.[21] The color white is accepted as the symbol of purity in many societies.[22] Periodic rebuilding of houses is often an example of house rituals. Ritual regulations also govern the spatial arrangement within the houses. Ritual principles may intertwine and dominate people's living spaces, who pursue life according to these principles.

The use of houses as sacred spaces for the performance of communal ceremonies is seen in south-east Asia, particularly among the Sa'dan Toraja.[23] Their noble houses have been used as sacred houses for communal ritual as well as residences. These houses symbolize family rank, and the rituals performed there strengthen the family's social prestige.[24] According to Waterson,[25] the origin-houses of Sumba are believed to have sacred powers and therefore they could be classified as temples; however, they are also ritual centers for certain clans who consider them as their houses. These houses contain the sacred heirlooms of the clan that allow contact with sacred ancestors. The rituals accompanying mortuary practices can also be considered within the realm of house ritual.[26] These rituals may include burying the deceased in particular parts of the house together with caches of

17 Baltalı Tırpan 2013, 472; Bourdieu 1973; 1977, 89; Lefebvre 1991, 69–73; Sahlins 1976, 35–36; 1985, ix.

18 Hodder 1994, 74.

19 Braithwaite 1982; Bradley 2005; Herbich and Dietler 1993, 27; Gillespie 2000; Plunket 2002.

20 Plunket 2002, 13.

21 See Donley 1982, 72; 1990.

22 Metcalf and Huntington 1991.

23 See Waterson 1990, 43–46.

24 Waterson 1990, 43–45.

25 Waterson 1990, 43.

26 Hodder 1990; Plunket 2002.

certain materials.[27] These rituals signify belief systems about the transformation of the deceased into ancestors. The spatial locations of these burials may signify a relationship of continuity between the living members of the house and their ancestors.[28]

The cross-cultural anthropological exploration of houses and their architecture illustrate that the common terminology that is used to interpret built spaces purely as 'domestic', 'secular', 'private', 'religious' and 'public' can be misleading. Many societies do not have a sharp separation between 'domestic/private' and 'public', and 'house' and 'temple', whereas these divisions exist in most western traditions. In different traditions, there is a continuum between public and private buildings, as well as between a temple and a house. Many functions may be fused within a single structure; in south-east Asian societies ritual functions are inseparable from a house's identity. We can see the fusing of house, granary, and ritual site into a single structure. A private house that is so defined according to traditional criteria can also become a public space at a given time, and certain rooms and units of the house can be used for public purposes. For example, we know that during the Ottoman period the judiciary court was held at the house of the judge until the 19th century. During judiciary activities, the space/house was transformed into a public space and experienced as such.[29] Therefore, meaning(s) of built spaces should not be treated as something fixed, unchanging and singular, since they are meaningful objects or forms that exist only through peoples' interactions with them. Buildings can sustain multiple meanings, different forms of interactions between people and different activities that are carried out at certain temporal contexts, which can give spaces a variety of meanings.

Houses and Ritual-Architectural Spaces in Tepe Gawra

As a case study, I will re-visit examples from Late Chalcolithic period tripartite houses from the northern Mesopotamian site of Tepe Gawra, Levels XII and XIA to illustrate how formal temple architecture of later periods (Levels XI, X, IX and VIII) developed out of house architecture and how houses and temples fuse multiple functions and meanings. I chose to look at structures from this extensively excavated site in northern Mesopotamia because of its deep, intact stratigraphy and wide horizontal exposures. To this end, I used Tobler's volume[30] on the Tepe Gawra excavations, field reports and line drawings of Tepe Gawra from the Uni-

27 Plunket 2002, 13.

28 Grove and Gillespie 2002, 13; Plunket 2002, 13.

29 Ergene 2003.

30 Tobler 1950.

versity of Pennsylvania Museum archives and Rothman's excellent volume [31] on Tepe Gawra providing object distribution analyses within the buildings.

Tepe Gawra is located 20 km northeast of Nineveh in northern Iraq (Fig. 1). It was a one-hectare site during the fourth millennium BC. [32] The excavations at the site provided a stratigraphic sequence from the 6th millennium BC to the mid-2nd millennium BC. The earliest levels belonged to the Halaf period, and preceding levels showed similarities to the southern Mesopotamian Ubaid material styles. The succeeding period chronologically corresponds to the Late Chalcolithic 1–3 periods of northern Mesopotamia, and it shows a distinct material cultural style. [33] The Late Chalcolithic levels of Tepe Gawra chronologically correspond to the Early and Early/Middle Uruk periods of southern Mesopotamia. [34]

The analysis of a sample of tripartite houses in Levels XII and XIA suggest that at Tepe Gawra formal religious architecture of later periods gradually developed out of tripartite house architecture. The standardized temple architecture at Tepe Gawra comes from later periods, such as Levels XI, X, IX and VIII. [35] These temples have eight major characteristics according to Rothman [36] and Tobler: [37] 1) tripartite floorplan with an entrance in front of the building; 2) niches usually placed in the back wall of the main room; 3) a platform or an altar in the center of the main room; 4) offering vessels or other votive items; 5) monumental size; 6) white plastered main room; 7) central location with respect to the other architectural remains of the settlement; and 8) a basin sunk in the floor. These main features are also observed in southern Mesopotamian temples from Ubaid and Uruk Periods, which also include other major features such as cardinal orientation, placement on a higher platform, and evidence of frequent rebuilding. [38]

A sample of tripartite houses from Levels XII and XIA reveal ritual-architectural elements of standardized temple architecture. In Level XII, there are five building complexes that have tripartite plans. [39] Tobler, who excavated and published the results, defined all these buildings as 'secular' since they contained ovens and household objects. [40] However, a close examination of the morphology of the buildings,

---

31 Rothman 2002.

32 Rothman 2002, 10.

33 Rothman 2002, 3; Speiser 1935, 30–35; Tobler 1950.

34 See Rothman 2002, 3, Table 1.1 for chronology.

35 See Rothman 2002; Tobler 1950, XXII.

36 Rothman 2002, 73–74.

37 Tobler 1950, 10.

38 See Heinrich 1982; Jawad 1965; Kubba 1987; Lundquist 1983.

39 See Rothman 2002, fig. 5.13.

40 Tobler 1950.

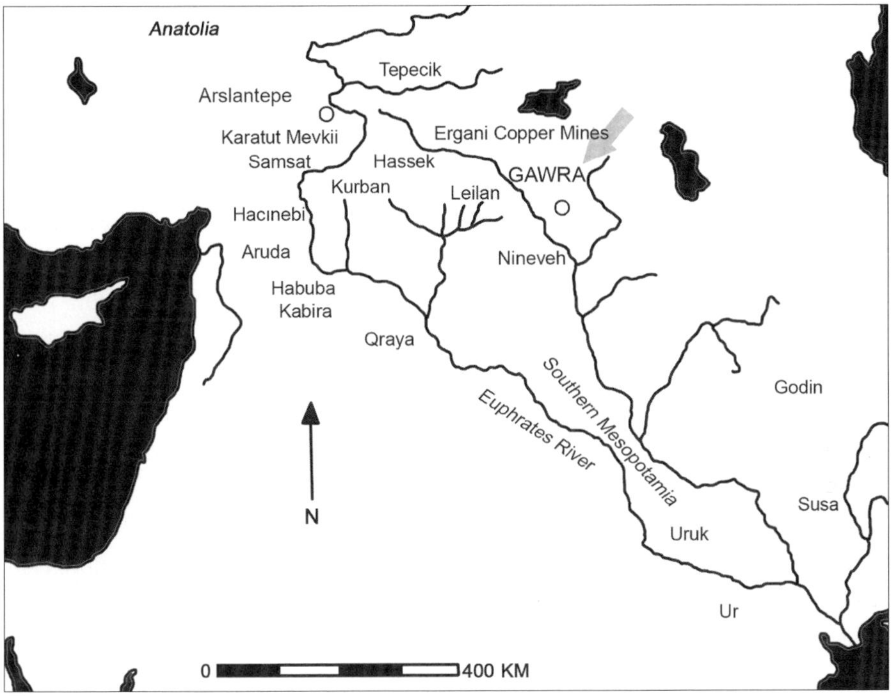

FIG. 1 Location of Tepe Gawra (modified after Stein 1998, fig. 11–1).

organization of space, decorative aspects and location of fixed and non-fixed elements show that they actually fall in-between the rigid categories of house and temple.

Building I is the largest structure in the excavated part of the town, with a 12.30 x 11.75 m external dimension.[41] It is located at the northeast where there was a major entrance to the town. The distribution of small objects within the building, such as spindle whorls, celts, pottery vessels, an obsidian core and implements, utilitarian bowls, a storage jar and a spatula along with an oven, suggest that the building was a house.[42] The building in terms of its formal tripartite plan, entrance system, decorative elements and features such as the white plastered walls and floors, niches at the rear wall of the main room, and the presence of a model hut, resembles standard temples of later periods.[43] These ritual-architectural elements suggest the house also had a religious significance encompassing ritual activities. In terms of use of space, the main room as a public area of the house fuses several different activities together. This is also supported by the findings of serving bowls,

41 Tobler 1950, 25–29, fig. 2.

42 Rothman 2002, 77; Tobler 1950, 28.

43 See Rothman 2002, 77; Speiser 1935; Tobler 1950.

a large pithos and the presence of a large bench at the back of the room.[44] Due to its large size (60.5 m^2) and high accessibility, the main room was the public part of the house where guests may have been received, and therefore the room may have housed public ritual ceremonies.

Tobler mentions the existence of a large number of sub-floor burials in the main room.[45] The house's association with sub-floor burials suggests its relation to death rituals and ancestor veneration. Although Tobler does not provide more information on the sub-floor burials, their presence under the main room may suggest that the deceased transformed into ancestors as a result of mortuary rituals by the living inhabitants of the house.

The room's material content also exhibited several spindle whorls suggesting small-scale household production of textiles. A flint core found in the room suggests household production of stone tools. The presence of personal items, such as a macehead and jewelry, suggest the residential status of the room. Two sealings were also found in the room, suggesting receipt of items sealed somewhere else and sent to the house.[46] In terms of its size and number of rooms, the house might have been a multi-family unit. Its solid, formal plan, large size, location at the main entrance of the town and the large, enclosed, open courtyard in front of it communicate the importance and the distinct status of the inhabitants of the house.

This building represents a house that fused several functions together, such as public gathering, ritual activities, mortuary (death-ritual) activities, domestic activities of food preparation and small-scale household production of textiles and stone tools. The deep private spaces of the house consist of the kitchen area with cooking facilities such as an oven, storage areas and the blocked room with a single sub-floor burial.[47] The strategic location of House I in the settlement, its size and the architectural elements and findings within suggest that the inhabitants of the house had an eminent social status. The special status of the inhabitants might have been authenticated by their access to ritual knowledge and activities. The several morphological changes the house experienced and the existence of sub-floor burials indicate that multiple generations lived in the house. The longevity of the house is also connected to the continuation of social memory and ancestral ties, which altogether suggest that the inhabitants had an important social status. The social status of the house was also communicated through its prominent location, formal plan, size and distinct architectural features that later became ritual-architectural elements of standardized temple architecture.

44 Rothman 2002, 77.

45 Tobler 1950, 25–29.

46 See Rothman 2002, 87, fig. 5.13.

47 Tobler 1950, 27–29.

House II also reveals a formal tripartite plan. It is located in the southeastern part of the town.[48] The major differences between this house and House I are its size (10 x 8.5 m) and entrance system. Like the first house, this house also presents a fusion of several different activities, such as ritual, mortuary, storage and domestic, indicated by small-scale textile production. It reveals many aspects of temple architecture, such as the location of niches at the back wall of the main room, the decoration of the main room with white plaster, a hut statue located in the main room, censers and the orientation of the building towards the cardinal points.[49] However, it also has the characteristics of a domicile, such as pottery vessels, spindle whorls, awls, needles, a spatula and a serving pot.[50]

The most interesting evidence about this house is that there was a jar containing a lapis and gold pin buried under the floor in one of the side rooms.[51] I suggest that this sub-floor find is a good example of a possible heirloom item, because it was not found lying around in the shallow spaces of the house. The fact that it was hidden beneath the floor of a room within a jar suggests that it was probably circulated at some point, because lapis lazuli (and also gold) was a trade material usually acquired from Afghanistan.[52] An ethnographic parallel of keeping sacred items in jars comes from the Native American tribe of Zuni, where valuable objects are kept in ceramic jars.[53]

The heirloom found in the house may suggest that the inhabitants had inalienable goods. The key attributes of inalienable objects are that they are not items of regular exchange transactions, they do not circulate, they are not produced in large quantities, they are often used in ceremonies of authentication and they can authenticate social identities that can be collective and/or individual.[54] The items can be produced from precious materials that come from long distances. According to Weiner, what is most important about the inalienable objects is the source of their authentication, since the objects derive their power from this source.[55] The properties of inalienable objects can be authenticated in cosmologies.[56] There is a correlation between the existence of ritual activities and symbolism and the inalienable objects in House II that may suggest that these items were ritually

48 See Rothman 2002, fig. 5.13.

49 Rothman 2002, 80; Tobler 1950, 28.

50 Rothman 2002, 78; Tobler 1950, 28.

51 Rothman 2002, 81.

52 Roaf 1990.

53 Bunzel 1932, 853.

54 Helms 1998; Weiner 1992, 100–102.

55 Weiner 1992, 100–101.

56 Weiner 1992, 102.

authenticated. Similar to House I, this house witnessed ritual activities and may have been occupied by several generations of families who might have authenticated their distinct status through their access to specific ritual knowledge and inalienable items.

In terms of mortuary data, Tobler mentions that the main room had a number of sub-floor burials.[57] One of those burials was a jar burial containing infant bones, and the jar was painted with a decoration that seems to represent a landscape.[58] The sub-floor burials and presence of heirloom valuables suggest the longevity of the house. It also suggests that multiple generations of inhabitants maintained or created a long-lasting differential status through keeping these heirlooms of social memory. According to ethnographic research in Tanimbar, heirloom valuables are perceived as connected to the founding ancestors, the origins of the house and to the sources of otherworldly power.[59] In a way, the heirlooms become the material embodiment of the house, as these items are closely associated with the history of the house and its inhabitants.

The tripartite houses of Level XII reveal a fusion of multiple activities, such as mortuary, food, textile and lithic production and consumption, guest and family gathering and ritual activities. However, the ritual significance of Houses I and II exhibit differences in terms of their material manifestation. These houses used visible ritual-architectural elements and symbols to signify ritual practice and knowledge. The rest of the houses in the settlement do not exhibit visible ritual-architectural elements. Therefore, I suggest that the inhabitants of Houses I and II communicated social difference through access to ritual, by which I mean the aspects of cosmological principles and ritual knowledge related to them might have been under the control of ritual specialists.

Level XIA stratigraphically superimposes Level XII. There are three tripartite buildings in this level.[60] The tripartite Building I is located on the northeast end of the site. In terms of size, this building is the largest of all the tripartite buildings (8.40 x 8.25 m). This tripartite building has an interesting type of entrance in which the side walls of the main room extend outwards, forming an external portico or porch (FIG. 2). The side rooms project outwards at the back part of the building. This building was accepted as a "formal temple" by the excavators since it is cardinally oriented and is similar to the later standardized temples,[61] however it does not have an altar and other features such as niches at the back wall and a basin

57 Tobler 1950, 28, 150.

58 See Tobler 1950, 150, fig. 309.

59 McKinnon 1991, 91.

60 See Rothman 2002, fig. 5.24.

61 Tobler 1950, 23–25.

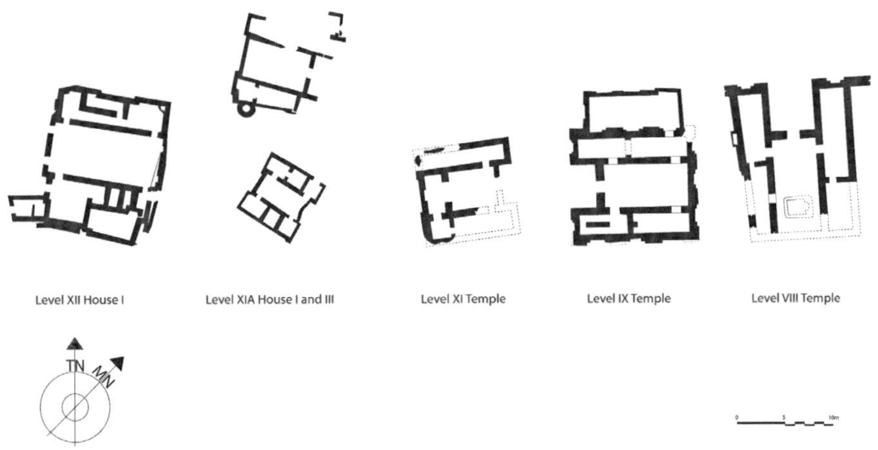

FIG. 2 Tepe Gawra Houses and Temples (modified after the courtesy of University of Pennsylvania Museum Archives).

that meet the criteria for temples.[62] Finds from the interior, such as lithics, twelve spindle whorls, three bone needles and a blade, suggest a specialized production activity.[63] Like the rest of the tripartite structures in this level, this building is attached to what I call long-room structures.[64] In this structure, a large oven and a pottery nest was found, indicating an existence of a specialized activity area within the building.[65] One of the flanking rooms also had an oven and serving dishes, suggesting food production and consumption activities.

As for the graves, 19 sub-floor burials were found in the area of the building complex, 16 of which were occupied by infants.[66] Nine of those burials were inside the building. They were mostly in the flanking rooms; only two were found in the main room.[67] One adult burial was under the southwestern corner of the main room. An infant burial was right below the main entrance to the main room. Only one of the burials had a differing grave good—an infant sub-floor burial that had white beads around the neck of the skeleton and "an ear ornament consisting of gold foil over a bitumen core."[68] The rest of the burials had ceramics as grave goods. The presence, location, and grave goods of burials within this building complex communicate several

62 Rothman 2002, 84.
63 Rothman 2002, 84.
64 Baltalı 2007, 115.
65 Rothman 2002, 84.
66 Tobler 1950, 101–102.
67 See Rothman 2002, 207, fig. A. 24.
68 Rothman 2002, 287.

messages: 1) the existence of the number of burials may suggest the longevity of the household; 2) death rituals took place in the house; 3) the significance of the ancestors associated with the house; and 4) grave goods showing inalienable possessions. The grave goods associated with a body can signify the possession of an inalienable item by the inhabitants of the house. The association of such goods as burial gifts may still signify the activeness of the inalienable possessions.[69] Grave goods can be considered inalienable possessions because the valuable item is obviously taken out of circulation and becomes a corporeal item of the deceased. Through the domestic ritual of burying the deceased, the living members of the house establish a spatial and temporal continuity between themselves and the dead.[70]

The formal architectural design, cardinal orientation and in-house sub-floor burials may communicate a specialized religious-ritual function, but this does not necessarily mean that the building's sole function was as a 'temple.' Rather, I suggest that it was a house that fused many functions together, such as ritual, burial-site, domestic functions and household production.

Conclusions

An examination of a sample of tripartite houses from Levels XII and XIA of Tepe Gawra illustrates that discrete categories of house and temple are very problematic since they prevent us from seeing the more complex overlapping dimensions of these built spaces. The houses discussed here are not just dwellings for people to live in, but they are places for public events, burial places, ritual sites, residential places and objectifications of cosmologies. These houses used architectural and decorative elements, as well as artifacts, indicating that rituals were practiced and symbolically expressed. The cardinal orientation, the tripartite plan with its particular entrance system and internal circulation pattern, the location of prayer niches at the back wall of the main room and white-plastered walls became formal elements of standardized temples in later periods of Tepe Gawra.[71] The analyses of houses in Levels XII and XIA suggest that at Tepe Gawra formal religious architecture of later periods appropriated and further canonized the ritual-architectural elements and cosmological symbolism detected in houses. Temples reveal formalization of religious ritual in the form of conventional temple architecture, thus signifying a standardized community religion.

The later period (Levels XI, X, IX, VIII) temples reveal common internal findings of storage bowls, flint blades and utilitarian bowls, as well as luxury ware, celts,

69 See Weiner 1992, 61.

70 Helms 1998, 34–41.

71 See Rothman 2002, 93, 100, fig. 5.26; Tobler 1950; Speiser 1935, fig. 2.

spindle whorls, seals, sealings, grinders, mullers, cooking ovens and personal items of jewelry. These findings suggest that formal temples also had domestic functions, such as food production, storage and consumption and small scale textile production that are "secular" in nature.[72] Interestingly, temples, like houses, continue the tradition of burying the dead underneath the floors of the main and flanking rooms.[73]

The tripartite architectural layout, organization and use of space, fixed and non-fixed internal architectural and decorative elements of the temples at Tepe Gawra have strong parallels in the site's house architecture. The symbolic relationship of temple and house can be seen in two interrelated ways: 1) the temple's overall space resembles house architecture, communicating the message of the house as the microcosm of the society and cosmic order; and 2) temples may have symbolically represented houses that have economic, residential and ritual qualities. Like the houses, temples may have symbolized sedentary life, domestication, and fertility, since they enclose activities of food processing, production and consumption and also enclose social units of society such as families and kin groups.[74] Similar to houses, temples were likewise burial sites of ancestors for the living.

The analysis of ritual-architectural elements within the houses shows that access to ritual knowledge and performance may have played an important role as the basis for social differences at Tepe Gawra.[75] Access to ritual, ancestor veneration, house continuity and possession of inalienable items may have been valued as signs of differential status within the society. Therefore, a further study of comparison of houses and temples may provide an important insight into the use of religious ritual in prestige systems and alignment of elite groups and religious ideologies through socio-political action in this important era of political centralization.

72 See Rothman 2002, 123–130.

73 Rothman 2002, 197–203.

74 Hodder 1990, 1994, 80–84.

75 See Baltalı 2007.

REFERENCES

Baltalı, S., *Architecture, Ritual Expression and Social Differentiation in Fourth Millennium North Mesopotamia.* Unpublished PhD Thesis, University of Virginia, 2007.

Baltalı Tırpan, S., "Architectural Spaces and Hybrid Practices in Mesopotamia" in *The Archaeology of Hybrid Material Culture: Occasional Papers No. 39. Center for Archaeological Investigations*, ed. by J. Card, 466–485. Carbondale: Southern Illinois University Press, 2013.

Bell, C., *Ritual Theory, Ritual Practice.* Oxford: Oxford University Press, 1992.

———. *Ritual Perspectives and Dimensions*. Oxford: Oxford University Press, 1997.

Bourdieu, P., "The Berber House" in *Rules and Meaning*, ed. by M. Douglas, 98–110. Suffolk: Penguin Modern Sociology Series, 1973.

———. *Outline of a Theory of Practice.* Cambridge: Cambridge University Press, 1977.

Bradley, R., *Ritual and Domestic Life in Prehistoric Europe*. London: Routledge, 2005.

Braithwaite, M., "Decoration as Ritual Symbol: A Theoretical Proposal and an Ethnographic Study in Southern Sudan" in *Symbolic and Structural Archaeology*, ed. by I. Hodder, 80–88. Cambridge: Cambridge University Press, 1982.

Bunzel, R.L., "Zuni Katchinas: An Analytical Study" in *7th Annual Report of Bureau of American Ethnology, 1929–1930,* 843–1108. Washington DC, 1932.

Carsten, J. and S. Hugh-Jones, *About the House: Levi-Strauss and Beyond*. Cambridge: Cambridge University Press, 1995.

Donley, L., "House Power, Swahili Space and Symbolic Markers" in *Symbolic and Structural Archaeology*, ed. by I. Hodder, 63–73. Cambridge: Cambridge University Press, 1982.

———. "A Structuring Structure: the Swahili House" in *Domestic Architecture and Use of Space*, ed. by S. Kent, 114–126. Cambridge: Cambridge University Press, 1990.

Ergene, B., *A Local Court, Provincial Society, and Justice in the Ottoman Empire: Legal Practice and Dispute Resolution in Çankırı and Kastamonu (1652–1744*). Leiden: Brill, 2003.

Flannery, K. V. and J. Marcus, "Cognitive Archaeology" in *Reader in Archaeological Theory*, ed. by D.S. Whitley, 35–48. London: Routledge, 1998.

Frangipane, M., *Yakındoğuda Devletin Doğuşu.* İstanbul: Arkeoloji ve Sanat Yayınları, 2002.

———. "Non-Urban Hierarchical Patterns of Territorial and Political Organization in Northern Regions of Greater Mesopotamia: Tepe Gawra and Arslantepe." *Subartu* 23 (2009): 135–148.

George, A.R., *House Most High: The Temples of Ancient Mesopotamia*. Indiana: Eisenbrauns, 1993.

Gillespie, S.D., "Maya 'Nested Houses': the Ritual Construction of Place" in *Beyond Kinship: Social and Material Reproduction in House Societies*, ed. by R. Joyce and S. D. Gillespie, 135–160. Philadelphia: University of Pennsylvania Press, 2000.

Helms, M., *Ulysses' Sail: An Ethnographic Odyssey of Power, Knowledge, and Geographical Distance*. Princeton: Princeton University Press, 1988.

———. *Access to Origins*. Austin: University of Texas Press, 1998.

Herbich, I. and M. Dietler, "Space, Time and Symbolic Structure in the Luo Homestead: An Ethnoarchaeological Study of 'Settlement Biography' in Africa" in *Actes du xii congrès international des sciences préhistoriques et protohistoriques*, ed. by J. Pavùk, 26–32. Nitra: Archaeological Institute of the Slovak Academy of Sciences, 1993.

Hodder, I., *The Domestication of Europe*. Oxford: Basil Blackwell, 1990.

———. "Architecture and Meaning: The Example of Neolithic Houses and Tombs" in *Architecture and Order: Approaches to Social Space*, ed. by M. Parker-Pearson and C. Richards, 73–85. London: Routledge, 1994.

Insoll, T., *Archaeology, Ritual and Religion*. London: Routledge, 2004.

Jawad, A.J., *The Advent of the Era of Townships in Northern Mesopotamia*. Leiden: Brill, 1965.

Jones, L., *The Hermeneutics of Sacred Architecture: Experience, Interpretation and Comparison. Volume one. Monumental Occasions*. Cambridge: Center for the Study of World Religions, 2000.

Joyce, R. and S. D. Gillespie, *Beyond Kinship: Social and Material Reproduction in House Societies*. Philadelphia: University of Pennsylvania Press, 2000.

Kubba, I., *Mesopotamian Architecture and Town Planning*. BAR International Series 367. Oxford: Archaeopress, 1987.

Lefebvre, H., *The Production of Space*. Oxford: Blackwell, 1991.

Levi-Strauss, C., *Anthropology and Myth: Lectures 1951–1982*. Oxford: Basil Blackwell, 1987.

———. "Maison" in *Dictionnaire de l'ethnologie at de l'anthropologie*, ed. by P. Bonte and M. Izard. Paris: PUF, 1991.

Lundquist, M. J., "What is a Temple? A Preliminary Typology" in *The Quest for the Kingdom of God: Studies in Honor of George E. Mendenhall*, ed. by H. B. Huffman, F. A. Spina and A. R. W. Green, 83–118. Indiana: Eisenbrauns, 1983.

McKinnon, S., *From a Shattered Sun: Hierarchy, Gender and Alliance in the Tanimbar Islands*. Winconsin: University of Wisconsin Press, 1991.

———. "The Tanimbarese Tavu: The Ideology of Growth and the Material Configurations of Houses and Hierarchy in an Indonesian Society" in *Beyond Kinship: Social and Material Reproduction in House Societies*, ed. by R. Joyce and S. D. Gillespie, 161–176. Philadelphia: University of Pennsylvania Press, 2000.

Metcalf, P. and R. Huntington, *Celebrations of Death. The Anthropology of Mortuary Ritual*. Cambridge: Cambridge University Press, 1991.

Pearson, M. P. and C. Richards, *Architecture and Order: Approaches to Social Space*. London-New York: Routledge, 1994.

Plunket, P., *Domestic Ritual in Ancient Mesoamerica. The Cotsen Institute of Archaeology. Monograph 46.* Los Angeles: UCLA Press, 2002.

Roaf, M., *Cultural Atlas of Mesopotamia and the Ancient Near East.* New York: Facts on File, 1990.

Rothman, M.S., *Tepe Gawra: The Evolution of a Small Prehistoric Center in Northern Iraq.* Philadelphia: University of Pennsylvania Museum of Archaeology and Anthropology, 2002.

Sahlins, M., *Culture and Practical Reason.* Chicago: University of Chicago Press, 1976.

———. *Islands of History.* Chicago: University of Chicago Press, 1985.

Speiser, E.A., *Excavations at Tepe Gawra. Vol. I.* Philadelphia: University of Pennsylvania Museum of Archaeology and Anthropology, 1935.

Tobler, A., *Excavations at Tepe Gawra. Vol. II.* Philadelphia: University of Pennsylvania Museum of Archaeology and Anthropology, 1950.

Waterson, R., *The Living House: An Anthropology of Architecture on South-East Asia.* Oxford: Oxford University Press, 1990.

———. "Houses and Hierarchies in Island Southeast Asia" in *About the House: Levi-Strauss and Beyond*, ed. by J. Carsten and S. Hugh-Jones, 47–68. Cambridge: Cambridge University Press, 1995.

Weiner, A., *Inalienable Possessions: The Paradox of Keeping while Giving.* Berkeley: University of California Press, 1992.

The Neolithisation of the Northeastern Corner of the Mediterranean

Cédric Bodet[1]

I am honored to express here my greatest esteem for Marie-Henriette and Charles Gates who introduced my fellow Bilkent students and me to the wonders of Near Eastern archaeology and offered us the privilege of an exciting fieldwork opportunity at Kinet Höyük, where Neolithic migrants to Cyprus may well have departed from.

Abstract

Cyprus was settled by several groups of farmers at a time when the Near Eastern agricultural economic model was still in its infancy on the mainland (Late PPNA/Early PPNB). These migrations have a wide-ranging impact on our perception of the early Neolithic of the Northern Levantine coastal area, long thought to be a no man's land. Quite the opposite, the data from the island allows the reconstruction, from an archaeo-ethnological perspective, of a primary and thriving neolithisation process for this territory. Consequently, although traditionally confined to the Middle Euphrates, the birthplace of farming (conceived here as a social system, and not as a mere technical innovation) deserves to be expanded to the Northwestern and the Central Levant, not only to make sense of otherwise incoherent archaeological data, but also to enlighten specific aspects of the social restructuration brought about by this new mode of production.

Introduction

Coastal areas tend to be densely populated because the sea is a transportation route, a climatic stabilizer and an inexhaustible tank of natural resources.[2] This is particularly accurate for settled hunter-gatherers and incipient farmers, spatially restricted

---

1 Arkeoloji Bölümü, Edebiyat Fakültesi, Muğla Sıtkı Koçman Üniversitesi, Kötekli Yerleşkesi, 48000, Muğla, Turkey.

2 Price and Gebauer 1995, 7.

modes of production took place in the 10th–9th millennia cal. BC (economically speaking, collecting must also be conceived as a mode of food production). The earliest cultivation practices have been recognized in the Euphrates basin during the second half of the Pre-Pottery Neolithic A (PPNA)[4] and the integration of animal herding dates to the Early Pre-Pottery Neolithic B (PPNB). By then, farming had become reliable and powerful and rapidly spread across Southwest Asia.[5]

Communities living in the coastal lands of the northeastern Mediterranean, not far from the formative zone of farming, are expected to have rapidly adopted the new way of life. However, this area has often been regarded as a backwater of the neolithisation process,[6] void of settled population up until the last centuries of the aceramic Neolithic, while Euphratean farming had already reached much more distant territories like Central Anatolia, the South Levant or Cyprus.

The Context

Geography

The territory understood here as Northwestern Levant comprises the fertile and environmentally heterogeneous strip of land located between the Mediterranean Sea to the West, the Syrian Desert to the East and the Hauran and the Pre-Taurus hills to the South and North, respectively (Fig. 1). Its geomorphology is shaped by the northern extremity of the African Rift Valley, locally materialized by the Bekaa, Orontes and Amuq valleys bordered by the Lebanon (West), anti-Lebanon (East), Ansariyeh and Amanus mountain ranges. At both ends of the Rift, the Ghûta oasis in the Damascene and the Çukurova Plain are also considered.

History of Research

The Early Neolithic in the area was first brought to light in the early 1970s by de Contenson's excavation of Tell Aswad, located in a southeastern suburb of Damascus. Since then, the Damascene has been included in the primary center of cereal cultivation of the 'Levantine corridor,'[7] though its PPNA date has recently been challenged by a new campaign led by Stordeur and Jammous. Full farming (plant cultivation and animal herding) seems to have started on the site in the earliest PPNB.[8] However, the Damascus basin is separated from the coast by both

4 Willcox 1999; Willcox and Stordeur 2012.

5 Harris 2002; Peter *et al.* 2005.

6 Cauvin 1997.

7 Bar-Yosef 1989, 58; 1998, fig. 5; Colledge *et al.* 2004.

8 Stordeur *et al.* 2010; Helmer and Gourichon 2008.

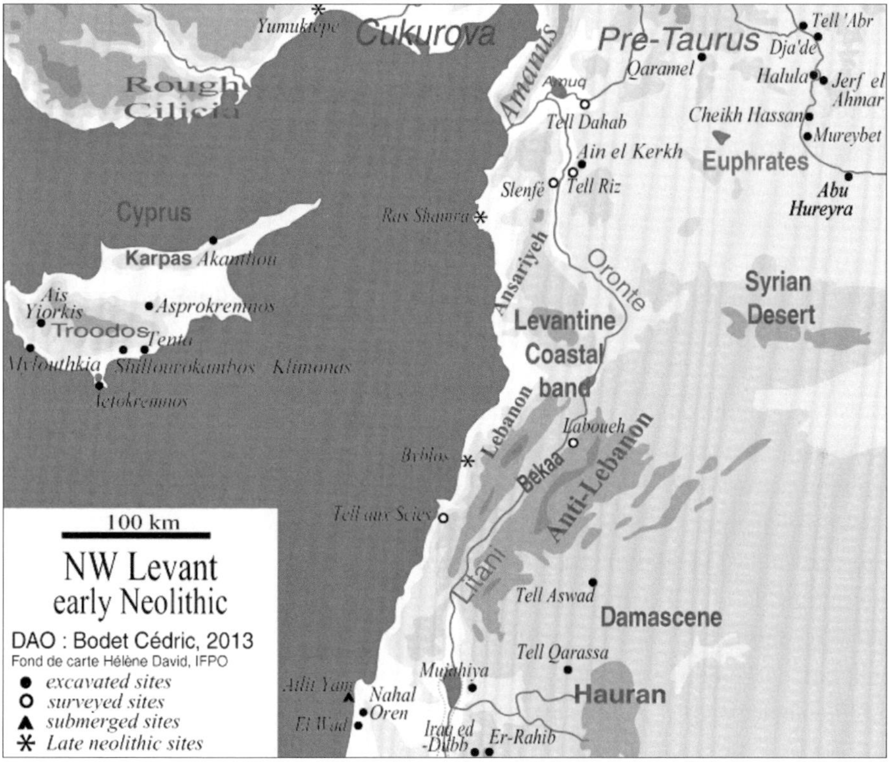

FIG. 1 LPPNA-EPPNB sites of the Northeastern Mediterranean area mentioned here.

Lebanese mountain chains and is completely integrated in the Southern Levantine cultural sphere.[9] The Neolithic of the rest of the NW Levant has remained largely unknown, expected to have been settled by Euphratean farmers at a late/final stage of the PPNB sequence (2nd half of the 8th millennium BC), with the sites of Ras Shamra, Byblos or Yumuktepe.[10]

Recently, a number of new elements have deeply altered this straightforward vision. First of all, the coastal vacuum is only felt in comparison with the site density of the Euphrates valley, where the construction of a series of dams immensely accelerated the pace of research,[11] but it is much less obvious in comparison with any other E/M PPNB *eq.*[12] area in Southwest Asia, including the Southern Levant.

9 Kuijt and Goring-Morris 2002.

10 Cauvin 1997, 209–212.

11 Bischoff and Pérouse 2003.

12 *Eq.*, or 'equivalent', refers to the Peneo supra-regional chronology (based on the Euphrates/NW Levant sequence, cf Table 1), used for interregional comparisons independently of local cultural sequences (here, especially between Cyprus and the Levant).

The low visibility of local sites can be explained by the fact that the entire Levantine coast has always been very densely populated, in recent history at least. Examples include, among many others, Les Sables, a rich Neolithic site which was destroyed by the expansion of Beirut, and the tell of Byblos, which was entirely covered by a modern village when Dunand [13] started to excavate it. Moreover, decades of wars in Lebanon halted subsequent research. [14] Finally, many sites in the Çukurova and the Orontes valleys are believed to be buried under a thick coat of river alluvium and those in the steep mountains to be badly eroded.

Environment

These parameters all have their importance, but are more or less common in archaeology. There is, however, one local event that radically erased all early Neolithic remains from the coast: the abrupt rise of the sea level following the Holocene climatic warming, [15] estimated to be at least 25 m for the span of the PPNB (120 m from the last glacial maximum onward) [16] and accounting for 2 to 40 km of submerged land. [17] The melting of the Scandinavian ice sheet took place mostly between 8500 and 7500 BC, [18] which implies that hypothetical coastal sites of the first half of the PPNB (and PPNA?) would not be visible today; recent underwater archaeological investigations off the Southern Levantine coast tend to show that they exist. [19] Consequently, it is hardly surprising that all Neolithic sites known near the coast (Ras Shamra, Byblos and Yumuktepe) pertain to the L/F PPNB, i.e. following the stabilization of the sea level. It is moreover significant that, at the very foundation of all these sites, a 'full farming' type of production (with morphologically fully domesticated plants and animals) is already in place, [20] showing that these populations probably inherited a long tradition of farming.

As a result, Cauvin's "réoccupation du littoral au PPNB Récent" (following an enigmatic earlier PPN vacuum) seems to be, in fact, the relocation of a number of coastal settlements pushed inland by the rising sea level. With this new perspective, it becomes reasonable to look for a radically different reality for the earliest Neolithic period of this area.

---

13 Dunand 1968, 13.

14 Yazbeck 2001, 41–43.

15 Peltenburg *et al.* 2000, 851–852; Peltenburg *et al.* 2001, 39, 56–59.

16 Dalongeville and Fouache 2005, 33–34.

17 Knapp 2002, 82.

18 Sanlaville 2000, 179.

19 *Infra*; Galili and Rosen 2010.

20 Helmer 1989, 111; Caneva 2001, 24; Caneva 2002, 121.

The Economy of Neolithic Societies of the Eastern Mediterranean, and the Culture of Populations Migrating to Cyprus[21]

Interestingly, it is the remote island of Cyprus which first and foremost necessitated a thorough reconsideration of the primary advent of farming on the Levantine coast. After the cold climatic episode of the Younger Dryas, Cyprus was still populated by Pleistocene fauna (pigmy hippos and pigmy elephants) without any endemic human population, let alone ephemeral incursions (such as Aetokremnos) by mainland hunter-gatherers during the Late Epipaleolithic.[22] In the Late PPNA *eq*, cereal cultivators make their first appearance (at Klimonas and possibly Asprokremnos) but do not seem to stay.[23] By 8500 BC onwards (E PPNB *eq*), a number of sites (Shillourokambos, Mylouthkia, Tenta, Ais Yiorkis) witness the permanent settlement of full-farming populations. It is absolutely remarkable that this migration[24] is contemporaneous with the advent of the first full-farming villages in the Fertile Crescent, such as Çayönü, Nevalı Çori and Dja'de.

The species brought onto the island to be farmed[25] are precisely the 'founder species' of the Neolithic Euphratean farming model,[26] namely barley, emmer, einkorn, (and pulses like lentil, flax, vetches, etc.), goat, sheep, cattle and pig. Most (if not all) of these species are exogenous[27] and were physically transferred, testifying of a high degree of resource-control prior to migration.[28] Cultivation and herding are clearly techniques upon which the experienced mainland farmers expected to rely on the island. Also, from their foundation onwards, the Cypriot villages display a high level of development, as shown by the mode of subsistence, the quality, size and organization of the built space, the complex naviform lithic

21 An article is dedicated to the appearance of the farming system in Cyprus in Peneo 2 (Bodet 2012), to which the reader is directed for more details.

22 Simmons 1999; Vigne and Buitenhuis 1999.

23 Vigne *et al.* 2012

24 Large-scale diffusion of farming generally proceeds through adoption by hunter-gatherers (*cf.* Bodet 2009 and 2012 for the Upper Euphrates and Central Anatolia). The Cypriot case is unique in the sense that farmers physically colonized a whole region.

25 The term "farmed" is deliberately chosen over "domesticated" to emphasize the anthropological aspect of the production, leaving aside its morphological (genetic) impact, which corresponds to another degree of production (*infra*, Bodet 2009). In fact, though they were farmed, Cypriot resources do not present obvious domesticated morphologies (Vigne and Buitenhuis 1999).

26 Harris 2002, 67; Bökönyi 1993.

27 Wild barley and wild pig were present on the island prior to the migration, but there is no evidence whether they are the origin of the species domesticated locally later on. See Bodet 2010a for further details.

28 Vigne *et al.* 2009.

industry, the obsidian, or the deep and elaborate water wells. The material culture on the island shows a clear tie with the contemporary Euphrates basin, but the distance and the agitated sea surrounding the island imply experienced sea-faring, and therefore coastal, communities as the source of the migrating population.[29] The dispersed locations of early Neolithic Cypriot sites (Fig. 1) as well as the uneven presence of certain resources like *Bos,* also suggest several and separate colonization events, departing from diverse points on the coast.

Demographic Growth

In southwest Asia, the PPNB economy is characterized by the establishment of an efficient and rather systematic mode of food production, effectively preventing food shortages. The outcome of this situation, backed by a sedentary context naturally reducing birth-spacing and infant mortality, is an unprecedented demographic growth.[30] However, high densities tend to be avoided by societies lacking the experience and the institutions related to the management of large groups. Also, once communities reach a certain size, certain farmers live far away from their cultivated plots and pastures,[31] a potential cause of internal tensions.[32] Because farming is viable by small production units, like the restricted family, a natural response to such situations is the frequent splitting of new couples from the core group to establish themselves further away.[33] On the Mediterranean coast, where the available land is limited by the sea[34] and where communities have a strong sea-faring tradition, uninhabited Cyprus was certainly an inviting land to spread to.

The demographic situation must be understood as the slow result of an accumulation in the long term, and does not represent, for the communities, anything like

29 Peltenburg *et al.* 2000.

30 Bellwood (2005, 15) calculated that the Neolithic transition could have caused a population growth from *ca.* 100,000 to 5 million people in the Near East, and a 1600% increase in the Levant. See also Davis *et al.* (1988) who point out that even a change in hunting practices among late Pleistocene hunter-gatherers certainly affected demography.

31 Fairbairn 2005, 205–206.

32 A higher population density leads to a redefinition of the producers' relation to the land and especially of the relation to each other regarding the land. A solution must then be adapted to the problem of intergenerational land redistribution. Among most agricultural societies, the social structure evolves towards the adoption of lineages, where land is inherited, generally by the elder male (Meillassoux 1991; Testart 1985; Dupuy 2004).

33 Meillassoux 1991, 100; Forest 1996a; Clastres 1997, 93, n. 11.

34 The ecological upheaval and the retreat of resources caused by the rising sea-level has been interpreted as the cause of the migration to Cyprus by Peltenburg *et al.* (2000, 852); I suppose that in the context of a search for land caused by the expansion of farming, the immersion of several kilometers of land accelerated the process.

an immediate threat to which a solution must be found in a hurry. The meticulous transportation of the community (and of the animals) indeed shows considerable preparation that could not have originated from a sudden turmoil or conflict. There is no demographic 'pressure,' but a matured deliberation from populations where the human density must be conceived as the booster of a most unusual move.

The Levantine Social Structures

If the migration is motivated by demographic expansion, it is very unlikely that the entire group (a tribe or a clan for example) would be physically involved, leaving 'its' territory behind to others. The split would concern only one fraction of the group, the rest remaining in place, and it would be conceived by all parts as a way to preserve the social and economic cohesion of the whole.

In primitive societies, marital alliances are processed according to what Levi-Strauss[35] calls the 'elementary' pattern, where partners are predefined and systematically exchanged in a reciprocal manner between the same subgroups: the 2 moieties, the 4 sections or the 8 subsections of the greater group.[36] Consequently, it is likely that individuals from all subgroups would be included in the migrating population, so as to reproduce the same system of alliance on the island. Later on, an effort would probably be undertaken to keep the biological and cultural bonds alive between the separate sections of the group, especially since such an operation widens the geographical and social scope of both groups:[37] for the group remaining on the mainland, the territory invested by the other half constitutes an opening for demographic congestions to come, and for the exiled group, the `motherland' remains a safety pool in case of accidental decline of animal, plant or even human resources (due to illness, food shortage, conflict, etc.). The connections between the Cypriot settlements and their coastal 'mother-villages' are thus expected to remain open. In order to illustrate the privileged nature of these relations, it is perhaps possible to establish a cautious analogy with Greek Iron Age mother-cities founding colonies in Asia Minor so as to relieve the local demography and extend their access to natural resources: both parts usually preserve, generation after generation, exclusive ties in trade, war or culture.[38]

To summarize our points, the colonization of Cyprus indicates that opulent, dense and strongly structured farming communities were established on the Eastern Mediterranean coasts by the Early PPNB at the latest. This local social and eco-

35 Lévi-Strauss 1967, 80–97.

36 As opposed to the 'complex' pattern where the partner is undetermined and where only restrictions are imposed (concerning a degree of proximity predefined by each society, but extending at least to the first degree parents: the 'incest prohibition').

37 Ghasarian 1996, 79–89.

38 Biers 1996, 110–111.

Table 1 Chronological chart of the NW Levantine sites discussed in the text (Northern tip of the Southern Levant).

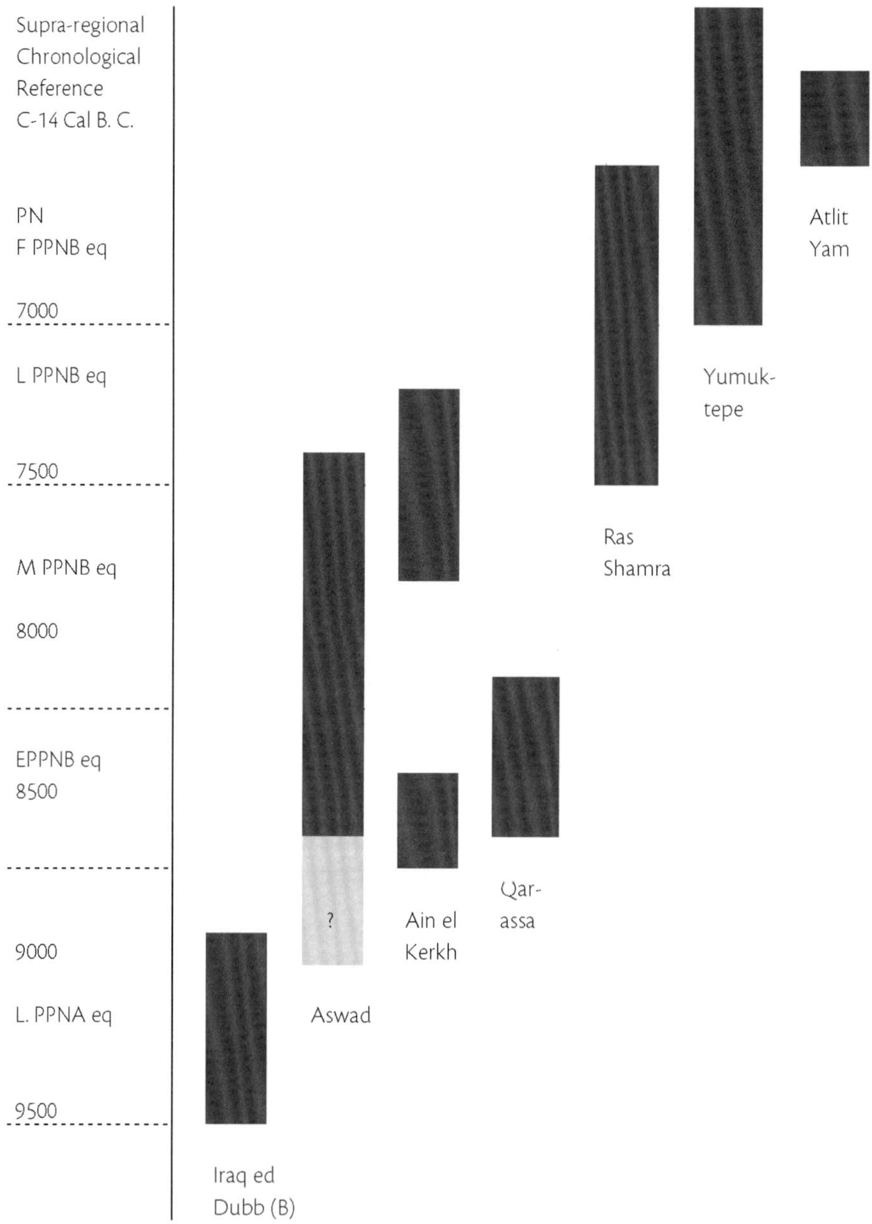

nomic development even seems largely initiated by their Late PPNA predecessors, as traces of cultivation of emmer wheat introduced from the Levant have been retrieved at Klimonas.[39] In the light of these recent discoveries coming from the island, it is now time to reevaluate the Northwestern Levantine archaeological data.

The Emergence of Farming on the Levantine Coast: An Archaeological Overview

The economic data of the coastal Neolithic sites is uneven and sporadic, but by comparison with neighboring regions, it is possible to formulate a general idea of local food production. This review focuses on the plausible territories of origin for the migration to Cyprus, so as to reconstruct the physical bond between both territories. The chronology of the sites discussed is represented in TABLE 1.[40]

In the Late PPNA, sedentism was widespread in the Northern extremity of the Southern Levantine coast (see FIG. 1), in particular at Nahal Oren, Michmoret, el Wad, and slightly more inland around the Sea of Galilee, at Mujahiya, 'Iraq ed-Dubb and possibly Er Rahib.[41] Large-scale storage of cereals and even incipient cultivation are likely at this early stage.[42]

Peltenburg *et al.*[43] note that the sea currents along the coast of Northern Palestine are favorable for transportation to Cyprus; this is also where, at Atlit Yam in particular, the characteristic water wells retrieved on the island have their best parallels (FIG. 2).[44] The latter site is one of several submerged Pre-Pottery Neolithic C (PPNC)/Pottery Neolithic (PN) sites located 200 to 400 m offshore (8–12 m deep, 4 ha in extension). These settlements are too late for the migration to Cyprus, but earlier sites are to be expected deeper and further offshore. Finally, the Levantine wild boars are as small as those retrieved in Cyprus, and, since no morphological domestication is attested for any other local domesticate, the island swine could possibly be of Palestinian origin. All these elements make the Southern Levant a possible candidate for the origin of the migration, in particular for the PPNA.

These elements are, however, neither conclusive nor exclusive of other territories. In spite of intense local investigations that uncovered many sites of earlier and later periods, the local Early PPNB, contemporary with the definitive migration of full-farmers to Cyprus, seems to be devoid of fully sedentary farming popula-

39 Vigne *et al.* 2012, 8847.

40 See Peneo 2, 2013 for the Cypriot chart.

41 Yeshurun *et al.* 2009; Kuijt 2002–2004, 4; Kuijt and Goring-Morris 2002, 382–385.

42 Colledge *et al.* 2004, 39.

43 Peltenburg *et al.* 2001, 46.

44 Galili and Rosen 2010, 47–48.

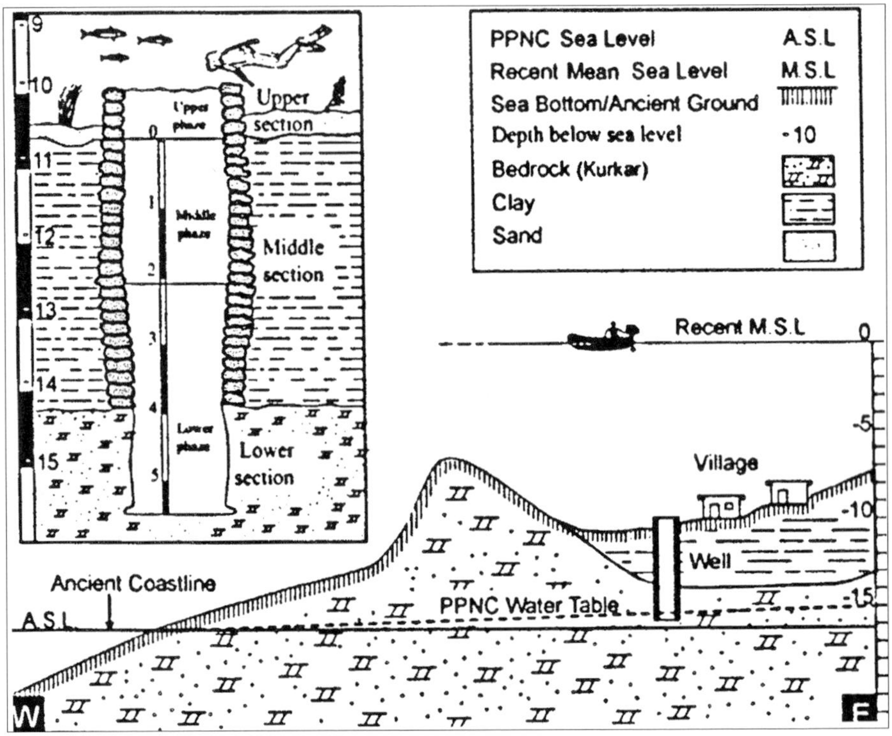

FIG. 2 Submerged neolithic villages (here, Atlit Yam) and their water wells, off the coast of the Southern Levant, featuring the present and ancient coastlines (After Galili and Rosen 2011, 49, fig. 4- NB. On p.48, the C-14 dates ranging from 8370–8210 cal BC must in fact be read BP; Galili, personal communication).

tions.[45] In particular, no sign of animal breeding, even of the proto-domestic type (without physical transformation), is attested in the Southern Levant before the middle of the Middle PPNB, at a time when an efficient version of the Neolithic mode of production diffuses from the North.[46] Also, the geographical distribution of the small sized swine, in particular its Northern limit, is also not well attested, as they have been encountered at Ras Shamra as well (*infra*). The analysis of the lithic industry finally seems to exclude Palestine as a primary origin for the migration.[47]

In conclusion, Palestine hardly fulfills the bio-geographical, cultural, demographic and economic conditions expected for the original territory of the Early PPNB Cypriot migrants.

45 Kuijt and Goring-Morris 2002, 382.

46 Horwitz and Lernau 2003; Horwitz *et al.* 1999, 69.

47 Coqueugniot 2003, 376.

Central Levant

Garfinkel[48] tried to correlate the stratigraphy of the coastal site of Byblos with the PPNB sequence of Jericho, but, with its 7th millennium calibrated radiocarbon date and its Amuq and Byblos points,[49] Byblos does not seem to have been founded much earlier than in the Late/Final PPNB (though an earlier settlement under the sea today cannot be excluded). However, slightly to the south, at the now-destroyed site of Tell-aux-Scies, Arimura[50] confidently argues for an Early PPNB date on the basis of the lithic technology. He also suspects the material culture of Laboueh, in the Bekaa Valley, to be roughly contemporary.

Next to this scanty data, Tell Aswad, just east of the Anti-Lebanon mountain chain, stands as a well known and abundant illustration of early Neolithic communities of the Central Levant. This site is located in the Ghûta, once a fertile oasis of the Damascene alluvial plain, featuring two or three lakes, marshes, and streams. Long thought to be PPNA, a recent campaign led by D. Stordeur post-dated it to the Early PPNB. At any rate, the new investigation confirmed the presence, in the Middle and most probably in the Early PPNB levels, of morphologically domestic *Capra, Ovis, Sus, Bos*[51] and cereals (emmer wheat, especially), mostly recovered as temper and basketry imprints on construction material.[52]

The wild ancestors of the animal and plant (sub)species found in Cyprus are all known in the wild in the Damascene. Wasse[53] showed in particular that *Capra* was an indigenous species of the Lebanese mountains. His assumption that Central Levant could constitute an independent center for caprine domestication is now fully supported by the reanalysis of Tell Aswad. At Early PPNB Tell Qarassa in the Hauran hills, the caprines and suid, still under study, are probably also under human control.[54] A similar picture can be drawn for cereals and other plants: pistachio, vetch, lentils and *Lathyrus*. Genetic analyses are even more explicit: according to Peltenburg *et al.*,[55] the seed assemblage of Mylouthkia (Cyprus) points to an origin in the "south-central Levant (upper Jordan Valley/Damascus Basin)." Willcox[56] prefers an origin in southeast Anatolia, but since this region has no access to the sea, the Cypriot cultivated plants would have certainly transited from the North/Central

48 Garfinkel 2004.

49 Dunand 1968, 15.

50 Arimura 2002, 2007.

51 Helmer and Gourichon 2005, 121–125, 133–136, 144.

52 Stordeur *et al.* 2010, 45–47; Colledge *et al.* 2004, 39.

53 Wasse 2001, 27–30.

54 Ibáñez *et al.* 2010; Gourichon, pers. comm.

55 Peltenburg *et al.* 2001, 850.

56 Willcox 2003, 236.

Levantine coast. He further notes that there are several centers for the emergence of cultivation, and that the Anatolian center cannot have been the only one.[57]

It is interesting to note that the Damascene was too dry to permit rain-fed agriculture. In spite of this, the seeds show no sign of desiccation, even those of plants very dependent on water, like linen and fig. It can be postulated that the marshes were drained and/or that the dry soil was artificially watered by some incipient irrigation system, possibly with the construction of rudimentary ditches. Edwards[58] recalls that systems to store and distribute spring water are known in the PPNB of the Southern Levant, as well as among many hunter-gatherers in ethnography. In any case, it is clear that the Central Levant hosts efficient full-farming communities in the earliest centuries of the PPNB.

Culturally speaking, in contrast with the Euphrates basin where the PPNA-PPNB transition is characterized by the advent of rectangular architecture,[59] the entire PPNB architectural sequence of the Damascene, from Early PPNB Tell Aswad to Late PPNB Tell Ramad, is dominated by elliptical and curved buildings.[60] This architectural conservatism is also characteristic of the contemporary Southern Levant[61] and of Cypro-PPNB sequences.

The Greater Ansariyeh Area

Ras Shamra is a major site on the coast of the Northern Levant, with a large Bronze Age exposure (Ugarit). The earliest layers, probably extending over several hectares but only known from two trenches, are traditionally dated to Late PPNB. However, one radiocarbon date and an Aswad point found just above the virgin soil (level VC) suggest an earlier foundation.[62]

More inland in the Orontes Valley, the site of Tell Ain el-Kerkh was also dated to the end of the PPNB when first investigated, in accordance with the regional chronology.[63] However, narrow naviform cores, Aswad points and other lithic

57 Willcox 2012.

58 Edwards 2010, 43.

59 We can note that this change, often explained as a technical innovation, in fact reflects the need, in this new domestic world revolving around the restricted family unit, to strongly differentiate the feminine and the masculine parts of the household (Bourdieu 1980; Meillassoux 1991; Forest 1996a). Such symbolical transformation, purely internal to each community, did not diffuse, and thus did not necessarily appear away from the Euphrates basin as fast as the farming techniques themselves.

60 Stordeur *et al.* 2010, 42, 55.

61 Kinzel *et al.* 2011, 44.

62 Arimura 2007, 149.

63 Iwasaki and Tsuneki 1999, 85, 91; Tsuneki *et al.* 2000.

features from the deepest layers show a strong similarity with the Early PPNB culture.[64] Five radiocarbon dates, roughly falling between 8700 and 8300 BC, later confirmed this date for the site foundation. Nearby, survey sites with similar characteristics, like Tell Riz, Tell Dahab in the Amuq Plain or Slenfé in the Ansariyeh Mountains may also pertain to this early horizon. Moreover, according to the specialists, and in spite of technological similarities with Dja'de, the local culture seems to be closer to the Damascene than to the Middle Euphrates sphere.[65]

The animal economy in what is termed here the greater Ansariyeh area shows a developed form of farming and a clear acquaintance with that of Cyprus, in particular when looking at the panel of species[66] and at the reduced size of *Sus*.[67] The high percentage of pigs in the early levels of Shillourokambos (Cypro-EPPNB) and Kerkh, gradually taking the place of non-domesticates like deer (and gazelle for the latter), shows a concern for resource management consistent with a context of recent sedentism. It can be noted that at Ras Shamra VC, the sheep subspecies, *Ovis aries*, is different from the *Ovis orientalis* found in Cyprus, but the latter is identified in other northern Levantine sites.[68]

As for plant foods, at Ain el-Kerkh, three cereals, pistachio and lentils are present. The gloss on the blades, probably serving as sickles, shows that cereal processing and cultivation were playing an important role early on.[69] Also the significant presence of chickpeas (*Cicer arietinum*) and Faba beans (*Vicia faba*) implies that such pulses were also consumed and possibly, for the former at least, already in the process of morphological domestication.[70] Tsuneki *et al.*[71] believe that these elements are not extremely convincing to postulate a direct physical link between Kerkh and Cyprus; minor variations in the plant cover between the Orontes Valley and the coast (where the migrating populations are supposed to originate) are indeed to be expected, but the overall economic correlation stands, making of the entire Northeastern Mediterranean region a homogeneous economic sphere.

---

64 Arimura 2002, 106.

65 Arimura 2007, 149; Coqueugniot 2003, 386–387; Coqueugniot 2004, 300; Stordeur *et al.* 2010, 53–55; Tsuneki *et al.* 2006, 48–62.

66 Tsuneki *et al.* 2006, 51–52.

67 Helmer 1989, 112–115; Helmer 1992, 97.

68 The exact subspecies of the sheep of Kerkh, Qarassa and Aswad could not be found in the publications but, if different from the widespread *orientalis*, it is assumed that this would have been mentioned, as Helmer did for Ras Shamra. Legge and Rowley-Conwy 2000, 424–425.

69 Arimura 2007, 149.

70 Tanno and Willcox 2006.

71 Tsuneki *et al.* 2006, 64–66.

The Çukurova Plain (and Central Anatolia)

The very fertile, warm and humid Çukurova Plain, the closest mainland plain to Cyprus where Vigne and Buitenhuis expect "very ancient and developed pre-ceramic establishments,"[72] stands as another good candidate for the origin of the migrants. The territory is a natural habitat for most resources found in Cyprus. Wild *Capra*, which prefers hilly landscapes, was probably roaming in the nearby Amanus Mountains and Rough Cilicia. The deer subspecies identified in Cyprus, the *Dama mesopotamica* or fallow deer, indicates an origin in the Levant, to which Çukurova is, ecologically speaking, close – remains of this subspecies are indeed known from the local Bronze Age horizon.[73]

However, no archaeological finds have yet been able to support the theory of such an origin, as the only local Neolithic site, Yumuktepe, dates to the Final PPNB.[74] It must be pointed out that the rise of the sea level, as well as the accumulation of alluvium brought by two big rivers (the Seyhan and the Ceyhan), probably had a more disastrous effect here than anywhere else. This observation can be extended to the narrow plain at the foot of the Amanus Mountains, where an early settlement somewhere offshore of Kinet Höyük cannot be ruled out. Moreover, it is significant that the earliest Cypriot sites are all located on the opposite side of the island compared to the Çukurova. Thus, if it happened to be an origin for the migrants, Çukurova certainly was not the only one. Equally due to a lack of investigation, we cannot say much about Rough Cilicia, the strip of mainland closest to the island: the rugged geomorphology is not well-suited for the suspected density and prosperity of the farmers in question, but it may have served as a transit place, as it is located just opposite the site of Akanthou, which possibly served as the redistribution center of Cappadocian obsidian on Cyprus.[75]

The Role of the Northwest Levant in the Advent of Farming

The Emergence of Farming Communities: A Theory

Farming can be regarded as a predetermined stage of human economic and social evolution, as it appeared entirely independently in several societies in the world before being adopted by nearly all humankind. The prime emergence of agriculture happened in rich ecosystems when the natural fertility was boosted by the advent of the warm Holocene climatic era. However, within permissive boundaries, the

72 Vigne and Buitenhuis 1999, 55–56.

73 Davis 2003, 260–261; Vigne and Cucchini 2005, 190.

74 Caneva 2001.

75 See Bodet 2010.

environmental context (resources, geomorphology and climate) only influences the rapidity of a process which remains intrinsically social in nature. This social maturity, outcome of a long evolution,[76] explains why previous warm climatic eras never witnessed the advent of farming, even in rich environments.[77]

This social evolution is the *longue durée* (Braudel's lengthiest time-span of historical sequence) of our analysis.[78] The extensive use of bows and arrows in the Upper Paleolithic fostered an individualized approach to food acquisition, at least compared to the strict egalitarian cooperation of the origins.[79] By the Epipalaeolithic, individuals seem to be ideologically sufficiently flexible and autonomous (from the group and its secular relations of production) to explore new economic approaches: the Natufians would probably have developed farming if not interrupted by the Younger Dryas. Against this long-term social background, the Holocene triggered an abundance of storable resources like cereals, on which the community could sustain itself all year long. At this point starts the first phase of the neolithisation process itself: these large storage structures enforce year-round sedentism, which, in turn, naturally impose a new approach to the procurement of local food resources.[80] Making use of their immense knowledge and familiarity with nature's resources and cycles, these communities, most probably the women,[81] slowly take the reproduction of suitable[82] resources under their control through incipient forms of sowing and penning. It must be noted that during this entire sequence, conscious aims are never being achieved by the actors, neither in sedentism nor in farming; it appears to be a multi-generational process of 'behavioral selection' (in a Darwinian sense) too slow to be perceived by the actors, but slowly transforming the society's *habitus*.[83]

---

76 Testart 1985.

77 Cook 2005; Bodet 2012, 282–284.

78 Smith 1992.

79 Testart 1985; 1987.

80 Testart 1982.

81 Forest 2006. On a side note, in primitive ideologies, men hunt and women give birth, as counterparts of a general exchange system. Women also usually gather plants, but this is a completely secondary mode of production, not restricted by rules, and this explains why the women, more than men, are inclined to 'play' with the plants or young animals born around the settlement (Testart 1985).

82 Suitable must be understood in behavioral terms, as resources do not all respond very well to domestication, but also ideologically, as a complete set of taboos and symbolical values shapes every primitive society's approach to the environment.

83 *Habitus* refers to "any habit, any form of practice, acquired –as opposed to given at birth– but embodied on the long term as permanent dispositions" (...) "something historical, tied to individual history". But "while a habit is mechanical and reproductive, *habitus* is a capacity of production which tends to reproduce its objective logic

Later on, once farming had become a widespread practice, a second phase started. One inevitable side-effect of farming is the production of surplus. This part of the food production left over after consumption can only hold a value in social relations. Indeed, ethnology shows that the combination of abundant food resources and dense clusters of pre-urban populations results in the emergence of some form of social competition, played out between influential individuals (chiefs or *big men*): the most notorious examples are the settled hunter-gatherers of the Pacific coast (NW America, Eastern Siberia) practicing the *potlatch* or the proto-agriculturalists of New-Guinea and Melanesia practicing the *kula* or other forms of 'gift / counter-gift' competition.[84] I have argued elsewhere that it is the intensive level of production[85] sustaining this social competition that causes the rapid genetic domestication of the farmed resources, especially of the animals, like in the Middle Euphrates Valley (in contrast, the comparatively loose production of Central Anatolian 'neo-farmers' or of farmers in unpopulated Cyprus, where social competition is absent, did not result in the physical domestication of the controlled animals, at least until the end of the Neolithic). Morphological domestication thus becomes, for us, a marker of intensity of food production and, therefore, for the social interactions at play.[86]

Socio-Economy of the Eastern Mediterranean Neolithic

In the archaeological material of Northern Mesopotamia, the sedentism phase correlates with the PPNA: this is when traces of accumulation of large amounts of storable plants (like club-rush), pre-domestic cultivation and wild animal, especially suid, management start to become visible.[87] With the PPNB, the second and more intensive socio-economic phase starts, characterized by large-scale plant and animal domestication, and the burgeoning of well-organized villages like Çayönü and Nevalı Çori, featuring possible traces of internal social disparity, though no stratification yet.[88] From the PPNA to the PPNB, this entire

but by transforming it; it is a transforming machine that makes us reproduce the social conditions of our own production, but in a relatively unforeseeable manner..." (Bourdieu 2002, 134–135).

84 Godelier 1996; Dupuy 2004; Testart 1982.

85 According to Dupuy (2004, 97), Sahlins has shown how, in pre-state societies, the degree of productivity and hierarchisation were tightly interdependent.

86 See Bodet 2010a; 2010b.

87 Savard *et al.* 2006; Rosenberg 2007; Vigne *et al.* 2009, 2–3; Willcox and Stordeur 2012.

88 Forest 1996b; Stordeur (2012) recognized an incipient form of such differentiation already at late PPNA Jerf el Ahmar (where some form of animal control is not excluded), which may be considered as an early instance of such modification of the internal social structure. See also Davis 1998; Hauptmann 2007.

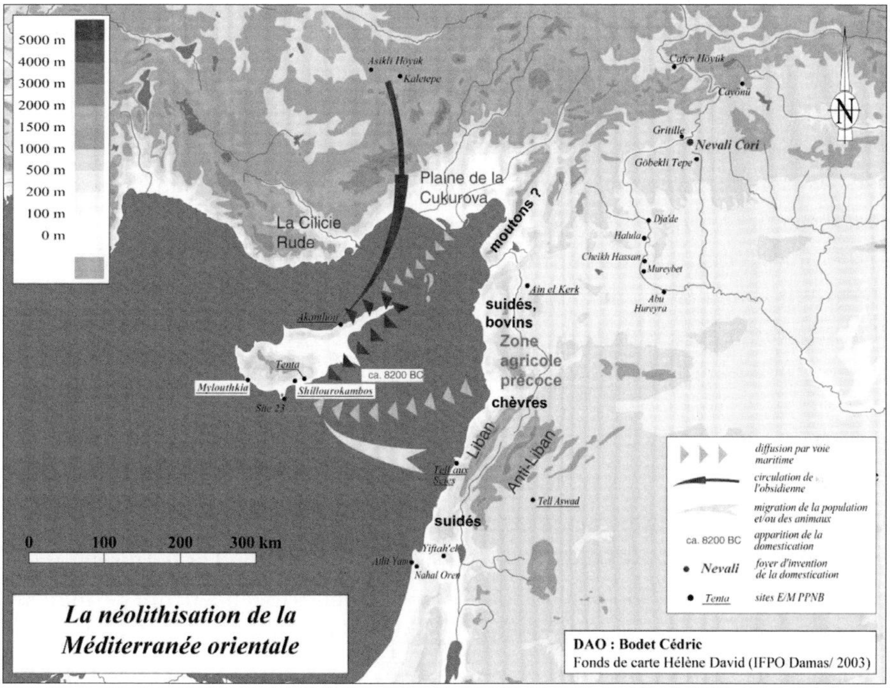

FIG. 3 Advent of farming in Eastern Mediterranean (After Bodet 2012, 492, fig. 157).

evolution can be followed in the Middle Euphrates River Valley (both Syrian and Anatolian), thus defined as a permissive area for the emergence of full-farming societies.[89]

Because the physical domestication of the resources implies an intensive form of production driven by social motives, the economic data from Tell Aswad, Tell Qarassa and Ain el-Kerkh tend to show that, already in the first half of the PPNB, the Northwest Levant witnessed internal thriving socio-economic interconnections and maybe some degree of inter-group competition. As new discoveries from Cyprus suggest, the roots of this development, with an early phase of storage, sedentism and a specific approach to wild foods are probably to be found in the local PPNA layers as well (at Aswad?). As suspected by Wasse, this opens the possibility for another independent center for the emergence of farming, almost contemporary with that in the Middle Euphrates.

However, this Levantine coastal area being technically (lithic industry, architecture), economically (full-farming), chronologically (at least partly) and physi-

89 Bodet 2012, 205–211.

cally (through the hills of the Pre-Taurus[90]) closely related to the communities of the Euphrates Valley, all the groups located between the Mediterranean coast and Northern Mesopotamia deserve to be integrated within a greater homogeneous cultural sphere (Fig. 3). Within this sphere, trying to identify one particular place and time for the 'invention' of agriculture[91] makes little sense before the evidence that the entire Northeastern Mediterranean region features all the environmental and human requirements for the beginning of the control of natural resources. We are thus in a position to say that the farming communities of the greater Northwestern Levant should be included within the 'permissive zone for incipient farming' of Western Mesopotamia (as opposed to the Tigris and Zagros centers).[92]

Kinship Structures

The advent of the farming mode of production addresses the question of the evolution of kinship structures. Social competition, understood as a cause of morphological domestication of natural resources, implies extended and permanent connections between separate groups, notably through gift exchange of prestigious objects such as obsidian. But primitive communities, which are entirely dependent on themselves for production and reproduction,[93] are not naturally inclined to open themselves up to foreign groups. In such a context, it is possible to ask whether the 'restricted kinship structure' (that is, an endogamous system of cross-cousin alliance), common among hunter-gatherers, did not begin to lose ground to the so-called 'generalized system' (exchange of women between more than two groups in a strict pattern), common in certain pre-state communities.[94] However, in a context of rapid population growth characterized by the splitting of new generations, a great number of individuals dispatched over a large area can be more or less closely related, and the generalized system scenario would not necessarily imply interaction with foreign groups. But those fascinating matters are to be addressed when the archaeological evidence allows a more secure use of the ethnological analogy.

---

90 The 'Pre-Taurus' is the hilly territory situated south of the Taurus piedmonts and north of the Jezirah steppe: Gaziantep, Urfa and Diyarbakır regions in terms of modern Turkish geography (Bodet 2012, 2).

91 See also Willcox 2012, 22–23 on the geographical origin of agriculture.

92 Bodet 2012.

93 Clastres 1997; Lévi-Strauss 1967.

94 Ghasarian 1996, Lévi-Strauss 1967.

REFERENCES

Arimura, M., “Tell Ain el Kerkh, site PPNB ancien dans le nord-ouest de la Syrie ? Etude préliminaire du matériel lithique des couches les plus anciennes.” *Orient-Express* 2002/4 (2002): 103–108.

———. “The Lithic Industry of the Early PPNB Layers at Tell Ain el-Kerkh, Northwest Syria” in *Systèmes techniques et communautés du Néolithique précéramique au Proche-Orient*, ed. by L. Astruc, D. Binder and F. Briois,137–151. Antibes: CEPAM, 2007.

Bar-Yosef, O., “The PPNA in the Levant – an Overview.” *Paléorient* 15/1 (1989): 57–63.

———. “On the Nature of Transitions: The Middle to Upper Palaeolithic and the Neolithic Revolution.” *Cambridge Archaeological Journal* 8/2 (1998): 141–163.

Bellwood, P., *First Farmers, the Origins of Agricultural Societies*. Malden: Blackwell, 2005.

Biers, W.R., *The Archaeology of Greece*. Ithaca: Cornell University Press, 1996.

Bischoff, D. and J.F. Pérouse, “La question des barrages et du GAP dans le sud est anatolien: patrimoines en danger?” *Les dossiers de l'IFEA* 3 (2003) : 3–60.

Bodet, C., “Remarks on the End of the Çayönü Culture.” *Orient-Express* 2002/2 (2002): 47–51.

———. “Emergences of Animal Husbandry in South West Asia: An Insight on Neolithic Social Structures.” *Peneo* 1 (2009): 1–25.

———. “Advent of Farming in Neolithic Cyprus: A Reflection of the Mainland, a Reflection on Society.” *Peneo* 2 (2010a): 1–27.

———. “The Ideological Gap, or the Diffusion of Neolithic Farming from the Middle Euphrates to Central Anatolia.” *Peneo* 3 (2010b): 1–24.

———. *L'apparition de l'élevage en Asie Antérieure: reflet des structures socio-économiques néolithiques*. Saabrücken: Edition Universitaires Européennes, 2012.

Bökönyi, S., “Domestication Models: The Anatolian-Mesopotamian and the Others in Southwest Asia” in *Archaeozoology of the Near East (1)*, ed. by H. Buitenhuis and A.T. Clason, 4–9. Leiden: Universal Book Services, 1993.

Bourdieu, P., *Le sens pratique*. Paris: Editions de Minuit, 1980.

———. *Questions de sociologie*. Paris: Editions de Minuit, 2002.

Caneva, I., “De Çayönü à Mersin: les premiers villageois de l'Anatolie du Sud Est” in *Les communautés villageoises du Proche Orient à l'Atlantique (8000–2000 avant notre ère)*, ed. by J. Guilaine, 13–34. Paris: Editions Errance, 2001.

———. “Ethnicity as a Form of Social Relationship Between Neolitihic Cilicia and Central Anatolia.” *The Neolithic of Central Anatolia*, ed. by F. Gérard and L. Thissen, 119–128. İstanbul: Ege Yayınları, 2002.

Cauvin, J., *Naissance des divinités, naissance de l'agriculture*. Paris: Editions du Centre National de la Recherche Scientifique, 1997.

Clastres, P., *Archéologie de la violence, la guerre dans les sociétés primitives*. Luxembourg: Editions de l'aube, 1997.

Colledge, S., J. Conolly and S. Shennan, "Archaeobotanical Evidence for the Spread of Farming in the Eastern Mediterranean." *Current Anthropology* 45 (2004): 35–58.

Cook, M., *A Brief History of the Human Race*. London: W. W. Norton & Company, 2005.

Coqueugniot, E., "Unité et diversité des industries lithiques taillées au Proche-Orient (Levant et Anatolie méridionale) du IXe au VIIe millénaire av. J.-C." in *Le Néolithique de Chypre*. Bulletin de Correspondance Hellénique: supplément 43, ed. by J. Guilaine and A. Le Brun, 374–387. Athens: École française d'Athènes, 2003.

———. "Les Industries lithiques du Néolithique Ancien entre Moyen Euphrate et Jézireh Orientale, réflexions sur deux voies évolutives" in *From the River to the Sea*, ed. by O. Aurenche, M. Le Mière and P. Sanlaville, 295–308. BAR International Series. Oxford: Archaeopress, 2004.

Dalongeville, R. and E. Fouache, "Les variations de la ligne de rivage en mer Méditerranée orientale du Pléistocène supérieur er de l'holocène récent." *Paléorient* 31/1 (2005): 27–38.

Davis, M.K., "Social Differentiation at the Early Village of Çayönü, Turkey" in *Light on Top of the Black Hill. Studies presented to Halet Çambel,* ed. by G. Arsebük, M. Mellink and W. Schirmer, 257–266. İstanbul: Ege Yayınları, 1998.

Davis, S.J.M., "The Zooarchaeology of Khirokitia (Neolithic Cyprus), including a view from the mainland" in *Le Néolithique de Chypre.* Bulletin de Correspondance Hellénique supplément 43, ed. by J. Guilaine and A. Le Brun, 253–268. Athen: École française d'Athènes, 2003.

Davis, S.J.M., R. Rabinovitch and N. Goren Inbar, "Quaternary Extinctions and Population Increase: The Animal Remains from Biq'at Quneitra." *Paléorient* 14/1 (1988): 96–105.

Dunand, M., *Byblos, son histoire, ses ruines, ses légendes*. Beyrouth: Institut Français du Proche-Orient, 1968.

Dupuy, F. *Anthropologie économique*. Paris: Armand Colin, 2004.

Edward, P.C., "Early Agriculture and Ditch irrigation." *Neo-Lithics* 2/10 (2010): 43–46.

Fairbairn, A., "A History of Agricultural Production at Neolithic Çatalhöyük East, Turkey." *World Archaeology* 37/2 (2005): 197–210.

Forest, J.D., *Mésopotamie, l'apparition de l'Etat,* VIIe-IIIe millénaires. Paris: Paris-Méditerranée, 1996a.

———. "Le PPNB de Çayönü et de Nevalı Çori: pour une approche archéo-ethnologique de la néolithisation du Proche-Orient." *Anatolia Antiqua* 4 (1996b): 1–31.

———. "Le processus de néolithisation proche-oriental : pour une archéologie sans frontiers." *Syria* 83 (2006): 125–138.

Galili, E. and N. Rosen, "Submerged Neolithic Settlements of the Mediterranean Carmel Coast and Water mining in the Southern Levant." *Neo-Lithics* 2/10 (2010): 47–52.

Garfinkel, Y., "Néolithique and Enéolithique Byblos in Southern Levantine Context. in *Neolithic Revolution, New Perspectives on SW Asia in Light of Recent Discoveries on Cyprus*, ed. by E. Peltenburg and A. Wasse, 175–188. Oxford: Council for British Research in the Levant, 2004.

Ghasarian, C., *Introduction à étude de la parenté*. Paris: Seuil, 1996.

Godelier, M., *L'énigme du don*. Paris: Fayard, 1996.

Harris, D.R., "Development of the Agro-Pastoral Economy in the Fertile Crescent during the Pre-Pottery Neolithic Period" in *The Dawn of Farming in the Near East. Studies in Early Near Eastern Production, Subsistence, and Environment* 6, ed. by R.T.J Cappers and S. Bottema, 67–83. Berlin: Ex Oriente, 2002.

Hauptmann, H., "Nevalı Çori ve Urfa Bölgesinde Neolitik Dönem: Genel bir Bakış" in *Türkiye'de Neolitik Dönem: Yeni Kazılar, Yeni Bulgular*, ed. by M. Özdoğan and N. Başgelen, 131–164. İstanbul: Arkeoloji ve Sanat Yayınları, 2007.

Helmer, D., "Le développement de la domestication au Proche-Orient de 9500 à 7500 BP: les nouvelles données d'El Kowm et de Ras Shamra." *Paléorient* 15/1 (1989): 111–121.

———. *La domestication des animaux par les hommes préhistoriques*, Paris: Dunod, 1992.

Helmer, D. and L. Gourichon, "Premières données sur les modalités de subsistance à Tell Aswad, fouilles 2001–2005 (Syrie, PPNB Moyen et Récent, Néolithique céramique ancien)." *Archaeozoology of the Near East* 8 (2008): 119–151.

Horwitz, L.K. and O. Lernau, "Temporal and Spatial Variation in Neolithic Caprine Exploitation Strategies: a Case Study of Fauna from the Site of Yiftah'el (Israel)." *Paléorient* 29/1 (2003): 19–58.

Horwitz, L.K., E. Tchernov, P. Ducos, C. Becker, A. von den Driesch, L. Martin and A. Garrard, "Animal Domestication in the Southern Levant." *Paléorient* 25/2 (1999): 63–80.

Ibáñez, J. J., A. Balbo, F. Braemer, L. Gourichon, I. Iriarte, J. Santana and L. Zapata, "The Early PPNB Levels of Tell Qarassa North (Sweida, Southern Syria)." *Antiquity* 84/325 (2010): online, [http://www.antiquity.ac.uk/projgall/ibanez325/].

Iwasaki, T. and T. Tsuneki, "Archaeological Investigations of the Rouj Basin, Idlib." *Annales Archéologiques Arabes Syriennes* 93 (1999): 83–92.

Kinzel, M., A. Abu-Laban, C. Hoffman Jensen, I. Thuesen and M.L. Jørkov, "Insights into PPNB Architectural Transformation, Human Burials and Initial Conservation Works: Summary on the 2010 Excavation Season at Shkârat Msaied." *Neo-Lithics* 1/11 (2011): 44–49.

Knapp, A.B., "Book Reviews: the Earliest Prehistory of Cyprus: from Colonization to Exploitation, ed. by Stuart Swiny" *Bulletin of the American Schools of Oriental Research* 328 (2002): 81–84.

Kuijt, I., "Pre-Pottery Neolithic A and Late Natufian at 'Iraq ed-Dubb, Jordan." *Journal of Field Archaeology* 29/3–4 (2002–2004): 291–308.

Kuijt, I. and N. Goring-Morris, "Foraging, Farming and Social Complexity in the Pre-Pottery Neolithic of the Southern Levant: A Review and Synthesis." *Journal of World Prehistory* 16/4 (2002): 361–439.

Legge, A.J. and P. A. Rowley-Conwy, "The Exploitation of Animals" in *Village on the Euphrates, from Foraging to Farming at Abu Hureyra*, ed. by A. Moore, G. Hillman and A.J. Legge, 423–471. Oxford: Oxford University Press, 2000.

Lévi-Strauss, C., *Les structures élémentaires de la parenté*. Paris: Editions Mouton, 1967.

Meillassoux, C., *Femmes, greniers et capitaux*. Paris: L'harmattan, 1991.

Peltenburg, E., S. Colledge, P. Croft, A. Jackson, C. Mc Cartney and M.A. Murray, "Agro-Pastoralist Colonization of Cyprus in the 10th Millennium BP: Initial Assessments." *Antiquity* 74 (2000): 844–853.

———. "Neolithic Dispersals from the Levantine Corridor: a Mediterranean Perspective." *Levant* 33 (2001): 35–64.

Price, T.D. and A.B. Gebauer, "New Perspectives" in *Last Hunters, First Farmers: New Perspective on the Prehistoric Transition to Agriculture,* ed. by T.D. Price and A.B. Gebauer, 3–19. Santa Fe: School of American Research Press, 1995.

Rosenberg, M., "Hallan Çemi" in *Türkiye'de Neolitik Dönem: Yeni Kazılar, Yeni Bulgular,* ed. by M. Özdoğan and N. Başgelen, 1–11. İstanbul: Arkeoloji ve Sanat Yayınları, 2007.

Sanlaville, P., *Le Moyen-Orient Arabe, le milieu et l'homme*. Paris: Nathan, 2000.

Savard, M., M. Nesbitt and M.K. Jones, "The Role of Wild Grasses in Subsistence and Sedentism: New Evidence from the Northern Fertile Crescent." *World Archaeology* 38–2 (2006): 179–196.

Simmons, A.H., *Faunal Extinctions in an Island Society: Pygmy Hippopotamus Hunters of Cyprus*. NewYork: Springer, 1999.

Smith, M.E., "Braudel's Temporal Rhythms and Chronology Theory in Archaeology." *Archaeology, Annales and Ethnohistory* , ed. by A.B. Knapp, 23–34. Cambridge, 1992.

Stordeur, D., "Les villages et l'organisation des groupes au Néolithique précéramique A, l'exemple de Jerf el-Ahmar, Syrie du Nord" in *Du village néolithique à la ville Syro-Mésopotamienne,* ed. by J.L.M. Fenollos. Coruña: Universidade da Coruña, Bibliotheca Euphratica, 2012.

Stordeur, D., D. Helmer, B. Jamous, R. Khawam, M. Molist and G. Willcox, "Le PPNB de Syrie du Sud à travers les découvertes récentes à tell Aswad" in *Hauran V: La Syrie Du Sud Du Néolithique À L'antiquité Tardive Recherches Récentes Actes Du Colloque De Damas 2007. Vol 1,* ed. by M. Al-Maqdissi, F. Braemer and J.-M. Dentzer, 41–68. Beirut: Institut français du Proche-Orient, 2010.

Tanno, K. and G. Willox, "The Origins of Cultivation of Cicer Arietinum L. and Vicia faba L.: Early Finds from Tell el-Kerkh, NW Syria, Late 10th Millennium BP." *Vegetation History and Archaeobotany* 15 (2006): 197–204.

Testart, A., *Les chasseurs-cueilleurs ou l'origine des inégalités*. Paris: Société d'Ethnographie, 1982.

———. *Le communisme primitif. I– Economie et idéologie*. Paris: Maison des Sciences de l'Homme, 1985.

———. "Game Sharing Systems and Kinship Systems Among Hunter-gatherers." *Man* 22 (1987): 287–304.

Tsuneki, A., J. Hydar, Y. Miyake, O. Maeda, T. Odaka, K. Tanno and A. Hasegawa, "Fourth Preliminary Report of the Excavation at Tell el-Kerkh (2000), Northwestern Syria." *Bulletin of the Ancient Orient Museum* XXI (2000): 1–36.

Tsuneki, A., M. Arimura, O. Maeda, K. Tanno and T. Anezaki, "The Early PPNB in the North Levant: A New Perspective from Tell Ain el-Kerkh, Northwest Syria." *Paléorient* 32/1 (2006): 47–71.

Vigne, J.-D. and H. Buitenhuis, "Les premiers pas de la domestication animale à l'ouest de l'Euphrate: Chypre et l'Anatolie Centrale." *Paléorient* 25/2 (1999): 49–62.

Vigne, J.-D. and T. Cucchini, "Premières navigations au Proche-Orient : les informations indirectes de Chypre." *Paléorient* 31/1 (2005): 186–194.

Vigne, J.-D., A. Zazzo, J.F. Saliège, F. Poplin, J. Guilaine and A. Simmons, "Pre-Neolithic wild boar management and introduction to Cyprus more than 11,400 years ago." *PNAS Early Edition* (2009): 1–4.

Vigne, J.-D., F. Briois, A. Zazzo, G. Willcox, T. Cucchi, S. Thiébault, I. Carrère, Y. Franele, T. Touquet, C. Martin, C. Moreau, C. Comby and J. Guilaine, "First Wave of Cultivators Spread to Cyprus at Least 10,600 Years Ago." *Proceedings of the National Academy of Sciences* 109/22 (2012): 8445–9.

Wasse, A., "The Wild Goat of Lebanon: Evidence for Early Domestication?" *Levant* 33 (2001): 21–33.

Willcox, G., "Agrarian Change in the Near East" in *The Prehistory of Food, Appetites for Change*, ed. by C. Gosden and J. Hather, 478–500. London: Routledge, 1999.

———. "The Origins of Cypriot Farming" in *Le Néolithique de Chypre. Actes du Colloque International Organisé par le Département des Antiquités de Chypre et l'Ecole Française d'Athènes. Nicosie 17–19 mai 2001.* Bulletin de Correspondance Hellénique Supplement 43, ed. by J. Guilaine and A. Le Brun, 231–238. Athens: École française d'Athènes, 2003.

———. "Domestication: pas d'origine unique pour l'agriculture." *La recherche* 461 (2012): 22–23.

Willcox, G. and D. Stordeur, "Large-scale Cereal Processing Before Domestication During the Tenth Millennium cal. BC in Northern Syria." *Antiquity* 86 (2012): 99–114.

Yazbeck, C., "Le Liban dans la Préhistoire, bilan des acquis et perspectives d avenir." *Orient Express* 1/2 (2001): 40–43.

Yeshurun, R., G. Bar-Oz and M. Weinstein-Evron, "The Role of Foxes in the Natufian Economy: A View from Mount Carmel, Israel." *Before Farming* 2009/1 (2009): 1–15.

Some Clay Finds from PPNB Gritille: Stamps, Sealings and Tokens

Christine Eslick — Mary M. Voigt[1]

"It was the best of times, it was the worst of times ..."[2] *Life on the Euphrates in the early 1980s was certainly not easy, but the company of a wonderful group of people made it bearable and sometimes exhilarating. This article is offered to Marie-Henriette and Charles with fond memories of the many months we spent together at Gritille, and with gratitude for their friendship in the ensuing years.*

Abstract

Recent research and publications on the final Pre-Pottery Neolithic (PPN) and earliest Pottery Neolithic (PN) in Anatolia and northern Syria have shed new light on some of the clay finds excavated in the later PPNB layers at Gritille in 1981–1984. Some unpublished finds, including stamps, sealings and tokens, are presented in detail, with discussion of the contexts in which they were found and implications for our understanding of the later PPNB in the upper Euphrates area.

---

1 C. Eslick: ceslick@bigpond.com; M.M. Voigt: mmvoig@wm.edu. The Gritille Project was sponsored by Bryn Mawr College, with the cooperation of the University of North Carolina and participation of the University of Pennsylvania Museum. It was funded through grants from the National Endowment for the Humanities (Grants RO-00227–81–1315 and RO-20934–82), the Metropolitan Museum of Art, the James F. Hanes Fund of North Carolina, the University Museum, and private donors. Richard S. Ellis is director of the project; we thank him for his help, most recently with the illustrations for this article. Mary M. Voigt was general supervisor of the Neolithic excavations and has overall responsibility for their publication; Christine Eslick is responsible for the small finds. Marie-Henriette Gates was assistant director of the project, field director for the 1983 and 1984 seasons and supervisor of Operation 17. Charles Gates was a supervisor in the Medieval trenches.

2 Charles Dickens, *A Tale of Two Cities*, Chapter 1.

covered an area of about 150 x 100 m and on the east side sloped steeply where it had been cut away by the river. The mound was excavated from 1981 to 1984 under the direction of Richard S. Ellis of Bryn Mawr College and has subsequently been flooded by the Atatürk Dam.[3]

The top of the mound was covered by a deep Medieval occupation, and the only trenches to reach prehistoric deposits were located in a long strip along the river edge of the site (Fig. 1).[4] The PPNB settlement was founded on virgin soil and extended at least 100 m from north to south; its east to west dimensions are unknown, the east side having been severely truncated by river erosion. The excavated PPNB deposit is *c.* 4 m deep and can be divided into two main phases: Lower Neolithic Gritille (Phases C, D and "Basal"), and Upper Neolithic Gritille (Phases A and B). In terms of material culture, these deposits are attributed to the final PPNB (PPNC).[5] Radiocarbon dates for Phase B (for which we have the best archaeological cal. sample) are in the first half of the 7th millennium cal. BC.[6]

Limited information on the layout of the Upper Neolithic settlement was obtained from the large trenches located at the southern end of the excavated area (Main Excavation Area, Operations 12/1, 16 and 17).[7] The best-preserved plan shows a cell-plan structure with an attached room (Buildings 1–2).[8] The long axis of the cell-plan structure was oriented east-west; further to the east was an open court, with another court located directly to its north. To the east of these courts lay an open area that sloped down toward the river. Thin layers of mud-brick decay from the structures to the west accumulated on this slope, along with some ash from pyrotechnic activities carried out within this open area (Fig. 2).

Small Clay Artifacts

In Lower Neolithic Gritille, clay items were rare. A small clay sphere and figurines were found, both classes having parallels in stone.[9] In Upper Neolithic Gritille, however, there was an explosion in the use of clay, with many more examples of the earlier types of objects, as well as new types, being produced.[10] These new types, some of which are the focus of this contribution, include baked clay stamp

3 Voigt and Ellis 1981; Ellis and Voigt 1982.

4 Voigt 1988, figs.2–7; for medieval, see Redford 1998.

5 Voigt and Ellis 1981, 93; Ellis and Voigt 1982, 325.

6 Voigt 1988, 227, table 1.

7 Voigt 1988, fig. 3–4.

8 Voigt 1988, fig. 8–9.

9 Voigt 1985, 16–18; Voigt 2000, 265–270.

10 Voigt 1985, 16–18; Voigt 2000, 265–270.

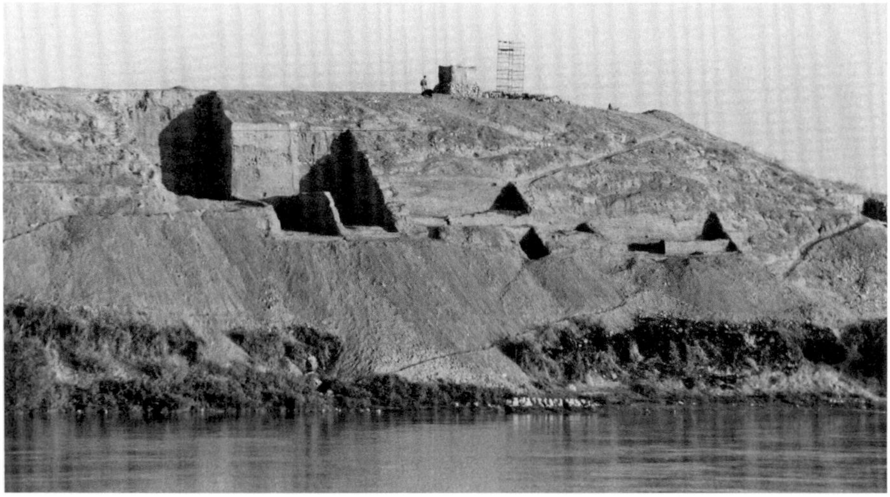

FIG. 1 East side of the mound, showing trenches with Neolithic deposits.

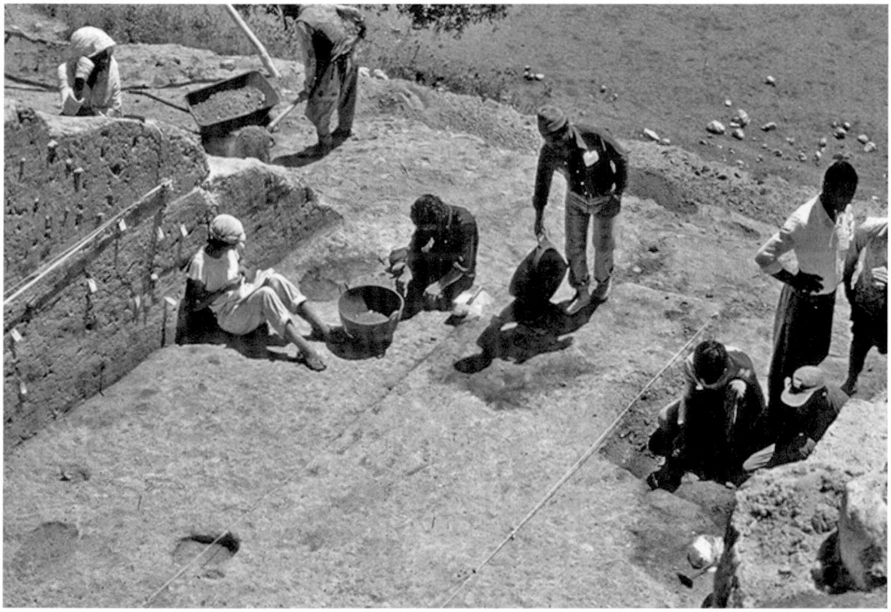

FIG. 2 Excavating an ashy surface in the east of Operation 16.

seals, clay sealings and a greater variety of tokens, as well as four small fragments of mineral-tempered baked clay vessels.[11]

Stamps

Among the most intriguing items found at Gritille were three that can be identified as stamps (Fig. 3). All were of baked clay and consisted of an elongated roll or stalk with one flat end forming the face on which a design was incised or impressed. The designs were a circle, a cross and a snake with triangular head. The snake stamp was the most elaborate, with the face extending out in a "tail" on which the end of the spiraling body and the triangular head of the snake were shown. Both the circle and snake stamps had a shallow groove around the stalk near the rounded end.

All the stamps come from Phase B, and all were recovered from a relatively small area within one trench (Operation 16). Two were associated with mud-brick architecture, from deposits that have been identified as mud-brick decay. The stamp with a circular impression on its face (GR83–174, GT6043) was recovered from the collapse of a house or courtyard wall of Building 3, dated late in Phase B.[12] The stamp with a snake design (GR83–448, GT9492) came from the same area, but within the collapse of an earlier architectural phase of Building 3. On the slope leading down to the west of this architectural complex were roasting pits and ash patches; the stamp with a cross (GR83–397, GT6132) was found in association with one of these pyrotechnic features, along with a large group of human and animal figurines.

GR83–174 (GT6043): Solid, swelling cylindrical stalk with one rounded end and opposing end flat. Circle impressed deeply into flat end causing knob-like protrusion in center. Part of flat end broken away. A shallow groove circles the stalk near the end. Dark gray baked clay. L. 3.964 cm; max. D. 1.503 cm; D. face 1.17 cm. Operation 16 locus 36 lot 74 (Phase B). Fig. 3.1.

GR83–397 (GT6132): Cylindrical stalk with one rounded end and one flat end that has a cross incised on it; pinched in slightly just above flat end. Black clay. L. 3.19 cm; max. D. 1.055 cm. Operation 16 locus 32 lot 82 (Phase B). Fig. 3.2.

GR83–448 (GT9492): Solid, cylindrical stalk with one rounded end and opposing end flat with cylinder extending out to accommodate the tail of the spiral

11 These sherds, three with a lightly burnished surface, fit well with the mineral-tempered pottery groups from other final PPNB and earliest PN sites in the Euphrates and Tigris basins: see Nieuwenhuyse *et al.* 2010.

12 Voigt 1985, fig. 7.

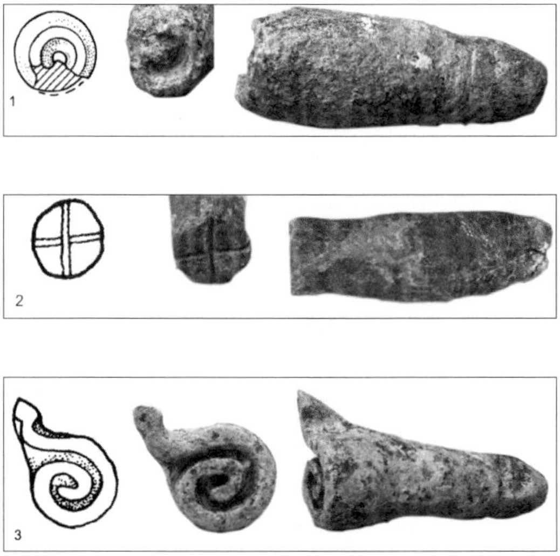

FIG. 3 Clay stamps
1. circle stamp, GR83–174
2. cross stamp, GR83–397
3. snake stamp, GR83–448

incised deeply into the face. On end of spiral a triangular shape represents head of the snake. A shallow groove circles the stalk near the end; within it is a shallow incised line. Very pale brown baked clay with mica flecks but no visible temper; matte surface. No wear on face. L. 3.485 cm; max. W. at face 2.065 cm; Th. 1.33 cm. Operation 16 locus 60 lot 197 (Phase B). FIG. 3.3.

Cylindrical or conical clay stamps of this type have been found over a wide area, although they are never common. Von Wickede listed four, two from late PPNB contexts at Jericho and Çayönü and two from early Pottery Neolithic deposits at Jarmo and Tell Halaf.[13] All were remarkably consistent in size (face diameter 2.5–3.0 cm) and design (spiral, whirl or concentric circles). The Jericho example was made from unbaked clay and bore a whirling pattern,[14] the Jarmo one was lightly baked with a deeply incised spiral,[15] the Tell Halaf stamp had a design of concentric circles formed by a groove near the edge and a deep impression in the center[16] and the Çayönü example has three concentric circles.[17] A comparable item with an incised design of two concentric circles with a dot in the centre was also found in the PPNB levels at Tell Halula. It was one of several cylindrical clay

13 Von Wickede 1990, 40, 66; for the dating of the Çayönü example to the Fourth Evolutionary Stage, or Final PPNB/PPNC, see Erim-Özdoğan 2011b, 191, 194, 224.

14 Kenyon 1955, 111, pl. XXIII:2; Kenyon and Holland 1982, 558, fig. 227:1, pl. VIIbB.

15 Morales 1983, 389, fig. 170:1.

16 Von Oppenheim 1943, 118, pls. 38:16, 114:14.

17 Morales 1990, 68–69, pl. 27:b. A slightly larger and rougher example (pl. 27:a) with double arch design may also belong to this group of stamps.

items found at this site: two were blank on the bottom and two were hollow.[18] Similar cylindrical items were produced in stone, as shown by the cylindrical stone stamp with an engraved design of two concentric circles found in a late PPNB deposit at El-Kowm 2-Caracol.[19]

Similar stamps, conical in shape with simple designs such as concentric circles, crosses and spirals, have been found at sites in central and western Anatolia. For example, Mersin-Yumuktepe, where the earliest stamps were on a floor dated 6445–6240 cal. BC[20]; Bademağacı EN II/4–3, *c.* 6400 BC[21]; Tepecik-Çiftlik[22]; and Ulucak Periods V and IV, from *c.* 6500–5800 cal. BC.[23] These sites have, however, also produced larger stamps with meandering and other elaborate designs, although it is increasingly recognized that these may be separate classes of items.[24] These western examples belong to the Pottery Neolithic, mostly to the second half of the 7th millennium, and are thus slightly later than the Gritille and other PPNB stamps. Exceptions are the stamps from Çatalhöyük levels VII-II,[25] occupation phases that may overlap with Gritille Phase B.[26] Some of the simpler of these have good parallels at Gritille. The earliest Çatalhöyük seal, no. 24, from level VII is cylindrical in form with a flat round face at one end on which is a design of two concentric circles with a dot in the centre. No. 26, also cylindrical and with a simple cross design, is unstratified, while no. 14, from level IV has a simple conical shape and cross on the face. Two others, nos. 21 and 22, from levels IV and VI, respectively, have a simple conical shape and spiral design on the flat face. The relationship of the stamps found in these central and western Neolithic sites to those of the PPNB sites further east is still unclear,[27] but a connection cannot be ruled out. The earlier examples so far, however, are all in the east.

---

18 Molist *et al.* 1996, 130, fig. 2:2, 4, 8, 9, fig. 3:1.

19 Stordeur *et al.* 1982, 39, fig. 16. The "nail headed inlays" from Çayönü with raised edge have a similar appearance but have been interpreted as inlays or nose studs and are earlier in date, coming mainly from the late Round and the Grill Building Subphases of the First Evolutionary Stage, 10th and 9th millennia cal. BC (Özdoğan 1999, 58, fig. 68; Erim-Özdoğan 2011b, 192–193, 222).

20 Caneva 2012, 5.

21 Umurtak 1999–2000, 1–20, fig. 3; Duru 2008, 106, fig. 189; Duru 2012, 19–20, figs. 70–72.

22 Bıçakçı *et al.* 2012, 103, fig. 56.

23 Çilingiroğlu 2009; Çilingiroğlu *et al.* 2012.

24 Caneva 2012, 5 and Duru 2012, 19; both scholars appear to see the larger stamps as pintaderas, and the conical ones with simple designs as seals; *cf.* Çilingiroğlu 2009 and discussion below.

25 Türkcan 2005, 175–185.

26 Cessford 2005, 99.

27 E.g., Erim-Özdoğan 2011b, 224; *cf* Türkcan 2005, 183–184.

Neolithic cylindrical and conical stamps have usually been explained as pintaderas, used for stamping decorative patterns on skin, leather, textiles or bread although, not unnaturally, evidence of such use has not survived.[28] Ç. Çilingiroğlu has suggested that at least some of the stamps from Ulucak in western Anatolia were used in textile production, as one, in particular, with a circular face and concentric circles (Stamp 1), was found in a building of Period IVb in association with loomweights and bone needles, as well as other domestic equipment.[29] This stamp also seemed to bear traces of red colored residue in its grooves. While this may suggest that some stamps were indeed used for patterning textiles, others may have had different uses.[30]

The earliest stamped impressions in Syria and southeastern Anatolia are on flat plaster plaques from Bouqras and el-Kowm. The Bouqras plaques (parts of at least seven were found in the 1976–1978 excavations) are from the earliest Pottery Neolithic (phases I and II, mid 7th millennium) and bear simple lozenge and zigzag patterns, apart from one round impression showing a caprid.[31] From PPNB layers at Tell el-Kowm 2 come a number of similar fragments.[32] The stamps that produced these impressions have not been found, but the designs are similar to those on the earliest stone stamps. Bouqras (level II, layer 4) also produced a jadeite seal with suspension hole and chevron design,[33] and from Ras Shamra level VC, from the end of the 8th millennium, came two steatite stamp seals with incised designs of a cross and cross-hatching respectively, and the steatite foot of a bovid (broken at the top) with incised cross-hatching on the base.[34] These stone stamps are of types certainly used as stamp seals in later periods. The purpose of the plaques remains unclear, but their occurrence at the same sites and with the same designs as the stone stamps makes some association with sealing likely.[35]

The earliest definite use of stamp seals for identification (impressions of stamps on clay sealings) comes from Sabi Abyad level 6 (Late Neolithic *c.* 6000 cal. BC), where the clay used to seal vessels bore on the outer surface impressions of stamp seals.[36] Although no actual stamps were found in this level, there

28 E.g., Mellaart 1967, pl. 121; Morales 1983, 369; von Wickede 1990, 66; Türkcan 2005, 182–183.

29 Çilingiroğlu 2009, 14–19, fig. 4.

30 Çilingiroğlu 2009, 19.

31 Akkermans *et al.* 1983, 356–357, pl. 42b,c.

32 Cauvin *et al.* 1979, 86, fig. 4: 2; Maréchal 1982, 223, figs. 3–4; Dornemann 1986, 17, pl. 21:7.

33 Contenson 1985, 347, fig. 19:3; Contenson and van Liere 1966, 185, pls. 8b:19, 13d.

34 Contenson 1977, 16–17, fig. 11; Contenson 1992, 96–97, fig. 125:14, 15, 18, pl. 88: 3, 4, 5.

35 Von Wickede 1990, 51.

36 Duistermaat 1996, 339–341.

can be no doubt that by this time stamp seals were in use to identify goods. At Sabi Abyad the impressions were preserved because the settlement burnt, and by chance the rooms in which these sealings had been stored were within the excavated area.

The designs used on the sealings at Sabi Abyad include a caprid (design A), zigzags (design B) and lozenges (design X), motifs also found on the plaster plaques at Bouqras and el Kowm.[37] There is thus continuity from PPNB into the early Pottery Neolithic in terms of iconography used on stamps, and it seems not unreasonable to suggest continuity of use too, with the plaques serving some form of identification purpose.

Where does this leave our cylindrical clay stamps? Among these earliest stamp seal impressions at Sabi Abyad is a design of concentric circles of the type used on the cylindrical stamps at Gritille and elsewhere (design W).[38] It occurs only once at Sabi Abyad but nevertheless shows this design was on a stamp used as a seal. The cross and the snake designs used on the Gritille stamps do not, however, occur on the Sabi Abyad sealings. Yet it is clear from this overview that the circle, cross and snake/spiral/whorl designs were part of a standard repertoire used over a wide area and for a considerable time. The most distinctive, the spiral/snake, was well established in Anatolia as early as the Epipaleolithic. For example, Epipaleolithic Hallan Çemi Tepesi has carved bone snakes,[39] and snakes appear at Göbekli Tepe.[40] A sculpted snake on the back of a male head was found at PPNB Nevalı Çori, located in the hills directly across the Euphrates from Gritille.[41] The link between snakes and male imagery has most recently been highlighted by Ian Hodder and Lynn Meskell.[42]

The prevalence of male imagery at PPNB settlements has also been emphasized by Hodder and Meskell, who cite the common occurrence of male figurines made of clay at Nevalı Çori.[43] At nearby and roughly contemporary Gritille, overt male and female symbolism is more or less balanced. In addition to the snake stamp, at least four modeled phalluses were found, made of stone, clay and *vaisselles blanches* (Fig. 4), and one small animal figurine has carefully depicted male

---

37 Duistermaat 1996, 358.

38 Duistermaat 1996, 357, figs. 5.6, 5.18:3.

39 Rosenberg 1994, 129, fig. 11:12.

40 E.g., on Pillars 1 and 5 from enclosure A and Pillar 33 in enclosure D: Hauptman 1999, fig. 34; Schmidt 1999, 13–15, pls. 5, 8:1; Schmidt 2011, fig. 9, 21.

41 Hauptman 1999, fig. 10; for a map showing the relationship between the sites see Özdoğan *et al.* 2011, 282.

42 Hodder and Meskell 2011.

43 Hodder and Meskell 2011, 240 with reference.

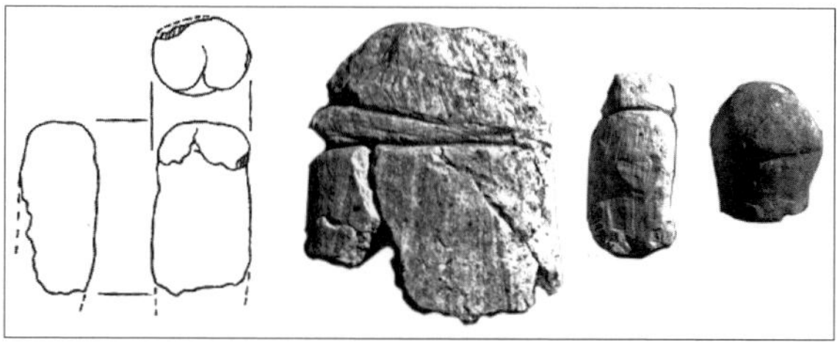

FIG. 4 Four of the phallic objects from Gritille Phase B (L to R): GR84–333 (clay); GR83–376 (*vaisselles blanches*); GR84–368 (chalky white limestone); GR83–412 (chalky white limestone).

genitalia.[44] These are counterbalanced by the circle stamp, which we suggest can be seen as a representation of females, and several animal figurines with sagging bellies that can be interpreted as an indication of pregnancy.[45] Human figurines do not depict primary sexual characteristics, with the exception of one pregnant female.[46] Another unique figurine has a snake-like, phallic head and torso, but heavy thighs suggesting a female lower body.[47]

Returning to the stamps from Gritille, it is reasonable to interpret the snake image as a male symbol and the circle image as a female image. Taking into account the fact that the stamps were deposited in the ruins of two successive houses, we follow a suggestion made by E. B. Banning that the symbol set does not just represent gender, but a social group, specifically a household or family.[48] Given the fact that the architectural sample at Gritille is very small and that the two stamps come from an unexcavated structure or its courtyard, any interpretation is wildly speculative, but given our preference for a gender balance in imagery at the site, we might suggest that symbols of both males and females were associated with this particular succession of households.

The cross stamp does not fit easily into an explanation of motifs based on gender symbolism, but it differs in a number of ways from the other two stamps and may represent a different kind of item. It is smaller, lacks the shallow groove around the end and, most importantly, was found in a different type of context. Interestingly, too, it has no parallels among the other PPNB and early Pottery Neolithic stamps of northern Syria/southeastern Anatolia, although it does have parallels to the west.

44 Voigt 2000, fig. 5d.

45 Voigt 2000, fig. 5:a-c.

46 Voigt 1985, fig. 13a-b.

47 Voigt 1985, fig. 12a-b.

48 Banning 2011, 253.

As for the ways in which these Gritille stamps, and the other PPNB clay stamps, were used, we still have no definite evidence. Stamps were being impressed on plaques in the PPNB period, but we have no evidence that small clay stamps were so used. Soon after PPNB time, stamps were used on sealings and, in western Anatolia, perhaps on textiles. The technique of stamping can be applied to many materials; in any place or period it may have been used on one material or many. Regardless of the way(s) in which the early stamps were used, the well-preserved snake motif on the Gritille stamp gives meaning to the spiral design used elsewhere, and, together with the circle stamps, shows the widespread and consistent use of gender symbolism on small items that were used by ordinary households.

Sealings

Nine pieces of shaped clay from the Neolithic layers at Gritille bore impressions; the best-preserved are presented here (Fig. 5). In two cases the impressions contained longitudinal striations made by some vegetal material. GR84–115 has four roughly parallel impressions on one side of the pellet; GR83–400 has a number of impressions on both flat faces. On both these objects the impressions could have been made by pressing a pellet of clay over grasses used to tie closed a bag or other container, in the case of GR83–400 with the ties then wound again over the clay. GR83–477 consisted of several fragments, one of which bore a clear impression with rounded section and irregularities that may indicate twisting. GR84–293 bore two deep impressions at right angles; the striations in the impressions suggest a wooden vessel,[49] while two examples (GR84–220B and GR83–401, not illustrated) were placed over a single strip with a smooth surface (leather?).

In all cases these clay items were baked. All the sealings with a clearly defined context were found in association with pyrotechnic features, all but one on the sloping surfaces with roasting pits and ash patches leading down toward the river. Given this distribution, it is almost certain that the sealings were accidentally fired, accounting for their preservation.

GR83–400 (GT8854): Flattened disk with impressions of grass-like pieces on both flat surfaces; broken away on one edge. Black baked clay. L. 4.492 cm; pres. W. 3.912 cm; max. Th. 1.826 cm. Operation 16 locus 38 lot 88 (Phase B). Fig. 5.1.

GR83–477 (GT4614): Fragments of shaped clay sealing. Across the corner of one piece is an impression with rounded shape; irregularities within it suggest the fiber was twisted. Baked. Operation 17 locus 9 lot 18 (Phase A). Fig. 5.4.

49 See e.g., Mellaart 1967, 215, fig. 55.

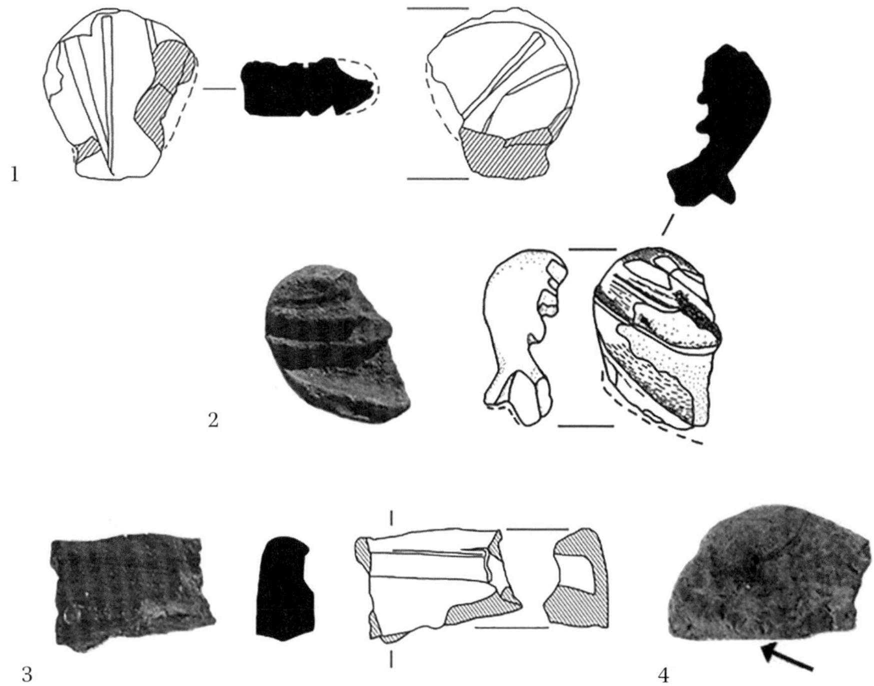

FIG. 5 Clay sealings.

1. clay with impressions on both faces, GR83–400
2. clay with deep vegetal impressions in one face, GR84–115
3. clay with impressions from wooden(?) rim, GR84–293
4. clay with impression across one corner, GR83–477

GR84–115 (GT16421): Carefully shaped disk with smooth convex surface marked with finger impressions and a pinch mark; other face has four deep parallel impressions that contain longitudinal grass-like striations. Minor damage on one edge. Hard, gritty, black baked clay. L. 3.15 cm; W. 2.17 cm; Th. 1.36 cm. Operation 12 locus 42 lot 49 (Phase A). FIG. 5.2.

GR84–293 (GT18936): Shaped piece of clay broken at both ends and on one side; one face is flat and the other bears a shallow longitudinal impression with a deeper rectilinear impression at one end. A slight ridge between the two impressions. Black baked clay. L. 2.43 cm; W. 1.58 cm; Th. 0.97 cm. Operation 17 locus 65 lot 104 (Phase B). FIG. 5.3.

Clay "sealings" such as these are found at many sites in final PPNB and early PN contexts, including Sumaki Höyük[50] and Çayönü.[51]

The purpose of sealing something can be twofold: clay can be used to block an opening in a container (in our case, perhaps a leather bag or a wooden vessel) in order to exclude air, water and animal pests, but clay that blocks an opening or is pressed against a covering can also be used to exclude people without authorization, that is, to make it obvious if the container has been opened. The sealing can be marked to identify the owner (e.g., by the use of a stamp seal), but the sealing itself may be sufficient in a given context (room or storage area) to indicate the property is only to be opened by certain persons or at certain times, and to show if it has been opened.[52]

As mentioned above, by *c.* 6000 cal. BC sealings were being used with seals to identify storage vessels. Hundreds were found at Sabi Abyad where clay had been pressed over baskets, ceramic vessels, stone vessels and leather bags to seal them, and the sealings also bore impressions of stamp seals, making their purpose clear.[53]

Most of the Gritille sealings appear to have been pressed against ties rather than used to block openings. Although they bear no indication of identification of a specific owner, they are an indication that property was being stored for opening by specific persons and/or at specific times. If the clay tokens that are found at PPNB sites were indeed used for recording, the presence of "special" property by the end of the period is not surprising.

Tokens

About fifty clay tokens and fragments of tokens were found in the Neolithic deposits at Gritille, as well as a number of tokens made from limestone. The clay tokens are unbaked or lightly fired. The clay is reddish-brown (unfired) or gray (fired), is often micaceous, and fine vegetable inclusions are usual. There is a limited range of shapes: spheres and part-spheres (33), disks (4), cones (5), rings (3) and cylinders (3), although there is some variation within each category. The surface is usually matte. A few have chips around the edges, the result of handling during use.

The spheres include proper spheres and ones that are rather flattened, these shapes merging so that the distinction was probably not intentional. About one-third were somewhat flattened (the precise number is unclear because many were fragmentary).

---

50 Erim-Özdoğan 2011a, 33–34, fig. 38:a-h.

51 Morales 1990, 66–67, pl. 26: i-k; Erim-Özdoğan 2011b, 224 "clay appliqué".

52 Duistermaat 1996, 341–342; von Wickede 1990, 29–34.

53 Duistermaat and Akkermans 1996, 17–44; Duistermaat 1996, 339–401.

Some were carefully shaped; others were less carefully made and are somewhat irregular in shape. Diameters range from 1.1 to 2.4 cm with occasional larger examples (GR83–312A and GR83–312B have diameters of 3.1 and 3.27 cm, respectively). Three examples (e.g., GR83–320A and GR83–385) have one flat face, forming a three-quarter sphere, and one (GR83–173) was a one-quarter sphere. No half-spheres were identified, although some of the fragmentary examples could have taken this form. One sphere (GR84–126) had an ovoid shape, which may or may not have been intentional.

The disks were all roughly lenticular in shape, but irregularly made. Of the cones, one (GR83–1) had slightly concave sides, two (GR84–77 and GR84–146) were very neatly made and one (GR84–220A) was elongated and pointed.

Only one ring token was identified, but there were many curved fragments that could have been parts of ring tokens, bent cone tokens, or arms/horns from figurines. Likewise the identification of some stalk-like clay pieces was uncertain, as they could have been broken parts of figurines, the tops of cylindrical stamps (see above) or cylinder tokens. Schmandt-Besserat includes cylindrical stamps such as the three we have discussed above among the PPNB tokens.[54] Türkcan has also suggested the small cylindrical stamps with shallow incised patterns at Çatalhöyük may have been tokens (he regards them as unsuitable for stamping),[55] but no other tokens have been identified at that site, and it is unlikely the eastern token system extended to the Anatolian plateau.[56]

Eight clay tokens are presented here to demonstrate the range found at Gritille (see Fig. 6). Type numbers refer to those of Schmandt-Besserat.[57]

GR83–1 (GT3612): Cone with sides slightly concave; base concave and top perhaps flat (recent break). Smooth, matte surface. Dark brown-gray baked clay. Max. Ht 1.85 cm, max. D. 2.41 cm. Operation 16 locus 1 lot 1 (balk cleaning) (Type 1:4). Fig. 6.5.

GR83–173 (GT6106): One-quarter sphere with irregular concavity in base. Light brown fired clay. Max. D. 1.58 cm; max. Th. 4.9 cm. Operation 16 locus 31 lot 78 (Phase B) (Type 2:30). Fig. 6.3.

GR83–198H (GT6429): Flattened sphere. Unfired clay, very fragile with quite large grit inclusions and possibly fine vegetal matter. Surface matte. D. 1.95–1.75 cm. Operation 16 locus 31 lot 87 (Phase B) (Type 2:1 but slightly flattened). Fig. 6.1.

---

54 See e.g., Schmandt-Besserat 1977, 139–142; 1992; 1994.

55 Türkcan 2005, 183.

56 Atalay 2005, 162–163.

57 Schmandt-Besserat 1992, 203–232.

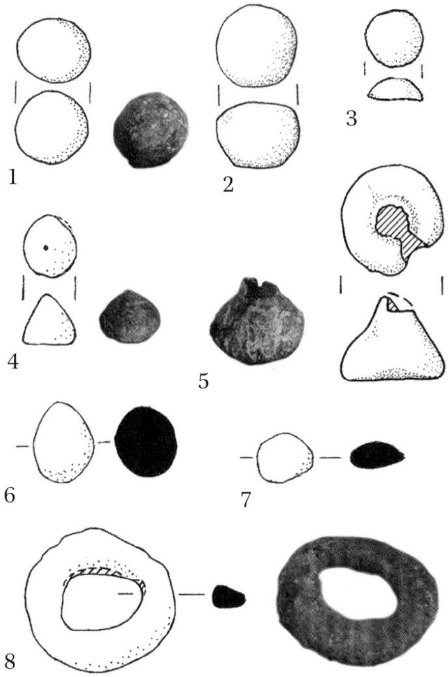

Fig. 6. Clay tokens.
1. flattened sphere, GR83–198H
2. three-quarter sphere, GR83–478
3. one-quarter sphere, GR83–173
4. small cone, GR84–77
5. cone with concave sides, GR83–1
6. ovoid, GR84–126
7. lenticular disk, GR84–220C
8. ring, GR84–147.

GR83–478 (GT8350): Three-quarter sphere. Gray fired clay. Surface matte. D. 2.45–1.87 cm. Operation 16 locus 38 lot 88 (Phase B) (Type 2:17). Fig. 6.2.

GR84–77 (GT16201): Cone, fairly regular shape, carefully made and base slightly concave. Dark gray baked clay with mica flecks. Ht 1.15 cm; D. base 1.4 cm. Operation 17 locus 16 lot 24 (Phase B) (Type 1:1). Fig. 6.4.

GR84–126 (GT16527): Irregularly shaped, ovoid to spherical token. Brown baked clay. Matte surface. D. 1.97–1.57 cm. Operation 17 locus 21 lot 39 (Phase B) (Type 2:1 or 6:1). Fig. 6.6.

GR84–147 (GT17307): Clay ring, irregular in shape, with irregular, flattened section. Dark gray baked clay. Smooth, grainy surface. Three additional ring fragments found with it. Ext. max. D. 3.67 cm; int. max. D. 2.03 cm; Th. 1.08 cm. Operation 17 locus 22 lot 57 (Phase B) (Type 16:17). Fig. 6.8.

GR84–220C (GT17879): Lenticular disk, irregularly shaped with one face smooth and one rough; part of edge flattened, so has teardrop shape in plan. Black fired clay. D. 1.44–1.25 cm; max. Th. 0.67 cm. Operation 17 locus 46 lot 82 (Phase B) (Type 3:3). Fig. 6.7.

Chronologically, almost all the tokens are from Phase B deposits, with a couple from Phase A; however, one irregular sphere (GR84–217, GT17177) was found in a Basal deposit. Spatially and functionally, most of the tokens were found on the sloping levels of collapse and ash that led down away from the western architectural units, and only a few were found in roasting pits or ash patches. Thus, unlike sealings (and figurines), the tokens were clearly curated, used after firing or without firing.

In four or five cases a number of tokens were found together in a group:

- A group of at least twelve spherical tokens, seven complete, or almost so, and fragments of at least five more, came from Operation 16 locus 31 lot 87 (GR83–198, GT6429). The shapes varied from proper spheres to flattened and ovoid. They range in size from *c.* 1.50 cm to 2.42 cm, with half (A-F) towards the smaller end and half (G-L) towards the larger end of the spectrum.
- Five clay items and fragments were found together in Operation 17 locus 46 lot 82, including a cone (GR84–220A, GT17879), two lentoid disks (GR84–220B and C), a curved piece that appears to have been from a ring token (GR84–220D), and an unidentifiable fragment.
- A clay ring and fragments of three other rings were found together (GR84–147, GT17307) in Operation 17 locus 22 lot 57.
- Two large spheres (GR84–312A and B, GT19408) were found together in Operation 12 locus 92 lot 137.
- An ovoid, flattened sphere (GR83–320A, GT7580) was found in Operation 16 locus 42 lot 143 with another (unidentifiable) fragment of shaped clay.

Tokens were used in settlements from Turkey to Iran from *c.* 8000 BC, and for the first four thousand years or so the system was remarkably stable, with plain spheres, cones, disks and cylinders forming the repertoire.[58] These are the types used at Gritille, with the addition of rings. As the earliest tokens appear at the same time as the first signs of cultivation and storage of cereals, their use as a means of counting or recording quantities of foodstuffs and numbers of animals appears established, especially as they continue to be used as part of later Mesopotamian temple accounting.[59] They are usually found in discard situations, suggesting they were produced as needed and then discarded.[60] The locations in which the Gritille tokens were usually found, the fact that they occur in groups, and the rare evidence of chips or use-wear all conform to Schmandt-Besserat's theory that these artifacts represent some kind of recording system.

58 Schmandt-Besserat 1992, 33–39; Schmandt-Besserat 1994, 13–17.

59 Schmandt-Besserat 1992, 168–170; Schmandt-Besserat 1994, 20.

60 Schmandt-Besserat 1992, 93.

Conclusion

The careful excavation and detailed recording of finds at Gritille and other recently excavated Neolithic sites are providing a more abundant sample of small fragile artifacts, as well as context information that can lead to better and more interesting interpretations of such finds.

The clay objects from Phase B at Gritille that have been presented here include components of a recording system that was in common use by the late PPNB period, an indication of an increasing need to keep track of goods and/or transactions. Tokens are the most visible and readily interpreted evidence of this system. The presence of sealings and possible use of stamps as emblems expands the evidence for the isolation of materials as the property of specific individuals or groups.

That the Gritille sample includes emblems easily linked to males (the snake) and females (the circle) suggests that gender was an important element in the definition of households or even multi-household groups that were of fundamental importance for early village communities in the Middle East.

REFERENCES

Akkermans, P. A., J. A. K. Boerma, A. T. Clason, S. G. Hill, E. Lohof, C. Meiklejohn, M. le Miere, G. M. F. Molgat, J. J. Roodenberg, W. Waterbolk-van Rooyen and W. van Zeist, "Bouqras Revisited: Preliminary Report on a Project in Eastern Syria." *Proceedings of the Prehistoric Society* 49 (1983): 335–372.

Atalay, S., "Domesticating Clay: The Role of Clay Balls, Mini Balls and Geometric Objects in Daily Life at Çatalhöyük" in *Changing Materialities at Çatalhöyük: Reports from the 1995–99 Seasons*. McDonald Institute Monographs and British Institute at Ankara Monograph 39, ed. by I. Hodder, 139–168. London: British Institute at Ankara, 2005.

Banning, E. B. Comment on I. Hodder and L. Meskell, "A 'Curious and Sometimes a Trifle Macabre Artistry'. Some Aspects of Symbolism in Neolithic Turkey." *Current Anthropology* 52:2 (2011): 252–253.

Bıçakçı, E., M. Godon and Y.G. Çakan, "Tepecik-Çiftlik" in *The Neolithic in Turkey. New Excavations & New Research 3: Central Turkey*, ed. by M. Özdoğan, N. Başgelen and P. Kuniholm, 89–134. İstanbul: Arkeoloji ve Sanat Yayınları, 2012.

Caneva, I., "Mersin-Yumuktepe in the Seventh Millennium BC: An Updated View" in *The Neolithic in Turkey. New Excavations & New Research 3: Central Turkey*, ed. by M. Özdoğan, N. Başgelen and P. Kuniholm, 1–29. İstanbul: Arkeoloji ve Sanat Yayınları, 2012.

Cauvin, J., M.-C. Cauvin and D. Stordeur, "Recherches préhistorique à El Kowm (Syrie). Première campagne 1978." *Cahiers de l'Euphrate* 2 (1979): 80–117.

Cessford, C., "Absolute Dating at Çatalhöyük" in *Changing Materialities at Çatalhöyük: Reports from the 1995–99 Seasons*. McDonald Institute Monographs and British Institute at Ankara Monograph 3), ed. by I. Hodder, 65–99. London: British Institute at Ankara, 2005.

Çilingiroğlu, A., Ö. Çevik and Ç. Çilingiroğlu, "Ulucak Höyük. Towards Understanding the Early Farming Communities of Middle West Anatolia: Contribution of Ulucak" in *The Neolithic in Turkey. New Excavations & New Research 4: Western Turkey*, ed.by M. Özdoğan, N. Başgelen and P. Kuniholm, 139–175. İstanbul: Arkeoloji ve Sanat Yayınları, 2012.

Çilingiroğlu, Ç., "Of Stamps, Loom Weights and Spindle Whorls: Contextual Evidence on the Function(s) of Neolithic Stamps from Ulucak, İzmir, Turkey." *Journal of Mediterranean Archaeology* 22/1 (2009): 3–27.

Contenson, H. de., "Le Néolithique de Ras Shamra V d'après les campagnes 1972–1976 dans le sondage SH." *Syria* 54 (1977): 1–23.

———. "La campagne de 1965 à Bouqras." *Cahiers de l'Euphrate* 4 (1985): 335–371.

———. *Ras Shamra-Ougarit 8: Préhistoire de Ras Shamra: les sondages stratigraphiques de 1955* à *1976.* Paris: Éditions Recherche sur les Civilisations, Diff. ADPF, 1992.

Contenson, H. de and W. J. van Liere, "Premier sondage à Bouqras en 1965: rapport préliminaire." *Annales Archéologiques Arabes Syriennes* 16 (1966): 181–192.

Dornemann, R.H., *A Neolithic Village at Tell el Kowm in the Syrian Desert*. Chicago: Oriental Institute of the University of Chicago, 1986.

Duistermaat, K., "The Seals and Sealings" in *Tell Sabi Abyad The Late Neolithic Settlement. Report on the Excavations of the University of Amsterdam (1988) and the National Museum of Antiquities Leiden (1991–1993) in Syria II*, ed.by P. M. M. G. Akkermans, 339–341. İstanbul: The Netherlands Institute for the Near East, 1996.

Duistermaat, K. and P.M.M.G. Akkermans, "Of Storage and Nomads. The Sealings from Late Neolithic Sabi Abyad, Syria." *Paléorient* 22/2 (1996): 17–44.

Duru, R., *From 8000 BC to 2000 BC. Six Thousand Years of the Burdur-Antalya Region*. Antalya: Suna ve İnan Kıraç Akdeniz Medeniyetleri Araştırma Enstitüsü, 2008.

———. "The Neolithic of the Lakes Region. Hacılar - Kuruçay Höyük - Höyücek - Bademağacı Höyük" in *The Neolithic in Turkey. New Excavations & New Research 4: Western Turkey*, ed. by M. Özdoğan, N. Başgelen and P. Kuniholm, 1–65. İstanbul: Arkeoloji ve Sanat Yayınları, 2012.

Ellis, R.S. and M.M. Voigt, "Excavations at Gritille, Turkey." *American Journal of Archaeology* 86 (1982): 319–332.

Erim-Özdoğan, A., "Sumaki Höyük. A New Neolithic Settlement in the Upper Tigris Basin" in *The Neolithic in Turkey. New Excavations & New Research 1: The Tigris Basin*, ed. by M. Özdoğan, N. Başgelen and P. Kuniholm, 19–60. İstanbul: Arkeoloji ve Sanat Yayınları, 2011a.

———. "Çayönü" in *The Neolithic in Turkey. New Excavations & New Research 1: The Tigris Basin*, ed. by M. Özdoğan, N. Başgelen and P. Kuniholm, 185–269. İstanbul: Arkeoloji ve Sanat Yayınları, 2011b.

Hauptmann, H., "The Urfa Region" in *Neolithic in Turkey. The Cradle of Civilization. New Discoveries*, ed. by M. Özdoğan and N. Başgelen, 65–86. İstanbul: Arkeoloji ve Sanat Yayınları, 1999.

Hodder, I. and L. Meskell, "A 'Curious and Sometimes a Trifle Macabre Artistry'. Some Aspects of Symbolism in Neolithic Turkey." *Current Anthropology* 52/2 (2011): 235–263.

Kenyon, K. M., "Excavations at Jericho, 1955." *Palestine Exploration Quarterly* 87 (1955): 108–117.

Kenyon, K.M. and T.A. Holland, *Excavations at Jericho 4.* London: Council for British Research in the Levant, 1982.

Maréchal, C., "Vaisselles blanches du Proche-Orient: El Kowm (Syrie) et l'usage du plâtre au Néolithique." *Cahiers de l'Euphrate* 3 (1982): 217–251.

Mellaart, J. *Çatal Hüyük. A Neolithic Town in Anatolia*. London: Thames & Hudson, 1967.

Molist, M., C. Barrachina and M. Gangonells, "Mobiliario Diverso" in *Tell Halula (Siria) un Yacimiento Neolítico del Valle Medio del Éufrates Campañas de 1991 y 1992*, ed. by M. M. Montaña, 125–133. Madrid 1996.

Morales, V.B., "Jarmo Figurines and Other Clay Objects" in *Prehistoric Archaeology along the Zagros Flanks*, ed. by L. S. Braidwood, R. J. Braidwood, B. Howe, C. A. Reed and P. J. Watson, 369–423. Chicago: Oriental Institute of the University of Chicago, 1983.

———. *Figurines and Other Clay Objects from Sarab and Çayönü.* Oriental Institute Communications 25. Chicago: Oriental Institute of the University of Chicago, 1990.

Nieuwenhuyse, O. P., P. M. M. G. Akkermans and J. van der Plicht, "Not So Coarse, Nor Always Plain—The Earliest Pottery of Syria." *Antiquity* 84 (2010): 71–85.

Özdoğan, A., "Çayönü" in *Neolithic in Turkey. The Cradle of Civilization. New Discoveries*, ed. by M. Özdoğan and N. Başgelen, 35–63. İstanbul: Arkeoloji ve Sanat Yayınları, 1999.

Özdoğan, M., N. Başgelen and P. Kuniholm, *The Neolithic in Turkey. New Excavations & New Research 2: The Euphrates Basin*. İstanbul: Arkeoloji ve Sanat Yayınları, 2011.

Redford, S., *The Archaeology of the Frontier in the Medieval Near East: Excavations at Gritille, Turkey.* Archaeological Institute of America, Monographs New Series 3. Philadelphia: University Museum Publication for the Archaeological Institute of America, 1998.

Rosenberg, M., "Hallan Çemi Tepesi: Some Further Observations Concerning Stratigraphy and Material Culture." *Anatolica* 20 (1994): 121–140.

Schmandt-Besserat, D., "The Beginnings of the Use of Clay in Turkey." *Anatolian Studies* 27 (1977): 133–150.

———. *Before Writing 1: From Counting to Cuneiform*. Austin: University of Texas Press, 1992.

———. "Tokens: A Prehistoric Archive System" in *Archives Before Writing Proceedings of the International Colloquium Orioli Romano, October 23–25, 1991*, ed. by P. Ferioli, E. Fiandra, G. G. Fissore and M. Frangipane, 13–28. Rome, 1994.

Schmidt, K., "Frühe Tier- und Menschenbilder vom Göbekli Tepe—Kampagnen 1995–1998. Ein Kommentierter Katalog der Grossplastik und der Reliefs." *İstanbuler Mitteilungen* 49 (1999): 5–21.

———. "Göbekli Tepe" in *The Neolithic in Turkey. New Excavations & New Research 2: The Euphrates Basin*, ed. by M. Özdoğan, N. Başgelen and P. Kuniholm, 41–83. İstanbul: Arkeoloji ve Sanat Yayınları, 2011.

Stordeur, D., C. Maréchal and M. Molist, "El Kowm 2-Caracol. Campagnes 1978, 1979, 1980. Stratigraphie et architectures." *Cahiers de l'Euphrate* 3 (1982): 33–49.

Türkcan, A. U., "Some Remarks on Çatalhöyük Stamp Seals" in *Changing Materialities at Çatalhöyük: Reports from the 1995–99 Seasons*. McDonald Institute Monographs and British Institute at Ankara Monograph 39, ed. by I. Hodder, 175–185. London: British Institute at Ankara, 2005.

Umurtak, G., "Some Observations about the Seals of the Neolithic and Early Chalcolithic Periods in the Burdur-Antalya Regions." *Adalya* 4 (1999–2000): 1–20.

Voigt, M.M., "Village on the Euphrates, Excavations at Neolithic Gritille in Turkey." *Expedition* 27/1 (1985): 10–24.

———. "Excavations at Neolithic Gritille." *Anatolica* 15 (1988): 215–232.

———. "Çatal Höyük in Context. Ritual at Early Neolithic Sites in Eastern and Central Turkey" in *Life in Neolithic Farming Communities. Social Organization, Identity, and Differentiation*, ed. by I. Kuijt, 253–293. New York: Springer, 2000.

Voigt, M.M. and R.S. Ellis, "Excavations at Gritille, Turkey: 1981." *Paléorient* 7 (1981): 87–100.

von Oppenheim, M.F., *Tell Halaf I*. Berlin 1943.

von Wickede, A., *Prähistorische Stempelglyptik in Vorderasien*. Munich: Profil, 1990.

Negotiating Peace, Enduring Conflict:
A Diachronic View on Prehistoric Warfare in the Eastern Aegean

Sinan Ünlüsoy[1] — *Çiler Çilingiroğlu*[2]

Marie-Henriette and Charles Gates (or "Mrs. and Mr. Gates," as we have always known them) have inspired and amazed us since our undergraduate days as deeply knowledgeable professors with the highest of scientific standards and work ethics. We find ourselves, not infrequently, recollecting fond memories of Bilkent with the Gateses, who always showed up early at the 8:40 class, read and commented on each and every paper we wrote, and respected and listened to what we had to say – regardless of how naive and silly it may have been. As instructors in our own universities now, we have both come to realize that it was the Gateses whom we took as virtuous examples for our teaching practices – with inevitable appreciation that it is extremely demanding to keep to the standards they set at Bilkent. Knowing that this article is insufficient to express our gratitude for everything they have taught us, we humbly dedicate it to the most decent and peaceful couple we have had the privilege to know.

Abstract

Prehistoric archaeology can offer valuable insights into the history of violence and warfare. However, archaeology as the study of material manifestations of past human societies has limited power when it comes to 'digging up' concepts and processes. By using selected archaeological criteria to discern evidence of raiding and warfare, we try to contextualize the changing role and importance of inter-societal violence for eastern Aegean (coastal West Anatolian) communities from the seventh to the late third millennium BC.

We argue that violence was an integral part of prehistoric living in all these ages, but as achievement-based societies were gradually replaced by rank societies, different modes

1 Department of Travel Management and Tourism Guidance, Yaşar University, Bornova 35100 İzmir, Turkey.

2 Department of Protohistory and Near Eastern Archaeology, Ege University, Bornova 35100 İzmir, Turkey.

of violence and violence related activities appeared. Most notably, the emergence of chiefly authorities in the Early Bronze Age, going hand in hand with a rising demand of sumptuous goods and accumulation of wealth at a few nodal sites, generated a system described as "competitive interaction" by Flannery and Marcus. Possible outcomes of these new social and economic conditions were organized raids, the possible emergence of a warrior group and an urgent need for effective defensive strategies, which all contributed to the transformation of these societies and their ideology. By highlighting the transformative power of violence, we suggest that one of the causes for the social evolution of communities dealt with here was their perpetual effort of negotiating peace and enduring conflict.

Introduction

Warfare has long been held as one of the most disgraceful elements in human societies with deep historical and evolutionary roots.[3] Enlightenment philosophers like Hobbes, Rousseau, Schiller and Goethe, among others, condemned wars, a chronic disease of Europe in the Middle Ages and afterwards. As a result, discussions about societal violence and conflict tend to revolve around the issue of 'being human.' There is a colossal question to be addressed by the Humanities: Is violence inherent to human nature? If yes, will it be ever possible to overcome the conscious and unconscious motives for violence?[4] In asking this question, philosophers like Hobbes and Rousseau felt they had to return to the origins and determine whether violence emerged in a unique instant in human history or whether it was always there with no specific historical circumstance to trigger its emergence. The difference in opinion is usually defined between the schools of thought of Hobbes and Rousseau, the former arguing for a timeless violence, hard-wired in human nature, and the latter for a defining historical moment that arrived with the emergence of private property.[5] Hobbes argues that in the hy pothetical natural condition, fear of death and need for security are the prime drives that shape human behavior which can therefore result in violent acts as a mean of protecting the 'self.'[6] Rousseau, on the other hand, does not readily follow Hobbes's hypothetical natural state by naming "compassion" as the true feeling constituting society even before there were rules, laws and proper language. Rousseau's famous passage on the creation of inequality and thus warfare is ever inspiring and challenging to the modern mind, which usually sees inequality and private property as ahistorical social conditions:

3 Einstein and Freud 1972.

4 Strachey 1957.

5 Dawson 1996, 1; Driessen 1999, 11.

6 Zelyüt 2013, 21–22.

> The first man who, having enclosed a piece of ground, bethought himself of saying *This is mine*, and found people simple enough to believe him, was the real founder of civil society. From how many crimes, wars and murders, from how many horrors and misfortunes might not any one have saved mankind, by pulling up the stakes, or filling up the ditch, and crying to his fellows: 'Beware of listening to this impostor; you are undone if you once forget that the fruits of the earth belong to us all, and the earth itself to nobody.'[7]

Prehistoric archaeology can offer valuable insights into the history, emergence and modes of inter-societal violence and warfare from the instant when the genus *Homo* began to produce tools. However, archaeology, as the study of material manifestations of past human societies, admittedly has limited power when it comes to 'digging up' concepts and processes. Archaeological clues collected in the field are mostly stripped of direct proof of intra- and inter-societal violence. Prehistoric research, then, has to turn to historical and ethnographic records to argue for or against the presence of violence. In this sense, prehistoric archaeology is susceptible to a variety of interpretations depending on the perspective of the researcher. Some researchers may interpret every single arrowhead, sling and fortification as 'clear' evidence of conflicts, whereas others could discover in the very same objects other functions and meanings not necessarily related to violence and conflict. Therefore, one has the impression that researchers arguing for prehistoric warfare are accused of justifying modern warfare, whereas archaeologists who deny its presence are accused of a "pacification of the past".[8] As a result, arguing for or supporting either position inevitably comes to mean having a political agenda.[9] It seems, unless it is demonstrated by direct evidence, i.e. mass burials of people carrying skeletal wounds and other traces of bodily injury, prehistorians will have a difficult time making a case for inter-societal violence or warfare.

In compliance with the ethnographic and historical record, we hold that violent acts existed in every era, but that there are very different modes and scales of, and both rational and irrational motives for, inter-societal violence in history.[10] For example, endemic warfare among native communities was recorded in the first European documents about New World societies.[11] Both egalitarian and rank societies studied from across the world show some form of violence against

7 Rousseau 1754, Part II.

8 *Cf.* Bernbeck 2010, 11; LeBlanc 2010, 40.

9 Dawson 1996, 2.

10 Armit *et al.* 2006, 2.

11 Keeley 1996; Eriksen 2001, 161–163; Flannery and Marcus 2012.

other groups. [12] There is, however, a blurred but important distinction between achievement-based and hereditary rank societies in terms of why and how raids were organized. In achievement-based groups, aggression and warfare were motivated by individual interests like gaining prestige, status, booty, access to important sources, revenge, etc., but there are also cases in which raids are organized in various tribal societies to intimidate neighboring groups and maintain political power or for ritual and symbolic purposes. [13] Rank societies tend to attack other groups for the chief's interests of territorial expansion and obtaining slaves. For instance, for an achievement-based society, a war captive would most likely be tortured and killed, while in a rank society headed by a chief, would be kept as a slave to be exploited as labor force. [14]

Different kinds and degrees of conflict and warfare are not always easy to recognize in archaeological data. The ambiguous character of archaeological evidence concerning raids and warfare led researchers to determine certain criteria for detecting prehistoric violence and conflict. Driessen, Ivanova and Molloy, among others, list different proxies in the archaeological record that might encapsulate information about conditions of peace and conflict. [15] The human remains, military hardware (weapons and armor), fortifications, settlement locations, burnt layers at sites, and iconographic and symbolic representations can be investigated for various indications of violence and conflict.

In this paper, we will explore archaeological evidence and indications for warfare in the eastern Aegean (or coastal western Anatolia) from the seventh to the end of the third millennium BC by using criteria defined in the above cited studies. We will be using the term 'warfare' to generically refer to inter-societal conflicts resulting in both offensive and defensive actions. In the eastern Aegean, past and present excavations provide immense information on multiple aspects of living and social, political and economical organization, but a diachronic investigation focusing on conflicts and warfare stretching from the Early Neolithic to the end of the Early Bronze Age (EBA) has never been attempted before (Fig. 1). We believe that the analysis of published data with this specific viewpoint engenders a novel understanding of eastern Aegean prehistoric communities and their social evolution through millennia. In what follows, we will examine the archaeological data in terms of certain criteria that provide insights and clues about the emergence, development and the nature of raids and warfare.

---

12 Eriksen 2001, 161–163; Flannery and Marcus 2012.

13 Redmond 1994; Flannery and Marcus 2012, 105, 170.

14 Flannery and Marcus 2012, 217–219.

15 Driessen 1999; Ivanova 2008; Molloy 2012, 91.

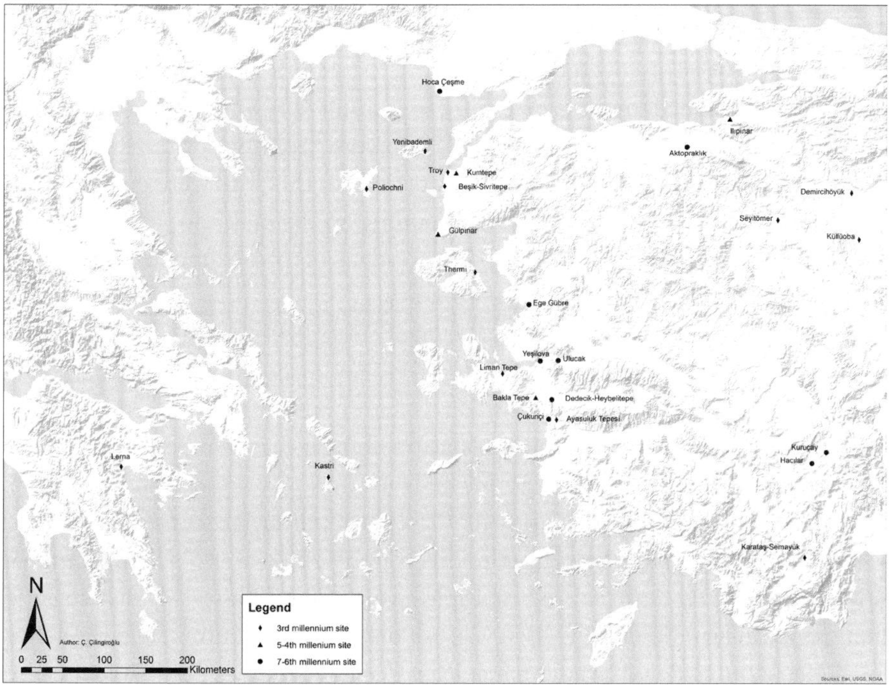

FIG. 1 Sites mentioned in the text.

Settlement Patterns and Fortifications

Foundation of a settlement on an easily defendable hilltop or the building of massive walls strengthened by towers and bastions are considered good indications of an external human threat.[16] There is, of course, controversy about the true nature and function of surrounding walls, towers and site locations. Some enclosure walls may not have a defensive character. They may have been built against wild animals, floods or simply as a symbol of group identity. The famous case of the Jericho tower, dating to the Pre-Pottery Neolithic, is a good example for this kind of discussion.[17]

In prehistoric western Anatolia, famous cases include Hacılar and Kuruçay. Mellaart describes Hacılar IIA-B (*ca.* 5800–5600 BC) as a "fortified village" surrounded by mud-brick walls 1.5–3 m thick; and Hacılar IA-B (*ca.* 5700–5600 BC) as a "fortress" built after intensive leveling activities, again surrounded by mud-brick walls 2 m thick.[18] According to Mellaart, however, the wall was a power symbol of

16 Driessen 1999, 16; LeBlanc 2010, 41.

17 Bar-Yosef 2010, 8.

18 Mellaart 1970, 75–76.

a ruler and had less of a defensive character.[19] Stone foundations of an enclosure wall have also been discovered at Kuruçay 11, a site in close proximity to Hacılar. The Kuruçay 11 settlement is evidently surrounded by a 26 m long and 1.1 m thick wall equipped with two semi-circular towers.[20] The excavator, Refik Duru, suggests that the northern and western portions of this wall were destroyed by successive flooding events.[21] Although flooding events may have had an impact on the building of an enclosure wall, the presence of towers implies a defensive purpose intended by the Kuruçay community.

Ditches are important structural elements that serve to protect settlements. Karul reports that the inhabitants of basal Hoca Çeşme, Aşağı Pınar 5 and Aktopraklık B built enclosure walls and ditches around their settlements.[22] There is, however, controversy over the true nature of these features. For example, the enclosure wall at Hoca Çeşme, a site located on a rock promontory, does not cover the area where defense is most needed.[23] The plastered surfaces of the ditch walls at Aşağı Pınar may have been used to divert and store water.[24] At Aktopraklık B, a site dated to *ca.* 5800 cal. BC, multiple layers of thick plastering may suggest that the main function of the ditch was not defensive in nature.[25] On the other hand, Keeley *et al.* firmly argue that at least V-shaped ditches can be universally associated with defensive purposes.[26] In this respect, at least, V-shaped ditches at Aşağı Pınar 5 need to be classified as defensive architecture.

Up until the early 6th millennium BC, except at Ege Gübre and possibly Çukuriçi,[27] no enclosing structures –indicated neither by positive nor negative remains– have been detected in the İzmir Region. More importantly, the selected locations of these early farming villages give no indication whatsoever of a constant human threat. Long-term extensive excavations at Ulucak and Yeşilova did not locate any enclosure walls or ditches surrounding the dwelling area.[28] Middle and Late Chalcolithic settlements at Kumtepe and Baklatepe likewise seem to be

19 Yakar 1994, 158.

20 Duru 2007, 336.

21 Duru 2007, 336.

22 Karul 2006.

23 Karul 2006, 480.

24 Karul 2006, 482.

25 Karul 2006, 481; Karul and Avcı 2013, 49–50.

26 Keeley *et al.* 2007: 58.

27 A ditch cutting Early Neolithic deposits at Çukuriçi has been recently identified. Its entire shape, depth and function remain elusive so far. Personal communication with B. Horejs 2014.

28 Çilingiroğlu *et al.* 2004; Çilingiroğlu, Çevik and Çilingiroğlu 2012, 142–145; Derin 2012.

devoid of enclosure walls and ditches.[29] One important exception comes from Gülpınar in southwest Troas, where an enclosure wall with four rows of river cobbles was discovered. The wall, which has a 5.5 m length, 75 cm preserved height and 55–60 cm thickness, was supported by five piers from the outside.[30] It seems to us that the construction technique and dimensions of this enclosure wall at Gülpınar does not suggest any defensive purpose.

At Ege Gübre, a late seventh millennium BC site north of İzmir, the settlement area is indeed delimited by walls. Here, the rectangular dwellings were built side by side around a large open courtyard. In the earlier phase, the 1.5–2 m thick wall with stone foundations and tower-like features were built along the northeastern axis of the settlement. During the later phase of the settlement, an even longer but narrower wall, *ca.* 70 m in length, was built on the eastern side of the settlement area. It is suggested that these walls had no defensive purposes; instead they were built to protect the settlement area from the floods of nearby stream.[31] Indeed, during excavations it was recorded that parts of this wall were damaged by silt deposits and repaired with larger cobblestones. Silty flood deposits are also observed on the profiles.[32] Ege Gübre shows that building of walls against environmental threats was practiced by early farmers, but there is no indication that the wall also served defensive purposes. Interestingly, even though flood events were also a major problem at the mid-seventh millennium site of Yeşilova on the Bornova Plain, excavations did not reveal any protection walls built for this specific purpose.[33]

When examining early farming villages in the seventh and early sixth millennia BC in terms of warfare, it is significant to underline the fact that they were in almost all cases founded on low-lying, flat alluvial plains close to freshwater sources. Both coastal and non-coastal sites, such as Ulucak, Yeşilova, Ege Gübre and Çukuriçi, were founded on alluvial plains without any natural geomorphological features providing immediate protection.[34] Only Dedecik-Heybelitepe has a favorable location in terms of protection, as it was founded on a slope overlooking the Torbalı Plain.[35] However, it would be premature to argue that the settlement's location is a function of defensive strategies. Middle Chalcolithic period sites, although the evidence is much patchier than the Neolithic period, do not show

29 Korfmann *et al.* 1995; Erkanal 2008.

30 Özgünel and Kaplan 2011; Kaplan *et al.* 2014, 136–137.

31 Sağlamtimur 2012, 199.

32 Sağlamtimur 2011.

33 *Cf.* Derin 2012, 179.

34 Çilingiroğlu, Çevik and Çilingiroğlu 2012, 139; Derin 2012, 177; Sağlamtimur 2011, 78; Galik and Horejs 2011, 85.

35 Lichter 2012, 133.

evidence for fortifications either. During these periods, we are not categorically denying acts of violence and raids. However, the societies in question do not seem to have felt the urge to take measures such as building massive enclosure walls or moving the settlements to higher, easily defendable areas.

Massive fortifications with towers and buttresses were built at the EB I coastal sites of Bakla Tepe, Troy, Yenibademli and Liman Tepe, implying a new type of political organization triggered by external threats across the Eastern Aegean at the very beginning of the third millennium BC.[36] At Liman Tepe, the massive EB I fortification wall was built using limestone slabs with regularly placed projections, the lower outer façade was covered with volcanic stones and the superstructure was possibly constructed from mud bricks.[37] Clearly, it is not only the eastern Aegean which experienced an ever-rising threat of attackers. Western Aegean communities, such as at Kastri on Syros and Lerna in the Argolid were also facing attacks, as suggested by their fortifications with regularly placed bastions.[38] Enclosure walls, although not as massive as at the eastern Aegean sites, were also a characteristic feature of inner west Anatolian EBA sites like Demircihöyük, Karataş and Küllüoba.[39]

At Troy, the earliest settlement was already built with an enclosure wall (Wall C), uncovered to a length of 13 m inside the Schliemann Ditch.[40] As the inner organization of the settlement changes and the size of the settled area increases, the fortification system is widened and rebuilt. The earliest massive fortification with 3.5 m preserved height, bastions and monumental gates, known as Wall IW, was constructed in the middle Troy I period.[41] Fortifications are strengthened and new monumental gates are built as the size of the settled area increases in the late EB I, EB II and EB III periods.[42] In Early Troy II, for instance, newly built fortifications, 300 m in length, incorporated regularly spaced bastions 3 m in width and projecting 2 m outwards from the walls. These massive construction activities at the site predate even the emergence of monumental architecture (or 'megara') in the citadel center.[43]

The pattern described above encourages us to suggest that the wealth of the elite was accumulated inside these walls, and there was apparently a constant danger of attack diverting the labor force to the protection of property, and welfare among those residing inside. The fact that fortifications were built before the elite

36 Şahoğlu 2008, 485; Ünlüsoy 2006, 135; Hüryılmaz 2002, 29; Erkanal 2008, 180.

37 Şahoğlu 2008, 487.

38 Broodbank 2001, 315; Broodbank 2014, 320.

39 Korfmann 1983; Efe 2007.

40 Ünlüsoy 2006, Abb. 1.

41 Ünlüsoy 2006, 136–137.

42 Ünlüsoy 2006, 138.

43 Ünlüsoy 2006, 139.

residences demonstrates the immediacy of danger and priority of safety. The walls with towers, buttresses and monumental gates would have given a clear message to potential attackers. Ivanova stresses that the construction of bastions, as opposed to building surrounding walls only, is a precaution taken by communities against organized attacks.[44] The hit-and-run raids of former times were being replaced by organized attacks including more people equipped with weapons.[45]

Another interesting fact implying an atmosphere of conflict and warfare during the EBA is the presence of a very few number of sites of continuous habitation from the early to the mid-third millennium BC. In the Troad, Troy is virtually the only known site where occupation is continuous from EB I to EB II and III, while EB I sites like Beşik-Sivritepe, Kumtepe, Çobantepe and Yeni Bademli (on Imbros) are apparently abandoned permanently during the first half of the third millennium BC. In the İzmir region, Çukuriçi and Yassıtepe, two EB I sites, were similarly abandoned before the mid-third millennium BC.[46] Ayasuluk Tepesi, a hilltop site very close to Çukuriçi, was settled from the Late Chalcolithic to the EB II period and abandoned afterwards until the beginning of the second millennium BC.[47] The Bakla Tepe EB I settlement was also possibly abandoned for some time and resettled again at the end of EB II.[48] A comparable pattern of site abandonment is observed in the Çivril Plain in inner-west Anatolia, albeit not from EB I to II, but from EB II to III. In this large alluvial plain, the quantity of sites decreases sharply with the EB III, during which some of the previously settled EB II sites are transformed into large nodal sites.[49]

It appears that Poliochni, Troy and Liman Tepe are the only known sites in the eastern Aegean that were continuously occupied from the early to mid to late third millennium BC, all with much improved fortification systems.[50] This pattern is a compelling indication of population concentrations at nodal sites across the Aegean to facilitate building of massive fortifications by concentrating labor force, on the one hand, and to intimidate anyone who would potentially attack the group, on the other.[51] Both real and perceived threats created group cohesion under the leadership of ruling elite, thereby generating new forms of social organization.[52]

---

44 Ivanova 2008, 227.

45 Ivanova 2008, 227.

46 Horejs 2009, 364; Derin and Caymaz 2014, 422–423.

47 Büyükkolancı 2009, 223; Konakçı 2015, 382.

48 Şahoğlu 2008, 486.

49 Dedeoğlu 2014, 23–24.

50 Cultraro 2004, Ünlüsoy 2006. Also see Massa 2014.

51 Ivanova 2008, 215–217.

52 See Frangipane 2010.

Burnt Horizons

Settlement-wide burnt horizons are one indication of raids, although fires can happen accidentally or be started deliberately. As Driessen puts it: "A layer of ashes represents an event, but, by itself, it elucidates neither the language, nor the home, of the fire-setter."[53] LeBlanc emphasizes that accidental fires rarely burn down whole settlements unless the houses are built of wood and other plant-based building materials.[54] Indeed, it is difficult to burn down a whole village of mud brick houses by accident.[55] Therefore, one needs to examine the state of the houses and house inventories after the fire event. If people did not have time to pack their things, the archaeologist may discover plenty of material culture *in situ*. Besides, the existence of hoards is considered to be one of the strongest signs for an expected human threat.[56]

During the 7th and 6th millennia BC, burnt horizons on settlement mounds are occasionally discovered. At Ege Gübre, there are no fire deposits, and the upper structures of the houses were not preserved at all.[57] The architectural remains at Çukuriçi VIII show that mud-bricks over stone foundations were not burnt,[58] while work at Çukuriçi IX is ongoing.[59] At Yeşilova, no major fire horizons are mentioned in the available literature. The house plans can only be discerned by the preservation of stone foundations. The upper structures of the dwellings are barely preserved.[60] As a result, none of the coastal sites in the İzmir Region seem to contain major fire horizons, which presents a striking contrast to the evidence from Ulucak summarized below.

At Ulucak, there are three main fire deposits in Levels Vb, Va and IVb. Other building phases also contain burnt deposits and houses, but it is difficult to assess the scale and intensity of those fires due to the limited area of excavations. Burnt deposits that are visible across several excavation areas display common characteristics. Entire buildings and walls have collapsed, the extremely high temperature of the fire caused ceramic sherds to deform,[61] items were all left inside the houses, and there are no skeletal remains to suggest that the fire was so sudden that people

53 Driessen 1999, 17.

54 LeBlanc 2010, 43.

55 LeBlanc 2010, 43.

56 Driessen 1999, 17.

57 Sağlamtimur 2011, 78.

58 Galik and Horejs 2011, 86.

59 Horejs 2012, 120.

60 Derin 2012, 180–181.

61 Çilingiroğlu 2012, 34.

could not evacuate the site in time.[62] Hoards are not reported inside the houses or below the floors to indicate that the threat was human. On the other hand, wood is one of the most frequently used building materials at the site along with mud-based materials.[63] Roofs were most probably covered with reeds and other plants as well as wooden beams. Houses were built close to each other, which would allow accidental fires to spread in a relatively short period of time. In such an instance, people can be saved, while their belongings should remain inside the houses. It proves impossible with the sole evidence of fire deposits at Ulucak to make a convincing case for forced fires as opposed to deliberate and accidental fires. The state of fire deposits at Ulucak suggest that these were accidental fires, perhaps except in the case of Level Va, where hundreds of sling missiles were stored inside the houses (see below).

As for the Chalcolithic, fire horizons are also an important feature of the Late Chalcolithic settlement at Bakla Tepe near İzmir. Here there are several superimposed fire deposits, and houses contained a lot of *in situ* remains to suggest that the fires were unexpected. Although the settlement is not fortified in this period, building of fortifications and a surrounding ditch in the following EB I period clearly indicates that the inhabitants at Bakla Tepe were driven to deal more effectively with continuing and perhaps increasing outside threats.[64] The EB I settlement at Çukuriçi likewise ended with a sudden fire event which is, however, interpreted rather as an earthquake, following which the site was completely abandoned.[65]

Fire horizons are repeatedly observed at EBA Troy. Although the EB I occupation of Troy was surrounded by enclosure walls and fire traces were identified occasionally, successive burnt settlements are more of a characteristic of late Troy I and Troy II building phases.[66] The fact that fire deposits were especially intense around the monumental gates points towards organized attacks.[67] As mentioned above, building of bastions was a major communal labor input in order to defend the site from what appears to be frequently organized attacks. In this respect, it is hardly surprising that rich hoards (the so-called "Troy Treasures") are associated with several occupation levels that were heavily burnt. Burnt destruction layers are also known from contemporary Poliochni Black-Blue, Thermi IIIA, Karaoğlan Mevkii, Seyitömer V and Kusura B/C.[68] All these findings together clearly indicate the frequent and organized nature of warfare during the EB II-III periods.

62 Çilingiroğlu and Çilingiroğlu 2007, 364, figs. 16, 19, 22.

63 Derin 2005, 88.

64 Şahoğlu 2008, 485.

65 Horejs 2009, 364.

66 Ünlüsoy 2006.

67 Ivanova 2008, 218.

68 Cultraro 2004; Ivanova 2008, 244; Bilgen 2011.

Contemporary sites in central Anatolia also provide evidence of hoarding before a sudden fire event. The so-called treasures from EBA Eskiyapar are probable cases for hoarding of valuable objects before a sudden fire event, presumably during a raid.[69] EB II-III, therefore, appears as a violent era in a larger geographical area. Organized attacks or hit-and-run raids are possible explanations for burnt sites.

Weapons and Military Paraphernalia

The presence and volume of finds that can be identified as 'weapons' and 'armour' in archaeological deposits, as well as related contextual information, provide valuable insights about the presence and type of threats. In prehistory, the most frequently used weapons that are well preserved are arrowheads, spearheads, maceheads and sling missiles. Potential armor before the use of metals in warfare prove very difficult to identify.

In prehistoric sites of western Anatolia, the most frequently encountered types of potential weapons are arrowheads and sling missiles. There is controversy over the true function(s) of these objects. Sling missiles and arrowheads were likely used in activities such as hunting and defense against wild animals to protect humans and domestic flocks. There are historical and ethnographic records that demonstrate such uses of the sling.[70] However, there is likewise ample evidence that both the bow and arrow and the sling were effective and much preferred weapons against human threats. For instance, slingers were an essential component of the Assyrian army. In Sennacherib's palace at Nineveh, the capture of Lachish in 701 BC is depicted on reliefs where slingers of the Assyrian army can be seen behind the archers in attacking positions.[71] Similarly, in Roman times, slingers, using cast lead slings of biconical shape, were an integral part of the auxiliary troops and were especially helpful during sieges.[72] We are inclined to suggest that in prehistory these objects were implemented in both defensive and offensive purposes against animal and human threats alike.

In the eastern Aegean, arrowheads are manufactured from flint or obsidian, whereas sling missles were either produced from rounded stones or unbaked clay. Unfortunately, the chipped stone assemblages from Ulucak, Ege Gübre and Çukuriçi, mentioned only briefly in publications, are still under study. Therefore, the presence and number of arrowheads in those assemblages remain unknown and cannot be included in the discussion.

69 Sazcı 2007, 360; Özgüç and Temizer 1993, 613; *contra* Bachhuber 2009.

70 Perlès 2001, 231.

71 Reade 1983, 47.

72 Paunov and Dimitrov 2000.

At Yeşilova, arrowheads produced from local flint are attested in the late 7th millennium BC deposits. However, their number is too low to suggest that these were intensively stored as weapons by the community. Nevertheless, because arrowheads are used in activities outside of the settlements (e.g. hunting or raiding) numbers found inside settlements are not necessarily a reliable measurement. Accordingly, it is reported that only nine examples were detected among the 3,192 chipped stones studied at Neolithic Yeşilova.[73] These arrowheads are *ca.* 4–5 cm in length and around 1 cm in width.[74] At Yeşilova, sling missiles likewise rarely appear in the assemblage. The early sixth millennium BC deposits yielded around ten spherical stone and one biconical clay sling missile.[75] Other than these, objects that may be interpreted as weapons are not known from the site. At Dedecik-Heybelitepe, the quantity of arrowheads is likewise very low. Only four pieces made out of silex were identified as arrowheads among 766 chipped stones collected during excavations.[76] As for sling missiles, only three examples of the biconical type were discovered during the field studies.[77] Similar to Yeşilova, the archaeological assemblage at Dedecik-Heybelitepe contains objects that were potential weapons, but there is insufficient evidence for mass production and storage of weapons at both sites. As a result, there is no unequivocal implication for the presence of an imminent threat in those sites.

In the İzmir Region, mass storage of weapons is attested at Ulucak. At the site's Levels V and IVs dated to *ca.* 6400–5700 cal. BC, hundreds of clay sling missiles have been discovered inside dwellings stored in piles. In fact, biconical and conical sling missiles are one of the most identified objects at the site. It is important to underline that hunting was not an important activity of the Ulucak inhabitants at this horizon, undermining the assumption that they were used in hunting activities.[78] As a result, the sling missiles may be indicative of an ever-present human threat. Mass storage of sling bullets is a frequent feature of seventh-sixth millennium BC sites on mainland Greece and the Lakes District as well. At Elateia, an Early Neolithic site in Thessaly, piles of biconical sling missiles were placed near hearths.[79] Accordingly, deposition of biconical sling missiles inside houses at Bademağacı, Höyücek and Hacılar[80] have been reported previously and

73 Derin *et al.* 2009, 13.

74 Derin 2012, res. 7.

75 Derin *et al.* 2009, fig. 31.

76 Herling *et al.* 2008, 28, 42; Abb. 18.

77 Herling *et al.* 2008, 26.

78 Çakırlar 2012, fig. 13.

79 Perlès 2001, fig. 11.1.

80 Duru 2008, res. 213a; Duru and Umurtak 2005, 112; Mellaart 1970, pl. 26.

were recently interpreted as signs of inter-societal conflicts as a result of negative impacts caused by the 8200 cal. BP rapid climate change event.[81]

The sling missiles at Ulucak are typically manufactured from clay wrapped around a small stone which can be seen clearly in broken missiles. Clay is then given the typical biconical or conical shape and smoothed. We would like to emphasize that the biconical shape is the optimal form for a sling bullet, providing more accuracy, higher velocity and longer range and was indeed the preferred type used during ancient Greek and Roman times.[82] Since at least three major occupation horizons at Ulucak experienced fierce fires, hundreds of sling missiles (n=600+) were fired and thus are very well preserved.[83]

Mass storage of sling missiles is detected in the houses of Ulucak Va. In Building 23, 294 sling missiles were found in a pile in the northeastern corner together with several loom weights. In Building 27, 54 sling missiles were stored in a pile in front of the southwestern wall of the building. In Building 28, 190 sling missiles were discovered in front of the western wall. Finally in Building 22, 30 sling missiles were placed close to the western wall of the building.[84] As a result, the Va occupation at Ulucak presents us with a good example of mass storage of potential weapons. It seems like the community was in expectation of or was preparing for a raid. Judging by the exceptionally good preservation of the material culture inside the houses due to a settlement-wide fire, the Ulucak community may have experienced a raid that left their houses in ashes. We should, however, mention again that there are no skeletal remains discovered in this level to support our scenario of a raid. Although the fire must have been sudden and unexpected for many portable objects to have been left inside the houses, people found sufficient time to evacuate their homes before they collapsed.

In the seventh and sixth millennium BC, arrowheads and sling missiles stand out as potential weapons of communities. The current state of research does not allow a detailed analysis and comparisons of objects that are potential weapons. Nevertheless, one can suggest that Yeşilova and Dedecik-Heybelitepe communities did not feel the urge to store large amounts of weapons and were seemingly not under an outside human threat. At Ulucak, the situation can be interpreted otherwise. The large amount of sling missiles and their mass storage in the houses can be potentially read as a sign of threat. Coupled by the fact that the settlement where sling missiles were stored was heavily burnt – albeit with no skeletal evidence – one can speculate that a raid was the cause of the sudden abandonment of the site.

---

81 Clare *et al.* 2008.

82 Korfmann 1973; Paunov and Dimitrov 2000, 46–47.

83 Korfmann *et al.* 2007, 43.

84 Korfmann *et al.* 2007, 42.

Same weapon types were used in the later prehistoric periods. Slings and arrowheads are known from Troy II-III, Poliochni, Demircihöyük, Küllüoba and other sites.[85] However, the most notable transformation following the Neolithic period is the introduction of mold-made metal weapons, such as maceheads, battle axes and daggers during the late 4th millennium BC. The earliest metal weapons from west Anatolia are the flat axes and daggers from Late Chalcolithic Bakla Tepe, Kuruçay and the Ilıpınar Cemetery.[86] Arsenical copper alloys of this period, as identified at Ilıpınar, were then gradually replaced by tin bronze objects by the mid-third millennium BC.[87] Parallel to this change, metal production techniques improved, enabling mass production of certain weapon types using molds.[88]

Related to this, the most important change in terms of warfare was the ever-growing importance of close combat weapons like maceheads, daggers, and so-called battle axes. Importantly, implementation of these types required discipline, group training and experience.[89] Therefore, transformation of weapon types may be construed as an indication of an emergent "warrior" status in society.[90] To sum up, technological advances in metal weapon production facilitated new social and economic forms during the EBA, which were revolutionary in terms of Aegean prehistory.

Symbolic Representations in the Art

Driessen suggests that iconography and artistic representation are among the most suitable tools for the archaeologist who is seeking to understand the state of violence and warfare in a given prehistoric society.[91] In the eastern Mediterranean, palace and temple walls, steles, seal impressions, wall paintings, rock-cut monuments and the like provide ample information about the wars and battles fought by state-run armies. However, finding any imagery related to human violence and aggression towards other humans prior to the late third millennium BC is impossible.

In the Epipaleolithic, incised pebbles from Öküzini show a cattle hunting scene.[92] If we step outside western Anatolia for a moment and examine the evi-

85 Ivanova 2008, 212, 240–241.

86 Fidan 2006, 92; Keskin 2010, 145.

87 Fidan 2006, 93.

88 Keskin 2010, 149–150.

89 Ivanova 2008, 252.

90 Ivanova 2007, 255.

91 Driessen 1999.

92 Otte *et al.* 1995, 941.

dence from the rest of Anatolia, we see that in the Neolithic and Chalcolithic periods, artistic representations do not depict raids or conflicts among humans. The scenes depicted or installations created usually contain wild animals in aggressive poses such as at Göbeklitepe or hunting scenes and abundant female and bull imagery as at Çatalhöyük.[93] Phalli and ithyphallic symbols from the Euphrates Basin constitute another major character of Pre-Pottery Neolithic art.[94] Stone plaques known from the Pre-Pottery Neolithic display either linear motifs or insects, as observed at Körtik Tepe in Diyarbakır.[95] Pottery with relief decorations at Tepecik-Çiftlik and Köşk Höyük, early 6th millennium sites on the Bor Plain in Niğde, depict plant gathering, milking, hunting and dancing scenes.[96] Clay stamps and painted pottery from the same era contain geometric and floral motifs with the occasional accompaniment of bucranium symbols.[97] Latmos's rock art in southwest Turkey, scattered accross the landscape in 170 localities, always depict multiple human figures in social scenes such as weddings, ritual dancing or family life.[98] In the following Middle and Late Chalcolithic periods, figurines and idols are mainly stylized depictions of single humans, mostly women with bent arms.[99]

In western Anatolia, a variety of images is found on figurines, pottery and stamps. The clay stamps display only geometric and floral shapes.[100] Clay vessels with female shapes are known from Ulucak IV.[101] Two pottery sherds from Ege Gübre shows in relief a man and a woman in action with arms stretched upwards.[102] Figurines from Ulucak, Ege Gübre and Yeşilova depict standing or sitting men and women without any attacking gestures or accompanying weapons.[103] Even animal figurines – mostly domestic livestock – show no aggressive postures whatsoever.[104]

Violent acts among humans or warriors are simply absent in the artistic expressions of transitional and early farmers. In our opinion, the apparent lack of conflicts

---

93 Schmidt 2012; Hodder 2006

94 Hauptmann 2007, fig. 25; Özdoğan 2011, fig. 25–26; Çelik 2010, fig. 10; also see Özdoğan 2001.

95 Özkaya and Coşkun 2011, 98.

96 Bıçakçı *et al.* 2012, 98; Öztan 2012, 39.

97 Mellaart 1970; Duru 2008; Lichter 2011.

98 Peschlow Bindokat and Gerber 2012, 71.

99 Takaoğlu 2006; Akdeniz 2010.

100 Çilingiroğlu 2009.

101 Çilingiroğlu 2012, pl. 38.

102 Sağlamtimur 2012, fig. 17b.

103 Çilingiroğlu *et al.* 2004, fig. 30; Derin *et al.* 2009, fig. 16; Sağlamtimur 2012, figs. 21–23.

104 Çilingiroğlu *et al.* 2004, fig. 31.

and fighting as a theme in art counts as an important indication of an absence of the ritualization of violence, warrior myths and cults. The social structure did not promote warriors as a significant class of individuals and raiding as a central activity of societal existence. It seems like the cosmological order was not based on human to human conflict; it was more concerned with an animistic perception of nature and human to human solidarity as exemplified in the above-cited imageries. Production and reproduction in a wild but slowly tamed universe were the central themes for the early farming communities across Turkey. The transformation from Göbeklitepe's aggressive wild animals to the harvesting and milking scenes of relaxed humans of Köşk Höyük reflect the true conversion of mindset from a foraging to farming way of living. Interestingly, none of those representations and cosmologies entails human-to-human violence.

Visual representations of human-to-human violence is absent in the Early Bronze Age as well. Artistic expressions showing the daily life and cosmology of Early Bronze Age societies are very rare in the eastern Aegean. The typical stone and marble idols depict extremely stylized human figures.[105] The pottery contains very occasional depictions of the human face.[106] To the best of our knowledge, humans with weapons or in attacking positions – a class of potential warriors – are not identified in the EBA in western Anatolia. None of the Troy treasures and, for that matter the Poliochni Treasure – though they include combat weapons – show humans in violent acts.[107]

In the Aegean, the earliest image hinting at violence and warriors originates from a seal showing fighting with daggers at EM III/MM I Crete (*ca.* 2200–1900 BC). Depictions of potential warriors with spears appear by MM II (*ca.* 1875–1750 BC) and become popular by LM I (*ca.* 1700–1600 BC).[108] So only with the LBA can a true warrior class be recognized in the archaeological record, especially when one considers the warrior burials with horses and weapons from mainland Greece.[109] Siege warfare and naval battles are depicted on various media as well, starting with the Late Helladic period.[110]

To conclude, as suggested by other described evidence above, warfare in a more organized form is clearly attested from the early third millennium BC onwards, and ever-increasing threats become apparent by the mid-third millennium BC, as suggested by the construction of heavy fortifications and bastions and the

105 Takaoğlu 2010.

106 Şahoğlu 2010, 141.

107 Ivanova 2008, 219.

108 Molloy 2012, 100. Absolute dates after Manning 2010, Table 2.1.

109 Georganas 2010, 305.

110 Papadopoulos 2006, 132–134.

introduction of short range weapons, along with the continuing use of arrows and slings. At this stage, although the societies are heavily investing in defending and attacking activities, they were not yet ritualizing warfare in a form visible in the archaeological record. That may be a major cause why artistic representations are not covering themes related to violence and warfare during the third millennium BC.

Discussion

Although raids were most probably an integral part of early farmers' lives, they were not as commonplace, well-organized and ritualized as during the later stages of the Bronze Age. Archaeologically, the presence of violence in early farming communities is indicated by potential weapons found ubiquitously at sites. Burnt levels, especially when they contain many portable objects along with stored weapons, can also be associated with raids.

Western Anatolian sites of the seventh and sixth millennia BC were founded on low-lying plains with no naturally defensible positions. Additionally, the archaeological record of fortifications and ditches for defensive purposes is inconclusive. The enclosure wall at Ege Gübre was arguably built against floods. The most convincing archaeological evidence for a raid originates from Ulucak Va, *ca.* 6100–6000 cal. BC, a settlement burnt heavily and suddenly with evidence for mass storage of sling missiles. Other than that, fire horizons may have resulted from forced fires, but the evidence is not that clear. Sling missiles and arrowheads discovered at western Anatolian sites, especially around the İzmir Region, can be interpreted as potential weapons used in human-to-human violent activities, along with hunting and defense against wild animals. The artistic expressions of early farmers do not contain fighting and raiding scenes. On the contrary, the pictorial language is composed of bull horns, domestic animals and women and men in varying postures, presumably representing themes like fertility, birth, male power and reproduction.

The life of early farmers in the eastern Aegean did not revolve around inter-societal conflicts; most probably they discovered effective ways of avoiding conflicts and negotiating peace by using mechanisms like gift exchange as long as this was a possibility.[111] The mechanisms that prevented social inequalities from becoming hereditary in those communities might have stopped centrally organized raids serving the political and economic interests of a ruler or a ruling class. As mentioned earlier, the ethnographic record shows that for achievement-based village societies, raiding was an integral part of everyday life. In such societies, violent actions were motivated by individual interests like gaining prestige, status, booty,

111 See also Özdoğan 2010 on southwest Asian Pre-Pottery Neolithic communities.

access to important sources, revenge, etc. We take here the liberty to speculate that perpetually moving, migrating and exploring new lands via land and sea during the entire Neolithic period may even be an epiphenomenon of conflict avoidance and peace negotiation.[112] In our opinion, rapid climate change and sedentary living with implications of territory and private property are not inevitable natural causes of inter-societal conflicts and warfare, and such circumstances may equally create cohesion, solidarity and sharing among communities to ensure long-term survival. Up until the early sixth millennium BC, the constant flow of vital raw materials, food, finished objects, techniques and ideas was secured by social mechanisms of solidarity and reciprocity that safeguarded peaceful relations. Only recurrent droughts and famines may have seriously undermined these solidarity networks based on mutual insurance.[113] The impact of such events is yet to be confirmed for the eastern Aegean.

A certain need for defense is discernible in the archaeological record with the Late Chalcolithic and EBA periods when settlement patterns dramatically changed. Labor-intensive construction activities for building heavy fortification walls, bastions and monumental gates accelerate with the EB I and EB II periods. Especially during the EB II, there is a concentration of populations at nodal sites, probably around a chiefly authority who provided security inside walls against frequent and organized raids. Settlements where the labor force was concentrated constructed massive walls and mass-produced weapons from bronze. A prestige goods economy, demanded and sustained by chiefly entities, both created and required war specialists, i.e. people whose subsistence partly or wholly depended on waging wars. Mold-made weapons are excellent material manifestations of increasing reliance on armed persons and the accelerating nature of intra- and inter-societal violence in these emerging social circumstances. Rising external threats, both real and perceived, arguably triggered the emergence of new forms of social organization.

Accumulation of wealth at a few sites is perhaps the most self-evident cause of organized violence. Much of the trade networks were a by-product of tireless demands of power and prestige-seeking chiefly lineages and their associates. Such an economic model motivated by the continuous mobility and acquisition of sumptuary items created an ever-growing visibility of social inequality. If chiefs did not share their wealth with the community in some form (redistribution, gift giving, feasting etc.), then communities themselves may have become restless in the wake of growing material injustice. Thus, it should be further investigated whether the organized attacks were coming from outside or from within these ranked political entities.

---

112 Rousseau 1754, Part II.

113 Fafchamps 1992, 166.

Chiefs, existing in a system of "competitive interaction" as described by Flannery and Marcus, were motivated by the mobility of sumptuary goods.[114] To keep these items in circulation and accumulate wealth, these rank societies triggered and supported enhanced organized warfare during the EBA. This type of organization and motive show a major contrast to the previous eras. Although, as outlined above, violence was present during the Neolithic and Early Chalcolithic periods, its organized use by a central figure to control and intimidate populations emerged by the third millennium BC.

The artistic representations are silent about warfare in both the eastern and western Aegean until the very end of the EBA. Therefore, one can suggest that the ritualization of warfare and the emergence of warrior cults had to wait until the second millennium BC.

To conclude, we find ourselves agreeing with both Hobbes and Rousseau. We believe that fear of death and need for security are indeed hard-wired in humans as a biological species, and these motives can lead to violent acts to protect the "self" as well as the group the "self" identifies himself/herself with.[115] However, human violence can go beyond being a simple act of protecting the self and close kin. Due to the complex cognitive structure and social environment of humans, motives for violent actions were sometimes directed by effective manipulation of basic fears and drives. In an achievement-based society, violence was still triggered over personal issues and property. In some cases, the whole group may have attacked another to show group solidarity for one offended person or family. As population size grew, kinship rules and morale were not enough to solve internal and external conflicts for a society to survive. Emergent leaders and their associates promised to provide security behind high walls, diverting massive labor force to building activities. This type of organization of labor engendered, perhaps not suddenly but gradually, at least two ranks in the society: the rulers and the ruled. To protect the interests of the ruler and his associates became the main motive for the ruled, who were, to use Rousseau's own words, "simple enough" to believe that economic production, at least partly, belonged to the chiefly authority in return for the services he provided. Trying to convey the idea that the rulers and the ruled are not naturally same, acquisition of sumptuous goods became an important index of the privileged. This made the society more complex, because the transport, production and protection of sumptuous goods created new social forms like 'merchants', 'craftsmen' and 'warriors.' In these conditions, the motive for the ruled was perhaps still to protect the self and close relatives; but for the chiefly authorities it was to protect the "new self" with its privileged social sta-

114 Flannery and Marcus 2012, Part III; Frangipane 2010, 84. Also see Earle 1997.

115 See Strachey 1957.

tus. Domination of one group in the society led to the accumulation of wealth in a few hands, which made social inequality all the more visible, triggering yet more violence and conflict both within the society and from the outside. Burnt layers, hoards, abandoned settlements, enhanced fortifications and increased production of metal weapons during the EBA may all be inevitable consequences of these developments. Although it is still challenging to grasp the details of this social and economic transformation in the eastern Aegean from the seventh to the late third millennium BC, the archaeological record examined in this paper demonstrates this general pattern.

Acknowledgements

We would like to express our sincere thanks to Mariya Ivanova, Yağmur Heffron and Canan Çakırlar for their valuable feedback on earlier versions of this paper.

REFERENCES

Akdeniz, E., "Kulaksızlar Atölyesinde Kilya Tipi Figürin Üretimi." *Olba* XVIII (2010): 1–19.

Armit, I., C. Knüseli, J. Robb and R. Schulting, "Warfare and Violence in Prehistoric Europe: an Introduction." *Journal of Conflict Archaeology* 2.1 (2006): 1–11.

Bachhuber, C., "The Treasure Deposits of Troy: Rethinking Crisis and Agency on the Early Bronze Age citadel." *Anatolian Studies* 59 (2009): 1–18.

Bar-Yosef, O., "Warfare in Levantine Early Neolithic. A Hypothesis." *Neo-Lithics* 1/10 (2010): 6–10.

Bernbeck, R., "A Scholastic Fallacy" *Neo-Lithics* 1/10 (2010): 11–12.

Bıçakçı, E., M. Godon and Y.G. Çakan, "Tepecik-Çiftlik" in *Neolithic in Turkey: New Excavations and New Research vol. 3*, ed. by M. Özdoğan, N. Başgelen and P. Kuniholm, 89–134. İstanbul: Arkeoloji ve Sanat Yayınları, 2012.

Bilgen, A.N., "Seyitömer Höyük" in *Karşıdan Karşıya (MÖ 3. binyılda Kiklad Adaları ve Anadolu)*, ed. by V. Şahoğlu and P. Sotirakopoulou, 208–213. İstanbul: Arkeoloji ve Sanat Yayınları, 2011.

Broodbank, C., *An Island Archaeology of the Cyclades*. Cambridge: Cambridge University Press, 2001.

———. *The Making of the Middle Sea*. London: Thames & Hudson, 2014.

Büyükkolancı, M., "Ayasuluk Tepesi ve St. Jean Anıtı 2007 Yılı Kazıları." *30. Kazı Sonuçları Toplantısı* (2009): 219–232.

Çakırlar, C., "Evolution of Animal Husbandry in Neolithic Central-West Anatolia, the Archaeozoological Record from Ulucak Höyük (*ca.* 7040–5660 cal. BC, İzmir, Turkey)." *Anatolian Studies* 62/1 (2012): 1–33.

Çelik, B., "Hamzan Tepe in the Light of New Finds." *Documenta Praehistorica* XXXVII (2010): 257–268.

Çilingiroğlu, A., Z. Derin, E. Abay, H. Sağlamtimur and İ. Kayan, *Ulucak Höyük: Excavations Conducted Between 1995 and 2002*. Ancient Near Eastern Studies, Supplement 15. Louvain: Peeters, 2004.

Çilingiroğlu, A. and Ç. Çilingiroğlu, "Ulucak" in *Türkiye'de Neolitik Dönem. Yeni kazılar, yeni bulgular*, ed. by M. Özdoğan and N. Başgelen, 361–372. İstanbul: Arkeoloji ve Sanat Yayınları, 2007.

Çilingiroğlu, A., Ö. Çevik and Ç. Çilingiroğlu, "Towards Understanding the Early Farming Communities of Central-Western Anatolia: Contribution of Ulucak" in *Neolithic in Turkey: New Excavations and New Research vol. 4*, ed. by M. Özdoğan, N. Başgelen and P. Kuniholm, 139–175. İstanbul: Arkeoloji ve Sanat Yayınları, 2012.

Çilingiroğlu, Ç., "Of Stamps, Loom Weights and Spindle Whorls: Contextual Evidence on the Function(s) of Stamps from Ulucak, İzmir, Turkey." *Journal of Mediterranean Archaeology* 22.1 (2009): 3–27.

———. *The Neolithic Pottery of Ulucak in Aegean Turkey. Organization of production, interregional comparisons and relative chronology*. BAR International Series 2426. Oxford: Archaeopress, 2012.

Clare, L., E.J. Rohling, B. Weninger and J. Hilpert, "Warfare in the Late Neolithic/Early Chalcolithic Pisidia, southwestern Turkey. Climate induced social unrest in the late seventh millennium calBC." *Documenta Praehistorica* XXXV (2008): 65–92.

Cultraro, M., "Island Isolation and Cultural Interaction in the EBA Northern Aegean: A Case study from Poliochni (*Lemnos*)." *Mediterranean Archaeology and Archaeometry* 4.1: 19–34.

Dawson, D., "The Origins of War: Biological and Anthropological Theories." *History & Theory* 35.1 (1996): 1–28.

Dedeoğlu, F., "Yukarı Menderes Havzası Bölgesel Yerleşim Analizi: Erken Tunç Çağında Sosyo-Ekonomik Örgütlenmedeki Değişim ve Dönüşüm Süreçleri" in *Yerleşim Sistemleri ve Mekan Analizi*, ed. by Ö. Çevik and B. Erdoğu, 19–42. İstanbul: Ege Yayınları, 2014.

Derin, Z., "The Neolithic Architecture of Ulucak Höyük" in *How did Farming Reach Europe?* ed. by C. Lichter, 85–94. İstanbul: Ege Yayınları, 2005.

———. "Yeşilova Höyüğü" in *Türkiye'de Neolitik Dönem. Yeni Kazılar, Yeni Bulgular vol. 4*, ed. by M. Özdoğan and N. Başgelen, 377–384. İstanbul: Arkeoloji ve Sanat Yayınları, 2007.

———. "Yeşilova Höyük" in *Neolithic in Turkey: New Excavations and New Research vol. 4*, ed. by M. Özdoğan, N. Başgelen and P. Kuniholm, 177–195. İstanbul: Arkeoloji ve Sanat Yayınları, 2012.

Derin, Z., F. Ay and T. Caymaz, "İzmir'in Prehistorik Yerleşimi, Yeşilova Höyüğü 2005–2006 Yılı Çalışmaları." *Arkeoloji Dergisi* XIII (2009): 1–52.

Derin, Z. and T. Caymaz, "İzmir'in Prehistorik Yerleşim Alanı, Yeşilova Höyüğü 2012 Yılı Çalışmaları." *35. Kazı Sonuçları Toplantısı* (2014): 419–433.

Driessen, J., "The Archaeology of Aegean Warfare" in *Polemos: Le Contexte guerrier en Egée à l'Age du Bronze. Actes de la 7ème Rencontre Egéenne Internationale*. Aegaeum 19, ed. by R. Laffineur. 11–19. Liège: Université de Liège, 1999.

Duru, R., "Göller Bölgesi Neolitiği" in *Türkiye'de Neolitik Dönem*, ed. by M. Özdoğan and N. Başgelen, 331–360. İstanbul: Arkeoloji ve Sanat Yayınları, 2007.

———. *MÖ 8000'den MÖ 2000'e, Burdur-Antalya Bölgesi'nin Altıbin Yılı*. Antalya: Suna ve İnan Kıraç Akdeniz Medeniyetleri Araştırma Enstitüsü, 2008.

Duru, R. and G. Umurtak, *Höyücek: 1989–1992 Yılları Arasında Yapılan Kazıların Sonuçları*. Ankara, 2005.

Earle, T., *How Chiefs Come to Power. The Political Economy in Prehistory*. Stanford: Stanford University Press, 1997.

Efe, T., "Küllüoba Kazıları ve Anadolu Tarihöncesi Araştırmalarına Katkısı" in *Studies in Honour of Refik Duru*, ed. by G. Umurtak, Ş. Dönmez and A. Yurtsever, 103–114. İstanbul: Ege Yayınları, 2007.

Einstein, A. and S. Freud, *Warum Krieg? Ein Briefwechsel.* Zürich: Diogenes, 1972.

Eriksen, T.,H., *Small Places, Large Issues. An Introduction to Social and Cultural Anthropology.* London: Pluto Press, 2001.

Erkanal, H., "Dei neuen Forschungen in Bakla Tepe bei İzmir" in *Proceedings of the International Symposium The Aegean in the Neolithic, Chalcolithic and the Early Bronze Age, 13–19 October 1997,* ed. by H. Erkanal, H. Hauptmann, V. Şahoğlu and R. Tuncel, 165–178. Ankara, 2008.

———. "Liman Tepe: New Light on Prehistoric Aegean Cultures" in *Proceedings of the International Symposium The Aegean in the Neolithic, Chalcolithic and the Early Bronze Age, 13–19 October 1997,* ed. by H. Erkanal, H. Hauptmann, V. Şahoğlu and R. Tuncel, 179–190. Ankara, 2008.

Fafchamps, M., "Solidarity Networks in Preindustrial Societies: Rational Peasants with a Moral Economy." *Economic Development and Cultural Change* 41.1 (1992): 147–174.

Fidan, E., "Waffen aus Metall von ihren Anfängen bis zum Ende der Frühen Bronzezeit aus dem inneren Westanatolien." *Colloquim Anatolicum* V (2006): 91–106.

Flannery, K. and J. Marcus, *The Creation of Inequality. How our Prehistoric Ancestors Set the Stage for Monarchy, Slavery, and Empire.* Cambridge: Harvard University Press, 2012.

Frangipane, M., "Different Models of Power Structuring at the Rise of Hierarchical Societies in the Near East: Primary Economy versus Luxury and Defence Management" in *Development of Pre-State Communities in the Near East,* ed. by D. Bolger and L.C. Maguire, 79–86. Oxford: Oxbow Books, 2010.

Galik, A. and B. Horejs, "Çukuriçi Höyük. Various Aspects of its Earliest Settlement Phase" in *Beginnings- New Research in the Appearance of the Neolithic between Northwest Anatolia and the Carpathian Basin,* ed. by R. Krauß, 83–94. Rahden: Deutschen Archäologischen Institut, 2011.

Georganas, I., "Weapons and Warfare" in *The Oxford Handbook of the Bronze Age Aegean,* ed. by E.H. Cline, 305–316. Oxford: Oxford University Press, 2010.

Hauptmann, H., "Nevali Çori ve Urfa Bölgesinde Neolitik Dönem: Genel Bir Bakış" in *Türkiye'de Neolitik Dönem. Yeni Kazılar, Yeni Bulgular,* ed. by M. Özdoğan and N. Başgelen, 117–132. İstanbul: Arkeoloji ve Sanat Tarihi, 2007.

Herling, L., K. Kasper, C. Lichter and R. Meriç, "Im Westen nichts Neues? Ergebnisse der Grabungen 2003 und 2004 in Dedecik-Heybelitepe." *Istanbuler Mitteilungen* 58 (2008): 13–65.

Hodder, I., *The Leopard's Tale, Revealing the Mysteries of Çatalhöyük.* London: Thames & Hudson 2006.

Horejs, B., "Metalworkers at the Çukuriçi Höyük? An Early Bronze Age Mould and a 'Near Eastern Weight' from Western Anatolia" in *Metals and Societies, Studies in Honour of Barbara S. Ottaway,* ed. by T. Kienlin and B.W. Roberts, 358–368. Bonn: Verlag Dr. Rudolf Habelt, 2009.

———. "Çukuriçi Höyük. A Neolithic and Bronze Age Settlement in the Region of Ephesos" in *Neolithic in Turkey: New Excavations and New Research vol. 4*, ed. by M. Özdoğan, N. Başgelen and P. Kuniholm, 117–131. İstanbul: Arkeoloji ve Sanat Yayınları, 2012.

Hüryılmaz, H., "Yenibademli Höyük: Kuzeydoğu Ege Denizi'nde bir Erken Tunç Çağı Yerleşmesi" *Hacettepe Üniversitesi Edebiyat Fakültesi Dergisi* 19.1 (2002): 27–44.

Ivanova, M., "Things Unfound: Patterns of Warfare in the Early Bronze Age Aegean and Thrace" in *Between the Aegean and Baltic Seas. Prehistory Across Borders.* Aegaeum 27, ed. by I. Galanaki, H. Tomas, Y. Galanakis and R. Laffineur, 249–256. Liège: Université de Liège, 2007.

———. *Befestigte Siedlungen auf dem Balkan, in der Ägäis und in Westanatolien, ca. 5000–2000 v. Chr., Tübinger Schriften zur Ur- und Frühgeschichtlicher Archäologie 8.* Münster: Waxmann, 2008.

Kaplan, D., T. Gürdal and A. Özdemir, "2012 yılı Gülpınar Kazıları (33. Yıl)." *35. Kazı Sonuçları Toplantısı*: 135–145.

Karul, N., "Kuzeybatı Anadolu'da Neolitik ve Kalkolitik Çağ Yerleşimlerinin Sınırlandırılması" in *Kültürlerin Yansıması, Hayat Erkanal'a Armağan*, ed. by E. Özgen and S. Günel, 479–485. İstanbul: Homer Kitabevi, 2006.

Karul, N. and M.B. Avcı, "Aktopraklık" in *Neolithic in Turkey: New Excavations and New Research vol. 5*, ed. by M. Özdoğan, N. Başgelen and P. Kuniholm, 45–68. İstanbul: Arkeoloji ve Sanat Yayınları, 2013.

Keeley, L., *War Before Civilization*. New York: Oxford University Press, 1996.

Keeley, L.H., M. Fontana and R. Quick, "Baffles and Bastions: The Universal Features of Fortifications" *Journal of Archaeological Research* 15.1 (2007): 55–95.

Keskin, L., "MÖ 3. Bin'de Batı Anadolu Sahil Kesimi Maden İşçiliği" in *Karşıdan Karşıya. MÖ 3. Bin'de Kiklad Adaları ve Batı Anadolu*, ed. by V. Şahoğlu and P. Sotirakopoulou, 144–153. İstanbul: Arkeoloji ve Sanat Yayınları, 2011.

Konakçı, E., "Ayasuluk Tepesi Orta Tunç Çağı Seramiği Üzerine Bir Değerlendirme" in *Mustafa Büyükkolancı'ya Armağan/Essays in Honour of Mustafa Büyükkolancı*, ed. by C. Şimşek, B. Duman and E. Konakçı, 381–404. İstanbul: Ege Yayınları, 2015.

Korfmann, M., "The Sling as a Weapon." *Scientific American* 229 (1973): 34–42.

Korfmann, M., Ç. Girgin, Ç. Morçöl and S. Kılıç, "Kumtepe 1993. Berichte über die Rettungsgrabung" *Studia Troica* 5 (1995): 237–289.

Korfmann, M., F. Dedeoğlu and M. Erdalkıran, "Ulucak Höyük Neolitik Dönem Sapan Taneleri" in *Refik Duru'ya Armağan*, ed. by G. Umurtak, Ş. Dönmez and A. Yurtsever, 41–50. İstanbul: Ege Yayınları, 2007.

LeBlanc, S.A., "Broader Implications." *Neo-Lithics* 1/10 (2010): 40–49.

Lichter, C., "Neolithic Stamps and the Neolithization Process. A Fresh Look at an Old Issue" in *Beginnings: New Research in the Appearance of the Neolithic between Northwest Anatolia and the Carpathian Basin*, ed. by R. Krauß. Rahden: Verlag Maria Leidorf, 2011: 35–46.

———. "Dedecik-Heybelitepe, Excavations at a Neolithic Settlement in the Torbalı Plain" in *Neolithic in Turkey: New Excavations and New Research vol. 4*, ed. by M. Özdoğan, N. Başgelen and P. Kuniholm, 133–138. İstanbul: Arkeoloji ve Sanat Yayınları, 2012.

Manning, S.W., "Chronology and Terminology" in *The Oxford Handbook of the Bronze Age Aegean*, ed. by E.H. Cline, 11–30. Oxford: Oxford University Press, 2010.

Massa, M., "Destructions, Abandonments, Social Reorganisation and Climatic Change in West and Central Anatolia at the End of the Third Millennium BC" in *Arkeoloji'de Bölgesel Çalışmalar Sempozyum Bildirileri YAS 4*, ed. by B. Erciyas and E. Sökmen, 89–123. İstanbul: Ege Yayınları, 2014.

Mellaart, J., *Excavations at Hacılar.* Edinburgh: Edinburgh University Press, 1970.

Molloy, B.P.C., "Martial Minoans? War as Social Process, Practice and Event in Bronze Age Crete." *The Annual of the British School at Athens* (2012) 107: 87–142.

Otte, M., I. Yalçınkaya, J.-M. Leotard, M. Kartal, O. Bar-Yosef, J. Kozlowski, I. López-Bayón and A. Marschack, "The Epi-Paleolithic of Öküzini cave (SW Anatolia) and its mobiliary art." *Antiquity* 69/266 (1995): 931–944.

Özdoğan, M., "The Neolithic Deity. Male of Female?" in *Lux Orientis: Archaeologie zwischen Asien und Europa. Festschrift für Harald Hauptmann*, ed. by R.M. Boehmer and J. Maran, 313–318. Rahden: Verlag Marie Leidorf, 2001.

———. "The Neolithic Medium: Warfare Due to Social Stress or State of Security through Social Welfare." *Neo-Lithics* 1/10 (2010): 54–55.

———. "Mezraa-Teleilat" in *Neolithic in Turkey: New Excavations and New Research vol. 2*, ed. by M. Özdoğan, N. Başgelen and P. Kuniholm, 203–260. İstanbul: Arkeoloji ve Sanat Yayınları, 2011.

Özgüç, T. and R. Temizer, "The Eskiyapar Treasure" in *Aspects of Art and Iconography: Anatolia and Its Neighbors, Studies in Honor of Nimet* Özgüç, ed. by M. Mellink, E. Porada and T. Özgüç, 613–628. Ankara: Türk Tarih Kurumu Basımevi, 1993.

Özgünel, C. and D. Kaplan, "2010 yılı Gülpınar/Smintheion Kazı Çalışmaları (31. Yıl)." *33. Kazı Sonuçları Toplantısı* (2011): 145–171.

Özkaya, V. and A. Coşkun. "Körtik Tepe" in *Neolithic in Turkey: New Excavations and New Research vol. 1*, ed. by M. Özdoğan, N. Başgelen and P. Kuniholm, 89–127. İstanbul: Arkeoloji ve Sanat Yayınları, 2011.

Öztan, A., "Köşk Höyük" in *Neolithic in Turkey: New Excavations and New Research vol. 3*, ed. by M. Özdoğan, N. Başgelen and P. Kuniholm, 31–70. İstanbul: Arkeoloji ve Sanat Yayınları, 2012.

Papadopoulos, A., "Cities Under Siege? A Look at Bronze Age Iconography" in *Symposium on Mediterranean Archaeology, Proceedings of the eighth annual meeting of postgraduate researchers,* BAR International Series 1514, ed. by J. day, C. Greenlaw, H. Hall, A. Kelly, L. Matassa, K. McAleese, E. Saunders and D. Stritch, 131–137. Oxford: Archaeopress, 2006.

Paunov, E. and D. Y. Dimitrov, "New Data on the Use of War Sling in Thrace." *Archaeologia Bulgarica* IV (2000): 44–57.

Perlès, C., *The Early Neolithic in Greece.* Cambridge: Cambridge University Press, 2001.

Peschlow-Bindokat, A. and C. Gerber, "The Latmos-Beşparmak Mountains. Sites with Early Rock Paintings in Western Anatolia" in *Neolithic in Turkey: New Excavations and New Research vol. 4,* ed. by M. Özdoğan, N. Başgelen and P. Kuniholm, 67–115. İstanbul: Arkeoloji ve Sanat Yayınları, 2012.

Reade, J., *Assyrian Sculpture.* London: British Museum Press, 1983.

Redmond, E.M., *Tribal and Chiefly Warfare in South America.* Ann Arbor: University of Michigan Museum, 1994.

Rousseau, J.-J., *Discourse on the Origin and Basis of Inequality Among Men* (*Discours sur l'origine et les fondements de l'inégalité parmi les hommes*), 1754. available in public domain: http://en.wikisource.org/wiki/Discourse_on_the_Origin_of_Inequality_Among_Men

Sağlamtimur, H., "Environmental Factors in the Neolithic Settlement of Ege Gübre" in *Beginnings: New Research in the Appearance of the Neolithic between Northwestern Anatolia and the Carpathian Basin,* ed. by R. Krauß, 77–82. Rahden: Deutsches Archäologisches Institut, 2011.

———. "The Neolithic Settlement of Ege Gübre" in *Neolithic in Turkey: New Excavations and New Research,* ed. by M. Özdoğan, N. Başgelen and P. Kuniholm, 197–225. İstanbul: Arkeoloji ve Sanat Yayınları, 2012.

Şahoğlu, V., "Liman Tepe and Bakla Tepe: New Evidence for the Relations Between the İzmir Region, the Cyclades and the Greek Mainland During the Late Fourth and Third Millennium BC" in *Proceedings of the International Symposium: The Aegean in the Neolithic, Chalcolithic and the Early Bronze Age, 13–19 October 1997,* ed. by H. Erkanal, H. Hauptmann, V. Şahoğlu and R. Tuncel, 483–501. Ankara, 2008.

———. "Batı Anadolu Sahil Kesiminde Erken Tunç Çağı Seramiği" in *Karşıdan Karşıya. MÖ 3. Bin'de Kiklad Adaları ve Batı Anadolu,* ed. by V. Şahoğlu and P. Sotirakopoulou, 136–143. İstanbul: Sabancı Museum, 2011.

Sazcı, G., *Troia Hazineleri.* İstanbul: AYGAZ Yayınları, 2007.

Schmidt, K., "Göbekli Tepe" in *Neolithic in Turkey: New Excavations and New Research,* ed. by M. Özdoğan, N. Başgelen and P. Kuniholm, 41–83. İstanbul: Arkeoloji ve Sanat Yayınları, 2012.

Strachey, A., *The Unconscious Motives of War.* London: Allen & Urwin, 1957.

Takaoğlu, T., "The Late Neolithic in the Eastern Aegean: Excavations at Gülpınar in the Troad." *Hesperia* 75.3 (2006): 289–315.

———. "Batı Anadolu'da Taş Kaplar ve İdoller" in *Karşıdan Karşıya. MÖ 3. Bin'de Kiklad Adaları ve Batı Anadolu,* ed. by V. Şahoğlu and P. Sotirakopoulou, 158–163. İstanbul: Sabancı Museum, 2011.

Ünlüsoy, S., "Vom Reihenhaus zum Megaron, Troia I bis Troia III" in *Troia - Archäologie eines Siedlungshügels und seiner Landschaft*, ed. by M. Korfmann, 133–144. Darmstadt: Zabern, 2006.

Yakar, J., *Prehistoric Anatolia, the Neolithic Transition and the Early Chalcolithic Transformation*. Jerusalem: Tel Aviv University, 1994.

Zelyüt, S., *Dört Adalı. Hobbes, Locke, Berkeley, Hume*. Ankara: Doğu Batı Yayınları, 2012.

PART 2

Early Bronze Age

Thoughts on Houses and Households in the Early Trans-Caucasian Culture: A View from Yanik Tepe in Northwestern Iran

Geoffrey D. Summers[1]

Marie-Henriette and Charles Gates participated in the final season of excavations at the great mound of Godin Tepe in western Central Iran directed by T. Cuyler Young Jr. between 1965 and 1973. Their tasks included supervision of the excavation of Godin Level IV levels belonging to the Early Trans-Caucasian (ETC) culture. A volume dedicated to the excavations at Godin Tepe has recently been published,[2] *as has my own volume on the ETC stratigraphy and architecture at Yanik Tepe in Iranian Azerbaijan.*[3] *I hope, then, that this modest contribution is timely, that it will revive interesting memories of excavations long past, and that it will stimulate new consideration of things Trans-Caucasian.*

Abstract

Spatial organization of Early Trans-Caucasian (ETC) agricultural villages have rarely been studied. Charles Burney's excavations at Yanik Tepe in Northwestern Iran conducted a generation ago provided rare glimpses over large areas of the third millennium BC settlement. At the same time, a seemingly abrupt change from round huts to agglutinative rectilinear building was documented in an otherwise conservative cultural assemblage that spanned more than one thousand years. After describing building techniques and materials, comparison is made between round buildings and square rooms. It is argued that, while at first sight this change appears to have been radical, closer analysis reveals that continuity in the design and function of both built and open spaces was greater than the differences. Remarks on aspects of houses and households are followed by brief conclusions that consider wider relevance.

1 Villa Bigorno, Coast Road, Pointe d'Esny, Mahébourg, Mauritius, Indian Ocean. I am indebted to Françoise Summers for improvements to the text and illustrations.

2 Gopnik and Rothman 2011. For a review that reveals something of the background to this unusual publication see Keall 2013.

3 Summers 2013.

Purpose

In recent years there has been an upsurge of interest in the archaeology of the house in relation to the emergence of the earliest permanent settlements in the Near East and Eastern Europe during the early Holocene. Current understanding suggests that there was a chronological progression of the very earliest permanent settlements from the Levant and North Syria through the highlands of Central Anatolia to Eastern Europe, together with some undefined role in this process played by islands in the Mediterranean Sea and submerged lands along its coasts. Regardless of the chronological disparity, markedly different geographies, and highly varied climate over these extensive lands, the settlements in question are generally termed "Neolithic" by archaeologists. This term recognises the twin developments of mixed farming and permanent settlement. Today it is commonly thought that ritual, and very often ritual connected with both the spiritual and the physical transition from life to death, was woven into fundamental changes in cognition and in society. Discoveries at Göbekli Tepe have demonstrated that the processes of change were well advanced in the Epipalaeolithic, completely predating the domestication of plants and animals.[4] The house, i.e. a structure or building in which people dwelt, can be seen as a material manifestation of these developments while the distribution of houses within a settlement should reflect, amongst other things, social relationships. Archaeology is relatively good at discerning how houses were constructed and what they were made of, as well as the identification of activities such as food preparation and cottage industry that took place in and around dwellings. Sometimes, although not in the ETC, excavation reveals burials beneath floors as well as human remains inside houses. Archaeology is less good, however, at discerning who built houses and who lived in them. One recently popular approach has been to examine not only the life of a particular house, but also ways in which houses might have been conscious creations of historical identity, sometimes over several generations. Ian Hodder has used the awkward term "history house" to emphasise such deliberate continuity. It is often assumed that these Neolithic houses were the dwellings of nuclear families, although this is not easily reconciled with recent evidence obtained from Çatal Höyük, particularly with regard to burial beneath floors. With regard to the Near East, if not Neolithic Europe, there are other possibilities.[5] The purpose of this paper is to review certain aspects of the reasonably extensive archaeological evidence from the ETC settlement of Yanik Tepe in Northwestern Iran in the light of ideas that have been advanced for these Neolithic houses.[6] Choosing to compare

4 Schmidt 2010.

5 Hodder 2013 with references. For a broader theoretical discussion of houses and households see Chapter 1 in Wesson 2008.

6 Summers 2013.

the Yanik Tepe houses with evidence from the earlier Neolithic period sites, rather than with contemporaneous Early Bronze Age sites in neighbouring areas, is justified by such similarities as the low level of settlement complexity and the transition at Yanik Tepe from circular to rectilinear buildings, a phenomena that can also be seen at the dawn of the Neolithic at sites in the Fertile Crescent. Discussion is restricted to this single site of Yanik Tepe, not least because excavation strategy resulted in exceptionally broad horizontal exposures in combination with recording of deep strata that span a considerable period of time.

Background to the ETC Culture

The term Early Trans-Caucasian was first coined by Charles Burney because it emphasised the vast geographic area over which the same conservative repertoire of pottery, architecture and settlement patterns is found.[7] Other terms commonly in use are Kura-Araxes, with implications for the heartland between the two rivers of the same name from whence it is often thought the bearers of this culture spread into the highlands of Eastern Turkey and Western Iran. In Turkey, the term Karaz, derived from the name of the type site on the Erzurum Plain, is frequently used. An extension of this culture, and presumably, therefore, a movement of the people who carried it, is found in the Southern Levant where it is termed Khirbet Kerak after the site of the same name.[8] Fig. 1 shows the approximate extent of the ETC as it is currently known.[9]

The culture is defined by an instantly recognizable corpus of pottery with a restricted range of shapes and distinctive decorative motifs that can be incised and excised, often white filled, or in relief, together with portable hearths and andirons. Domestic architecture, both curvilinear and rectilinear, is typified by freestanding structures in ETC I and II which at some settlements in Northwestern Iran developed into an agglutinative rectilinear style in ETC III. Contrary to earlier opinions which placed an importance on transhumance and nomadic elements within ETC culture,[10] it is now clear that that the great majority of ETC sites were settled agricultural villages practicing mixed farming. It need hardly be emphasised that over such a huge and diverse area, ratios of livestock to cereals, patterns of animal husbandry, the choice of crops and the role of irrigation will have varied greatly. None of this is to deny a role for some form of transhumance, especially perhaps in the rugged highlands of the Van region, but even there small agricultural villages

7 Burney and Lang 1971.

8 Papers in Greenberg *et al.* 2009.

9 For other maps of the ETC see Batiuk 2013.

10 For example Cribb 1991.

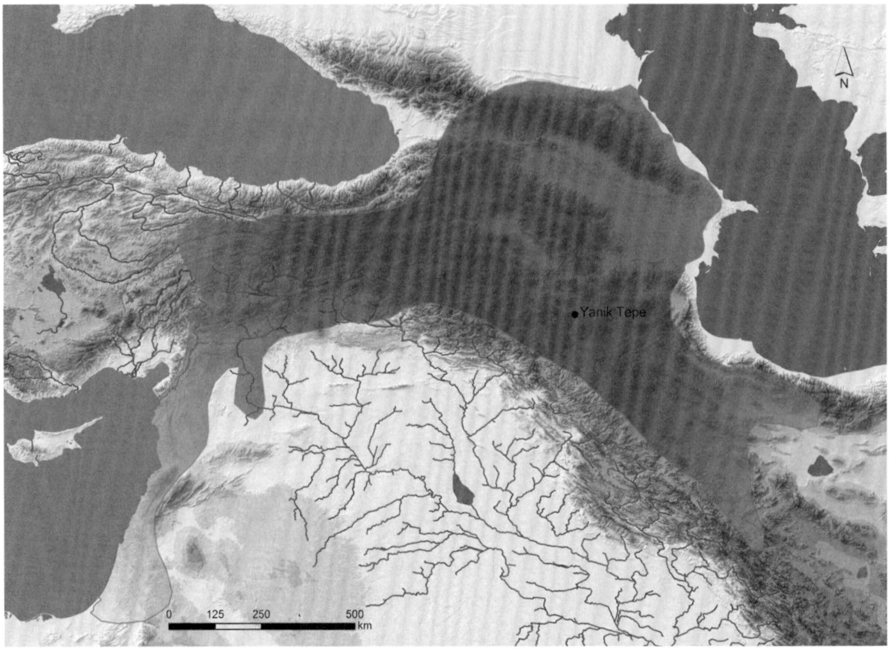

FIG. 1 Map showing the approximate extent of the ETC culture in grey tone with the position of Yanik Tepe (after a map prepared by Michele Massa).

such as Dilkaya and Karagündüz appear to have been the norm. One recent study has placed great emphasis on the role of ETC wine production,[11] but this is not substantiated by excavations at Yanik Tepe or other, much smaller exposures at Haftavan Tepe and elsewhere in Northwestern Iran. Limited archaeobotanical investigations at Haftavan, in the ETC II Level VIII and the Middle Bronze Age Level VII did not yield any grape seeds.[12] Some sites were occupied for very long periods, in a number of instances perhaps approaching one and a half millennia. No ETC sites appear to have attained any status greater than that of a village, either in terms of size or complexity. Most seem not to have been provided with defensive walls, although some, such as Shengavit, apparently were, and there was a substantial stone and mudbrick wall at Yanik Tepe constructed for some public purpose.[13] The most carefully excavated and the most comprehensively published site containing extensive ETC levels is Arslantepe, close to the Euphrates River

11 Batiuk 2013.

12 Investigations, unpublished, by the present author. For Haftavan see Burney 2012 with references.

13 New evidence for Shengavit is courtesy of Mitchell Rothman, for Yanik Tepe see Summers 2013.

just above modern Malatya. However, this exceptional settlement is located on the fringe of what, in this context, can be usefully called Greater Mesopotamia. Certainly in the preceding Chalcolithic periods, Arslantepe looked towards the south.[14] It was from this vantage point that Giulio Palumbi made his influential study, and from whence, until Antonio Sagona's work at Sos Höyük near Erzurum, the only long and secure sequence of radio-carbon dates had been obtained.[15] In the Caucasus, until only a few years ago, there were but two synthetic studies easily available to western scholars, a chapter written by Charles Burney in *The Peoples of the Hills* and Sagona's published dissertation.[16] Both of these works were hampered by reliance on such local chronologies and sequences, generally of relatively short-lived sites, as were proposed by local archaeologists in what were then the Soviet Republics.[17] Iran was largely disregarded for want of publications. Since the collapse of the Soviet Union, things have greatly improved with a considerable amount of excavation in progress over much of the region.

In addition to the realisation that the ETC was characterised by permanently settled farming villages, with no significant settlement hierarchy, earlier assumptions that the core ETC zone was both an important source of metals and a focal area of developments in metallurgy have not been sustained. With reference to metals, it is to be noted that very recent discoveries of a huge Early Bronze Age "palatial" building on the central Anatolian Plateau, at Kültepe, ancient Kanesh, and a similar building at Yassı Höyük, near Kırşehir, point to substantial interaction with North Syria and the northern Jezirah. These connections were in place long before the Middle Bronze Age trading system with Assur on the Tigris that, for the most part, has been revealed by cuneiform texts rather than by architecture and artefacts. This corridor of trade presumably ran to the south of the main ETC zone of occupation, but did not prevent ETC settlements arising in the Amuq, such as at Tabara el Akrad,[18] nor distinctive elements moving down into the Levant.[19]

Yanik Tepe

Only one excavated and published ETC site located in Northwestern Iran provides sufficient areal exposure to permit at least some discussion of the layout of the settlement, Yanik Tepe, excavated by Charles Burney over three seasons from

14 Papers in Frangipane (ed.) 2012.

15 Palumbi 2008; Sagona 1984 and 2000.

16 Burney and Lang 1971; Sagona 1984.

17 Sagona 2010.

18 Hood 1951.

19 Greenberg and Goren 2009.

1960 to 1962 (FIG. 1). Although the settlement mound covered some eight or more ha and rose to a height of about 16.5 m above the modern plain, only a portion of this area was built up at any one time during the long duration of the ETC settlement. The earliest area of ETC settlement was situated on the lower slopes of the older mound, the latest centred around the summit. Following a break at the end of the late Chalcolithic period came a long sequence of occupation divisible into ETC II and ETC III by a total change from freestanding circular huts with external annexes and bins to agglutinative rectilinear buildings, some of which possessed an upper story (FIGS. 2-4). These two periods were probably separated by a brief hiatus, as shown on one of the drawn sections reproduced here as FIG. 5. The stark difference in building forms notwithstanding, there is strong evidence for cultural continuity between these two periods. Continuity is seen not only in the ceramic repertoire but, more significantly, in the continued tradition of constructing elaborate in-built kitchen ranges (FIG. 6 & FIG. 7), and more generally in the activities that took place inside both circular huts and the later rectangular rooms. External activities seen in the earlier period presumably moved up onto the flat roof spaces in the second. The start of ETC II, which it is useful to define as the foundation of the earliest ETC village at Yanik Tepe, is probably to be put at around 3000 BC or a little earlier, while the final abandonment at the end of ETC III fell well into the second millennium BC. In this minimal chronological scheme, ETC I settlements lay to the north of the Urmia Basin, within but not necessarily confined to, the Kura-Araxes Valley.[20] In both periods, buildings were continually revamped, and were often rebuilt on the wall stubs of their forerunners. The round buildings of ETC II were sometimes totally rebuilt in almost exactly the same position, in some instances four times or more, before new huts were built on a different area of the village. The agglutinative nature of the ETC III architecture assured a large measure of spatial continuity throughout the sequence, and more substantial walls and roofs were less prone to fire and, in any case, required less frequent restructuring.

House Construction, Revamping, Materials and Manpower

The walls of the round huts at Yanik Tepe were constructed of sun dried mudbricks bonded with mud mortar. In some instances the vertical walling appeared to curve slightly inwards as it rose, thus indicating the curve of the wattle and daub superstructure that rested on the wall tops. Round buildings with a diameter of 5 m would have required about 60 bricks for a single course of the circumference. If the wall was 1 m in height the number of mudbricks required would have be

20 For one view of ETC origins see Kiguradze and Sagona 2003.

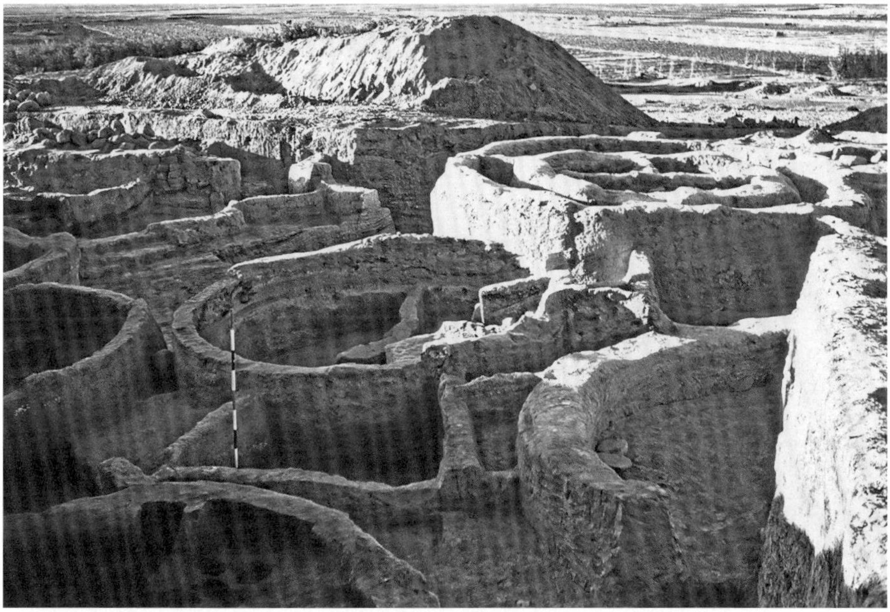

FIG. 2 Excavation of ETC II circular huts at Yanik Tepe: looking northwest with Circle 4 at centre and a silo, Circle 1, at upper right.

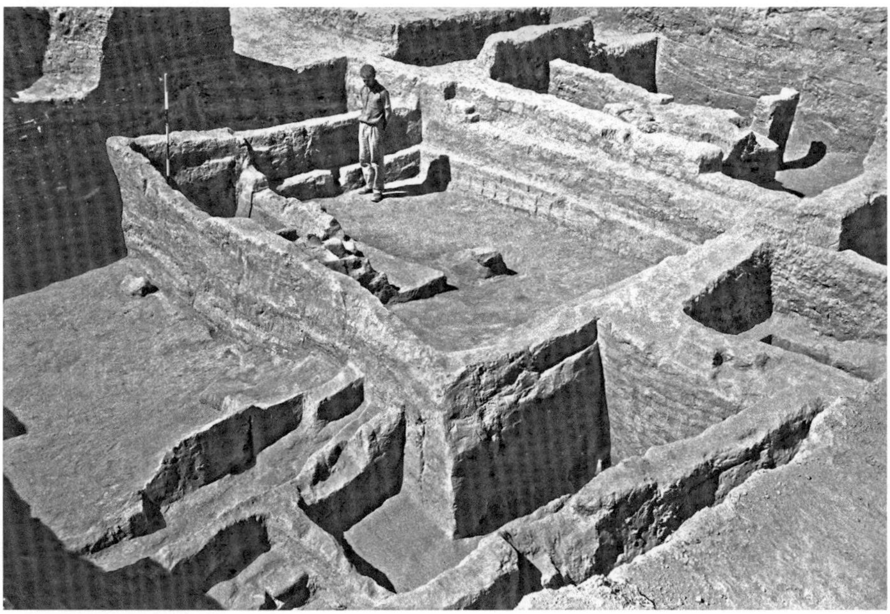

FIG. 3 A view of the agglutinative rectilinear buildings at Yanik Tepe. The figure stands in Room 5, with Room 9 in the foreground.

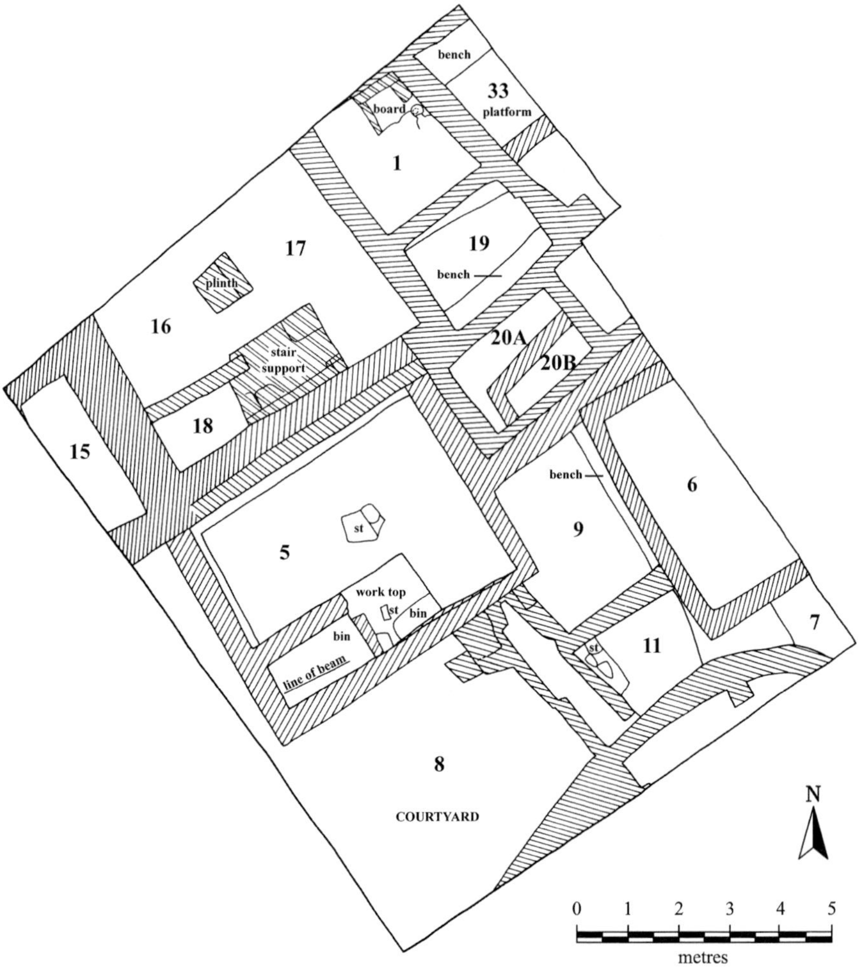

FIG. 4 Plan of ETC III Level 10 Trench L4/1 at Yanik Tepe (after Summers 2013).

about 600. Total manpower required for the manufacture of that number of bricks would have been in the order of 120 man hours, or about a week of work for a family.[21] In practice, such a task was doubtless spread over a longer time, if only because mudbricks had to dry in the sun for at least several days. Thus, construction would have been interspersed between other activities, with building being done in summer once harvests were gathered in. Additional materials included reeds, wattles and mud for the superstructure, as well as timber for the central post. Reeds grew not far from the site, but they had to be cut, transported with

21 Akar 2013 provides an order of magnitude.

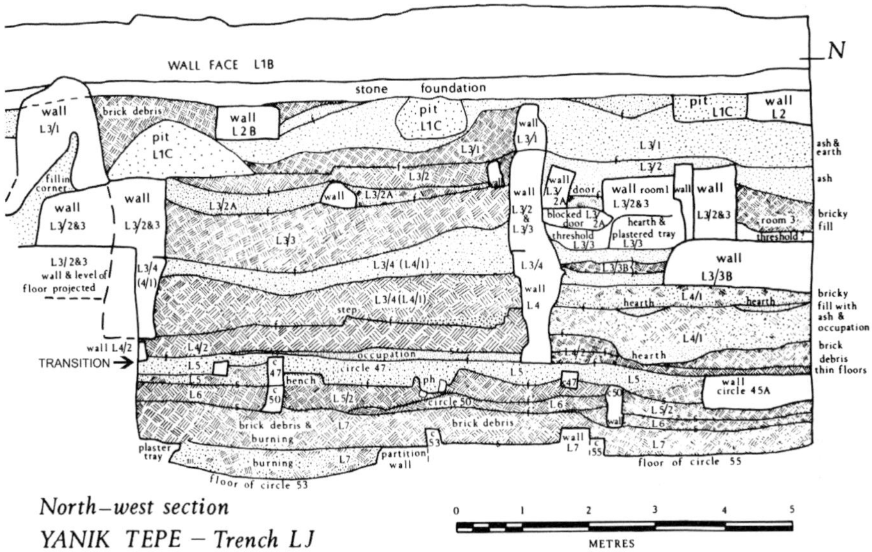

FIG. 5 North-west section of Trench LJ on the summit of the mound with the transition from circular to rectilinear buildings indicated (adapted from Summers 2004 Figure 3).

animal power, stacked and dried. Suitable branches for wattles would also have been found close by. Where a base was needed for the central post, an old, worn, quernstone was often employed. The short-lived ETC II defensive wall, whether a town wall or a substantial enclosure within the settlement, was partly constructed from river boulders, perhaps brought from as far as 10 km away. Construction of this large wall, over at least two phases, demonstrates an availability of animal traction to bring river boulders over several kilometres on ox-drawn carts or sleds. The same mode of transport could also have been employed to bring straw, reeds, branches and large timbers.

External surfaces gradually rose, mainly as a consequence of midden-like accumulations of refuse and building activities. Thus, hut floors came to be at lower elevations than the ground outside. In itself, this difference in level between internal and external surfaces seems not to have been a problem, rainwater and snowmelt being kept at bay by high thresholds. The length of life of an individual building is not easy to assess. Each hut underwent its own lifecycle, with some houses being substantially revamped on several occasions. Such building renewal often involved raising internal floors, construction of new kitchen ranges and alterations of other internal features such as benches and partitions. The mud coating applied to wattle or wicker roofs would have needed frequent maintenance. Additionally, substantial raising of the floor level, something that was not uncommon, probably went hand in hand with provision of a new roof and, very possibly, the raising of wall tops. Touching hut walls made no provision for overhanging eaves to direct water away from wall faces. Revamping would have been less demanding of labour than complete rebuilding, but in some cases houses were totally rebuilt more or less precisely on the stubs of demolished mudbrick walls from the previous phase. That continuity of dwelling space might have been a deep-rooted cultural concern, or a practical necessity related to availability of space, or both, could be indicated by tolerance of inconveniences associated with renewal rather than building on a vacant plot. Reconstruction of a house doubtless necessitated temporary relocation of occupants and belongings. At other times, such as in the aftermath of a considerable fire, old building lines were ignored, with, in some instances, replacement huts erected in a different area of the village leaving the fire damaged area vacant.

The rectilinear houses, hardly larger in floor area, were different not only in shape and configuration, but also in that some parts had an upper story. Building them took greater effort: taller walls needed greater quantities of mudbricks, while flat roofs required beams and rafters in addition to reeds and mud. Central supports comprised piers built of mudbrick rather than timber posts, these being necessary to support the ends of substantial beams and rafters above rooms too broad to be spanned by a single beam. Stairs and ladders were installed, since access to rooms was only from above. Thus the amount of labour involved in constructing these rooms was considerably greater than that needed for even the largest of the circular buildings. Walls were at least 2.5 m in height, so that the number of bricks required for a room measuring 5 by 4 m would have been around 1,450, with additional bricks needed for a central pier. This number approaches two and a half times the quantity required for a 5 m diameter round house which would have had almost the same floor area.

From this foregoing discussion, three things emerge. Firstly, ETC building at Yanik Tepe does not seem to have necessitated skills that were beyond the capabilities of its occupants, or the community on which they could draw. Secondly, the defensive wall demonstrates a capacity for limited community activity. Thirdly, building does not seem to have been confined by the line of an encompassing wall around the settlement, thus repeated rebuilding on wall stubs of previous huts is not obviously explained by absence of available space within the settlement.

Round Huts and Square Rooms

A broad survey of ETC settlements would reveal variations in building form, including circular, rectilinear with rounded corners, freestanding rectilinear and agglutinative rectilinear. The origins of the circular architecture seen at many sites has not (yet) been found in late Chalcolithic settlements anywhere within the vast ETC zone, let alone in the Kura-Araxes region that is most probably the homeland of the culture.[22] It may thus be asked why large circular buildings with mudbrick walls, sometimes (although not at Yanik Tepe) set on stone footings, should have been selected for the first ETC II phase of settlement at Yanik Tepe. Likewise, it can be asked why the tradition of round buildings that had lasted for well over half a millennium should suddenly have been abruptly abandoned in favour of agglutinative rectilinear rooms. This second question is not seeking to explain the hiatus, although that issue too requires a resolution, but rather it seeks to understand why the change might have been preferred.

One place to begin this discussion is with the possible advantages of round buildings. At the outset it should be made clear that there is no evidence to support the discredited idea that the ETC round buildings at Yanik Tepe represent the translation of what had not very long before been nomadic or transhumant pastoralist shelters into permanent village buildings. The earliest ETC Yanik buildings had floor areas almost as large as any in later levels. Furthermore, walls were built of sun dried mudbrick, hardly a building material most suited to frequent moving of the settlement. With regard to some of the practical benefits, firstly, they permit the covering of a floor area of some 19 m^2 in a shape that is not constrained by the normal 3 m roof span dictated by readily available timber. Secondly, the internal space is divisible into semicircles or quadrants that could be considered advantageous in a space that was used for both food preparation and consumption as well as for sleeping. It is true that as much as one fifth of the circumference of the wall could be taken up by the kitchen range, and also that the placement of the doorway would have made some positions within the rooms more attractive than others, but those considerations would perhaps take on somewhat more significance inside a rectangular room where axiality was more apparent. At a more practical level, the effort required for construction of a circular hut was not huge. The required number of sun dried mudbricks could be produced with ease, while acquisition of other building materials would not have been especially arduous. It is not, however, enough to argue that shortage of roofing timber alone would have been sufficient reason for choosing to build circles with lightweight wattle and daub roofs. The construction of these roofs, like the tradition of making mudbricks, was brought to the settlement by ETC newcomers. We are faced, then, with a balance between cultural choice related to geometries of space, building traditions, and the practicalities of acquiring building materials.

22 Of course there are many Neolithic and early Chalcolithic settlements within the Caucasus and Trans-Caucasus region that have circular buildings, but late Chalcolithic buildings were not round. For one recent summary see Sagona 2011.

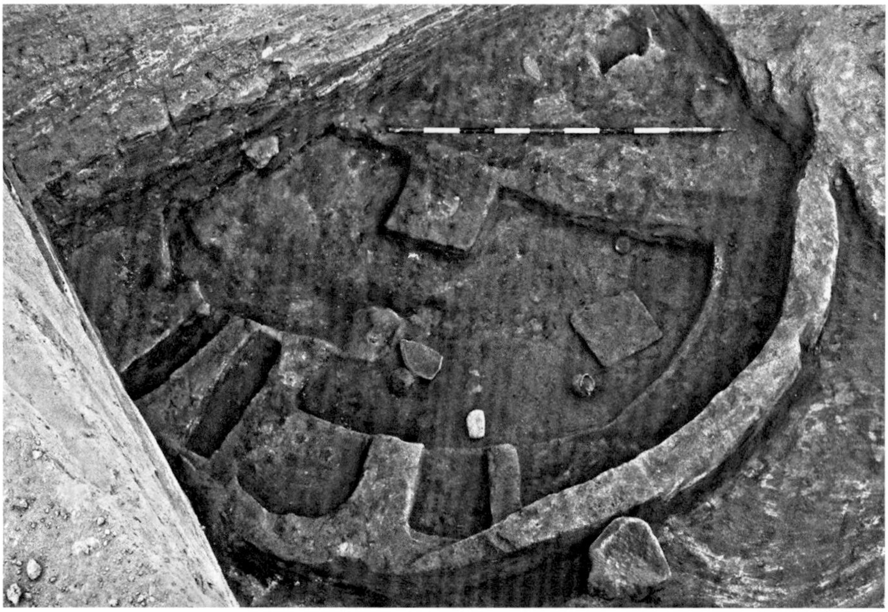

Fig. 6 The ETC II kitchen range in Circle 45, Yanik Tepe.

On a different tack, possible disadvantages of round buildings are worth considering. In the larger circles, height would have been restricted by the length of available timbers for a central post, while the pitch of the superstructures had to be such that the mud covering would not slide off when wet. Circumference walls were little more than 1 m tall, with the result that there was no standing room for adults around the extremities of these huts. The risk of fire was not inconsiderable, with the ever present danger that sparks from an oven or hearth would catch the roof alight. In winter these buildings would have been cold.

Agglutinative rectangular rooms offered some obvious advantages. Desirable thermal properties, meaning coolness in summer and warmth in winter, are an obvious benefit. In spatial terms, upper floors and flat roofs could be used for storage, protected from domestic animals, rising damp and vermin. In summer, roofs could be used for drying, as well as many domestic activities such as preparing food, processing dairy produce, weaving, and many aspects of daily life. Inside rooms bedding could be laid out against walls and perpendicular to them, rather than radially, as could many things to be stowed or stored. One downside would have been the effort expended in building, even though the greater part of this could be offset over the longer term by less frequent need to repair and rebuild.

It would seem, then, that rectilinear agglutinative building had significant advantages over circular huts. This being the case, it is pertinent to ask why it might have been that it took so many generations before the change took place. That question, in turn, might make us think what caused the sudden hiatus between the two levels, as well as the ways in which that cause, or those causes, may have directly impacted the change in architectural style. These questions seem to be unanswerable with the limited evidence currently available. There might, however, be another way of approaching this issue, and that is to examine more closely how significant the differences between the two styles were in terms of the concepts and use of space.

At ETC III Yanik Tepe, room shapes were either broad rectangles or squares. Central brick piers were employed to overcome maximum widths that are normally constrained by the optimal 3 m spans of timber beams obtained from fast growing trees. Thus the shift from curved to straight walls did not entail such a radical shift in either the total area of floor space within a room, nor in the layout of built ranges, benches and less permanent furnishings. Round houses with central wooden posts were replaced by square rooms, often with central brick piers. The major difference, presumably advantageous, was the flat roof that could be utilised as elevated external space. A second advantage would have been improved thermal qualities of adjacent rooms with party walls. At first glance it might seem that patterns of circulation between huts on the one hand and adjacent rooms on the other were considerably altered by a change from open ground to rooftop. However, a closer look at the spaces between and entrances into round buildings shows that movement was constricted by the necessity to go around or over bins and also by descent into huts by means of steps from elevated thresholds set high in, or at the top of, the mudbrick walling. Circulation over rooftops with entry via stairs or ladders might not, therefore, have been so very different from moving around between round houses.

As already mentioned, many round buildings contained built in kitchen ranges, the most elaborate of which comprised gypsum-plastered trays with central lips and space beneath to accommodate the knees of women kneading dough to make thin flat bread and similar preparation of food, stoves with compartments that could be filled with glowing stones, closed ovens for roasting or baking, *tandır*s and hearths on which pots could be boiled (Figs. 6-7). These were normally to the right of the doorway on entry. Very similar and equally sophisticated ranges were found in some of rectilinear rooms of the ETC, indicating that there were no major changes in the use of roofed space.

Building Continuity and Discontinuity

As already noted, many of the ETC II round houses, i.e. huts containing built in kitchen ranges, and other circles, were revamped more than once, not infrequently

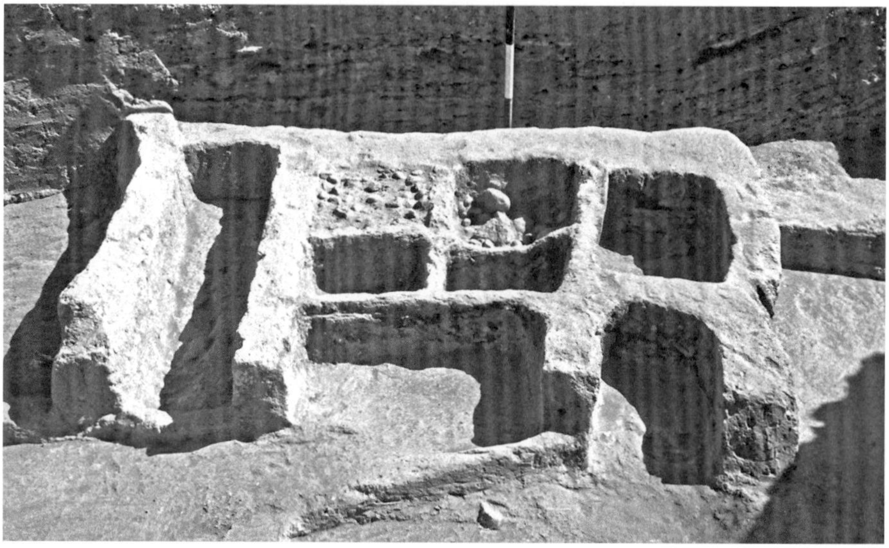

Fig. 7 The ETC III kitchen range in Trench K/4, Yanik Tepe.

rebuilt in precisely the same place on several occasions. There are obvious practical advantages in constructing new walls on the stubs of old, not least of which is reduction of subsidence. Such reasoning might offer one explanation as to why the base of the large silo, Circle 42, which had grown over several phases and subphases, was replaced by a round house, labelled 42D (Fig. 8), constructed on its stub. The house was rebuilt at least three times. In very many other instances, however, new circles were built with no regard for foundations, these being hardly necessary given the light weight of the superstructure. Confines of space offer, perhaps, a better explanation for continuity of building plot. While it would seem that there was plenty of empty space on other parts of the mound where it would have been possible to construct a new house, such an action would imply that the house and its occupants was an independent social unit, such as a nuclear family might be. Rebuilding on the same spot, despite increasingly crowded construction of external bins and additional circles, suggest that there were other social reasons, as well perhaps as socio-economic and political ones, for attachment to place. On the other hand, when a group of buildings was badly damaged or destroyed by one of the not infrequent accidental fires, an event that necessitated replacement of several houses, no attempt was made to erect new huts on the walls of the damaged buildings. Thus such social, psychological, political or ancestral ties that might have influenced decisions to build a replacement house directly on the walls of the old could be totally ignored when new clusters of huts were constructed, whether at different locations within the settlement or, once levelled after the fire, on the same ground.

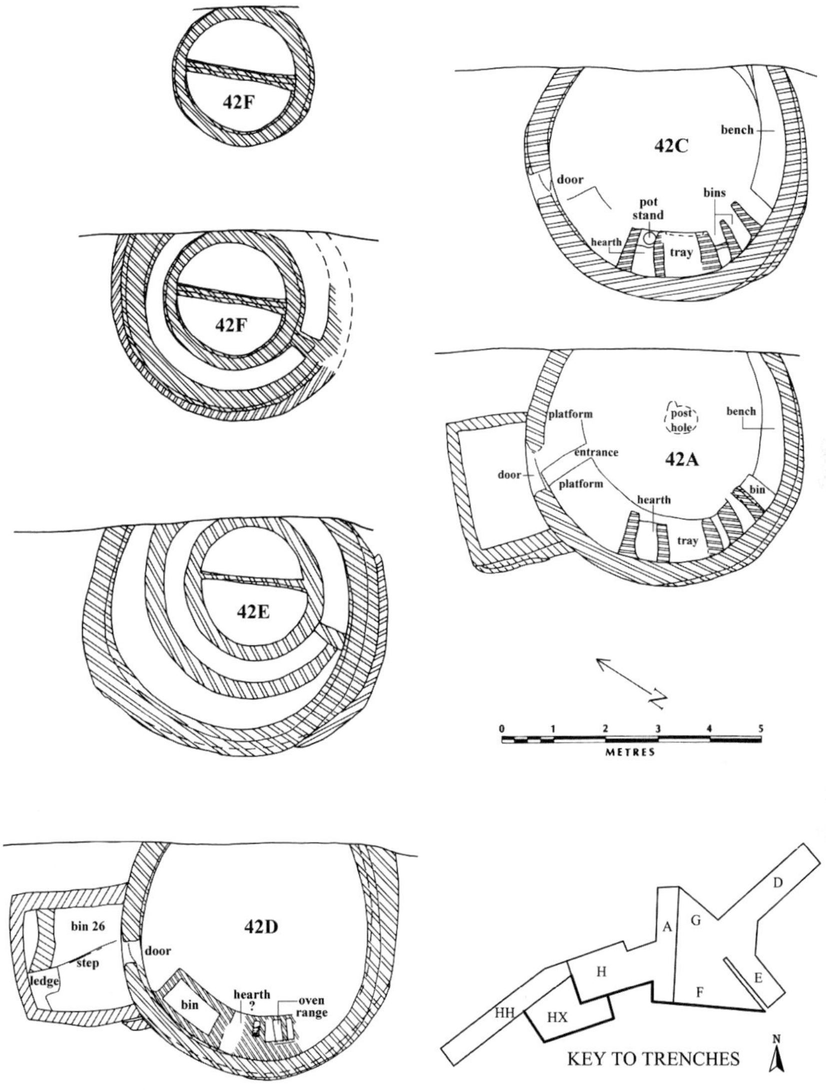

FIG. 8 Building continuity of Circle 42 in Trench HX, with three phases of silo, F-E, followed by three of round houses, D-A (adapted from Summers 2013).

Rectilinear buildings of ETC III were agglutinative. Individual rooms with in-built kitchen ranges could be seen as the equivalent of the earlier round houses, while other rooms could have functioned in the same way as circular huts that did not contain kitchens. One point to be made here is that individual rooms had individual life histories. Because these structures were more substantial than the round buildings, and much less prone to fire, repairs and refurbishment was necessary only when timber beams required replacement or mudbrick walling failed.

Spatial Distribution of Round Buildings

At Yanik Tepe the most extensive exposure of round buildings that were all in use at the same time was Level 15 (Figs. 9-11).[23] These plans represent a large exposure of a burnt level at Yanik Tepe where excavation was halted. To some extent, these plans represent a conflation of phases. This was the only ETC level in which a portion of a large wall, defensive in nature, was uncovered. Elsewhere it has been suggested that this wall enclosed an area at the centre of the city, possibly set aside for cultic purposes, rather than following a circuit around the settlement.[24] The true purpose hardly matters for the discussion here, which focuses on spatial distribution of circular buildings and enclosed spaces. However, the massive stone and mudbrick wall does demonstrate a capacity for organisation of labour for communal ends.

Looking at the plan (Figs. 10-11), several things are striking. Most obvious is the large silo comprising two concentric walls with spaces divided into compartments by radial walls. There were no doors or openings through the wall, access being from above. This structure grew in size over several phases. No traces of contents were found, but it seems reasonable to assume that the main function was storage of grain. Between Circles 12 and 17 at the southwest, is a stretch of wall with a central gated entrance, marked by an arrow on Fig. 11, that gave access into an open yard. At the north, built against Circle 13 and running to the north of Circle 11, are hints of a further stretch of an enclosing wall. In a later phase, before the huts shown on the plan were destroyed by a fire, the defensive wall seems to have turned northwards to bound the west side of this area of the settlement, as reconstructed in Fig. 10. It is not unlikely that there was some kind of boundary to the west of Circles 12 and 13 in the earlier phase. Looking now at the other huts, they seem to surround the silo, Circle 1. Those huts with built in kitchen fittings, Circles 13, 11, 10, 2, 4 and 16 clockwise from top left, together with Circle 20 at bottom right, are taken to have been houses. The spaces between these houses were crammed with small walled yards or annexes and built bins. It is possibly significant that Circles 12 and 17, located at either side of the entrance, were not provided with internal built features. Doorway positions were not established in either hut. Doorways were found in four houses, Circles 11, 2, 4 and 16. These entrances are indicated by arrows on the plan. No house opened directly into the yard in front of the silo, suggesting that this restricted space might have been used for storing such things as hay and winter fuel, and perhaps also for occasional penning of young animals. Whatever uses this space was put to, there is no indication that it was for shared or communal activities, such as food preparation and

23 See Summers 2013 for the levels and stratigraphy.

24 Summers 2013.

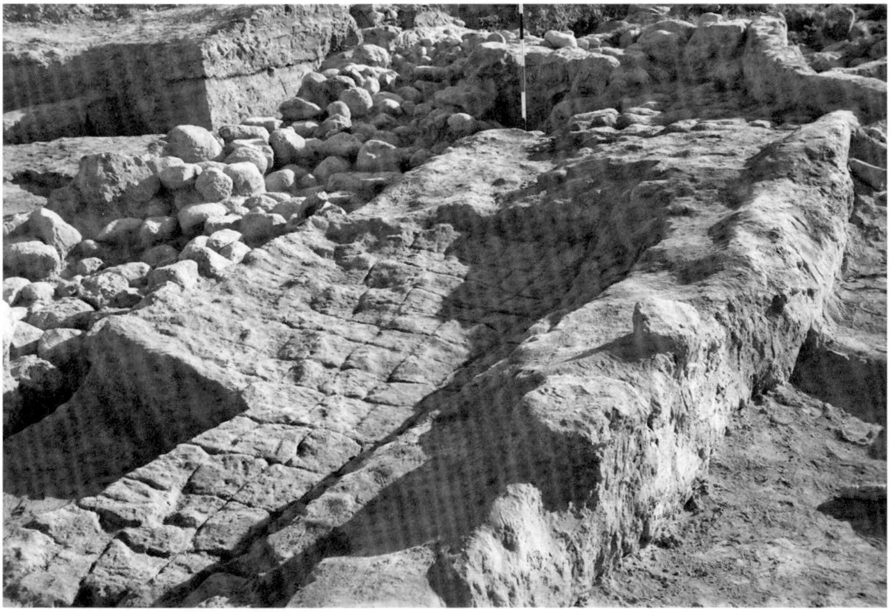

FIG. 9 The defensive wall, perhaps enclosing a central area within the settlement, built of large river cobbles and mudbricks.

cooking, regularly performed by occupants of the houses. More surprising, perhaps is that the entrances to the houses face away from each other (FIG. 11). There is no conformity in the direction which the house entrances face, each appearing to be secluded, almost hidden. In some cases entry would seem to have involved crossing low built bins that were presumably filled and covered. Generally the thresholds were set high in the mudbrick walls with internal steps down to floor level. It is worth repeating here that circulation over ETC III rooftops of differing elevations, and descent into rooms via stairs or ladders, was no different. Restricted circulation and access would, therefore, seem to have been a significant cultural trait shared by the inhabitants of Yanik Tepe over many centuries. One crucial question is who lived in the houses and how were they related to one another.

Houses and Households at Yanik Tepe

The comments that follow are restricted to discussion of the archaeological evidence from Yanik Tepe. The houses at Yanik, both round and rectilinear, were permanent. They can be identified, and indeed may be defined, by their complex installations for food preparation. The grinding of grain and kneading of dough are attested by quern stones and built in plastered trays with knee space beneath, while differ-

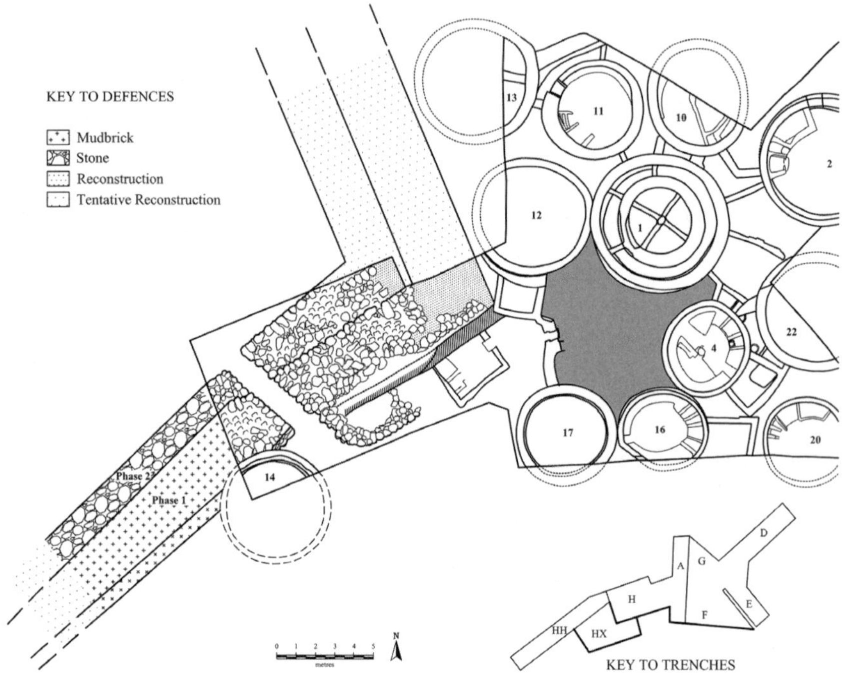

FIG. 10 Plan of Level 15 at Yanik Tepe with the line of the defences reconstructed and the enclosed yard in grey (adapted from Summers 2013).

ent types of hearths and ovens indicate various types of cooking, such as broiling and roasting. Internal division found in many of the round houses, together with mudbrick platforms and benches, bears witness to other activities. These can be assumed to have included food consumption, sleeping and normal day to day activities. Craft production, such as basketry and weaving, is highly likely, although no specific evidence was recorded at Yanik.[25] Additionally, these houses should be considered as comprising more than the buildings themselves. The round houses often had annexes or yards physically demarcated by low walls, but whether or not they were roofed is unclear. Also appended to house exteriors were built bins of mud or mudbrick. These features must be considered as an integral part of the house, with seasonal variation in the types and intensities of activity for which they were used. All of the bins were found to be empty. In ETC III, many of these same outdoor activities took place in upper floor rooms and on flat roofs, although external bins continued to be used. These houses, then, were dwellings in which people lived

25 Such activities are attested elsewhere in the ETC, e.g. at Karagündüz Höyük north of Lake Van and at Godin Tepe: Kozbe 2004; Rothman 2011.

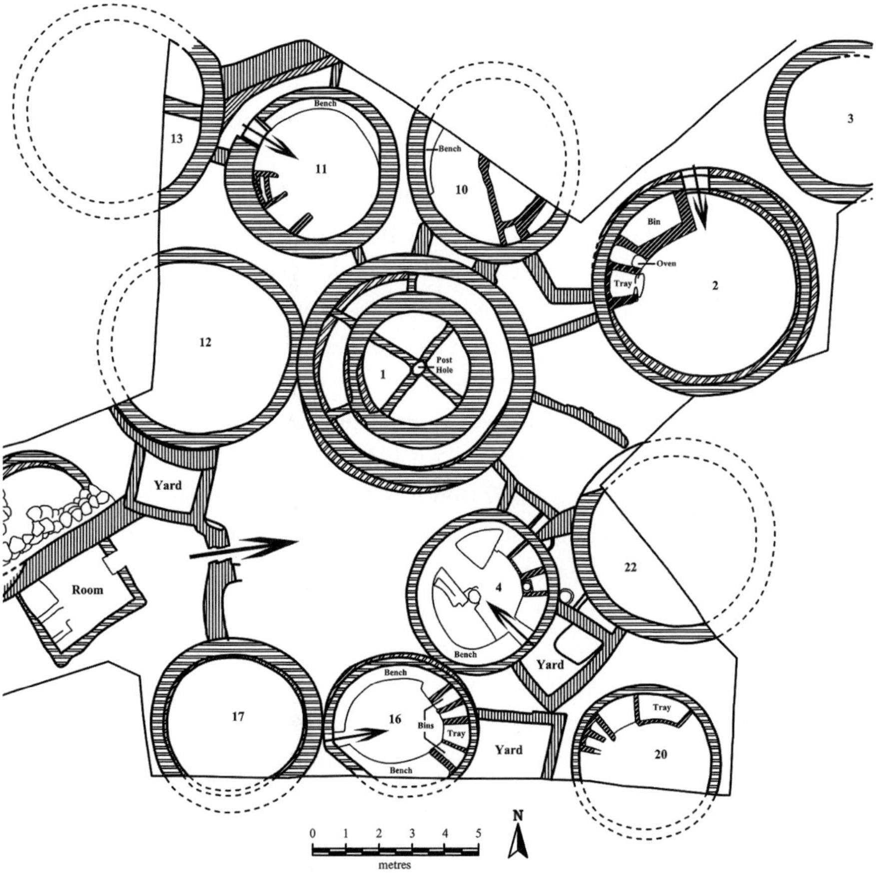

FIG. 11 Plan of Level 15 at Yanik Tepe with entrances to houses marked by arrows.

year-round. With regard to the ETC II period of circular huts, it can be seen that many buildings, some of them as large or larger than the biggest houses, were devoid of kitchen fittings or other indications of domestic activity. Similar non-domestic spaces are more difficult to discern in the following period because the upper floors were not preserved. At Yanik Tepe there is no evidence of ritual activity having taken place in the round houses. While this is not to deny the crucial symbolic importance of these buildings and their fairly standardised built in kitchen ranges, there were no shrines, nor any objects of obviously, or even vaguely, ritual associations. Also absent, as at all ETC sites, were burials beneath the floors.[26]

26 Thus the "house concept" discussed by Düring (2007) and the analysis he undertakes is not directly comparable with Yanik.

"Households", rather than houses or dwellings, are very much more difficult to define.[27] There is, however, no better single word that can be substituted. Households need not be restricted to a particular structure or structures, nor to definable built or enclosed space, and their essence is not material. Rather, households are domestic socioeconomic groups that usually include kin, but which are not necessarily synonymous with family. Members of a household may include, for instance, unrelated dependents or slaves. To be useful in prehistoric archaeology, any definition has to go beyond seeing the household as relating only to production and consumption.[28] Prehistoric households are, therefore, extremely difficult to define on the basis of archaeological evidence. The point here is to question the idea or assumption that individual round houses at Yanik Tepe, and by implication elsewhere within the ETC culture, each represent the dwelling of an individual family.[29] They might, but they might not. An added complication is that households are usually multi-generational, but it would be fruitless to try to link generational family history to the life history of a particular house at Yanik Tepe.

One approach might be to consider that houses were female domains, each dominated by a mother and her children with, perhaps an elder relative. Houses would, in this case, have been places where food was prepared, babies suckled and children raised. Male activities might frequently have been performed in the larger of the huts that were devoid of cooking facilities. This possibility does not, however, offer much help with the question of family structure and kinship. It is possible to suggest that the huts around the open space that was dominated by the silo formed dwelling units of an extended or composite family, rather than being the houses of individual nuclear families. Tempting though this scenario might be, it remains no more than one possible interpretation of incomplete evidence.

Concluding Remarks

One fundamental problem concerning the huge geographic area over which the ETC spread, its longevity and its cultural conservatism, must be some explanation of why there was no obvious development of complexity involving a development of urbanism and state formation that typified its neighbours in Mesopotamia, North Syria and Central Anatolia. As shown by excavations at Arslantepe near Malatya, as well as the spread of Khirbet Kerak ware into the Levant and occasional occurrence of unmistakably ETC pottery in the northern fringes of the Jazireh, there was some

27 Complexities in defining houses and households are illustrated by the definitions offered by the United Nations for the purpose of international statistical comparisons: http://unstats.un.org/unsd/demographic/sconcerns/fam/fammethods.htm.

28 Sahlins 1973. See the discussion by Wilk 1991.

29 See, for instance, the discussion by Düring and Marciniak 2006.

level of interaction with the more advanced states to the south. ETC conservatism would seem to have involved conscious rejection of complexity. An alternative to organised religion centred around priesthoods and temples must have had some relevance. On the other hand, the broad pattern of agricultural villages is not so very different from what is apparent over the earlier part of the Chalcolithic and Early Bronze Age in northern Central Anatolia and the Balkans. In Anatolia from the time of the Aceramic Neolithic and in the Balkans from the arrival of Neolithic farming, archaeologists have generally understood houses to have been homes centred around hearths. However, it is salutatory that burials beneath floors at Çatal Höyük caution against simple correlation between occupants, "houses" and placement of the dead.[30] One purpose of this article has been to ask if these Anatolian/Balkan models of Neolithic houses and households can be applied to the ETC, or whether the evidence from Yanik Tepe in particular might offer different interpretations.

Archaeological evidence for continuity of physical space, and particularly dwellings, that reflect wider socio-economic concepts of long-lived households is to be seen, to choose the best known examples, at the Central Anatolian Neolithic sites of Aşıklı Höyük and Çatal Höyük. Ian Hodder and others have seen this continuity of place as a reflection or an embodiment of a sense of history, for which the term "history house" has been used.[31] Similar multi-rebuildings of houses on the stubs of their predecessors are found at Yanik Tepe, examples of which are illustrated in Fig. 8. The extent to which this continuity at Yanik was cultural, symbolic or pragmatic was discussed above. The shifting of areas of settlement within the village following fires, as well as the massive stone and mudbrick wall that was not in existence for more than two phases within the lengthy ETC II occupation, perhaps favour the pragmatic view over a conscious sense of the past. Other parallels with Aşıklı Höyük and Çatal Höyük might also be worth consideration. The change at Aşıklı Höyük from round huts to rectangular rooms and, at Çatal Höyük, the circulation of people over rooftops with descent into rooms from above are notable examples. We may ask if these similarities are little more than coincidence separated by millennia and by geography, or whether these relatively egalitarian, or weakly hierarchical, communities shared common solutions to common problems. At Çatal Höyük, as at Yanik Tepe, it is extremely difficult to gain insights into kinship systems, families and households from the archaeological evidence. Models built from ethnographic studies of modern tribal societies, briefly discussed elsewhere,[32] are seductive, but may lead down entirely false trails.

30 Hodder 2013.

31 Valuable discussions by Hodder (2013) and Wesson (2008) contain a wealth of references.

32 Summers 2013.

To conclude in a positive vein, the evidence from Yanik Tepe can be employed to address broader cultural issues within the Trans-Caucasus and the Ancient Near East. Such questions take us beyond mundane archaeological analysis of stratigraphies, description of buildings and ceramics, and the study of landscapes that, however fascinating these may be in their own right, should not be an end in themselves. If this paper has achieved anything I hope it will stimulate further studies of the ETC culture and encourage renewed excavation with a focus on horizontal exposure that might clarify some of the issues raised.

REFERENCES

Akar, M. http://www.alalakh.org/mudbricks2008.asp visited 22 October 2013.

Batiuk S.D., "The Fruits of Migration: Understanding the 'Longue Duree' and the Socio-economic Relations of the Early Transcaucasian Culture." *Journal of Anthropological Archaeology* 32 (2013): 449–477.

Burney, C.A., "Haftavan Tepe." *Encyclopaedia Iranica* Vol. XI, Fasc. 5 (2012): 531–533. Available at: http://www.iranicaonline.org/articles/haftavan-tepe

Burney, C. and D.M. Lang, *The Peoples of the Hills, Ancient Ararat and Caucasus*. London: Weidenfeld and Nicolson, 1971.

Cribb, R., *Nomads in Archaeology*. Cambridge: Cambridge University Press, 1991.

Düring, B. S., "The Articulation of Houses at Neolithic Çatalhöyük, Turkey" in *The Durable House: House Society Models in Archaeology*, ed. by R. A. Beck, Jr., 130–153. Center for Archaeological Investigations, Occasional Paper No. 35. Carbondale: Southern Illinois University Press, 2007.

Düring B.S. and A. Marciniak, "Households and Communities in the Central Anatolian Neolithic." *Archaeological Dialogues* 12 (2006): 165–187.

Frangipane, M. (ed.) *Fifty Years of Excavations and Researches at Arslantepe-Malatya (Turkey). A Contribution to the Study of the Earliest Centralised Societies, Proceedings of the International Conference held in Rome on 5–7 December, 2011 to Celebrate the 50th Anniversary of the Sapienza University Expedition at Arslantepe.* Origini 34, 2012.

Gopnik, H. and M.S. Rothman, *On the High Road: The History of Godin Tepe, Iran*. Bibliotheca Iranica: Archaeology, Art and Architecture Series, 1. Co-published with the Royal Ontario Museum. Costa Mesa, 2011.

Greenberg, R. and Y. Goren (eds.) *Transcaucasian Migrants and the Khirbet Kerak Culture in the Third Millennium BCE*. Tel Aviv University 36/2, 2009.

Hodder, I., "From Diffusion to Structural Transformation: the Changing Roles of the Neolithic House in the Middle East, Turkey and Europe" in *Tracking the Neolithic House in Europe: Sedentism, Architecture and Practice, One World Archaeology*, ed. by D. Hofmann and J. Smyth, 349–362. New York: Springer, 2013.

Hood, S., "Excavations at Tabara el Akrad." *Anatolian Studies* 1 (1951): 113–147

Keall, E.J., "Review of 'On the High Road. The History of Godin Tepe, Iran'." *Iranian Studies* 46 (2013): 135–138.

Kiguradze, T. and A. Sagona, "On the Origins of the Kura-Araxes Cultural Complex" in *Archaeology in the Borderlands: Investigations in Caucasia and Beyond*, ed. by A. T. Smith and K. Rubinson, 38–94. Los Angeles: The Cotsen Institute of Archaeology Press, 2003.

Kozbe, G., "Activity Areas and Social Organization within Early Trans-Caucasian Houses at Karagündüz Höyük, Van" in *A View from The Highlands: Studies in Honour of Charles Burney*, ed. by A. Sagona, 35–53. Leuven: Peeters, 2004.

Palumbi, G., *The Red and Black: Social and Cultural Interaction between the Upper Euphrates and the Southern Caucasus Communities in the Fourth and Third Millennium BC*. Rome: Studi di Preistoria Orientale (SPO) Volume 2, 2008.

Rothmann, M. S., "Migration and Resettlement: Godin Period IV" in *On the High Road: The History of Godin Tepe, Iran*, ed. by H. Gopnik and M. S. Rothman. Bibliotheca Iranica: Archaeology, Art and Architecture Series, 1. California: Mazda co-published with the Royal Ontario Museum, 2011.

Sagona, A.G., *The Caucasian Region in the Early Bronze Age*. British Archaeological Reports International Series 214. Oxford: British Archaeological Reports, 1984.

———. "Sos Höyük and the Erzurum Region in Late Prehistory: A Provisional Chronology for Northeastern Anatolia" in *Chronologies des pays du Caucase et de l'Euphrate aux IVe-IIIe millenaires*, ed. by C. Marro and H. Hauptmann, 329–373. Institut français d'etudes anatoliennes d'Istanbul, Varia Anatolica XI. Paris 2000.

———. "Past and Present Directions in the Archaeology of the Transcaucasus." *TÜBA-AR* 13 (2010): 143–157.

———. "Anatolia and the TransCaucasus. Themes and Variations *ca.* 6400–1500 BCE" in *The Oxford Handbook of Ancient Anatolia 10,000–323 BCE.*, ed. by S. R. Steadman and G. McMahon, 684–703. Oxford: Oxford University Press, 2011.

Sahlins, M., *Stone Age Economics*. Chicago: Aldine Transaction, 1973.

Schmidt, K., "Göbekli Tepe-The Stone Age Sanctuaries: New Results of Ongoing Excavations with a Special Focus on Sculptures and High Reliefs." *Documenta Praehistorica* 37 (2010): 239–256.

Summers, G.D., "Yanik Tepe and the Early Trans-Caucasian Culture: Problems and Perspectives" in *A View from The Highlands: Studies in Honour of Charles Burney*, ed. by A. Sagona, 617–643. Leuven: Peeters, 2004.

———. *Yanik Tepe, Northwestern Iran. The Early Trans-Caucasian Period. Stratigraphy and Architecture*. Leuven: Peeters, 2013.

Wesson, C.B., *Households and Hegemony: Early Creek Prestige Goods, Symbolic Capital, and Social Power*. Lincoln: University of Nebraska 2008.

Wilk, R., "The Household in Anthropology: Panacea or Problem." *Reviews in Anthropology* 20 (1991): 1–12.

The Late Early Bronze Age Regional Catastrophe: a View from Cilicia

Tevfik Emre Şerifoğlu [1]

It is a great honour and pleasure to have the opportunity to contribute to this important publication prepared in honour of Marie-Henriette and Charles Gates. Marie-Henriette Gates was the first person to introduce me to archaeological methods and theories, and Charles Gates was the person from whom I learned basic excavation techniques almost two decades ago. I thank these two exemplary figures in our field wholeheartedly for all their efforts training us (their students) and for their continuous support.

Abstract

Archaeological excavations conducted at sites in various parts of the Middle East recorded destruction layers dated approximately to the 24th century BC, which corresponds to the end of the EB II in Anatolia and EB III in Syria-Palestine. These events seem to have resulted in a cultural and possibly economic change manifested in new pottery types and architectural traditions. In this article I will be evaluating the relevant evidence from Cilician sites and try to interpret the reasons and outcomes of these regional phenomena through an interregional perspective.

Introduction

The archaeological evidence shows that many settlements in Greece, Anatolia, Syria and Mesopotamia witnessed a devastating destruction at end of the EB II period (approximately 2300 BC). Most of these sites were re-settled, but the EB III cultural material bear important changes which point to a change in lifestyle.

1 Department of Archaeology, Bitlis Eren University, Rahva Yerleşkesi, Beş Minare Mah., Ahmet Eren Bulv. 13000 Bitlis, Turkey.

The destruction of sites like Lerna,[2] Eutresis[3] and Ayia Irini[4] in Greece, Troy[5] and Beycesultan[6] in western Anatolia and Karaz[7] and Bayburt-Pulur Höyük[8] in eastern Anatolia was linked by many scholars to the arrival of Indo-Europeans, which would be Greek-speaking populations in Greece and Luwians in Anatolia, or a massive movement of various different groups to these areas.[9] The abandonment of the southwestern Anatolian settlement of Bademağacı[10] in this period and the destruction that occurred at Kültepe at the very beginning of the EB III period were probably linked to this same phenomenon.[11] Around the same time, major settlements including Ugarit[12] in northern Syria and Tell Leilan, Chagar Bazar, Tell Brak and Tell Mozan in northern Mesopotamia were gradually abandoned,[13] and many sites including Khribat Al-Batrawi,[14] Tell Beth Shean[15] and Jericho[16] in Jordan and Palestine were destroyed or abandoned,[17] which show that this was a period of regional catastrophe that cannot be simply explained by a massive invasion of outsiders. It should also be noted that this period of destruction corresponds to the end of the Old Kingdom Period in Egypt.[18]

The situation in Cilicia, which is located in between all these major cultural regions, was not very different. Tarsus and Kinet Höyük of Cilicia Pedias and Kilise Tepe of Cilicia Trachea are the best-studied sites in Cilicia for this period, even though only a small portion of the late Early Bronze Age occupational levels could be exposed at all three sites. Tarsus and Kilise Tepe were both destroyed by a big fire at the end of the EB II period, after which the local material culture went

2 Wiencke 2000, 660.

3 Hood 1986, 59.

4 Caskey 1986, 25.

5 Blegen *et al.* 1950; Korfmann and Kromer 1993; Joukowsky 1996.

6 Lloyd and Mellaart 1962, 56–58.

7 Koşay and Turfan 1959; Ceylan 2001, 74.

8 Kökten 1945, 481–486.

9 Blegen 1928; Mellaart 1958; Caskey 1960; Lloyd and Mellaart 1962, 61; Gimbutas 1963; 1973; Drews 1988, 18–20; Wiencke 1989; Rutter 1995; Maran 1998.

10 Umurtak 2011, 213.

11 Özgüç 1964, 35.

12 Yon 2006, 16.

13 Weiss 2012, 5–10.

14 Nigro and Sala 2009, 373–375.

15 Mazar 1997.

16 Prag 1986.

17 Kenyon 1966.

18 Murnane 1995, 697–698.

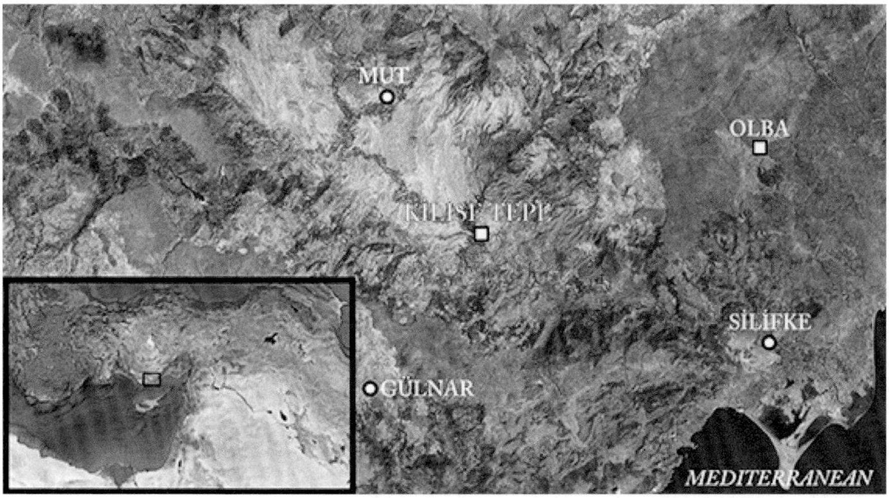

FIG. 1 Map of the Göksu Valley.

through a radical change, which manifests itself with new pottery forms at Tarsus and with a change in both pottery and architectural traditions at Kilise Tepe.[19] On the other hand, although the town was not destroyed at the end of the EB II period, Kinet Höyük also witnessed some cultural changes at the beginning of the EB III period, best manifested by a change in architectural building techniques.[20]

Kilise Tepe in between Central Anatolia and Cilicia Pedias

Kilise Tepe is the largest mound located in the Göksu Valley, through which one of the main ancient routes linking the Mediterranean coast and Cilicia Pedias to central Anatolia passed (FIG. 1). The Early Bronze Age levels were first investigated between 1994 and 1998, and work resumed in 2007, to be completed with one final season in 2011. Unfortunately, the Early Bronze Age levels could only be exposed in a small area, which is located on the northwestern slope of the mound (FIG. 2).

The Early Bronze Age at Kilise Tepe is represented by six major building periods, which correspond to EB II and III (phases f, g, h, i, j and k).[21] The area that was excavated seems to be a residential quarter at the northwestern edge of the mound at the end of the EB II period, which is represented by two rooms, one having a hearth at its centre (FIG. 3). The walls of this building, which were covered with a

19 Goldman 1956, 32, 61, 131; Jackson, Postgate and Şerifoğlu 2013, 5–6.

20 Gates 2009, 352–354; 2011, 183–184.

21 Şerifoğlu 2012; Jackson, Postgate and Şerifoğlu 2013, 5–6.

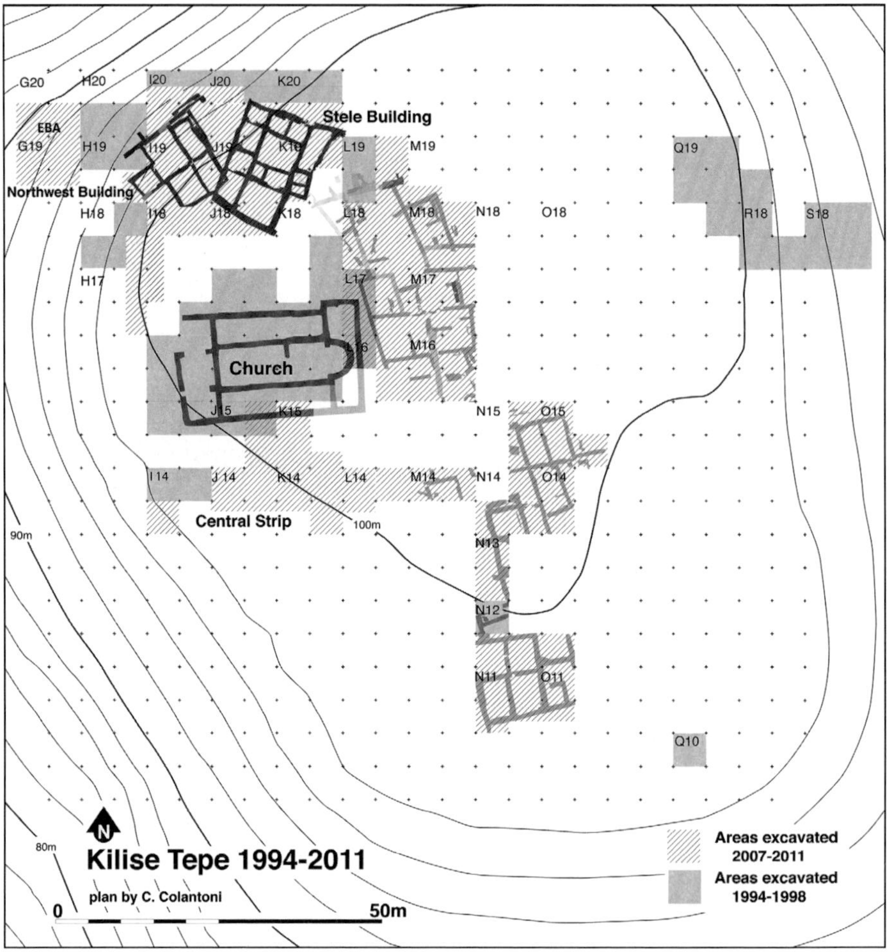

Fig. 2 Plan of Kilise Tepe, showing the excavated areas.

thick layer of plaster, had stone foundations and mudbrick superstructures. Two walls at the southwestern side of the building, which were almost completely built out of stone, were almost 1.5 m high and these, together with the walls possibly belonging to another structure just to the west of this building, have a different character, and were either built in this way to stop soil erosion or were a part of a defensive structure with thick, high walls (Fig. 4). A stone mould and the relatively high number of copper items found at this level indicate that there might have been a small scale metalworking industry present at the site.

The pottery traditions of this period are closely related to central Anatolian traditions, but also shared some elements with Cilicia Pedias. The most popular wares were the red and black burnished ware, the scored ware and the metallic

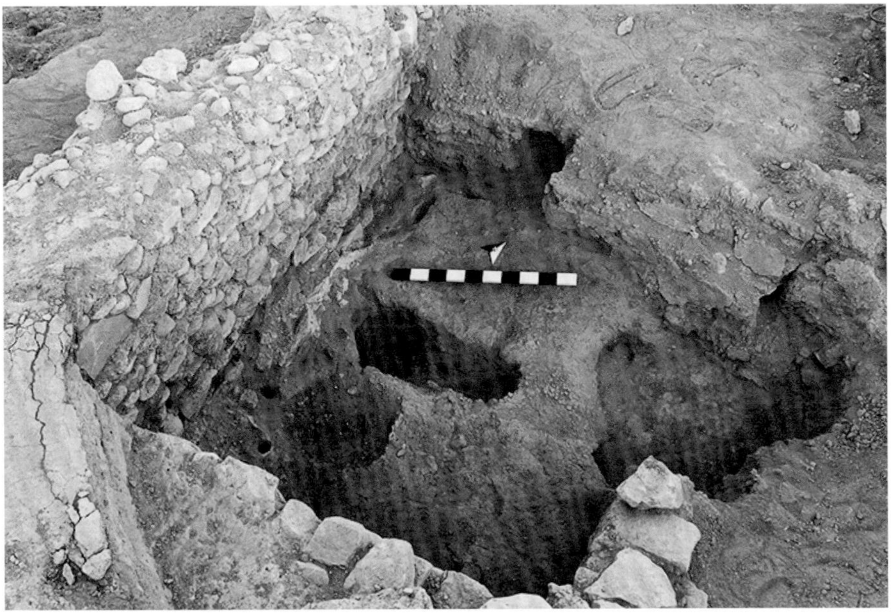

FIG. 3 The Early Bronze Age II room (Kilise Tepe, level Vg).

ware, which were all handmade. The red and black burnished ware tradition, which is represented by bowls and small pots with a light grey-coloured soft paste, a thick slip and a lustre burnish, was very popular in central Anatolia,[22] whereas the other two were in use in both central Anatolia and Cilicia Pedias. Metallic ware pots, trefoil jugs and bowls with a red or brown slip on their thin walls, show great similarities to examples reported from the Konya Plain and Cilicia Pedias.[23] On the other hand, examples of scored ware pottery, by which we refer to medium and large size pots and bowls with shallow striation marks on their surfaces, were even reported from Troy I and IIa–d,[24] and therefore represent a widespread tradition of EB II Anatolia.

Level Vg was destroyed by a fierce fire, which resulted in the collapse of the whole EB II building complex, leaving thick destruction debris behind. The inhabitants of the following level (level Vf), which corresponds to the beginning of EB III, did not spend any time removing the rubble, and they simply covered the destruction debris with a thick layer of clay plaster and started building new

22 Symington 2007, 297.

23 Garstang 1953, fig. 122; Goldman 1956, fig. 247; Mellaart 1963, 228f, figs. 6, 14–17; Özten 1989, 409f.

24 Blegen *et al.* 1950, 53f., figs. 252, 409–410.

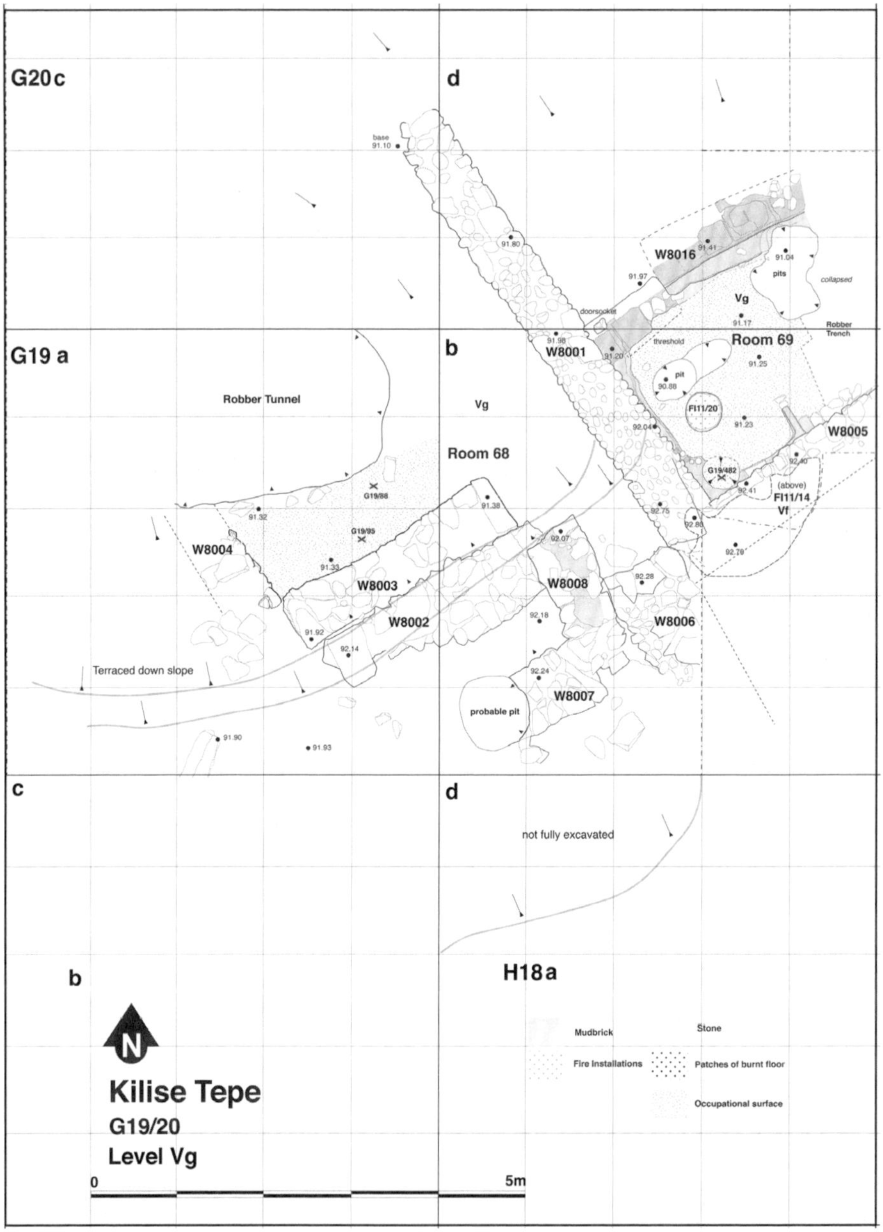

FIG. 4 Plan of Level Vg.

buildings and features on top of that (FIG. 5). A large circular oven, with a diameter of almost 2 m, was built on top of the Vg building, and a large multi-room building was constructed only about 1 m south of this oven (FIG. 6). Although no direct evidence that would reveal the function of the oven could be found, the

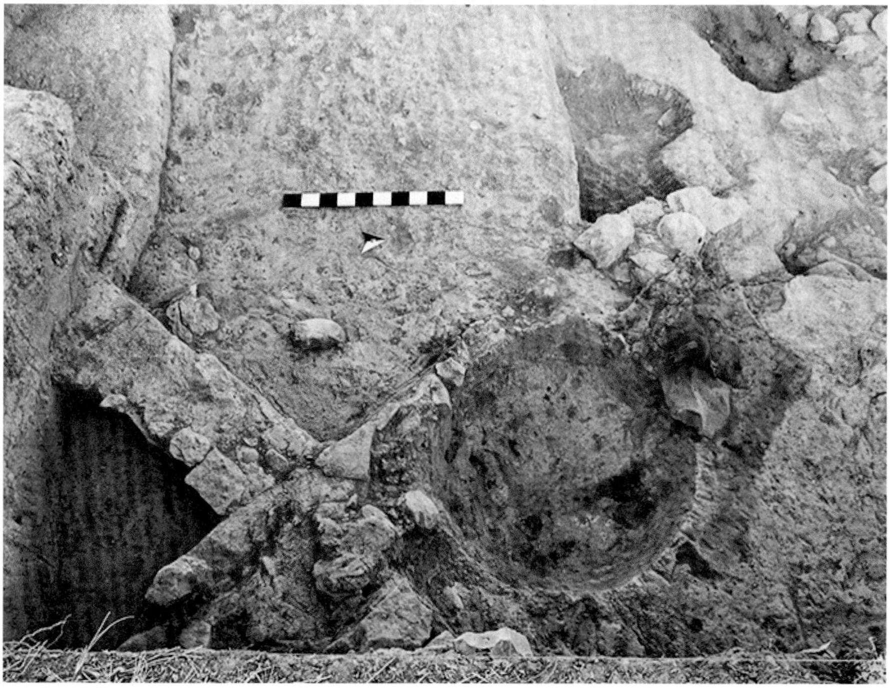

FIG. 5 The earliest Early Bronze Age III architecture (Kilise Tepe, level Vf-Phase 4)

size and the shape imply that it may have been used to fire pottery. It should also be mentioned that the walls of the newly constructed building followed a different general alignment than the Vg structures, reflecting a break from the earlier architectural tradition.

There was also a radical change in pottery traditions at this level. The only EB II pottery tradition that survived into this period was the red and black burnished ware, but the examples from this period have a less shiny surface, and the tradition, which had lost its popularity, gradually disappeared from the pottery repertoire. Some new pottery types which need to be mentioned include the orange ware, the yellowish brown ware and the smeared wash ware variation of the latter, of which a great majority were wheel-made.

The fine grit tempered and well fired orange ware bowls, which had a simple straight or simple incurving rim or an S-shaped profile, pots, jugs and juglets usually had a red, yellowish red, reddish brown, light brown or pale brown slip, and the pale or light brown slipped examples usually had a brown, reddish brown or red coating or paint covering their rims. Some of the pots also had a vertical fluting on their shoulders, and pottery with other forms could be decorated with horizontal grooves applied below their rims.

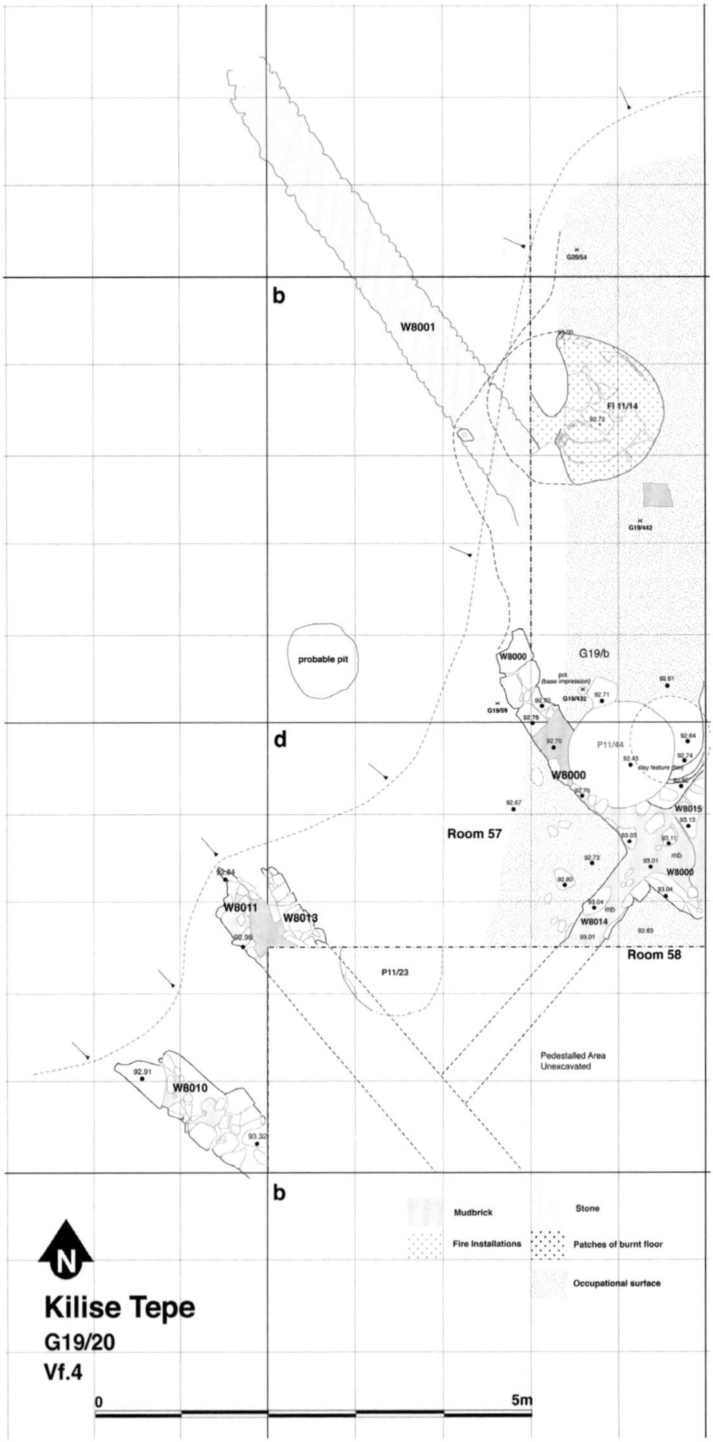

FIG. 6 Plan of Level Vf-Phase 4.

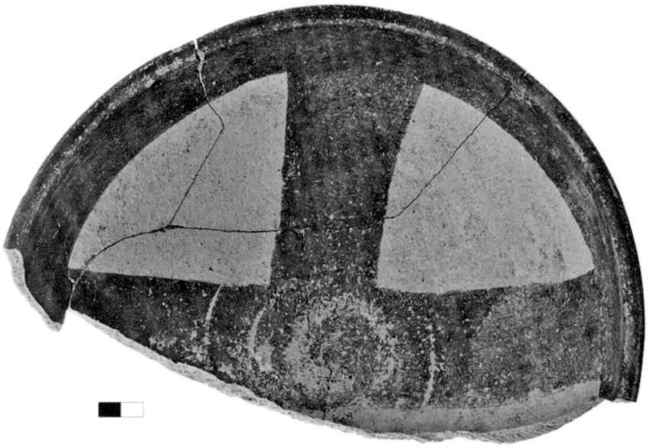

FIG. 7 A red-cross bowl from Kilise Tepe, level Vf-Phase 4.

The earliest examples of red-cross bowls found at Kilise Tepe were manufactured mainly using this ware (FIG. 7). Red-cross bowls were very popular in both western Anatolia and Cilicia at the end of the Early Bronze Age, as manifested by examples from various sites.[25] These bowls, which were usually slipped with a yellowish red clay, had red painted rims and a cross painted on their interior surfaces. Besides numerous sherds, a half-complete example was found in the area between the new building and the oven mentioned above.

Yellowish brown ware was the second most popular pottery type of this period. Bowls with a simple incurving rim or with an S-shaped profile and a flaring rim, jars with externally thickened or flaring rims, platters, and small and medium sized pots, which were manufactured using this ware, usually had a brown coating on their exterior and could be decorated with grooves or incised geometric decorations, like triangles, on their shoulders.

An important variation of this ware was the smeared wash ware. Bowls, platters and medium to large size pots of this type, which were smeared with a slip, have surface colours which vary slightly from dark to reddish brown, as the slip has different thicknesses at different parts of the surface. Smeared wash ware is one of the main denominators of the EB IV period in northern Syria, which is contemporary with the EB III period of Anatolia, and was in use in Cilicia Pedias during this same period.[26] The examples found at Kilise Tepe can be local imitations of this ware, but the unusual forms of some of the examples, when the rest of the Kilise Tepe pottery repertoire is considered, imply that they may well be imports (FIG. 8).

One interesting find from the earliest phase of level Vf was a double spouted jug, which was found lying on the floor, in the area between the oven and the

25 Lamb 1937, 17, fig. 6:1a-c; Goldman 1956, fig. 273:445; Lloyd and Mellaart 1962, 236, fig. P.64:23, 26; Korfmann 1983, 292; Easton 2002, 324; Symington 2007, 308.

26 Goldman 1956, 145; Braidwood and Braidwood 1960, 415–417, 447–450; Kühne 1976, 95–97; Mazzoni 1985, 9; Rova 1989; Akkermans and Schwartz 2003, 244.

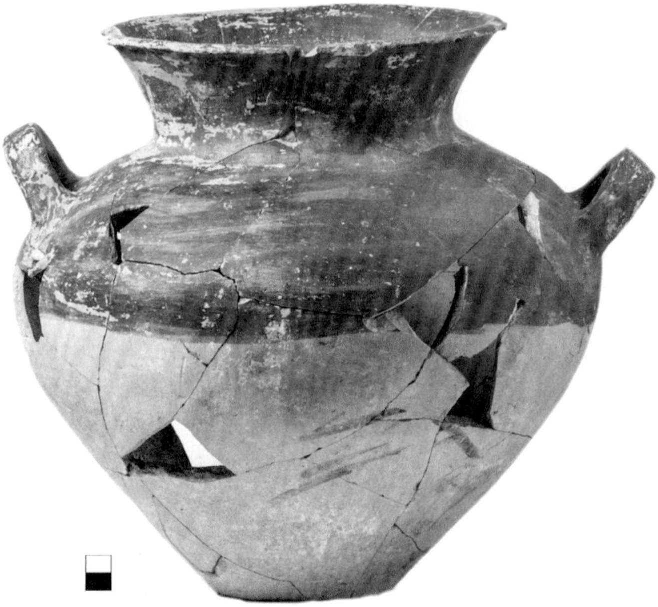

Fig. 8 A smeared wash ware pot from Kilise Tepe, level Vf-Phase 4.

newly constructed building (Fig. 9). This is the only example of a vessel with this form found at Kilise Tepe and represents a cultural tradition which appeared in this period but did not continue afterwards. Examples of double spouted vessels were reported from several western Anatolian sites, including Troy, Beycesultan, and Yortan, so this can be seen as a local tradition of that part of Anatolia, which managed to infiltrate into Cilicia Trachea in this period.[27] Interestingly, multi-spouted vessels also became popular in Cyprus in this period—and remained so during the Middle Bronze Age—and the tradition may have spread there from Cilicia Trachea or directly from western Anatolia through maritime trade.[28]

In general terms, the pottery traditions of the earliest phase of EB III indicate that Cilicia Trachea developed close cultural relations with western Anatolia during this period. This is best manifested by the red-cross bowls and the double spouted vessel mentioned above. However, as reflected by the popularity of the smeared wash ware pottery tradition, contacts with Syria were also intensified, which may have been formed through Cilicia Pedias, but also through a maritime route directly linking this area to northwestern Syria.

The new level Vf building and the oven went into disuse after only a short period of time, and by the next phase of level Vf, this part of the mound was an open space workshop area. In fact, this part of the mound continued to be used

27 Schliemann 1880, No.358–359; Lloyd and Mellaart 1962, 241; Kâmil 1982, 48, 105.

28 Spiteris 1970, 34–35, 42–43, 56–57.

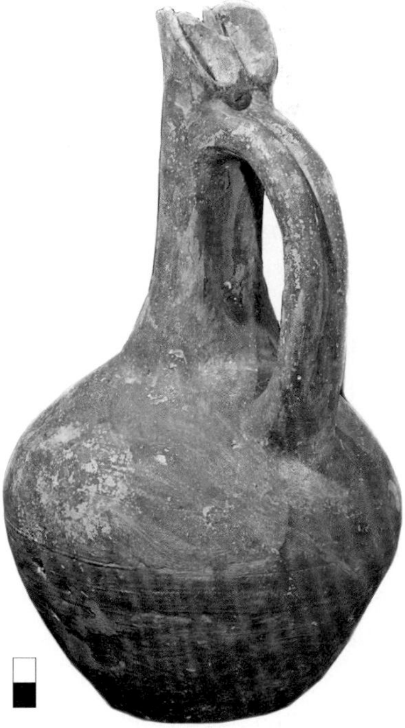

FIG. 9 A double spouted jug from Kilise Tepe, level Vf-Phase 4.

in this way until the second half of the MBA, with fire installations and clumsy workspace division walls. The level Vf pottery traditions mentioned above did not lose popularity until the beginning of the MBA, and therefore one cannot talk about cultural discontinuity, and the change in the function of the area can only be explained with a reduction in settlement size. The high numbers of spindle whorls recovered from level Ve, which is the transitional phase between the Early and Middle Bronze Ages, imply that the site had an active textile industry at the very end of the Early Bronze Age.

The Political and Economic State of Mesopotamia, Syria and Anatolia at the End of the Early Bronze Age

The regional catastrophe, which manifested itself in the form of either destruction or abandonment of sites all across the eastern Mediterranean region, was linked by many scholars to a radical climatic change that occurred in the northern hemisphere during this period.[29] In this scenario, some sites were abandoned as the EBA cities could no longer sustain themselves because the seasonal agricultural production was interrupted as a result of the lack of rainfall, which triggered a

29 Weiss, *et al.* 1993; Weiss 1997; Cullen *et al.* 2000; Staubwasser and Weiss 2006.

movement back to the earlier village based economy, and some other sites were destroyed by groups in movement, which could be either nomads or previously urban communities that had to leave the areas they were living in, looking for places with more favourable climatic conditions to continue their lives.

Although this may have been the situation, the archaeological evidence implies that we are not actually looking at one great regional event that took place during a specific period, i.e. the end of the EB II, but a set of linked events, and even a process that probably spanned several centuries, that includes adaptation to the changing climatic conditions, attempts to develop and expand the zone of inter-regional trade, and warfare between competing, emerging powers.

Where Syria and Mesopotamia are concerned, the period we are looking at saw the emergence and the expansion of the Akkadian Empire, which managed to control the whole Mesopotamian plain for almost two hundred years.[30] The formation of this empire could well have been an attempt to adapt to the degrading climatic conditions in southern Mesopotamia at a time when the local city-states were rapidly growing economically and did not only need to sustain the increasing population but were also in need of raw materials, which were required by the ruling elites to display their wealth and to continue to assume power. However, during this same period, there were newly emerging powers in northern Mesopotamia and Syria, which controlled not only the routes that provided the essential raw materials to southern Mesopotamia but also the fertile areas that could still produce high amounts of agricultural products to sustain the local population.[31] Therefore, it would not be illogical to think that the newly emerging Akkadian elites living in the Sumerian cities of southern Mesopotamia, which were weakened by the changing economic conditions and constant battles amongst themselves, saw the opportunity and united under Sargon to take control, in the hope of increasing their wealth and saving southern Mesopotamia from a total economic collapse.

In this respect, Sargon may have simply followed the duty ordained to him by the Akkadian elites, and, after uniting southern Mesopotamia, he marched north to take control of the fertile northern Mesopotamian plains and the major trade routes mentioned above. This grand project was continued by the Akkadian rulers following him, and Naram-Sin even marched further to the north in an attempt to directly control the actual raw material sources.[32] To achieve these goals, Akkadians had to impose power over a vast area, either through warfare, as

30 Akkermans and Schwartz 2003, 277–282.

31 Akkermans and Schwartz 2003, 268–277.

32 Unger and Naab 1934; Weiss 2002, 22; Frahm and Feinberg 2013, 1129–1132.

seen in the case of Ebla,[33] or by utilising treaties, as seen in the case of Urkesh.[34] The Akkadians managed to turn the Khabur plain into a large agricultural zone feeding the southern Mesopotamian cities, and by exerting power over northern Syria, they managed to control the major trade routes linking Anatolia and the Mediterranean coast to Mesopotamia.[35]

Around this same period, Anatolia witnessed the emergence of numerous powerful polities, whose economic growth was probably linked to the exploitation of local metal sources and control of the trade routes linking eastern Europe and the Aegean and Black Sea coasts to Syria and Mesopotamia.[36] The central Anatolian polities, which probably also fought amongst themselves to extend their political presence to neighbouring areas, accumulated great wealth during this period, which is best manifested by the elite burials at Alacahöyük.[37] Meanwhile, another set of polities was growing in power in western Anatolia, which owed their wealth to the trade contacts they had with the Aegean islands, Greece and the Balkans.[38]

Towards the end of the Early Bronze Age, many Anatolian settlements were either viciously destroyed or witnessed a reduction in size.[39] Around the same period, many sites in northern Mesopotamia and Syria were gradually abandoned,[40] and other sites in Palestine were either destroyed or abandoned.[41] At the very end of the EBA, the degraded climatic conditions finally also resulted in the collapse of the northern Mesopotamian economy, which was caused by the disruption of agricultural activities as a result of the decreasing annual precipitation. This triggered the collapse of the Akkadian Empire, as it could no longer sustain its population, its army and its elites.[42] The Akkadian Empire was then replaced by the Kingdom of Ur III in southern Mesopotamia, which had to struggle to protect its borders and maintain its fragile economy during its one century long existence.[43]

33 Pettinato 1976, 44; Matthiae 1978; Milano 1995, 1228.

34 Buccellati and Buccellati 1997, 92–93; 2000, 139; 2002; Bryce 2009, 752–753.

35 Koliński 2007, 360; Ristvet *et al.* 2004; McMahon 2013, 470–472.

36 Düring 2011, 289–296.

37 Arık 1937; Koşay and Akok 1944; Sagona and Zimansky 2009, 213–216.

38 Şahoğlu 2005; Düring 2011, 287–289.

39 Mellaart 1958; Mellink 1986.

40 Akkermans and Schwartz 2003, 282–287; Ristvet and Weiss 2005; Koliński 2011.

41 Ritter-Kaplan 1984; Richard 1987, 34–40; Mazar 1997.

42 Westenholz 1999, 55–59.

43 Sallaberger 1999, 121–336.

The Political Scene in Anatolia at the End of the Early Bronze Age

Looking at the events that took place in the whole region in a chronological perspective, it would be wiser to think that these did not occur simultaneously, but were a result of a series of incidents that spanned a period of time. As already mentioned before, at the end of the Early Bronze Age, both central Anatolia and western Anatolia had a set of polities, which were competing to extend their spheres of influence, to grow their economies and to increase their wealth. These polities were probably formed and gained power during the EB II period, as at this point in history, the level of socio-economic organization and technology allowed them both to exploit the metal sources of Anatolia efficiently and also develop advanced metal industries.[44] The exploited sources and possibly the worked metal artefacts could be traded to distant areas with a good profit, and the opportunities Anatolia could provide also attracted merchants from the neighbouring regions to here.

The legends about the expeditions of Sargon and Naram-Sin into central Anatolia, whether or not they reflect actual events, provide a good idea about the political situation in central Anatolia during this period. The legend of *Šar-Tamhari*, which was written and told centuries after the actual events, informs us about the military expedition of Sargon to central Anatolia.[45] According to the legend, Mesopotamian traders whose trade activities were being disrupted by the local Kingdom of Purušhanda, appealed to Sargon to open the way between Mesopotamia and Anatolia by punishing this kingdom. The legend claims that Sargon managed to capture the hostile Kingdom of Purušhanda and secured the trade link between the two areas.

Other ancient documents also written centuries after the actual events, mention another Akkadian expedition to central Anatolia, this time by Naram-Sin.[46] These texts inform us about a general uprising in central Anatolia and northwestern Syria. Naram-Sin had to conduct a military expedition to this area to suppress this uprising by defeating a coalition of 17 city-states. These ancient texts clearly indicate that central Anatolia and northwestern Syria were ruled by numerous city-states in this period, which could unite against a common enemy if there was a common cause to defend, and the archaeological evidence does support this view. The excavations in central Anatolia have revealed that many settlements started to develop during the EB II and reached a level of higher complexity at the beginning of the EB III period. The inhabitants of Alişar already felt the necessity

44 Sagona and Zimansky 2009, 200–210.

45 Güterbock 1964; Westenholz 1997, 102–139; Haas 2006, 68–71, CTH 310. For a discussion about an Old Assyrian version of the legend found at Kültepe-Kanesh see Alster and Oshima 2007, and Westenholz 2007.

46 Westenholz 1997, 246–258; Haas 2006, 72–76, CTH 311.

to build a fortification wall around the settlement during the EB II period,[47] which was later enhanced, and Alacahöyük witnessed the rise of an elite class probably during this period which manifested itself with the rich burials of the following EB III period.[48] A fortification wall was built around Çadır Höyük in the EB III period,[49] and both Acemhöyük and Kültepe seem to have achieved a certain level of social complexity during this period.[50]

The archaeological evidence clearly shows that the situation in western Anatolia was not different from central Anatolia in this period. The trade contacts with the Aegean Islands, Greece, the Balkans and central Anatolia resulted in the formation of wealthy city-states across the region during the EB II period.[51] The developments in metallurgy and metal trade were probably the driving force for the fast economic and political growth of these polities, where the ruling elite, who were at the top of the newly formed social hierarchy, accumulated great wealth.[52] The excavations at various sites have shown that the EB II settlements, which quickly grew in size, were defended by fortification walls, which shows that there was some sort of competition between the city-states which may have caused them to fight for power from time to time.

It seems like the western Anatolian polities reached the peak of their power at the very end of the EB II and the beginning of the EB III period, which may have resulted in some alliances amongst them in this period, although local conflicts must still have occurred. This is best manifested by the expansion of western Anatolian cultural influence to the neighbouring areas. The change in pottery and architectural style at Küllüoba in northwest central Anatolia,[53] and the appearance of northwestern Anatolian cultural material and architectural elements in Thrace at the very end of the EB II period[54] are good indications of this. It should be noted that no sites in these neighbouring areas were reported to be attacked or destroyed in this period, which clearly shows that these changes were the result of an expansion of the western Anatolian sphere of cultural influence.

On the other hand, the abandonment of some western Anatolian settlements in this period were perhaps not a result of a regional catastrophe or economic

47 Von der Osten 1937, 116–118, 208–214.

48 Arık 1937; Koşay and Akok 1944.

49 Steadman 2011, 245.

50 Özgüç 1966, 52.

51 Şahoğlu 2005; Sagona and Zimansky 2009, 194–198; Steadman 2011, 238–241.

52 Renfrew 1967; Stos-Gale *et al.* 1984; Şahoğlu 2005, 352–352; Düring 2011, 274–278.

53 Fidan 2012, 25.

54 Özdoğan 2011, 221.

collapse, but were caused by the movement of populations to developing regional centres, which were constantly growing in size. The abandonment of the southwestern Anatolian settlement of Bademağacı for the time being[55] and Karataş-Semayük turning into a more organized settlement with better built structures, accompanied by innovations in pottery technology,[56] can be seen as proofs of these developments in this region.

In fact, something similar to these events in western Anatolia was happening in Greece in this same period, probably as a result of the same fast growing economic system and the newly emerging socio-political system. For instance, Lerna in the Argolid provides some interesting information about the socio-political and cultural developments on the mainland. Technical studies conducted on the pottery of Lerna IV have shown that these mainly followed the traditions of the EB II period of central Greece.[57] This is probably because the socio-political developments in that area resulted in an expansion of the sphere of cultural influence of a political entity that emerged in central Greece. Lerna went through a harsh destruction in the EB III period, which was explained mainly by the arrival of new, hostile groups in this area, but this may well be a result of a conflict between the local city-states or between groups of allied polities which were trying to expand their areas of political and commercial control.

Cilicians seem to have adapted quickly to the new economic and political order in Anatolia and Syria during the EB II period, as it was situated at a strategic location sandwiched just in between these greater cultural regions. All the major settlements seem to have grown into regional centres, probably of local polities controlling the hinterland surrounding them and the main trade routes passing through their land. This is not only manifested by the increasing size of the settlements but also by the fortification walls built around them, which hint at the existence of a level of concern for their security, fearing an attack that may come either from the neighbouring polities or from other political entities in the neigbouring regions. Fortification walls were built around Tarsus and Kinet Höyük during the EB II period and the thick walls unearthed at the northwestern edge of Kilise Tepe may also belong to a defensive structure of some sort.[58] It should be indicated that building fortification walls was a general trend in the whole region in this period, which was also seen at the *Kranzhügel* settlements of the neighboring northern Syria.[59]

55 Umurtak 2011, 213.

56 Mellink 1984, 104–105.

57 Rutter 1995, 650.

58 Goldman 1956, 21–25; Gates 2008, 284–285; 2009, 354.

59 Cooper 2006, 76–78.

The concerns of the inhabitants of these Cilician settlements were not in vain, as Kilise Tepe and Tarsus were attacked and destroyed at the end of the EB II period. Kinet Höyük was not attacked in the same vicious way, but some burning traces on walls imply that the site was affected to some degree by these same events. The architectural traditions changed drastically at Kinet Höyük at the beginning of the Early Bronze III period, with a shift from entirely mudbrick structures to buildings with stone foundations and mudbrick superstructures, but the pottery traditions mostly survived.[60] However, at Tarsus the post-destruction pottery traditions were understood to be radically different from what were popular during the EB II period, whereas the architectural layout remained the same.[61] On the other hand, at Kilise Tepe a more radical change was observed, and both the architectural layout and the pottery traditions went through important changes after the destruction. In general terms, the strong central Anatolian cultural influence was replaced by a west Anatolian influence, which is best manifested by the post-destruction pottery traditions of Tarsus and Kilise Tepe, but some trends also hint at close contacts with northern Syria.

Destruction in Cilicia: was it an Invasion of a Foreign Group or an Aftermath of a Regional Conflict?

The varying cultural responses of the inhabitants of the Cilician sites to the destruction imply that the invading groups attacked these settlements with different aims. It looks like the invaders wanted Kilise Tepe to become a solid part of their political and economic system and at least some of them settled here, changing the local socio-cultural structure. The reason for invading Tarsus was slightly different, and here they probably wanted to exert some control over the local population by settling some western Anatolians here, dragging Tarsus into their sphere of political and cultural influence. On the other hand, it seems like Kinet Höyük was not a direct target, but the invaders wanted to exert a level of political influence over this southeastern edge of Cilicia as well, probably to have some control over the land and sea routes which this settlement was located on. The change in architectural traditions is a sign of increasing cultural influence over this area.

The current evidence implies that the destruction of Cilician sites at the end of the EB II period was a result of an organized combined attack of western Anatolian powers on this region. Taking the political system present in Anatolia during this period into account, this can be seen as an attempt to secure the trade connections western Anatolia had with northern Syria and probably also with

60 Gates 2008, 284–285; 2011, 183–184.

61 Goldman 1956, 21–25.

Cyprus. It can be speculated that the connection was blocked for some reason by central Anatolian powers, which were competing with western Anatolians over the control of the main trade routes. This combined attack must have allowed the western Anatolians to open the way between western Anatolia and Syria using an alternative route passing through the Göksu Valley and other routes in Cilicia Trachea, and having a strong political presence in Cilicia must have allowed them to monopolise the trade link with Cyprus.

The EB II period did not only witness a rise in political complexity in Anatolia and the neigbouring regions, but also a boom in metallurgy, and therefore, the trade networks of the period seem to have mostly served to appease the needs of this developing industry.[62] Cilicia Trachea and Cyprus are regions which are both relatively rich in copper sources.[63] Unfortunately, it is still not clear whether the Cilician sources were in use or not in this period, but at least it is clear that with the EB II period a complex metal industry made its appearance very suddenly in Cyprus, both exploiting the local sources and also importing raw materials from Anatolia.[64] Another important source of copper was the Ergani-Maden mines,[65] and the central Anatolian polities must have had the monopoly over the trade of copper from this source to western Anatolian.

Strangely enough, Cyprus seems to have been disconnected from the metal trade network around 2300 BC, and the local metal industry collapsed, not to be re-established until the MBA.[66] It is hard to guess whether this happened before or after the destruction of the Cilician sites, but a post-destruction date is more probable, as that period witnessed an overall collapse of the regional economies.

Taking all the evidence into account, a scenario can be suggested for what may have happened in Cilicia at the end of the EB II period (Fig. 10). The combined western Anatolian army probably marched into the Göksu Valley through Karaman after passing through the southwestern edge of the Konya plain, in order to cut the connection of the rival central Anatolian polities with the Mediterranean coast, because the central Anatolians were blocking the eastern Anatolian route and the western Anatolians could not risk also losing their connection with Syria and Cyprus.

After conquering Kilise Tepe, the western Anatolians must have marched into Cilicia Pedias through the coast and also conquered Tarsus. No destruction was reported from the Amuq,[67] so this expedition must have ended once the western

---

62 Sagona and Zimansky 2009, 200–210.

63 Wagner and Öztunalı 2000.

64 Spiteris 1970, 62–64; Renfrew 1972, 338; Nakou 1995, 1–2; Broodbank 2000, 292–293.

65 Wheeler *et al.* 1975, 34; Muhly 1977, 73, 79.

66 Webb *et al.* 2006, 282.

67 Braidwood and Braidwood 1960, 396–397.

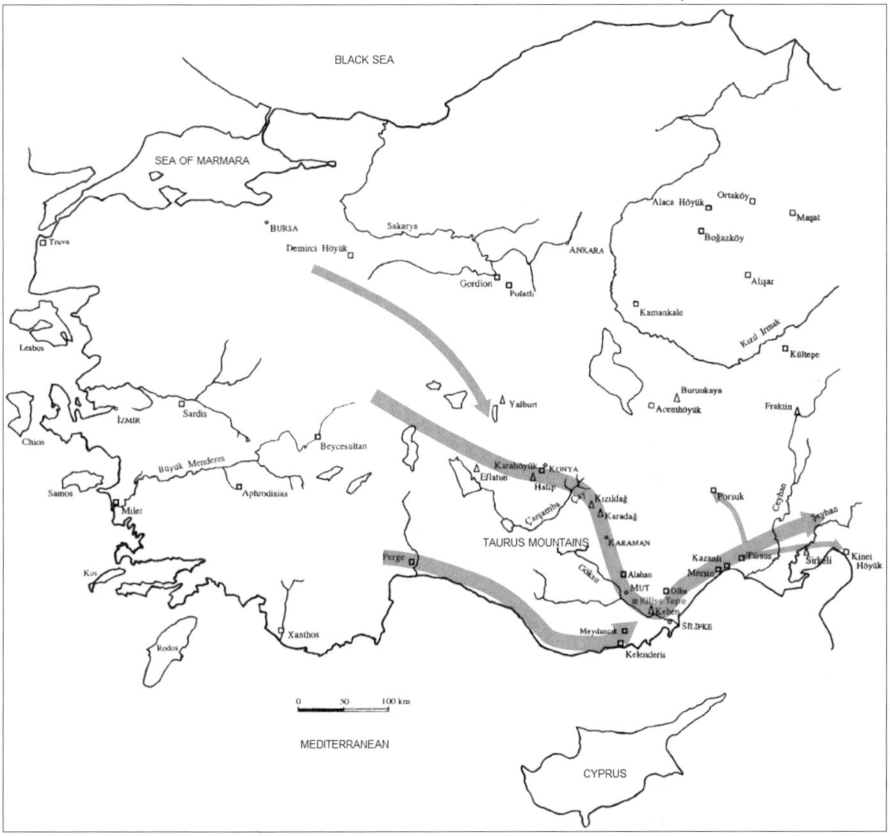

FIG. 10 Map showing the proposed advance routes of western Anatolians.

Anatolians managed to exert full control over Cilicia, probably following a minor raid also to Kinet Höyük. This expedition allowed them to open and secure a new route allowing the Ergani-Maden copper to flow into western Anatolia through northwestern Syria and the Cypriot copper through Cilicia. The disappearance of the red-black burnished ware from the pottery repertoire of the Amuq sites in the EB III period is a sign of success of this expedition, as this can be seen as proof of weakening relations between northwestern Syria and central Anatolia.[68] The expedition may have also allowed the western Anatolians to open a new route to reach the Göltepe-Kestel sources[69] to obtain the precious tin they required for the metal industry, which were also in the hands of central Anatolians until that point.

68 Braidwood and Braidwood 1960, 429.

69 Yener 2000; 2008.

However, things did not go as planned after the conquest. At Kilise Tepe new buildings were quickly constructed, and the archaeological material from Tarsus and Kilise Tepe show that new trade contacts were formed both with Syria and western Anatolia, which indicates that the trade network could be activated. However, this did not last long, and, together with the collapse of the Akkadian Empire and the Mesopotamian and northern Syrian economies, the trade network also lost its function. The connection of western Anatolia with Syria and Cyprus was gradually lost, and the whole region entered a period of economic depression that was to end only with the MBA.

Conclusion

The regional catastrophe witnessed at the end of the Early Bronze Age was probably not a sudden event that occurred throughout the Middle East, but was a process that was triggered by the rise of complex political entities, a developed economy and an interregional trade system, which both emerged and collapsed because of a change in climatic conditions across the region. Therefore, the destruction and abandonment of numerous settlements at the end of the EB II and at the beginning of the EB III periods did not have one specific reason but was caused by different phenomena at different parts of the ancient Near East.

The climatic conditions did not deteriorate at the end of the Early Bronze Age at a level that would result with the collapse of the local economies in Anatolia, Cyprus or Greece, unlike Mesopotamia and Syria, where the political entities like the Akkadian Empire emerged as a response to the changing climatic conditions and collapsed because it could not tolerate it any more. However, as the economic system in Anatolia was very much connected to and relied on Syria and Mesopotamia, the economic and political collapse of the systems there resulted in an economic depression in Anatolia as well.

The destruction in Cilicia was probably not caused by immigrants or marauding invaders who were looking for new lands to settle after they had to leave their homelands because of the climatic changes or because they were pushed out by other groups. These settlements were destroyed because of a regional conflict between Anatolian polities, which were competing to secure their control over certain parts of the interregional trade network. As these polities grew stronger economically, the tension between them increased, and especially the trade of copper which were acquired from the sources in Ergani-Maden and Cyprus, and tin acquired from Göltepe-Kestel, became central issues, as copper and tin were essential needs of the growing economies and were also required by the elites, who saw these metals and the level of control over their trade as a sign of prestige.

A combined systematic attack of western Anatolian polities in Cilicia was probably the last episode of a series of events that took place in Anatolia, which finally allowed them to secure the connection to Syria and Cyprus, warding off the central Anatolian threat. However, they did not know that an overall economic collapse was waiting for them, and this precarious attempt was to be in vain. Only with the establishment of a new political and economic order with the Middle Bronze Age, when the climatic conditions improved and new kingdoms emerged in Mesopotamia, Anatolia was once again to see a thriving economy and the establishment of new complex political entities.

REFERENCES

Akkermans, P. M. M. G. and G.M. Schwartz, *The Archaeology of Syria: From Complex Hunter-Gatherers to Early Urban Societies* (c.16,000–300 BC). Cambridge: Cambridge University Press, 2003.

Alster, B. and T. Oshima, "Sargonic Dinner at Kaneš: The Old Assyrian Sargon Legend" *Iraq* 69 (2007): 1–20.

Arık, R.O., *Les fouilles d'Alaca Höyük: Entreprises par la Société d'Histoire Turque. Rapport préliminaire sur les travaux en 1935*. Ankara, 1937.

Blegen, C. W., *Zygouries: A Prehistoric Settlement in the Valley of Cleonae*. Cambridge: American School of Classical Studies, 1928.

Blegen, C. W., Caskey, J. L., Rawson, M. and J. Sperling, *Troy. General Introduction: The First and the Second Settlements*. Vol.1. Princeton: Princeton University Press, 1950.

Braidwood, R.J. and L.S. Braidwood, *Excavations in the Plain of Antioch. Volume 1: The Earlier Assemblages, Phases A-J*. Chicago: University of Chicago Press, 1960.

Broodbank, C., *An Island Archaeology of the Early Cyclades*. Cambridge: Cambridge University Press, 2000.

Bryce, T., *The Routledge Handbook of the Peoples and Places of Ancient Western Asia: the Near East from the Early Bronze Age to the Fall of the Persian Empire*. New York: Routledge, 2009.

Buccellati, G. and M. K. Buccellati, "Urkesh: The First Hurrian Capital." *Biblical Archaeologist* 60/2 (1997): 77–96.

———. "The Royal Palace of Urkesh. Report on the 12th Season at Tell Mozan/Urkesh: Excavations in Area AA, June-October 1999." *Mitteilungen der Deutschen Orient-Gesellschaft zu Berlin* 132 (2000): 133–183.

———. "Tar'am Agade, Daughter of Naram-Sin, at Urkesh" in *Of Pots and Plans*, ed. by L. Al-Gailani Werr, J. Curtis, H. Martin, A. McMahon, J. Oates, J. Reade, G. Cadogan: 11–31. London: NABU, 2002.

Caskey, J.L., "The Early Helladic Period in the Argolid." *Hesperia* 29 (1960): 285–303.

———. "Did the Early Bronze Age End?" in *The End of the Early Bronze Age in the Aegean*, ed. by G. Cadogan, 9–30. Leiden: Brill, 1986.

Ceylan, A., "1999 Yılı Erzincan ve Erzurum Yüzey Araştırmaları." *Araştırma Sonuçları Toplantısı* 18/2 (2001):71–82.

Cooper, L., *Early Urbanism on the Syrian Euphrates*. New York: Routledge, 2006.

Cullen, H. M., de Menocal, P. B., Hemming, S., Hemming, G., Brown, F. H., Guilderson, T. and F. Sirocko, "Climate Change and the Collapse of the Akkadian Empire: Evidence from the Deep Sea." Geology 28/4 (2000): 379–382.

Drews, R.,*The Coming of the Greeks: Indo-European Conquests in the Aegean and the Near East*. Princeton: Princeton University Press, 1988.

Düring, B. S., *The Prehistory of Asia Minor*. Cambridge: Cambridge University Press, 2011.

Easton, D.F., *Schliemann's Excavations at Troia 1870–1873*. Mainz am Rhein: Zabern, 2002.

Fidan, E., "Küllüoba İlk Tunç Çağı Mimarisi." *Masrop* 7 (2012): 1–44.

Frahm, E. and J.M. Feinberg, "Empires and Resources: Central Anatolian Obsidian at Urkesh (Tell Mozan, Syria) During the Akkadian Period." *Journal of Archaeological Science* 40 (2013): 1122–1135.

Garstang, J., *Prehistoric Mersin: Yümük Tepe in Southern Turkey. The Neilson Expedition in Cilicia*. Oxford: Clarendon Press, 1953.

Gates, M.-H., "2006 Season at Kinet Höyük (Yeşil-Dörtyol, Hatay)." *Kazı Sonuçları Toplantısı* 29/2 (2008): 281–298.

———. "2007 Season At Kinet Höyük (Yeşil-Dörtyol, Hatay)." *Kazı Sonuçları Toplantısı* 30/2 (2009): 351–368.

———. "2009 Season at Kinet Höyük (Yeşil-Dörtyol, Hatay)." *Kazı Sonuçları Toplantısı* 32/3 (2011): 182–195.

Gimbutas, M.,"The Indo-Europeans: Archaeological Problems." *American Anthropologist* 65/4 (1963): 815–836.

———. "The Destruction of Aegean and East Mediterranean Urban Civilization around 2300 BC" in *Bronze Age Migrations in the Aegean. Archaeological and Linguistic Problems in Greek Prehistory: Proceedings of the First International Colloquium on Aegean Prehistory*, ed. by R. A. Crossland and A. Birchall, 123–139. Sheffield: Noyes Press, 1973.

Goldman, H., *Excavations at Gözlü Kule, Tarsus. Volume II: From the Neolithic through the Bronze Age*. Princeton: Princeton University Press, 1956.

Güterbock, H. G., "Sargon of Akkad Mentioned by Hattusili I of Hatti." *Journal of Cuneiform Studies* 18 (1964): 1–6.

Haas, V., *Die hethitische Literatur*. Berlin: De Gruyter, 2006.

Hood, S., "Evidence for Invasion" in *The End of the Early Bronze Age in the Aegean*, ed. by G. Cadogan, 31–68. Leiden: Brill, 1986.

Jackson, M.P.C., Postgate, J.N. and T.E. Şerifoğlu, "Kilise Tepe 2011 Yılı Kazıları." *Kazı Sonuçları Toplantısı* 34/2 (2013): 5–24.

Joukowsky, M.S., *Early Turkey: An Introduction to the Archaeology of Anatolia from Prehistory through the Lydian Period*. Dubuque: Kendall Hunt Publications, 1996.

Kâmil, T., *Yortan Cemetery in the Early Bronze Age of Western Anatolia*. Oxford: British Archaeological Reports, 1982.

Kenyon, K.M., *Amorites and Canaanites*. London: Oxford University Press, 1966.

Kökten, K., "Kuzey-Doğu Anadolu'nun Prehistoryasında Bayburt Çevresinin Yeri." *Ankara Üniversitesi Dil ve Tarih-Coğrafya Fakültesi Dergisi* 3/5 (1945): 465–505.

Koliński, R., "The Upper Khabur Region in the Second Part of the Third Millennium BC." *Altorientalische Forschungen* 34/2 (2007): 342–369.

———. "On Grain, Bones, and Khabur Collapse." *Folia Praehistorica Posnaniensia* 16 (2011): 201–217.

Korfmann, M.,"Red Cross Bowl: Angeblicher Leittyp für Troja V" in *Beiträge zur Altertumskunde Kleinasiens: Festschrift für Kurt Bittel*, ed. by R.M. Boehmer and H. Hauptmann, 291–297. Mainz am Rhein: Verlag Philipp von Zabern, 1983.

Korfmann, M. and B. Kromer, "Demircihöyük, Beşiktepe, Troia—eine Zwischenbilanz zur Chronologie dreier Orte in Westanatolien." *Studia Troica* 3 (1993): 135–146.

Koşay, H. Z. and K. Turfan, "Erzurum-Karaz Kazısı Raporu." *Belleten* 23 (1959): 339–413.

Koşay, H.Z. and M. Akok, *Ausgrabungen von Alaca Höyük. Ein Vorbericht über die im Auftrage der Türkischen Geschichtskommission im Sommer 1936 durchgeführten Forschungen und Entdeckungen*. Ankara, 1944.

Kühne, H., *Die Keramik vom Tell Chuera und ihre Beziehungen zu Funden aus Syrien-Palästina, der Türkei und dem Iraq*. Berlin: Mann, 1976.

Lamb, W., "Excavations at Kusura near Afyon Karahisar." *Archaeologia* 86 (1937): 1–64.

Lloyd, S. and J. Mellaart, *Beycesultan. Volume I, The Chalcolithic and Early Bronze Age Levels*. London: British Institute of Archaeology at Ankara Publication, 1962.

Maran, J., *Kulturwandel auf dem griechischen Festland und den Kykladen im späten 3.Jt. v. Chr.* Bonn: Habelt, 1998.

Matthiae, P., "Tell Mardikh: Ancient Ebla." *American Journal of Archaeology* 82/4 (1978): 540–543.

Mazar, A., "Four Thousand Years of History at Tel Beth-Shean: An Account of the Renewed Excavations." *Biblical Archaeologist* 60/2 (1997): 62–76.

Mazzoni, S., "Elements of the Ceramic Culture of Early Syrian Ebla in Comparison with Syro-Palestinian EB IV." *Bulletin of the American Schools of Oriental Research* 257 (1985): 1–18.

McMahon, A., "North Mesopotamia in the Third Millennium BC" in *The Sumerian World*, ed. by H. Crawford, 462–477. New York: Routledge, 2013.

Mellaart, J., "The End of the Early Bronze Age in Anatolia and the Aegean." *American Journal of Archaeology* 62/1 (1958): 9–33.

———. "Early Cultures of the South Anatolian Plateau." *Anatolian Studies* 13 (1963): 199–236.

Mellink, M.J., "The Prehistoric Sequence of Karataş-Semayük." *Kazı Sonuçları Toplantısı* 6 (1984): 103–106.

———. "The Early Bronze Age in West Anatolia: Aegean and Asiatic Correlations" in *The End of the Early Bronze Age in the Aegean*, ed. by G. Cadogan, 139–152. Leiden: Brill, 1986.

Milano, L., "Ebla: A Third-Millennium City-State in Ancient Syria" in *Civilizations of the Ancient Middle East*, Vol.II. ed. by J.M. Sasson, J. Baines, G. Beckman and K. S. Rubinson 1219–1230. New York: Charles Scribner's Sons, 1995.

Muhly, J.D., "The Copper Ox-Hide Ingots and the Bronze Age Metals Trade." *Iraq* 39/1 (1977): 73–82.

Murnane, W.J., "The History of Ancient Egypt: An Overview" in *Civilizations of the Ancient Middle East*, Vol.II. ed. by J.M. Sasson, J. Baines, G. Beckman and K. S. Rubinson, 691–718. New York: Charles Scribner's Sons, 1995.

Nakou, G., "The Cutting Edge: A New Look at Early Aegean Metallurgy." *Journal of Mediterranean Archaeology* 8/2 (1995): 1–32.

Nigro, L. and M. Sala, "Preliminary Report on the Fourth Season of Excavation by "La Sapienza" University of Rome at Khirbat al-Batrāwī in upper Wādī az-Zarqā', 2008." *Annual of the Department of Antiquities of Jordan* 53 (2009): 371–384.

Özdoğan, M., "Kanlıgeçit." *Arkeoatlas* 2011/01: 220–221.

Özgüç, N., "Excavations at Acemhöyük." *Anadolu* 10 (1966): 29–53.

Özgüç, T., "Yeni Araştırmaların Işığında Eski Anadolu Arkeolojisi." *Anadolu* 7 (1964): 23–42.

Özten, A., "A Group of Early Bronze Age Pottery from the Konya and Niğde Region" in *Anatolia and the Ancient Near East, Studies in Honor of Tahsin Özgüç* ed. by. K. Emre, M. Mellink and N. Özgüç, 407–418. Ankara: Türk Tarih Kurumu Basımevi, 1998.

Pettinato, G., "The Royal Archives of Tell Mardikh-Ebla." *The Biblical Archaeologist* 39/2 (1976): 44–52.

Prag, K., "The Intermediate Early Bronze-Middle Bronze Age Sequences at Jericho and Tell Iktanu Reviewed." *Bulletin of the American Schools of Oriental Research* 264 (1986): 61–72.

Renfrew, C., "Cycladic Metallurgy and the Aegean Early Bronze Age." *American Journal of Archaeology* 71/1 (1967): 1–20.

———. *The Emergence of Civilisation: The Cyclades and the Aegean in the Third Millennium BC*. London: Methuen, 1972.

Richard, S., "Archaeological Sources for the History of Palestine: The Early Bronze Age: The Rise and Collapse of Urbanism." *The Biblical Archaeologist* 50/1 (1987): 22–43.

Ristvet, L., Guilderson, T. and H. Weiss, "The Dynamics of State Development and Imperialization at Third Millennium Tell Leilan, Syria." *Orient Express* 21/2 (2004): 94–99.

Ristvet, L. and H. Weiss, "The Hābūr Region in the Late Third and Early Second Millennium BC" in *The History and Archaeology of Syria*, Vol. 1. ed. by. W. Orthmann, 1–26, Saarbrücken: Saarbrücken Verlag, 2005.

Ritter-Kaplan, H., "The Impact of Drought on Third Millennium BC Cultures on the Basis of Excavations in the Tel Aviv Exhibition Grounds." *Zeitschrift des Deutschen Palästina-Vereins* 100 (1984): 2–8.

Rova, E., "Die sogenannte 'Smeared-Wash Ware': Ein Beitrag zur Syrischen Keramik des III. Jahrtausends v. Chr." *Baghdader Mitteilungen* 20 (1989): 139–196.

Rutter, J.B., *Lerna. A Preclassical Site in the Argolid. Vol.3, The Pottery of Lerna IV.* Princeton: American School of Classical Studies, 1995.

Sagona, A. and P. Zimansky, *Ancient Turkey*. New York: Routledge, 2009.

Şahoğlu, V., "The Anatolian Trade Network and the Izmir Region during the Early Bronze Age." *Oxford Journal of Archaeology* 24/4 (2005): 339–361.

Sallaberger, W., "Ur III-Zeit" in *Mesopotamien. Akkade-Zeit und Ur III-Zeit*, ed. by A. Westenholz and W. Sallaberger, 117–390, Göttingen: Academic Press Fribourg, 1999.

Schliemann, H., *Ilios: The City and Country of the Trojans: the Results of Researches and Discoveries on the Site of Troy and Throughout the Troad in the Years 1871–72–73–78–79*. New York, 1880.

Şerifoğlu, T. E., "Kilise Tepe Erken Tunç Çağı Çalışmaları." *Kazı Sonuçları Toplantısı* 33/1 (2012): 375–388.

Spiteris, T., *The Art of Cyprus*. New York, 1970.

Staubwasser, M. and Weiss, "Holocene Climate and Cultural Evolution in Late Prehistoric-Early Historic West Asia." *Quaternary Research* 66/3 (2006): 372–387.

Steadman, S.R., "The Early Bronze Age in the Plateau" in *The Oxford Handbook of Ancient Anatolia*, ed. by S. R. Steadman and G. McMahon, 229–259. Oxford: Oxford University Press, 2011.

Stos-Gale, Z.A., Gale, N.H. and G.R. Gilmore, "Early Bronze Age Trojan Metal Sources and Anatolians in the Cyclades." *Oxford Journal of Archaeology* 3/3 (1984): 23–44.

Symington, D., "The Early Bronze Age Pottery" in *Excavations at Kilise Tepe, 1994–98, From Bronze Age to Byzantine in Western Cilicia*, ed. by N. Postgate and D. Thomas (eds.), 295–318. London: McDonald Institute for Archaeological Research, 2007.

Umurtak, G., "Bademağacı." *Arkeoatlas* 2011/01: 213.

Unger, E. and J.P. Naab, *Pir Hüseyin'de Naram-Sin Steli'nin Keşfi*. İstanbul, 1934.

Von der Osten, H.H., *The Alishar Hüyük, Seasons of 1930–32*. Chicago: Oriental Institute of the University of Chicago, 1937.

Wagner, G.A. and Ö. Öztunalı, "Prehistoric Copper Sources in Turkey" in *Anatolian Metal I*, ed. by Ü. Yalçın, 31–67. Bochum: Deutsches Bergbau Museum, 2000.

Webb, J.M., Frankel, D., Stos, Z.A. and N. Gale, "Early Bronze Age Metal Trade in the Eastern Mediterranean. New Composition and Lead Isotope Evidence from Cyprus." *Oxford Journal of Archaeology* 25/3 (2006): 261–288.

Weiss, H., Courty, M.-A., Wetterstrom, W., Guichard, F., Senior, L., Meadow, R. and A. Curnow, "The Genesis and Collapse of Third Millennium North Mesopotamian Civilization." *Science* (New Series) 261/5124 (1993): 995–1004.

Weiss, H., "Late Third Millennium Abrupt Climate Change and Social Collapse in West Asia and Egypt." *NATO ASI Series* 49 (1997): 711–723.

———. "Akkadian: Akkadian Empire" in *Encyclopedia of Prehistory*, Volume 8: South and Southwest Asia, ed. by P. N. Peregrine and M. Ember 21–23. New York: Springer, 2002.

———. "Quantifying Collapse: The Late Third Millennium Khabur Plains" in *Seven Generations Since the Fall of Akad*, ed. by H. Weiss, 1–24. Wiesbaden: Harrassowitz, 2012.

Westenholz, A., "The Old Akkadian Period: History and Culture" in *Mesopotamien. Akkade-Zeit und Ur III-Zeit*, ed. by A. Westenholz and W. Sallaberger, 15–118. Göttingen: Academic Press Fribourg, 1999.

Westenholz, J.G., *Legends of the Kings of Akkade*. Winona Lake: Eisenbrauns, 1997.

———. "Notes on the Old Assyrian Sargon Legend Author(s)." *Iraq* 69 (2007): 21–27.

Wheeler, T.S., Maddin, R. and J.D. Muhly, "Ingots and the Bronze Age Copper Trade in the Mediterranean: A Progress Report." *Expedition* 17/4 (1975): 31–39.

Wiencke, M.H., "Change in Early Helladic II." *American Journal of Archaeology* 93/4 (1989): 495–509.

———. "Lerna" in *The Oxford Handbook of the Bronze Age Aegean*, ed. by E. H. Cline, 660–670. Oxford: Oxford University Press, 2000.

Yener, K.A., *The Domestication of Metals: The Rise of Complex Metal Industries in Anatolia*. Leiden: Brill, 2000.

———. "The Dynamics of Local Provisioning of Tin during the Early Bronze Age" in *Ancient Mining in Turkey and the Eastern Mediterranean*, ed. by Ü. Yalçın, H. Özbal and A. G. Paşamehmetoğlu, 57–64, Ankara: Atılım University, 2008.

Yon, M., *The City of Ugarit at Tell Ras Shamra*. Winona Lake: Eisenbrauns, 2006.

Early Bronze Age Graves and Burial Customs in Mezraa Höyük

Derya Yalçıklı[1]

Abstract

Salvage excavations carried out at Mezraa Höyük, located south of the Şanlıurfa/Birecik district and on the eastern side of the Euphrates River, have established a settlement sequence stretching from the Late Chalcolithic (Late Uruk) to the Early and Middle Bronze Ages, the Iron Age and the Medieval Period (11th and 13th centuries CE). The Early Bronze settlement at Mezraa Höyük spans the entire 3rd millennium BCE. Architectural levels dating to the EB I-II have been identified on the southeastern slope, and those dating to the EB III/IV were found in the east and on the summit in the northeast areas on the höyük. A cemetery area for the EBA has not been determined, but all structures belonging to this period are associated with numerous cist, pithos and cooking pot graves. These graves, which can be dated to the early and late stages of the EBA, point to a continuous and unique burial tradition in the region.

Introduction

Mezraa Höyük is one of several archeological sites within the Karkamış Dam Lake Basin. It is situated on the east side of the Euphrates, within the borders of the town of Mezraa, 7 km south of Birecik, in the Şanlıurfa Province (Fig. 1). The höyük was discovered by G. Algaze and his team during their survey expeditions that took place between 1987–1990.[2] As part of the Salvage Project of the Archaeological Heritage of the Ilısu and Carchemish Dam Reservoirs, and with the support of the Middle East Technical University's Center for Research and Assessment of the Historic Environment (METU-TAÇDAM), excavations were carried out in 2000 and 2002. Another salvage campaign was conducted with the support of the Ministry of Culture and Tourism between 2005 and 2007.[3]

Excavations were carried out in three areas: the East and Southeast Slopes and

1 Department of Archaeology, Çanakkale Onsekiz Mart University, Çanakkale, Turkey.

2 Algaze *et al.* 1994, 48, fig. 7 No. 51.

3 Yalçıklı 2009; Yalçıklı ve Tekinalp 2002; 2003; 2004a; 2004b; 2011.

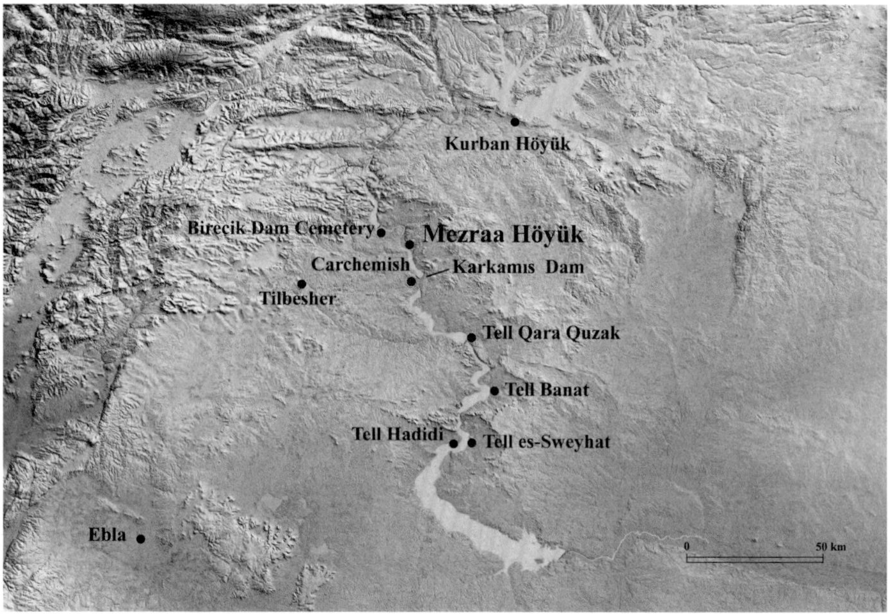

FIG. 1 Map showing the location of Mezraa Höyük.

the Summit in the northeast (FIG. 2). As a result of these excavations, architectural levels dated to the Late Uruk, Early and Middle Bronze Ages, the Iron Age and the Medieval Period (11th and 13th centuries CE) were identified. The existence of a long sequence that covers the entire 3rd millennium BCE has also been determined. Architectural levels from EB I-II have been uncovered in the Southeast Slope, and those from EB III/IV were unearthed from the east and the Summit area. During our work on the höyük, we have not encountered a cemetery from the EBA. Yet, we have come across pit, pithos, and composite graves (see below), as well as burials inside cooking pots. We have found graves within architectural levels on the Southeast and East Slopes, but there were no graves dated to EBA architectural levels around the Summit area.

Southeast Slope

This area is situated on the steep southeast slope of the höyük facing the Euphrates. This area is considered to be of importance due to its Late Chalcolithic (Late Uruk) and early EBA levels. In other parts of the höyük, these levels lie under MBA and Medieval layers.

A big landslide on the south side of the höyük, possibly as a result of a change in the Euphrates' riverbed that took place around the middle of the 3rd millennium

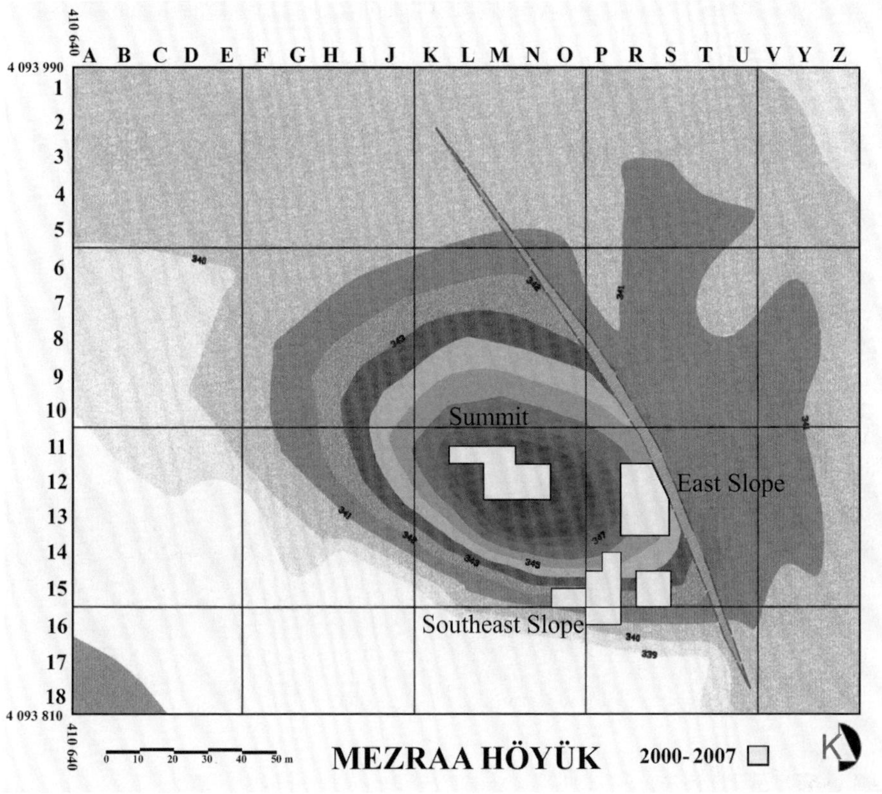

FIG. 2 Topographical map of Mezraa Höyük.

BCE, has destroyed some parts of the slope. Although we cannot estimate the entire extent of this landslide, it did have a considerable impact on the architectural levels dated to Late Chalcolithic Age and EB I-II. The southern walls of structures dated to EB I-II have been destroyed. The ongoing erosion on the steep slope is causing further damage. It is understood that Mezraa Höyük used to cover a much greater land area during the first half of the EBA, before the erosion.

Seven of the nine architectural levels discovered on the southeast slope are dated to the EBA. Among these architectural levels, Level II is dated to EB III/IV; Level III to the end of EB I and the beginning of EB II; and Levels IV-VIII are dated to EB I. In these architectural levels a limited part of structures with walls facing northwest and southeast were discovered. These structures were usually built on limestone foundations that have two rows, with mudbrick walls and compact, white-plastered earth floors. Although no complete plan of these structures is available, we assume that they are rectangular and had multi-room spaces. In the Southeast area, pithos graves, cooking pot and composite grave types have been

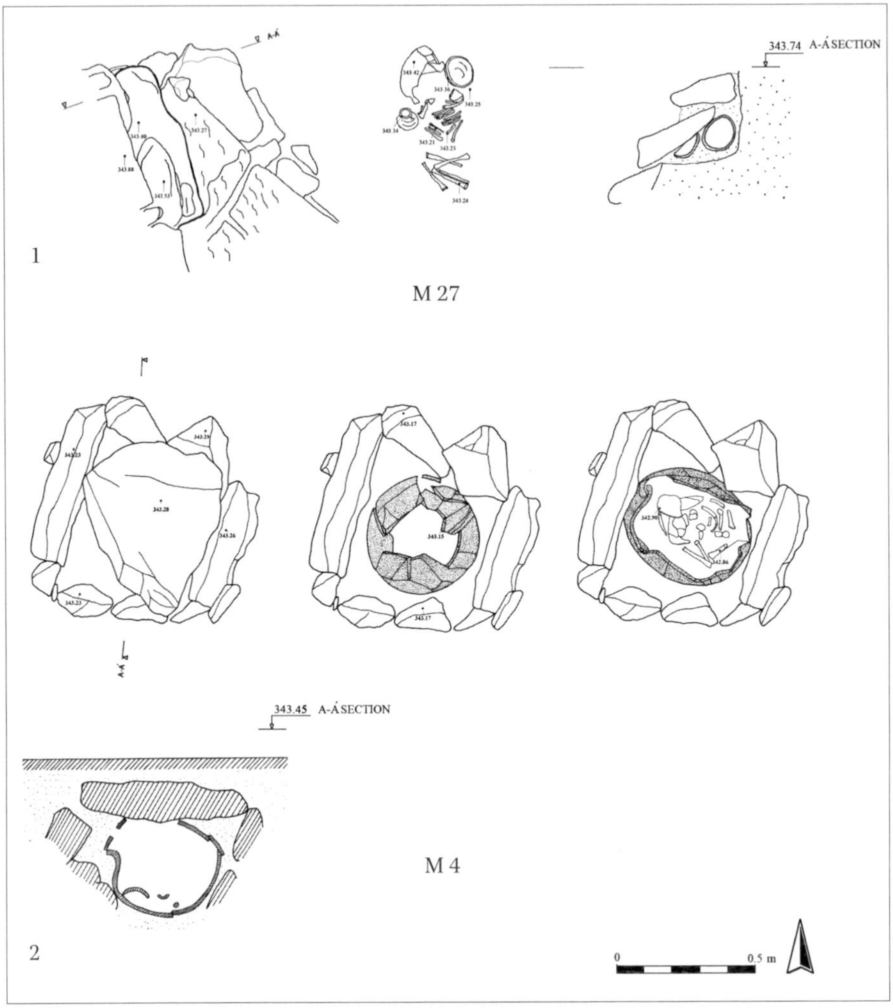

FIG. 3 Graves, M 27, 4

located. According to Mezraa Höyük's phasing, these graves have been dated to EB I (Levels IV-VIII), except for a pithos grave which cannot be assigned to an architectural level but belongs to EB III/IV.

East Slope

This area is situated on the edge of a cross section that is 40 m long and 4 m high, created by the removal of soil in order to enlarge the agricultural field. This area includes four architectural levels belonging to EB III/IV, underlying five architectural levels of the MBA and the Medieval periods. Intense Medieval occupation has considerably damaged two of the MBA architectural levels below. Structures dating to a late phase of the EBA were situated to the northwest and southeast. These structures have mudbrick walls on foundations of two- or three-rowed limestones and include surfaces paved with flat stones, as well as tamped earth floors. In these densely settled architectural levels of VII and VIII, three graves have been unearthed.

Burial Types

Pit Burials

These are simple pits dug into the ground, into which the body is placed.[4] There are two such graves at Mezraa Höyük, both found in a storeroom in the East area, Level VII, and dated to the second half of the 3rd millennium BCE. These graves were situated below floors on the edge of the western wall (M 27) and at the corner of the southwestern (M 15), respectively.

M 27 contains the remains of a child aged 1–2 years. (Fig. 3.1, Fig. 5.1). This grave is different from the others because of its stone slab. The skeleton was found lying in the hocker position along a north-south axis, with its head facing west. There were two bowls placed on each side of the head, a bottle (Fig. 7.1), and one bronze needle placed on the chest. M 15 contained the remains of a newborn, covering an area of 23 x 19 cm.[5] The skeleton was laid in an east-west direction in the hocker position, with the head facing north. There were not any burial goods around the skeleton. It is understood that after the body was placed inside the grave, it was simply covered with earth.

Such graves have been in use since the Paleolithic.[6] Parallels exist from both the Chalcolithic[7] and the EBA.[8]

---

4 Carter and Parker 1995.

5 The work on skeletal remains has been conducted by Professor Yılmaz Selim Erdal from the Department of Anthropology at Hacettepe University. I would like to thank him for the information he provided on the age and sex of the skeletons.

6 Nadel 1995; Belfer-Cohen 1995.

7 For Tell el Judeideh, see Braidwood and Braidwood 1960, 135–136; for Tell Kurdu, see Braidwood and Braidwood 1960, 174, pl. 79.E; for Gedikli-Karahöyük, see Alkım 1967a, 5, fig. 2; for Samsat, see Özgüç 2009, 99; for Tell Chagar Bazar, see Mallowan 1936, 17–18.; for Tell Leilan, see Schwartz 1988, 9, fig. 9,11.; for Tell Hammam et-Turkman, see Van Loon 1988, 144, pl. 62a.

8 For Gedikli-Karahöyük, see Alkım 1967b, 464 ; for Oylum Höyük, see Özgen 1993, 467 ; for Titriş Höyük, see Algaze *et al.* 1992, 38; for Gritille, see Ellis 1983, 245; 1984, 119; for Samsat, see Özgüç 1986, 221; 2009, 75, 82,85, fig. 345, 358–360; for Gre Virike, see Ökse 2001, 272; 2006, 4; for Tell el Judeideh, see Braidwood and Braid-

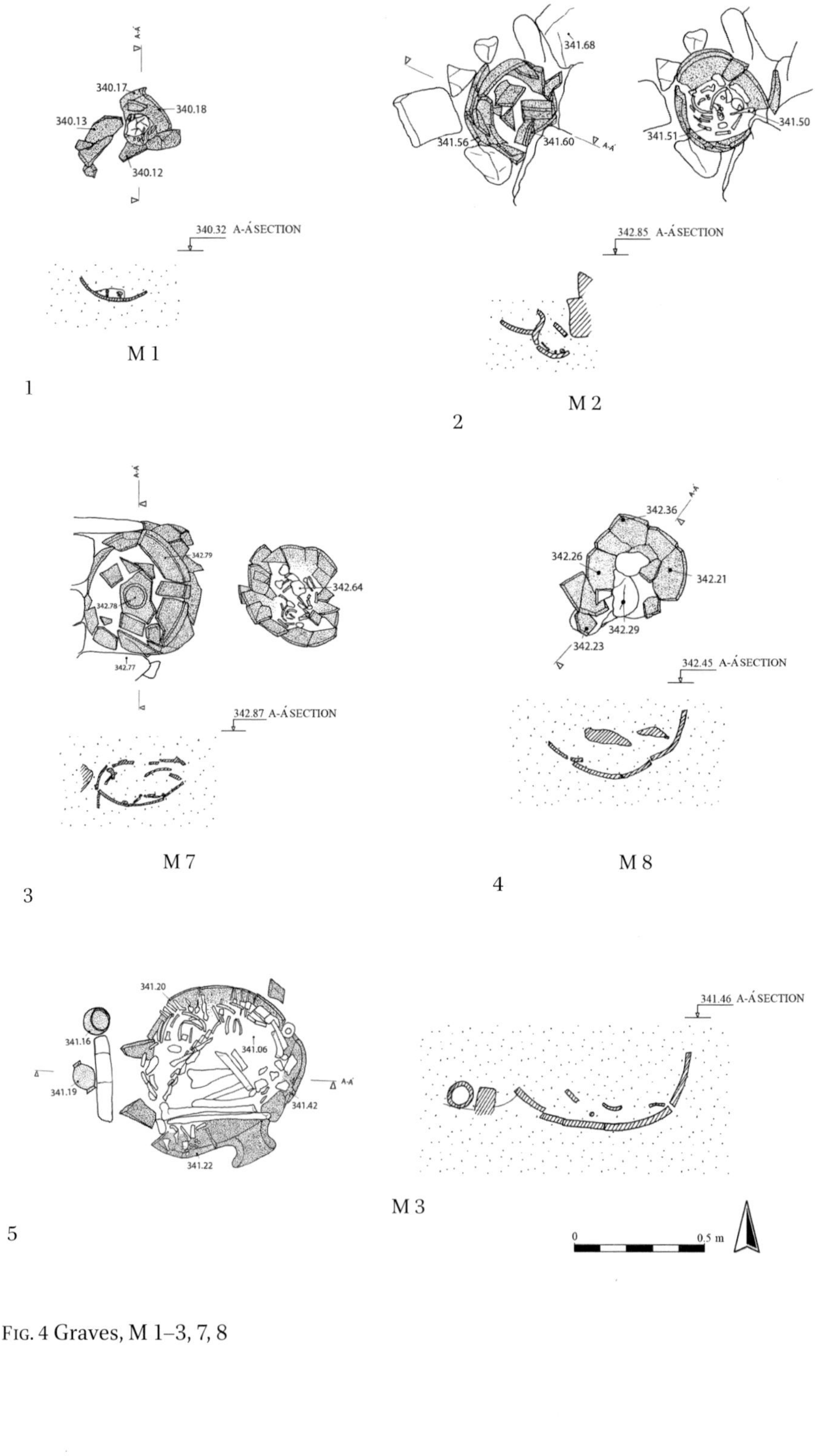

FIG. 4 Graves, M 1–3, 7, 8

Cooking Pot and Pithos Burials

This type of grave, for which the size of the vessel is determined by that of the occupant, are sealed with a stone or another vessel.[9] In Mezraa Höyük, there are seven graves of this type: six cooking pots and one pithos.

Cooking Pot Burials

The most basic example of this type of grave was excavated in trench P 16 where the slope of the höyük meets the level of the plain. This grave (M 1), which belongs to Level VII and is dated to EB I, was preserved by coincidence in an area otherwise disturbed by the intense Medieval occupation.[10] Measuring 31 x 26 cm, M 1 consists of pieces of three different jars and a single bowl (Fig. 4.1, Fig. 5.2). Although the upper part of the grave was damaged, the remains of a newborn laid in the hocker position were found. The biggest pottery fragment that formed the grave was placed at the bottom. The head of the skeleton was placed on the rim fragment with the head facing west. This grave is a basic application of the cooking pot grave type.

Another structure measuring 7.20 x 5.10 m, dated to EB I, was identified in Level VI in trench P 15. One cooking pot grave (M 2) was found at the foundation level of the western wall[11] (Figs. 4.2, Fig. 5.3), probably belonging to an early phase (b) in this particular location. The grave was surrounded by little pieces of stone. The pot was put in place almost vertically with its wide mouth, covered by an upside-down bowl, opening facing northwest. (Fig. 7.3). A newborn had been laid in the hocker position inside, with its head placed near the opening of the pot, facing west. Since the pot was positioned almost vertically, the bones had accumulated at the bottom.

In trench P 15, another structure of Level V with heavily damaged upper layers was exposed. Its foundation walls are so badly damaged that its plan could not be reconstructed. Two pot graves (M 7, M 8) have been discovered under the foundation stones.[12] One of the graves (M 7) is in good condition but the other one was damaged (M 8). The well-preserved grave was detected in the southwest of the structure, 10 cm below the floor (Fig. 6.1). The opening of the grave pot, which was positioned almost vertically, was closed with a bowl (Fig. 7.4), and wet clay was applied during this process. The skeleton of an infant aged 9–12 months

---

wood 1960, 343, 395, figs. 197, 201; for Tell Leilan, see Schwartz 1988, 15, 22–23; for Tell Shiyukh Tahtani, see Sconzo 2007, 274; for Tell Germayir, see Mallowan 1937, 124–126; for Tell Arbit, see Mallowan 1937, 126; for Tell Hammam et-Turkman, see Van Loon 1988, 144–145; for Tell Chagar Bazar, see Mallowan 1936, 18, fig. 4; for Tell Tawi, see Kampschulte and Orthman 1984, 63–74, fig. 13.

9 Carter and Parker 1995, 106–107.

10 Yalçıklı and Tekinalp 2002, 163.

11 Yalçıklı and Tekinalp 2002, 163, fig. 10c.

12 Yalçıklı and Tekinalp 2003, 176; 2004a, 117, fig. 9.3–4.

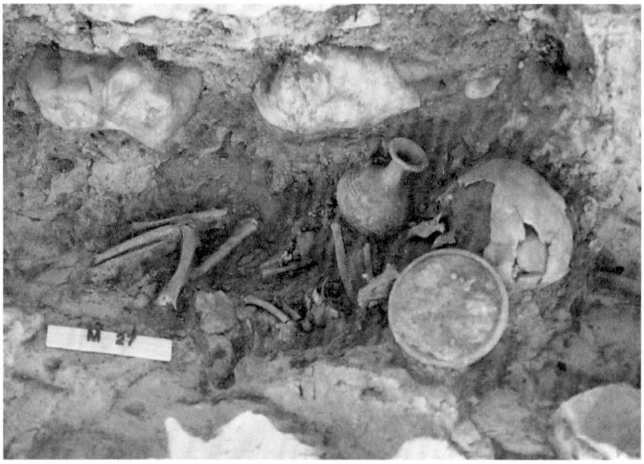

FIG. 5.1 Grave, M 27

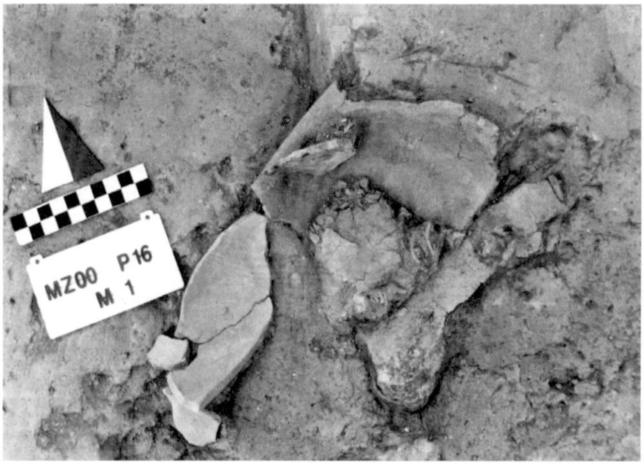

FIG. 5.2 Grave, M 1

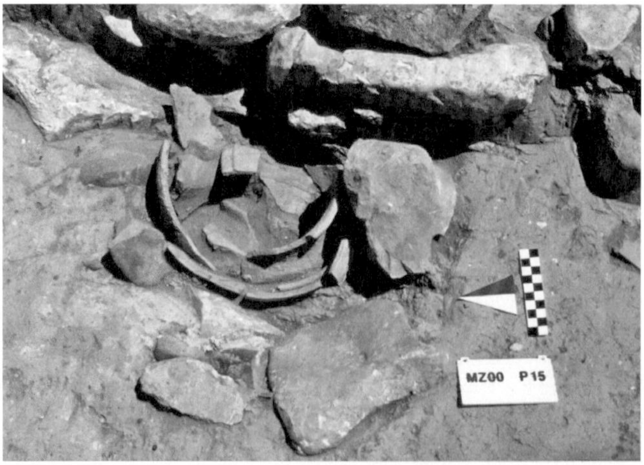

FIG. 5.3 Grave, M 2

was found inside, lying in the hocker position along an east-west axis and facing south. Around its neck was a necklace made from limestone beads.

Along the slope, close to the surface, the lower part of a second pot grave (M 8) associated with the same structure has been preserved (Fig. 4.4). Some skeletal remains could be recovered, but the position or direction of the body could not be determined.

On the east side of the höyük, in trench R13, another part of the Level VIII structure dated to EB III/IV was uncovered. Another cooking pot grave (M 29) under the floor of this structure was encountered (Fig. 6.2).[13] For this grave a glazed cooking pot with a triangular handle at the rim (Fig. 8.1) was used. The mouth of this pot was closed with a base sherd with its broken edges smoothed. We assume that this three-footed base was used to close the jar grave of a child. Also, next to this pot, a rattle made of baked clay was discovered. The skeleton of a newborn was placed inside the pot in the hocker position, lying along the southeast-northwest axis, with its head near the opening of the pot, facing west.

We encounter the earliest examples of this grave type in the Neolithic around the Carchemish region,[14] and now Mezraa Höyük is included in this group as well. Other earlier examples, both from the Chalcolithic[15] as well as from the EBA,[16] are found at numerous sites.

Pithos Burials

A medium-sized pithos grave (M 3), damaged at its southeastern tip, was found at the end of a wall (Fig. 4.5) in trench O 15 on the southeast slope of the höyük.[17]

13 Yalçıklı 2009, 133, fig. 8.

14 Woolley 1914, 88.

15 For Tell el Judeideh, see Braidwood and Braidwood 1960, 258, pl. 79.C; for Gedikli-Karahöyük, see Alkım 1967a, 5; 1968, 408; for Samsat, see Özgüç 1988, 294; 2009, 96, 99, fig. 392–393; for Tepe Gawra, see Tobler 1950, 98–125; Peasnall 2001, 171–234; for Tell Leilan, see Schwartz 1988, 8–9.

16 For Carchemish, see Woolley and Barnett 1952, 215; for Şaraga Höyük, see Sertok and Kulakoğlu 2001, 456; for Gre Virike, see Ökse 2001, 272; 2002, 249, fig. 19; 2006, 11–12, figs. 22, 33; for Tilbeşar, see Kepinski-Lecomte and Ergeç 2001, 134; for Hacınebi, see Stein 1998, 183–184; for Titriş Höyük, see Algaze *et al.* 1992, 38–39; Honca and Algaze 1998, 106–109, fig. 13; for Hassek Höyük, see Behm-Blancke 1984, 53–54; for Horum Höyük, see Tibet *et al.* 1999, 223; for Lidar Höyük, see Hauptmann 1983, 96; for Tell el Judeideh, see Braidwood and Braidwood 1960, 343, fig. 228, 3–4, 11; for Oylum Höyük, see Özgen and Carter 1991, 262; Özgen 1993, 467; Özgen *et al.* 1994, 97–98; for Gedikli-Karahöyük, see Alkım and Alkım 1966, 12; for Tell Hadidi, see Dornemann 1979, 138; for Tell Leilan, see Shwartz 1988, 14; for Tell Jerablus Tahtani, see Peltenburg 1999, 100; for Tell Shiyukh Tahtani, see Falsone and Sconzo 2012, 175–176; for Chagar Bazar, see Mallowan 1936, 17–18.

17 Yalçıklı and Tekinalp 2002, 163.

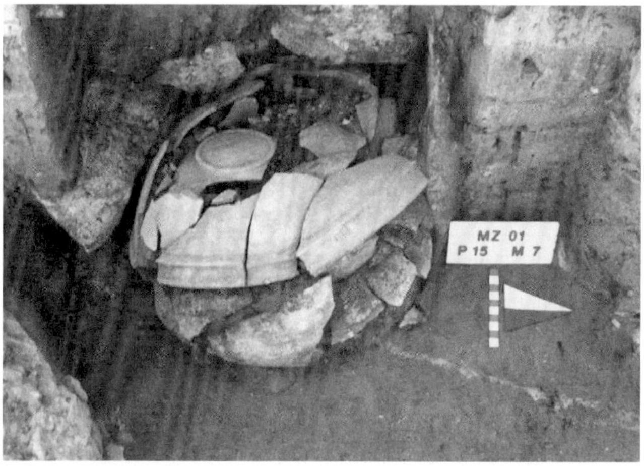

FIG. 6.1 Graves, M 7

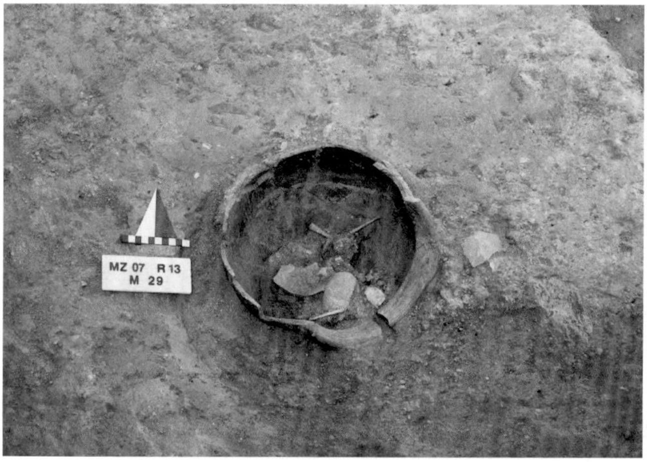

FIG. 6.2 Grave, M 29

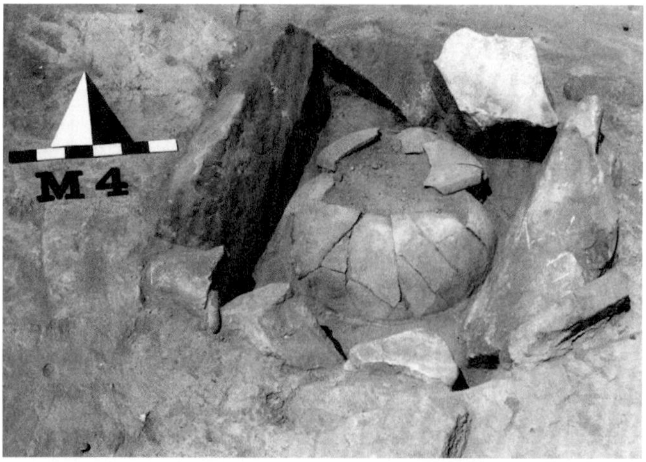

FIG. 6.3 Grave, M 4

The pithos, lying along a southeast-northwest axis, was found collapsed *in situ*, surrounded by stones. It contained the body of a woman aged 35–40, laid in the hocker position with her face towards the southwest. There were a spouted vessel and a bowl on the west side. These finds are dated to EB III/IV. Any possible relation between this grave of an adult and the surrounding structures has not yet been established.

Pithos graves from the surrounding areas are attested as early as the Chalcolithic [18] and continue into the EBA. [19]

Composite (Stone Cist and Cooking Pot) Burials

The term "cist" refers to graves constructed with flat stones arranged to form a rectangular box with no opening. [20] We use the term "composite" for the new kind of grave encountered in Mezraa Höyük, which consists of a stone cist containing a pot burial.

In Mezraa Höyük, the composite burial type is represented with one example (M 4) recovered on the Southeast Slope in trench P 15 (Figs. 3.2, Fig. 6.3). The grave, dated to EB I (Level IV), lies along a northeast-southwest axis and is connected to the walls marking the southeast and southwest edges of a structure. [21] It was placed 10 cm below a floor belonging to the later phases of the structure. Measuring 1.10 x 0.86 m, it was sealed with a flat stone. A cooking pot, covered with a wide-mouth jug and supported by small stones, was found inside the cist, placed along a southwest axis. The jug itself was leaning at a 45 degree angle, with its mouth towards the northeast. The body of possibly a 1-year-old was laid in the hocker position along the northeast-southwest axis with its head near the opening of the vessel. The necklace around its neck consists of onyx and limestone beads (Figs. 7.2, Fig. 7.5).

We see the earliest examples of cist graves from the Chalcolithic Period in this region at Tepe Gawra, [22] while comparanda increase considerably for the EBA. [23]

---

18 For Oylum Höyük, see Özgen 1993, 467–472, figs. 1–2; Özgen and Helwing 2003, 64, fig. 3; for Gedikli-Karahöyük, see Alkım 1967a, 5–6.

19 For Carchemish, see Woolley and Barnet 1952, 215–216; for Gre Virike, see Ökse 2004, 188–189 fig. 24; 2006, 12–13 Figs. 15–17; for Hassek Höyük, see Behm-Blanke 1984, 56 fig. 9; for Titriş Höyük, see Algaze *et al.* 1992, 38–39; Honca and Algaze 1998, 106–109 fig. 14; for Oylum Höyük, see Özgen and Carter 1991, 262; Özgen *et al.* 1994, 97–98; Özgen *et al.* 1997, 59–62 Figs. 14.1–2, 16.1; for Samsat,, see Özgüç 2009, 101; for Jerablus Tahtani, see Peltenburg 1999, 100, for Tell Shiyukh Tahtani, see Falsone and Sconzo 2012, 175–176.

20 Carter and Parker 1995, 106.

21 Yalçıklı and Tekinalp 2003, 175–176; 2004a, 116.

22 Peasnall 2001, 171–234.

23 For Carchemish, see Woolley and Barnett 1952, 218; for Gre Virike, see Ökse 2002, 248; 2006, 7,11, Figs. 11, 31; for Şaraga Höyük, see Sertok and Kulakoğlu 2002,

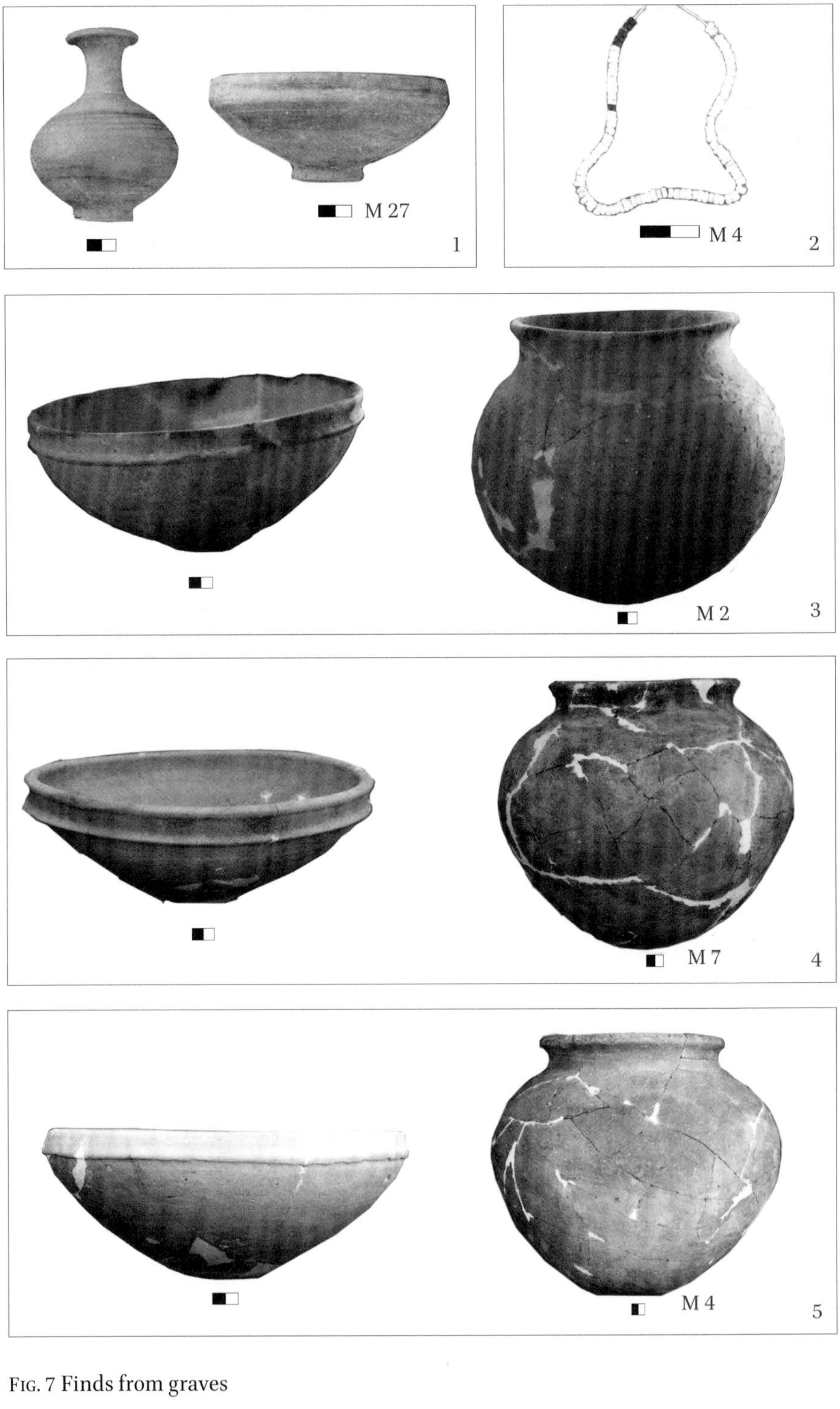

FIG. 7 Finds from graves

Composite graves similar to those found at Mezraa were also recovered at the nearby Birecik Dam Cemetery[24] and Tell Qara Quzak.[25]

Grave Types in the Early Bronze Age

At Mezraa Höyük, graves belonging to EB I make up 62%, whereas those belonging to EB III/IV are at 38% (Fig. 8.2a). Among those graves, the ratio of cooking pot and pithos graves (78%) to pit burials (22%) is significant (Fig. 8.2b). Cooking pot graves alone constitute 56%. Both pithos and composite graves belong to the smallest group, each making up 11%.

Most of the EBA graves in Mezraa Höyük are part of an intramural tradition. A pithos grave (M 3) of EB III/IV belonging to an adult is an exception. This grave is situated on the heavily eroded south side of the höyük where the steep slope prevented settlement until the Medieval period. The excavation area has been expanded here in an attempt to locate a possible extramural cemetery, but no other graves have been recovered so far. When we take the position of intramural graves into consideration, it is understood that preferred locations were near walls, rather than in the centre of rooms. There were no traces of fire observed in or around any of the graves.

Among the graves found in Mezraa Höyük, there are a total of four intact jar graves. Due to the damaged condition of the others, we have only a limited amount of information. One of the four graves is dated to EB III/IV, and the rest are dated to EB I. The graves dated to EB I are covered with a wide jar, and the other one is covered with a tripod base. It is significant that all the jars and pots used in these graves are daily wares used during the early period of the EBA and described as "standard ware."[26] The grave pots for this particular grave are round-bodied, wheel-made with a flaring rim, with exterior surface colors ranging from reddish brown to black. Dimensions of pots in this group vary between 29–36.5 cm in height, 32–41 cm in body diameter, and 20–26.5 cm for rim diameter. One pot from EB III/IV is handmade with a triangle handle (see above), has a black color

356–357, fig. 4; for Tilmen Höyük, see Alkım 1962, 455–456, figs. 28, 30; for Lidar Höyük, see Hauptmann 1984, 227–228; for Titriş Höyük, see Algaze *et al.* 1995, 20, fig. 12; Matney and Algaze 1995, 46; Algaze 1997, 125, fig. 6–7; Honca and Algaze 1998, 104–107, figs. 2–4; for Hacınebi, see Stein 1998, 183–185, fig. 6; for Horum Höyük, see Tibet *et al.* 1999, 223; for Birecik Dam Cemetery, see Sertok and Ergeç 1999, 89, figs. 3, 5; for Til Barsip, see Thureau-Dangin and Dunand 1936, 108–109, pl. XXXII.1–2; for Tell al-Abd, see Bounni 1979, 55; for Tell Tawi, see Kampschulte and Orthmann 1984, 75–80, figs. 18–20.

24 Sertok and Ergeç 1999, 89–90, fig. 6.C, D.

25 Olávarri and Valdés Pereiro 2001, 20, pl. VIII.

26 Orthmann and Rova 1991, 71.

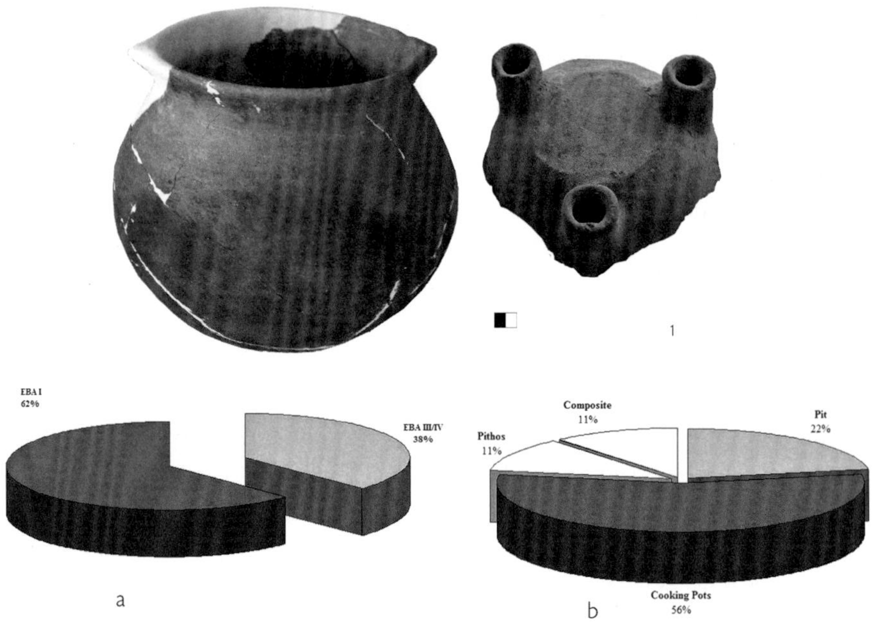

		BOWL		POT		
burial		height (cm)	rim diameter (cm)	height (cm)	body diameter (cm)	rim diameter (cm)
M 2	EBA I-II	12.5	29.5	29.3	32.5	23.5
M 4	EBA I-II	12.1	29.3	36.5	40.8	26.5
M 7	EBA I-II	11.7	32.7	29.2	32.0	20.3
M 29	EBA III-IV	—	—	25.0	24.4	25.0

Fig. 8 Finds from M 29 and distribution.

and is glazed. Its length and body diameter are around 25 cm (Fig. 8.3), which could easily fit a newborn or even a 1 year-old.

It is understood that among the jars that belong to EB I, flat bottomed and thickened rim "standard ware" type jars were used to close the mouths of the grave pots (Fig. 8.3). Our findings indicate that pots with 12 cm depth and bowls with 30 cm rim diameter were preferred to cover grave pots.

Two pit burials we unearthed from the bottom of the structure dated to EB III/IV show us that such graves were part of the intramural burial tradition. Some differences between pit burial styles of a newborn and a 1–2 year-old buried at the same location is noteworthy. The presence of two ceramic pots, a pin placed on the chest, which was used for fastening the wrapping around the body, and the closing of the grave with a stone slab all show us that a little more care was shown for the burial practice for the older child.

In cooking pot graves, the bodies were placed with their heads near the rim of the pot and legs towards the bottom. It is observed that during the decomposition process, the skull and the bones tend to collect at the bottom of the pot. The rim of cooking pot grave M 2 was plastered with mud and its lid shut tightly. This shows us that the pot was originally empty during the burial and was later filled with earth when it was cracked or broken.

We encounter early examples of cooking pot graves in Northern Syria and Southeast Anatolia during the Chalcolithic Period, and cist graves appear from the beginning of the EBA. During the early phases of EB I at Mezraa Höyük, we come across a composite burial type. The most distinct feature separating this kind of grave from cooking pot burials, which are otherwise surrounded by stones, is the enclosing cist formed by vertically placed flat stones and its stone cover. We see that jars and pots used in composite graves have the same form as those used in cooking pot graves. It is observed that a necklace, similar to that left in a cooking pot grave (M 7) as a personal ornament, has also been found in a composite grave as well. We see the most similar application of composite graves at the Birecik Dam Cemetery, 13 km northeast of Mezraa Höyük, and at Tell Qara Quzak, 40 km south of Mezraa Höyük. The composite graves at Birecik Dam Cemetery follow an extramural burial tradition, whereas graves at Mezraa Höyük belong to an intramural tradition.

It has been observed that during the EBA, in a large area across Mesopotamia and Syria, intramural burial traditions were widespread.[27] In this period, different grave types have been observed around the Euphrates region.[28] Various grave types including pits and chamber graves can be observed within this tradition. It is significant that there has been an increase in the number of graves that reflect this kind of tradition, especially in EB III/IV. In Mezraa Höyük, the intramural tradition continues throughout the EBA without any interruption.

27 Orthmann 1980; Peltenburg 1995; Carter and Parker 1996; Laneri 1999.

28 For Titriş Höyük, see Laneri 1999, 229; 2007, 250–259; 2011; for Hassek Höyük, see Behm-Blancke 1984, 53, 54; for Carchemish, see Woolley 1952, 215; for Gedikli-Karahöyük, see Alkım 1967b, 464; for Tell Chagar Bazar, see Mallowan 1936, 18, fig. 4; for Tell Jerablus Tahtani, see Peltenburg 1995, 7–15; for Tell Hadidi, see Dornemann 1979, 117–132.

Conclusion

Mezraa Höyük graves all belong to the individual grave type.[29] With the exception of one grave, all EBA graves found in Mezraa Höyük belong to the tradition of intramural burials for newborns or 1–2 year-olds. Therefore it is assumed that throughout the EBA, adults were buried outside the settlement. Unfortunately, we have not been able to determine a burial area around Mezraa Höyük so far.

All the graves we have dated to EB I are intramural and consist of the cooking pot type. In EB III/IV, the new practice of using pit graves began; cooking pots also continued to be used, but to a lesser extent. Although we could determine a standard size for the cooking vessels used for graves during the EB I, a similar analysis is not possible for EB III/IV due to the small number of graves.

The common feature in all graves is that the dead have been placed in the hocker position. The orientation of the body and the pots are the same throughout, except for the direction the skeletons are facing. Besides two examples, facing north (M 15) and south (M 7), all bodies face west or southwest. This could be identified as a shared aspect for different grave types. In general, no grave goods other than necklaces that some children wore around their necks were recovered. Even though it is not possible to determine the sex of the children, those with necklaces are possibly girls. In graves belonging to EB III/IV, no personal belongings were found other than little bottles, bowls and a rattle. These types of grave goods were left outside pithos and pot graves. The bronze needle found on the chest of a skeleton indicates that the deceased had been wrapped with some cloth or buried with his/her clothes.

It has been observed that grave construction and the burial process for children aged 1–2 years have been carried out with more care and attention compared to the graves for newborns. This significant difference could be a sign of increased emotional sensitivity towards children who have died at a relatively older age. This situation is also visible in one newborn grave in EB I, constructed by gathering various pottery sherds and in another newborn grave, which consists of a single pit situated in the EB III/IV storage room.

Composite graves were in use both for intramural and extramural burial traditions during the early phase of the EBA. It is quite difficult to explain the reason behind this type of common usage. For example, one grave consisting of a stone cist and a large pithos has been found in the cemetery dated to the 2nd millennium at Panaztepe in Western Anatolia.[30] This example shows us that we could come across similar practices in different regions and periods. T. Özgüç

---

29 See Orthmann 1980, 100 for individual *vs.* collective graves in the third millennium BCE.

30 Erkanal 1993, 497–498.

notes the practice of composite graves, during a later period, placing pot graves inside cists in Poland and east Germany, locations rather far from the Euphrates.[31]

The question of how to interpret the widespread usage of composite graves still needs an answer. Does the usage of two different types in a single grave mean some kind of 'togetherness' for different belief groups/communities? Özgüç, taking into consideration the fact that cist and jar graves are found together in many grave sites, stated that this could reflect a common situation that gathers different grave types at one place. However, he does not favor the idea of 'togetherness' of different societies at one place.

Carter and Parker have stated that cist and pithos graves were intensively used during the EBA in Anatolia and in the Euphrates region, and that cist graves might be related to the arrival of Proto-Hurrian communities.[32] Cooper, who has analyzed the distribution of the graves found in the Euphrates region, drew attention to the fact that cist graves have been concentrated around the upper Euphrates, whereas shaft graves concentrate around the central Euphrates region. According to Cooper, when written sources are taken into consideration, we see that there were two different societies active in the region, and that shaft graves in the south may be connected with the Amurru, i.e. Semitic groups.[33] Despite such discussions and theories, there is not yet any consensus on which groups may have been represented by the graves in the region. Since this type of grave has no parallels in the Euphrates region, it may be said that this is a new local type which emerges in the Carchemish region during the early phases of the EBA.

The three different grave types attested in the early and late phases of the EBA in Mezraa Höyük show greater differences within this particular region than among intramural grave types found in other regions. In general, it can be observed that evidence for intramural burial traditions during the early phase of the EBA is scarce but tends to increase for the later phase. On the other hand, Mezraa Höyük, which shows us that the intramural tradition was in use during the 3rd millennium BCE without interruption, has a unique position.

31 T. Özgüç 1948, 38.

32 Carter and Parker 1995, 113.

33 Cooper 2006, 249–250; 2007, 66–68.

REFERENCES

Algaze, G., "Excavations at Titriş Höyük: The 1995 Season." *Kazı Sonuçları Toplantısı* (1997) 28/1: 121–135.

Algaze, G., R. Breuninger and J. Knudstad, "The Tigris-Euphrates Archaeological Reconnaissance Project: Final Report of the Birecik and Carchemish Dam Survey Areas." *Anatolica* 20 (1994): 1–96.

Algaze, G., P. Goldberg, D. Hońça, T. Matney, A. Mısır, A. Miller Rosen, D. Schlee and L. Somers, "Titriş Höyük, A Small EBA Urban Center in Southeastern Anatolia: The 1994 Season." *Anatolica* 21 (1995): 13–63.

Algaze, G., A. Mısır, T. Wilkinson, E. Carter and R. Gorny, "Şanlıurfa Museum / University of California Excavations and Surveys at Titriş Höyük, 1991: A Preliminary Report." *Anatolica* 28 (1992): 33–60.

Alkım, U.B., "Tilmen Höyük Çalışmaları (1958–1960)." *Belleten* XXVI-103 (1962): 447–499.

———. "İslahiye Bölgesi Araştırmaları Gedikli ve Kırışkal Höyük Kazıları (1967)." *Türk Arkeoloji Dergisi* XVI-2 (1967a): 5–13.

———. "İslahiye Bölgesi Araştırmaları ve Gedikli Höyük Kazısı." *Belleten* XXXI-123 (1967b): 462–468.

———. "İslahiye Bölgesi Araştırmaları, Gedikli ve Kırışkal Höyük Kazıları." *Belleten* XXXII-127 (1968): 407–412.

Alkım, U.B. and H. Alkım, "Gedikli (Karahöyük) Kazısı Birinci Ön Rapor." *Belleten* XXX/117 (1996):

Behm-Blancke, M.R., "Hassek Höyük Vorläufiger Bericht über die Ausgrabungen in der Jahren 1981–1983." *Istanbuler Mitteilungen* 34 (1984): 31–65.

Belfer-Cohen, A., "Rethinking Social Stratification in the Natufian Culture: The Evidence from Burials" in *The Archaeology of Death in the Ancient Near East*, ed. by S. Campbell and A. Green, 9–16. Oxford: Oxbow Books, 1995.

Bounni, A., "Preliminary Report on the Archeological Excavations at Tell al-'Abd and 'Anab al-Safinah (Euphrates) 1971–72" in *Archeological Reports from the Tabqa Dam Project-Euphrates Valley, Syria*, ed. by D. N. Freedman, 49–61. Boston: American Schools of Oriental Research, 1979.

Braidwood, R.J. and L.S. Braidwood, *Excavations in the Plain of Antioch I, The Earlier Assemblages Phases A-J.* Chicago: The Oriental Institute of the University of Chicago, 1960.

Carter, E. and A. Parker, "Pots, People and the Archaeology of Death in Northern Syria and Southern Anatolia in the Latter Half of the Third Millennium BC" in *The Archaeology of Death in the Ancient Near East*, ed. by S. Campbell and A. Green, 96–116. Oxford: Oxbow Books, 1995.

Cooper, L., *Early Urbanism on the Syrian Euphrates.* London: Routledge, 2006.

———. "Early Bronze Age Burial Types and Social-Cultural Identity with the Northern Euphrates Valley" in *Euphrates River Valley Settlement. The Carchemish Sector in the Third Millennium BC*, ed. by E. Peltenburg, 55–70. Oxford: Council for British Research in the Levant, 2007.

Dornemann, R.H., "Tell Hadidi: A Millennium of Bronze Age City Occupation" in *Archaeological Reports from the Tabqa Dam Project-Euphrates Valley, Syria*, ed. by D. N. Freedman, 113–151. Cambridge: American Schools of Oriental Research, 1979.

Ellis, R., "Gritille, 1982." *Anatolian Studies* 33 (1983): 244–246.

———. "The Gritille Project." *Kazı Sonuçları Toplantısı* 5 (1984): 117–119.

Erkanal, A., "1991 Panaztepe Kazısı Sonuçları." *Kazı Sonuçları Toplantısı* 14/1 (1993): 495–502.

Falsone, G. and P. Sconzo, "Tell Shiyukh Tahtani, Syria: Report of the 2006–09 Seasons" in *Proceedings of the 7th International Congress of Archeology of the Ancient Near East (7ICAANE)*, ed. by R. Matthews, 167–190. Wiesbaden: Harrasowitz, 2012.

Hauptmann, H., "Lidar Höyük 1981." *Türk Arkeoloji Dergisi* 26/2 (1983): 93–110.

———. "Lidar Höyük 1983." *Anatolian Studies* 34 (1984): 226–228.

Honca, M.D. and G. Algaze, "Preliminary Report on the Human Skeletal Remains at Titris Höyük: 1991–1996 Seasons." *Anatolica* 24 (1998): 101–141.

Kampschulte, I., W. Orthmann. *Gräber des 3. Jahrtausends v. Chr. im Syrischen Euphrattal, 1. Ausgrabungen bei Tawi 1975 und 1978.* Bonn: Habelt, 1984.

Kepinski-Lecomte, C. and R. Ergeç, "Researches III Tilbeshar." *Kazı Sonuçları Toplantısı* 22/1 (2001): 133–136.

Laneri, N., "Intramural Tombs: A Funerary Tradition of the Middle Euphrates Valley During the IIIrd Millennium BC." *Anatolica* 25 (1999): 221–236.

———. "Burial Practices at Titriş Höyük, Turkey: An Interpretation." *Journal of Near Eastern Studies* 66/4 (2007): 241–266.

———. "A Family Affair: The Use of Intramural Funerary Chambers in Mesopotamia During the Late Third and Early Second Millennia BCE." *Archeological Papers of The American Anthropological Association* 20/1 (2011): 121–135.

Mallowan, M.E.L., "The Excavations at Tall Chagar Bazar and an Archaeological Survey of the Habur Region, 1934–5." *Iraq* 3 (1936): 1–85.

———. "The Excavations at Tall Chagar Bazar and an Archaeological Survey of the Habur Region. Second Campaign, 1936." *Iraq* 4 (1937): 91–177.

Matney, T. and G. Algaze, "Urban Development at Mid-Late Early Bronze Age Titris Höyük in Southeastern Anatolia." *Bulletin of the American Schools of Oriental Research* 299/300 (1995): 33–52.

Nadel, D., "The Visibility of Prehistoric Burials in the Southern Levant: How Rare are the Upper Palaeolithic / Early Epipalaeolithic Graves?" in *The Archaeology of Death in the Ancient Near East*, ed. by S. Campbell and A. Green, 1–8. Oxford: Oxbow Books, 1995.

Ökse, A.T., "Gre Virike 1999 Kazısı / Excavations at Gre Virike, 1999" in *Salvage Project of the Archaeological Heritage of the Ilısu and Carchemish Dam Reservoirs, Activities in 1999*, ed. by N. Tuna, J. Öztürk and J. Velibeyoğlu, 263–307. Ankara: Middle East Technical University, 2001.

———. "Gre Virike 2000 Kazısı / Excavations at Gre Virike in 2000" in *Salvage Project of the Archaeological Heritage of the Ilısu and Carchemish Dam Reservoirs, Activities in 2000*, ed. by N. Tuna and J. Velibeyoğlu, 241–285. Ankara: Middle East Technical University, 2002.

———. "Gre Virike 2001 Kazısı / 2001 Excavations at Gre Virike" in *Salvage Project of the Archaeological Heritage of the Ilısu and Carchemish Dam Reservoirs, Activities in 2001*, ed. by N. Tuna, J. Greenhalgh, and J. Velibeyoglu, 179–226. Ankara: Middle East Technical University, 2004.

———. "Early Bronze Age Graves at Gre Virike (Period II B): An Extraordinary Cemetery on the Middle Euphrates." *The Journal of Near Eastern Studies* 65/1 (2006): 1–37.

Olávarri, E. and C. Valdés Pereiro, "Excavaciones en Tell Qara Quzaq: Campañas IV-VI (1992–1994)" in *Tell Qara Quzaq II. Campañas IV-VI (1992–1994)*, ed. by G. Del Olmo Lete, J.-L. Montero Fenollós and C. Valdés Pereiro, 13–76. Barcelona, 2001.

Orthmann, W., "Burial Customs of the 3rd Millennium BC in the Euphrates Valley" in *Le Moyen Euphrate: Zone de contacts et d'échanges*, ed. by J. C. Margueron, 97–105. Leiden: Brill, 1980.

Orthmann, W. and E. Rova, *Gräber des 3. Jt. v. Chr. im syrischen Euphrattal. 2. Ausgrabungen in Wreide*. Saarbrücken: Harrassowitz, 1991.

Özgen E., "An Early Bronze Age Burial at Oylum Höyük Near Kilis" in *Studies in Honor of Nimet* Özgüç. *Aspects of Art and Iconography. Anatolia and its Neighbors*, ed. by M. J. Mellink, E. Porada, T. Özgüç, 467–472. Ankara: Türk Tarih Kurumu, 1993.

Özgen, E. and E. Carter, "Oylum Höyük, 1989." *Kazı Sonuçları Toplantısı* 12/1 (1991): 259–268.

Özgen, E., B. Helwing, "On the Shifting Borders Between Mesopotamia and the West: Seven Seasons of Joint Turkish-German Excavations at Oylum Höyük." *Anatolica* 29 (2003): 61–85.

Özgen, E., B. Helwing, B. and H. Tekin, "Vorläufiger Bericht über die Ausgrabungen auf dem Oylum Höyük." *Istanbuler Mitteilungen* 47 (1997): 39–90.

Özgen, E., H. Tekin and H.K. Ensert, "Oylum Höyük 1991 ve 1993 Kazı Çalışmaları." *Kazı Sonuçları Toplantısı* 16/1 (1994): 95–107.

Özgüç, N., "Samsat 1984 Yılı Kazıları." *Kazı Sonuçları Toplantısı* 7 (1986): 221–227.

———. "Samsat Kazıları 1987." *Belleten* LII/202 (1988): 291–294.

———. *Samsat Sümeysat, Samosata Kumaha, Hahha, Hahhum: Bir Başkent ve Kalenin Uzun Yaşamının 6000 Yıllık Döneminden Kesitler.* Ankara: Türk Tarih Kurumu, 2009.

Özgüç, T., *Ön Tarih'te Anadolu'da Ölü Gömme Âdetleri.* Ankara: Türk Tarih Kurumu, 1948.

Peasnall, B.L., "Appendix: Burials from Tepe Gawra, Levels VIII to XIA/B" in *Tepe Gawra: The Evolution of a Small, Prehistoric Center in Northern Iraq*, ed. by M. S. Rothman,

171–234. Philadelphia: University of Pennsylvania Museum of Archaeology and Anthropology, 2001.

Peltenburg, E.J., "Tell Jerablus Tahtani 1992–1996: A Summary" in *Archaeology of the Upper Syrian Euphrates. The Tishrin Dam Area*, ed. by G. del Olmo Lete and J. L. Monlero Fenollós, 97–105. Barcelona, 1999.

Peltenburg, E.J., S. Campbell, P. Croft, D. Lunt, M. Murray and M. Watt, "Jerablus-Tahtani, Syria, 1992–4: Preliminary Report." *Levant* 27 (1995): 1–28.

Schwartz, G. M., *A Ceramic Chronology from Tell Leilan. Operation I.* New Haven: Yale University Press, 1988.

Sconzo, P., "Collapse or Continuity? The Case of the EB-MB Transition at Tell Shiyukh Tahtani" in *Société humaines et changment climatique á la fin du troisième millénaire: une crise a-t-elle eu lieu en haute Mésopotamie?*, ed. by C. Marro and C. Kuzucuoğlu, 267–309. Paris: De Boccard, 2007.

Sertok, K. and R. Ergeç, "A New Early Bronze Age Cemetery. Excavations Near the Birecik Dam, SE Turkey. Preliminary Report (1997–98)." *Anatolica* 25 (1999): 87–107.

Sertok, K. and F. Kulakoğlu, "Şaraga Höyük 1999 Yılı Kazısı Sonuçları / Results of the 1999 Season Excavations at Şaraga Höyük" in *Salvage Project of the Archaeological Heritage of the Ilısu and Carchemish Dam Reservoirs, Activities in 1999*, ed. by N. Tuna, J. Öztürk and J. Velibeyoğlu, 453–486. Ankara: Middle East Technical University, 2001.

———. "Şaraga Höyük 2000" in *Salvage Project of the Archaeological Heritage of the Ilısu and Carchemish Dam Reservoirs, Activities in 2000*, ed. by N. Tuna and J. Velibeyoğlu, 351–381. Ankara: Middle East Technical University, 2002.

Stein, G.J., "1996 Excavations at Hacınebi Tepe." *Kazı Sonuçları Toplantısı* 19/1 (1998): 179–207.

Thureau-Dangin, F. and M. Dunand. *Til-Barsib,* Paris, 1936.

Tibet, A., C. Marro and R. Ergeç, "Horum Höyük: 1997 Çalışmaları." *Kazı Sonuçları Toplantısı* 20/1 (1999): 219–240.

Tobler, A.J., *Excavations at Tepe Gawra II. Levels IX-XX.* Philadelphia: American Schools of Oriental Research, 1950.

Van Loon, M.N., *Hammam et-Turkman I, Report on the University of Amsterdam's 1981–84 Excavations in Syria I, II.* Istanbul, 1988.

Woolley, C.L., "Hittite Burial Customs." *Liverpool AAA* 6 (1914): 87–98.

Woolley, C.L. and R. D. Barnett, *Carchemish, Part III: The Excavations in the Inner Town and the Hittite Inscriptions, Report on the Excavations at Jerablus on Behalf of the British Museum.* London: British Museum Press, 1952.

Yalçıklı, D., "Mezraa Höyük 2007 Yılı Kazısı." *Kazı Sonuçları Toplantısı* 30/2 (2009): 129–134.

Yalçıklı, D. and M. Tekinalp, "Mezraa Höyük 2000 Yılı Kazıları / Mezraa Höyük Excavations 2000" in *Salvage Project of the Archaeological Heritage of the Ilısu and*

Carchemish Dam Reservoirs, Activities in 2000, ed. by N. Tuna and J. Velibeyoğlu, 159–210 Ankara: Middle East Technical University, 2002.

———. "Mezraa Höyük 2000–2001 Yılı Kurtarma Kazıları." *Kazı Sonuçları Toplantısı* 24/1 (2003): 171–178.

———. "Mezraa Höyük 2001 Yılı Kazıları / Mezraa Höyük Excavations 2001" in *Salvage Project of the Archaeological Heritage of the Ilısu and Carchemish Dam Reservoirs, Activities in* 2001, ed. by N. Tuna, J. Greenhalgh, and J. Velibeyoğlu, 107–160. Ankara: Middle East Technical University, 2004a.

———. "Mezraa Höyük 2002 Yılı Kurtarma Kazıları." *Kazı Sonuçları Toplantısı* 25/1 (2004b): 377–386.

———. "Mezraa Höyük 2002 Yılı Kazıları / The 2002 Excavations Season at Mezraa Höyük" in *Salvage Project of the Archaeological Heritage of the Ilısu and Carchemish Dam Reservoirs, Activities in 2002* (Vol. 1), ed. by N. Tuna and O. Donan, 119–155. Ankara: Middle East Technical University, 2011.

Anyone Out There?
Looking for Life in Early 3rd Millennium Central Anatolia

Thomas Zimmermann [1]

For Marie-Henriette and Charles—örnek hoca, örnek dost, örnek insanlar.

Abstract

The Central Anatolian plateau was, and still is, a key region to understanding the economical, social and ideological dynamics of the EBA in Western Asia at large. Reference sites like Alaca Höyük, Eskiyapar and Horoztepe yielded a stunning array of precious objects testifying to the emergence of elites who were controlling and benefitting from crucial resources along the interregional trade routes. And it is exactly these sites which are playing the lead in a still unsolved riddle: the rich and versatile archaeological evidence of the third millennium's second half is contrasted by the literally pitch black earlier 500 years. The architecture and material culture of the excavated EBA sites, mainly clustered around modern Ankara and Çorum, are indeed all conventionally dated to the second half of, if not the late, third millennium BC. This chronological assessment, leaving the first half-millennium in Central Anatolia awkwardly devoid of human activity, stands further in gross disarray with recent chronological revisions of the neighboring Black Sea littoral and its hinterland. This contribution aims to reassess the current chronological dilemma in the light of new scientific data from the "Hatti heartland" and its neighboring regions.

---

1 Department of Archaeology, Bilkent University, 06800 Ankara, Turkey.
I am indebted to Julian Bennett for proofreading the manuscript; any shortcomings and Bavarianisms are solely the author's responsibility.

> [T]he greater part of modern Turkey, and especially the region more correctly described as Anatolia, shows no sign whatever of habitation during the Neolithic period.[2]

Thus wrote Seton Lloyd in 1956, the eminent archaeologist and long term director of the British Institute of Archaeology at Ankara, giving his impression of a barren, lifeless pre-Bronze Age Anatolian landscape, only to be debunked a few years later by the discovery of Neolithic Çatal Höyük. However, this vast, seemingly hostile region with its harsh, cold winters,[3] especially the northern Central Anatolian part, indeed remained a wallflower of the research agenda for many generations of fieldworkers—the iconic Hattusha and Alişar excavations may count as the proverbial exceptions to the rule. That said, prehistoric archaeology in this very region experienced an unprecedented boom in research activity in the 1930s and 1940s,[4] coinciding with the intellectual dynamics of the evolving young Turkish republic: sites like Etiyokuşu, Ahlatlıbel, Koçumbeli and certainly Alaca Höyük were not mere attempts to reveal the still rather fragmentarily known (Early) Bronze Age heritage of Central Anatolia proper; they were considered political benchmarks for the 'Anatolist' approach to a reawakened national identity debate—with Turkish roots to be sought in the indigeneous Hattian and Hittite cultures of the Anatolian heartland, as opposed to the smoldering debris of long-gone Ottoman splendour.[5] Here, the "royal" graves of Alaca Höyük, excavated by the first generation of "modern" Turkish archaeologists, yielded a breathtaking variety of masterfully accomplished metal objects. Some of the abstract and zoomorphic ceremonial standards associated with the burials made a swift career as Turco-Hattian and (too) often mistakenly labeled "Hittite" icons—on chocolate bars of a major Turkish sweets producer—and also as the long-term municipal symbol of modern Ankara,[6] until it fell victim to revisionist policies.

So far, so good. After decades of intensive surveying and extensive excavations, one would think the chronological framework for Central Anatolia in the third millennium BC should be safe and sound. One could not be further off the mark. An EB I period seems to be nonexistent in the western and northeastern Kızılırmak catchment area for too many EBA sites, and, rather surprisingly, not many seem discomfited by this. To begin with, a critical revision of the data so far

2 Lloyd 1956, 53.

3 Lloyd 1956, 3.

4 Özdoğan 1998, 116–119.

5 Özdoğan 1998; Erimtan 2008.

6 Zimmermann 2008a, 509–511.

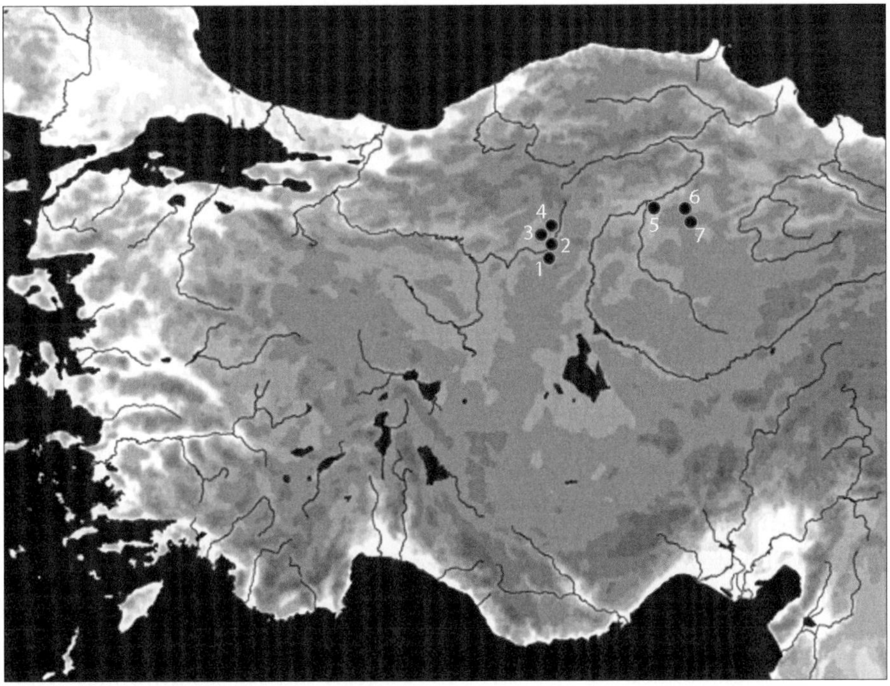

FIG. 1 Map showing important findspots mentioned in the text: 1) Ahlatlıbel 2) Koçumbeli 3) Etiyokuşu 4) Karaoğlan 5) Resuloğlu 6) Kalınkaya 7) Alaca Höyük.

accumulated might help approach the issue more thoroughly (FIG. 1). Admittedly, the much intensified archaeological activities in the wake of the Turkish Republic's foundation, especially in the vicinity of Ankara and Çorum, highlighted the previously entirely obscure material record of pre-Hittite times.

However, the subsequent publications of these key sites are largely too simple, fragmentary and even partly contradictory to be of any substantive value as a means to better understand the cultural dynamics of the EBA in Central Anatolia. So, for Ankara and its environs, the by far best presented site is Etiyokuşu, published comprehensively by Şevket Kansu in 1940.[7] Up to three occupation layers (I-III in area A, two layers in area B and only one horizon in area C)[8] could be distinguished, all with rather dispersed, unfortunately badly preserved, architecture. Two major building types transpired, basically rectangular structures and round installations, the latter presumably used for storage and disposal.[9] The finds and features of Ahlatlıbel, which

7 Kansu 1940.

8 Schachner 1999, 135.

9 Kansu 1940; Schachner 1999, 135, fig. 68.

presumably can be attributed only to one large building complex or "manor" belonging to a local ruler,[10] were never fully published; the site presumably incorporates several layers (at least one "older" stratum), however their exact number remains obscure. The situation for neighboring Koçumbeli is by no means better: only a small fraction of the (probably) completely excavated settlement was ever published, and only a rather sketchy, confusing cut-out of the already limited domestic building remains was made accessible in print.[11] Even worse, the proclaimed overall number of detected layers hovers between two and four. According to the original publication, the material culture from Karaoğlan, at least, is attested to represent only the EB II. Remzi Oğuz Arık's expedition from 1937 to 1948 further revealed some rather sketchy and inconclusive, presumably agglutinating, architecture.[12] A building with massive foundations and one round structure stand out against remaining architecture, however the ceramic inventories are much too similar in all cases to allow for a functional, let alone chronological distinction.[13]

Travelling further to the west, another old, single-season expedition, that at Polatlı in 1949, is the only other endeavour that has revealed Early Bronze Age occupation levels in this region on anything approaching a substantial scale. The short campaign conducted there in 1949 by Seton Lloyd and Nuri Gökçe—the results of which were promptly published in 1951[14]—identified more than 30 (!) separate occupation layers, grouped by the excavators into four major phases, representing the "Copper Age"[15] (levels I–X and XI–XV); a period encompassing the early second millennium BC (levels XVI–XXII); and finally the "true" Hittite period (levels XXIII–XXXI), evidently referring to the era from the 17th century BC onwards.[16] However, the excavator's correlation with assemblages not only from neighboring sites like Ahlatlıbel and Etiyokuşu, but also with those of remote centres like Alişar, Troy and Tarsus, would push finds and features of the lower so-called "Copper Age" levels towards the final quarter of the third millennium BC.

Traversing the Central Anatolian landscape northeast towards Alaca Höyük, a site weighty with meaning ever since its initial excavation, the situation hardly

10 Bittel 1936/37; Schachner 1999, 98.

11 Tezcan 1966; Schachner 1999, 151–152.

12 Arık 1948; Schachner 1999, 151.

13 Schachner 1999, 151.

14 Lloyd and Gökçe 1951.

15 The "Copper Age" mentioned here (and repeatedly in may other contemporary articles) actually refers to phenomena one would nowadays define as belonging to the third millennium BC, hence EBA (but not necessarily EB I) contexts. The term is owed to the contemporary (and now profoundly revised) understanding of sociocultural and technological developments in later prehistory.

16 Lloyd and Gökçe 1951, 23–24.

changes. The magnificent burial assemblages there, published originally in a series of monographs,[17] overshadow the scarce domestic remains from the Early Bronze Age.[18] The latter, despite all efforts, do not allow for any conclusive reconstruction of complete building units—apart from a few roughly rectangular compartments. That said, although the EBA at Alaca Höyük extends over four layers (8–5 in the domestic settlement sequence), only the strata of the late and final EBA (layers 6 and 5) were ever published.[19] Needless to say that this scholarly negligence further distorted and cemented the idea of a Central Anatolian Early Bronze Age restricted to the second half of the third millennium.

The aforementioned burials, however, were taken—after having been inconclusively linked to Eurasian traditions[20]—as a typical example for Hattian culture in the later third millennium BC by generations of archaeologists. The famous abstract and zoomorphic "standards" were especially subject to a quite colourful debate regarding their technology, meaning, and needless to say, their value as chronological markers.[21] The complex stratigraphic situation of the burials, however, was subject to discussion until rather recently[22]— the outcome, not surprisingly, once again favours a traditional chronological positioning in the advanced or late third millennium BC.[23] In fact, a cross-regional scrutiny of the associated metal artifacts shows that from both a typological and technological point of view, the luxurious assemblages have very little, if anything, in common with contemporary casting traditions known from either the northwest (the (in)famous Troy treasures),[24] or the Mesopotamian southeast (Ur III objects from the royal burials), with probably the exception of a few selected jewelry items.[25] That said, the few "Mesopotamianizing"

17 Arık 1937; Koşay 1938; Koşay 1951.

18 An unpublished Ph.D. Thesis (Gürsan-Salzmann 1996) attempted to reappraise the domestic structures of the EBA occupation; unfortunately the major questions concerning spatial organization and reconstructable dwelling patterns remain unsolved.

19 *Cf.* Schachner 1999, 98–99.

20 This was above all attempted by W. Orthmann (1967) and G. Mansfeld (2001) with different examples from Caucasian and Eurasian contexts, but using a similar line of reasoning. This approach was eventually debunked due to chronological incompatibility (Zimmermann 2008a; Düring 2011, 293–294); however, recent developments might necessitate reappraisal (*cf. infra*).

21 *Cf.* Gonnet-Bağana 1967; Börker-Klähn and Krafzik 1986; Korfmann 1986; Baltacıoğlu 2006; Zimmermann 2008a with bibliography.

22 *Cf.* Özyar 1999; Gerber 2006.

23 For a synoptic account see Zimmermann 2008a, 511–512; Düring 2011, 290–294; Steadman 2011, 246–247; *cf.* Bachhuber 2011 for a considerably earlier dating of the burials.

24 *Cf.* Tolstikov and Treijster 1996, 231–236.

25 *Cf.* Maxwell-Hyslop 1971, 44–45.

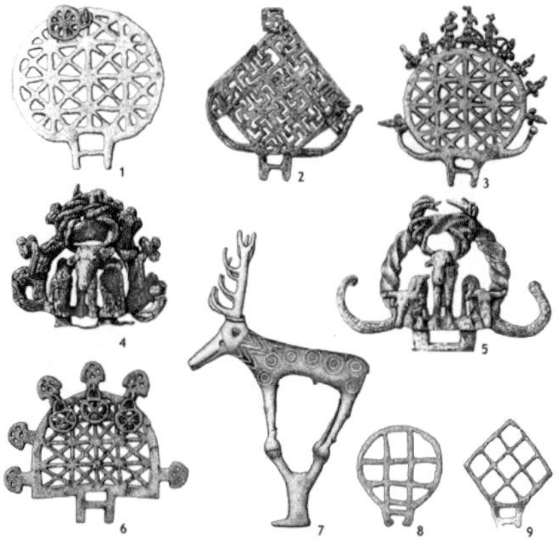

FIG. 2 Ceremonial standards from Alaca Höyük burials (after Müller-Karpe 1974, not to scale)

casting resemblances once again seem to be tempting enough to chronologically moor the burials in the later quarters of the third millennium BC.[26]

This is, roughly drawn, the picture we have today: a Central Anatolian landscape, vibrant in the second half of the third millennium BC, a focus on technological innovations and emerging elites—but virtually void and deserted from 3000 to 2500 BC. Can this be true? One recent article has already tried to challenge the traditional late dating of Central Anatolian EBA pottery assemblages,[27] focusing specifically on the debated assemblages from the vicinity of Ankara (*cf. supra*) to drag their chronology down into the first half of the third millennium. However, a stylistic comparison with material from such a remote site as Demircihöyük on the Eskişehir plain, which might have undergone adaptations and transformations at a different pace from the EBA sites of Central Anatolia proper, has to remain a working hypothesis as long as no reliable scientific database is established to finally come to terms with a still highly vulnerable chronology.

Hope for fresh, much needed scientific dates to eventually correct this impression now rests on the excavation of the Bronze Age levels of Resuloğlu (Sungurlu, Uğurludağ), about 90 km to the west of Alaca Höyük, which could yield the backbone for the trustworthy regional radiocarbon chronology which is so desperately needed. The ceramic material thus far processed and published from the cemetery and the very recently excavated EBA strata from the nearby mounds render, especially with their diagnostic dark-faced, grooved wares, the impression of an occupation starting no earlier than EB II and extending into the early decades of the second millennium BC.[28]

26 Tolstikov and Treijster 1996, 230; Treister [sic!] 2002.

27 Bertram 2008.

28 Yıldırım 2006; 2011.

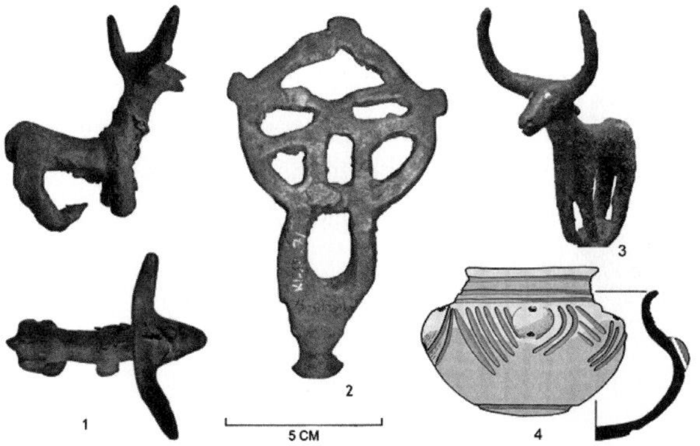

Fɪɢ. 3 Ceremonial items and a grooved "EBA III" cup from Kalınkaya-Toptaştepe. 3–4: not to scale (drawings and photographs by Ben Claasz Coockson).

To this we can add the small settlement and cemetery of Kalınkaya-Toptaştepe, a literal stone's throw from Alaca Höyük, and another small piece of the jigsaw to help fill in the still sketchy picture of Early Bronze Age rural settlements. Partly excavated in two short campaigns in 1971 and 1973 and recently reappraised by the author, the partially disturbed Early Bronze Age cemetery here yielded versatile, if rather equivocal metal assemblages for a fine-tuned chronology including miniature versions of Alaca-type bull statuettes (Fɪɢ. 3.1, Fɪɢ. 3.3) and a coarse, probably unfinished ceremonial standard (Fɪɢ. 3.2) that once again would, conservatively speaking, rather testify to a date at the very end of the third millennium BC[29] (an observation supported by the associated typical dark-faced pottery with grooved decoration (Fɪɢ. 3.4).

The pottery from the test trench on the mound itself (which is currently under analysis and reevaluation) likewise has a EB II-III appearance, albeit with some notable exceptions: bowls or "fruitstands" with conical pedestals and thin-walled S-profiled vessels with incised sawtooth motifs retain a Late Chalcolithic, late fourth millennium heritage (Fɪɢ. 4.1, Fɪɢ. 4.3), while a conical jug with "whirling" grooves (Fɪɢ. 4.2) definitely does not fit in the known typological setup of a "late" Early Bronze Age.[30] Unfortunately, the preserved documentation and excavation diaries do not allow for a more precise statement on the stratigraphic and, ultimately, the chronological embedding of the domestic Kalınkaya material.

Enter the new radiocarbon dates for some Alaca Höyük burials: metal ferrules from burials A and S, although excavated in the 1930s, still contained a sufficient amount of wood to be C14-dated with admittedly surprising—or even perhaps

29 Zimmermann 2007a, 16–22.

30 See Schoop 2005, 38–43, pl. 5,11; 6,1.3 for parallels.

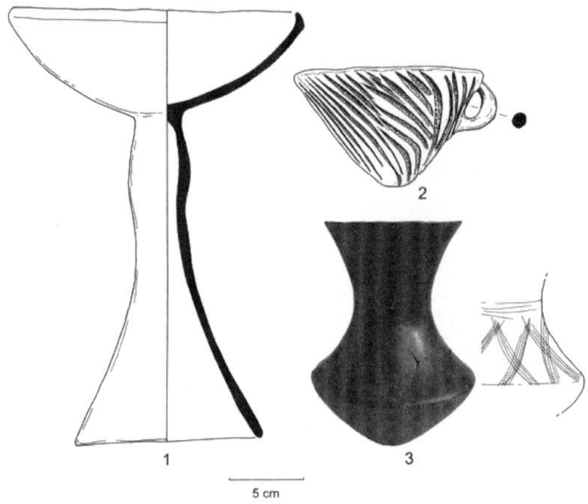

FIG. 4 Presumably Chalcolithic/ EB I (?) pottery from Kalınkaya-Toptaştepe (drawings and photograph: Ben Claasz Coockson)

comforting[31]—preliminary results. Two calibrated dates range within the 2500 BC cal. zone, a third, rather high date pushes at least burial S back to a stunning 2850 BC cal.[32] To be sure, the dates currently available are too few in number and not immune to the objection that anything stored in a dusty museum storeroom for more than 70 years could not be declared definitively free from any contaminating effects. If accepted however, the resulting chronological, but above all methodological, landslide would be substantial indeed and would bury anything Early Bronze Age academia has become fond of –be it itinerant metal-smiths trained in Mesopotamia or the overall mechanisms in the emergence of elites in the second half of the third millennium BC.[33]

Admittedly, it is too early to rewrite the Central Anatolian Early Bronze Age chronology from scratch, but let us briefly reconsider a few possible phenomena to explain the 'early third millennium void.' Either layers corresponding to the early third millennium BC have not yet been located at any site; or, the chronological range of layers containing diagnostic material was miscalculated or not sufficiently associated with strata from neighboring regions; or, the current traditional dating of key features like the Alaca Höyük burials is utterly wrong; or, recalling Seton Lloyd's account of the Neolithic, no human communities set foot on Central Anatolian turf for about 500 years for one reason or another. Since the first and last possibilities seem overburdened by too many presuppositions which demand awkward models for explanation, the remaining ones—*lex parsimoniae* in action!—need to be considered.

31 Yalçın 2011.

32 Yalçın 2011, 64.

33 For a critical review see also Zimmermann 2009.

The recent dramatic, however indispensable, re-dating of the İkiztepe cemetery on the Black Sea coast from the late third into the mid-late fourth millennium BC is an instructive example on how self-deluding frameworks largely based on typo-chronological vicious circles have to inevitably succumb to secure data, once secure data becomes available.[34] Typological and archaeometric observations on metal assemblages retrieved from the border zone between Northern Anatolia and the Black Sea littoral suggest a much more southerly extent of Pontic casting traditions, as attested at İkiztepe—and eventually a much earlier date than the currently advocated late third millennium paradigm.[35] The Anatolian highlands have still to be peopled for the early third millennium. The number of inhabitants dwelling in the currently absent EBA I might steadily increase, in sync with new scientific datasets, and an undogmatic view towards safer and more sound typological paradigms.

34 Welton 2010, esp. 530–550. The official, late date of the İkiztepe burials and selected objects from the domestic layers was challenged several times in the past (Parzinger 1993, 236–238; Thissen 1993; Schoop 2005, 315–322; Lichter 2006; Zimmermann 2007b; 2008b). However, with the these utterly important results, first presented at a workshop on "Western Anatolia before Troy," 22–24 November 2012 in Vienna, Austria, the refutation of a late third millennium dating now has a much more solid scientific foundation to rest on.

35 İpek and Zimmermann 2007; Zimmermann and İpek 2010.

REFERENCES

Arık R.O., *Alaca Höyük Hafriyatı. 1935'deki Çalışmalara ve Keşiflere Ait İlk Rapor.* Ankara: Türk Tarih Kurumu, 1937.

———. "Karaoğlan Höyüğü Bakır Çağı Mimarlığından Özellikler." *III. Türk Tarih Kongresi* (1948): 47–59.

Bachhuber, C., "Negotiating Metal and the Metal Form in the Royal Tombs of Alaca Höyük in North-Central Anatolia" in *Interweawing Worlds. Systemic Interactions in Eurasia, 7th to 1st Millennia BC*, ed. by T. C. Wilkinson, S. Sherratt and J. Bennet, 158–174. Oxford: Oxbow Books, 2011.

Baltacıoğlu, H., "Güneş Kursları, Alaca Höyük ve Arinna" in *Cultural Reflections, Studies in Honour of Hayat Erkanal*, ed. by A. Erkanal-Öktü *et al.*, 129–137. İstanbul: Homer Yayınevi, 2006.

Bertram, J., "Ahlatlıbel, Etiyokuşu, Koçumbeli—Zur Neubewertung der Ankara-Gruppe." *TÜBA-AR* 11 (2008), 73–84.

Bittel, K., "Beiträge zur kleinasiatischen Archäologie. Die prähistorische Siedlung bei Ahlatlıbel." *Archiv für Orientforschung* 11 (1936/37), 38–47.

Börker-Klähn J. and U. Krafzik, "Zur Bedeutung der Aufsätze aus Alaca Höyük." *Die Welt des Orients* 17 (1986), 47–60.

Düring, B.S., *The Prehistory of Asia Minor. From Complex Hunter-Gatherers to Early Urban Societies.* Cambridge: Cambridge University Press, 2011.

Erimtan, C., "Hittites, Ottomans and Turks: Ağaoğlu Ahmed Bey and the Kemalist Construction of Turkish Nationhood in Anatolia." *Anatolian Studies* 58 (2008), 141–171.

Gerber, C., "Zur Stratigraphie der Fürstengräber von Alaca Höyük: Neue Einsichten in ein altes Problem" in *Cultural Reflections, Studies in Honour of Hayat Erkanal*, ed. by A. Erkanal-Öktü *et al.*, 379–388. İstanbul: Homer Yayınevi, 2006.

Gonnet-Bağana, H., "Le disque solaire Hittite d'après les documents archéologiques." *Anadolu (Anatolia)* 11 (1967), 161–166; 167–196.

Gürsan-Salzmann, A., *Alaca Höyük: A Reassessment of the Excavation and Sequence of the Early Bronze Age Settlement.* Unpublished Ph.D Thesis (Ann Arbor 1996).

İpek Ö. and T. Zimmermann, "Another Glimpse at 'Hattian' Metalwork?—A Group of Bronze Age Metal Items from Bekaroğlu Köyü, District of Çorum, Turkey." *Anatolia Antiqua* 15 (2007), 49–58.

Kansu, Ş.A., *Türk Tarih Kurumu Tarafından Yapılan Etiyokuşu Hafriyatı Raporu 1937.* Ankara: Türk Tarih Kurumu, 1940.

Korfmann, M., "Die 'grosse Göttin' in Alaca Höyük." *IX. Türk Tarih Kongresi* (1986): 153–163.

Koşay, H.Z., *Alaca Höyük Hafriyatı. 1936'daki Çalışmalara ve Keşiflere Ait İlk rapor.* Ankara: Türk Tarih Kurumu, 1938.

———. *Türk Tarih kurumu Tarafından Yapılan Alaca Höyük Kazısı. 1937–1939'daki Çalışmalara ve Keşiflere Ait İlk Rapor.* Ankara: Türk Tarih Kurumu, 1951.

Lichter, C., "Varna und İkiztepe: Überlegungen zu transpontischen Kulturbeziehungen im 5. und 4. Jahrtausend." *Cultural Reflections, Studies in Honour of Hayat Erkanal*, ed. by A. Erkanal-Öktü et al., 526–534. İstanbul: Homer Yayınevi, 2006.

Lloyd, S., *Early Anatolia. A Description of Early Civilization in Asia Minor, as Revealed by the Last Half Century of Excavating and Exploration.* London: Harmondsworth, 1956.

Lloyd S. and N. Gökçe, "A New Investigation of Second and Third Millennium Stratigraphy in Anatolia." *Anatolian Studies* 1 (1951), 21–75.

Mansfeld, G., "Die 'Königsgräber' von Alaca Höyük und ihre Beziehungen nach Kaukasien." *Archäologische Mitteilungen aus Iran und Turan* 33 (2001), 19–61.

Maxwell-Hyslop, K.R., *Western Asiatic Jewellery c. 3000–612 BC*. London: Methuen Young Books, 1971.

Müller-Karpe, H., *Handbuch der Vorgeschichte. Dritter Band Kupferzeit. Dritter Teilband Tafeln.* München: C. H. Beck, 1974.

Orthmann, W., "Zu den 'Standarten' aus Alaca Hüyük." *Istanbuler Mitteilungen* 17 (1967), 34–54.

Özdoğan, M., "Ideology and Archaeology in Turkey" in *Archaeology under Fire. Nationalism, Politics and Heritage in the Eastern Mediterranean and Middle East,* ed. by L. Meskell, 111–123. London: Routledge, 1998.

Özyar, A., "Reconsidering the 'Royal' Tombs of Alacahöyük: Problems of Stratigraphy According to the Topographical Location of the Tombs." *TÜBA-AR* 2 (1999), 79–85.

Parzinger, H., *Studien zur Chronologie und Kulturgeschichte der Junstein-, Kupfer- und Frühbronzezeit zwischen Karparten und Mittlerem Taurus. RGF 52*. Mainz: Philipp von Zabern, 1993.

Schachner, A., *Von der Rundhütte zum Kaufmannshaus. Kulturhistorische Untersuchungen zur Entwicklung prähistorischer Wohnhäuser in Zentral-, Ost- und Südostanatolien.* BAR International Series 807. Oxford: Archaeopress, 1999.

Schoop, U.-D., *Das anatolische Chalkolithikum. Eine chronologische Untersuchung zur vorbronzezeitlichen Kultursequenz im nördlichen Zentralanatolien und den angrenzenden Gebieten.* Remshalden: Verlag Bernhard Albert Greiner, 2005.

Steadman, S. R., "The Early Bronze Age on the Plateau" in *Ancient Anatolia. 10,000–323 BCE,* ed. by S. R. Steadman and G. T. McMahon, 229–259. Oxford: Oxford University Press, 2011.

Tezcan, B., *1964 Koçumbeli Kazısı. Koçumbeli Excavation in 1964.* Ankara: Türk Tarih Kurumu, 1966.

Thissen, T., "New Insights in Balkan-Anatolian Connections in the Late Chalcolithic: Old Evidence from the Turkish Black Sea Littoral." *Anatolian Studies* 43 (1993), 207–237.

Tolstikov, W.P. and M.J. Trejster, *Der Schatz aus Troia. Schliemann und der Mythos des Priamos-Goldes.* Stuttgart/Zürich: Belser, 1996.

Treister, M., "The Relative and Absolute Chronology of the Trojan Treasures" in *Mauerschau. Festschrift für Manfred Korfmann*, ed. by R. Aslan *et al.* 245–258. Remshalden-Grunbach: Bernhard Albert Greiner, 2002.

Welton, M.L. *Mobility and Social Organization on the Ancient Anatolian Black Sea Coast: An Archaeological, Spatial and Isotopic Investigation of the Cemetery at İkiztepe, Turkey.* Unpublished PhD Thesis, Near and Middle Eastern Civilizations, University of Toronto (Toronto 2010).

Yalçın, Ü., "Alacahöyük İlk Tunç Çağı Kral Mezarları Üzerine" in *Çorum Kazı ve Araştırmalar Sempozyumu*, ed. by Ö. İpek, 55–64. Çorum, 2012.

Yıldırım, T., "An Early Bronze Age Cemetery at Resuloğlu, near Uğurludağ, Çorum. A Preliminary Report of the Archaeological Work Carried out between Years 2003–2005." *Anatolia Antiqua* 14 (2006), 1–14.

———. "Resuloğlu Kazısı ve Anadolu Arkeolojisi'ne Katkıları" in *Çorum Kazı ve Araştırmalar Sempozyumu*, ed. by Ö. İpek, 11–28. Çorum, 2011.

Zimmermann, T., "Kalınkaya-Toptaştepe, eine chalkolithisch-frühbronzezeitliche Siedlung mit Nekropole im nördlichen Zentralanatolien: Die Grabfunde der Kampagnen von 1971 und 1973." *Istanbuler Mitteilungen* 57 (2007a), 7–26.

———. "Anatolia and the Balkans, Once Again—Ring-Shaped Idols from Western Asia and a Critical Reassessment of Some „Early Bronze Age" Items from İkiztepe, Turkey." *Oxford Journal of Archaeology* 26 (2007b), 25–33.

———. "Symbols of Salvation?—Function, Semantics and Social Context of Early Bronze Age Ritual Equipment from Central Anatolia." *ANODOS—Studies of the Ancient World 5–6* (2008a), 509–520.

———. "Kultureller Austausch im südosteuropäisch-türkischen Schwarzmeergebiet vom 5. bis zum 3. Jahrtausend v. Chr.—Annäherungen an ein chronologisches und forschungsgeschichtliches Dilemma" in *Festgabe 40 Jahre Lehrstuhl für Vor- und Frühgeschichte der Universität Regensburg 1968–2008. Regensburger Beiträge zur Prähististorischen Archäologie Bd. 20*, ed. by P. Schauer, 461–479. Regensburg: Akademie Verlag, 2008b.

———. "Frühmetallzeitliche Eliten zwischen Ostägäis und Taurusgebirge im 3. Jahrtausend v. Chr.—Versuch einer kritischen Bestandsaufnahme" in *Aufstieg und Untergang. Zwischenbilanz des Forschungsschwerpunktes, Studien zu Genese und Struktur von Eliten in vor- und frühgeschichtlichen Gesellschaften*, ed. by M. Egg and D. Quast, 1–29. Mainz: Römisch Germanisches Zentralmuseum, 2009.

Zimmermann, T. and Ö. İpek, "The "Hattian" Metal Assemblage from Bekaroğlu Köyü—An Archaeometrical Footnote." *Anatolia Antiqua* 18 (2010), 31–34.

PART 3

Middle and Late Bronze Ages

Late Middle Bronze Age International Connections: An Egyptian Style Kohl Pot from Alalakh

Murat Akar[1]

Marie-Henriette and Charles Gates are two of the most prominent scholars in their fields of Near Eastern, Anatolian and Classical Archaeology. Being their student in the Bilkent University Archaeology and History of Art department has been the greatest opportunity of my life. I am proud to have been their student and feel very special to have been part of the Kinet Excavation Team! Thus it is an honor to contribute this paper on the subject of international connections in the late Middle Bronze Age with a focus on Tell Atchana, ancient Alalakh in the Amuq, the neighboring region to Cilicia, where Marie-Henriette and Charles Gates focus their research. It is also an honor to contribute with a topic from Alalakh, the site where Marie-Henriette Gates did her doctoral dissertation research.

Abstract

This paper presents a stone vessel carved in the Egyptian style found during the new excavations at Tell Atchana, ancient Alalakh in the Amuq Valley of Hatay. This vessel, a stone kohl pot, is part of an increase in foreign imports and artistic trends at Alalakh during the final decades of the Middle Bronze Age that reflects the signs of early internationalism in the Eastern Mediterranean Late Bronze Age.

Introduction

The internationalism that is ultimately the defining characteristic of the Late Bronze Age (*ca.* 1650–1200 BC, hereafter LBA) has its roots in the changing political and commercial dynamics observed towards the end of the Middle Bronze

1 M. Akar, Mustafa Kemal University, Faculty of Science and Literature, Department of Archaeology, Hatay/TURKEY, muratakr@gmail.com.
I would like to thank K. Aslıhan Yener, Mara Horowitz and Tara Ingman for their thoughtful comments and help on the editing.

Age (*ca.* 2000–1650 BC, hereafter, MBA).[2] The final decades of the MBA witnessed the establishment of long distance inland and maritime networks reflected in the increase of intrusive elements in material culture, local adaptation of foreign technological and stylistic approaches, and in the ways of presenting symbolic and ideological values. In that respect, the Amuq Valley of Hatay is an ideal geographic location to observe cross-cultural interactions, being located in the confluence buffer zone between Anatolia, the Near East, and the Levant. The evidence acquired from the excavations conducted at Tell Atchana by Sir Leonard Woolley in the 1930s and 40s has already proven the validity of this statement with the wide variety of artifacts reflecting cross-cultural interactions.[3]

Alalakh was the capital city of the territorial kingdom of Mukish as part of the larger extent of the Amorite Kingdom of Yamkhad based at Aleppo.[4] At the end of the MBA, the kingdom's organization consisted of small agricultural centers nested within a central system, and its economy was based on agriculture.[5] Yet Alalakh, as the capital, was also located in a very advantageous position with access to major land routes from Anatolia and the Levant. Its connection to the Mediterranean maritime network through the coastal site of Sabuniye[6] at the mouth of the Orontes gave it the character of an inland harbor town. Alalakh seems to have started benefiting more from its geographical location towards the end of the MBA.

The early stages of internationalism at Alalakh first appear in Period 7 (Level VII)[7] when both architectural forms and artifact assemblages included significant amounts of 'foreign elements' as the products of long distance trade, political and social interactions. In a number of cases where foreign styles were locally adopted, Alalakh's royal court seems to have brought artisans and craftsmen with diverse unique skills from abroad, thus creating a cosmopolitan production industry during the lifespan of Alalakh Period 7.

---

2 This paper follows the date ranges based on Middle Chronology.

3 Woolley 1955.

4 Klengel 1992.

5 Magness-Gardiner 1994, 37; Zaccagnini 1997, 341.

6 Pamir 2013.

7 "After an exhaustive correlation of the new excavation results with Woolley's stratigraphy, a new phasing system is in preparation that is based on the numbers assigned by Woolley using Roman numerals, but written in Arabic numerals to be clear where we have independently phased a new context or rephased a Woolley context. The numbers assigned to major phases remains the same; e.g. Level VII Palace is now Level 7, and Level IV Palace is now Level 4. [...] the designation "local phase" refers to the stratigraphy in the individual squares (excavations units) that begin with the number 1 at the top of each sequence, whereas "Period" refers to the site-wide sequence." Yener 2013a, 13.

Pre-Period 7 Material Culture

Being part of the Amorite horizon, the majority of the MBA levels of Alalakh (Woolley's Levels XVI-VIII) present a dominant inland Northwest Syrian character both in architecture and material culture.[8] The data in hand defining the early MBA sequence originated from the two soundings (Great Stratification Pit and Temple Sounding) conducted by Sir Leonard Woolley, where the fragmentary evidence is neither enough to attempt a historical reconstruction nor to fully comprehend the nature of the MBA settlement.[9] Thus, the recent Koç University excavations directed by K. Aslıhan Yener with co-assistant directors Murat Akar and Mara Horowitz have the goal of establishing reliable new data sets concerning, among other things, the MBA sequence of the settlement.[10] Several excavation units located in various districts of the settlement are progressively descending toward the early MBA levels.[11]

The ceramic data acquired from Woolley's and recent excavations imply a strong continuity in the choices of shapes and minimal foreign impact in the development of artistic choices in pottery production for the majority of the MBA levels.[12] While the bulk of the assemblage is dominated by plain Simple Ware traditions, the distinct Syro-Cilician ware appears to be a common form widely diffused at Alalakh, as well as in Northwest Syria and Cilicia, as the result of early interregional encounters.[13] Sporadic appearances of Syro-Cilician ware in Central Anatolian contexts, including Kültepe[14] and Acemhöyük,[15] signify the extent of these early connections.

Apart from the ceramic collections, other types of artifacts in Woolley's deep pre-Period 7 exposures are minimal in number and variety due to the limited size of the excavation area. Distinct chronological markers such as stone vases are absent from the collection, except for one fragment retrieved from Period XI.[16] The terracotta figurines[17] of Woolley's MBA levels are stylistically similar to each other and seem to provide a consistent tradition over a long period. Overall, the earlier MBA levels at Alalakh show the general characteristics of Northwest Syrian material culture.

8 Woolley 1955, 304–305; Heinz 1992.

9 Woolley 1955, 10–90; Batiuk and Horowitz 2010.

10 Yener 2013a.

11 At this stage, the pre-Period 7 stratigraphic data has only been acquired from two squares located in the courtyards of the Period 7 and Period 4 palaces (Squares 32.57, 33.32).

12 Woolley 1955; Heinz 1992.

13 Bagh 2003; Bulu in press.

14 Özgüç 1955, 460, fig.29.

15 Öztan 2008, 27, fig 1a/b.

16 Woolley 1955, 292.

17 Woolley 1955, 244.

Period 7

Period 7 welcomes a number of new stylistic and technological advancements in production technologies and artistic expressions. This is best observed in the architectural decorative elements found in the palace. The use of cement was first applied during the construction of the palace and temple floors,[18] while the well preserved wall painting fragments discovered in the rooms of the palace (5, 11, 12, 13)[19] indicates the interest of Alalakh's royal court in innovative stylistic expressions.[20] The appearance of wall paintings at Alalakh,[21] Qatna,[22] Mari,[23] Tel Kabri,[24] Tell Sakka,[25] Tell Burak[26] and Tel el Dab'a[27] are generally accepted as a product of a Mediterranean *koine,* but the mechanisms of interactions between distinct cultural zones are still under discussion. While the possibility of royal patronage is still a plausible explanation for travelling Minoan artisans, exchange of craftsmen,[28] technologies or stylistic expressions based on the current state of evidence,[29] there is disagreement as to whether the Levantine frescoes should be considered Minoan, considering the earlier appearances of wall paintings in the Near East.[30] More evidence on painting practices from the Near East may alter the West-to-East Aegeocentric[31] vision in the future.

A cylinder seal impression with a bull leaping scene found on an envelope fragment from the Alalakh Period 7 Palace archives[32] is another pictorial presentation of a festival game or ritual activity widely diffused over a large geographical area, including the Aegean, Anatolia and Syria, Egypt and the Levant.[33] First appearing in the Period 7 Palace, bull leaping as a subject continued to be embraced at Alalakh during the LBA.[34]

---

18 Woolley 1955, 225. No earlier building phases with cement floors have been discovered during the new round of excavations.

19 Woolley 1955, 99–103.

20 Woolley notes that the earliest use of fresco decoration dates back to Level IX at Alalakh.

21 Woolley 1955, 228–232

22 Pfälzner (in collaboration with von Rüden) 2008.

23 Parrot 1937.

24 Niemeier and Niemeier 1991; 2002.

25 Taraqji 1999.

26 Kamlah and Sader 2010.

27 Bietak 2007.

28 Zaccagnini 1983.

29 Woolley 1955; Niemeier and Niemeier 2000: 96.

30 Niemeier and Niemeier 2000; Koehl 2013.

31 Sherratt 1994; von Rüden 2013, 74–74.

32 Collon 1975, 60–61, fig.11.

33 Collon 1994, 81; Sipahi 2005.

34 Yener 2008.

Ivory production gained significant importance during the span of Period 7 under the likely patronage of the royal court and maintained its popularity during the LBA.[35] The elephant tusks found in the storage rooms of the Period 7 palace and hundreds of inlays and appliques define the considerable extent of the production capacity reached at the site.[36]

Alalakh Period 7 also yields a number of artifacts that express the skills and quality achieved in stone craftsmanship. Commonly accepted as depicting Yarim-Lim,[37] the bust found in the Period 7 Temple is a remarkable example of the Old Syrian sculptural tradition.[38] Found in the same context, an Egyptianizing bust[39] with its diverse style, as well as various composite statue fragments such as eye sockets, beard and hair pieces,[40] may signify the implementation and adaptation of different artistic styles and practices by Alalakh sculptors.

The stone workshop found in Woolley's Period 4 Palace, Courtyard 22 sounding (stratigraphically associated with Period 7) provides further evidence of a stone working industry at Alalakh.[41] The single burnt room context exposed in the sounding yielded a cache of artifacts including unfinished obsidian vessels, raw materials and various stone tools, providing a snapshot of the stages of stone vessel production.[42] However, obsidian vessels were very limited in the overall assemblage of Period 7 (and also in other periods). Sparks correctly argues that there would have been no suspicion of a local obsidian workshop if the evidence was only limited to the two other obsidian vessels[43] found in the temple and palace, which have neither stylistic correlations with the ones found in the workshop nor with the Amuq region in general. Her conclusion was that the Atchana workshop's operation was limited in time prior to its destruction and its products very highly individual in form, serving an elite group.[44]

Woolley also points out the possibility of manufacturing highly individual forms with foreign attributes in local workshops by judging the unfinished

35 Yener 2007, 152.

36 Woolley 1955, 288. The identification of raw materials for ivory objects from Period 7, whether elephant or hippopotamus, is still unclear; see Caubet 2013.

37 Woolley 1955, 235: AT 47/74.

38 Woolley 1955, 235.

39 Woolley 1955, 235: AT 47/62.

40 Woolley 1955, 235–236: AT 47/78, AT 47/90, AT 47/77, AT46/155, AT47/79.

41 Sparks 2001, 96.

42 Sparks 2001, 94–95.

43 Woolley 1955, 294: AT 48/41, AT 39/135.

44 Sparks 2001, 96–97.

condition of the Cretan style columnar red marble lamp, which had been found in a later Period 2 context, but possibly belongs to Period 7 based on its form.[45]

Accordingly, Period 7 should be regarded as the renaissance of Alalakh when various technological advancements and artistic styles in different production industries were brought under the sponsorship of the royal family. This would have called for the necessity of the exchange of artists and craftsmen from different regions and cultures.[46]

An Egyptian Style Kohl Pot from the Slope Cemetery of Alalakh

An Egyptian style kohl pot (AT 14614), found during the course of new excavations on the eastern slope of the tell in Sq. 45.45 (Fig. 1), adds to the repertoire of foreign style artifacts from the late MBA of Alalakh. Ongoing excavations in Sq. 45.44 (10 x 10 m) in close proximity to Woolley's 'Private Houses' have been progressively descending through LB I into MB II levels. The excavations revealed five local phases of architecture documenting successive re-buildings of the city wall from Local Phase 5 to 2 (MB II-LB I).

The city wall exterior—the entire eastern slope itself—was used as the cemetery of the settlement. Belonging to different ages and sexes, eighty-eight inhumation burials dated from MB II to LB I were found within the limits of Sq. 45.44 and in the adjacent Sq. 45.45 located to the east.[47] The squares immediately to the north, 45.71 and 45.72, also yielded fifty-eight individuals.[48] Apart from an elite white-plastered tomb found in Sq. 45.71,[49] the graves on the eastern slope mostly seem to belong to the commoners of Alalakh. Eastern slope excavations revealed that there was indeed an extramural cemetery for the settlement, contra Woolley's statement in his final publication that local burial traditions were restricted to intra-site practices.[50]

From MB II to LB I, the majority of the eastern slope burials contained one or two cups, including Simple Ware S-curved 'shoulder goblets,' as grave goods.[51] This typical MBA vessel type continued to be used as a burial gift throughout the LB I (1650–1400 BC), emphasizing conservative practices in the choice of burial

45 Woolley 1955, 295.

46 Zaccagnini 1983.

47 Ingman 2014.

48 Boutin 2010, 111.

49 Yener and Yazıcıoğlu 2010, 24; Yener 2013b.

50 Woolley 1955, 201.

51 See Ingman 2014, 195–196: Table 10 for distribution of closed and open vessel shapes.

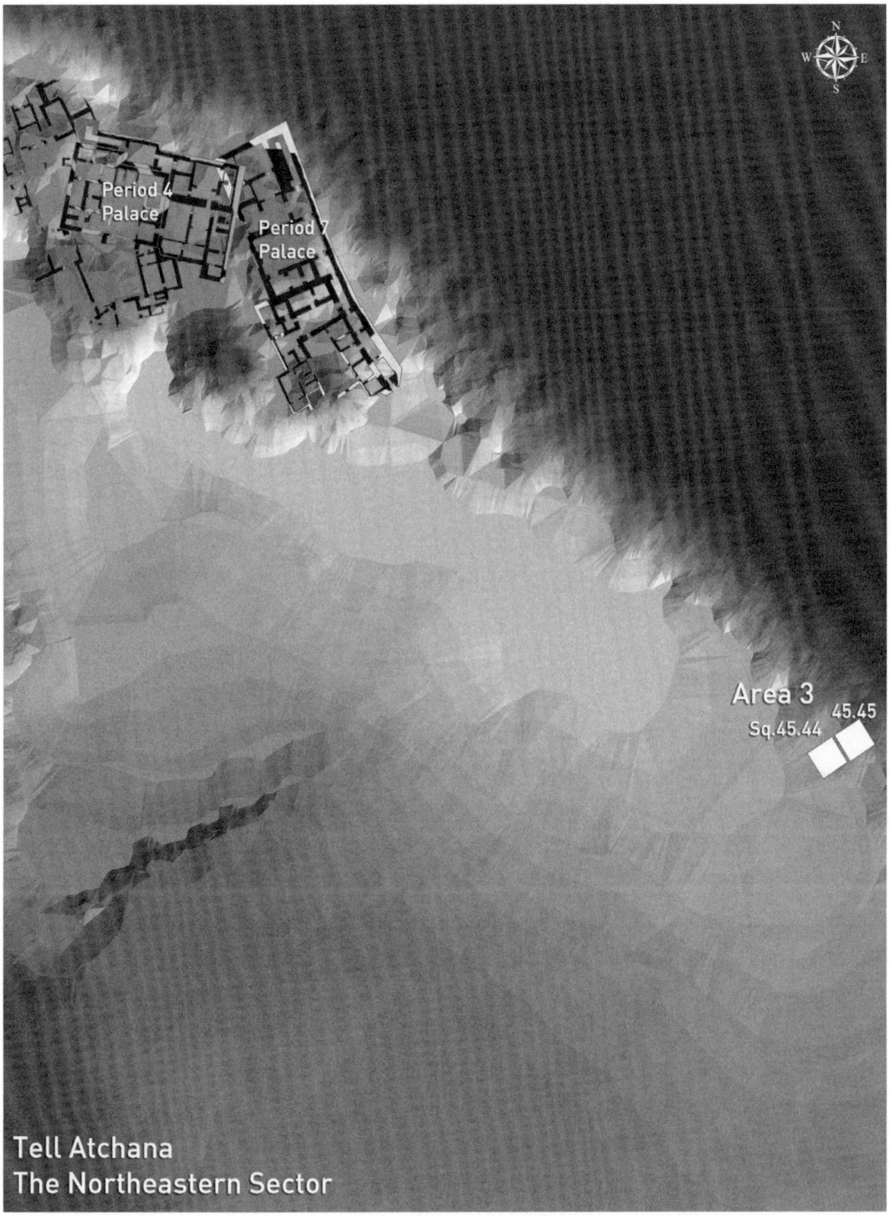

FIG. 1 Map showing the location of Area 3 squares 45.44 and 45.45.
Drawn by Murat Akar.

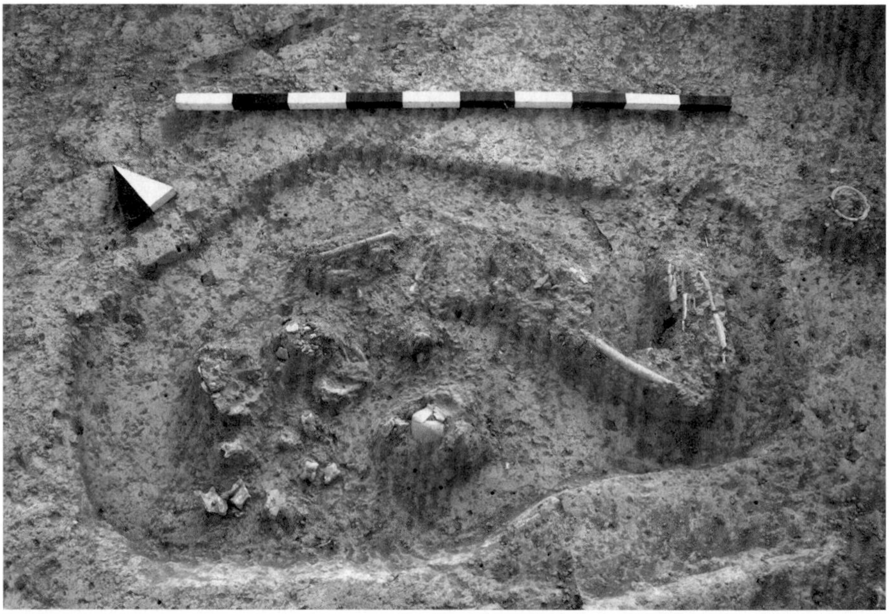

FIG. 2 The infant inhumation burial L.44. Photograph by Murat Akar.

assemblages among the common people of Alalakh.[52] Ornaments such as necklaces, bracelets, anklets and pins were few in number. A few of the graves yielded terracotta anthropomorphic and zoomorphic figurines.[53]

In the eastern slope, the continuous use of space as a cemetery from at least the late MBA through the late LB I ultimately affected the preservation quality of the burials, where in most cases one burial cuts another due to the shallowness of the deposition. Adding the erosion factor caused by the slope itself, the graves suffered from post-depositional disturbance.

In Sq. 45.45, a stone vessel with its lid was found in the slope fill-wash in close proximity to the edge of the limits of the excavation area along the slope, belonging to Period 7 or 6 (at 95.815 meters above sea level). Even though the vessel was out of context, it is highly probable that it was part of a gift group belonging to one of the burials in the near vicinity. Based on proximity, elevation, and the finding of the vessel intact with its lid, it is likely to be associated with burial L.44, an infant inhumation oriented in a NW-SE direction inside a cut measuring 1 x 0.5 m (FIG. 2). The burial itself also suffered from erosion due to its proximity to the slope; the bones were found in a very fragmentary and incomplete condition.

52 Pers. Com., Mara Horowitz.

53 See Ingman 2014, 109: Table 7 for the distribution of grave goods.

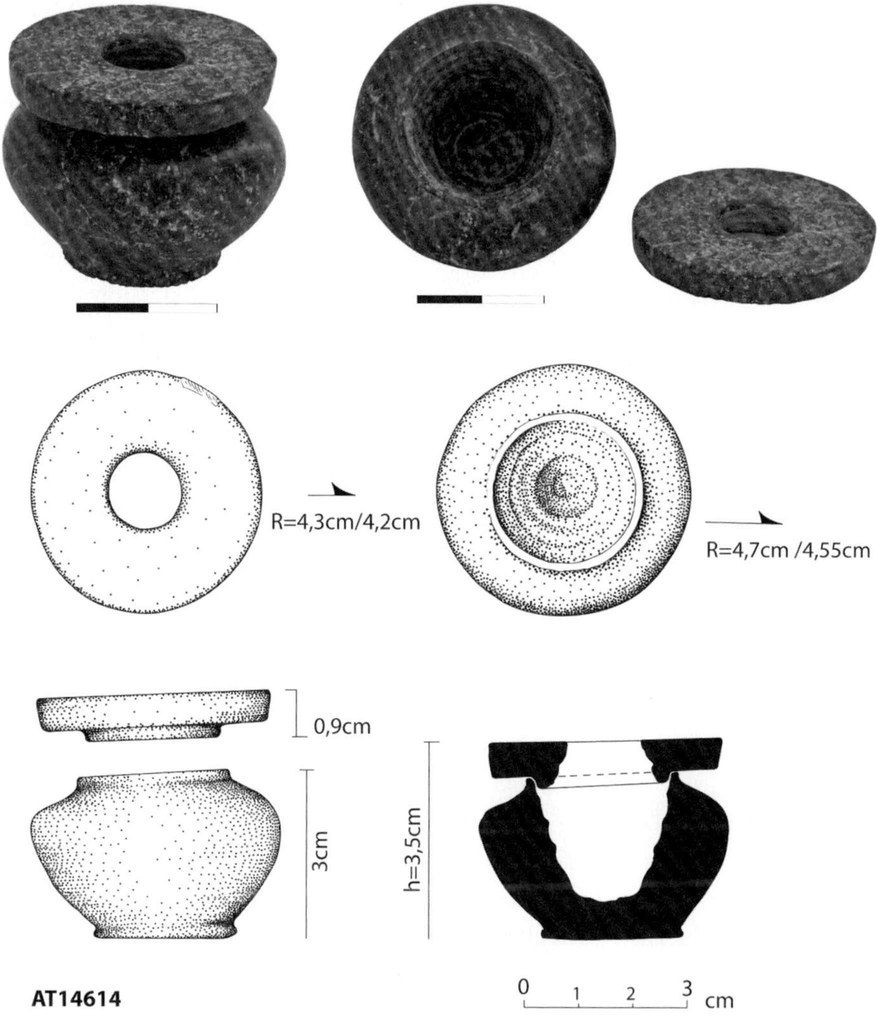

FIG. 3 The Egyptian style kohl pot AT 14614. Photo by Murat Akar, drawings by Ayça Sarıönder.

A number of grave goods, including a Simple Ware biconical cup (AT 14670), eight *astragalii* from a sheep or goat (AT 14650), a small worked stone (AT 14682) and a Syrian Brown-Grey Burnished Ware piriform juglet (AT 14615), were found in the burial. In comparison to other graves found on the eastern slope, it is a rich assemblage.[54]

54 Ingman 2014, 432.

The Kohl Pot (AT 14614)

The vessel has the shape of an Egyptian kohl pot (Fig. 3). Carved from a black stone,[55] it has a squat shouldered form (3 cm h., 4.7 cm max. dia.) with a flat rimmed base (2.6 cm dia.) and a slightly flared rim (2.9 cm dia.). The inside of the vessel was drilled out (2,4 cm max. dia.). The lid (0.9 cm h., 4.3 cm dia.) has a perforation in the center (1.3 cm dia.) which was opened with a drill; the underside is carved to create a projecting ring that sits inside the vessel. A final polishing was applied to both the vessel and the lid. Except for a small chip on the lid, possibly made in antiquity, the vessel is complete. No residue was visible inside by visual observation. Typologically, it falls into the Egyptian Middle Kingdom kohl pot family.[56]

Stone vessel production was a widespread industry in Egypt from the early Pre-dynastic period onwards.[57] Found in various shapes, different raw materials were used in their production. Uses of stone vessels varied from daily purposes to cult practices.[58] In Egyptian Middle Kingdom courtly and provincial tombs, kohl pots were the dominant preferred type of stone vessel for both females and males.[59] At Alalakh, various other Egyptian Style stone vessels were found in the residential context of the Period 7 palace, as well as in the enigmatic shaft burial located in the southern wing of the Palace in Room 17.[60]

Kohl was a common cosmetic in Egypt. Whether the vessel was used with its primary intent to store kohl at Alalakh or as an exotic object itself to be placed in a burial is currently unclear. It also is difficult to identify an origin for AT 14614, or any of Alalakh's Egyptian style vessels, since they are representatives of the larger Eastern Mediterranean aesthetic taste from the late MBA onwards.[61] The object could have also been produced in a Levantine workshop[62] or in one of the stone workshops at Alalakh, which were clearly capable of replicating or adapting Egyptian stone vessel carving and drilling technology based on other examples of stone vessels found at the site.[63]

---

55 Possibly black serpentine.

56 Petrie 1935, 665–667, pl. XXIX, 711, pl. XXX; Aston 1994, 145: shape 157a; Bevan 2007, 206.

57 Shaw 2012, 62.

58 Sparks 2003, 39.

59 Aston 1994, 51–73; Bevan 2007, 100.

60 Woolley 1955, 295: pl. LXXX.

61 Woolley correctly categorize the Egyptian style vessels as ".... the product of Middle East koiné, that partial but real uniformity of culture which, thanks to international trade, derived from and extended over Egypt, Syria, the Aegean, and Mesopotamia." (1955: 292). See also Sparks 2003, 40.

62 See Sparks 2001 for an overview of the Levantine stone workshops.

63 Bevan 2007, 56.

Conclusion

Alalakh Period 7 shows numerous signs that it was no longer only a provincial agrarian society with inland city characteristics but instead had become part of the larger Eastern Mediterranean economy, where the system was never exclusively oriented around agriculture and economic self-sufficiency. The production and circulation of goods and materials has defined the vitality of this period.[64] In that respect, the relatively high number of foreign and foreign-style artifacts and the technological enhancements observed in Period 7 contexts can be regarded as the harbinger of early internationalism. These artifacts were primarily sponsored and controlled by the royal court. Yet some were sporadically found in non-royal contexts, as in the case of an Egyptian style stone vessel in a commoner's burial at Alalakh (Period 7 or 6). This finding may emphasize that the acquisition of prestigious exotic products, or domestically made imitations and adaptations, was not only limited to the royal house but accessible to other members of the Alalakh society, who also started to benefit from these early international interactions.

64 Horden and Purcell 2000, 123; Yener 2007, 152; Akar 2009, 3.

REFERENCES

Akar, M., "The Role of Harbour Towns in the Re-Urbanization of the Levant in the Middle Bronze Age (1800–1600 BC). Perspectives from Cilicia and the Amuq Plain of Hatay." *Archatlas,* February 2010, Edition 4 (2009). http://www.archatlas.org/workshop09/works09-akar.php.

Aston, B. G., *Ancient Egyptian Stone Vessels: Materials and Forms.* Heidelberg: Heidelberger Orientverlag, 1994.

Bagh, T., "The Relationship between the Levantine Painted Ware, Syro-Cilician Ware and Khabur Ware and the Chronological Implications" in *The Synchronization of Civilizations in the 2nd Millennium BC. Proceedings of the Sciem 2000-Euroconference, Haindorf 2–7 of May 2001.*, ed. by M. Bietak, 221–238. Vienna: Verlag der Österreichischen Akademie der Wissenschaften, 2003.

Batiuk, S.D. and M. Horowitz, "Temple Deep Sounding Investigations 2001–2006" in *Tell Atchana, Ancient Alalakh. Volume 1. 2003–2004 Excavation Seasons*, ed. by K. A. Yener, 161–168. İstanbul: Koç University Press, 2010.

Bevan, A., *Stone Vessels and Values in the Bronze Age Mediterranean.* Cambridge, New York: Cambridge University Press, 2007.

Bietak, M., "Introduction: Context and Date of the Wall Paintings" in *Taureador Scenes in Tell-El Dab'a (Avaris) and Knossos*, ed. by M. Bietak, N. Marinatos and C.Palivou, 13–43. Vienna: Verlag der Österreichischen Akademie der Wissenschaften, 2007.

Boutin, A.T., "The Burials" in *Tell Atchana, Ancient Alalakh. Volume 1. 2003–2004 Excavation Seasons*, ed. by K. A. Yener, 111–117. İstanbul: Koç University Press, 2010.

Bulu, M., forthcoming. "A Syro-Cilician Pitcher from a Middle Bronze Kitchen at Tell Atchana, Ancient Alalakh" in *Overturning Certainties. Festschrift Presented to K. Aslıhan Yener for Her 40 Years of Field Archaeology in the Eastern Mediterranean*, ed. by M. Horowitz, Ç. Maner and A. Gilbert. Leiden: Brill.

Collon, D., *The Seal Impressions from Tell Atchana/Alalakh.* Kevalaer: Butzon & Bercker, 1975.

———. "Bull-Leaping in Syria." *Egypt and Levant* IV (1994): 81–88.

Heinz, M., *Tell Atchana/Alalakh: Die Schichten VII–XVII.* Alter Orient Und Altes Testament Band 41. Kevelaer: Verlag Butzon & Bercker, 1992.

Horden, P. and N. Purcell, *The Corrupting Sea. A Study of Mediterranean History.* Oxford: Blackwell, 2000.

Ingman, T., *Mortuary Practices at Tell Atchana, Ancient Alalakh in the Middle and Late Bronze Ages.* Unpublished M.A. Thesis, Koç University, 2014.

Kamlah, J. and H. Sader, "Deutsch-libanesische Augrabungen Auf Tell El- Burak südlich von Sidon. Vorbericht nach der siebten Kampagne 2010." *Zeitschrift des Deutschen Palästina-Vereins* 126, no. 2 (2010): 93–115.

Klengel, H., *Syria: 3000 to 300 B.C.: A Handbook of Political History.* Berlin: Akademie Verlag, 1992.

Magness-Gardinier, B., "Urban-Rural Relations in the Bronze Age Syria. Evidence from Alalah Level VII Palace Archives" in *Archaeological Views from the Countryside: Village Communities in Early Complex Socities*, ed. by G.M Schwartz and S.E. Falconer, 37–47. Washington: Smithsonian Institution, 1994.

Niemeier, B. and W.-D. Niemeier, "The Frescoes in the Middle Bronze Age Palace Tel Kabri: The 1986–1993 Excavations Seasons" in *Tel Kabri: The 1986–1993 Excavations Seasons*, ed. by Aharon Kempinski, 254–285. Tel Aviv: Emery and Claire Yass Publications in Archaeology, 2002.

Niemeier, B. and W-D. Niemeier, "Minoan Artisans Travelling Overseas: The Alalakh Frescoes and the Painted Plaster Floor at Tel Kabri, Western Galilee" in *Thalassa. L'egée préhistorique et la mer. Actes de la troiseme rencontre égeenne internationale del l'universite de Liege, Calvi, Corse (23–25 Avril 1990)*, ed. by R. Laffineur and L. Basch. Aegaeum, 189–200. Liege: Université de Liege, 1991.

Özgüç, T., "Excavations at Kültepe Level II Finds." *Belleten* XIX, no. 76 (1955): 453–461.

Öztan, A., "Some New Finds from Acemhöyük" in *Fundstellen: Gesammelte Schriften zur Archäologie und Geschichte Altvorderasiens* ad honorem *Hartmut Kühne*, ed. by D. Bonatz, R. M. Czichon and F. J. Kreppner, 25–29. Wiesbaden: Harrassowitz Verlag, 2008.

Pamir, H., "A Late Bronze-Iron Age Port Settlement on the Northeastern Mediterranean Coast" in *Across the Border: Late Bronze-Iron Age Relations between Syria and Egypt. Proceedings of a Symposium Held at the Research Center of Anatolian Studies, Koç University, İstanbul, May 31-June 1, 2010*, ed. by K.Aslıhan Yener. Leuven: Peeters, 2013.

Parrot, A., "Les Peintures Du Palais De Mari." *Syria* 18, no. 4 (1937): 325–354.

Petrie, W. M. F., *Funeral Furniture and Stone and Metal Vases*. London: British School of Archaeology in Egypt, 1937.

Pfälzner, P. in collaboration with C. von Rüden, "Between the Aegean and Syria: The Wall Painting from the Royal Palace of Qatna" in *Fundstellen: Gesammelte Schriften zur Archäologie und Geschichte Altvorderasiens* ad honorem *Hartmut Kühne*, ed. by D. Bonatz, R.M. Czichon and F.J. Kreppner, 95–118. Wiesbaden: Harrassowitz Verlag, 2008.

Shaw, I., *Ancient Egyptian Technology and Innovation. Transformations in Pharaonic Material Culture*. London: Bloomsbury Academic, 2012.

Sherratt, S., "Comment on Ora Negbi, 'the Libyan Landscape' from Thera: A Review of Aegean Enterprises in the Late Minoan Ia Period." *Journal of Mediterranean Archaeology* 7, no. 2 (1994): 237–240.

Sipahi, T., "Hüseyindede'den Hitit Tasvir Sanatı İçin Yeni Bir Sahne" in *V. Uluslararası Hititoloji Kongresi Bildirileri. Çorum 02–08 Eylül 2002*, ed. by A. Süel, 661–678. Ankara: Nokta Ofset, 2005.

Sparks, T.R., "Stone Vessel Workshops in the Levant: Luxury Products of a Cosmopolitan Age" in *The Social Context of Technological Change: Egypt and the Near East, 1650–1550 BC*, ed. by A. J. Shorthland, 93–112. Oxford: Oxford Books, 2001.

———. "Egyptian Stone Vessels and the Politics of Exchange (2617–1070 BC)" in *Ancient Perspectives on Egypt*, ed. by R. Matthews and C. Roemer, 39–239. Great Britain: UCL Press, 2003.

Taraqji, A.F., "Nouvelles decouvert sur les relations avec l'egypte a Tel Sakka et a Keswe, dan la region de Damas." *Bulletin de la Société Française d'Egyptologie* 144 (1999): 27–43.

von Rüden, C., "Beyond the East-West Dichotomy in Syrian and Levantine Wall Painting" in *Critical Approaches to Near Eastern Art*, ed. by M. Feldman, 55–78. Berlin: de Gruyter, 2013.

Woolley, C.L., *Alalakh: An Account of the Excavations at Tell Atchana in the Hatay, 1937–1949.* Report of the Research Committee of the Society of Antiquaries of London 18. London: Society of Antiquaries, 1955.

Yener, K.A., "Tell Aççana Höyük'te Bulunan Miken Boğa Atlama Krateri" in *Festschrift for Muhibbe Darga*, ed. by E. Konyar. İstanbul: Koç Vakfı Yayınları, 2008

———. "New Excavations at Alalakh: The 14th–12th Centuries BC" in *Across the Border: Late Bronze-Iron Age Relations between Syria and Anatolia. Proceedings of a Symposium Held at the Research Center of Anatolian Studies, Koç University, İstanbul May 31-June 1, 2010*, ed. by K.A.Yener, 11–36. Leiden: Peeters, 2013.

———. "A Plaster Encased Multiple Burial at Alalakh: Cist Tomb 3017" in *Amilla the Quest for Excellence. Studies in Honor of Guenter Kopcke in Celebration of His 75th Birthday*, ed. by R. B. Koehl, 263–279. Philadelphia, Pennsylvania: INSTAP Academic Press, 2013.

Yener, K.A. and G.B. Yazıcıoğlu, "Excavation Results" in *Tell Atchana, Ancient Alalakh. Volume 1. 2003–2004 Excavation Seasons*, ed. by K. A. Yener, 11–32. İstanbul: Koç University Press, 2010.

Zaccagnini, C., "Patterns of Mobility among Ancient Near Eastern Craftsmen." *Journal of Near Eastern Studies* 42 (1983): 245–264.

———. "Economic Aspects of Land Ownership and Land Use in Northern Mesopotamia and Syria from 3rd Millennium to the Neo-Assyrian Period" in *Urbanization and Land Ownership in the Ancient Near East*, ed. by M. Hudson and B. A Levine. Cambridge, MA: Peabody Museum of Archaeology and Ethnology, 1997.

A White Painted Pendant Line Style Jug Fragment from Tatarlı Höyük

Özlem Oyman-Girginer[1]

Abstract

Tatarlı Höyük (Fig. 1a) is located 24 km east of Ceyhan in the province of Adana. The mound, which stands out with its dimensions and its location among the ancient settlements in the Cilician Plain, was first discovered by M.W. Seton-Williams during the Cilician survey in 1951.[2] During the course of the Ceyhan Survey in 2005, this mound was visited by a team that included myself under the direction of K. Serdar Girginer.[3] The excavations of Tatarlı Höyük,[4] which began in 2007, again under Girginer's direction, suggest that an uninterrupted settlement from the Chalcolithic to the Hellenistic Period existed on this mound.[5] In this paper, a fragment of a White Painted Pendent Line Style (*WP PLS*) jug unearthed on a stone paved surface dating to the Middle Bronze Age (MBA) will be discussed. It is one of the earliest artifacts that show Cypro-Anatolian connections in the 2nd millennium BC. This find will be presented here with respect to interrelations between different regions in the Eastern Mediterranean and its chronological implications.

Introduction

The stone paved area (Fig. 1b), which was exposed in trenches BA 187 and AZ 187 located to the east of the Tatarlı Höyük citadel and to the west of monumental Building A, produced artifacts providing important evidence. The 25 m^2 portion of this stone pavement uncovered thus far was destroyed party due to Hellenistic pitting. This pavement was covered with a thin but compact soil floor. Almost 18 m^2 of this area was elaborately arranged by flat and bulky stones. A deep basalt

1 Çukurova Üniversitesi Arkeoloji Bölümü, Balcalı Mahallesi Sarıçam/Adana, Turkey.

2 Seton-Williams 1954, 128–129, 170, no. 39.

3 Girginer 2007, 177.

4 Girginer and Oyman-Girginer et.al. 2010; Girginer and Oyman-Girginer et al. 2011; Girginer 2012 and Girginer and Oyman-Girginer et al. 2014.

5 Especially apart from the 2nd Millennium BC bullae, cylinders and stamp seals, for prehistoric seals see Girginer and Collon 2014 and Ünal and Girginer 2010.

offering vessel (?) was placed in the middle of the stone-paved floor. At first, the Hellenistic pits created difficulties in finding an undisturbed context to help date the architecture of Building A correctly. However, excavations of the 2013 season prove that the stone pavement in question still continues in patches under Building A. So, it became clear that this pavement belongs to an earlier phase of this building. The material discovered on the stone pavement also presents evidence for the dating of these architectural remains.

On the northern part of the stone pavement in trench AZ 187, during the season of 2011, eight bird-shaped vessels, a ring-shaped vessel, a bull rhyton [6] and a fragment of a handle with an "ankh" sign were unearthed. An associated female figurine has parallels with those from Kinet Höyük, [7] Alalakh, [8] Tilmen Höyük, [9] Sirkeli Höyük [10] and other Syrian settlements. [11] The *WP PLS* jug fragment from Tatarlı Höyük, which is the focus of this paper, was found on the southern part of the stone pavement, located in trench BA 187.

The fragment in question has a round outflaring rim and a cylindrical narrow neck. The oval-sectioned handle runs from the mouth to the neck (Fig. 2a-c). It has a fine, well-fired, cream-colored fabric, was self-slipped (5Y 8/2), and the polish on the surface has been partially preserved. Painting was applied to the interior of the mouth, on the handle and on the body of the jug. The painting on the handle was applied as five alternating oblique stripes. On the body there are six vertical stripes alternating with a wavy line. The wavy lines were painted in reddish brown (5YR 4/4), but the stripes and vertical lines have a darker color (7.5YR 2.5/1). These colors were applied in dull tones, and it seems that the colors are partly worn off. P. Åström points out that the earlier versions of this style were painted with bright red colors, but the later ones have a dull black color. [12] So, we suggest that the fragment from Tatarlı Höyük is certainly one of the later versions of *WP PLS*.

6 These archeological artifacts will be published by the Tatarlı Höyük team.

7 Gates 2000, 82, 98, fig. 7, n.8.

8 Woolley 1955, 244 pl. LIV; Yener-Yazıcıoğlu 2010, 237, A03-R1023 (topsoil); 239, A03-R1284+A03-R1328 (Period: MBIIC). Similar figurines were also discovered in the settlements of the Amuq Plain, Tell Judaidah and Chatal Höyük, see Pruß 2010, 20–21, 57–58, pl. 4–5.

9 Duru 2003, 26, pl. 36 n.1,3

10 Novak-Kozal 2013, 417, 428, pl. 12; Kozal-Novak 2013, 235.

11 *Zincirli* (von Luschan 1943, 62, pl.76, 34a-b), *Hama* H (Fugmann 1958, 90, pl. 10, fig.110, 117, 124; Badre 1980, 164–165, pl. 1, Nr. Hama 12, 19), *Ebla* (Matthiae 1965, 185, pl. 73.1; Marchetti 2001, 349 no. 260, 351 no. 298, pl. 114; Badre 1980, 206, pl. 12 Nr. Mardikh 18, 218 pl. 14, Nr. Mardikh 75), *Tell Afis* (Michele and Pedrosi 2012, 173, fig. 3).

12 Popham 1963, 89.

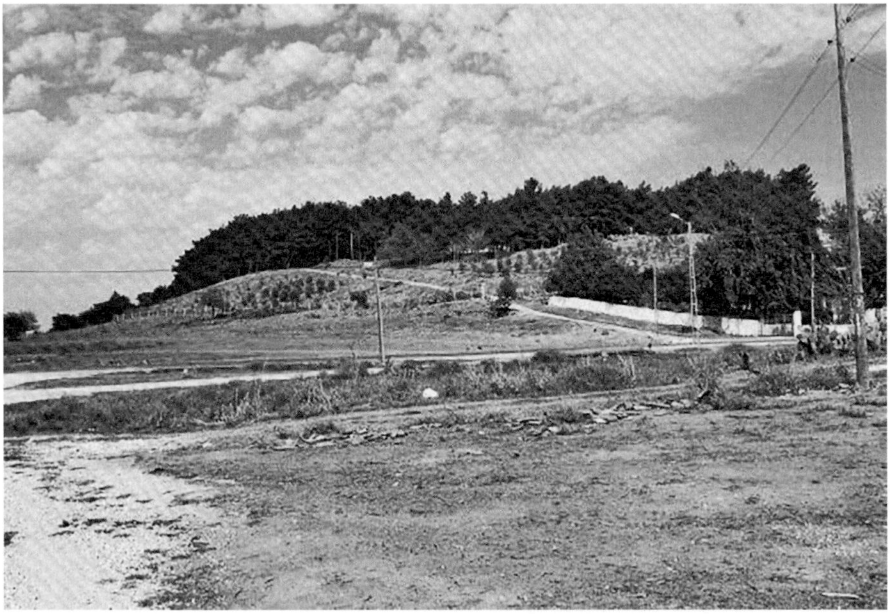

FIG. 1A The view from the southeast of Tatarlı Höyük.

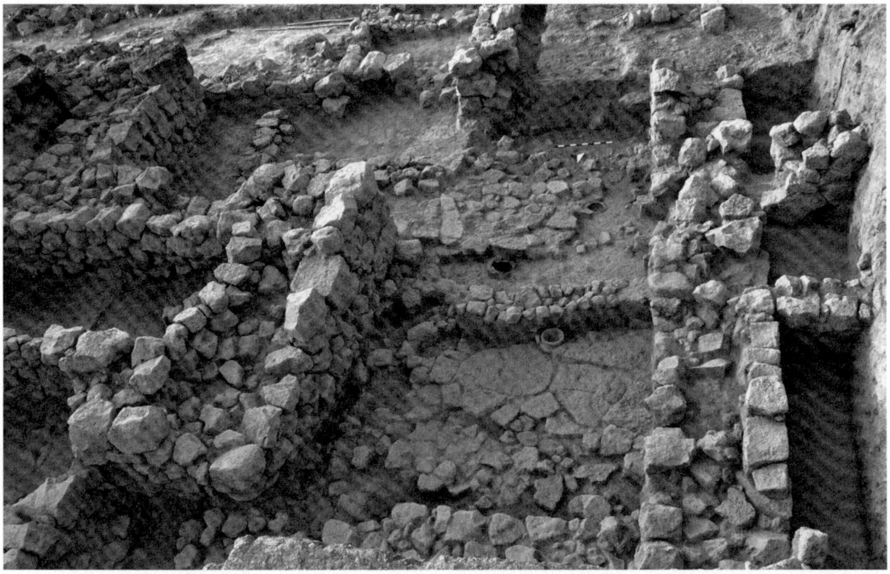

FIG. 2B The stone-paved area in the west of Building A.

WP PLS examples have been discovered in Cyprus, Crete,[13] Egypt, the Eastern Mediterranean and Anatolia. However, the number of Anatolian examples is quite limited, so this sherd of *WP PLS* unearthed in Tatarlı Höyük is very important in this respect. *WP PLS* is very common in Tell el-Dab'a in Egypt. One of the three most popular styles among *White Painted Wares* (*WP*) in Egypt is *WP PLS.*[14] Here, this ware makes its first appearance in layer G and becomes more common in layer E/1, but its quantity reduces from layer D/3 onwards. The latest occurrence of the ware is in layer D/2.[15] Layers G and F of Tell el-Dab'a are dated to the 13th Dynasty, so they were approximately contemporary with the last phase of MB II and the transitional phase to MB IIB.[16] According to M. Bietak, *WP PLS* makes its first appearance in *ca.* 1720 BC in Tell el-Dab'a and was widespread between 1630–1600 BC, finally disappearing by 1580 BC. W. G. Dever dates layer F of Tell el-Dab'a to the first half of the 18th century BC, and layer D/3 to 1575 BC. He also suggests that layer E/1 is probably dated to 1675–1625 BC. On the other hand, S. W. Manning proposed another date for layer D/3: 1640–1600 BC. In general, it seems that the maximum timespan for the layers including the artifacts in *WP PLS* could be assigned to 1725–1575 BC.[17]

A fragment of a jug in *WP PLS* was also unearthed in Kahun in Egypt. W.M.F. Petrie pointed out that it was found together with a number of ceramics from the 12th dynasty in a deep chamber.[18] This fragment with a round outflaring rim and a cylindrical neck was partially preserved. It has an oval-sectioned handle running from mouth to neck. This jug is well-fired, has light brown fine clay including sporadic medium sized grit. Its light brown outer surface was finished with a light polish, and a colored decoration including black and blackish brown designs applied to the inside of the mouth, the turning point of the handle, around the neck and on the shoulder.[19] P. Åström suggests that this fragment is not a later version of *WP PLS*, so it cannot be assigned to an earlier period than the middle of Middle Cypriot II.[20]

13 Maguire 2009, 47, 223, no. ZAK 817; Popham 1963, fig.1, pl. 26a. This fragment of *WP PLS* was unearthed in Zakro. Museum no: Heraklion Museum Box 72 Gamma.

14 Maguire 2009, 26, 93–99, fig. 26–27 (DAB 1–34 belong to this group. It seems that DAB 82–96 belong to *WP PLS* or WP Cross Line Style).

15 Maguire 2009, 41, tab. 3 (According to the table, from the G layer of Tell el Dab'a there was 1 *WP PLS*, 1 from F layer, 8 from E/1 layer, 8 from D/3 layer and 1 from D/2 layer). Furthermore see: Merrillees 2002.

16 Papadimitriou 2013, 114; Hein 2009, 30, fig. 4.1; Maguire 2009, 84.

17 Merrillees 2002, 3; Dever 1997, 295, fig. 9.4; Manning 1999, 189, fig. 36.

18 Petrie 1891, 10, pl. I:18; Gjerstad 1926, 304–305.

19 Merrillees 2002, 3, fig. 1–2 (British Museum, Department of Egyptian Antiquities, No: 50765, the neck of a jug); Maguire 2009, 173, KAH 391.

20 Åström 1972, 212, no. 7.

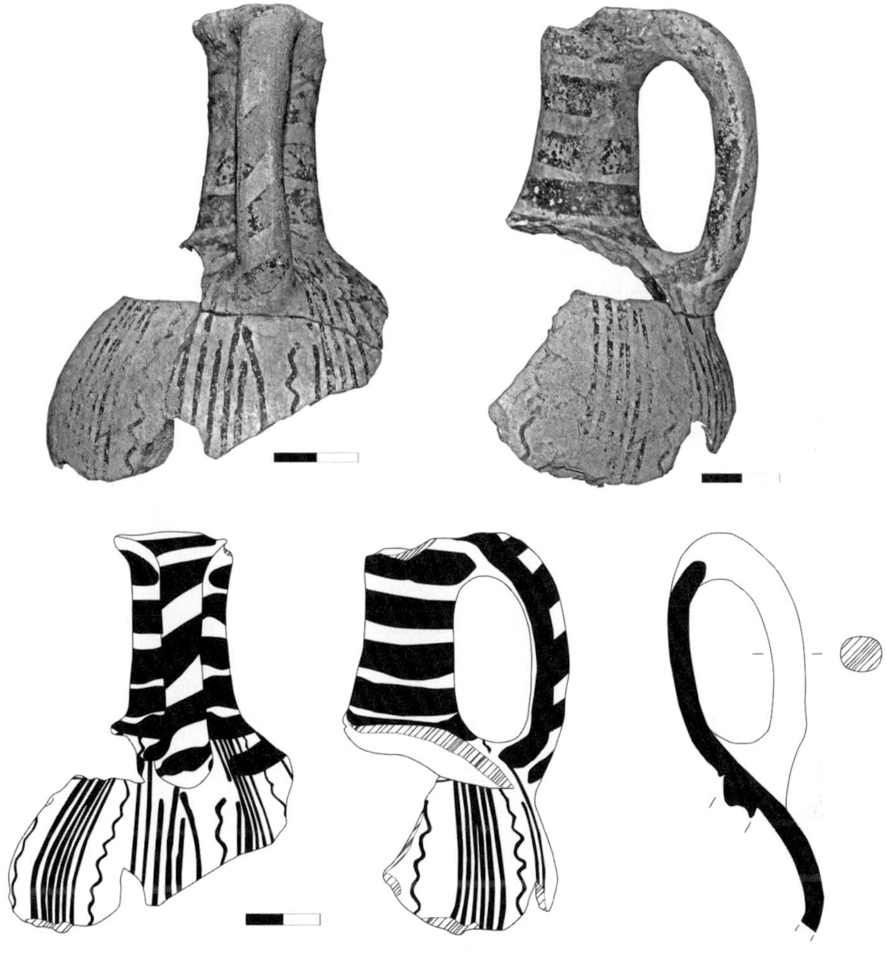

FIG. 2 A Fragment of Jug WP PLS (Drawing: Ebru İncaman; Photo: M. Ali Öngen)

The ancient Syrian settlements where this ware appears are listed as follows: Tell Daruk,[21] Qal at Er-Rus,[22] Kassabine,[23] Majjdalouna,[24] Ras Shamra,[25]

21 Maguire 2009, 174, fig.13, DAR 396; Oldenburg and Rohweder 1981, 32, 95, fig. 39 (Period: M/LBA Layer 26).

22 Maguire 2009, 174, fig.13, QAL 403–404; Ehrich 1939, 47, no. 7 (from Layer 2 and Layer 3); Åström 1972, 215.

23 Maguire 2009, 175, fig. 13, KAS 410; Åström 1966, 139, and no. 2.

24 Maguire 2009, 175, fig. 13, MAJ 413; Chéhab 1940, 50, fig. 3e.

25 Maguire 2009, 175–176, fig.13, RSH 416–421; also see; Schaeffer 1949, pls. XXXIX, XLIII.4; fig. 100.19; fig. 100.25; 131.3; fig. 108.19–20; 131.8,6; fig. 102.3; 131.9, fig. 131.10; Frankel 1974, fig. 19c; Maguire 1990, ill.65, RSH 326.

Sarepta[26] and Tell Sukas.[27] The *WP PLS* from Ras Shamra was discovered in the second layer of this ancient settlement.[28] One of the jugs[29] belongs to MB II or early MB III. According to C.F.A. Schaeffer, MB II is probably dated to 1900–1750 BC, and MB III to 1750–1600 BC.[30] Both jugs from Tomb LXXXV belong to MB II or early MB III.[31] Another jug in *WP PLS* was discovered in a tomb in Majjdalaouna in the northeast of Sidon. The jug in question was found next to *White Slip* and *Base Ring* wares. M. Chéhab dated this tomb, including many archeological artifacts, to a period from 16th century BC to 15th century BC,[32] but it seems that this jug is probably dated to an earlier period than 1600 BC.[33]

WP PLS also appears in Achzib,[34] Ain Shems (Beth Shemesh),[35] Tell el-Ajjul,[36] Akko,[37] Tell Dan,[38] Dhahrat el-Humraiya,[39] Gezer,[40] Ginosar,[41] Hazor,[42] Tel

26 Maguire 2009, 182, fig. 13, SAR 469–472; Pritchard 1975, 86–87, no.2, fig. 51:2; Anderson 1979, 791.1, pl. 29.1, 763, pl.21.7, 771, pl. 23.28, 776, pl. 24.27.

27 Maguire 2009, 183–184, fig.13 SUK 479–487; Thrane 1978, 51.10, fig. 55 context, fig.4 plan 3 (MBA), 51–52.19, fig.56, 54.170, figs. 43–44 and 62; Buhl 1983, 52.259, pl. XIV (Period H), 52.262 (Period F), 52.263, 52.264 (Period A), 52.265 (Period H), 52.266 (surface), pl. XVI.

28 Åström 1972, 214.

29 Åström 1972, 214–215; Schaeffer 1949, fig. 102.3, 131.10; Maguire 2009, 176, RSH 417.

30 Åström 1972, 214–215.

31 Åström 1972, 215; Schaeffer 1949, fig. 108. 19–20, fig. 131. 8,6; Maguire 2009, 176, RSH 421.

32 Åström 1972, 215; Chéhab 1940, 50, fig. 3.e; Maguire 2009, 175, fig.13, MAJ 413.

33 Åström 1972, 215.

34 Maguire 2009, 186, ACH 500; Oren 1975, fig.4: 90.

35 Maguire 2009, 186, AIS 503 (MBIIA) -504 (MBIIB); Grant 1929, 126–127, no. 649; Grant and Wright 1938, 97, pl. XXIV:8; Åström 1972, 213.

36 Maguire 2009, 186, AJJ 506; Maguire 1990, ill.1, row 1; 121 row 2.4.

37 Maguire 2009, 201, AKK 621–624 (MBIIA); Dothan 1976, fig.8: 1–2, 6, 10.

38 Maguire 2009, 204, DAN 650–651; Biran 1986, fig. 8: top left and left middle.

39 Maguire 2009, 204–205, DHA 652–661; Ory 1948, 79, 86, pl. XXXII: 3–6, 8–9, 19–21, 24, fig.4–5.

40 Maguire 2009, 207, GEZ 676 (pre-MBIIC)-677; Macalister 1912, vol III, pl. CXLV:1, vol II, 172; Dever *et al.* 1974, pl. 20:39; Åström 1972, 213.

41 Maguire 2009, 208, GIN 692 (MBIIA/B to MBIIB); Epstein 1974, fig. 15:9.

42 Maguire 2009, 208, HAZ 693–694 (MBIIB); Yadin *et al.* 1961, pl: CCLXXXVII: 23, CCCXII: 5.

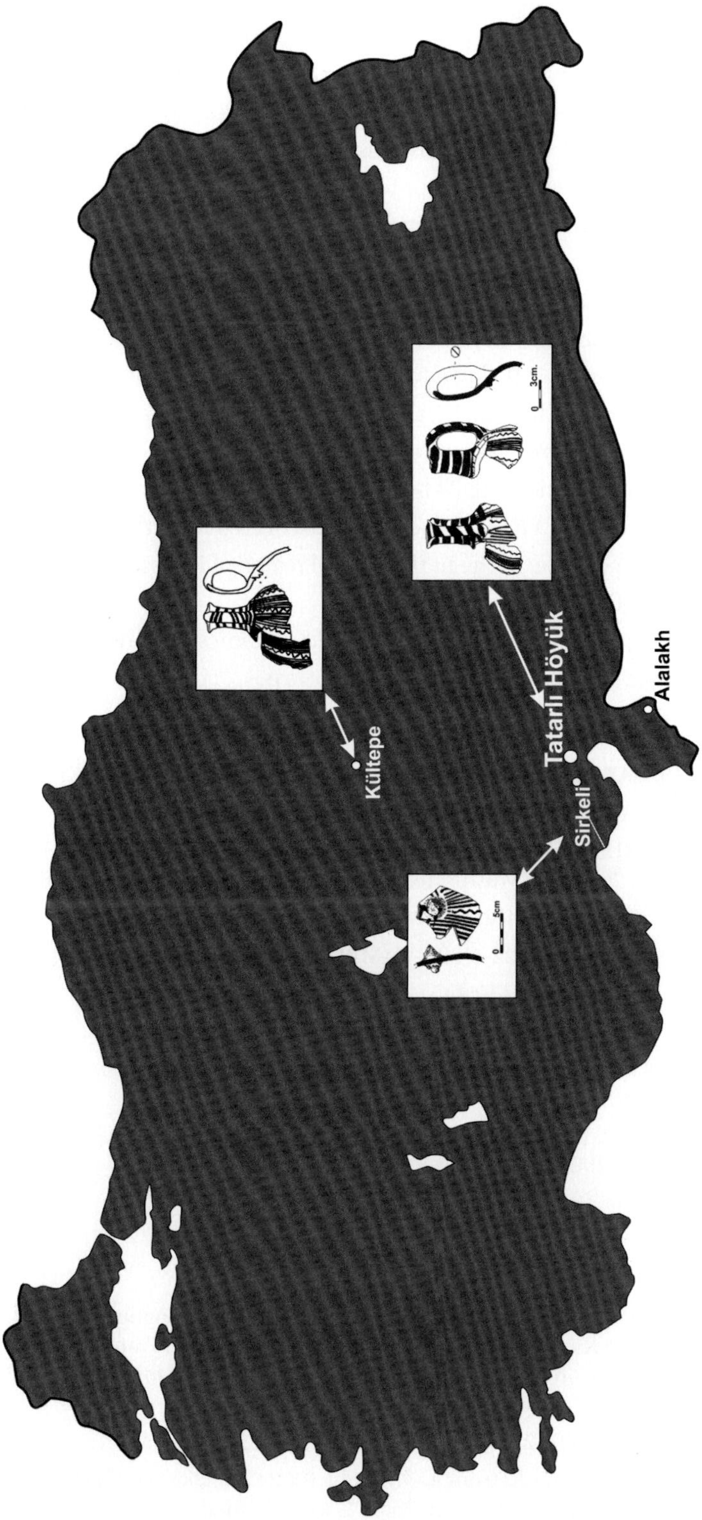

FIG. 3 The distribution of WP PLS in Anatolia.

Jerishe,[43] Tel Kabri,[44] Lachish,[45] Megiddo,[46] Tell Nami,[47] Tel Megadim,[48] Atlit[49] and Yiftahel.[50] One of the fragments from Gezer was ascribed to Macalister's Second Semitic period (*ca.* 1800–1400 BC).[51] Another fragment of a *WP PLS* jug was unearthed in Tomb 3, later called Tomb 13, in Ain Shems; this fragment was first dated to 1900 BC, but then it was assigned to the middle or to the end of the 17th century BC.[52] Another fragment was also discovered in Ain Shems VI. E. Grant and G. E. Wright suggested that this layer is dated to the 19th–18th centuries BC. The layer in question is probably not later than the 18th century BC.[53] *WP PLS* examples from Megiddo were unearthed in a number of tombs, such as Tombs 3076, 3110, 3128, and 4107. Tombs 3128 and 4107 belong to Megiddo XII, dated to 1770–1700 BC. However, it seems that Tombs 3076 and 3110 belong to Megiddo XI; these tombs are dated to 1750–1650 BC. Another fragment in the same style was found in Megiddo X and consequently dated to 1650–1550 BC. A small jug from Tomb 24 belongs to MB II/LB I.[54] Another ancient settlement where a great deal of *WP PLS* vessels were discovered recently is Dhahrat el-Humraiya, 13 km south of Jaffa, in the in the coastal region of Palestine. The jugs in question are dated to MB II.[55]

The ancient settlements in Cyprus, where *WP PLS* ceramics were discovered, are listed as follows: Kalopsidha,[56] Dhiorios Aloupotrypes,[57] Dhenia,[58] Galino-

43 Maguire 2009, 209, JER 707–709 (MBIIA); Geva 1982, fig. 32: 11–12, 14.

44 Maguire 2009, 210, KAB 718; also see; Maguire 1987, fig. 9:5; Maguire 1990, ill.2.

45 Maguire 2009, 213, LAC 736 (MBII-III); Tufnell 1958, 197–198, pl.79: 813.

46 Maguire 2009, 214–215, MEG 752–757, pl. 12:2–3, pl. 15:3; Guy 1938, pl.103:10, 48–50; Loud 1948, pl. 26:13, 17 (MBIIB), 16, pl. 34:12 (MBIIA/B), pl. 46:11 (MBIIC).

47 Maguire 2009, 220, NAMI 802 (MBIIA); Artzy and Marcus 1992, fig. 4:2.

48 Wolff and Bergoffen 2012, 421–422, fig 3:1–7 (MBIIA)

49 Mazar and Ilan 2014, 120–122, fig.10:4–5.

50 Maguire 2009, 221, YIF 811, fig. 49.2; Maguire 1990, ill.1; Barda and Braun 2003, fig. 9/3.

51 Åström 1972, 213; Macalister 1912, vol.II, 172, vol. III, pl. CXLV:1; Maguire 2009, 207, GEZ 677.

52 Åström 1972, 213; Grant 1929, 126–127, No. 649 (tomb 3); Grant and Wright 1938, 101 (tomb 13); Maguire 2009, 186, AIS 504.

53 Åström 1972, 213.

54 Åström 1972, 214.

55 Åström 1972, 214.

56 Åström 1966, 83; Maguire 1990, 53, Tab. 2, App. III Tab. C (T.11); Gagne 2012, 184, App. 1, fig. 927–936. The Kaopsidhaian ones were unearthed only in Trench 9. Some of them include a decoration with one wavy line between three or four horizontal lines, but a few of them were decorated with double wavy lines.

57 Frankel *et al.*, 1976, 36, pl. VIII.2 row 3; Maguire 1990, 53, 132–133, Tab. 2.

58 Maguire 1990, 52, 165, Tab. C.; Åström and Wright 1962, 227–228. The fragments belonging to WP PLS and WP IV groups in Tomb G were defined.

porni,[59] Kythrea,[60] Ayia Paraskevi,[61] Lapithos,[62] Nitovikla,[63] Lambertis[64] and Yeri.[65]

Besides Tatarlı Höyük, *WP PLS* has been discovered in only a few other Anatolian settlements (Fig. 3). These settlements are Kültepe, Sirkeli Höyük and Alalakh. It should be pointed out that the fragmentary small jug from Kültepe Ib enables us to examine chronological links with the Eastern Mediterranean region in the MBA.[66] The Kültepe Ib layer must be assigned to a date that cannot be later than the 10th year of the reign of Samsuiluna. This period is ascribed to 1785–1785 BC in high chronology; to 1740–1739 BC in middle chronology; or to 1676–1675 BC in low chronology. K. R. Veenhof suggested that the level in question with this find should probably be dated to a timespan between 1750/1745–1685/1680 BC.[67] According to the recent revised eponym list studies of Barjamovic, Hertel and Larsen, the destruction of Kültepe II occurred in 1835/1832 BC. Also, according to the same list, the last date for this period is 1718 BC.[68]

Another example of the ware was recovered during the Sirkeli Höyük excavations carried out between 1992 and 1997 by B. Hrouda. E. Kozal suggests that this artifact probably belongs to the earliest group of Cypriot finds from the 2nd millennium BC in Cilicia. The one from Sirkeli Höyük was found on a stone pavement in Trench 16.2 associated with Amuq-Cilician and Plain Wares that date to the MB II period.[69]

Alalakh is another settlement where a similar type of vessel was discovered. The sherd was defined by C. Epstein. This piece that is in the Antakya Museum was ascribed to Alalakh VIII. This well-polished sherd has a copper-red decoration.[70] L. Woolley described this piece as "one painted sherd, red on orange clay...

59 Maguire 1990, 53, Tab. 2; Gagne 2012, 181 App. 1, fig. 924. According to Gagne, this jug in the Ashmolean Museum (no. 1953.832) was probably produced in Kythrea or Kalopsidha.

60 Maguire 1990, 53, Tab. 2, App. III, Tab. C (T.1); Gagne 2012, 141, App. 1, figs. 367–377.

61 Gagne 2012, 171, App. 1, figs. 789–794, 798. Gagne points out that the decorative combination of the straight and the wavy lines on the vessels from Ayia Paraskevi is an oriental style, but it shows different characteristics than the usual PLS.

62 Maguire 1990, 52–53, Tab. 2, App. III, Tab. C (Lapithos T.18A)

63 Maguire 1990, 53, Tab. 2, App. III, Tab. C.

64 Maguire 1990, 53, Tab. 2, App. III, Tab. C. (T.38, T.21)

65 Maguire 1990, 53, Tab. 2, App. III, Tab. C.

66 Åström 1989, 15–16, fig.1; Åström 1987, 62, fig. 2; Maguire 2009, 47, 222 no. KUL 813.

67 Merrillees 2002, 5; Veenhof 2000, 149.

68 Bajramovic, Hertel and Larsen 2012, 91–97.

69 Kozal 2013, 217, fig. 1

70 Merrillees 2002, 5; Popham 1963, 90, n.7.

burnished after painting."[71] However, there is no drawing of the sherd in question. R.S. Merrillees suggested that this sherd can confirm the date of the piece from Kültepe. According to M.-H. Gates, the most probable date for Alalakh VIII is 1720–1650/1630 BC.[72] However, Bergoffen and Heinz could not locate this piece.[73] Bergoffen states that the first samples of Cypriot ceramics at Atchana come from the VI and V strata.[74] The only example of *WP PLS* at Atchana is a body sherd, which belongs to a closed cup. It is made of pink (7.5 YR 7/3) fabric, burnished, with a light grey (10 YR 7/2) slip and dark grey (10 YR 4/1) paint.[75]

The jug fragment from Tatarlı Höyük is a new point on the Anatolian map showing particularly the distribution of *WP PLS*. This fragment can be placed into the same historical period, for which the same ware has been found in various settlements. This find is from the 17th–16th centuries BC, and the other artifacts, which were discovered on the stone paving, also support this suggestion. The recent excavations at Tatarlı Höyük are promising, as they will provide evidence to help scholars to establish chronological connections with neighboring cultures, and thus shed light on the history of Kizzuwatna as well.

71 Merrillees 2002, 5; Woolley 1955, 313.

72 Merrillees 2002, 5; Gates 1987, 75; *cf.* Heinz 1992, 208.

73 Bergoffen 2005, 37.

74 Bergoffen 2005, 14.

75 Bergoffen 2005, 83, pl. 2d.

REFERENCES

Anderson, W.P., "A Stratigraphic and Ceramic Analysis of the Late Bronze and Iron Age Strata of Sounding Y at Sarepta (Sarafand, Lebanon)," PhD Thesis, University of Pennsylvania, 1979.

Artzy, M. and E. Marcus, "Stratified Cypriote Pottery in MB IIa Context at Tell Nami," in *Studies in Honor of Vassos Karageorghis*, ed. by G.C. Ioannides, 103–110. Nicosia: The Society of Cypriot Studies, 1992:

Åström, P. and G. Wright, "Two Bronze Age Tombs at Dhenia in Cyprus." *Opus Athenaium* 4 (1962): 225–276.

Åström, P., *Excavations at Kalopsidha and Ayios Iakovos in Cyprus*, Studies in Mediterranean Archaeology 2. Lund: Astrom Editions, 1966.

———. *The Swedish Cyprus Expedition, The Middle Cypriote Bronze Age*. Vol. 4, Part 1B. Lund: Berlingska Boktryckeriet, 1972.

———. "The Chronology of the Middle Cypriote Bronze Age" in *High, Middle or Low? Acts of an International Colloquium on Absolute Chronology Held at the University of Gothenburg 20th–22nd August 1987,* Part 1, 57–66, ed. by P. Åström, Göteborg, 1987.

———. "Early Connections between Anatolia and Cyprus" in *Anatolia and the Ancient Near East: Studies in Honor of Tahsin Özgüç*, 15–17, ed. by K. Emre, B. Hrouda, M.J. Mellink, and N. Özgüç. Ankara: Türk Tarih Kurumu Basımevi, 1989.

Badre, L.E., *Les figurines anthropomorphes en tere cuites à l'age du bronze en Syrie.* Paris: Geuthner, 1980.

Barda, L. and E. Braun, "Tomb 1 of the Second Millennium BCE at Yiftah'el, Lower Galilee." ᶜ*Atiqot* 44 (*2003*): 67–95.

Bajramovic, G., T. Hertel and M.T. Larsen, *Ups and Downs at Kanesh, Chronology, History and Society in the Old Assyrian Period.* Leiden: The Netherlands Institute for the Near East, 2012.

Bergoffen, C.J., *The Cypriot Bronze Age Pottery from Sir Leonard Woolley's Excavations at Alalakh* (*Tell Atchana*). Vienna: Verlag der Österreichischen Akademie der Wissenschaften, 2005.

Biran, A., "The Dancer from Dan, the Empty Tomb and the Altar Room", *Israel Exploration Journal* 36 (1986): 168–187.

Buhl, M.-L., *Sukas VII. The Near Eastern Pottery and Objects of other Materials from the Upper Strata*. Kobenhavn: Munksgaard, 1983.

Chéhab, M., "Tombes pheniciennes, Majdalouna." *Bulletin du Musée de Beyrouth* 4 (1940): 37–53.

Dever, W.G. et al. *Gezer II : Report of the 1967-70 Seasons in Fields I and II.* Jerusalem : Hebrew Union College/Nelson Glueck School of Biblical Archaeology, 1974.

Dever, W.G., "Settlement Patterns and Chronology of Palestine in the Middle Bronze Age" in *The Hyksos: New Historical and Archaeological Perspectives*, ed. by E.

Oren, University Museum Monograph 96, 285–301. Philadelphia: University of Pennsylvania Museum Publication, 1997.

Dothan, M., "Akko: Interim Excavation Report, First Season, 1973/4." *Bulletin of the American Schools of Oriental Research* 224 (1976): 1–48.

Duru, R., *Tilmen, A Forgotten Capital City: The Story of a 5400 Year Old Settlement in the Islahiye Region-Southeast Anatolia.* İstanbul: TURSAB, 2003.

Ehrich, A.M.H., *Early Pottery of the Jebeleh Region.* Philadelphia: The American Philosophical Society, 1939.

Epstein, C., "Middle Bronze Age Tombs at Kefar Szold and Ginosar." *Atiqot* 2–6 (1974): 13–39.

Frankel, D., *Middle Cypriot White Painted Pottery: An Analytical Study of the Decoration,* Studies in Mediterranean Archaeology 42, Göteborg: Astrom Editions, 1974.

Frankel, D. R. Hedges and H. Hatcher, "Chemical Analysis of Middle Cypriote White Painted Ware Sherds in the Ashmolean Museum, Oxford." *Report of the Department of Antiquities Cyprus* (1976): 35–42.

Fugmann, E., *Hama. Fouilles et recherches 1931–1938 II-1, L'architecture des périodes pré-Hellénistiques.* Kopenhagen: Nationalmuseet, 1958.

Gagne, L.A.C., *Middle Cypriot White Painted Ware: A Study of Pottery Production and Distribution in Middle Bronze Age Cyprus.* PhD Thesis, Toronto, 2012.

Gates, M.H., "Alalakh and Chronology Again" in *High, Middle or Low? Acts of an International Colloquium on Absolute Chronology Held at the University of Gothenburg 20th–22nd August 1987,* Part 2, 60–86, ed. by P. Åström, Göteborg,1987.

———. "Kinet Höyük (Hatay, Turkey) and MB Levantine Chronology." *Akkadica* 119–120 (2000): 77–101.

Geva, S., *Tell Jerishe: the Sukenik Excavations of the Middle Bronze Age Fortifications,* QEDEM 15, Jerusalem, 1982.

Girginer, K.S., "2005 Yılı Adana (Ceyhan) ve Kayseri (Develi) Yüzey Araştırmaları." *24. Araştırma Sonuçları Toplantısı* 2 (2007): 173–196.

———. "Excavations at Tatarlı Höyük in 2011." *ANMED, News of Archaeology from Anatolia's Mediterranean Areas* 10 (2012): 110–114.

Girginer, K.S. and D. Collon, "Cylinder and Stamp Seals From Tatarlı Höyük." *Anatolian Studies* 64 (2014): 59–72.

Girginer, K.S. et al., "Tatarlı Höyük (Ceyhan) Kazısı: İlk İki Dönem." *31. Kazı Sonuçları Toplantısı* 3 (2010): 453–476.

———. "Excavations at Tatarlı Höyük in 2009 and 2010." *ANMED, News of Archaeology from Anatolia's Mediterranean Areas* 9 (2011): 128–135.

———. "2012 Tatarlı Höyük Kazıları." *35. Kazı Sonuçları Toplantısı* 2 (2014): 182–196.

Gjerstad, E., *Studies on Prehistoric Cyprus.* Uppsala: The Swedish Cyprus Expedition, 1926.

Grant, E. *Beth Shemesh,* Haverford Collection, 1929.

Grant, E. and G.E. Wright, *ᶜAin Shems Excavation Part IV (Pottery)*, Haverford Collection, 1938.

Guy, P.L.O., *Megiddo Tombs*. Chicago: University of Chicago Press, 1938.

Hein, I., "A Contribution from Tell el-Dab'a/Ezbet Helmi to the Cyprus Connection" in *Egypt and Cyprus in Antiquity, Proceedings of the International Conference, Nicosia, 3–6 April 2003*, 29–39, ed. by D. Michaelides, V. Karageorghis and R. Merrillees. Oxford: Oxbow Books, 2009.

Heinz, M., *Tell Atchana/Alalakh: Die Schichten VII–XVII*, Alter Orient und Altes Testament Band 41. Kevelaer: Verlag Butzon & Bercker, 1992.

Kozal, E., "Exploring Sirkeli Höyük in the Late Bronze Age and its Interregional Connections" in *Across the Border: Late Bronze-Iron Age Relations Between Syria and Anatolia*, ed. by K. A. Yener, Ancient Near Eastern Studies Supplement 42, 213–219. Leuven: Peeters, 2013.

Kozal, E. and M. Novak, "Sirkeli Höyük. A Bronze and Iron Age Urban Settlement in Plain Cilicia" in *Anatolian Metal VI*, ed. by Ü. Yalçın, 229–238. Bochum, 2013.

Loud, G., *Megiddo II, Seasons of 1935–39, Plates*. Chicago: University of Chicago Press, 1948.

Macalister, R.A.S., *The Excavations of Gezer, 1902–5 & 1907–9*, vols. I-III. London: J. Murray, 1912.

Maguire, L.C., "Imported Cypriot Pottery from Middle Bronze Age Levels at Kabri" in *Excavations at Kabri: Preliminary Report of 1986 Season*, 44–51, ed. by A. Kempinski. Tel Aviv, 1987.

———. *The Circulation of Cypriot Pottery in the Middle Bronze Age."*Unpublished PhD Thesis, University of Edinburg, 1990.

———. *The Cypriot Pottery and its Circulation in the Levant. Tell El-Dabᶜa XXI*. Vienna: Austrian Academy of Sciences Press, 2009.

Manning, S.W., *A Test of Time: The Volcano of Thera and the Chronology and History of the Aegean and East Mediterranean in the Mid Second Millennium BC*. Oxford: Oxbow Books, 1999.

Marchetti, N., *La coroplastica Eblaita e Siriana nel Bronzo Medio*. Materiali e Studi Archeologici di Ebla 5. Roma: Arbor Sapientiae, 2001.

Matthiae, P., *Missione archeologica italiana in Siria. Rappoto preliminare della campagna 1964*. Roma: Centro di Studi Semitici, 1965.

Mazar, E. and D. Ilan, "A Middle Bronze Age Tomb at 'Atlit'." *Atiqot* 79 (2014): 111–130.

Merrillees, R.S., "The Relative and Absolute Chronology of the Cypriote White Painted Pendent Line Style." *Bulletin of the American Schools of Oriental Research* 326 (2002): 1–9.

di Michele, A. and M.E. Pedrosi, "Fortification and Burial Grounds in Tell Afis (Syria) between Middle Bronze Age and Late Bronze Age" in *Broadening Horizons 3, Conference of Young Researchers Working in the Ancient Near East*, 169–182,ed. by F.B. Tema- M.B. Garcia *et al.* Barcelona: Universitat Autonoma de Barcelona, 2012.

Novak, M. and E. Kozal, "Sirkeli Höyük 2011 Yılı Çalışmaları." *34. Kazı Sonuçları Toplantısı* 1 (2013): 413–428.

Oldenburg, E. and J. Rohweder, *The Excavations at Tall Daruk (Usnu?) and ᶜArab al-Mulk (Paltos)*. Copenhagen: Munksgaard, 1981.

Oren, E., "The Pottery from the Achzib Defence System, Area D: 1963 and 1964 Seasons." *Israel Exploration Journal* 25 (1975): 211–225.

Ory, J., "A Bronze Age Cemetery at Dhahrat el Humraiya." *Quarterly of the Department of Antiquities in Palestine* 13 (1948): 75–89.

Papadimitriou, N., "Regional or 'International' Networks? A Comparative Examination of Aegean and Cypriot Imported Pottery in the Eastern Mediterranean." *TALANTA* XLIV (2013): 92–136.

Petrie, W.M.F., *Ilahun, Kahun and Gurob*. London: D. Nutt, 1891.

Popham, M., "Two Cypriot Sherds from Crete." *Annual of the British School at Athens* 58 (1963): 89–93.

Pritchard, J.B., *Sarepta: A Preliminary Report on the Iron Age*. Philadelphia: Museum of the University of Pennsylvania, 1975.

Pruß, A., *Die Amuq-Terrakotten, Untersuchungen zu den Terrakotta-Figuren des 2. und 1. Jahrtausends v.Chr. aus den Grabungen des Oriental Institute Chicago in der Amuq-Ebene,* Subartu XXVI. Turnhout: Brepols, 2010.

Schaeffer, C.F.A., *Ugaritica II, Mission de Ras Shamra*. Paris: Librairie orientaliste Paul Geuthner, 1949.

Seton-Williams, M.V., "Cilician Survey." *Anatolian Studies* 4 (1954): 121–174.

Thrane, H., *Sukas IV. A Middle Bronze Age Collective Grave on Tall Sukas*. Cophenagen: Publications of the Carlsberg Expedition to Phoenicia 5, 1978.

Tufnell, O., *Lachish IV. The Bronze Age*. London-New York: Oxford University Press, 1958.

Ünal, A. and K.S. Girginer, "Tatarlı Höyük Kazılarında Bulunan 'Anadolu Hiyeroglifli' Damga Mühür Baskısı" in *Veysel Donbaz'a Sunulan Yazılar. DUB.SAR.E.DUB.BA.A,* 275–281, ed. by Ş. Dönmez. İstanbul: Ege Yayınları, 2010.

Veenhof, K.R., "Old Assyrian Chronology." *Akkadica* 119–120 (2000): 137–150.

von Luschan, F., *Ausgrabungen in Sendschirli 5. Die Kleinfunde von Sendschirli,* ed. by W. Andrae. Berlin: De Gruyter, 1943.

Wolff, S.R. and C. Bergoffen, "Cypriot Pottery from MBIIA Loci at Tel Megadim." *Orbis Biblicus et Orientalis* 255 (2012): 419–430.

Woolley, C.L., *Alalakh: An Account of the Excavations at Tell Atchana in the Hatay, 1937–1949*. Report of the Research Committee of the Society of Antiquaries of London 18. London: Society of Antiquaries, 1955.

Yadin, Y. Y. Aharoni *et al., Hazor III-IV: An Account of the Third and Fourth Seasons of Excavations, 1957–1958 (Plates)*. Jerusalem: Israel Exploration Society, 1961.

Yener, K.A. and B. Yazıcıoğlu, "Appendix B: Small Finds Catalogue" in *Tell Atchana, Ancient Alalakh. Volume 1. 2003–2004 Excavation Seasons*, ed. by K. A. Yener, 215–283.

Hittite Gods Abroad: Evidence for Hittite Diplomatic Activities?

Hermann Genz[1]

Abstract

During the Late Bronze Age the Hittite Empire was one of the global players in the ancient Near East. Relations with neighboring political entities are mainly attested through historical records, especially in the cuneiform archives from Boğazköy-Hattuša, but also from various other sources in the ancient Near East and Egypt. It is therefore quite interesting to note that the material evidence for contacts between the Hittites and their neighbors is surprisingly meagre, especially when compared to the ubiquity of Mycenaean and Cypriot pottery or Egyptian objects in the Eastern Mediterranean. One of the most prominent groups of Hittite objects attested outside Central Anatolia, besides Hittite seals, comprise small figurines of Hittite deities, often executed in precious materials. As the author finds it difficult to accept these as objects of trade, it is suggested here that these items should be interpreted as the personal protective deities of Hittites traveling abroad, most likely envoys on diplomatic missions.

Introduction

According to Late Bronze Age (LBA) texts from the Hittite realm and various other LBA political entities in the Ancient Near East, it is clear that the Hittites, throughout the second half of the 2nd millennium BC, were part of the international political system[2]; in fact during the Empire Period they were one of the global players in the Near East. On the other hand, the material evidence for contacts of the Hittites with their neighbors is surprisingly meagre. In comparison with the wide distribution of various Egyptian artifacts[3] and Mycenaean[4] or Cypriot pottery[5] in the LBA Eastern Mediterranean and the Near East, the distribution

1 Department of History and Archaeology, American University of Beirut, Riad El Solh, Beirut, 11072020, Lebanon.

2 Bryce 1998; Klengel 1999.

3 Hasel 1998, 91–117; Higginbotham 2000, 74–128; Cline 2009, 31–47.

4 Leonard 1994; van Wijngaarden 2002.

5 Åström 2001; Karageorghis 2001; Cline 2009, 60–67.

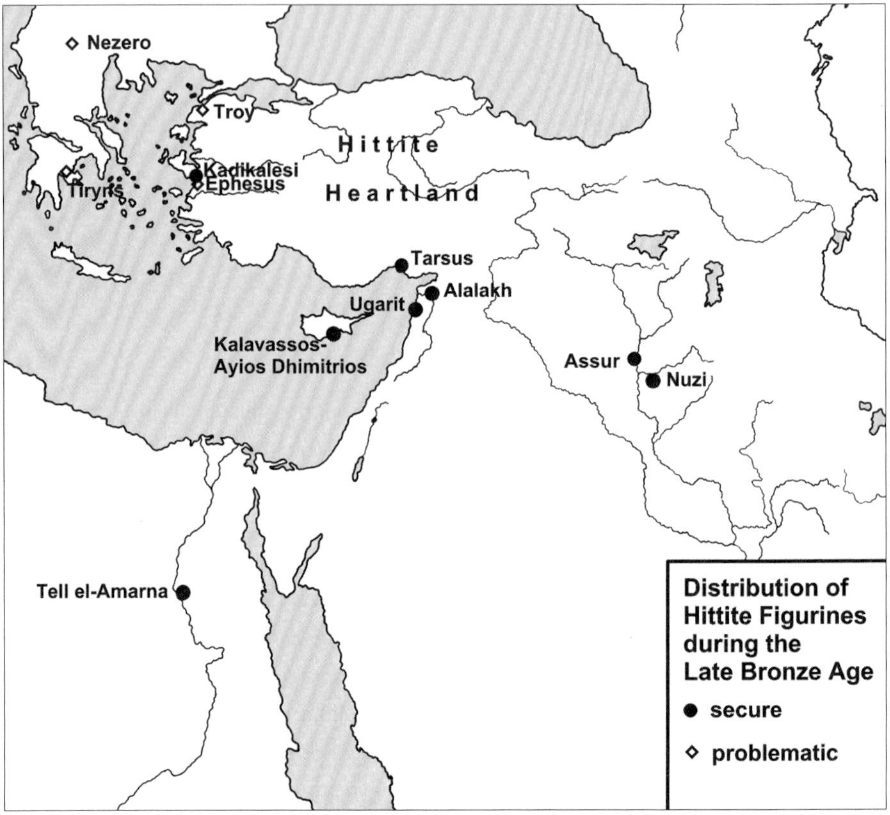

FIG. 1 Distribution of Hittite and allegedly Hittite figurines outside of Central Anatolia

of Hittite artifacts outside of the Hittite heartland is rather negligible.[6] In fact, the majority of Hittite artifacts found outside of the Hittite heartland consist of seals[7] and small figurines of Hittite deities (FIG. 1). It is the latter with which this paper is concerned.

Hittite Figurines

Before we actually can embark on a study of the Hittite figurines found outside Central Anatolia, first it needs to be defined how Hittite figurines differ from comparable objects from neighboring regions. This is a crucial problem, as unfortunately up to now no detailed catalogue of Hittite figurines has been compiled.

6 Genz 2006; Genz 2011.

7 Gorny 1993; Jablonka 2006; Genz 2011.

General overviews on Hittite figurines are provided by Bossert,[8] Bittel,[9] Seeden[10] and Bryce.[11] The finds from Boğazköy have been discussed in detail by Bittel[12] and Boehmer.[13] For the more recent finds from the Upper City, preliminary publications are provided by Neve.[14] A small bronze figurine of a seated goddess was found at Alaca Höyük.[15] Many more Hittite figurines are known from various sites in Central Anatolia, but as most of these unfortunately are surface finds or entirely without provenance,[16] they are only able to add to our knowledge of the iconography of Hittite deities, and contribute nothing to issues such as chronology and contextual interpretation. Almost all extant Hittite figurines depicting deities are rather small, whereas we have hardly any examples of the monumental sculpture that is attested in textual sources.

In addition to the figurines, the numerous depictions of Hittite deities on rock reliefs[17] and detailed descriptions of cult images in Hittite texts[18] are valuable sources for the study of the Hittite pantheon.[19]

Hittite figurines are made of a wide range of materials, are shown in different postures, and with different attributes. Yet a number of elements seem to be characteristic for Hittite figurines, especially the prominent noses and the large ears. High conical caps, often adorned with horns, and upturned shoes are found on many, but not all, examples.

However, given our incomplete knowledge of Hittite figurines, it is no wonder that a number of them from various sites in the Eastern Mediterranean and the Near East previously identified as Hittite have to be discounted or remain doubtful (Fig. 1). These items will be briefly mentioned below, but will not be taken into account for the discussion. Below follows the catalogue of undoubtedly Hittite figurines outside Central Anatolia.

8 Bossert 1942, 61–63.

9 Bittel 1976, 146–149, 159.

10 Seeden 1980, 129–130.

11 Bryce 2002, 156–162.

12 Bittel 1957.

13 Boehmer 1972, 68–70, 171–173; 1979, 29–31, 44–45.

14 Neve 1992, abb. 81–82, 94, 228.

15 Koşay 1951, 24 and pl. LVII.

16 Alp 1961; Ekiz 1995; 1997; 1998; 1999; 2000; İlaslı 1993; Kulaçoğlu 2000; Özgüç 1949; 1999.

17 Bittel *et al.* 1975; Kohlmeyer 1983; Ehringhaus 2005; Seeher 2011.

18 Von Brandenstein 1943; Güterbock 1943; Rost 1961; 1963; Haas 1994, 491–506.

19 Haas 1994.

Catalogue

I. The West (Aegean and Western Anatolia)

I.i. Kadıkalesi near Kuşadası: Bronze figurine of a smiting god with high conical cap. Legs broken off. Preserved height 7.8 cm. Unstratified, found in a Byzantine context.[20]

Canby has identified a fragmentary silver statue from Nezero in Thessaly as Hittite,[21] but Seeden and Cline dispute this identification.[22] The same is true for the figurine of a smiting god from Tiryns,[23] which Cline identifies rather as Syro-Palestinian.[24] A figurine from Troy,[25] while exhibiting Hittite influence, is interpreted rather as a product of a local workshop. A unique figurine from Ephesos showing a standing male in front of a spouted vessel has been interpreted as being of Hittite origin,[26] but doubts remain due to the unique character of the find.[27]

II. Cilicia, Syria and Northern Mesopotamia

II.i. Tarsus: Figurine made of rock crystal, showing a male in a long garment. The hat, presumably made of some other material, is missing. Height 6 cm. Found in a layer containing mainly Late Bronze but also some Iron Age pottery. No identification with a specific deity has been suggested.[28]

II.ii. Alalakh: Lapis lazuli pendant from the cella of the temple, Level II. Statue of a female figure, dressed in a long garment. The lower legs are broken off. The hat, presumably made of some other material, is missing. No scale provided, but rather small.[29]

II.iii. Ugarit (Fig. 2.1): Electrum triad of figures on a plinth: Two male figurines in long robes and high caps flank a figurine with a bull's head and an anthropomorphic body. A loop is attached to the back of the central figure. Height, 3.3 cm.[30]

---

20 Akdeniz 2004.

21 Canby 1969.

22 Seeden 1980, 122; Cline 1991, 135.

23 Canby 1969.

24 Cline 1991, 138.

25 Mellink and Strahan 1998.

26 Hanfman 1962.

27 Schachner and Meriç 2000, 97 and n.35; Akdeniz 2004, 27–28.

28 Goldman 1956, 342–344 and fig. 456.

29 Woolley 1955, 81 and pl. LXIXl.

30 Schaeffer 1956, 94–95 and fig. 113.

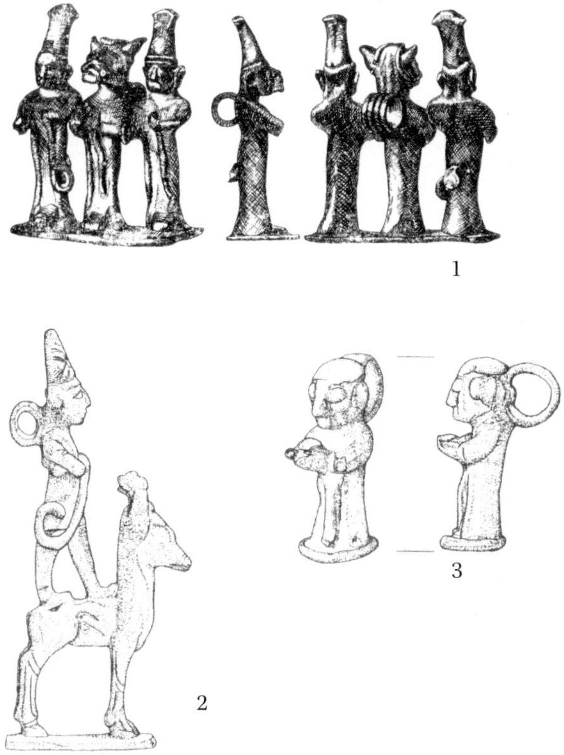

Fig. 2

1 Electron triad from Ugarit (after Schaeffer 1956, fig. 113);
2 Silver figurine from Kalavassos-Ayios Dhimitrios (after Genz 2011, fig. 5.1);
3 Silver figurine from Tell el-Amarna (after Genz 2011, fig. 5.2)

II.iv. Assur: Lapis lazuli relief, showing a male figure in a short tunic and a conical cap, carrying a hare and a bird of prey. Legs are broken off. Preserved height 2.25 cm. Found in the postament of the Ištar temple in Assur in a context dated to the 13th century BC.[31] Identified as the god of the wilderness.[32]

II.v. Nuzi: Small figurine probably made of ivory. The figurine wears a horned crown and a cutaway coat. Only one foot has a shoe, while the second one is bare. In her hands the figurine carries an axe and an unidentified object. Height: 8.2 cm. Found in the cella of Temple A, Stratum II.[33] Identified as Ištar.[34] Traditionally Stratum II has been dated to the 15th century BC, based on a clay tablet bearing the seal impression of Šauštatar.[35] However, Stein argues that the seal of Šauštatar

31 Andrae 1924, 9–10 and pl. 8:1; Bossert 1942, 60 and fig. 595; Güterbock 1943, 315; von der Osten-Sacken 1988, 65.

32 Güterbock 1943, 315; von der Osten-Sacken 1988, 65.

33 Mellink 1964.

34 Mellink 1964, 162–163.

35 Mellink 1964, 155.

was used as a dynastic seal, and therefore dates Stratum II from the mid-14th to the 13th centuries BC.[36]

III. Cyprus

III.i. Kalavassos-Ayios Dhimitrios (Fig. 2.2): Silver figurine of a god with a short tunic and a high conical cap, carrying a curved staff, standing on a stag. Height 6.2 cm. A loop is attached to the back of the figurine. From tomb 12. The tomb contained the skeletons of three infants and one child of 5–6 years, as well as seven pottery vessels, 49 *astragalii* and a gold earring, in addition to the figurine.[37] The figurine has been identified as the god of the wilderness.[38]

IV. Egypt

IV.i. Tell el-Amarna (Fig. 2.3): Silver figurine of a male in a long dress and with a flat golden cap, holding a bowl or a loaf of bread in his extended right hand. Height 2.86 cm. Found in a jar with gold and silver ingots and scrap silver buried in the courtyard of House T36.63, in the northern suburb of Tell el-Amarna. The contents of the jar are interpreted either as a jeweler's hoard or a thief's loot.[39]

Discussion

The figurines listed in the catalogue above can be identified as representations of Hittite deities with reasonable certainty, although in many cases the identification with specific deities of the Hittite pantheon is not possible. Most of these statues were made of precious materials, such as electrum, silver, lapis lazuli, rock crystal or ivory. Another common feature is their extremely small size, never exceeding 10 cm in height, which makes them easily portable. Moreover, several of the statues (Ugarit, Kalavassos-Ayios Dhimitrios, Tell el-Amarna) have loops on their backs, suggesting that they were worn as pendants. Bell provides a list of further Hittite statuettes with suspension loops.[40] The statuettes seem to have been worn frequently, as suggested by traces of heavy wear on the loop of the statuette from Tell el-Amarna.[41]

Despite the fact that they were made of precious materials, the small size of the figurines precludes the idea that they were objects of trade or official diplo-

36 Stein 1989.

37 South 1997, 163 and pl. XV:1; Kozal 2002, 657.

38 Kozal 2002, 653.

39 Bell 1986.

40 Bell 1986, 146.

41 Bell 1986, 145.

matic gifts. We do have textual evidence that statues of deities were exchanged: for instance, statues of gods were brought from Ahhiyawa and Lazpa to Hatti to cure the speech affliction of Muršili II.[42] A similar case is attested in EA 23,[43] where the Mitannian king Tušratta sends an image of Šauška of Niniveh to Egypt to assist in healing Amenhotep III. However, in these cases, larger images presumably were involved. In the Amarna letters statues are frequently mentioned as diplomatic gifts, for instance in EA 26 and EA 41.[44] Unfortunately it remains unclear whether these are statues of deities or not. In cases where the weight of objects is provided, like in EA 41,[45] the quantities of gold or silver are quite considerable, making it highly unlikely that the extremely small statues discussed here were part of the diplomatic gift exchange.

It is suggested here to interpret these statues as the personal protective deities of Hittites traveling abroad. The small size of the statues suggests that they were personal items, and the loops attested in several cases make it most likely that they were worn as pendants.

In the textual sources, Hittite merchants are hardly attested,[46] making it unlikely that these items can be interpreted as reflecting Hittite trade activities. Moreover, the generally valuable materials suggest that these statues were the possessions of high-ranking individuals. While this does not necessarily rule out merchants, it is more plausible to identify the owners of these statues as Hittite officials, who are widely attested in the textual sources as envoys or emissaries.[47] It is certainly not a coincidence that many of these items were found in important political centers such as Ugarit, Assur and Tell el-Amarna. How the objects ended up in these places is of course entirely a matter of speculation. Due to their small size, such objects in rare cases may have been lost. In the cases of Alalakh, Nuzi and Assur, where the statues were found in temples, they may have been deposited as offerings to ensure safe travel or success in the diplomatic missions. In some cases we know that negotiations dragged on for a considerable time,[48] so some of the envoys may have died abroad. In other cases the contexts provide even less clear information. The statuette from Tell el-Amarna was found in a hoard of scrap metal, ready for recycling.[49] How the statuette from Kalavassos-Ayios Dhimitrios

42 Bryce 2002, 168.

43 Moran 1992, 61–62; Haas 1994, 346.

44 Moran 1992, 84–90 and 114–115.

45 Moran 1992, 114.

46 Klengel 1979; Hoffner 2001; Bryce 2002, 87–97; Genz 2011, 322.

47 Genz 2011, 323; for general comments see Oller 1995.

48 Oller 1995, 1470.

49 Bell 1986, 150–151.

came to be included in a child's tomb remains a complete enigma. There is definitely no further Hittite material from the tomb. The examples from Tarsus and Kadıkalesi unfortunately come from disturbed contexts, thus nothing can be said about their original context.

Traveling to foreign destinations was certainly seen as a challenge, not only by the Hittites. In addition to the actual dangers of the voyage such as storms or brigands,[50] the travelers had to face many unknown encounters such as incomprehensible languages, unfamiliar customs, or strange food, not to mention the additional stress placed on diplomatic envoys concerning the success of their respective missions. It is therefore not surprising that travelers would have tried to ensure divine protection. The most prominent example is the case of Wen-Amun, an Egyptian priest who during the 21st Dynasty had to travel from Karnak to Byblos to obtain cedar wood for the temple of Amun. He took a statue of Amun-of-the-Road on his journey.[51] Archaeological evidence may be provided by the discovery of a statue of a goddess on the Uluburun ship, which has been interpreted as the ship's protective goddess.[52]

The Hittites are known as a deeply religious people,[53] and for several kings the personal protective deities are known, for instance Ištar for Hattušili III[54] or Šarruma for Tudhaliya IV.[55] It certainly can be assumed that other high-ranking Hittites adhered to the same custom.[56] In this respect it is certainly interesting to add a note on the identification of the deities depicted. Both the statues from Assur and from Kalavassos-Ayios Dhimitrios depict the God of the Wilderness, which is widely seen as a protective god.[57] The same is possibly true for the triad from Ugarit.[58]

In conclusion, the wide geographical distribution of small statues of clearly Hittite origin should most likely be interpreted in the light of Hittite diplomatic activities, where these items served as the protective deities for Hittite envoys and messengers. The same interpretation certainly holds true also for Hittite seals, which have an even wider distribution outside the Hittite heartland.[59] As these

50 Oller 1995, 1467.

51 Wilson 1969, 26.

52 Pulak 1997, 246.

53 Bryce 2002, 134–162.

54 Bryce 2002, 146.

55 Haas 1994, 391; Bryce 2002, 137.

56 Bryce 2002, 148.

57 Von der Osten-Sacken 1988; Haas 1994, 452–454.

58 Haas 1994, 480.

59 Gorny 1993; Singer 1995; Jablonka 2006.

seals do not only contain the names, but often also the titles of their owners, a strong case can be made to identify them as belonging to high-ranking officials, precisely the group from which envoys and emissaries were chosen.[60]

60 Singer 1995, 91–91.

REFERENCES

Akdeniz, E., "Kuşadası Kadıkalesi Kazısında Bir Hitit Heykelciği." *Olba* 9 (2004): 21–56.

Alp, S., "Amasya Civarında Bulunan Bir Hitit Heykelciği ve Diğer Hitit Eserleri." *Anatolia* 6 (1961): 191–216.

Andrae, W., *Hethitische Inschriften auf Bleistreifen aus Assur.* Leipzig: WVDOG, 1924.

Åström, P., *The Chronology of Base Ring Ware and Bichrome Wheel-made Ware*. Stockholm: The Royal Academy of Letters, History and Antiquities, 2001.

Bell, M.R., "A Hittite Pendant from Amarna." *American Journal of Archaeology* 90 (1986): 143–151.

Bittel, K., "Einige Funde hethitischer Plastik" in *Boğazköy III. Funde aus den Grabungen 1952–1955,* ed. by K. Bittel, 29–31. Berlin: Abhandlungen der deustchen Orientgesellschaft 2, 1957.

———. *Die Hethiter. Die Kunst Anatoliens vom Ende des 3. bis zum Anfang des 1. Jahrtausends vor Christus.* Munich: Beck, 1976.

Bittel, K., J. Boessneck, B. Damm, H. G. Güterbock, H. Hauptmann, R. Naumann and W. Schirmer, *Das Hethitische Felsheiligtum Yazilikaya* (*Boğazköy-Hattuša IX*). Berlin: Gebrüder Mann Verlag, 1975.

Boehmer, R. M., *Die Kleinfunde von Boğazköy* (*Boğazköy-Hattuša VII*). Berlin: Gebrüder Mann Verlag, 1972.

———. *Die Kleinfunde aus der Unterstadt von Boğazköy* (*Boğazköy-Hattuša X*). Berlin: Gebrüder Man Verlag, 1979.

Bossert, H. T., *Altanatolien. Kunst und Handwerk in Kleinasien von den Anfängen bis zum völligen Aufgehen in der griechischen Kultur.* Berlin: Bovon, 1942.

Bryce, T. R., *The Kingdom of the Hittites*. Oxford: Oxford University Press, 1998.

———. *Life and Society in the Hittite World.* Oxford: Oxford University Press, 2002.

Canby, J. V., "Some Hittite Figurines in the Aegean." *Hesperia* 38 (1969): 141–149.

Cline, E. H., "Hittite Objects in the Bronze Age Aegean." *Anatolian Studies* 41 (1991): 133–143.

———. *Sailing the Wine-Dark Sea: International Trade and the Late Bronze Age Aegean* (BAR International Series 591). Oxford: British Archaeological Reports, 2009.

Ehringhaus, H., *Götter Herrscher Inschriften. Die Felsreliefs der hethitischen Großreichszeit in der Türkei.* Mainz am Rhein: Verlag Philipp von Zabern in Wissenschaftliche Buchgesellschaft, 2005.

Ekiz, H. H., "Afyon Müzesi'nde Bulunan bir Hitit Heykelciği." *Anadolu Medeniyetleri Müzesi 1994 Yıllığı* (1995): 159–163.

———. "Ankara Anadolu Medeniyetleri, Çorum, Karaman ve Konya Müzeleri'nde Bulunan Bazı Tanrı Heykelcikleri." *Anadolu Medeniyetleri Müzesi 1996 Yıllığı* (1997): 161–172.

———. "Özel Bir Koleksiyonda Bulunan Bir Grup Tanrı Heykelciği." *Anadolu Medeniyetleri Müzesi 1997 Yıllığı* (1998): 79–93.

———. "Gaziantep Müzesi'nde Bulunan Hayvan Üstünde Duran İki Tanrı Heykelciği." *Anadolu Medeniyetleri Müzesi 1998 Yıllığı* (1999): 131–140.

———. "Anadolu Medeniyetleri Müzesi'nde Bulunan Üç Hitit Heykelciği." *Anadolu Medeniyetleri Müzesi 1999 Yıllığı* (2000): 65–75.

Genz, H., "Hethitische Präsenz im spätbronzezeitlichen Syrien: die archäologische Evidenz." *Baghdader Mitteilungen* 37 (2006): 157–167.

———. "Foreign Contacts of the Hittites" in *Insights into Hittite History and Archaeology* (*Colloquia Antiqua 2*), ed. by H. Genz and D. P. Mielke, 301–331. Leuven: Peeters, 2011.

Goldman, H., *Excavations at Gözlü Kule, Tarsus II. From the Neolithic through the Bronze Age*. Princeton: Princeton University Press, 1956.

Gorny, R. L., "The Biconvex Seals of Alişar Höyük." *Anatolian Studies* 43 (1993): 163–191.

Güterbock, H.G., "Eti Tanrı Tasvirleri ile Tanrı Adları / Hethitische Götterdarstellungen und Göttemamen." *Belleten* 7 (1943): 273–293, 295–317.

Haas, V., *Geschichte der hethitischen Religion* (HdO I, 15). Leiden: Brill, 1994.

Hanfmann, G.M.A. ,"A 'Hittite' Priest from Ephesus." *American Journal of Archaeology* 66 (1962): 1–4.

Hasel, M.G., *Domination and Resistance. Egyptian Military Activity in the Southern Levant, ca. 1300–1185 BC*. Leiden: Brill, 1998.

Higginbotham, C.R., *Egyptianization and Elite Emulation in Ramesside Palestine. Governance and Accommodation on the Imperial Periphery* (Culture and History of the Ancient Near East Vol. 2). Leiden: Brill, 2000.

Hoffner, H.A., "Some Thoughts on Merchants and Trade in the Hittite Kingdom" in *Kulturgeschichten. Altorientalische Studien für Volkert Haas zum 65. Geburtstag*, ed. by T. Richter, D. Prechel and J. Klinger, 179–189. Saarbrücken: Geburtstag, 2001.

İlaslı, A., "A Hittite Statue Found in the Area of Ahurhisar" in *Aspects of Art and Iconography: Anatolia and its Neighbors. Studies in Honor of Nimet Özgüç*, ed. by M. J. Mellink, E. Porada and T. Özgüç. 301–308. Ankara: Türk Tarih Kurumu Basımevi, 1993.

Jablonka, P., "Emar und Troia: Zur Verbreitung hethitischer Hieroglyphensiegel." *Baghdader Mitteilungen* 37 (2006): 511–529.

Karageorghis, V. (ed.). *The White Slip Ware of Late Bronze Age Cyprus*. Österreichische Akademie der Wissenschaften, Denkschriften XX. Vienna: Verlag der Österreichischen Akademie der Wissenschaften, 2001.

Klengel, H., "Handel und Kaufleute im hethitischen Reich." *Altorientalische Forschungen* 6 (1979): 165–174.

———. *Geschichte des hethitischen Reiches* (HdO I, 34). Leiden: Brill, 1999.

Kohlmeyer, K., "Felsbilder der hethitischen Grossreichszeit." *Acta Praehistorica et Archaeologica* 15 (1983): 7–53.

Koşay, H. Z. *Alaca-Höyük Kazısı 1937–1939.* Ankara: Türk Tarih Kurumu Basımevi, 1951.

Kozal, E., "Hethitische und hethitisch beeinflußte Objekte aus Zypern" in *Mauerschau. Festschrift für Manfred Korfmann*, ed. by R. Aslan, S. Blum, G. Kastl, F. Schweizer and D. Thumm, 651–661. Remshalden-Grunbach: Bernhard Albert Greiner, 2002.

Kulaçoğlu, B., "Anadolu Medeniyetleri Müzesi Altın Serpuşlu Gümüş Tanrı Heykelciği." *Anadolu Medeniyetleri Müzesi 1999 Yıllığı* (2000): 125–130.

Leonard, A., *An Index to the Late Bronze Age Aegean Pottery from Syria and Palestine.* Studies in Mediterranean Archaeology 114. Jonsered: Paul Aströms Forlag, 1994.

Mellink, M. J., "A Hittite Figurine from Nuzi" in *Vorderasiatische Archäologie. Studien und Aufsätze Anton Moortgat zum fünfundsechzigsten Geburtstag gewidmet von Kollegen, Schülern und Freunden*, ed. by K. Bittel, E. Heinrich, B. Hrouda and W. Nagel, 155–164. Berlin, 1964.

Mellink, M.J. and D. Strahan, "The Bronze Figurine from Troia Level VIIa." *Studia Troica* 8 (1998): 141–149.

Moran, W.L., *The Amarna Letters.* Baltimore: Johns Hopkins University Press, 1992.

Neve, P., *Hattuša. Stadt der Götter und Tempel.* Mainz am Rhein: Philipp von Zabern in der Wissenschaftlichen Buchgesellschaft, 1992.

Oller, G.H., "Messengers and Ambassadors in Ancient Western Asia" in *Civilizations of the Ancient East III*, ed. by J. M. Sasson, 1465–1473. New York: Charles Scribner's Sons, 1995.

Özgüç, N., "Dövlek Köyü'nden (Şarkışla İlçesi) Getirilen Eti Heykelciği." *Türk Tarih Arkeologya ve Etnografya Dergisi* 5 (1949): 45–52.

Özgüç, T., "The Metal Figurines of Two Hittite Gods" in *Essays on Ancient Anatolia, Bulletin of the Middle Eastern Culture Center in Japan XI,* ed. by T. Mikasa, 23–38. Wiesbaden: Harrassowitz Verlag, 1999.

Pulak C., "The Uluburun Shipwreck" in *Res Maritimae: Cyprus and the Eastern Mediterranean from Prehistory to Late Antiquity*, ed. by S. Swiny, R. L. Hohlfelder and H. W. Swiny, 233–262. Atlanta: American Schools of Oriental Research, 1997.

Rost L., "Zu den hethitischen Bildbeschreibungen, 1. Teil." *Mitteilungen des Instituts für Orientforschung* 8 (1961): 161–217.

———. "Zu den hethitischen Bildbeschreibungen, 2. Teil." *Mitteilungen des Instituts für Orientforschung* 9 (1963): 175–239.

Schachner, A. and R. Meriç, "Ein Stempelsiegel des späten 2. Jahrtausends v. Chr. aus Metropolis in Ionien." *Studi Micenei ed Egeo-Anatolici* 42 (2000): 85–102.

Schaeffer, C. F. A., "Matériaux pour l'étude des relations entre Ugarit et le Hatti." *Ugaritica* 3 (1956): 1–96.

Seeden, H., *The Standing Armed Figurines of the Levant.* Prähistorische Bronzefunde 1.1. Munich: Beck, 1980.

Seeher, J., *Götter in Stein gehauen. Das hethitische Felsheiligtum von Yazılıkaya.* Istanbul: Ege Yayınları, 2011.

Singer, I., "A Hittite Seal from Megiddo." *Biblical Archaeologist* 58 (1995): 91–93.

South, A. K., "Kalavassos-Ayios Dhimitrios 1992–1996." *Report of the Department of Antiquities of Cyprus 1997* (1997): 151–173.

Stein, D., "A Reappraisal of the 'Šauštatar Letter' from Nuzi." *Zeitschrift für Assyriologie und Vorderasiatische Archäologie* 79/1 (1989): 36–60.

van Wijngaarden, G.J., *Use and Appreciation of Mycenaean Pottery: In the Levant, Cyprus and Italy* (*ca. 1600–1200 BC*). Amsterdam: Amsterdam University Press, 2002.

von Brandenstein, C.G., "Hethitische Götter nach Bildbeschreibungen in Keilschrifttexten." *Mitteilungen der Vorderasiatisch-Ägyptischen Gesellschaft* 46/2 (1943).

von der Osten-Sacken, E., "Der kleinasiatische Gott der Wildflur." *Istanbuler Mitteilungen* 38 (1988): 63–81.

Wilson, J.A., "Egyptian Myths, Tales and Mortuary Texts" in *Ancient Near Eastern Texts Relating to the Old Testament,* ed. by J. B. Pritchard, 3–36. Princeton: Princeton University Press, 1969.

Woolley, L., *Alalakh. An Account of the Excavations at Tell Atchana in the Hatay, 1937–1949.* London: Society of Antiquaries, 1955.

"A Goatherd Shall Not Enter!"
Observations on Pastoralism and Mobility in Hittite Anatolia

N. İlgi Gerçek[1]

It is my honor to present this contribution to Marie-Henriette and Charles Gates in gratitude for the instruction and guidance I received from them as a student at Bilkent University and ever since.

Abstract

Mobile pastoralists are well documented in the history of Anatolia, where the natural environment, especially in its mountainous regions, presents the ideal conditions for the existence of various forms of mobile pastoralism. Historically attested forms of mobility range from transhumance—where only part of the population moves seasonally with the herds—to more intensive forms of pastoral nomadism. Although the importance of pastoralism for the economy of Hittite Anatolia is undisputed, the degree to which pastoralism was accompanied by mobility has not been explored. In secondary literature, mobility has traditionally been mentioned mainly in connection with the Kaška of the Black Sea region. Scholars have portrayed the Kaška as a tribally organized (semi-)nomadic population, and considered them to be the antithesis of the agrarian Hittite state in their social, political, and economic organization. This contribution investigates mobility and pastoralism in Hittite Anatolia with the aim of better understanding their role in Hittite economy and politics. It reconsiders the extent to which mobility accompanied pastoral activities in the Hittite heartland and its peripheries, and explores the strategies employed by the Hittite state in their interactions with mobile population groups. Hittite texts will form the focus of the analysis, especially the agreements with peripheral populations, administrative letters from Maşat Höyük, and the recently published land donation documents (*Landschenkungsurkunden*).

1 Department of Ancient Languages and Cultures, Faculty of Letters, İstanbul University, Ordu Cad. No. 196, 34459 Laleli, İstanbul, Turkey.
I thank the Center for Canon and Identity Formation (University of Copenhagen) for the post-doctoral fellowship that made this research possible. I also thank Gary Beckman for reading and commenting on a draft of this paper. All oversights and errors are my own. Abbreviations follow the *Chicago Hittite Dictionary*.

Introduction

Mobile pastoralists are well documented in the history of Anatolia, where the natural environment, especially in its mountainous regions, presents ideal conditions for pastoralist and agrarian economies.[2] Mobile pastoralism as a subsistence strategy is thought to have existed in this region since prehistoric periods.[3] Still, while mobile pastoralism has become a sub-field in its own right in Assyriology, this topic has remained an underexplored area in Anatolian studies, particularly Hittitology.[4]

Despite the dearth of economic documents from Hittite archives, it is fairly clear that pastoralism was an important component of the Hittite economy.[5] The prevalent assumption in Hittitological literature is that pastoralism was not accompanied by mobility in the Land of Ḫatti (i.e., the core territory of the Hittite state corresponding roughly to the central Anatolian plateau), and that only certain populations on the peripheries of Ḫatti practiced mobile pastoralism.[6] As a subsistence strategy and way-of-life, mobile pastoralism has traditionally been associated with the Kaška of the Black Sea region, and with population groups

2 The best-documented period of mobile pastoralism in Anatolia starts with the large-scale movement of Turkic mobile pastoralists into this region during the 11th century CE. Southern Anatolia and the Lake District, the eastern and southeastern highlands, as well as the mountainous areas of the Black Sea Region have been, and still are to some extent, inhabited by Türkmen, Yörük, Kurdish, and Zaza pastoralists; Yakar 2006, 45.

3 According to Yakar (2006, 46), these conditions existed in Anatolia since the early Holocene, and diverse subsistence strategies such as agriculture and mobile pastoralism may have existed together as early as the Neolithic period. Similarly, Schachner 2012, 30.

4 Also noted in Simon 2010, 545. The most important contributions on this topic are Simon 2010; Yakar 1990, 2000, 2006, 2008. Archaeological investigations of mobile pastoralism in Bronze Age Anatolia appear to have focused on eastern and southeastern Anatolia; see Yakar 2006, 53–58 with further references; Simon 2010 (on southern Anatolia during the LBA). For archaeological investigations of mobile pastoralism in other periods in Anatolia see Cribb 1991; Bernbeck 2008; Düring 2011; Hammer 2014.

5 For the place of pastoralism in Hittite economy and culture, see Beckman 1988; Schachner 2012; Yakar 2000. Beckman's article predates the publishing of the Maşat Höyük texts (treated in detail below), which brought to light more evidence on pastoralism in Ḫatti. In his recent contributions to the study of Hittite economy, Klengel (2005, 2006, 2007) treats the place of animal husbandry and hunting within the Hittite economy. His discussion revolves more around the types of animals kept, their uses, and their prices. His only remark on the question of mobility is that sometime in the 3rd millennium BCE, an economic system similar to the *yayla* pattern was developed in Anatolia as a consequence of human impact on the natural environment, through which the forests and vegetation gave way to grasslands or steppes due to intensive use of forests.

6 Beckman 1988, 40–41. Beckman maintains that in Ḫatti, animals were kept in close proximity to or on the peripheries of the settled areas, what he calls "close-in grazing."

inhabiting the mountainous regions of Southern Anatolia (known in historical sources as Kizzuwatna, Tarḫuntašša, and Lukka). However, the textual and archaeological evidence pertaining to mobility and pastoralism in Hittite Anatolia, admittedly scarce and scattered, has not been investigated methodically.[7] Several assumptions and generalizations concerning mobile pastoralists have not been substantiated either by textual or archaeological evidence.[8]

This study collects and analyses Hittite textual evidence pertaining to mobility and pastoralism, some well known in secondary scholarship, and some less thoroughly studied. It investigates the role of (mobile) pastoralism in the Hittite economy and politics, and explores the Hittite state's interactions with pastoralists. The ultimate aim of this contribution is to provide a base for further study of pastoralism and mobility in LBA Anatolia. After a brief explanation of some terms and concepts employed in the discussion, I will examine Hittite terminology related to (nomadic) tribes; the textual evidence on pastoralism in the Black Sea region and southern Anatolia (corresponding to Tarḫuntašša, Kizzuwatna, and Lukka[9]); and finally, the evidence from the land donation documents, which mainly concern central Anatolia.

Mobile pastoralism (or pastoral nomadism) is a specialized herding occupation which necessitates the movement of the whole or a part of a community with the herds.[10] In recent years, anthropologists have moved away from rigorous typological classification of mobile pastoralists in favor of a view of mobile pastoralism as a continuum of social and economic activities. These activities may range from intensive pursuit of pastoral activities to emphasis on agricultural production.[11] In this study, I use "mobile pastoralism" as a general category subsuming various types of pastoralist strategies. Transhumance is a general term used to indicate seasonal movement with herds, and vertical transhumance indicates that the movement is occurring in mountainous areas.[12] In Anatolian contexts, the seasonal occupation

7 Though Yakar uses textual information from a variety of different sources in his valuable study *Ethnoarchaeology of Anatolia* (2000), his discussion of mobile pastoralism relies more on ethnographic data.

8 Simon (2010) makes a similar observation on the presumed tribal organization and nomadism of "the Lukka people."

9 Lukka will be left out of the discussion due to the scarcity of textual evidence, see Simon 2010.

10 For terminology related to pastoral nomadism see Khazanov 1994, 17–25; Wendrich and Barnard 2008, 7–10.

11 Szuchman 2009, 3; Wendrich and Barnard 2008, 8–9.

12 Wendrich and Barnard 2008, 7–8. Some scholars maintain that transhumance and *yayla* pastoralism are not inherently nomadic, and that the key variable in determining mobility is the participation of the community in the movement of the herds; Yakar 2000, 192–198; Khazanov 1994, 22–23.

of the highlands for pasturage and small-scale agriculture is often called *yayla* (Turkish for plateau) pastoralism (and agriculture).[13]

The Hittite Word for (Nomadic) Tribe?

The logogram ÉRIN.MEŠ *ŠUTU*[14] and its possible Hittite equivalent *latti-* are commonly thought to denote "tribe" or "tribal troop(s)," and possibly "nomadic tribes."[15] The meaning of the word is derived from the logogram's connection—first proposed by Güterbock—to mobile pastoralist groups called *Sutû*, who appear notably in Mari texts.[16] Güterbock suggested that when the Hittites adopted this term, it no longer referred to the *Sutû* of northern Syria, but meant, more generally, "tribe" or "tribal troop." The connection between (ÉRIN.MEŠ) *ŠUTU* and *latti-* was established through the discovery of two duplicate ritual fragments (see below), in which *latti-* in one fragment (KBo 53.36 3'-4') corresponded to ŠU-TUM in the other (KUB 46.46 + Bo 4171 obv.? 13'-14').[17] This ŠU-TUM was then interpreted by Hoffner to be the same as (ÉRIN.MEŠ) *ŠUTU*. Thus, the CHD renders *latti-*/(ÉRIN.MEŠ *ŠUTU*) as "1. tribal troop(s), tribe(?) 2. (a feature of the Exta)."[18] Puhvel, on the other hand, has translated the word as "nomad population, nomad military (unit); nomad roaming ground, habitat; local region (in extispicy)" in the HED, with no further justification.[19]

The correspondence between *latti-* and (ÉRIN.MEŠ) *ŠUTU*, which is also supported by the similarities in how they are used in extispicy,[20] is plausible. However, I find the rendition of *latti*/*ŠUTU* as "tribe" or "tribal troop" (with or without the

---

13 Khazanov 1994, 23–24; Schachner 2012, 30–31; Yakar 2000, 220.

14 ÉRIN.MEŠ *ŠUTU* has the variant spellings ÉRIN.MEŠ *Š/S/ZUTE* in the Deeds of Šuppiluliuma, which are standardized to ÉRIN.MEŠ *ŠUTU* in the Annals of Muršili. For a history of scholarship on ÉRIN.MEŠ *ŠUTU* see Hoffner 1979.

15 *Cf.* Beal 1992, 103–107 (see below). On *latti-*/ÉRIN.MEŠ *ŠUTU* see, CHD L s.v. *latti-;* HED L s.v. *latti-*; Hoffner 1979; Beal 1992, 104–108.

16 Güterbock 1956, 62, n. c. On the *Sutû*, see Heltzer 1981.

17 The fragments belong to a ritual for the Sun-goddess of the Earth (CTH 448). For a recent edition see Görke 2012, www.hethiter.net, under CTH 448.2.2.1.

18 The CHD (L, pp. 48–49) suggests that *latti-*/*ŠUTU* bands may have consisted of nomads (thanks to the logogram's connection to the Suteans), however, the suggestion seems to apply only to the Kaška.

19 CHD L, s.v. *latti-*; HED L, s.v. *latti-* (Puhvel 2001, 64–67). Puhvel even suggests that *latti-* comes from the same root as Greek *νομάδ-* (2001, 66). In his review of HED L, Hoffner (2003, 623) has criticized Puhvel for his treatment of *latti-*, noting that the examples used have already been listed in CHD L, and that they "contribute nothing to establishing either the etymology or the morphology of the word."

20 Hoffner 1979, 264; Schuol 1994, 284.

connotation "nomadic") misleading, and in numerous contexts, inappropriate. "Tribe" is a contested category in the social sciences, implying a distinct socio-political organization, economy, and kinship structure whose presence is not warranted by the available evidence.[21] The contexts in which the word *latti-* and the logogram (ÉRIN.MEŠ) *ŠUTU* appear, as well as their restricted distribution, urges us to interpret their usage and meaning differently.[22]

The logogram (ÉRIN.MEŠ) *ŠUTU*, attested more frequently than *latti-*, appears primarily in the Deeds of Šuppiluliuma and the Annals of Muršili;[23] less frequently in oracle reports and letters;[24] and once in a fragmentary ritual for the Sun-goddess of the Earth. It is used in all clear contexts (with one possible exception mentioned below) in reference to fighting units. In most instances it refers to Kaška fighting units.[25]

The word *latti-*, on the other hand, is attested once in a letter from Maşat Höyük (HKM 46), and twice in *taknaz dā-* (literally "taking from the earth") and substitute rituals for the Sun-goddess of the Earth:

> 1. The enemy has crossed (the frontier?) in two places in large numbers. One *latti* crossed at the town Išteruwa; one *latti* crossed at the town Zišpa.[26]
>
> 2. When one is finished, one writes his *latti* on [2 wooden tablets].[27]

---

21 Kamp and Yoffee 1980, 88–89; Parkinson 2002; Szuchman 2009, 4–5; Porter 2012. The problem has also to do with the definition of the term "tribe," which has been used in two main ways in the social sciences: one usage refers to a non-hierarchical society on an evolutionary trajectory of political systems (emphasizing its political characteristics), and the other refers to groups bound by a kinship structure within or on the peripheries of states; Emberling 1997, 306. In Hittitological literature the use of the term "tribe" is not accompanied by any explanation, but seems to refer loosely to societies without central political institutions.

22 The attestations of ÉRIN.MEŠ *ŠUTU* and *latti-* in extispicy will not be taken into account in the following discussion, since they do not give us any clues about their meaning.

23 For the Deeds of Šuppiluliuma (CTH 40) see Güterbock 1956; del Monte 2009; for the Annals of Muršili II (CTH 61.I and 61.II) see Goetze 1933; Grélois 1988. Note that both texts were composed during the reign of Muršili II.

24 For the attestations, see CHD L s.v. *latti-*, 47–49 and HED L s.v. *latti-*, 64–66.

25 The ÉRIN.MEŠ *ŠUTU* featured in the Annals of Muršili II were employed in the Hittite army. The term seems to have been used in reference to troops of Arzawa as well.

26 HKM 46 3–7: *ka-a-ša-kán* LÚ.KÚR *pa-an-ga-ri-it* / 2 *AŠ-RA za-a-i*[*š*] *nu-kán* 1-*iš* / *la-at-ti-iš I-NA* ^{URU}*Iš-te-ru-wa* / *za-a-iš* 1-*iš-ma-kán la-at-ti-iš* / *I-NA* ^{URU}*Zi-iš-pa za-iš*. For text and translation see Alp 1991, 200–203, 324; Hoffner 2009, 174, with further references. The letter goes on to describe how the enemy has vanished without a trace.

27 KUB 17.18 iii 14–15: GIM-*an-ma ze-en-*⸢*na-an-zi nam-ma*⸣ *la-at-ti-en-š*[*i*$^{?}$*-in*$^{?}$] / [*I-NA* 2 GIŠ.ḪUR *g*]*ul-ša-an-zi*. "When they are finished" (iii 14) refers to the first four days of

3.a. [...h]is *latt*[*i*...] his *latti* [...].[28]
b. [...] his *ŠUTU* in front [...] he places his *ŠUTU* in front [...].[29]

In HKM 46 (1) *latti-* refers to two large groups of the enemy. These groups were most likely raiding parties, since they were considered a threat: in lines 15–17 of the same letter, Adad-bēlī, the writer of the letter, asks the king to send a lord so that the countryside would not be damaged by the enemy.[30]

In ritual contexts (2, 3.a and b), *latti-* has been translated as "tribe" ("Stamm," "Sippe").[31] Taracha has suggested that *ŠUTU/latti-* refers to the "Ahnenfiguren," which identify the substitute as "members of the family," and which play an important role in *taknaz dā-* and substitute rituals.[32] Indeed, the function of *latti-* in the ritual seems to be to identify the ritual patient. However, the specific meaning "tribe" is derived not from the context, but from the assumption that *ŠUTU* means "tribe." "Group" or "(extended) family" might be more appropriate translations here.

Finally, in trying to understand the denotation of *latti-*/ÉRIN.MEŠ *ŠUTU*, it is important to note that neither is used to refer to Kaška groups in any of the agreements Hittite kings concluded with them (CTH 138–140, see below). In other words, ÉRIN.MEŠ *ŠUTU* or *latti-* are not used to identify social groupings among the Kaška.[33]

Based on the evidence presented above, I suggest that when the term ÉRIN. MEŠ *ŠUTU* entered the Hittite writing system, it referred to contingents of soldiers (i.e., troops) consisting of mercenaries.[34] As Beal suggested, it is possible that

---

the ritual, described in the preceding paragraphs. The lines that follow (iii 15–21) reveal that the one tablet is bound to a sheep and one to a goat, after which a pit is dug out. The sheep and goat are placed (bound and alive) into pits for the Sun-goddess of the Earth and the male Sun-god respectively.

28 KBo 53.36 3'-4'.

29 KUB 46.46 (Bo 760) + Bo 4171 13'-14': [...]x *a-pé-el ŠU-TUM pé-ra-an* 14') [...*a-p*]*é-el ŠU-TUM pé-ra-an ti-an-zi*. We may find the same expression, though in fragmentary context, in Bo 3385 i 4'-5': [*apē*]*l ŠUTUM* [*peran*] *ti*[*anzi*]; see Taracha 2000, 111–112.

30 Hoffner (2009, 174) notes that the two *latti*s of the enemy may have been pastoralists leading their flocks to summer pastures. Hoffner's alternative interpretation is based on his assumption that the Kaška were "sedentary pastoral communities"; more on the Kaška below.

31 Taracha 2000, 111–112; Görke 2012 (in her online edition of CTH 448.2.1.1 and 448.2.2.1; www.hethiter.net).

32 Taracha 2000, 111–112.

33 In the agreements the Hittite rulers concluded with them, groups of Kaška men (LÚ. MEŠ) or Kaška troops (ÉRIN.MEŠ) are identified by their "towns" (URU), including important cities such as Kammama or Turmitta.

34 This happened sometime during the reign of Šuppiluliuma I, who established Hittite control in northern Syria and Mesopotamia; Hoffner 1979, 261. Already in the 14th

these troops "were armed, fought and/or dressed differently than other soldiers."[35] Provided that the correlation between ÉRIN.MEŠ *ŠUTU* and *latti-* is correct, we may ascribe to these terms the general meaning "group, troop," possibly with the connotation "(extended) family."[36]

Another term to consider is the logographically written LÚ(.MEŠ) (GIŠ) ZA.LAM.GAR, often rendered as "tent man/people," "tent attendant," or "nomadic populations."[37] Though this term may refer to mobile pastoralists in Mesopotamian contexts,[38] in Hittite documentation it seems rather to be a professional designation, probably denoting a type of craftsperson or official.[39] In CTH 263, a protocol for the Palace Gatekeeper, LÚ ZA.LAM.GAR is listed among the GIŠTUKUL men who reside in the palace;[40] and in CTH 269, a royal decree concerning social and economic matters, the LÚ ZA.LAM.GAR is listed alongside other officials and tradesmen.[41] In CTH 106.A (Bo 86/299 i 76), the treaty between Tudḫaliya IV and Kurunta, the LU.MEŠ ZA.LAM.GAR appear in a long list of professionals resident in the frontier district of Tarhuntašša, summarized as "šarikuwa groups (auxiliaries?), craftsmen and agricultural workers."[42] In CTH 428.1, a fragment of the military oaths, the LÚ.MEŠ GIŠZA.LAM.GAR-*TIM* appear as participants in a

---

century, "*Sutû*" had started to be used as a generic term for predominantly (though not exclusively) mobile pastoralist communities that inhabited the peripheries of urban and agricultural zones, who were often hired as mercenaries; Singer 2011, 12; Heltzer 1981, 83, 93. It is therefore probable that when ÉRIN.MEŠ *ŠUTU* was integrated into the Hittite writing system, it designated mercenary units recruited from communities who inhabited the fringes of centralized states. The Hittites seem to have encountered the *Sutû* first as foes and probably eventually employed them as mercenaries; we may compare this with Ḫattušili III who is reported to have fought alongside *Aḫlamu* against Shalmanezer I of Assyria; see Grayson 1987, 184.

35 Beal 1992, 107–108. Beal (1992, 103–108) has further suggested that the function of the *ŠUTU* was "doing one thing while the troops are doing something else" and has defined them as "light troops."

36 Schuol (1994, 284) suggests that *latti-* may have been used in Hittite extispicy as the translation of a Mesopotamian term or concept. She offers *kiṣru* ("knot" or "contingent of soldiers, troops"; CAD K s.v. *kiṣru*) or *kiṣirtu* ("congestion, stricture" or "contingent of soldiers"; CAD K s.v. *kiṣirtu*) as possible Akkadian equivalents of *latti-*.

37 E.g., Pecchioli-Daddi 1982, 133; Otten 1988, 15; Beckman 1999, 116; Kitchen and Lawrence 2012, 615; Miller 2013, 91, 123. In KBo 5.11 i 15 (CTH 263) LÚ GIŠZA.LAM.GAR is given as the logographic equivalent of the Hattic word *dāgulrunāil*; see Miller 2013, 90–91.

38 See CAD K s.v. *kuštāru*; Heltzer 1981, 6, n. 37.

39 See CAD K s.v. *kuštāru*; CAD Z s.v. *zaratu*. For the professional title LÚ GIŠZA.LAM.GAR in Hittite documentation, see Pecchioli-Daddi 1982, 133.

40 KBo 5.11 i 15; Miller 2013, 88–97.

41 IBoT 3.73 2'; Miller 2013, 122–125.

42 Bo 86/299 i 84: ÉRIN.MEŠ *ša-ri-ku-wa-aš* EN.MEŠ ŠU-*TI* LÚ.MEŠ GIŠTUKUL GÍD.DA-*ya*.

ritual. Based on these attestations and the frequent use of tents in Hittite rituals, we may suggest that this profession had something to do with their production or their use in rituals.[43]

To conclude, the Hittite language does not seem to have a word for "nomad" or "nomadic tribe." As we shall see in the textual evidence presented below, Hittite sources referred to those who were preoccupied with pastoralism as "herdsmen," distinguishing them according to the type of animal.[44] Still, different types of mobility and pastoralism, as well as their significance to the Hittite economy *can* be documented from Hittite textual evidence. In the sections that follow, I will examine the evidence pertaining to mobile pastoralism in Hittite Anatolia, focusing on the Black Sea region, southern Anatolia, and the land donation documents.

The Black Sea Region and the Kaška

The inhabitants of the central Black Sea region, a diverse group of people often referred to as "Kaška men" (LÚ.MEŠ ^{URU}Kaška) in Hittite sources, have traditionally been portrayed in Hittitology as mobile pastoralists.[45] The argument that the Kaška were semi-nomadic pastoralists was first articulated by E. von Schuler, based on the following points:[46] 1) the Kaška simply abandoned their settlements rather than defend them when the Hittite army attacked, and the destruction of their settlements did not have a significant effect on their livelihood;[47] 2) the

43 For the use of tents in rituals see Popko 1980, 101–104.

44 On herding and herdsmen in Ḫatti, see Beckman 1988.

45 On the Kaška and their interactions with the Hittite state, see von Schuler 1965; Glatz and Matthews 2005; Singer 2007; Zimansky 2007. A detailed treatment of the Kaška may be found in my University of Michigan dissertation *The Kaška and the Northern Frontier of Ḫatti* (2012), now in preparation for publication as a monograph in the series "Studies in Ancient Near Eastern Records" (De Gruyter). Somewhat differently from previous work on the Kaška, I argue that in Hittite sources the term "Kaška" refers to diverse groups of people with different types of economic and socio-political organization, lifestyles, and cultural traits. These groups were made up of indigenous populations of the Black Sea region, deported communities from elsewhere in Anatolia, as well as fugitives, who withdrew from the Hittite state or remained outside of its direct control.

46 Von Schuler 1965, 75–78.

47 One wonders if the claims of Hittite rulers to have "burnt down" or "destroyed" settlements or their territories are to be taken literally. Such claims appear often, but as was mentioned by von Schuler, the destruction does not appear to affect the Kaška. And moreover, the same towns appear to have been resettled shortly thereafter. We may compare the claims of having burnt down or destroyed towns to rare instances in which the Hittite king threatens to consecrate a certain town to a god. In the latter case, the threat of destruction seems much more real, which may suggest that "burning down" towns is only a literary motif. For example, in Year 2 of the Exten-

presumed southward expansion of Kaška territory throughout the history of documentation can only be explained as migratory movements necessitated by a pastoralist lifestyle; and most importantly 3) the designation of Kaška fighting units as ÉRIN.MEŠ *ŠUTU* (i.e., mobile pastoralists, see above). Recent scholarship describes them as predominantly pastoralist communities who were involved in agriculture to some degree, and who practiced seasonal vertical transhumance, moving seasonally from winter settlements at lower elevations to summer settlements/campsites close to highland pastures.[48]

The Middle Hittite Kaška agreements, the corpus of letters from Maşat Höyük, and the annals of Hittite kings provide numerous references that concern pastoralism, demonstrating that it was a crucial component of the economy of north-central Anatolia, not only among Kaška groups, but also in Hittite-controlled territories.[49] Furthermore, the available evidence does not imply a drastic difference between Kaška and Hittite communities, in either the economic significance of pastoralism or specific practices. The only textual reference that seems to present pastoralism as a defining trait of the Kaška comes from the Annals of Muršili II (CTH 61.II). It is part of the narrative that describes the rise and territorial expansion of the Kaška ruler Piḫḫuniya. The text describes how "he (i.e., Piḫḫuniya) took the entire territory of Ištitina and turned it into his *grazing grounds*" after entering Zazišša and taking control of the Upper Land.[50] Alternatively, the Kaška are described in Muršili II's Hymn and Prayer to the Sun-goddess of Arinna (CTH 376.A), as "swineherds and weavers of linen."[51] Pig-rearing and flax cultivation are not conducive to a mobile lifestyle, and most scholars view this as a derogatory description of the Kaška.[52]

---

sive Annals of Muršili II, Muršili II threatens the inhabitants of Kammama and a town whose name is broken that he will dedicate Palḫuišša to the Storm God and coerces them to do his bidding. On burning towns *cf.* Ünal 1983, 164–180.

48 Yakar 2000, 283–302. See also Glatz and Matthews 2005, 59; Zimansky 2007, 168; Hoffner 2009, 174.

49 For the agreements with the Kaška (CTH 137–140), see von Schuler 1965, 109ff; Kitchen and Lawrence 2012, 355–364, 1039–52 (note that the translations in Kitchen and Lawrence closely follow von Schuler's edition); Gerçek 2012 (University of Michigan doctoral dissertation).

50 KBo 3.4+ iii 71–72: KUR [URU]*Iš-ti-ti-na-ma-za ḫu-u-ma-an da-a-aš / na-at-za a-pé-el ú-i-ši-ya-u-wa-aš pé-e-da-an i-ya-a-at*. Von Schuler (1965) sees this passage as an indication that Kaška mobility was motivated by the search for pastures.

51 KUB 24.4 (CTH 376) i 26: *na-at* [LÚ.MEŠ]SIPAD.ŠAḪ *e-še-er Ù* [LÚ.MEŠ]*E-PÍ-IŠ* GAD.ḪI.A *e-še-er.*

52 Singer 2002, 49; Freu 2005; Beckman 2013, 204. Glatz and Matthews (2005, 31–32) have argued that this may be a realistic description of Kaška economic activities, drawing attention to the history of pig-rearing and flax cultivation in the Black Sea region. The narrative context of this reference lends support to Glatz and Matthews'

Much of our evidence, especially from the annals, concerns pillage and raids targeting livestock. It is evident that this was an activity carried out by both the Kaška and the Hittite state. Aside from the annals, which record numerous formulaic references to the Hittite king carrying off cattle, sheep, and deportees as booty in the wake of successful campaigns, the Maşat Höyük correspondence provides ample evidence for raids targeting herds.[53] In ABoT 60 (9'-15'), a Hittite official informs the king that the enemy,[54] 7000 in number, has attacked Tarittarā, taking away shepherds, oxherds, and cattle. In HKM 10 (37–38), it is reported that the enemy has taken 40 cattle and 100 sheep. In HKM 36 (3–9), it is stated that the enemy is positioned near sheepfolds (TÚR.ḪI.A). Similarly, we find out from HKM 17 (18–20) that Hittite officials are planning an attack on sheepfolds in the vicinity of the (enemy) town Marišta after a reconnaissance of the territory. The Kaška agreements, too, mention the possibility of such raids. In one of the agreements (CTH 138.3.A, passage cited below) the allied Kaška are warned against mingling their own herds with those of the enemy, since in the case of a Hittite raid the allies' animals would be carried off along with those of the enemy.

Pastoralism was an important element in the peaceful interactions between the Hittite state and the allied Kaška who were bound by agreement. Corresponding paragraphs in the agreements CTH 138.1.A and CTH 138.3.A contain numerous provisions concerning herdsmen, grazing rights, and the movement of cattle and sheep. These passages demonstrate that the allied Kaška were not just given grazing rights in Hittite controlled territory, but appear to have been employed by the Hittite state as herdsmen. This can best be seen in CTH 138.3.A (ii 21'-28'):

> Because you are allies, the cattle [and sheep] of Ḫatti [and your cattle] and sheep are mixed together, and the cowherds and shepherds [pasture] together. But if an enemy attacks, we shall hold you alone responsible. [...] you indeed drive (the animals) here. The cowherds and shepherds [...] If

argument: "Moreover, those lands which belong to Ḫatti, the Kaška land—they were swineherds and weavers of linen—Arawanna, Kalašma, Lukka, and Pitašša, have declared themselves free from the Sun-goddess of Arinna. They discontinued the payment of their tributes and began to attack Ḫatti." An ethnic description or an anthropological observation on the Kaška society seems out of place in this context. It seems more likely that this remark on the Kaška was intended to describe the role or importance of the Kaška for the Sun-goddess of Arinna, in order to illustrate how the Sun-goddess herself is affected by their defiance—a type of argument commonly attested in Hittite prayers. In short, we may interpret this line as an indication that groups of Kaška were employed in the service of the Sun-goddess of Arinna as "swineherds and weavers."

53 See HKM 25; 8; 10; 17; 36; ABoT 60.

54 The consensus opinion is that "the enemy" frequently mentioned in the Maşat letters was groups of Kaška; Giorgadze 2005.

> they kill anyone, either one man, or one [ox, or one sheep], you shall replace them (i.e. the men) and [you shall replace the] cattle [and sheep] of Ḫatti as well. You shall give three men for one man, you shall also give [three oxen for one ox] and you shall give three [she]ep for one sheep.[55]

According to this passage, not only were the cattle and sheep of Ḫatti and allied Kaška grazing together, but also the Kaška were held responsible for Hittite herds in the case of an enemy attack. In the paragraphs that follow (KUB 26.19 ii 29'-39'), unfortunately in rather fragmentary context, the Kaška bound by agreement are warned against encouraging the hostile Kaška to carry off animals and kill herdsmen, and against dividing up the cattle among themselves (i.e., the allies and the Kaška who were not allies).

Hittite sources, especially the Kaška agreements (CTH 138.1.A and CTH 138.3.A), refer to Kaška herdsmen alongside Hittite herdsmen as a subgroup of specialists who were entrusted with the care of the animals. Further documentation for specialist herdsmen comes from the Deeds of Šuppiluliuma. The text mentions that when the Hittite king is confronted by "the entirety of the (Kaška) enemy" (which probably meant very high numbers), "the shepherds [had come to] help" the enemy.[56]

The mention of sheepfolds in the Maşat documents near both Hittite-controlled and "enemy" towns indicates that the animals (at least in some regions and for part of the year) were kept enclosed in the vicinity of settlements. At other times, probably during the warmer months, the animals were in the care of herdsmen, who sought pastures in the countryside outside the towns and at higher elevations.

There is an undeniable degree to which Hittite sources depict the inhabitants of the central Black Sea region as mobile people. This is best illustrated in the Maşat correspondence and the annals. The "enemy" mentioned in the Maşat letters (i.e., the Kaška) is constantly on the move, has superior knowledge of the terrain, and has the ability to appear and vanish suddenly despite their large numbers. Numerous letters report that the enemy "has come," "is going/on the move" or "has disappeared." Consider the following examples:[57]

---

55 KUB 26.19 ii 21'-28': ^{LÚ}*ták-šu-la-aš-za ku-it šu-meš nu ŠA* KUR ^{URU}*Ḫa-at-ti* GU4.ḪI.A U[DU.ḪI.A *šu-me-en-za-an-na* GU4.ḪI.A] / UDU.ḪI.A *an-da i-[mi]-ya-an-za nu* $^{\text{LÚ.MEŠ}}$SIPAD.GU4 $^{\text{LÚ.MEŠ}}$SIPAD.UDU *ták-ša-a[n ú-e-ši-ya-an-da-ri]* / *ma-a-an* ^{LÚ}KÚR-*ma w[a-a]l-aḫ-zi ú-e-ša šu-me-eš-pát ḫar-ú-e-ni* [...] / *šu-me-eš-pát u-un-n[a]-at-te-ni* $^{\text{LÚ.MEŠ}}$SIPAD.GU4-*ya* $^{\text{LÚ.MEŠ}}$SIPAD.UDU x[...] / *ma-a-na-aš-ta ku-na-an-zi-ya ku-in-ki na-aš-šu* 1 LÚ *na-aš-ma* ⌜1⌝ [GU4 *na-aš-ma*? 1 UDU] / *nu a-pu-u-uš-ša šar-ni-ik-te-ni ŠA* KUR ^{URU}*Ḫa-at-ti-ya* G[U4.ḪI.A UDU.ḪI.A *šar-ni-ik-te-ni*] / *A-NA* 1 LÚ EGIR-*an* 3 LÚ.MEŠ *pí-iš-kát-te-ni A-NA* 1 GU4-*ya* [3 GU4 *pí-iš-kát-te-ni*] / *IŠ-TU* 1 UDU 3 [UD]U-*pát pí-iš-te-ni.*

56 KUB 19.11+ obv. 14': $^{\text{LÚ.MEŠ}}$SIPAD.UDU-*ya an-da wa-ar-ri*; Güterbock 1956, 63; del Monte 2009, 14–16.

57 Translations follow those in Hoffner 2009 with minor modifications.

> 1. Concerning what you wrote to me, saying: "The enemy has come. He pressed the city Ḫapara on that side and the city Kašepura on this side. But he himself passed through, and I don't know where he went." And was that enemy enchanted that you didn't recognize him?[58]
>
> 2. Because the enemy marches into the land at any moment, you should locate him somewhere and attack him.[59]
>
> 3. The enemy is going to Marišta.[60]
>
> 4. The enemy is moving *en masse* at night—sometimes six hundred, sometimes four hundred of the enemy—and is reaping crops.[61]

Also relevant to the question of mobility is the following paragraph:

> [No] one shall settle in a city belonging to Ḫatti [on his own authority]. Now, a Kaška man who, within a territory$^{?}$, [occupies] a city on his own authority, [is] His Majesty's en[emy...]. And he (His Majesty) will fight him. (CTH 138.1.A rev. 86'-87')[62]

The annals, too, corroborate this picture. There are numerous references to Kaška people—the entire population with their animals and presumably movable property—abandoning their towns and fleeing before the advancing Hittites to seek refuge on mountains or in other such places out of the reach of the Hittite army.[63] Moreover, both the Maşat correspondence and the annals also make numerous references to Kaška groups mobilized in order to attack Hittite territory. However, in both the annals and the Maşat correspondence, the contexts in which we find instances of Kaška mobility seem to be raids and military campaigns, that is, situations in which the Kaška were either attacking or retreating. Our sources unfortunately do not reveal to what degree mobility was a significant element in the lifestyles of the people who inhabited this region.

58 HKM 6 3–14.

59 HKM 8 12–17.

60 HKM 17 15–16.

61 HKM 25 6–10.

62 KUB 23.77a (+) 86'-87': *ŠA* KUR ^{URU}*Ḫa-at-ti-ya-az* ⸢URU⸣-*a*[*n* ZI-*it le-e k*]*u-iš-ki e-ša-r*[*i*] ⸢*ki-nu-un-za-kán*⸣ *ku̯-iš* ⸢x x⸣-*ri*$^{(?)}$ *an-da* / LÚ ^{URU}*Qa-aš-ga* ZI-*it* URU-*an* [*e-ša-ri*$^{?}$ *na-aš A-NA*] ^{d}UTU-*ŠI* ^{LÚ}K[ÚR]-x ⸢*na*⸣-*an za-aḫ-ḫi-e-iz-zi*.

63 See years 13, 14, 15, 16, 18 of the Extensive Annals of Muršili II.

The evidence presented here demonstrates that pastoralism was a crucial component of the economy of the central Black Sea region during the LBA. However, the inhabitants of this region—including the Kaška—also pursued agricultural activities and lived in settlements that ranged from small villages mentioned no more than once in Hittite texts to towns that date back to the Old Assyrian period (e.g., Turmitta).[64] Whereas the care of animals was entrusted to specialist herdsmen who led them to distant pastures for part of the year, entire communities could move to inaccessible locations at higher elevations in times of conflict with the Hittite state.

Southern Anatolia

The mountainous regions of Southern Anatolia have been—and continue to be—home to mobile pastoralist groups throughout most of their recorded history.[65] The most important information concerning pastoralism in Southern Anatolia during the LBA comes from Hittite treaties concluded with Kizzuwatna and Tarḫuhtašša.

Paragraphs 5'-8' of the Padatiššu Treaty (between an unnamed Hittite King and Paddatiššu of Kizzuwatna, CTH 26)[66] concern the movement of mobile pastoralists across the frontier zone.[67]

> §5 [If (the population of) a settle]ment of the Great King, with its "women,"[68] its goods, its large and small cattle, sets out and enters the Land of Kizzuwatna, [Paddatiššu] must seize them and return them to the Great King.[69]

64 For the agricultural pursuits of the Kaška, see the Maşat letters HKM 19, 47, ABoT 60. See also the references in the Annals of Muršili II to Kaška gathering crops (unaware of the advancing Hittite army), the destruction or plunder of Kaška crops by the Hittite army, and the delivery of wine and grain as tribute from Kaška territory; von Schuler 1965, 77.

65 On mobile pastoralism in southern Anatolia (Tarḫuntašša and Lukka) during the LBA, see Simon 2010.

66 For text and translation, see Beckman 1999: 11–13; Kitchen and Lawrence 2012, 293–298; Wilhelm 2014 (www.hethiter.net, under CTH 26). The translations from Akkadian follow Beckman 1999 with some modification.

67 Since fugitives are treated earlier in the text (§§ 1'-2'), it is fairly certain that the communities in question here are not fugitives.

68 Wilhelm (2014, www.hethiter.net, under CTH 26) argues that the translation "women" of MUNUS.NITA.MEŠ (e.g., in Beckman 1999) is inaccurate: "MUNUS.NITA steht hier und im folgenden nicht für NITLAM4 (*ḫīrtu*), es handelt sich vielmehr um einen Kollektivbegriff für Frauen und Männer mit Sklavenstatus."

69 KUB 34.1 14'-15'. Lines 15'-16' lay down the same stipulations for the Great King.

§6 [If some]one from the Land of Ḫatti falsely reports: "The (population of a) settlement, with its "women" [and its goods], has set out and has entered the Land of Kizzuwatna," but the (population of a) settlement with its "women" [and its goods] has [no]t set out, and if there are those in the settlement busy with herding, [then whatever] trustworthy m[an] of Ḫatti Paddatiššu may ask for an oath, [will swear an oath about this], and the "women" must be returned.[70]

§7 [If] ox[herds] go down from Ḫatti into the frontier district of Kizzuwatna, a thief [among them?] who steals something must make twofold restitution to his victim and pay thirty shekels of silver. [If he] does [not] pay [the thirty shekels of silver], then he is a thief, and must be…[71] [If a man from Ḫatti who is] not an oxherd goes (into the Land of Kizzuwatna) to steal,[72] he must be put to death.[73]

We may derive from the Paddatiššu Treaty the following observations illustrating the economic significance of pastoralism in southern/southeastern Anatolia (the frontier districts of Ḫatti and Kizzuwatna) during the late Old Kingdom: The paragraphs prohibiting the movement of the entire population of a settlement from the territory of one polity to the other (§§5'-6') and those concerning the return of fugitives (§§1'-2') show that the rulers of Ḫatti and Kizzuwatna sought to restrict cross-frontier mobility. However, concessions were made for herdsmen, who were allowed entry into the treaty partner's territory. We may even suggest that laws against theft were more lenient for pastoralists (§§ 7'-8').

The Hittite rulers Ḫattušili III and Tudḫaliya IV (*c.* 1267–1237 BCE) concluded a series of treaties with Ulmi-Teššup/Kurunta, the ruler of the appanage kingdom Tarḫuntašša.[74] A central concern in both treaties is the (re)organization and delim-

70 KUB 34.1, 18'-22'. Lines 22'-26' lay down the same stipulations for the Great King.

71 The punishment for failure to compensate depends on how one interprets the verb *ú-wa-ab-ba-tu-šu* (rev. 29'), which has been linked previously to the verbs *abātu* 'to destroy' or *ebētu* 'to bind'; Wilhelm 2014 (www.hethiter.net), with further references.

72 I follow Wilhelm's (2014, www.hethiter.net) restoration and interpretation of line 30'. Beckman (1999, 13) translates "and the oxherd goes to the thief"; CAD (R, p. 308), on the other hand, interprets *ana šarrāqi illak* as "the cowherd becomes a thief."

73 KUB 34.1, 30'-33'. Paragraph 8 (lines 34'-37') lay down the same stipulations for the Great King.

74 For the Ulmi-Teššup Treaty (CTH 106.B), see van den Hout 1995; Beckman 1999, 109–113; Kitchen and Lawrence 2012, 631–642. For the Bronze Tablet (CTH 106.A), see Otten 1988; Beckman 1999, 114–124; Kitchen and Lawrence 2012, 609–630.

itation of the frontier district of Tarḫuntašša (i.e., the land of the Ḫulaya River).[75] Resources important for pastoralism—salt licks, mountain pastures, and water sources—play a central role in the (re)organization of the frontier district.[76] The treaty also brings regulations to the movement of herdsmen in the frontier district and their access to the district's natural resources:

> That which is the frontier district of the Land of Tarḫuntašša—it is the land of the Ḫulaya river—(even) a goatherd shall not enter! And if they drive (their animals) from the land of the Ḫulaya River to the great salt lick rock (*:lapani :waniya*),[77] they shall not take away his salt lick rights. They are given to the king of Tarḫuntašša, and he shall always take the salt. My father, Ḫattušili, gave to Kurunta, king of the land of Tarḫuntašša, the cities of Šarmana, Pantarwanta, and Maḫrimma, together with fields, meadow, sheep pasturage, all the salt lick, and I, My Majesty, Tudḫaliya, Great King, have also given it to him. No other person shall encroach on the salt of Šarmana.[78]

The focus on salt licks, sheep pasturage, and the movements of goatherds testifies to the prevalence of mobile pastoralism in this region. That some of the terminology related to pastoralism was Luwian (i.e., *:lapana-*), may further suggest that at least some of the mobile pastoralist communities were Luwian speakers.[79]

Mobile Pastoralism in the Land Donation Documents

We have little information on mobile pastoralism in the central Anatolian plateau—the territory that constituted the Hittite heartland. Ethnographic information suggests that this territory was suitable only for *yayla* pastoralism of short distance and duration.[80] Some evidence pertaining to mobile pastoralism

75 Hawkins 1995, 50, n.166.

76 KBo 4.10+ (The Ulmi-Teššup Treaty, CTH 106.B) i 15'-37'; Bo 26/299 (The Bronze Tablet, CTH 106.A) i 14-ii 20.

77 In his recent treatment of this passage Simon (2010: 551), following CHD (L s.v. *:lapana-*) adopts the older, now outdated, translation of *:lapana-* as "summer pasture." The meaning of the word *:lapana* has been established by Watkins (1997) as "salt lick." See also HED L s.v. *lapana-* "saltlick."

78 Bo 26/299 (CTH 106.A) ii 4–15. See also the corresponding lines in the Ulmi-Teššup Treaty, KBo 4.10+, i 33'-35'; translation follows Beckman 1999, 114–124 with minor modifications.

79 With Simon 2010, 545.

80 Yakar 2000, 220.

in central Anatolia may be found in the land donation documents (*Landschenkungsurkunden*), which were introduced during the early years of Telipinu's reign and fell out of use sometime around 1400 BCE.[81] Since land donations mention animals, herdsmen, pastures, and fields located in highland areas, they shed some light on the role of pastoralism in Hittite economy.

A number of land donations included different types of pasturage.[82] The most common type of pasture was the Ú.SAL(-*LUM*), often used to refer to the pastures used for cattle, located near rivers or canals.[83] More significant for the question of mobile pastoralism are the attestations of "winter and summer pastures for sheep" (*ri-it ku-ṣi di-ši* UDU.ḪI.A)[84] and "summer [pasturage] for cattle" ([*ri-i*]*t di-ši* GU4),[85] which document the practice of seasonal transhumance and long-distance grazing.[86] Also attested are the Hittite terms *wešiya-* "pasture"[87] and *wellu-* "grassland, meadow."[88] Herdsmen and animals are occasionally part of land donations.[89] Finally, a few land donations mention fields located on mountains (A.ŠÀ *ša* ḪUR.SAG).[90] References to "winter and summer pasturage," as well as agricultural fields located at higher elevations connected to towns and villages, are indicative of *yayla*-type pastoralism and agriculture in Hittite Anatolia.

The land donation documents relevant to the question of mobile pastoralism appear to involve regions in the central Anatolian plateau as well as the mountainous regions in its peripheries. Bo 90/758 mentions "winter and summer pastures for sheep," along with the "shepherds of the House (of the town) Uḫḫiwa."[91] Uḫḫiwa was located in the vicinity of Wašḫaniya in the southwest of Kaneš (Kültepe).[92]

81 Rüster and Wilhelm 2012.

82 Rüster and Wilhelm 2012, 78–86.

83 Nr. 91 (KBo 5.7) rev. 22, 20, 48 in Rüster and Wilhelm 2012, 231–244. Ú.SAL *alalešša*(*r*), may have been a type of pasture as well; Rüster and Wilhelm 2012, 83–84.

84 Nr. 30 (Bo 90/758) obv. 2 in Rüster and Wilhelm 2012, 162–165.

85 Nr. 7 (2064/g) obv. 2 in Rüster and Wilhelm 2012, 108–113.

86 Rüster and Wilhelm (2012, 164) note that Tudḫaliya IV's donation document for Šaḫurunuwa (CTH 225, KUB 26.50 obv. 7'f. + KBo 22.58 7'f.) mentions pasturage for different types of animals (cattle, sheep, and horse pasturage).

87 Nr. 91 (KBo 5.7) rev. 10, Rüster and Wilhelm 2012, 231–244.

88 Nr. 91 (KBo 5.7) rev. 1, Rüster and Wilhelm 2012, 231–244.

89 Rüster and Wilhelm (2012, 85) note that most of the animals are mentioned in the lengthy land donation document of Arnuwanda and Ašmunikal (Nr. 91); for a table of the animals mentioned in the land donation documents, see p. 86.

90 E.g., Nr. 22 (Bo 90/732) rev. 60 and Nr. 47 (KBo 32.185) obv. 20 in Rüster and Wilhelm 2012, 140–150, 200–204.

91 Nr. 30 in Rüster and Wilhelm 2012, 162–165.

92 Forlanini 2009, 49–50, n. 70, cited in Rüster and Wilhelm 2012, 164, note to l. 7.

Two land donations, Bo 90/732 and KBo 32.185, mention mountain fields located in the region around Tapikka (Maşat Höyük), in the Tokat province in north central Anatolia.[93] KBo 5.7, on the other hand, involves pastures and grasslands in southern Anatolia.[94]

Conclusions

The records of the Hittite state show that seasonal vertical transhumance (or *yayla* pastoralism) was a prevalent subsistence strategy in LBA Anatolia, especially in the Black Sea region and southern Anatolia, but also in parts of the central Anatolian plateau. In these regions, specialist herdsmen maintained the herds on distant pastures for part of the year, while the majority of the population led a sedentary life; for other parts of the year, animals were kept in enclosures closer to the settlements. Herdsmen and flocks were an essential component of agricultural estates, temples, and royal mausoleums.[95]

Some communities inhabiting the Black Sea region (including the Kaška) and the highlands of southern Anatolia appear to have pursued animal husbandry more intensively, which necessitated higher degrees of mobility. Hittite kings regularly employed specialist herdsmen from these regions, but sought to monitor their movements, and, in some cases, restrict their access to certain resources. It is evident from the corpus of letters from Maşat Höyük and the treaties discussed above that Hittite rulers perceived mobility as a threat. Indeed, the state was frequently involved in conflicts with the Kaška, who appear to have used mobility as a strategy to remain outside the control of the Hittite state.

Hittite sources referred to pastoralists as "herdsmen" and further classified them according to the type of animal. The Hittite language does not appear to have had a word for "nomad" or "(nomadic) tribe." It is also interesting to note that we do not find derogatory descriptions of pastoralists in Hittite sources.

Finally, we may mention some of the socio-political and environmental factors that may have affected subsistence strategies in Hittite Anatolia. Aside from the feasibility of a range of mobile pastoralist subsistence strategies in Anatolia, economic and political pressure from the state, competition over natural resources, and unstable climatic conditions which affected agricultural productivity[96] may

93 Nr. 22 and Nr. 47 in Rüster and Wilhelm 2012, 140–150, 200–204.

94 Nr. 91 in Rüster and Wilhelm 2012, 231–244.

95 See Beckman 1988, 35.

96 Schachner (2010, 670–671) demonstrates (based on the work of W.-D. Hütteroth), that although Central Anatolia is considered to be suitable for rain-fed agriculture, precipitation can fluctuate quite dramatically. Hütteroth's work (Hütteroth and Höhfeld 2002, 86–90, cited in Schachner 2010, 670–671) has shown that in a 34-year

have compelled parts of the population in Anatolia to focus more intensively on pastoralism and inhabit increasingly marginal ecologic zones.[97]

Land donation documents imply that already during the Old Kingdom, Hittite rulers had begun to exercise stricter control over the ownership and use of arable land, pastures, meadows, and forested areas in order to maximize the productive potential of the land. A Middle Hittite historical fragment concerning the freeing of pasturage by the Hittite king reveals how pastoralists were affected by economic pressure from the state:

> From the presence of His Majesty he (?) return[ed], and he spoke to me as follows: "His Majesty has releas[ed] the fields." I (spoke) as follows: "Whatever field he has released, I have freed from (my) ha[nd(?)]." For the sake of the cattle (and) sheep of the poor man he has released it—so that the cattle (and) sheep of the poor man will survive. Because the fields of *aliya* are not dear to His Majesty, but the field of a man is dear [to him], he will finally restrain(?) that one. Now he has releas[ed] it for the sake of the poor man.[98]

Similar dynamics (i.e., increasing state control over, or involvement with, pastoralism) may be observed in the Maşat correspondence, which documents the competition over economic resources between the Hittite state and the groups they called "Kaška," as well as the Empire Period accords with Tarḫuntašša, which gave its ruler Kurunta the sole rights over crucial resources.

---

period of observation (between 1928–1961), only eight years had average crops, and only eleven had "good" crops.

97 Schachner (2012, 32) has suggested that state control over the population was weaker in pre-19th century CE Anatolia in comparison to Egypt and Mesopotamia, since climatic conditions in Anatolia in general were equally conducive for agriculture, and people could move to other regions when state control intensified. Indeed, stipulations concerning (the return of) fugitives and cross-frontier population movement feature in most Hittite treaties.

98 KUB 48.106, 7'-14'. This section has been treated in Beckman 1988, 36–37, n. 30–31, with further references. Translation follows Beckman, with minor modifications.

REFERENCES

Alp, S., *Hethitische Briefe aus Maşat Höyük*. Ankara: Türk Tarih Kurumu Basımevi, 1991.

Beal, R.H., *The Organisation of the Hittite Military*. Heidelberg: Carl Winter Universitätsverlag, 1992.

Beckman, G.M., "Herding and Herdsmen in Hittite Culture" in *Documentum Asiae Minoris Antiquae. Festschrift für Heinrich Otten zum 75. Geburtstag*, ed. by E. Neu and C. Rüster, 33–44. Wiesbaden: Harrassowitz Verlag, 1988.

———. *Hittite Diplomatic Texts*. 2nd ed. Atlanta: Scholars Press, 1999.

———. "Foreigners in the Ancient Near East." *Journal of the American Oriental Society* 133 (2013): 203–115.

Bernbeck, R., "An Archaeology of Multisited Communities" in *The Archaeology of Mobility: Old World and New World Nomadism*, ed. by H. Barnard and W. Wendrich, 43–77. Los Angeles: The Cotsen Institute of Archaeology Press, 2008.

Cribb, R., *Nomads in Archaeology*. Cambridge: Cambridge University Press, 1991.

del Monte, G., *Le Gesta di Suppiluliuma, L'opera storiografica di Mursili II re di Hattusa*. Pisa: Pisa University Press, 2009.

Düring, B., "Millennia in the Middle? Reconsidering the Chalcolithic of Asia Minor" in *Oxford Handbook of Ancient Anatolia* ed. by S. R. Steadman and J. G. McMahon, 796–812. Oxford: Oxford University Press, 2011.

Emberling, G., "Ethnicity in Complex Societies: Archaeological Perspectives." *Journal of Archaeological Research* 5 (1997): 295–344.

Forlanini, M., "On the Middle Kızılırmak, II" in *Central-North Anatolia in the Hittite Period: New Perspectives in Light of Recent Research,* ed. by F. Pecchioli Daddi *et al.*, 39–69. Rome: Herder, 2009.

Freu, J., "Les 'barbares' gasgas et le royaume hittite" in *Barbares et civilisés dans l'antiquité*, ed. by S. Aufrère *et al.*, 61–99. Paris: L'Harmattan, 2005.

Gerçek, N. İ., *The Kaška and the Northern Frontier of Ḫatti*. PhD.Unpublished PhD Thesis, University of Michigan, 2012.

Giorgadze, G. G., "'Feind' und 'Ansiedeln' in den hethitischen Texten aus Maşat-Höyük" in *V. Uluslararası Hititoloji Kongresi Bildirileri, Çorum 02–08 Eylül 2002. Acts of the Vth International Congress of Hittitology, Çorum, September 02–08, 2002,* ed. by A. Süel, 371–376. Ankara, 2005.

Glatz, C. and R. Matthews, "Anthropology of a Frontier Zone: Hittite-Kaska Relations in Late Bronze Age North-Central Anatolia." *Bulletin of the American Schools of Oriental Research* 339 (2005): 21–39.

Goetze, A., *Die Annalen des Muršiliš*. Leipzig, 1933.

Grayson, K. A., *Assyrian Rulers of the Third and Second Millennia BC (To 1115 BC)*. Toronto: Toronto University Press, 1987.

Grélois, J.-P., "Les annales décennales de Mursili II (CTH 61, I)." *Hethitica* 9 (1988): 17–145.

Güterbock, H. G., "The Deeds of Suppiluliuma as Told by His Son, Mursili II." *Journal of Cuneiform Studies* 10 (1956): 41–68, 75–98, 107–130.

Hammer, E., "Local Landscape Organization of Mobile Pastoralists in Southeastern Turkey." *Journal of Anthropological Archaeology* 35 (2014): 269–288.

Hawkins, J.D., *The Hieroglyphic Inscription of the Sacred Pool Complex at Hattusa (SÜDBURG)*. Wiesbaden: Harrassowitz Verlag, 1995.

Heltzer, M., *The Suteans*. Naples: Istituto Universitario Orientale, 1981.

Hoffner, H.A., "The Hittite Word for 'Tribe'" in *Studia Mediterranea Piero Meriggi Dicata*, ed. by O. Carruba, 261–266. Pavia: Aurora Edizioni, 1979.

———. "On a Hittite Lexicographic Project." *Journal of the American Oriental Society* 123 (2003): 617–625.

Hütteroth, W.-D. and V. Höhfeld, *Türkei*. Darmstadt: Wissenschaftliche Buchgesellschaft, 2002.

Kamp, K.A. and N. Yoffee, "Ethnicity in Ancient Western Asia during the Early Second Millennium BC: Archaeological Perspectives and Ethnoarchaeological Prospectives." *Bulletin of the American Schools of Oriental Research* 237 (1980): 85–104

Khazanov, A.M., *Nomads and the Outside World* trans. by Julia Crookenden. 2nd ed. Madison: University of Wisconsin Press, 1994.

Kitchen, K.A and P.J.N. Lawrence, *Treaty, Law and Covenant in the Ancient Near East. Part 1: The Texts.* Wiesbaden: Harrassowitz Verlag, 2012.

Klengel, H., "Studien zur hethitischen Wirtschaft: Einleitende Bemerkungen." *Altorientalische Forschungen* 32 (2005): 3–22.

———. "Studien zur hethitischen Wirtschaft, 2: Feld- und Gartenbau." *Altorientalische Forschungen* 33 (2006): 2–21.

———. "Studien zur hethitischen Wirtschaft, 3: Tierwirtschaft und Jagd." *Altorientalische Forschungen* 34 (2007): 154–173.

Miller, J.L., *Royal Hittite Instructions and Related Administrative Texts.* Atlanta, 2013.

Otten, H., *Die Bronzetafel aus Boğazköy. Ein Staatsvertrag Tutḫaliyas IV.* Wiesbaden: Harrassowitz Verlag, 1988.

Parkinson, W.A., "Introduction: Archaeology and Tribal Societies" in *The Archaeology of Tribal Societies,* ed. by W. A. Parkinson, 1–12. Oxford: Oxbow Books, 2003.

Pecchioli-Daddi, F., *Mestieri, professioni e dignità nell'Anatolia ittita.* Rome: Edizioni dell'Ateneo, 1982.

Popko, M., "^{GIŠ}ZA.LAM.GAR in den hethitischen religiösen Texten." *Rocznik Orientalistyczny* 41 (1980): 101–104.

Porter, A., *Mobile Pastoralism and the Formation of Near Eastern Civilizations: Weaving Together Society.* Cambridge: Cambridge University Press, 2012.

Puhvel, J., *The Hittite Etymological Dictionary. Volume 5: Words Beginning with L.* Berlin: De Gruyter, 2001.

Rüster, C. and G. Wilhelm, *Landschenkungsurkunden hethitischer Könige*. Wiesbaden: Harrassowitz Verlag, 2012.

Schachner, A., "M.Ö. 16. Yüzyıl: Hitit Anadolusu'nda bir Dönüm Noktası" in *VII. Uluslararası Hititoloji Kongresi Bildirileri,* ed. by A. Süel, 661–692. Ankara, 2010.

———. "Orta Anadolu'da Coğrafya ve Ekonomi: Hititlerin Bıçak Sırtındaki İmparatorluğu." *Colloquium Anatolicum* 11 (2012): 25–54.

Schuol, M., "Die Terminologie des hethitischen SU-Orakels. Eine Untersuchung auf der Grundlage des mittelhethitischen Textes KBo XVI 97 unter vergleichender Berücksichtigung akkadischer Orakeltexte und Lebermodelle, II." *Altorientalische Forschungen* 21 (1994): 247–304.

Simon, Z., "Das Problem des luwischen Nomadismus" in *Proceedings of the 6th International Congress on the Archaeology of the Ancient Near East. May 5th–10th 2008, "Sapienza"- Università di Roma,* ed. by P. Matthiae *et al.*, 545–556. Wiesbaden: Harrassowitz Verlag, 2010.

Singer, I., *Hittite Prayers*. Atlanta: Society of Biblical Literature, 2002.

———. "Who were the Kaška?" *Phasis* 10 (2007): 165–181.

———. *The Calm before the Storm. Selected Writings of Itamar Singer on the End of the Late Bronze Age in Anatolia and the Levant.* Atlanta: Society of Biblical Literature, 2011.

Szuchman, J., "Integrating Approaches to Nomads, Tribes and the State in the Ancient Near East" in *Nomads, Tribes, and the State in the Ancient Near East: Cross-Disciplinary Perspectives*, ed. by J. Szuchman, 1–13. Chicago: Oriental Institute of the University of Chicago, 2009.

Taracha, P., *Ersetzen und Entsühnen. Das mittelhethitische Ersatzritual für den Großkönig Tuthalija (CTH *488.4) und verwandte Texte.* Leiden: Brill, 2000.

Ünal, A., "Untersuchungen zur Terminologie der hethitischen Kriegsführung, I. 'Verbrennen, in Brand stecken' als Kriegstechnik" in *Festschrift Annelies Kammenhuber*, ed. by G. Frantz-Szabó, 164–180. Rome, 1983.

van den Hout, Th.P. J., *Der Ulmitešub-Vertrag. Eine prosopographische Untersuchung.* Wiesbaden: Harrassowitz Verlag, 1995.

von Schuler, E., *Die Kaškäer: Ein Beitrag zur Ethnographie des alten Kleinasien.* Berlin: De Gruyter, 1965.

Watkins, C., "Luvo-Hittite *: lapan(a)-*" in *Studies in Honor of Jaan Puhvel. Part One. Ancient Languages and Philology,* ed. by D. Disterheft, M. Huld and J. Greppin, 29–35. Washington D.C.: Institute for the Study of Man, 1997.

Wendrich, W. and H. Barnard, "The Archaeology of Mobility: Definitions and Research Approaches" in *The Archaeology of Mobility: Old World and New World Nomadism*, ed. by H. Barnard and W. Wendrich, 1–21. Los Angeles: The Cotsen Institute of Archaeology Press, 2008.

Yakar, J., "Transhumance and the Question of Nomadism in Early Anatolia" in *X. Türk Tarih Kongresi. Ankara, 22–26 Eylül 1986. Kongreye Sunulan Bildiriler II*, 597–606. Ankara, 1990.

———. *The Ethnoarchaeology of Anatolia: Rural Socio-Economy in the Bronze and Iron Ages*. Tel Aviv: the Institute of Archaeology of Tel Aviv University, 2000.

———. "Traits of Nomadic People: Ethnoarchaeological and Archaeological Research in Turkey" in *Die Sichtbarkeit von Nomaden und saisonaler Besiedlung in der Archäologie. Multidisziplinäre Annäherungen an ein methodisches Problem*, ed. by S. R. Hauser, 45–63. Halle, 2006.

———. "The Archaeology of the Kaška" in *VI Congresso Internazionale di Ittitologia: Roma, 5–9 settembre 2005*, ed. by A. Archi and R. Francia, 817–827. Rome, 2008.

Zimansky, P., "The Lattimore Model and Hatti's Kaska Frontier" in *Settlement and Society: Essays Dedicated to Robert McCormick Adams*, ed. by E. C. Stone, 157–173. Los Angeles: Cotsen Institute of Archaeology Press, 2007.

Anatolian Lead Figurines: A Stocktaking

Yağmur Heffron[1]

It is truly an honour to be dedicating this article to Bayan Gates, who introduced me to the ancient Near East, and Charles Bey, who taught me how to read images. I consider it a tremendous piece of luck to have had such extraordinary teachers, to whom I am ever grateful for continuing to inspire, encourage, and improve me. Close to finishing this article, I discovered that Kutlu Emre's seminal Anatolian Lead Figurines and Their Stone Moulds *was indeed very well known to Bayan Gates, or "Miss Marie-Henriette Carre at Yale University who went over the English text."*[2] *I would like to think this an auspicious detail in my choice of topic. Incidentally, the irony of presenting some of the most inelegant pieces of ancient Near Eastern art to two exceptionally graceful people, is not lost on me.*

Abstract

Anatolian lead figurines belong to a distinct category of small-scale mould-made objects attested throughout an extensive geography stretching from Troy in the northwest to Sippar in the southeast. Their notable concentration in Anatolia, particularly in early second millennium BC, is undoubtedly connected to Assyrian trade, which sets the historical background for stylistic and iconographic comparisons with the Syro-Mesopotamian milieux. To date, Anatolian lead figurines have been catalogued in great detail,[3] their production and place in the exchange networks put into consideration,[4] and their stylistic trends examined and classified.[5] Save for the earliest commentaries,[6] however, the iconography and symbolic significance of these remarkable objects have received

1 Department of History, University College London, Gower Street, London WC1E 6BT, UK.

2 Emre 1971, xii.

3 Emre 1971.

4 Canby 1965, 2003.

5 Marchetti 2003.

6 Emre 1969; 1970; 1971.

little detailed discussion. Consequently, the place of Anatolian lead figurines within the broader iconographic repertoire of religio-magical meaning remains underexplored. This article offers a vantage point for a more holistic treatment of Anatolian lead figurines by integrating previous efforts and formulating new interpretations.

Introduction

Anatolian lead figurines belong to a group of small-scale mould-made objects, coined as "trinkets,"[7] attested across an extensive geography as far northwest as Troy and as far southeast as Sippar.[8] The earliest known examples are dated to the third millennium BC.[9] During the first half of the second millennium BC, lead figurines and the stone moulds used in their manufacture display a notable concentration in south-central Anatolia.[10]

Their average dimensions (height *ca.* 5.5 cm, width *ca.* 2.5 cm) characterise lead figurines essentially as miniatures while their average thickness (*ca.* 0.3 cm) and flat, unworked backs indicate these were objects intended for frontal viewing. In addition to representational (mostly anthropomorphic, occasionally zoomorphic) figurines, the repertoire of mould-made lead trinkets includes a great variety of decorative geometric shapes, some certainly intended as items of personal adornment (pendants, earrings, pins or hair decoration), while others can be identified as stamp seals.[11]

Lead figurines were manufactured with the use of stone moulds (ranging between 5–9 cm in height; 3–5 cm in width; 1–2 cm in thickness), which are indicative of the relatively simple and inexpensive manufacture of mass-produced goods. The physical qualities of lead, an extremely malleable metal with a fairly low melting point (327.46 °C = 621.43 °F) and a high resistance to corrosion, are particularly well suited to small-scale metallurgy with a potentially sizeable output of easily affordable objects. Lead trinkets, therefore, can be described as modest items of popular consumption.

The wide geographic distribution and the temporal tenacity of lead trinkets likewise attest to the popularity of these objects, although differences of meaning and function would certainly have existed over time and space. Marchetti contextualises early trinket manufacture generally in terms of "Early Bronze Age urbanisation, probably in the area between southeastern Anatolia and northern

7 Canby 1965.

8 Emre 1971, 1.

9 Canby 2003, 171.

10 Emre 1971, 3.

11 Canby 1965, 44.

Mesopotamia,"[12] specifically "the marked increase in metallurgical production which took place in the Levant and Anatolia during Early Bronze IV."[13] By the MBA, trinket manufacture—now concerned solely with figurines rather than stamps, jewellery, and the like—concentrates in Anatolia, as northern Mesopotamia gradually ceases to be "a significant area of production."[14]

It is in the early second millennium BC that lead trinkets—mainly of the figurine variety—and moulds become highly conspicuous in the archaeological record of Anatolia, pointing to a surge of popularity in the region. The apparent intensification in the manufacture and circulation of lead figurines can be situated within the historical context of the *kārum* period, at a time when Assyrian mercantile activities in Anatolia place the region in close contact with the Syro-Mesopotamian milieux.[15] There is little doubt that the evidently intensified circulation of lead trinkets in Anatolia was a direct result of interregional contacts established by *kārum* period trade.[16] Once these contacts diminish by late 17th century BC,[17] so do lead figurines disappear from the archaeological record,[18] further confirming the direct link between trinket production and the *kārum* network. In fact the emergence of trinkets during the third millennium can likewise be contextualised with an earlier incarnation of a comparable system of interregional communication.[19] As to *why* such a peculiar class of object a) emerges in the first place; and b) proves so tenacious in the specific context of long-distance exchange, only to disappear once the systems of exchange are rearranged, deserves a closer examination. To this end, this article offers an exploration of the extent of multiple and sometimes overlapping uses to which lead figurines may have been put. Both in terms of craft production and symbolic meaning, it is important to acknowledge that lead figurines make up a particularly versatile group of objects, and appreciate the highly diverse "social lives,"[20] they certainly would have had.

12 Marchetti 2003, 411.

13 Marchetti 2003, 391.

14 Marchetti 2003, 411.

15 See Michel 2011 for a recent overview of the *kārum* period; see also Kulakoğlu 2011 for Kültepe-Kaneš, centre of the Anatolian *kārum* network.

16 Emre 1969, 169–170.

17 According to Barjamovic, Hertel and Larsen's (2012) reappraisal of the *historical* chronology of the *kārum* period, Level Ib ends in 1690 BC (Middle Chronology), the point beyond which textual sources are no longer attested, and so Assyrian trade is assumed to have ended. Occupation in Kültepe's Lower Town continues for Level Ia, a final, atextual period of occupation, estimated to have ended in 1650 BC (Kulakoğlu 2014; 87).

18 Marchetti 2003, 412.

19 Canby 1965, 53; Marchetti 2003, 411.

20 After Appadurai 1986.

A detailed and holistic examination of lead figurines from this perspective holds great potential to reflect previously unconsidered complexities of ideational exchange during the *kārum* period.

Archaeological Contexts

The known archaeological contexts of Anatolian lead figurines tend to be of lay characters, suggesting that the primary setting for the use of these objects was largely outside the public/official domain and instead belonged to the private/domestic sphere.[21] Published lead figurines from Kültepe-Kaneš, for instance, are all associated with residential areas, found *in situ* on floors, recovered from household debris,[22] or from street fill.[23] The distribution of lead figurines from Boğazköy (in its early second millennium BC incarnation as the modest-sized *kārum* Hattuš) also follows the same trend pointing towards a domestic use for lead figurines.[24] Likewise in Acemhöyük, find-spots are recorded within residential areas.[25]

Nonetheless, lead figurines were not entirely excluded from public/official settings. Three figurines from Alişar come from the so-called Complex I, a large structure divided into small compartments by thick walls without any detectable windows or doors. Based on the absence of fire installations, domestic utensils and other indicators of residential function, the excavators have interpreted this structure as a "community storehouse."[26] The find-spots of the Alişar figurines from Complex I are perhaps more indicative of a temporary context of storage than a final context of use, suggesting these objects were regulated commodities of exchange. Yet another Alişar figurine, representing a woman with a round headdress (presumably a goddess), was found in the foundations of the "palace" in M/11.[27] Such a location points to the well-attested ancient Near Eastern tradition of selecting magically potent objects and/or materials as foundation deposits for the purpose of consecrating a special building or providing it with a means of supernatural protection.[28] The Alişar foundation figurine belongs to a specialised context of use which, unlike an ordinary architectural space in which human activity took place, is inaccessible. Once deposited, the figurine could no longer

21 Heffron 2011, 223ff.

22 Emre 1971, 16.

23 Emre 1993, 171.

24 Boehmer 1979, 37–38.

25 Emre 1971, 7; N. Özgüç 1966, 26.

26 Schmidt 1931, 74f, fig. 108; Emre 1971, 10.

27 Emre 1971, 24; von der Osten 1937, 193, 456, fig. 512.

28 See Ellis 1968.

be handled, manipulated, or even seen—the end of the figurine's social life until its discovery by archaeologists. Nonetheless, although the single episode of ritual deposition may have removed the figurine from circulation, its magical efficacy was presumably thought to be continuous.

It is striking that extant lead trinkets of known Anatolian provenience are not attested in burial contexts, whereas they have indeed been found in Old Assyrian, as well as Ur III period, graves in Aššur.[29] Miscellaneous lead objects, such as circlets, sheets and even vessels, on the other hand, are part of the funerary assemblage in various Anatolian sites during the Early and the Middle Bronze Ages.[30] There are two possible exceptions to this apparent rule of excluding representational lead objects from graves. One is a small, highly worn lead object[31] found inside a stone cist grave from the 17th century phase of the extramural cemetery at Ilıca near Afyon.[32] Although its form is vaguely reminiscent of the schematic so-called Anatolian idols of the EBA, its poor state of preservation makes it difficult to say conclusively whether it was intended as a figural representation or served simply as an ornament, counterweight, or similar. The second lead object from a funerary context is undoubtedly a figurine, albeit broken, recovered from a Level Ia pithos grave from Kültepe.[33] Seeing as this figurine has not been categorised as a funerary gift, but ascribed to the "filling of pithos grave Nr. 5," it may well be intrusive.

As for moulds, two from Kültepe are attributed to a metal workshop, one having been recovered in association with crucibles and other equipment for small-scale metallurgy.[34] The remaining three moulds were evidently part of ordinary household assemblages.[35]

Previous Research

Lead figurines first received scholarly interest as early as the mid-19th century and have generated discussion since.[36] J. V. Canby's "Early Bronze 'Trinket Moulds'"[37] is the first synthetic analysis of the stone moulds used in the production of lead trinkets, and by extension, the trinkets themselves. The key significance of Canby's

29 Moorey 1994, 295.

30 E.g. in Alişar, Akyurt 1998: 66.

31 Akyurt 1998, 47, fig. 57-h.

32 For the Ilıca cemetery, see Orthmann 1967.

33 Emre 1993, 174, fig. 5, pl. 33–2; see below also.

34 See Emre 1971, 16, with references.

35 See T. Özgüç 1950, 53–54; Emre 1971, 16.

36 See Emre 1971, 2–3 for a more detailed account of early research on lead figurines.

37 Canby 1965.

approach is that she evaluates trinket production in accordance with the wide geographic distribution and the large variety of styles of trinkets and trinket moulds. The circulation of both classes of object during the EBA certainly covered a considerable geographic span indicative of an extensive communication network along which these items travelled.[38] The further intensification of trinket production in the MBA is no doubt due to the flourishing of the *kārum* trade network, of which lead trinkets are rightly described as a hallmark.[39] Canby also draws attention to the conspicuous variety of Mesopotamian, Cilician, Central Anatolian and Aegean influences in the EBA trinket repertoire—a trait also true for the MBA.[40] What is also remarkable about this repertoire is that it can often be seen on a single one-part mould, the peculiarities of which have been noted by Canby:

> This [one-part] mould differs from the general [two-part] type in two ways which have a significant bearing on how and where it was used. First, in the unusually large number of negatives crowded on to the small surface; and second, in the variety of wares which could be made from the piece. Neither peculiarity would be easy to understand if the piece came from an urban metal shop. Both could be explained if the piece had belonged to an itinerant smith. The care taken to make frugal use of a stone which was not in itself valuable would be worthwhile to a travelling smith who wanted to economize on the weight and bulk of his luggage. The preference for a general variety over specialties in one line of objects would also suit an itinerant smith. The probability that lead which is simple to handle [...] was used in the mould lends further weight to this theory.[41]

Drawing on stylistic comparisons between the inventory of negatives with well-attested artistic traditions of the EBA, Canby thus makes a compelling case for the possible route taken by itinerant smiths who were presumably travelling with caravans going "from north Mesopotamia to Cilicia, north to the Halys region and down to the west part of the Konya plain, then up to the Troad."[42] This likely route is not dissimilar to that followed by Assyrian merchants of the *kārum* period.[43] Canby further notes, "most of the Anatolian areas visited contain rich silver

38 See also Bittel 1933, 39–40.

39 Moorey 1994, 295.

40 Emre 1971; Marchetti 2003.

41 Canby 1965, 52.

42 Canby 1965, 53.

43 Seeing as explicit references to Cilicia remains unattested in Kültepe texts, it is possible that 2nd millennium contacts between this region and central Anatolia (otherwise suggested, for instance, by the MBA pottery of Tatarlı Höyük, Éric Jean,

mines,"[44] suggesting a similarity of focus between third millennium BC exchange and the *kārum* period network. From a metallurgical perspective, the acquisition and working of silver are intimately linked with lead-working (see below), further supporting the idea that lead trinkets may well be a diagnostic by-product of long-distance trade in which silver was of prime importance. Having established the significance of lead figurines as popular objects of exchange across several culture zones—across which imagery and styles travelled from their places of origin into new contexts—Canby postulates that buyers of lead trinkets would have adopted and developed new and different tastes,[45] to which craftsmen responded by imitation[46] or hybridization.[47]

Thus emerges an attractive paradigm for contextualizing the manufacture and exchange of lead trinkets during the *kārum* period. The peculiar nature of EBA trinkets whose distribution seems to have relied significantly on itinerancy offers a plausible explanation for the veritable surge in the popularity of these items during the *kārum* period, when a highly complex trade network was in place. That being said, significant differences between the third and second millennium BC repertoires—not only of lead trinkets but also of stone moulds—are indicative of change in the patterns of manufacture and consumption.

A notable difference between the crowded moulds of the EBA and those from the *kārum* period is that the latter were used only for the production of figurines.[48] This significant reduction of variety, coupled with the use of entire moulds for single items, attests to a more specialised mode of production focusing perhaps on the particular tastes of a single market. Presumably the itinerant production of the late third millennium BC began to give way to (but was not necessarily replaced by) a more settled context of metallurgical activity. Archaeological evidence for on-site production of lead figurines in multi-purpose metal workshops at *kārum* period sites such as Kültepe and Acemhöyük is certainly indicative of such a change.

To date, Emre's *Anatolian Lead Figurines and Their Stone Moulds* remains the only detailed catalogue of all extant figurines and moulds available for study at the time of publication. This catalogue is particularly useful in providing the precise find-spots for excavated figurines and moulds, information which is not always available in the published excavation records themselves. The iconographic/

---

personal communication) may have continued outside, or at least peripheral to, the *kārum* network.

44 Canby 1965, 53–54.

45 Canby 1965, 52–53.

46 Canby 1965, 59.

47 Canby 1965, 51.

48 Canby 1965, 49, n.56.

stylistic classifications extend beyond figurine types to individual attributes (such as items of clothing, objects carried by the figures, or accompanying animals) of each type, establishing parallels and highlighting divergences on various levels.[49] While a small number of later finds have received some attention,[50] a considerable number of lead trinkets and moulds cited in preliminary excavation reports[51] or on museum display[52] illustrate the growing extent of finds awaiting comprehensive analysis. A renewed effort towards collecting new finds under an exhaustive catalogue is therefore much needed.

Marchetti's examination of style and regional schools of production, which relies a great deal on Emre's catalogue, also presents previously unpublished finds from outside Anatolia.[53] In the light of this updated repertoire, Marchetti identifies several schools of production, based on distinct stylistic traits: The so-called "classic" and "elegant" groups attributed to workshops of Kültepe-Kaneš; the "Alişar group," "south-eastern Anatolian workshops," "Anatolian moulds of various styles," "the group with the 'master of animals' subject," "the 'Eblaite' and north-Syrian groups," and finally the "northern Mesopotamian workshops."[54] Admittedly, Marchetti's criteria for isolating distinct schools are not equally elucidated for each category, some being defined primarily on stylistic grounds, others grouped thematically. Nonetheless, the existence of regional workshops/schools, which developed their own stylistic trademarks and perhaps also thematic specialisations, is compelling. Significantly, Marchetti also attributes the flourishing of regional workshops to the "thriving commercial network" during the period corresponding to the *kārum* Ib phase of Kültepe-Kaneš; and consequently their decline to the collapse of the *kārum* network and the reformulation of trade patterns with the emergence of the Hittite state.[55] Again, the emphasis rests on the evident dependence of lead trinket manufacture on an interregional network of communication operating along a specific route and/or with specific goals of exchange.

Notably absent from all previous discussions is a focused and purposive evaluation of the symbolic meanings of lead figurine imagery, particularly of anthropomorphic figurines. As a general classification, Emre rightly ascribes a

---

49 See for example Emre 1971, 74–74, figs. 37–38 for typological charts for headdresses.

50 N. Özgüç 1976; Toklu 1976; Emre 1993.

51 E.g. Acemhöyük, see Öztan 2001; 2002; 2003; 2004; 2005; 2007; 2008; 2009.

52 A small collection comprising a stone mould and five figurines from Kaman Kalehöyük, for instance, can be seen at the site museum.

53 Marchetti 2003.

54 Marchetti 2003.

55 Marchetti 2003, 412.

protective function to lead figurines to do with domestic cults,[56] an interpretation also maintained by Bittel.[57] Emre also suggests a link between the divine beings represented by figurines and personal/family deities attested in Kültepe texts (e.g. "your god," "our god," "gods of our fathers").[58] This proposal does in fact tally with references to "figurine of the dead (made) of lead" (NU ÚŠ *ša* A.BAR),[59] which must belong to an associated constellation of ideas based on the protective and intermediary qualities of ancestors.[60]

While Emre's preliminary identifications of individual types have established a firm point of reference, they do require further exploration and discussion. The general understanding of the cast (!) of characters in lead figurine iconography as divine/protective beings is certainly valid, but their distinctive individual attributes remain underexplored. Were these high deities of a formal pantheon, or simply heroes of 'folk belief'? Did they hold a special significance in certain contexts and/or for particular people or groups? To what extent can the symbolism of lead figurines be deduced from the iconographic and stylistic parallels in other media, such as terracotta or metal figurines in the round, clay plaques, or cylinder seals? Can any figure be equated with specific divine beings named in contemporary texts or identified as the forerunners of divinities known from later sources? Are there plausible thematic links uniting lead figurines as representatives of a particular level of supernatural existence, natural phenomena, or urban society? How can their evident exclusion from burial contexts in Anatolia be interpreted? Ultimately, a considered and careful approach to the possible range of meanings for the symbolism of lead figurines is an essential step in accounting for the ubiquity of these items. The symbolic meanings attached to lead figurines must have been crucial to the boom in their popularity during the *kārum* period.

Preliminary identifications have of course been suggested for some of the more conspicuous characters of the lead figurine repertoire. Among single figures, Emre identifies the male deity holding a crook and in association with a caprid as the Mesopotamian god Amurru.[61] Whether the divine female often shown accompanying this god represents Amurru's Mesopotamian consort Ašartu, or else a local Anatolian goddess, however, is moot.[62] Otherwise, Emre's identifications remain

56 Emre 1971, 82.

57 Bittel 1976, 97.

58 Emre 1971, 82.

59 Moorey 1994, 295.

60 Marchetti (2003, 410) briefly mentions divinised royal ancestors of Old Syrian iconography but does not suggest a comparable identification for the divine types in Syro-Anatolian lead figurine imagery.

61 Emre 1971, 140–141.

62 Emre 1971, 141–142.

limited to *types*, such as the axe-bearing deity being described as a weather-god; or the figure with a scimitar ("sickle-like weapon") as a netherworld deity.[63] As for the popular theme of pairing a male figure wearing a horned conical hat with a female figure in an elaborate headdress, Bittel avoids naming names (see below) but concludes, "daß ein Götterpaar gemeint ist, darf als sicher gelten."[64] By extension, those couples accompanied by children are described as a "divine family,"[65] but the implications of child imagery within the lead figurine pantheon are not addressed. Is this a child-divinity, or a visual metaphor for human worshippers placing themselves under divine (or ancestral) protection? Or are we to read the "divine family" as a generic auspicious emblem for fertility, procreation, and generational continuity?

Much of the lead figurine identifications draw on the contemporary *kārum* period glyptic repertoire and its Syro-Mesopotamian parallels, as well as later Hittite art, highlighting notable similarities in the manner and divine attributes of each recognisable type. Marchetti also draws attention to another sphere of comparison: "In order to set the production of Syro-Anatolian lead figurines more satisfactorily in a historical perspective, it seems necessary to compare it with contemporary production of metal figurines and other forms of visual art."[66]

Ultimately, however, all discussions regarding the divine character and attributes of the various beings represented in the lead figurine repertoire echo Bittel's cautious warning: "Die Gottheiten mit bestimmten Namen zu benennen, wird man noch nicht wagen."[67] An in-depth discussion of the nature and implications of the lead figurine 'pantheon' is yet to be produced. Of particular interest for such a discussion are the potential shifts in meaning for given (stock-) themes represented by different but seemingly interchangeable characters. For the divine pair or the divine family, for example, the female element is variously represented by the nude Syrian type[68] or else dressed in an ankle-length or long, patterned skirt,[69] sometimes in clear imitation of the Mesopotamian flounced robe.[70] Such variations on what appears to be a single theme raise the question of whether these 'goddess' types are to be understood as wholly separate beings or different aspects of the same divine personality. A particularly challenging task for a detailed evaluation of the potential range of symbolic associations for individual

63 Emre 1971, 142–145.

64 Bittel 1976, 97.

65 Emre 1971, 65–66.

66 Marchetti 2003, 408.

67 Bittel 1976, 97.

68 Emre 1971, pl. III/2–3.

69 Emre 1971, pl. X/2–6.

70 Emre 1971, pl. XI/2.

types and themes is to differentiate between visual codes which may be conveying fundamental differences in meaning, and those which are simply the result of stylistic preference. Ultimately, this avenue of investigation ought to be situated within a rigorous interpretative framework exploring the range of functions for which lead figurines were intended. Whether these items were simply decorative items, apotropaic charms, or indeed both, will have a bearing on evaluating their underlying symbolism, which in all likelihood changed according to context. An equally significant point of consideration is the potential means by which lead trinket imagery may have travelled between different cultural zones as well as smaller pockets of regional tastes. To this end, a closer scrutiny of the context of craft production is necessary.

Craft Production of Lead Figurines and Stone Moulds

Lead trinkets were produced using open or closed moulds, the latter being more common for single moulds with multiple negatives and requiring dowel holes drilled onto the casting surface. The shallow negatives on the casting surface are carved to an average depth of 0.3 cm, producing a rather two-dimensional effect for the finished product. Each negative is equipped with its own conical pour-channel fanning out to an average width of 1 cm at the edge of the mould. Canby reconstructs the casting of lead trinkets in two-part closed moulds as follows:

> [The closing half of a two-part mould] must have had corresponding holes which would have permitted it to be dowelled tightly against this [i.e. carved] surface while the metal was poured in and allowed to solidify. It would presumably have had the air vents missing on our piece and perhaps corresponding pour channels [...] It would have been otherwise flat since none of the objects to be cast from it required a back surface. During the casting operation the mould must have been propped up in a bed of sand or earth or held by the hand.[71]

This seems a fairly straightforward method easily followed in the context of itinerancy, but equally well suited to settled workshop production. Both modes were presumably current during the early second millennium BC. As noted above, the establishment of a complex and sophisticated trade network in the *kārum* period would have encouraged the activities of itinerant craftsmen, who presumably continued in this line of business from the third into the second millennium BC. A notable aspect of lead trinket production in the *kārum* period, however, is the

71 Canby 1965, 43.

presence of archaeologically detectable workshops pointing to on-site production. Not surprisingly, the most compelling evidence comes from Kültepe-Kaneš (see above), which, as the focal point of the *kārum* network, also seems to have established itself as a major centre of lead trinket production and/or distribution.[72]

Contemporary residents of Acemhöyük too appear to have engaged in the production of lead objects. Reports on several seasons mention lead circlets in contexts suggestive of metalworking, i.e. in association with fire installations, crucibles, blowpipes and moulds, as well as metal slag and fragments of bronze pins, weapons and other utensils.[73] No finished objects made of lead, however, are recorded for these contexts, which may be indicative of an auxiliary role for lead in more general metallurgical pursuits. The presence of lead in mixed metallurgical contexts could be indicative of its alloying with copper, for which Moorey presents "three possible reasons: to ease the filling of complex moulds; to lower the temperature to assist the casting of several objects from one melt; and to increase the weight available."[74] Another likely metallurgical pairing is of course between lead and silver, especially in Anatolia, rich in deposits of both.[75] In fact, the earliest metallurgical acquaintance with silver may well have taken place in the course of lead exploitation. At any rate, seeing as silver was one of the principal raw materials drawing Assyrians into Anatolia, it is by no means a coincidence that a small (side?) industry of lead trinket production flourished in the wider context of interregional exchange involving a considerable movement of silver from Anatolia into north Mesopotamia.

Canby, however, questions whether lead figurines in Anatolia were at all the products of local workshops, on the basis that they "look most foreign when compared to the full-bodied, sculptured quality of contemporary Anatolian arts".[76] Perhaps it is unfair to expect full compliance with canonical Anatolian traits from a category of objects with a veritable mixed background. While markedly un-Anatolian looking pieces are certainly part of the repertoire, the large ears, predominant flat noses, and round eyes of a considerable number of figurines are very much at home in Anatolian art.[77] Also, Canby's assertion that "the figurines [...] were found only in the houses of Assyrian merchants"[78] is inaccurate, as the

72 Also note that the number of published figurine moulds found in Kültepe-Kaneš exceeds the total number of moulds from contemporary settlements at Boğazköy, Alişar, Acemhöyük, and Konya-Karahöyük.

73 Öztan 2002, 42; 2004, 233; 2005, 93; 2006, 550f; 2008, 516f; 2009, 331.

74 Moorey 1994, 293.

75 Lehner and Yener 2015, 531.

76 Canby 2003, 173.

77 See, for instance, Emre 1971, pl. VI.

78 Canby 2003, 173.

ethnicity of house owners is not known for all cases, so trinket moulds cannot be conclusively assigned to one particular group. More importantly, Canby ignores the presence of lead figurines and moulds in workshops, which is clear evidence of on-site production. What seems crucial here is to distinguish one-part crowded moulds, which certainly do fit the model of travelling metal smiths; and two-part moulds for single figures better suited to but not exclusive to on-site production.

As the contextual associations of stone moulds in Kültepe and Acemhöyük show, the production of lead figurines belonged to a general sphere of metalworking, presumably carried out by professionals who also produced bronze tools and weaponry, and perhaps also worked with silver. It does not necessarily follow, however, that the production of the moulds for casting lead figurines was exclusively confined to this same sphere. Topçuoğlu, for instance, has drawn attention to the stylistic similarities between the manner in which details, particularly of dress, are rendered both for lead figurines and in contemporary cylinder seals.[79] The use of schematic linear patterns for figurines is well attested in the figurine tradition. In glyptic, Alexander attributes similar stylistic traits, such as herringbone or curvilinear patterns, to native Anatolian seals.[80]

Such parallels are not surprising, considering, as Topçuoğlu observes, that the craft skill of carving miniature negatives in stone is not only fundamental to seal-cutting but also used for trinket moulds, and may well have constituted a shared expertise between two spheres of production.[81] Insofar as the parallels between stone moulds and cylinder seals rest on the use of striations, it is important to note that while an Anatolian glyptic style developed gradually during the course of the *kārum* period as "designers grasped the nature of the cylinder seal, mastered its design problems, and introduced Anatolian themes and motifs," geometric patterning was already a well-established aspect of Anatolian art, stretching well back into the third millennium and attested in a variety of media,[82] including trinket moulds. It is not at all implausible that the pronounced use of geometric patterning entered seal-cutting via mould production, nor that the first Anatolian seal-cutters could originally have been trained in the manufacture of trinket moulds. This potential set of relationships introduces yet another context in which influences may have circulated between local and foreign traditions. Considering the transmission of styles and techniques specifically among cylinder seal engravers, Alexander postulates a vertical continuity from master to apprentice.[83]

79 Topçuoğlu 2013.

80 Alexander 1979, 576–577.

81 Topçuoğlu 2013.

82 Alexander 1979, 576.

83 Alexander 1979, 616–617.

The potential role of seal-cutters in the trinket industry, and *vice versa,* has significant implications not only for the organisation of production or in terms of visual influences, but also on the transmission of craft skills and canons of style. If (at least some) mould producers were also seal-cutters, this would ascribe moulds to the sphere of a stone-worker's craft, isolating it from that of figurines, a metal-worker's craft. In turn, the production of moulds and the production of cast figurines would be affected by any social, economic, perhaps even ethnic differences that may have existed between the two specialties. Separate traditions of production for moulds and trinkets would also introduce an extra link in the commercial chain ending with the consumer, thus affecting the market value of both moulds and figurines as commodities. Last but not least, as seal-cutters and metal-smiths would have been trained in and exposed to different iconographic traditions, canons, and conventions, whether a mould was produced by one or the other craft specialist could have significant bearing on the choice and rendering of images created. It is therefore crucial to hold trinket imagery against not only the background of contemporary glyptic traditions, but also to industries of metal and even clay, as proposed by Marchetti (see above). It is also significant that Marchetti attributes sandstone moulds to non-professional production,[84] suggesting that amateurs could also carve their own moulds (and presumably cast their own figurines).

As for the manufacture of lead figurines themselves, a sphere of craft production with which it shares notable traits is that of Old Babylonian terracotta plaques, a category of object also with third millennium BC antecedents that reached peak popularity in the first half of the second millennium BC. Although lead figurines belong principally to a Syro-Anatolian milieu and Old Babylonian plaques are very much a south Mesopotamian specialty, the technical, stylistic and thematic similarities between these two seemingly disparate ventures suggest a possible exchange of techniques and ideas between the two craft specialties. Terracotta plaques are flat slabs of fired clay with relief decoration on the front, and blank on the back. Though larger than lead figurines, they tend to be no bigger than the palm of a hand, and can easily be classified as miniatures. Cast into one-piece open moulds, terracotta plaques belong to the realm of mass production, using the readily available and highly versatile medium of clay, which becomes extremely durable once baked. Being thus highly suitable for the easy and inexpensive production of small-scale goods for popular consumption, the use of clay for making plaques is not unlike that of lead in trinket manufacture. In terms of archaeological context, Old Babylonian plaques are also firmly rooted in the private/domestic sphere, reinforcing their interpretation as objects of popular consumption in non-elite, non-officialised settings.

84 Marchetti 2003, 403.

Admittedly, both the formal and contextual similarities between lead figurines and terracotta plaques can be explained simply by similar methods of manufacture being used for a similar purpose of producing inexpensive items for popular consumption, without necessarily predicating that the two industries were in contact. Certain stylistic and thematic parallels, however, do raise the possibility of transfer of ideas between the two. Canby has already noted the parallels between Anatolian lead figurines and terracotta plaques.[85] In particular, the frontal male-female pairs in lead figurine iconography are highly similar to those of the plaque repertoire. Both in lead and on terracotta plaques, this well-attested duo is characterised by a rigid, formal posture, with no apparent interaction but clearly intended to be read as a single iconographic unit. While some lead figurines showing the so-called divine pair appear rather clumsy in comparison to their counterparts in clay,[86] there are also neat examples in which the rendering of the flounced robe and other details are so similar to terracotta plaques[87] that one wonders if the craftsman was working from a model! Another notable parallel with plaque imagery is the nude female, a long-standing favourite across the ancient Near East. The manner in which she emerges in the lead figurine repertoire is of a distinctly Syrian type, which suggests an alternative route she may have followed from the medium of clay to that of lead. Emre has also suggested a parallel between a partial Kültepe figurine showing an unusual variation on the 'divine family' theme (it comprises only one 'parent' who also happens to be male and holds his 'children' at an awkward position),[88] and two terracotta plaques showing a presumably divine female figure holding a small child across each shoulder.[89] The overall subject matter of these plaques, however, is far too complex[90] to postulate a convincing link with the typical motif of children being held by or associated with divine characters of the lead figurine repertoire.

It is important to acknowledge that the quintessential tradition of Syrian plaques,[91] though with palpable origins in the Old Babylonian production technology of open moulds,[92] has its own set of symbolic meanings and ritual function quite separate from those of Old Babylonian plaques. According to Moorey, "As

85 Canby 1965, 49, n.56.

86 Compare Emre 1971, pl. X-4 with Barrelet 1968, pl. LXXVII-790.

87 Compare Emre 1971, pl. XI-2 with Woolley and Mallowan 1976, pl. 82–161.

88 "In contrast to the goddesses who usually hold their children at waist level, the god's hands are at breast level and he carries the little girls by holding and supporting the soles of their feet" (Emre 1993, 174).

89 Van Buren 1933–1934; see also Opficius 1961, 252.

90 See Black and Green 1992, 234.

91 See Badre 1980.

92 Moorey 2003, 34.

[the technology of open moulds] was used there almost exclusively for nude female images, without any sign of the wide range of motifs produced with it in Babylonia, this would appear to have been no more than a technological transfer."[93] The singular focus of Syrian plaque imagery is indeed conspicuous, suggesting a deliberate singularity of focus on female symbolism, meaningful perhaps in the context of "popular rituals of women"[94] but at any rate quite distinct from the varied apotropaic repertoire of protective/auspicious beings[95] on Babylonian plaques. The link, therefore, between Syrian plaques and lead trinkets, as represented by the typical nude female, may well have been established as a separate line of contact.

Considering the Social Lives of Lead Figurines and Stone Moulds

The single most important aspect of lead trinkets to be acknowledged is their sheer versatility of use and associated meaning. The following discussion explores some of the categories under which they would have functioned as commodities, based on the understanding that "a commodity is a thoroughly socialised thing."[96] More specifically, Appadurai defines a commodity as *"any thing intended for exchange,"*[97] a definition to which lead trinkets fit particularly well not only in their inherent characteristics, but also the wider context of interregional circulation within which they existed. The term "trinket," coined by Canby and used throughout this article, is particularly apt for lead figurines because it conveys an ambiguity, an open-endedness of purpose in keeping with the versatility of this class of artefact. It would be erroneous to expect a rigid set of predetermined functions from lead trinkets, which could easily be put to a great variety of uses. This is primarily due to the physical qualities of lead itself, lending itself to a wide range of purposes, attested both archaeologically and in texts.[98]

Some of the more 'practical' uses of lead trinkets are immediately obvious. On one side of a mould purchased in İzmir is the negative of a pair of small tweezers[99] attesting to the use of stone moulds for manufacturing small implements. Quite a few of the abstract geometric patterns inside square or circular frames would have been intended to produce stamp seals.[100] While some of the linear patterns on

93 Moorey 2003, 34.

94 Moorey 2003, 23.

95 Assante 2002, 8.

96 Appadurai 1986, 3.

97 Appadurai 1986, 9, italics original.

98 Moorey 1994, 121.

99 Canby 1965, pl. IX-c.

100 Canby 1965, 43ff.

these seal designs were used much more widely than the confines of Anatolia and Cilicia, Canby stresses that "their use on metal seals is a characteristic Anatolian phenomenon."[101] Trinket moulds also produced spindle whorls,[102] again with good Anatolian parallels in clay.[103] Equally frequently, abstract geometric designs carved on trinket moulds were intended to produce jewellery or ornaments such as pins, earrings or pendants,[104] with parallels in gold and silver at Ur, Tell Brak, and Mari.[105] As for figural pendants, these represented various animals including a lion, a caprid (?), stylised double-headed bovines or birds atop a quadruple spiral.[106] A beak-spouted vessel, handle no doubt intended as a pendant loop, attested on two moulds,[107] is a faithful replica of EBA types.[108] Beak-spouted pitchers remain an Anatolian favourite also throughout the second millennium BC, during which period they are also conspicuous in religious iconography as libation vessels.[109] It is likely that the choice of beak-spouted pitchers as pendants was related to the use of actual vessels in ritual settings, perhaps identifying the wearer as a devout libation-pourer, or as someone who has taken part in a sacred ceremony and/or been to a sacred location. The circulation of lead trinkets in pilgrimage (?) markets is certainly an attractive possibility[110] in keeping both with the role of itinerancy in their production and circulation, as well as with the amuletic character of the lead trinket repertoire as a whole.

As for anthropomorphic imagery, the term "figurine" is useful as a descriptive category, but does not necessarily indicate *precise* function. While it is fairly clear that a stamp seal is for sealing, a whorl for spinning, and jewellery for wearing, what does one *actually do* with a lead figurine? As apotropaia, miniatures such as lead figurines would have been very well suited to being worn on one's person. Just as non-representational ornaments in precious metals were imitated in the trinket repertoire, figurines could also have been inexpensive alternatives to gold pendants mentioned in *kārum* period texts. In a Kültepe letter (Kt 2001/k 325a-b), for instance, a certain Ziki, who happens to be an *ugbabtum* priestess, is mentioned

101 Canby 1965, 43, with references.

102 Emre 1971, 45.

103 Canby 1965, 48, n. 52–54.

104 Canby 1965, 44.

105 Aruz 2003, 258; see Emre 1971, pl. II-1.

106 Canby 1965, 42; Emre 1971, 46–48.

107 Emre 1971, 48, nos. 37, 38.

108 Canby 1965, 46, fig. 1.

109 N. Özgüç 1965, 13ff, pl. XXIV 71, 73; see also Müller-Karpe 2002, 258, figs. 1, 3.

110 I was struck by this idea on a visit to the Scottish National Museum in Edinburgh when I encountered an AD 14th century stone mould for a "pilgrim's badge" of St. Andrew on display there.

as the owner of "jewellery in the shape of a gold figurine of a deity" (DINGIR*li ša* KÙ.GI *ša* a-bi$_4$-*ša šu-ku-ta-ša*).[111] The practice of fashioning divine images as gold pendants is also attested for the Hittite period.[112] An immediate problem is that lead figurines are not equipped with loops or hooks to indicate they were worn as pendants. An alternative means of wearing lead figurines on one's person would have been to sew them onto clothing, as suggested by Van Buren.[113] This possibility is firmly refuted by Emre, however, on account of the rudimentary 'platforms' on which many of the lead figurines stand indicate that these objects were intended to rest on or against a surface.[114] The most compelling example for this is a Kültepe mould showing a winged god standing on a 'table,' the back legs of which extend diagonally outwards.[115] Such an awkward rendering of this simple form disagrees with the skilful way in which the figure itself has been depicted. Presumably once the figurine was cast, the table legs were meant to be bent—easy to do with lead—to form an actual table which could thus stand firmly on a surface, bending the figure at the ankles would then allow it to stand upright.

From a production point of view, for those figurines with an interactive aspect there would have been an intermediate period of latency after initial casting and before final display. If the figurine were to be transported prior to sale or use, it would be far easier to keep it in this stage. Did the saleability or value of figurines diminish once they were modified and thus no longer in mint condition? Was the manipulation of the figurine the final stage of its production process and accordingly carried out by the metal-smith, or did it mark the beginning of its use life, meant for the consumer to perform? Did the transformation of a flat figurine into a freestanding piece hold any symbolic value? From a functional point of view, once set up, freestanding lead figurines (especially those standing on tables!) could easily receive offerings. Miniature cult scenes arranged inside clay vessels[116] are certainly part of the contemporary repertoire of ritual objects. More importantly, if lead figurines were intended to be propped up against a vertical surface or made to stand upright by means of a fold-out platform, this suggests that the primary relationship of these objects were not to a *person* wearing them, but to a *setting* in which they were placed. As small, portable objects, lead figurines could easily have been moved from one place to another, creating *ad hoc* ritual settings and/ or apotropaic zones according to the desires and needs of their owners.

111 Albayrak 2004, 11.

112 Darga 1992.

113 Van Buren 1954, 110.

114 Emre 1971, 82; see, for instance, Emre 1971, pl. X, 2a-c.

115 Emre 1971, XV 1a-b.

116 See T. Özgüç 1994 and 1999.

On the protective function of lead figurines, Emre has intuitively raised the question whether the raw material of lead itself may have been significant.[117] There is in fact compelling evidence from Hittite texts to support this postulation. The inherent magical quality attributed to lead seems to have served specially to seal channels communicating with the underworld so as to prevent undesirable forces from reaching the world above. In other words, lead was regarded as an apotropaic material through which evil forces could not pass. An incantation (KUB 33.66 obv ii 9 ff) gives a long list of the various evils to be trapped inside a bronze cauldron sealed with lead:

> *a-ru-ni-ma* URUDU-*aš pal-ḫa-eš ki-an-da-*[*ri*] *iš-tap-pu-ul-li-iš-mi-it* A.GAR5-*aš nu-kán* [*i-da-a-lu*] *an-da da-iš ta-ar-pí-in da-iš pár*$^{?}$-[ ]*da-iš e-eš-ḫar da-iš ḫa-pa-an-zi d*[*a-iš*] DIRIG *da-iš iš-ḫa-aḫ-ru da-iš* [...] *da-iš lúm*$^{?}$*-pa-an da-iš kam-ma-ra-*[*an da-iš*] *ḫur-di da-iš i-na-an d*[*a-iš*]
>
> In the sea copper (=bronze?) cauldrons are set. Their lids (are of) lead. And [evil(?)] he put therein, the evil demon (*tarpin*) he put, [...] he put, bloodshed he put, *hapanzi* he p[ut], sorrow he put, tears he put, [...] he put, grief he put, fog (?) [he put], cursing (?) he put, disease he p[ut].[118]

It is worth noting that included in the list of evils in this text is *tarpiš*, a demon comparable to the Mesopotamian *šēdu*, whose counterpart *lamassu* in turn corresponds to Hittite *annariš*.[119] Like *lamassu* and *šēdu* in Mesopotamia, Hittite *annariš* and *tarpiš* are often referred to as a pair, in which case they tend to be viewed as benevolent; when *tarpiš* appears alone, however, he does so as a malevolent demon, which is also how *šēdu* is perceived singly.[120] The reference to *tarpiš* therefore further highlights the apotropaic quality of lead, which evidently kept away not only generic maladies such as plague and bloodshed, but also the more precise, personalised agents of evil. A similar passage comes from the *Telipinu Myth* (KUB 17 rev IV 14–19):

> *ḫa-a-aš-ta* ^{LÚ}NI.DUH 7 ^{GIŠ}IG *a-ap-pa ḫu-it-ti-ia-at* 7 ^{GIŠ}*ḫa-at-ta-lu*
> *kat-ta-an da-an-ku-i ták-ni-i* ZABAR *pal-ḫi ar-ta iš-tap-pu-ul-li-iš-me-et*
> A.GAR$_5$-*aš za-ak-ki-iš-me-iš* AN.BAR-*aš ku-it an-da-an pa-iz-zi na-aš-ta*
> *nam-ma ša-ra-a Ú-UL ú-iz-zi an-da-da-an ḫar-ak-zi*
> *Ù ŠA* ^{d}*Te-li-pí-nu kar-pí-in kar-di-mi-ia-at-ta-an*
> *wa-aš-du-ul ša-a-u-ar an-da e-ep-du na-at a-ap-pa le-e ú-iz-zi*

117 Emre 1971, 81.

118 Hoffner 1968, 65.

119 Hoffner 1968, 64.

120 Hoffner 1968, 64.

> The Gatekeeper opened seven doors, he drew back seven bolts.
> Beneath the black earth bronze cauldrons are set, their lids
> (Are of) lead, their latches (are of) iron, that which goes inside, it
> Henceforth does not come up, inside it vanishes
> And the wrath of Telipinu, the cause of anger,
> The sin, the fury, let it (=the cauldrons) hold inside! And it shall not come back again.[121]

The Hattic origin of the *Telipinu Myth* is a strong indication that the belief in apotropaic qualities of lead was already in existence in Anatolia before the myth was committed to writing by Hittite scribes. In other words, such a belief would have been contemporary with the lead figurines of the early second millennium BC. If so, the widespread practice of depositing lead circlets in Anatolian graves in the second millennium BC could also be considered as an act of magical significance, presumably in order to filter undesirable netherworld forces which would have been given unintended release through the digging of a grave, or more simply to ensure that the dead remained clear of the world of the living. The deposition of the Alişar figurine in the 'palace' foundations (see above) also belongs to the same constellation of ideas linking lead to magical protection.

As a highly versatile metal, the commodity value of lead itself as a raw material is also significant. Even as cast objects, the value of lead trinkets would have been determined to a great extent by the ever-present possibility of being melted down and recycled into a completely new and different existence. Especially small-scale objects would have had permanent latency as raw material. In other words, the social lives of lead trinkets could have been a complex series of multiple 'reincarnations.' The potential currency value for lead trinkets in and of themselves was recognised by Canby, who suggests these items may well have been "more negotiable if shaped into trinkets."[122]

Although not equally as versatile as lead trinkets, the moulds used in their manufacture would also have been meaningful in a wide range of contexts. For the purposes of the modern scholar, trinket moulds have principally served to examine the production technology for lead figurines.[123] In this respect, the contrast between the crowded moulds Canby attributes to itinerant metal-working and those with single figures is but one example of how different modes of production can provide crucial information otherwise unattainable from the products themselves. Marchetti's observation, for instance, that the preference of softer

121 Translation from transliteration in Mazoyer 2003, 51.

122 Canby 1965, 53.

123 See Opitz 1933.

stone for moulds may be linked to amateur (or occasional) production[124] could not have been made by studying the figurines alone. The social life of moulds was not, however, confined solely to their primary function as production equipment. Indeed, Marchetti has already noted that moulds travelled as widely as the figurines, seeing as moulds carved in the characteristic traits of one workshop/group can be encountered much farther afield.[125] The presence of at least two moulds from Kültepe-Kaneš in storage rooms[126] with no association to metal production is also significant in this regard, suggesting that moulds may have been treated as merchandise. One of these moulds was found in a Level Ib house storeroom[127] and the other evidently kept alongside the tablet archive of the house owner,[128] suggesting that the mould may have been considered an object of considerable value and importance.

It is safe to assume that, in addition to moulds that travelled as part of the professional equipment of itinerant metal-smiths, there would have been moulds which travelled as items of trade. In most part, the commodity value of stone moulds within exchange circuits were presumably determined by their principal consumers, namely metal-smiths. From the latter's perspective, important considerations would have been the weight and durability of the stone, and the variety and quality of the carved negatives. If catering for a conservative market, the smith's preference would have been towards well-established themes in familiar styles. Alternatively, demand for more exotic trinkets would have rendered 'foreign' moulds more desirable. Ready-made, rather than self-produced, moulds could also have been exchanged as style guides or become style guides in the context of exchange. It is also likely that moulds became curios in and of themselves, being traded for sheer novelty value, and may even have even come to acquire magico-symbolic associations of their own. Two stone moulds from Old Assyrian levels in Aššur, associated with a temple context,[129] suggest these objects may have held a votive value. Perhaps they were dedicated by metal-smiths or merchants as thanks offerings after a successful Anatolian journey?

Finally, moulds would easily have made construction material in the form of spolia, as was evidently the case for a broken sandstone mould recycled for a Level III wall of the lower town at Acemhöyük.[130]

124 Marchetti 2003, 403.

125 Marchetti 2003, 411.

126 Emre 1971, 16–17.

127 Emre 1971, fig. 9.

128 Emre 1971, fig. 3.

129 Andrae 1922, 84, pl. 29, pl. 55a-b.

130 N. Özgüç 1976, 552.

Conclusion

Anatolian lead figurines and their stone moulds remain as intriguing as ever, and will no doubt continue to generate scholarly interest not simply in and of themselves, but as unique indicators of change and continuity in imagery, magico-religious practices, and artisanal production in a complex network of interregional connections. The sheer versatility of lead miniatures; the range of stylistic and iconographic influences they display; and their multi-faceted contexts of production, use, and meaning make these objects a highly valuable source for *kārum* period studies as a whole. In utilising such a source, it is vital to recognise the wide extent to which lead trinkets and trinket moulds could have had multiple uses, circulating within a complex world of long-distance trade and cross-cultural exchange, their commodity values shifting and adapting to different phases of their social lives. The production of cast lead miniatures is uniquely tied to hybridities of skill, style, and meaning.

It is quite striking that the lead trinket industry in Anatolia, despite its evidently multifarious nature, appears to have failed to survive beyond the *kārum* system of exchange. Just as the beginnings of this particular strand of image production can be ascribed to interregional links between north Mesopotamia and the Anatolian plateau in the late third millennium BC, so can its end be attributed to that of the *kārum* network. In this respect the production, use, and circulation of lead figurines could very well be contextualised in terms of the dynamics of mechanical reproduction of images as discussed by D. Wengrow, who traces the origin of hybrid beings in iconography to the development of mechanical technologies of image (re-)production.[131]

While Wengrow's focus rests particularly on the emergence of fantastical combination creatures ("monsters") at the cusp of urbanism, the underlying principles of his model are also applicable to the production of lead figurines. Wengrow identifies seals as the fundamental technical means which allowed, for the first time, the effortless creation of identical images *ad infinitum*. Although relatively more complex, the production of lead miniatures also operates on a similar principle in that it too allows continuous (re)production. More to the point is the emphasis on the "links between large scale distributions of images and the growth of commercial and political networks."[132] Another pertinent drive for the creation and dissemination of hybrid images are "periods of intensified exposure to outside influence,"[133] which tallies well with the peculiarities of *kārum* period trade within which lead trinkets circulated. A closer examination of the circumstances of the

131 Wengrow 2014.

132 Wengrow 2014, 16, 60.

133 Wengrow 2014, 54.

manufacture, exchange, use, meanings, and the final disappearance of *kārum* period lead trinkets can and ought to be treated as part of greater diachronic trends of change beyond the immediate confines of the early second millennium. The potential of this class of objects to offer new solutions to old problems and raise new questions is by no means exhausted, and awaits renewed interest and rigour.

Acknowledgements

This article began life many years ago, but took its present form during the Anniversary Fellowship I held at the McDonald Institute for Archaeological Research, University of Cambridge, between 2013–2015. As always, I would like to thank Nicholas Postgate for suffering numerous early drafts *ca.* 2009, and my co-editors, Emre Şerifoğlu and Eric Jean, for helping me tidy up the current version, *ca.* 2014. I am also grateful to İlgi Gerçek for looking over the Hittite.

REFERENCES

Akyurt, İ.M., *M.Ö. 2. Binde Anadolu'da Ölü Gömme Adetleri.* Ankara: Türk Tarih Kurumu, 1998.

Albayrak, İ., "'She Will Live, Eat and Be Anointed Together with Them' *ušbat aklat u paššsat ištīšunu*" in *Assyria and Beyond: Studies Presented to Mogens Trolle Larsen*, ed. by J. G. Dercksen, 9–20. Leiden: Nederlands Instituut voor het Nabije Oosten, 2004.

Alexander, R.L., "Native Group Cylinder Seal Engravers of Karum Kanish Level II." *Belleten* 43 (1979): 573–618.

Andrae, W., *Die archaischen Ischtar-Tempel in Assur.* Leipzig: J. C. Hinrichs, 1922.

Appadurai, A., "Introduction: Commodities and the Politics of Value" in *The Social Life of Things*, ed. by A. Appadurai, 3–63. Cambridge: Cambridge University Press, 1986.

Aruz, J., "Mould for Jewelry, Seals and Amulets" in *Art of the First Cities: The Third Millennium BC from the Mediterranean to the Indus*, ed. by J. Aruz and R. Wallenfels, 257–258. New York: Metropolitan Museum of Art, 2003.

Assante, J., "Style and Replication in 'Old Babylonian' Terracotta Plaques: Strategies for Entrapping the Power of Images" in *Ex Mesopotamia et Syria Lux: Festschrift für Manfried Dietrich zu seinem 65. Gebrurtstag* (AOAT 281), ed. by O. Loretz, K. A. Metzler and H. Schaudig, 1–29. Münster: Ugarit-Verlag, 2002.

———. "The Lead Inlays of Tukulti-Ninurta I: Pornography as Imperial Strategy" in *Ancient Near Eastern Art in Context: Studies in Honor of Irene J. Winter by Her Students*, ed. by J. Cheng and M. H. Feldman, 369–407. Leiden: Brill, 2007.

Badre, L., *Les figurines anthropomorphes en terra cuite à l'Age du Bronze en Syrie.* Paris: Paul Geuthner, 1980.

Barjamovic, G., T. Hertel and M. T. Larsen, *Ups and Downs at Kanesh: Chronology, History and Society in the Old Assyrian Period.* Leiden: Nederlands Instituut voor het Nabije Oosten, 2012.

Barrelet, M.-T., *Figurines et reliefs en terre cuite de la Mésopotamie antique I: Potiers, termes de métier, procédés de fabrication et production.* Paris: Paul Geuthner, 1968.

Bittel, K., *Prähistorische Forschung in Kleinasien* (*Istanbuler Forschungen* 6). Istanbul: Universum-druckerei, 1934.

———. *Die Hethiter: Die Kunst Anatoliens vom Ende des 3. bis zum Anfang des 1. Jahrtausends vor Christus.* München: Beck, 1976.

Black, J. and A. Green, *Gods, Demons and Symbols of Ancient Mesopotamia.* London: The British Museum, 1992.

Boehmer, R. M., *Die Kleinfunde aus der Unterstadt von Boğazköy: Grabungskampagnen 1970–1978* (*Boğazköy-Hattuša* 10). Berlin: Gebr. Mann, 1979.

Canby, J. V., "Early Bronze 'Trinket' Moulds." *Iraq* 27/1 (1965): 42–61.

———. "A Figurine from Urkesh: A 'Darling' from Troy to Mesopotamia." *Iraq* 65 (2003): 171–173.

Darga, M., *Hitit Sanatı*. İstanbul: Akbank Kültür ve Sanat Kitapları, 1992.

Ellis, R.S., *Foundation Deposits in Ancient Mesopotamia*. New Haven: Yale University Press, 1968.

Emre, K., "Kültepe Menşeli Yeni bir Kalıp." *Belleten* 33 (1969): 163–170.

———. "Eine neue Gussform aus Kültepe." *Zeitschrift für Assyriologie* 60 (1970): 134–147.

———. *Anadolu Kurşun Figürinleri ve Taş Kalıpları / Anatolian Lead Figurines and Their Stone Moulds*. Ankara: Türk Tarih Kurumu, 1971.

———. "New Lead Figurines and Moulds from Kültepe and Kızılhamza" in *Aspects of Art And Iconography: Anatolia and Its Neighbours. Studies in Honor of Nimet Özgüç*, ed. by M. J. Mellink, E. Porada and T. Özgüç, 169–177. Ankara: Türk Tarih Kurumu, 1993.

Heffron, Y., *Household Rituals in Middle Bronze Age Anatolia: An Archaeological-Textual Study*. Unpublished PhD Thesis, University of Cambridge, 2011.

Hoffner, H.A., "Hittite *tarpiš* and Hebrew *terāphîm*." *Journal of Near Eastern Studies* 27/1 (1968): 61–68.

Kulakoğlu, F., "Kültepe-Kaneš: A Second Millennium BCE Trading Center on the Central Plateau" in *The Oxford Handbook of Ancient* Anatolia, ed. by S. Steadman and G. McMahon, 1012–1030. Oxford: Oxford University Press, 2011.

———. "Kanesh after the Assyrian Colony Period: Current Research at Kültepe and the Question of the End of the Bronze Age Settlement" in *Current Research at Kültepe-Kanesh: An Interdisciplinary and Integrative Approach to Trade Networks, Internationalism, and Identity*, ed. by L. Atıcı, F. Kulakoğlu, G. Barjamovic, A Fairbairn, 85–94. Atlanta, Lockwood Press, 2014.

Lehner, J.W. and K.A. Yener, "Organization and Specialization of Early Mining and Metal Technologies in Anatolia" in *Archaeometallurgy in Global Perspective: Methods and Syntheses*, ed. by B.W. Roberts and C.P. Thorton, 529–557, New York: Springer, 2015.

Mazoyer, M., *Télipinu: le dieu au marécage: Essai sur les mythes fondateurs du Royaume hittite*. Paris: L'Harmattan, 2003.

Marchetti, N., "Workshops, Trading Routes and Divine Figures: On the Early Middle Bronze II Syro-Anatolian Lead Figurines." *Orientalia NS* 72 (2003): 390–420.

Michel, C., "The *Kārum* Period on the Plateau" in *The Oxford Handbook of Ancient Anatolia*, ed. by S. Steadman and G. McMahon, 313–336. Oxford: Oxford University Press, 2011.

Moorey, P.R.S., *Ancient Mesopotamian Materials and Industries: The Archaeological Evidence*. Oxford: Clarendon Press, 1994.

———. *Idols of the People: Miniature Images of Clay in the Ancient Near East*. Oxford. Oxford University Press, 2003.

Müller-Karpe, A., "Die Keramik des Mittleren und Jüngeren hethitischen Reiches" in *Die Hethiter und ihr Reich*, 256–263. Bonn: Kunst- und Ausstellungshalle der Bundesrepublik Deutschland GmbH, 2002.

Opficius, R., *Das Altbabylonische Terrakottarelief.* Berlin: De Gruyter, 1961.

Opitz, D., "Altorientalische Gußformen" in *Aus fünf Jahrtausenden morgenlandischer Kultur: Festschrift Max Freiherrn von Oppenheim zum 70 Geburtstage, gewidmet von Freunden und Mitarbeitern* (*AfO* Beiband I), 179–215. Berlin, 1933.

Orthmann, W., *Das Gräberfeld bei Ilıca.* Wiesbaden: F. Steiner, 1967.

Özgüç, N., *Kültepe Mühür Baskılarında Anadolu Grubu / The Anatollian Group of Cylinder Seal Impressions from Kültepe.* Ankara: Türk Tarih Kurumu, 1965.

———. "Acemhöyük Kazıları / Excavations at Acemhöyük." *Anadolu / Anatolia* 10 (1966): 1–52.

———. "An Ivory Box and Stone Mould from Acemhöyük." *Belleten* 40 (1976): 555–560.

Özgüç, T., *Türk Tarih Kurumu Tarafından Yapılan Kültepe Kazısı Raporu 1948.* Ankara: Türk Tarih Kurumu, 1950.

———. "A Figurine of a God from Anatolia in the Hermitage Museum in Leningrad" in *Florilegium Anatolicum*: *Mélanges offerts* à *E. Laroche*, 291–296. Paris: Éditions E. de Boccard, 1979.

———. "A Cult Vessel Discovered at Kanish" in *Beiträge zur altorientalischen Archäologie und Altertumskunde: Festschrift für Barthel Hrouda zum 65. Geburtstag*, ed. by P. Calmeyer and B. Hrouda, 221–227. Wiesbaden: Harrassowitz Verlag, 1994.

———. "Vases Used for Ritual Purposes from Eskiyapar" *Essays on Ancient Anatolia* (*BMECCJ* 11), ed. T. Mikasa, 1–22. Wiesbaden: Harrassowitz Verlag, 1999.

Öztan, A., "1998–1999 Acemhöyük Kazıları." *Kazı Sonuçları Toplantısı* 22/1 (2001) 119–128.

———. "2000 Yılı Acemhöyük Kazıları." *Kazı Sonuçları Toplantısı* 23/2 (2002): 327–334.

———. "2001 Yılı Acemhöyük Kazıları." *Kazı Sonuçları Toplantısı* 24/1(2003): 39–48.

———. "2002 Yılı Acemhöyük Kazıları." *Kazı Sonuçları Toplantısı* 25/1 (2004): 231–238.

———. "2003 Yılı Acemhöyük Kazıları." *Kazı Sonuçları Toplantısı* 26/2 (2005): 91–104.

———. "2005 Yılı Acemhöyük Kazıları." *Kazı Sonuçları Toplantısı* 28/2 (2007): 549–560.

———. "2006 Yılı Acemhöyük Kazıları." *Kazı Sonuçları Toplantısı* 29/3 (2008): 515–524.

———. "2007 Yılı Acemhöyük Kazıları." *Kazı Sonuçları Toplantısı* 30/3 (2009): 329–342.

Schmidt, E.F., *Anatolia through the Ages: Discoveries at the Alişar Mound 1927–29* (OIC 11). Chicago: The Oriental Institute, 1931.

Toklu, G., "Acemhöyük'te Bulunan Bir Kurşun Figürin Grubu." *Belleten* 40 (1976): 561–564.

Topçuoğlu, O., "A Look behind the Scenes: Seal Carvers of Ancient Kanesh as Artists and Artisans." Paper delivered at the 1st Kültepe International Meeting, Kayseri, September 2013.

Van Buren, E.D., "A Clay Relief in the Iraq Museum." *Archiv für Orientforschung* 9 (1933–1934): 165–171.

———. "Seals of the Second Half of the Layard Collection." *Orientalia* 23 (1954): 97–113.

Von der Osten, H.H., *The Alişar Hüyük: Seasons of 1930–1932* (OIP 29). Chicago: The Oriental Institute, 1937.

Wengrow, D., *The Origin of Monsters: Image and Cognition in the First Age of Mechanical Reproduction.* Princeton: Princeton University Press, 2014.

Woolley, L. and M. Mallowan, *Ur Excavations VII: The Old Babylonian Period*, ed. by T. C. Mitchell. London: The British Museum.

Pot-marks as a Feature of Interregional Connectivity at Tell Atchana-Alalakh: Evidence from the 2006–2012 Excavations

Mara T. Horowitz[1]

An important and long-overdue discussion on pre-firing incised pot-marks from Anatolia was begun by Marie-Henriette Gates based on the recovery of a destroyed store-room at Kinet Höyük where pot-marks were especially prevalent.[2] *Throughout her distinguished career, Marie-Henriette Gates has contributed tremendously to the archaeology of Anatolia and Syria. Her exemplary fieldwork at the important site of Kinet Höyük together with Charles Gates is particularly relevant to my research on Amuq ceramics, and I would like to dedicate this piece on the pot-mark tradition of Tell Atchana to her on the occasion of this Festschrift.*

Abstract

The pre-firing marking of ceramic vessels in the eastern Mediterranean Bronze Age is a topic that generates a wide variety of interpretations. This paper presents a body of previously unpublished pot-marks from Tell Atchana, ancient Alalakh, and considers patterns of their use in the Middle and Late Bronze Ages. The marks occurring at Alalakh are very similar to those at other sites in Syria and Anatolia and, with an inception date in the early 16th century BC, they begin to be found at approximately the same time as marks at many of the sites in Anatolia and well before the expansion of the Kingdom of Hatti into areas beyond the central

1 Purchase College, SUNY, 735 Anderson Hill Road, Purchase, NY 10577, USA.
The author would like to thank Aslıhan Yener, Murat Akar, Gül Bulut, and the crew of the Alalakh Excavation Project. Special thanks to my assistants Müge Bulu Akar and Jessica Sue Wiles. Postdoctoral fellowships for the study of local ceramics at Tell Atchana were provided by the Fund for Amuq Valley Archaeological Expeditions and by the Research Center for Anatolian Civilizations, Koç University, Istanbul. Thanks also to the editors of this volume for their hard work and support.

2 Gates 2001, 139.

of Alalakh, as opposed to other parts of the city, strongly associates marking practices with an industry of currently unknown organization supplying large amounts of pottery to a central authority, although the exact meaning of the signs remains open to interpretation. The apparent disappearance of these pot-marks at Alalakh by the mid-14th century BC seems to indicate that a change in the local ceramic industry occurred concurrent with the arrival of Hittite political administration that obviated the need for pot marking.

The topic of pot-marks is an interesting one with the potential to illuminate the economic, political, and cultural lives of the people who made them.[3] For ceramics specialists, the subject adds another possible layer of interpretation to the usual system of typologies based on ware, shape, decoration, function, and technical analyses. This paper addresses pre-firing incised pot-marks at Tell Atchana-Alalakh in the context of interregional connections and modes of ceramic production in the Late Bronze Age (LBA).

The new excavations at Tell Atchana, ancient Alalakh, have produced a large body of ceramic and contextual data that is allowing the first methodical study of the occurrence of pot-marks at the site. This preliminary analysis reveals that Atchana's pot-marks are strongly concentrated in the palace-area (Area 1, see Fig. 1) sample dating to the Late Bronze I (LB I), and are very rare in contemporary non-palatial contexts and in the Late Bronze II (LB II) period. Only one pot-mark is currently known from the Middle Bronze Age (MBA), and that from the final occupation phase before the outset of the LBA. This pattern of pot-mark occurrence, while preliminary in nature, suggests that the administrative center of Alalakh in LB I (including the 'Niqmepa Palace' excavated by Woolley[4]) was the primary recipient of marked pottery. This paper considers several explanatory models for this pattern of marked pottery.

Pot-marks in Theory and Application

Many uses have been proposed for pot-marks, from banal and practical to ritual and sacred.[5] In the ancient Near East, pot-marks have been inconsistently studied. Pot-marks have sometimes been compared to contemporary forms of writing in order to assign them at least a phonetic value, if not a further derived meaning. The marks appearing on Cypriot pottery have had the most attention paid, perhaps because of ongoing interest in deciphering the Cypro-Minoan script(s) of the island.[6]

3 Hirschfeld 2008, 120.

4 Woolley 1955.

5 Gates 2001; Glatz 2012; Hirschfeld 2002, 2008.

6 Hirschfeld 2008, 120.

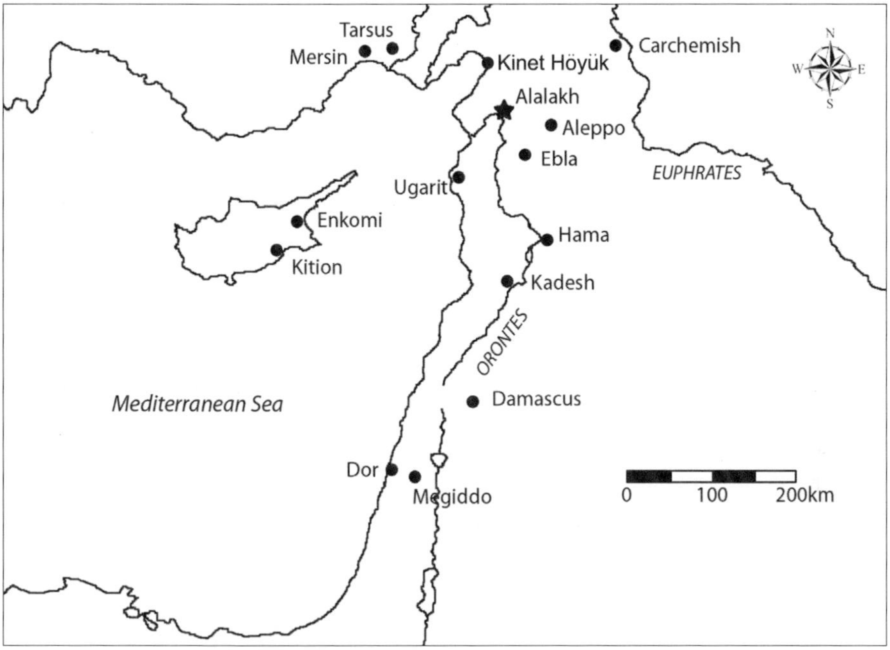

FIG. 1 Map of the Northeast Mediterranean (M. Horowitz)

On the mainland, approaches differ to the pre-firing marks on pots, a tradition that occurred in diverse regions such as Egypt, the Levant, Syria, and Anatolia in many parts of the Bronze Age.[7] In Anatolia, pre-firing pot-marks have been compared to the Luwian hieroglyphic script to search for both for phonetic and symbolic values[8] and for numeric values perhaps representing vessel volume.[9] However, the use of very similar pot-marks in southeastern Anatolia and the Amuq before the first evidence for the Luwian script in the Anatolian plateau would seem to contradict the theory that the marks derived from the script.[10]

Pre-firing pot-marks have also been interpreted as a way to mark a particular batch of pottery being either the product or property of a particular individual or institution. Gates suggested that the symbols were not part of a script or invested with any greater meaning, but were only used and interpreted by those within the pottery workshops.[11] A suggestion was made by Archi and

7 Glatz 2012, 11–15.

8 Müller-Karpe 1998; Mielke 2006.

9 Seidl 1972; Müller-Karpe 1988.

10 See Glatz 2012, fig. 2.

11 Gates 2001, 140–141.

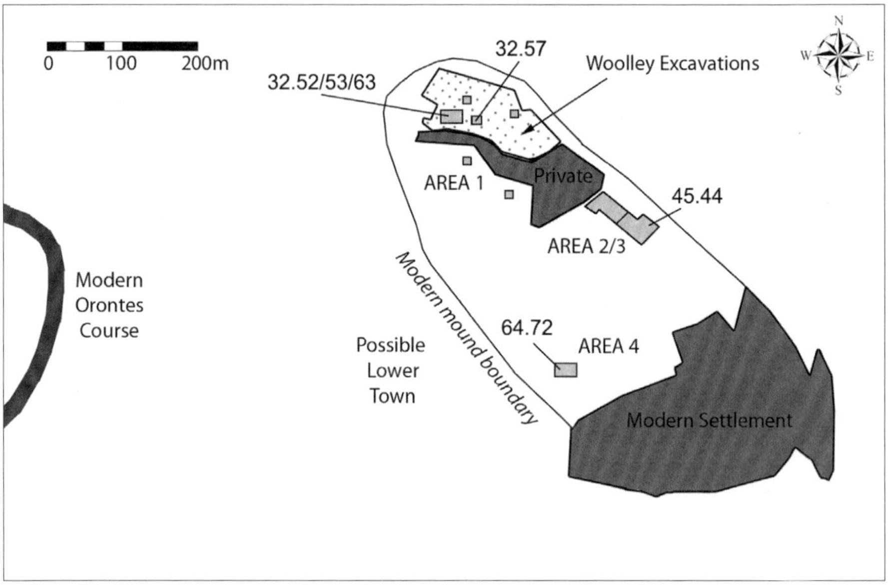

FIG. 2 Plan of Tell Atchana-Alalakh (M. Horowitz)

Venturi that the pot-marks on large storage jars at Tell Afis were related to 'storage and distribution of primary goods and foodstuffs.'[12] Both of these interpretations associate the marking with a system of highly centralized political management, in particular the Hittite Empire. Alternatively, Griffin's study at Korucutepe concluded that the pot-marks found there were intended to distinguish the work of different potters using a common kiln[13] and not as a system of bureaucratic or imperial management.

Unfortunately, the general lack of reliable data (publication of contextualized finds, large sample sizes) on pot-marks in Syria, the Levant, and Anatolia makes analysis of trends in marking and possible economic-political interpretations difficult. A recent publication by Glatz[14] has synthesized much of the available information and generated a typology and catalog of pre-firing pot-mark signs occurring at sites across Anatolia that have sufficiently published their ceramics. A similar study building on this work for the sites of Syria and neighboring regions is badly needed. This paper presents new data on pot-marks from Alalakh to contribute to the discussion on the interrelationship between potters' marking practices, the organization of production, interregional contacts, and political structure in the LBA of the ancient Near East.

12 2013, 218; see also Venturi 2013, 232.

13 Griffin 1980.

14 Glatz 2012.

Tell Atchana-Alalakh

Tell Atchana is the site of the ancient city of Alalakh, located on a bend of the Orontes River on the southern side of the Amuq Plain. Originally excavated by Sir Leonard Woolley in the 1930s and 40s, new excavations directed by Aslıhan Yener since 2001 have greatly expanded our knowledge of the city's history and material culture. The city's chronological periods are now known to stretch from Amuq J (Early Bronze IV) through to the Iron II period.[15] Alalakh was, during the Middle and Late Bronze Ages, the largest site in the Amuq and is known to have served as the seat of a minor king during much of that period.[16] Both the city and the surrounding territory between the Amanus Mountains and the craggy hills of northwestern Syria are sometimes referred to as Mukish.[17]

This paper focuses on LB I at Atchana (*c.* 1600–1400,[18] Periods[19] 6–4). Alalakh's political situation in the early LB I is still uncertain. Following the destruction of the city and its hegemonic overlord at Aleppo by Hittite raids, there is new evidence for a time of recovery before the arrival of the Mitanni imperial expansion.[20] In this period the seeds were already sown for a new Late Bronze material culture which, while clearly rooted in the preceding era, began to exhibit clearly new cultural traits, such as ceramic forms associated with dining and the appearance of pre-firing incised pot-marks. In LB IIa (c.1400–1300 BC, Periods 3–1[21]), an increase in site-wide ceramic homogeneity (in ware and form) and the final abandonment of a number of Middle Bronze-rooted wares and forms could suggest a shift in the dynamics of production, in terms of craft organization, demand, and political administration.

Pot-marks in Woolley's Catalog

Woolley's excavations at Atchana (1936–1939, 1946–1949) produced a huge collection of ceramics coming mostly from the area in and around the palaces and

15 Yener *at al.*, forthcoming.

16 Yener 2010.

17 Von Dassow 2008; Yener 2010.

18 This paper uses the Middle Chronology throughout and is not intended to make any statement about the absolute dating of Alalakh, which is still under study.

19 Woolley used the term 'Level' and Roman numerals in his site phasing; the new excavations have created site-wide 'Periods' whose numbering, given in Arabic numerals, is largely synchronous with Woolley's system. Thus, Level IV is now Period 4. Minor modifications and re-phasing will be discussed in Yener *et al.*, forthcoming.

20 Yener *et al.*, forthcoming.

21 Period 1 at Alalakh begins in the late 14th century BC and continues into the 13th century, although new evidence reveals that most of the city mound was not inhabited after c.1290 BC. The Temple of Alalakh, Woolley's 'Ishtar Temple,' definitely continued through at least the reign of Hattusili III. Further study is needed.

adjacent temples at the northern end of the site (now Area 1). Woolley's collections span a time period of over a thousand years, from the earliest (Level XVII, Amuq J, c.2200–2000 BC) to the latest[22] (Level O, 12th–9th century BC/Amuq N and O). A variety of pot-marks were noted in Woolley's final publication[23] ranging from simple lines to more elaborate symbols. There are a total of eight incised marks illustrated by Woolley.[24] These are described as "maker's marks."[25] He mentions that these maker's marks occurred on "several plates (Type 3a) and a saucer (Type 6b) from the Niqmepa palace" (see Fig. 3.1–2) and that they appeared "on the base of the vessels."[26]

Unfortunately Woolley does not indicate whether all eight of the illustrated marks occurred only on these types, or only in the Niqmepa palace (Level IV); nor does he state if there is only the one example of each mark, or if there were many and only one representative was chosen for the publication. The illustrations do not give profiles, so it is impossible to study the curvature and angle of the sherds. It is also not clear whether by 'on the base' Woolley meant actually on the base, or merely anywhere on the underside of the plates and saucer. He also does not mention any closed vessels being marked. Woolley's illustrated marked sherds are not indicated as being oriented in any particular or consistent direction.

The two shapes mentioned by Woolley as being marked, Types 3a and 6b,[27] are not precisely equivalent to types in the new Atchana typology. Type 3a is a wide plate[28] of the curved profile variety; the V-shaped plate that is so common at Atchana actually does not appear in Woolley's type list/catalog, apparently because he condensed his types from over 350 created in the field to 168 for the publication.[29] Thus, several varieties of plates came to be represented by the curved variety alone. The illustrated example in Woolley (see Fig. 3.1) is nearly 40cm wide.

The plate of V-shaped type was found to be the most commonly marked vessel in the new excavations. The stratified examples of marked plates recovered

22 Woolley encountered a variety of features he termed 'Level O' which he did not attempt to date, see Woolley 1955. Based on reanalysis of Woolley's ceramic collection, these features are likely contemporary to the Iron I-II remains now recovered by the Yener excavation in Area 1.

23 Woolley 1955.

24 Woolley 1955, PL.CVIII: m; see fig. 3.3–10.

25 Woolley 1955, 352.

26 Woolley 1955, 352.

27 Woolley 1955, PL. CIX: 3a, 6b.

28 The plate in the Atchana typology (Type 3) is defined as having a radius at least twice the length of the vessel height. Vessels with these measurements form a discrete natural group in the Atchana ceramic corpus.

29 Woolley 1955, 320.

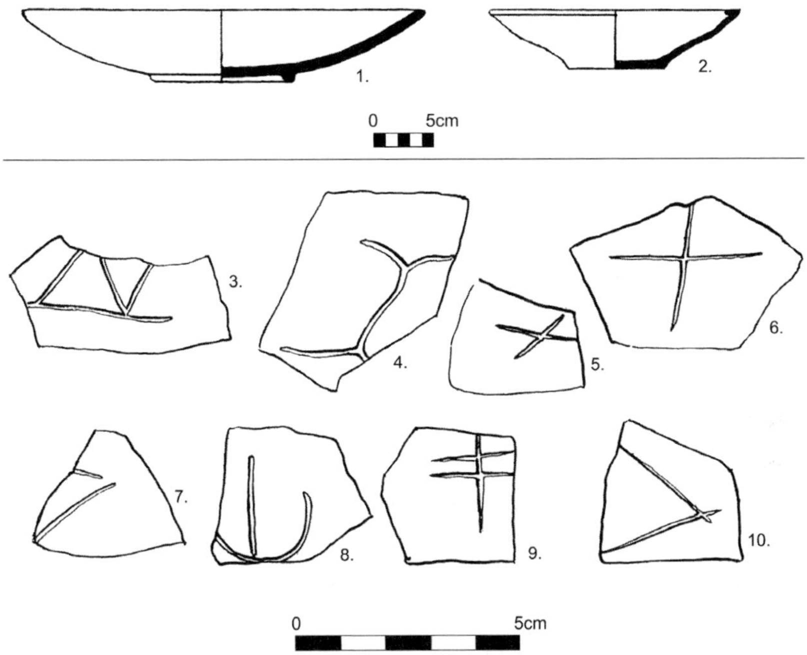

FIG. 3 Woolley 1955 types and pot-marks

1 Woolley Type 3a
2 Woolley Type 6b
3 Incomplete pot-mark, three strokes of a zig-zag attached to a horizontal line.
4 Incomplete pot-mark, vertical line branching into two 'horns' at top and bottom.
5 X-motif pot-mark, angles uneven (horizontal angles are obtuse, vertical angles acute).
6 X-motif pot-mark
7 Incomplete pot-mark, two lines converging but not meeting.
8 Vertical stroke, meeting a semicircle line at the bottom .
9 Vertical stroke crossed by two horizontal strokes.
10 V-shaped pot-mark, lines crossing slightly past the point.

in 2006–2012 are all from Site Periods 6, 5, and 3; the new excavations do not yet have a sample from Period 4 in Area 1. As mentioned, the plate does not occur in the Middle Bronze levels at Atchana, Period 7/Level VII and earlier.

The type called a "saucer" by Woolley (Type 6b, see FIG. 3A.2) is about 20cm wide and has a flat base. It is listed as 'always plain.'[30] No such vessel shape has been found in the 2006–2012 excavations. There are eight examples of Type 6b listed in

30 Woolley 1955, 322.

Woolley's analysis of types by Level, which is of limited use since it only included whole or nearly whole vessels.[31] There is one Type 6b from Level I, one from Level III, four from Level IV, and two from Level V.[32] Woolley did not specify which maker's mark appeared on an example of Type 6b or from what Level it originated.

Pot-marks in the New Excavations

Major categorizations of the corpus from the Woolley excavations by ware (macroscopically determined) and shape typologies have been previously attempted and discussed.[33] As senior ceramicist in the new Alalakh Excavations, the author completed a two-year study to create a modern typological system for the Atchana ceramics, allowing for the first time a reliable sequence to be built. The recent excavations have generated a new body of whole and fragmentary ceramics numbering in the hundreds of thousands. The various local plain and decorated ceramic wares have been re-classified as the 'Simple Ware Group' based on similarities in their form, fabric, and manufacture as observed macroscopically.

The name 'Simple Ware' is widely used for the local plain wheel-made ware of the northwest Syrian and Amuq region.[34] This ceramic tradition is part of a broad regional material culture horizon with a long lifespan deriving from the first wheel-made plain ceramics of the Uruk period.[35] The Simple Ware of the MBA and LBA is a plain-surfaced, wheel-made pottery of well-processed, variably sandy calcareous fabric.[36] The ware has a broad and multi-purpose repertoire of forms including pitchers, jugs, jars, bowls, plates, cups, stands, and other domestic shapes.[37] Under the umbrella of the Atchana Simple Ware Group are decorated traditions including Red Slip, Grey Burnished, Syro-Cilician painted style, 'Banded Ware' painted style, and 'Late Bronze Geometric Ware' painted style.[38] Pot-marks have not been found at Atchana on decorated ceramics, only on plain Simple Ware and in one case, on cookware.

While pot-marks do occur on jar shoulders and jug handles, the most common place to encounter a pot-mark at LB I Atchana is on the underside of a large

31 Woolley 1955, 321, n.2.

32 Parts of Woolley's Level Vb will be re-phased as Period 4a; with the 'Niqmepa Palace' as 4b. Yener *et al.*, forthcoming.

33 See Swift n.d.; Williams and Hassert 1978; McClellan 1989; Heinz 1992.

34 Braidwood and Braidwood 1960.

35 Braidwood and Braidwood 1960, Mazzoni 2002b; Mazzoni 2002a; Nigro 2002; Horowitz 2015.

36 Mazzoni 2002b; Nigro 2002; Mullins 2010.

37 Horowitz 2015.

38 Horowitz 2015.

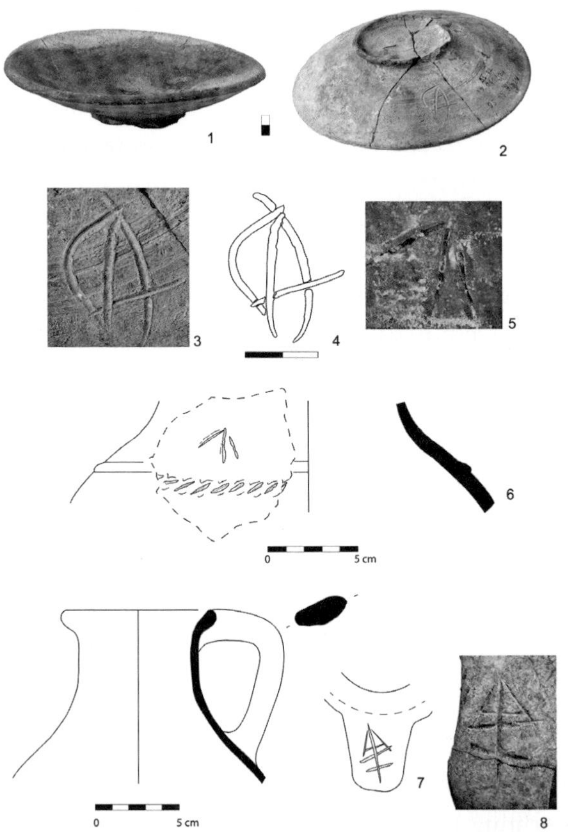

FIG. 4 Previously unpublished pot-marks from the Woolley excavation and from the 2006–2012 excavations at Tell Atchana-Alalakh.
1–4. ATP 1948 no.7650, marked as Level IV. V-shaped plate with four-stroke pot-mark.
5–6. AT18686.1: Three-stroke pot-mark
7–8. ATWD-1501, marked as Level IV. Six-stroke pot-mark

V-shaped plate in plain Simple Ware (see FIG. 4.1–2). These plates were first introduced in the transitional period between the MB II and LB I, becoming a very common part of LB assemblages at the site.[39] They are primarily large, between 28–32cm in diameter, though smaller versions do occur sporadically. A variety of rim and base types occur on the plate in LB I and LB IIa. The most common simple rim is straight or slightly thickened with a somewhat flattened end. Rolled-in rims also occur regularly, and there is a continual scattering of other rim types throughout the LB. Ring, flat, and concave bases all occur. In the latter part of the LB IIa a rounded bottom is introduced, but it never becomes common at the site, and the large local plate with flat or ring base continues in use well into the Iron Age at both Atchana and Tell Tayinat.[40]

Unfortunately, due to the wide range of shape and ware typologies used across Anatolia and Syria for Bronze Age ceramics, and the wide variety of counting and

39 Horowitz 2015.

40 While traditionally treated as separate sites, Atchana and Tayinat seem to be part of the same larger site complex located only about 800m apart (Yener *et al.*, forthcoming).

recording methods for sherd collections, it is only possible to make a comparison in the broadest terms between the frequency of marked vessels at different sites.[41] In the discussion that follows the catalog below, quantitative analyses of overall frequency of pot-marks within the sherd collection at Atchana are presented and compared to those sites presented by Glatz.[42]

Catalog of Pot-Marks

This catalog presents a selection of pot-marks from the Yener excavations of 2006–2012. Preparation for publication of this material is ongoing, and some of the recorded pot-marks have not yet been processed and illustrated. There are 18 pot-marks recorded from 2006–2012. One square, 32.57, produced 12 of them from its early and middle LB I levels (Periods 6–5, Levels VI-V). A contemporary square, 45.44, produced one pot-mark from an un-phased burial and one from a transitional Middle/Late Bronze phase equated with Period 7/Period 6. Four squares (32.53, 32.63, 32.62, and 64.72) produced one each from post-LB I contexts, but only two of these can be considered secure. Twelve of these pot-marks appear in the following catalog, but all are included in the following analysis.

AT18686.1 Square 45.44, Loc 97, Lot 670, Phase 5 Site Period 7/6

This mark consists of a V with the pointed end facing upwards toward the rim of the vessel, and a third line forming another V with the right-hand line of the primary V (Fig. 4.5-6). The third line converges with the point of the primary V but does not actually intersect. The mark is about 2 x 2.25 cm and is located on the shoulder of a round-bottomed cook-pot in the Middle Bronze style, with a shoulder slashed band relief and a dark brown fabric tempered with crushed calcite or limestone (Mineral Ware). Context is inside a mud brick wall that was in use around the time of the transition from Period 7 to 6, but cannot yet be dated more closely. The mark is comparable to Glatz Type 4.[43]

AT6893.7 Square 32.57, Loc 103, Lot 473, Phase 3a Site Period 6

The mark consists of a small V, bisected by a line, evoking the silhouette of a pair of calipers (Fig. 6.4). The strokes of the V are inconsistent, beginning at the tips and fading out before the point of the V, which is marked by a separate gouge. The crossing line is also broken, apparently begun on one side beyond where the sherd breaks, and skipping a bit before crossing the first line of the V and ending

41 E.g. Glatz 2012, Table 3.

42 Glatz 2012.

43 Glatz 2012, fig. 2.

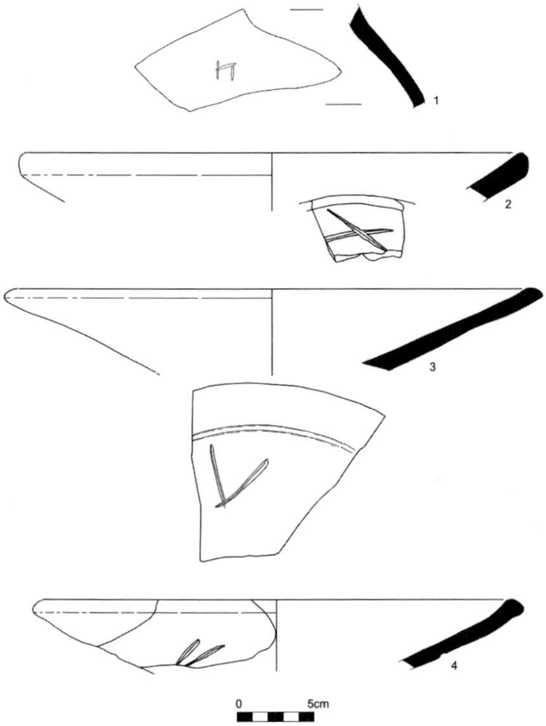

FIG. 5 Pot-marks from the 2006–2012 excavations at Tell Atchana-Alalakh.
1 AT0780.1: Aleph-shaped pot-mark
2 AT1264.77: X-shaped pot-mark
3 AT1437.35: V-shaped pot-mark
4 AT1437.36: V-shaped pot-mark

almost exactly on the second stroke of the V. The vessel form is uncertain; the slight curvature might indicate a plate or shallow bowl, made in plain Simple Ware. Context is a street deposit. Not represented in Woolley 1955 or among the types shown in Glatz 2012, FIG. 2.

AT7331.2 Square 32.57, Loc 123, Lot 504, Phase 3b Site Period 6

This sign is cut off at both ends, and so may have been a V or an X, or something more elaborate (FIG. 6.6). It consists of two deeply incised lines converging until they almost meet before the break. The shape of the vessel cannot be determined, though the straight vessel wall strongly suggests a V-shaped plate. The ware is Simple Ware.

AT9636.1 Square 32.57, Loc 157, Lot 615, Phase 3d Site Period 6

A small V, applied 'sideways' with respect to the vessel rim (FIG. 6.7). The curvature of the sherd may suggest the shoulder of a closed Simple Ware vessel. This mark seems to have been drawn in one stroke with perhaps an angle-pointed tool, beginning at the lower end and continuing through the point to the upper end to finish with an inward bend. The line thins dramatically in the course of the lower line. The surface of the vessel seems to have been smoothed after the impression of the mark, giving it almost the appearance of a stamp mark. Dimensions *c.* 1 cm x 1 cm. Not represented in Woolley 1955 or Glatz Fig 2.

AT6915.1 Square 45.44, Loc 53, Lot 237, Phase 0[44] Site Period 5/6/earlier

A small V, applied to the shoulder of a closed plain Simple Ware vessel with the point facing downward and strokes quite wide at the center of the lines, evoking a pair of rabbit ears (Fig. 6.5). The lines are deeply incised and drawn from the tips down to the point, with one line extending slightly past the point. The sherd was recovered from the fill soil in an LB I human burial, one of many just beyond and downhill of the contemporary town wall. This is the only pot-mark found in Square 45.44's LB I contexts, despite it having several phases of a pottery workshop on the inside of the town wall, although it was in the fill of the grave and so could have been from an earlier date than the LB I like many of the stray sherds from the city slope cemetery.

The wasters and fragments found in the nearby workshop contexts, which date to Atchana Periods 6 (late) and 5, are very much in the local MB tradition (Horowitz 2015). The characteristic LB plates are not common in this square, are generally smaller than the 30cm standard, and do not occur among the wasters piled in one corner of the workshop area. Resembles Woolley 1955, Pl. CVIII: m-8 (see Fig. 3.10). Comparable to Glatz Type 2, but inverted.

AT0780.1 Square 32.57, Loc 28, Lot 62, Phase 2a Site Period 5

The mark is small, about 1.5 x 1.5 cm, and resembles a Hebrew 'aleph' oriented upright on the shoulder of a closed plain Simple Ware vessel (Fig. 5.1). This sign does not appear in Woolley's published corpus from 1955. It is formed of three strokes, the two parallel lines made first and then crossed by the third line, made from the top of the right-hand vertical line to the middle of the left-hand vertical line. The sherd is from the shoulder/neck area of a closed Simple Ware vessel showing some interior reworking by hand, not uncommon in local jars, jugs, and pitchers. Context is a floor deposit in a kitchen/workshop room. Not represented in Woolley 1955, but comparable to Glatz Type 12, the mark from Kinet Höyük.

AT1437.35 Square 32.57, Loc 27, Lot 125, Phase 2b Site Period 5

A large V-shaped mark applied to the underside of a plain Simple Ware plate (Fig. 5.3). The lines overlap slightly at the point of the V. The depth of the lines

44 The abundant burials in the east slope below the town wall are dated by their relationship to the MB II-LB I town wall sequence but not phased according to the stratigraphy of Square 45.44 within the town wall.

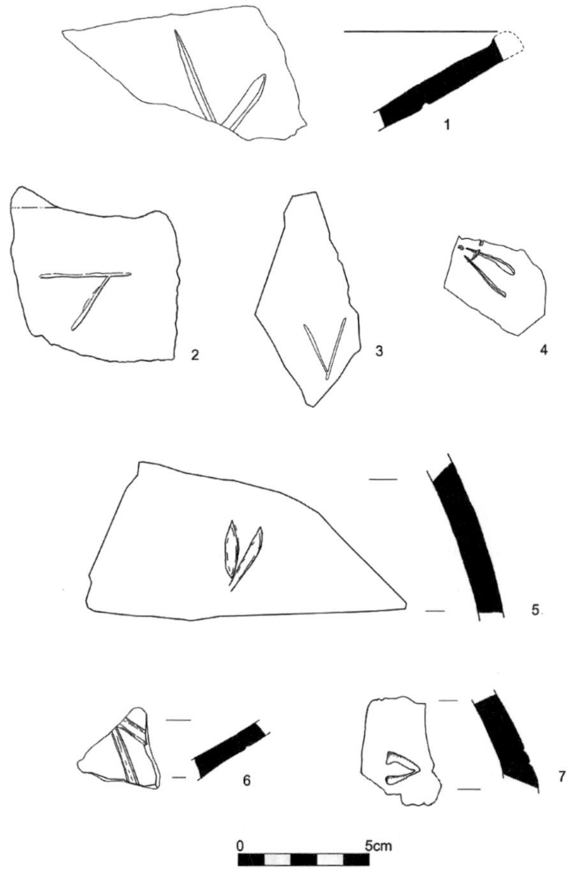

FIG. 6 Pot-marks from the 2006–2012 excavations at Tell Atchana-Alalakh.
1 AT1698.1: V or X-shaped pot-mark
2 AT1752.14: V-shaped pot-mark
3 AT6752.10: V-shaped pot-mark
4 AT6893.7: V-shaped pot-mark with crossing line
5 AT6915.1: V-shaped pot-mark
6 AT7331.2: Incomplete pot-mark, possibly a V or X
7 AT9636.1: V-shaped pot-mark

suggests they were made beginning at the outer points of the V. The two parallel gouges following the line of the plate rim do not appear to be intentional, rather the result of something sharp dragged along during the wheel-throwing process. Total size c.2.75cm tall and 2.75cm wide. Context is a building fill layer below a floor. Resembles Woolley 1955, Pl. CVIII: m-8 (see FIG. 3.10). Comparable to Glatz Type 2, but inverted.

AT1437.36 Square 32.57, Loc 27, Lot 125, Phase 2b Site Period 5

Similar to the previous entry and coming from the same context, this V applied to the underside of a plain Simple Ware plate is somewhat narrower (FIG. 5.4). The tip of the V is missing where the sherd is broken, therefore the sign could actually have been an X if the lines continued past where they meet. Again the lines appear to have been drawn from the tips down toward the point, giving a 'rabbit-ears' effect. Total size c.2cm wide and at least 3cm long. Similar to Woolley

1955, Pl. CVIII: m-8 (see Fig. 3.10). Context is a building fill layer below a floor. Comparable to Glatz Type 2, but inverted.

AT1698.1 Square 32.57, Loc 38, Lot 148, Phase 2b Site Period 5

The mark is incompletely preserved, possibly a large V or X. It is applied to the underside of a V-shaped plain Simple Ware plate with rolled-in rim (Fig. 6.1). One line is thicker than the other, perhaps because they were drawn beginning from opposite ends. This might suggest the motif is an X rather than a V. Total size c.5cm between line tips, 4cm length preserved. Context is a mixed deposit (floor and trash accumulation). Could be comparable to Woolley 1955, Pl. CVIII. m-8 (see Fig. 3.5, Fig. 6, or Fig. 10), and to Glatz Type 2, 7, or 8.

AT1752.14 Square 32.53, Loc 12, Lot 80, Phase 2a Site Period 3

This mark is similar to a V, but one line extends past the point where the lines join (Fig. 6.2). The mark is applied to the underside of a V-shaped plain Simple Ware plate with a thickened rim (partly preserved). The longer line of the V parallels the rim of the vessel, making the mark 'sideways'. The mark is similar to Woolley 1955, Pl. CVIII: m-8 (see Fig. 3.10), except for the extended line past the point, though the orientation of that mark is uncertain. Context is a floor deposit belonging to a building below the Woolley Fortress (Level II). Similar to Glatz Type 2, but rotated 90 degrees and with extended line past the point.

AT6752.10 Square 64.72, Loc 40, Lot 162, Phase 3b Site Period 3

This V-shaped mark is applied to the exterior of a closed vessel with a very fine, atypical Simple Ware fabric (Fig. 6.3). The orientation is uncertain due to re-working on the interior, obscuring the wheel-marks. The mark is unusually shallow. It is drawn from the tips down toward the point, with one line extending slightly past the joining point. Total size c.2.5cm long and 1.75cm wide. Context is the floor of a building with domestic and small-scale workshop areas. The mark is similar to Woolley 1955, Pl. CVIII: m-8 (see Fig. 3.10). Comparable to Glatz Type 2, but orientation uncertain.

AT1264.77 Square 32.63, Loc 13, Lot 8, Phase 1 Site Period 0 (Topsoil interface)

An X inscribed just under the rim of a plain Simple Ware plate (Fig. 5.2). The lower points of the X are cut off where the sherd breaks. It is difficult to tell in which direction the incision strokes were made. Unfortunately this is not a secure context, and the sherd may date to any part of the LB or even the Iron Age. Dimensions are c.3.5cm max horizontally, *c.* 2cm maximum vertically. Very similar to Woolley 1955, Pl. CVIII: m-3 depending on orientation (see Fig. 3.5-6). Comparable to Glatz Type 8.

Two New Pot-marks from the Woolley Collections

In the course of preparations for the Alalakh exhibit at the new Hatay Museum, two previously unpublished pot-marks were discovered and are presented here for the first time. Pending the completion of a detailed study of Woolley's unpublished collection at the Alalakh Excavations depot, the unnumbered vessel below has been assigned a temporary number. The only information on the find locations is a grid number (GG) in the case of no. 7650, otherwise both pieces are marked with the Roman numeral 'IV' indicating Woolley's Level IV.

ATP 1948 no.7650 Marked as Level IV Site Period 4

The mark is applied to the underside of a plain Simple Ware V-shaped plate (Fig. 4.1-4). It consists of four lines, applied in a clearly visible sequence. The first is a clearly incised long curved line, approximately perpendicular to the rim, about 4cm in length. Next, a line was applied from near the lower end of the first, crossing it and proceeding in an arc back toward the top of the mark but not converging. A third line was applied crossing both previous lines closer to the top of the mark, parallel to the vessel rim. Finally, a fourth line begins at the lower end of the second line and converges with its upper end. This mark does not appear in Woolley's catalog or the new catalog presented above. Dimensions are c.4 x 3cm. Not comparable to Woolley or Glatz Fig. 2 types.

ATWD-1501 Marked as Level IV Site Period 4

The mark is applied to the upper part of the handle of a plain Simple Ware jug (Fig. 4.7-8). The mark consists of six lines forming a complex arrow-like shape. The first three lines were arranged to form an A with the point facing 'upwards' toward the rim. Two more lines roughly parallel to the crossing line of the A were added below, and then a long central line was placed from the point of the A down across all three perpendicular lines. Dimensions are c.3 x 2 cm. This mark does not appear in Woolley's catalog. Not directly comparable to Glatz Fig. 2; the top triangular section resembles Type 10 examples from Boğazköy-Hattusa, Alaca Höyük, Mersin-Yumuktepe and Kinet Höyük, but with an extended middle stroke crossed by another line.

A Tree-Motif Pot-mark or Decoration

In some cases, it is difficult to tell whether a mark was meant to be a decoration or to communicate another form of information, as was presumably the case with the catalog presented above. The Middle Bronze tradition at Alalakh made liberal use of incised decoration in a wide variety of motifs and while most create horizontal bands of decoration on a vessel, individual or separate motifs do also occur. The

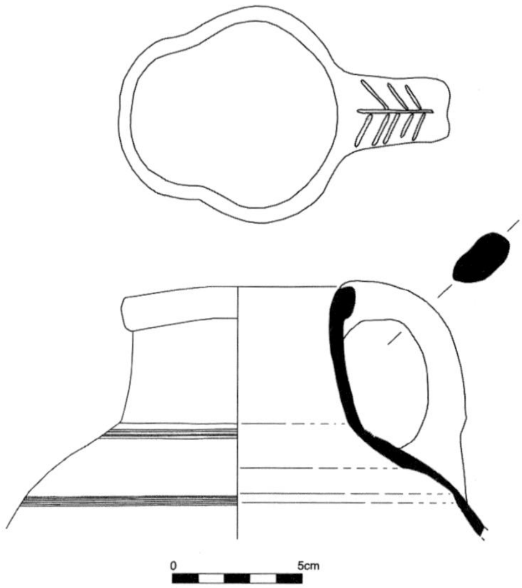

FIG. 7 Trefoil pitcher, AT10770.1: Tree-shaped incised mark.

piece presented below falls in between the categories of pot-mark and decoration. On the one hand, the design is incised on the handle of a pitcher in the same location as other pot-marks. On the other, the motif resembles the typical painted decoration on handles of pitchers in the Syro-Cilician tradition of the MBA.[45] The piece has not been included in the analytical section below.

AT10770.1 Square 32.57, Loc 65, Lot 662, Phase 2b Site Period 5

The mark is applied to the upper part of the handle and consists of a long vertical line with shorter lines rising diagonally from it (FIG. 7). There are three lines on the right side and five on the left. The mark resembles a stylized tree or branch. The center line was drawn first with a pointed tool, the branches drawn from the center line outwards. The vessel form is a necked pitcher with trefoil spout on a folded rim. The shoulder and shoulder-neck join of the pitcher are marked with horizontal combing. Context is a pit fill. The mark resembles Glatz Type 6, found at Boğazköy and Alaca Höyük. The mark does not appear in Woolley.

Patterns of Pot-marks in The New Excavations

Pot-marks are relatively rare in the archaeological assemblages of Atchana, clustering in certain phases and parts of the site. Estimating the rate of marked vessels is difficult since most of the assemblages are sherd scatter. An approximate measure

45 See Heinz 1992.

of marked vessels per stratigraphic phase was created for this study using an average ratio of total sherds to MNI[46] from the ongoing Atchana Context Study.[47] On average, the MNI per context is less than the total sherd count by about a factor of five. Thus, the estimate of marked vessels per phase in Square 32.57 (a 9x9m area) was calculated by totaling the sherds that could be associated exclusively with a phase, and then multiplying by 5.

TABLE 1 - Estimates of pot-marked vessel frequency by sherd count for Atchana Square 32.57, sub-phases 4–2a

Local Phase	Period/Level	# pot-marks	Total sherds	% marked	x5 = estimate of marked vessel rate
4	6 (VI)	0	n/a	0	0%
3d	6 (VI)	1	15723	0.006	0.032%
3c	6 (VI)	0	n/a	0	0%
3b	6 (VI)	2	7930	0.030	0.150%
3a	6 (VI)	1	19404	0.005	0.025%
2c	5 (V)	2	7595	0.030	0.150%
2b	5 (V)	3	7359	0.040	0.200%
2a	5 (V)	3	8972	0.030	0.150%

The rate of pot-marks by sherd count in the six of 32.57's eight sub-phases where pot-marks occur (dating to the early and middle parts of the LB I) is comparable to that reported from excavations at Kuşaklı-Sarissa (0.04%) and Boğazköy-Hattusa (0.01%).[48] The estimated marked-vessel frequency numbers using the MNI-to-sherd count ratio are also low in phases where pot-marks occur, ranging from 0.032 to 0.200. This is less than the calculated rates of pot-marks by vessel count (MNI) at Kuşaklı (4.4%) and Boğazköy (1.2%), but it is also from a smaller sample and using a different system for calculating MNI than that used at other sites.[49] These frequency estimates generated from Kuşaklı and Boğazköy are also not directly comparable to the 32.57 Period 6 and 5 estimates from Atchana because

46 The MNI calculation formula at Atchana is based on a batching system that distinguishes sherds belonging to individual vessels (unrelated rims, bases, and handles are all counted, but with wheel-made plain ware it can be especially difficult to associate rims and bases) and not counting groups of undifferentiated body sherds. Thus, the MNI numbers should be considered likely to be higher than reality.

47 The Atchana Context Study system combines sherds, samples, and other artifacts from all the loci and lots making up a particular deposit into a numbered 'context', and studies them together.

48 Glatz 2012, 15–16; see also Müller-Karpe 1988; Mielke 2006.

49 See Glatz 2012, 16.

they refer to larger time periods. A breakdown of pot-mark frequency by count at 12 sites in the time periods MB, LB I, LB II, and the 12th century BC can be found in Glatz[50] but the rates per period are not computed and the total sherd count per period is not provided.

The average estimated rate of pot-marks per vessel based on this system for 32.57 Period 6 is 0.041% and for Period 5 is 0.16%. A rate for the entire LB I period cannot be computed for Atchana at this time because a new sample has yet to be acquired from Period IV/Level 4. A rate could not be calculated for the single recovered pot-mark from contemporary LB I phases in Square 45.44 because the context was the fill of a grave not closely phased within the Period 5–6 remains to which it belongs. None of the Period 5 pottery workshop wasters in 45.44 contained pot-marks. Thus Square 45.44, located beyond the palace area, produced one pot-mark from a 9x9m area loosely dating to Periods 5–6 (LB I) and one pot-mark from a wall of the transitional Period 7 (final MB) to Period 6, the assemblages of which have not yet been subject to a full analysis or final phasing. In contrast, 32.57 produced 12 pot-marks from the same excavation area size for Periods 5–6 and none from Period 7.

Though the Atchana samples are still small to be making broad comparisons, the numbers can give a preliminary indication that the palace area in Periods 5 and 6 had a rate of pot-marks 12 times higher than one contemporary non-palatial area. The overall rate of pot-marks at excavated LB I contexts from Atchana is currently impossible to calculate due to the incomplete data in Woolley's publication of Level IV (Period 4), the later part of the LB I.

In the LB IIa, pot-marks are very rare at Atchana. There are only two from secure contexts, one in 32.53 (Area 1) and one in 64.72 (Area 4). Both of these contexts date to Period 3 (c.1400–1330/BC) at the site, an era lying between the destruction of Period 4's 'Niqmepa Palace' and the construction of the massive 'Hittite Fortress' in Period 2.[51] The structure of local administration is not well known for this era. The local dynasty of Idrimi may have continued for a time, to be replaced by Hittite hegemony in the 1350s BC or later.[52] The sizeable new excavations from Periods 2 and 1 at Atchana have revealed no pot-marks in secure contexts in a sample size six times greater than that of Periods 6, 5, and 3. It seems evident that beginning in or just after the Amarna period, potters at Alalakh were no longer marking their wares. This is in contrast to many sites in Anatolia, as well as Tell Afis, which seem to show a peak in pot-marks the 14th and 13th centuries.[53]

50 Glatz 2012, fig. 4.

51 See Yener 2013; Akar 2013; Yener *et al.*, forthcoming.

52 See Woolley 1955; von Dassow 2008.

53 Glatz 2012, fig. 4; Archi and Venturi 2013, fig. 6.

Pre-firing pot-marks were already in use at Boğazköy and Korucutepe in the 20th century BC, followed by Yanarlar in the 19th century BC.[54] Ten other sites in Anatolia begin to use pot-marks at or slightly later than 1600 BC, as Atchana currently seems to. Three sites, Kuşaklı, İmikuşağı, and Korucutepe, seem to abandon their pot-mark tradition after about 1400–1350 BC, as Atchana does, while Yanarlar's tradition disappears around 1600 BC. This pattern seems to show that pre-firing pot-marks cannot be exclusively associated with a universal Hittite imperial management strategy, although it is of course possible that Hittite management policies varied depending on the existing structure and particular priorities at different sites. It is also possible that pot marking simply served different purposes at different times and locations.

In order to establish if there is an order in which varying sites and regions began to use pot-marks generally, and particular symbols specifically, and thus what the region of origin might be, a thorough study of sites in Syria and the Levant should be undertaken. It would also be productive to compare the evidence for internal political and economic organization at sites with pre-firing pot-marks in order to investigate whether there is a specific correlation between such organization and the use of pot-marks.

Conclusions

Understanding the chronology, use, and interregional distribution of pre-firing pot-marks in the ancient Near East is important to the study of the organization of production and connects directly to strategies of economic and political management, both local and imperial. Alalakh's destruction, and the destruction of Aleppo, in the late 17th / early 16th century BC marked the end of the 'Amorite' or 'Old Syrian' period in Syria and the beginning of a period in which first the Mitanni Empire and then the Hittite Empire came to dominate the area. The political situation in the Amuq in the earlier part of the LB I is not well understood, and it is in this time (Period 6) that the pre-firing pot-marks first appear at Alalakh. New ceramic forms, particularly the large V-shaped plate, were adopted into the local repertoire of Alalakh at that time, and these are the most likely form to be marked. Similar plates first appear at a wide variety of Syrian and Cilician sites at the MB/LB boundary,[55] and also at sites in Canaan and Egypt,[56] perhaps as part of a new international form of dining.[57] Demand for plates seems to have been

54 Glatz 2012, fig. 5.

55 Mazzoni 2002; Horowitz 2015.

56 See Killebrew 2004.

57 Horowitz 2015.

particularly high in the institutions of authority at Alalakh where large amounts of food would have been regularly provided and consumed.

As proposed by Glatz,[58] the mode of production may have been the determining factor as to whether pot marking was employed by the potters. It is of course possible for managers in an imperial system to employ local independent producers without reorganizing them, placing large orders for plain wheel-made ware from multiple potters to supply official facilities. The potters might mark their wares if they used the same firing facilities, or to identify their products as proof of delivery to powerful clients.

The clustering of pot-marks in the new sample from the LB I (Periods 6–5–4) palace and temple area of Alalakh may be related to the form of production that was supplying pottery for the local administrative power of the site, known in Period 4 to be a king residing in a palatial-administrative complex. However, without more data from contemporary ceramic production areas, it is not yet possible to define the ceramic production system of LB I Alalakh as independent (self-organized) or attached (organized by and dependent on administrators). There is always the possibility that both modes were in operation simultaneously.

The widespread use of pot-marks, and the similarity of some of Atchana's pot-marks to those of many sites in Syria and Anatolia that were not linked by a single government, could suggest the movement of itinerant potters or the expansion of their protégés who specialized in new and difficult-to-make forms like the large V-shaped plate that was newly in demand across large regions. The spread of the plate and its associated dining habit, as well as the plain wheel-made aesthetic,[59] testifies to the wide sphere of cultural interaction and participation in the 16th century BC. As such, we might consider the late MBA and LB I-II pot-marks of the Anatolian and Syrian regions as a sign of a fundamental regional connectivity among potters underlying the ethno-linguistic diversity, political expansions, and conflicts endemic to the region throughout that period.

58 Glatz 2012, 34.

59 See Horowitz 2015 for a discussion of how the increase and spread of plain wheel-made ware in the LBA may have been less about the mode of production and more about an aesthetic associated with the powerful societies of Mesopotamia, the Levant, and Egypt.

REFERENCES

Akar, M., "The Late Bronze Age Fortresses at Alalakh: Architecture and Identity in Mediterranean Exchange Systems" in *Across the Border: Late Bronze – Iron Age Relations Between Syria and Anatolia. Proceedings of a Symposium held at the Research Center of Anatolian Studies, Koç University, Istanbul, May 31-June 1, 2010*, ed. by K. A. Yener, 37–60. Leuven: Peeters, 2013.

Archi, A. and F. Venturi, "Tell Afis in the Thirteenth Century BCE: Under the Rule of the Hittites." *Near Eastern Archaeology* 76 (2013): 4.

Braidwood, R and L. Braidwood, *Excavations in the Plain of Antioch: The Earlier Assemblages Phases A-J*. University of Chicago Oriental Institute Publications 61. Chicago, 1960.

Gates, M.-H., "Potmarks at Kinet Höyük and the Hittite Ceramic Industry" in *La Cilicie: Espaces et Pouvoirs Locaux (2e millénaire av. J.-C.-4e siècle ap. J.-C.). Actes de la table ronde internationale d'Istanbul, 2–5 Novembre 1999*, ed. by É. Jean, A. M. Dinçol and S. Durugönül, 137–157. Varia Anatolica 13. Paris: De Boccard, 2001.

Glatz, C., "Bearing the Marks of Control? Reassessing Pot Marks in Late Bronze Age Anatolia." *American Journal of Archaeology* 116: 1 (2012): 5–38.

Griffin, E., "The Middle and Late Bronze Age Pottery" in *Korucutepe: Final Report of the Universities of Chicago, California (Los Angeles), and Amsterdam in the Keban Reservoir, Eastern Anatolia 1968–1970*, ed. by M. N. van Loon, 3–109. Amsterdam: North Holland Publishing Company, 1980.

Heinz, M., *Tell Atchana Alalakh : die Schichten VII-XVII*. Alter Orient und Altes Testament 41. Kevelaer; Neukirchen-Vluyn: Butzon & Bercke; Neukirchener Verlag, 1992.

Hirschfeld, N., "Marks on Pots: Patterns of Use in the Archaeological Record at Enkomi" in *Script and Seal Use on Cyprus in the Bronze and Iron Ages*, ed. by J. S. Smith, 49–109. Colloquia and Conference Papers 4. Boston: Archaeological Institute of America, 2002.

———. "How and Why Potmarks Matter." *Near Eastern Archaeology* 17: 1/ 2 (2008): 120–129.

Horowitz, M. T., "The Evolution of Plain Ware Ceramics at the Regional Capital of Alalakh in the Second Millennium BC" in *Plain and Simple? The Production, Use and Social Significance of Plain Pottery Traditions in the Early Complex Societies of the East Mediterranean and Near East*, ed. by C. Glatz. Walnut Creek. California: Left Coast Press, 2015.

Killebrew, A., "New Kingdom Egyptian-Style and Egyptian Pottery in Canaan: Implications for Egyptian Rule in Canaan during the 19th and Early 20th Dynasties" in *Egypt, Israel, and the Ancient Mediterranean World: Essays in Honor of Donald B. Redford*, ed. by G. N. Knoppers and A. Hirsch, 309–343. Probleme der Ägyptologie 20. Leiden: Brill, 2004.

Mazzoni, S., "The Ancient Bronze Age Pottery Tradition in Northwestern Central Syria" in *Céramique de l'Âge du Bronze en Syrie I*, eds. M. Al-Maqdissi, V. Matoian and C. Nicolle, 69–80. Bibliothèque archéologique et historique 161. Beyrouth: Inst. Français d' Archéologie du Proche-Orient, 2002a.

———. "Late Bronze Age Pottery Production in Northwestern Central Syria" in *Céramique de l'Âge du Bronze en Syrie I*, eds. M. Al-Maqdissi, V. Matoian, and C. Nicolle, 129–150. Bibliothèque archéologique et historique 161. Beyrouth: Inst. Français d' Archéologie du Proche-Orient, 2002b.

McClellan, T., "The Chronology and Ceramic Assemblages of Alalakh" in *Essays in Ancient Civilization Presented to Helene J. Kantor*, eds. B. B. Williams and A. Leonard Jr., 181–212. SAOC 47. Chicago IL, 1989.

Mielke, D.-P., *Die Keramik vom Westhang*. Kuşaklı-Sarissa 2. Rahden: Marie Leidorf, 2006.

Müller-Karpe, A., *Hethitische Töpferei in der Oberstadt von Hattuša: Ein Beitrag zur Kenntni spät-großreichszeilicher Keramik und Töpfereibetriebe unter Zugrundelegung der Grabungsergebnisse von 1978–82 in Boğazköy*. Marburg: Hitzeroth, 1988.

Müller-Karpe, A., "Untersuchungen in Kuşaklı 1997." *MDOG* 130 (1998): 93–174.

Mullins, R., "The Middle and Late Bronze Age Pottery from Tell Atchana (Alalakh) 2003–2004 Seasons" in *Tell Atchana, Ancient Alalakh. Volume 1. 2003–2004 Excavation Seasons*, ed. by K. A. Yener, 51–62. Istanbul: Koç University Press, 2010.

Nigro, L., "The Middle Bronze Age Pottery Horizon of Northern Inner Syria on the Basis of the Stratified Assemblages of Tell Mardikh and Hama" in *Céramique de l'Âge du Bronze en Syrie I*, eds. M. Al-Maqdissi, V. Matoian and C. Nicolle, 97–116. Bibliothèque archéologique et historique 161. Inst. Beyrouth: Français d' Archéologie du Proche-Orient, 2002.

Pucci, M., "The Chatal Höyük Publication Project: A Work in Progress" in *Proceedings of the 6th International Conference on the Archaeology of the Ancient Near East*, Vol. 1, 567–580. Wiesbaden: Harrassowitz Verlag, 2010.

Seidl, U., *Gefäßmarken von Boğazköy. Boğazköy-Hattusa 8*. Berlin: Gebr. Mann, 1972.

Smith, J.S. (ed.), *Script and Seal Use on Cyprus in the Bronze and Iron Ages*. Colloquia and Conference Papers 4. Boston: Archaeological Institute of America, 2002.

Swift, G. F., Jr. n.d. *The Pottery of the 'Amuq Phases K to O, and its Historical Relationships*. Unpublished PhD Thesis, Chicago: University of Chicago, 1958.

Venturi, F., "The North Syrian Plateau Before and After the Fall of the Hittite Empire: New Evidence from Tell Afis" in *Across the Border: Late Bronze – Iron Age Relations Between Syria and Anatolia, Proceedings of a Symposium at the Research Center of Anatolian Civilizations, Koç University, İstanbul May 31 – June 1, 2010*. Ancient Near Eastern Studies, Supplement 42, ed. by K.A. Yener. Leuven: Peeters, 2013.

von Dassow, E., *State and Society in the Late Bronze Age : Alalah under the Mitanni Empire*. Studies on the Civilization and Culture of Nuzi and the Hurrians 17. Bethesda Md.: CDL Press, 2008.

Williams, B. and S. Hassert, "Some Aspects of the Excavations at Tell Atchana, Part I: A Critical Review of Pottery from Levels XVII-VII." *Serapis* 4(1977–1978): 41–56.

Woolley, C. L., *Alalakh: An Account of Excavations at Tell Atchana in the Hatay, 1937–1949.* Reports of the Research Committee of the Society of Antiquaries of London 18. Oxford: Society of Antiquaries, 1955.

Yener, K. A., ed. *Tell Atchana, Ancient Alalakh. Volume 1. 2003–2004 Excavation Seasons.* Istanbul: Koç University Press, 2010.

Yener, K. A., "New Excavations at Alalakh: The 14th – 12th Centuries BC" in *Across the Border: Late Bronze – Iron Age Relations Between Syria and Anatolia. Proceedings of a Symposium held at the Research Center of Anatolian Studies, Koç University, Istanbul, May 31-June 1, 2010,* ed. by K. A. Yener, 11–36. Leuven: Peeters, 2013.

Yener, K.A., M. Akar and M.T. Horowitz (eds.), *Tell Atchana, Ancient Alalakh, Volume II. Excavations at Alalakh 2006–2010: The Late Bronze II Levels,* Forthcoming.

The Bay of İskenderun Landscape Archaeology and Survey Project: Dutlu Tarla and Dağılbaz Höyük — Three Millennia of Settlement in the İskenderun Plain

Ann E. Killebrew[1] — *Brandon R. Olson*[2] — *Gunnar Lehmann*[3]

Abstract

Between 2004 and 2009 the Bay of İskenderun Landscape Archaeology and Survey Project conducted six seasons of survey, focusing on the Issos, İskenderun, and Arsuz Plains. In the course of our work, 200 archaeological sites were documented in this previously underexplored region of Cilicia. Our surveys revealed that two neighboring sites, Dutlu Tarla and Dağılbaz Höyük, served as the principal settlements in the İskenderun Plain during most of the Bronze and Iron Ages. Considered together, they dominated the human landscape of this region for nearly three millennia. In our contribution in honor of Marie-Henriette and Charles Gates, we present the results of our investigation at these two sister sites and their role in the İskenderun Plain. We also critique the various approaches we employed during the course of our investigations at these sites, which included both extensive and intensive survey methodologies.

Introduction

From earliest times, the Cilician Plain (Cilicia Pedias ["Flat Cilicia"] or Çukurova) of Asia Minor served as a vital link between East and West. Geographically, Cilicia Pedias is enclosed by three imposing mountain ranges rich in timber—the Taurus, Anti-Taurus and Amanus Mountains. Three major rivers—the Cydnus (Tarsus Çay), the Sarus (Seyhan), and the Pyramus (Ceyhan)—and a number of smaller rivers and streams originating from the mountains provide abundant water to Çukurova.

---

1 The Pennsylvania State University, Classics and Ancient Mediterranean Studies, Jewish Studies and Anthropology, 108 Weaver Building, University Park, PA 16802, USA.

2 Boston University, Department of Archaeology, 675 Commonwealth Avenue, Boston, MA 02215, USA.

3 Department of Bible, Archaeology and Ancient Near Eastern Studies, Ben-Gurion University, P.O.B. 653, Beer Sheva 84105, Israel.

cultural lands, pasturage, wetlands, harbors, and communication routes for millennia. The plain itself consists of a collection of smaller inter-connecting fertile coastal plains. The Bay of İskenderun and its associated plains comprise the easternmost region of Cilicia, an area that has served throughout history as a geographic, cultural, and political interface between Cilicia, Asia Minor's largest and most fertile coastal flatlands, and the northern Levantine regions of present-day southern Turkey and northern Syria.

Eighteenth and nineteenth century travelers to the region, along with explorers, archaeologists, and historical geographers, provide the first modern documentation of Cilicia's historical sites and landmarks.[4] However, in spite of these scattered studies of the region, southeastern Cilicia Pedias remained archaeologically underexplored with few systematic large-scale surveys or excavations. The Bay of İskenderun Landscape Archaeology and Survey (henceforth BILAS) Project attempts to address this lacuna. Comprising 1,100 km^2 of the eastern coast of the İskenderun Gulf in the Turkish province of Hatay, BILAS (2004–2009) has documented nearly 200 archaeological sites in southeastern Cilicia. The survey area, bordered on the north by Erzin and its environs, to the east by the Amanus Mountains (or Nur Dağları ["Mountains of Light"]), and the south by Arsuz and its hinterland, encompasses the Bay of İskenderun's Issos, İskenderun, and Arsuz Plains (Fig. 1). In this contribution to the Festschrift honoring Marie-Henriette and Charles Gates, we present the twin sites of Dutlu Tarla and Dağılbaz Höyük situated in the İskenderun Plain. It is especially fitting to present these two sites, which were first identified and documented by Ann E. Killebrew, Gunnar Lehmann and Marie-Henriette Gates during the course of this survey project. We offer it with thanks and appreciation to Marie-Henriette and Charles Gates for their invaluable archaeological guidance, generous assistance and hospitality, and cherished friendship, which they extended to the authors of this chapter during the past decade.

Description of the Project

The BILAS Project[5] began in 2004 under the direction of Ann E. Killebrew (The Pennsylvania State University), Gunnar Lehmann (Ben-Gurion University of the

4 E.g. Chammas 1931; 1933; Gjerstad 1934; Seton-Williams 1954; Gough 1956; Tobin 2004; and especially Hellenkemper and Hild 1986; Hild and Hellenkemper 1990 for a compilation of the primary and secondary sources.

5 This survey is also known as the Mopsos Survey Project, thus named in honor of the legendary Greek who founded cities in Cilicia after the Trojan War. One of the project goals is to redress the lack of archaeological information about this region's human landscape and specifically examine archaeological identities in a region that has been a cultural crossroads since prehistoric times.

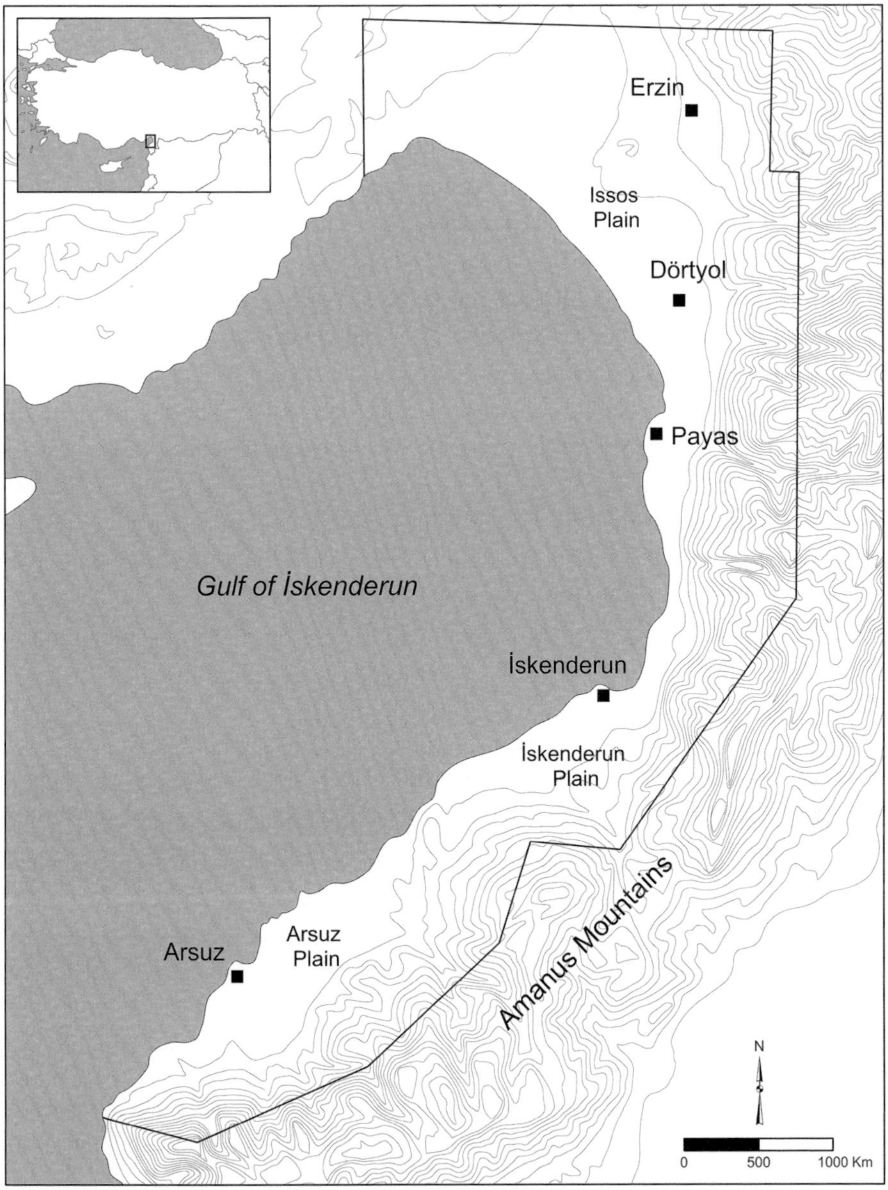

FIG. 1 Map of the Bay of İskenderun and location of the BILAS Project.
Graphics by B. R. Olson. © Mopsos/BILAS Project.

Negev) and Marie-Henriette Gates (Bilkent University). Six seasons of pedestrian survey were conducted (2004–2009), representing the first large-scale, multi-season, and systematic investigation of this region.[6] Included among the goals of this survey were the creation of an inventory of archaeological sites in an area experiencing rapid urban and commercial development and the investigation of the plains encircling the Bay of İskenderun as an interface of cultural exchange between the greater Mediterranean world and the Levant.

The project employed both extensive and intensive survey methods in order to identify and map archaeological sites and features across the survey area. Due to security concerns, the current geopolitical situation and modern development, approximately one-third of the survey area was inaccessible. The extensive methods of survey and documentation adopted by our project included visiting sites described in historical sources and/or earlier traveler accounts,[7] site identifications from previous targeted or small-scale surveys[8] and information obtained by interviewing local inhabitants, which proved to be an especially invaluable resource for locating ancient settlements. Not infrequently, sites were discovered by chance when traveling from one area to another, often clearly visible from the modern road. For each identified site, team members systematically surveyed the area collecting a representative sample of surface artifacts. One of the senior team members identified its spatial extent by mapping site boundaries based on artifact scatter with a hand-held GPS unit. Additional documentation included ground and satellite photography, the creation of detailed topographic maps when relevant and the compilation of oral histories and textual references to the site when possible. Artifacts were washed, identified and registered. Diagnostic finds, mainly consisting of pottery rims, handles, bases, and body sherds with distinctive fabrics and decorations, were drawn and photographed. All spatial

6 Lehmann *et al.* 2006; Lehmann, Killebrew and Gates 2008; Killebrew, Lehmann and Gates 2009; Killebrew and Lehmann 2010; Killebrew 2011. The Bay of İskenderun (Mopsos) Landscape Archaeology and Survey Project has been funded in part by grants from The Pennsylvania State University (2004–2009), the National Geographic Society (2007), the Loeb Classical Library Foundation (2009) and Dumbarton Oaks (2010). Publication research has been partially funded by an American Research Institute in Turkey (ARIT) fellowship (2008), a Fulbright Senior Research Fellowship (2010–2011, Fulbright Scholar Program), and a National Endowment of the Humanities fellowship (2014–2015). The project directors express their sincere thanks and gratitude for this support. We also take this opportunity to thank the Ministry of Culture and Tourism's Department of Cultural Affairs and their representatives (Güner Sağir [2004], Nihal Metin [2005], Gökhan Bozkurtlar [2006], Sevim Yıldız [2007], Zerrin Akdoğan [2008] and Binnur Çabuk Karadağ [2009]) who provided invaluable assistance and guidance during the course of the survey.

7 E.g. Chammas 1931; 1933.

8 Özgen and Gates 1993; Seton-Williams 1954; Steadman 1994.

data and chronological information for each site were recorded on paper forms, in a Microsoft Access database and in GIS.

Limited intensive pedestrian survey methods were also employed for representative landscapes, or collection units, which were selected using high-resolution satellite imagery. Collection units for pedestrian transect survey were selected based on field conditions including areas without noticeable modern disturbances (e.g. intrusive development), the presence of landfills or other identifiable features capable of adversely affecting visibility and artifact distribution. Other collection units were established in the vicinity of archaeological sites identified by extensive survey methods as outlined above. The size and shape of the collection units were typically based on modern landscape features (e.g. field boundaries, road systems, property boundaries, etc.) in an attempt to maintain geographic homogeneity within each unit. Surveyors walked through collection units in evenly spaced transects whenever possible, varying between 10–30 m. depending on visibility and field conditions. The BILAS team recorded all features and collected diagnostic artifacts from the surface. Areas with high artifact densities were identified as sites, assigned unique site numbers and documented on paper and digitally as described above. Once the field team surveyed the site and completed the requisite forms, survey continued within the collection unit. All spatial data and chronological information for each collection unit were also recorded on paper forms, in a Microsoft Access database and in GIS. Over six field seasons, the project intensively surveyed 24.15 km^2 (a roughly 3% sample of the approximately 736 km^2 of surveyable area), walked 228 collection units and identified, recorded and collected a representative sample of material culture from 200 archaeological sites within the boundaries of the BILAS Project.[9]

The İskenderun Plain

The İskenderun, or Alexandretta, Plain is one of three sub-plains in the survey area and is the focus of this Festschrift contribution. It is bordered on the east by the Amanus Mountains and extends from the Syrian Gates/Pillars of Jonah southwards to a narrow Amanic spur that reaches the Mediterranean Sea. Due to its geography, this 95 km^2 plain has played an important role in the history of the region. In addition to its natural harbor, the main Asia Minor/Syrian overland route crosses this plain through the Syrian Gates and continues southeastward towards the Amuq Plain and northern Syria via the Belen Pass, one of the few accessible routes over the Amanus Mountains.

9 For preliminary reports, see Lehmann *et al.* 2006; Lehmann, Killebrew and Gates 2008; Killebrew, Lehmann and Gates 2009; Killebrew and Lehmann 2010; and Killebrew 2011.

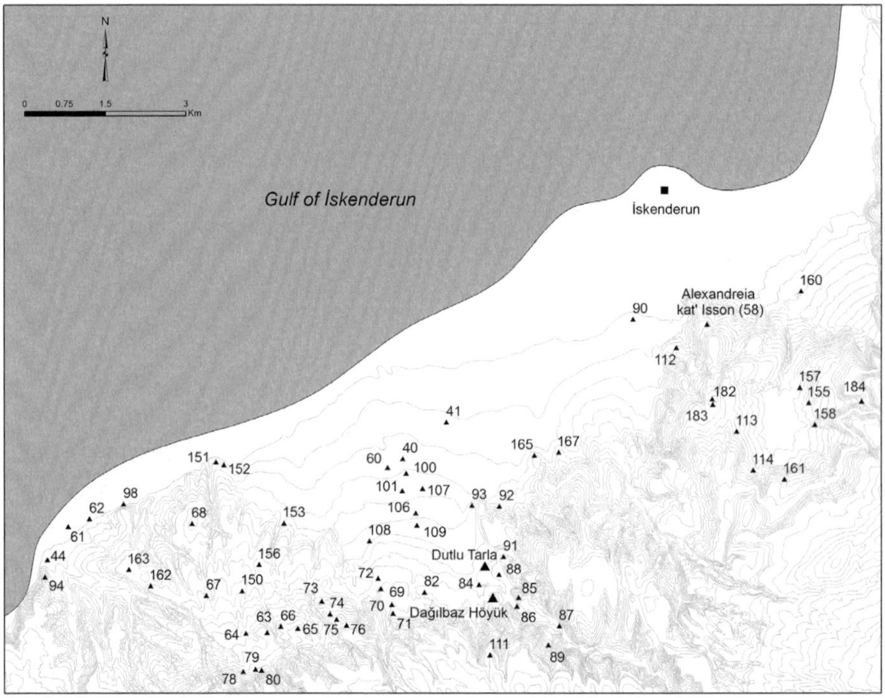

FIG. 2 Sites documented by the BILAS Project in the İskenderun Plain and location of Dağılbaz Höyük (Site 45) and Dutlu Tarla (Site 83), each indicated by a large triangle, and Alexandreia kat'Isson (Site 58). Graphics by B. R. Olson. © Mopsos/BILAS Project.

The BILAS Project identified nearly 70 archaeological sites on this plain (FIG. 2), ranging from the Early Bronze through Ottoman periods in date. Of these documented sites in the İskenderun Plain, two neighboring sites—Dağılbaz Höyük (Site 45) and its adjacent "lower city" Dutlu Tarla (Site 83)—served as the dominant settlements, especially during the Bronze through Persian periods. Within a 4 km^2 range of Dağılbaz Höyük and Dutlu Tarla, six small, additional architectural features or sites (nos. 82, 84, 85, 86, 88 and 91) were identified during intensive pedestrian survey of this area (FIG. 3).

Site 84 is an old stone bridge straddling a tributary of the Belen River (Bahçedere) that separates Dağılbaz Höyük and Dutlu Tarla. The bridge, which is attributed to the "Franks" (i.e. the Crusaders) by villagers, is still used by local farmers who cultivate their fields on these two sites. To the west of Dağılbaz Höyük (Site 45), a scatter of Hellenistic-Late Roman (*c.* 323 BCE-638 CE) period pottery and roof tiles marks a small settlement (Site 82) on the summit of an uncultivated hill.

Four sites were documented in close proximity to the east of Dutlu Tarla and Dağılbaz Höyük. Site 91, a small Hellenistic period cemetery, is the northernmost

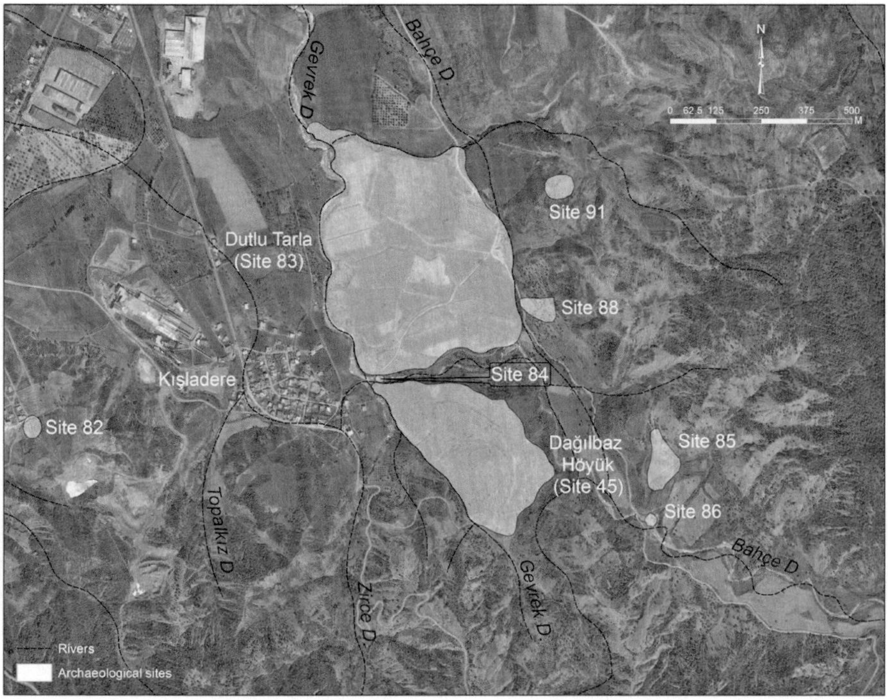

FIG. 3 General setting of Dağılbaz Höyük and Dutlu Tarla and sites in their vicinity. Satellite image provided by Digital Globe. Graphics by B. R. Olson. © Mopsos/BILAS Project.

of these. Several recently looted cist tombs were visible on the surface—the result of illicit excavations. The site is littered with human bones, a scatter of pottery and large broken tiles that originally covered Hellenistic tile graves. To the south and on the eastern bank of the Bahçedere, a concentration of roof tiles and Hellenistic-Late Roman sherds were recorded at Site 88. A wall, identified as a possible terrace and a boundary wall or the remains of a former irrigation channel, along with the walls of structures, are visible on the surface.

To the east of Dağılbaz Höyük, two additional sites within the 4 km^2 range were documented. Site 85 is an abandoned village situated on top of a hill. It was identified on maps as Sıfın by M. Hartmann, H. Kiepert and R. Dussaud, which was still inhabited in the late 19th century.[10] Currently, the only standing structures on the site are two Alawite shrines (*türbe*). Stone foundations of additional buildings, together with Hellenistic-Late Roman, Ottoman and modern pottery and roof tiles, are also visible today. Just to the south of Site 85 and to the east of

10 Hartmann 1894, 528.

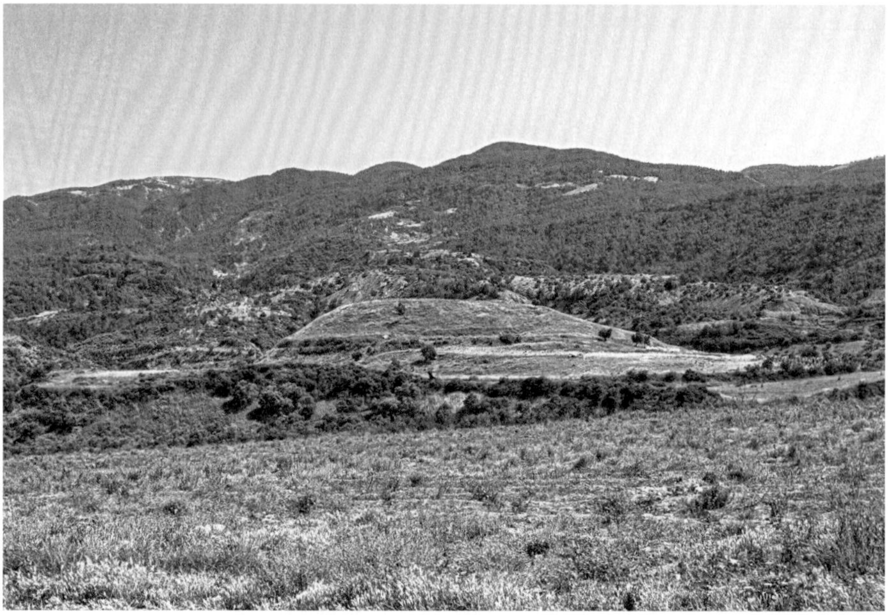

FIG. 4 View of Dağılbaz Höyük, looking south from Dutlu Tarla.
Photo by A. E. Killebrew. © Mopsos/BILAS Project.

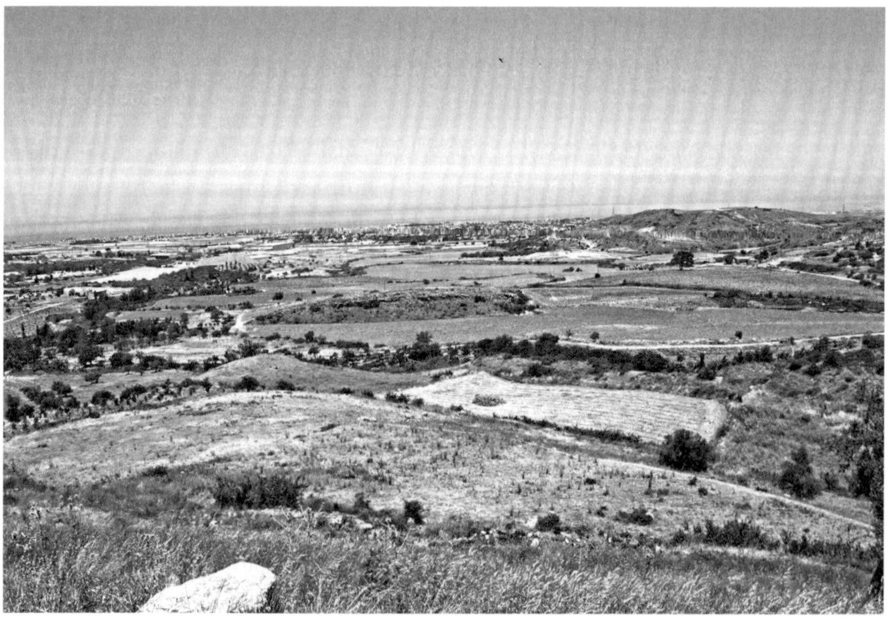

FIG. 5 View of Dutlu Tarla, looking north from Dağılbaz Höyük.
Photo by A. E. Killebrew. © Mopsos/BILAS Project.

Site 45 is Site 86, a ruined bridge (Sıfın Köprüsü), which originally spanned the Bahçedere and probably dates to the Ottoman period.

Dağılbaz Höyük and Dutlu Tarla

General Description and Survey Methodology

The impressive and commanding mound of Dağılbaz Höyük (Fig. 4) lies approximately 7.3 km southwest of the modern city center of İskenderun. The site is situated *c.* 500 m east of the small village of Kışladere in a well-watered area. The site is bounded by the Amanus Mountains in the south, the Bahçedere to the east (though appreciable artifact densities stopped just west of the Bahçe) and the Gevrekdere, a seasonal stream (Fig. 3). Dağılbaz consists of two landforms, a höyük measuring 3.8 ha in size and a fairly level plain measuring approximately 7.5 ha that extends northwest, north and east of the höyük. At 3.8 ha, Dağılbaz is the largest höyük documented by BILAS. Today, parts of the mound are covered in thick brush and used by herders for grazing, with the base of the höyük periodically cultivated.

Dutlu Tarla lies immediately north of Dağılbaz. The two sites are separated by a branch of the Bahçedere. Dutlu encompasses an even more impressive area measuring 27 ha in size and consists mainly of a flat, fertile plain that is regularly cultivated (Fig. 5). It is also bounded by the Bahçe and Gevrek streams to the east and west respectively (Fig. 3).

Dağılbaz Höyük and Dutlu Tarla were first documented as archaeological sites by the BILAS team in 2006. Due to their prominent role in the region, they were resurveyed in 2007 and 2009. During the 2006 and 2007 surveys, each site was subdivided into sections based on general physical features. At Dağılbaz, the major divisions included the summit, the slopes and the lower flanks of the site, features that were further sub-divided into smaller units. Teams consisting of one or two individuals were assigned to each sub-section. At the larger and flatter Dutlu Tarla, transects were walked based largely on modern agricultural fields. Most notably, physical conditions at each site varied from season to season. Throughout our multi-year study, some areas were under cultivation certain years while other fields were fallow, often overgrown with dense brush. Local field conditions present on the designated survey day were the single most significant factor impacting survey results. Recently ploughed fields were rich in surface artifacts, while overgrown or fallow areas of the sites yielded very little pottery. Artifacts visible on the surface were collected, washed, analyzed, dated and counted according to type. After recording the artifact numbers, body sherds were discarded at the site of origin and diagnostics were saved for additional study.

In an attempt to document these two sites in greater detail, Dağılbaz Höyük and Dutlu Tarla were resurveyed in 2009. A detailed topographic map was created by employing a total station, and a systematic survey of both sites was conducted using a "dog leash" method, which utilized a 10 m long string that rotated around a central axis and created a circular survey area with a diameter of 20 m. The primary goal of this approach was to more accurately map the distribution of artifact scatters on the surface, in addition to tracing the occupation and use patterns of both sites over time.

Having determined the site boundaries in previous survey seasons, 50 x 50 m grids were overlaid onto both sites. Half of these grid units were selected as collection units, and randomly assigned points were generated for each selected grid square. GPS coordinates were then assigned to each point. Groups of two-person field teams employed a hand-held GPS unit to identify the GPS point in the field, marked it and attached the "dog leash" to the point and collected all artifacts within the circular unit. A total of 29 collection units were surveyed at Dağılbaz Höyük and 50 at Dutlu Tarla. The areas surveyed account for roughly 9% of the total area at Dağılbaz (an 11.3-ha site) and 6% at Dutlu (a 2-ha site). All finds were cleaned and analyzed, and specific sherd counts for each unit based on time period were entered into a Microsoft Excel database. The survey data were then imported into ArcMAP, and pottery density rasters were created using interpolation to examine settlement patterns

Survey Results

The preliminary results of three seasons of survey at Dağılbaz Höyük and Dutlu Tarla enable us to begin to reconstruct an archaeological history of these two sites and their hinterlands. Their settlement history is reflected in the pottery collected on their surfaces. Though the archaeology of the Bay of İskenderun is still relatively unknown, these unstratified ceramic assemblages can be dated via comparison with unpublished evidence from the well-stratified contexts at Kinet Höyük recently excavated by M.-H. Gates, the large-scale excavations at Gözlü Kule (Tarsus) on the western edge of the Cilician Plain, [11] and with excavated sites in the Amuq Plain. [12] The survey also documented a number of key physical features. At Dağılbaz Höyük, the 200 x 100 m summit of the mound is protected on all sides by steep slopes. Large boulders exposed by illicit excavations at the crest of the höyük were likely part of a monumental structure. Several stone walls, visible in modern cuts into the slope of the mound, may have served as fortifications. Along its lower flanks, ancient agricultural terraces are preserved.

11 Goldman 1950; 1956.

12 See e.g. Braidwood and Braidwood 1960; Woolley 1955; Heinz 1992; Yener 2010.

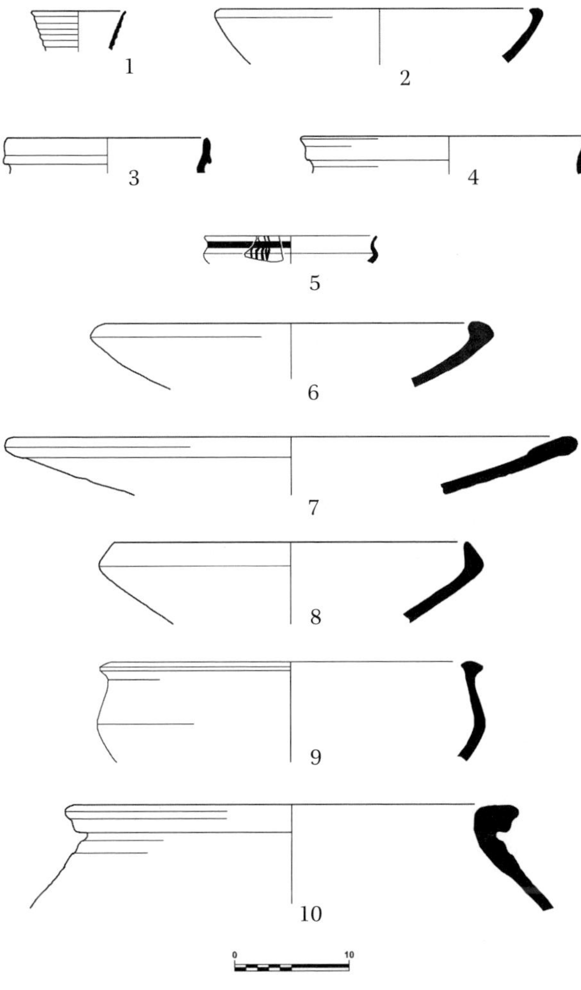

FIG. 6 Early Bronze-Late Bronze Age Pottery from Dağılbaz Höyük. Graphics by G. Lehmann. © Mopsos/BILAS Project.

Figure number	Registration number	Vessel form	Period
6.1	MS3 S45 202–13	cup	Early Bronze Age IVA
6.2	MS3 S45 169–1	bowl	Middle Bronze Age
6.3	MS3 S45 202–18	cooking pot	Middle Bronze Age
6.4	MS3 S45 262–13	cooking pot	Middle Bronze Age
6.5	MS4 S45 308–9	bowl	Middle Bronze Age
6.6	MS3 S45 178–8	bowl	Middle Bronze Age
6.7	MS3 S45 186–1	platter	Late Bronze Age
6.8	MS4 S45 262–3	bowl	Late Bronze Age
6.9	MS4 S45 308–4	deep bowl	Late Bronze Age
6.10	MS4 S45 208–1	storage jar	Late Bronze Age

These terraces reflect an effective land reclamation and soil retention scheme that originated in antiquity and continues today. An irrigation ditch runs along the southern side, and sections of stone walls have been identified on the slopes.

At Dağılbaz Höyük, sherds and flints indicate that the earliest settlement commenced with the Early Bronze Age (EBA) (Fig. 6.1).[13] Though occupied during the EBA, the principal settlement during this period was at the adjacent and neighboring Dutlu Tarla (see below).

The Middle Bronze Age (MBA) is well-represented at Dağılbaz Höyük (Fig. 6.2–6, Fig. 7.1). Incurved bowls (Fig. 6.2, Fig. 6.6) have parallels at Alalakh Strata VIII-X.[14] The cooking pots (Fig. 6.3–4) have close parallels at Alalakh Stratum VIII.[15] A painted bowl (Fig. 6.5) resembles similar vessels at Alalakh Strata VII-VIII.[16] Among the Middle Bronze finds is a typical female figurine of the period (Fig. 7.1). As the figurine shows no indication of a pudendum, it is best identified with female figurines of Type IB in Pruß's study of Syrian figurines, equivalent to Badre's Type MAIS 2.[17] Pruß dates figurines of this type to the MB I and the beginning of MB II.

Late Bronze Age (LBA) Dağılbaz Höyük was a flourishing regional center. The pottery includes standard Hittite platters, deep bowls and storage jars (Fig. 6.6–10).[18] Among the survey finds at Dağılbaz Höyük was also the lower part of a leg, including the hoof, of a Hittite bull figurine (Fig. 7.2). Such bull figurines were a typical representation of ritual, spouted zoomorphic vessels in the Hittite period. They usually appear as a pair of bulls and were found in public buildings and temple contexts during the early stages of the Hittite Empire. They are believed to represent Hurri and Sheri, the two bulls pulling the chariot of the storm god Teshup.[19] The discovery of such figurines at Dağılbaz Höyük suggests the presence of a Hittite sanctuary at the site. The storage jar handle with a seal impression bearing Anatolian hieroglyphic signs dates to an early phase of the Hittite Imperial period (Fig. 7.3). The impression was found on the lower western slopes of the site and has been dated to the 15th–14th centuries BCE.[20]

The later settlement history of Dağılbaz Höyük is marked by the presence of Late Helladic IIIC ceramics of the 12th century BCE found at the surface on

---

13 See e.g. Braidwood and Braidwood 1960, fig. 313.

14 Heinz 1992, pl. 17:5–9; 34:16; 54:5; 55:7.

15 Heinz 1992, pl. 22:39–41.

16 Heinz 1992, pl. 3:13; 20:27.

17 Pruß 2010, 50–56; Badre 1980, 47–50.

18 See e.g. Goldman 1956, fig. 390: L and N; Gates 2001, figs. 3:3, 5; 8:1–11.

19 Aruz, Benzel and Evans 2008, 79, 189.

20 D'Alfonso and Killebrew 2011.

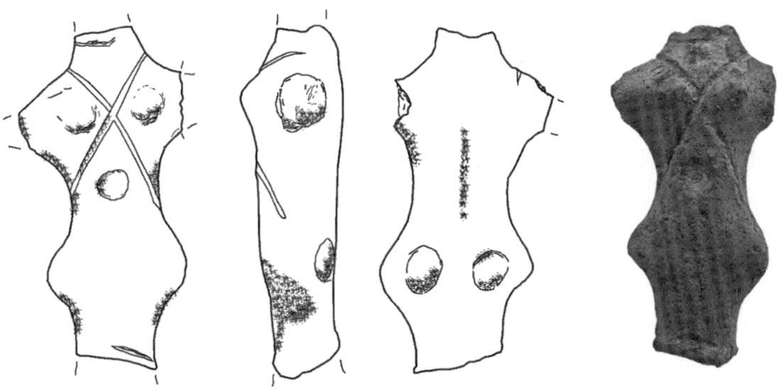

1 MS3 S45 213–1

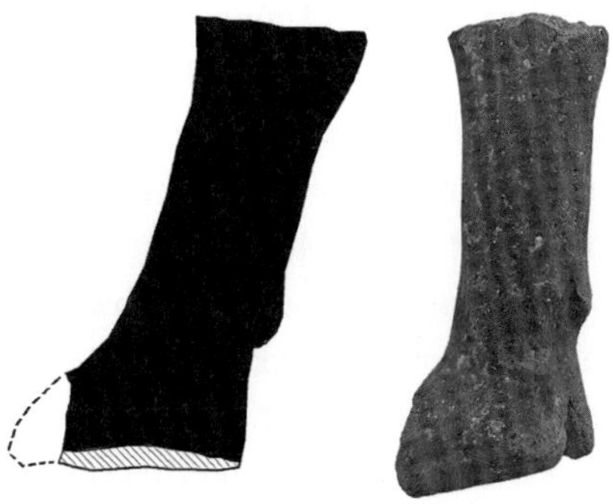

2 MS3 S45 194–1

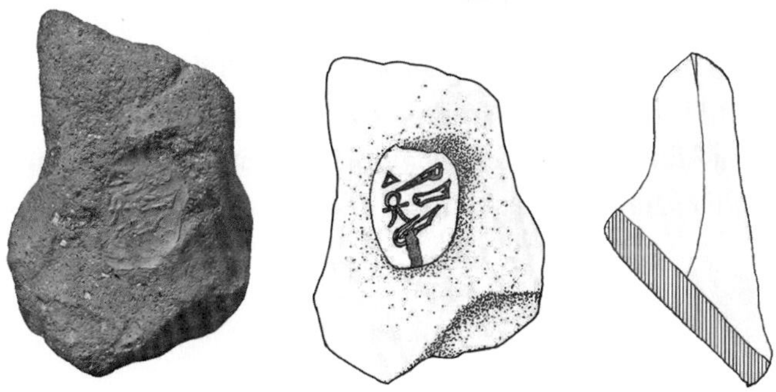

3 MS6 S45 646–4

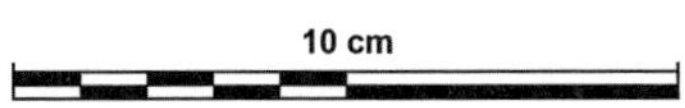

Fig. 7 Finds from Dağılbaz Höyük

1 Middle Bronze female figurine

2 Fragmentary leg of a Hittite bull figurine

3 Late Bronze I seal impression with Anatolian hieroglyphic signs stamped on a storage jar handle. Graphics for nos. 1 and 2 by G. Lehmann, photos for nos. 1 and 2 by A. E. Killebrew and photo for no. 3 by B. R. Olson. © Mopsos/BILAS Project.

top of the mound.[21] There is also a sherd of a Proto-White Painted (or White Painted I) amphoroid krater or amphoriskos of the 11th century BCE. The few Iron Age sherds collected on the mound suggest that the site was at best modest in size during the 12th century BCE through the Persian period, when we note an increase in the number of sherds. The pottery, especially the appearance of significant numbers of basket handle amphorae suggests renewed settlement during the Late Persian or early Hellenistic periods that continued through the early Roman period.

The adjacent site of Dutlu Tarla slopes gently down from south to north. Today the site is under cultivation and consists of agricultural fields, fallow fennel fields and lemon tree groves. The Early Bronze period, mainly EB III, was the dominant era of the site's occupation. Especially large concentrations of third-millennium pottery were recovered from most of the surface area of Dutlu Tarla. Smaller quantities of Persian, Hellenistic, Roman, Late Roman and Byzantine-period pottery were collected in the northwestern area of the site, along with significant quantities of pottery slag, suggesting the presence of a potter's workshop. Based on the survey findings, the majority of the ceramics found at Dutlu Tarla date to the EBA (Fig. 9.1-7), reflecting the site's dominant role in the İskenderun Plain during much of the third millennium BCE. The parallels in the Amuq Plain date to Amuq Phases H and I, EB II-IVA.[22] No sherds dating to the Middle Bronze through Iron Ages were identified, suggesting that the site was abandoned until the Persian and Hellenistic periods. The latest activity documented at the site dates to the Late Roman/Byzantine period (Fig. 9.8).

21 Lehmann 2013, 298; fig. 7.2.

22 Braidwood and Braidwood 1960, Figs. 286, 310–311.

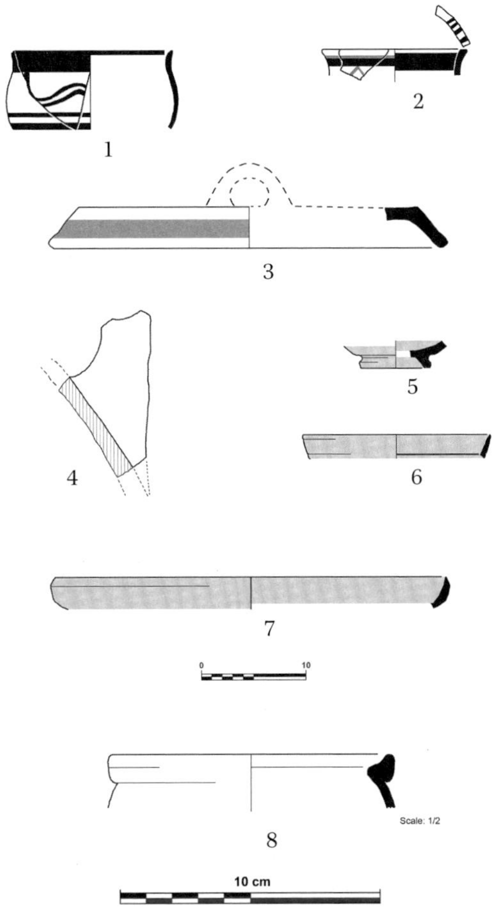

FIG. 8 Iron I through Early Roman Pottery from Dağılbaz Höyük. Graphics by G. Lehmann. © Mopsos/BILAS Project.

Figure number	Registration number	Vessel form	Period
8.1	MS3 S45 178–1	bell-shaped bowl	Late Helladic IIIC
8.2	MS3 S45 201–15	amphoroid krater or amphoriskos	Proto-White Painted or White Painted I
8.3	MS3 S45 183–1	lid	Persian period
8.4	MS3 S45 211–2	handle of basket-handle amphora	Persian period or early Hellenistic
8.5	MS3 S45 178–19	ESA cup (Hayes Form 22)	Hellenistic-Early Roman
8.6	MS4 S45 262–34	ESA vertical rim	Hellenistic-Early Roman
8.7	MS3 S45 183–2	ESA up-turned plate	Hellenistic
8.8	MS4 S45 307–2	cooking pot	Hellenistic

ESA = Eastern Sigillata A

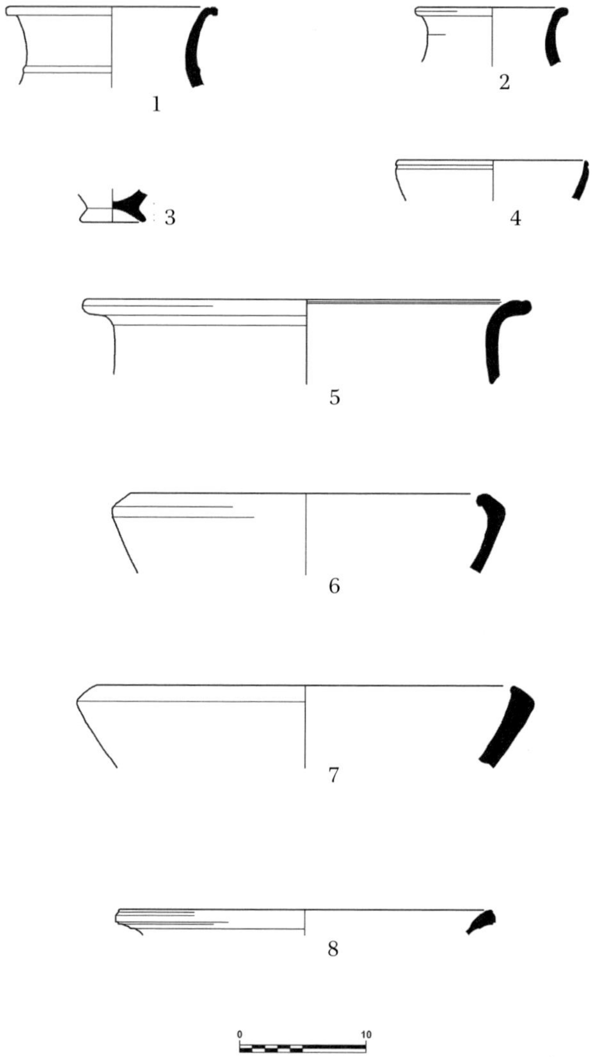

FIG. 9 Early Bronze and Late Roman Red Ware Pottery from Dutlu Tarla. Graphics by G. Lehmann. © Mopsos/BILAS Project.

Figure number	Registration number	Vessel form	Period
9.1	MS4 S83 314–2	jar, reddish yellow	Early Bronze Age
9.2	MS4 S83 317–13	jar	Early Bronze Age
9.3	MS4 S83 312–1	cup, brittle orange	Early Bronze Age
9.4	MS4 S83 317–11	bowl	Early Bronze Age
9.5	MS4 S83 548–7	deep bowl	Early Bronze Age
9.6	MS4 S83 166–11	deep bowl	Early Bronze Age
9.7	MS4 S83 314–6	deep bowl, misfired	Early Bronze Age
9.8	MS4 S83 316–11	red-slipped bowl	Late Roman

Conclusions

The survey data from Dağılbaz Höyük and Dutlu Tarla lead to several conclusions. Methodologically, the time consuming dog leash survey at Dağılbaz Höyük did not yield useful results. This was due to several factors including poor site visibility, especially dense vegetation and weed overgrowth, as well as modern activities at the site, such as agricultural fields in the process of being harvested. Previous seasons of survey produced superior results when field conditions were better. The dog leash survey at Dutlu Tarla, where visibility was good, confirmed that the Hellenistic-Late Roman/Byzantine period settlement was most prominent in the northeastern section of the site. Early Bronze pottery was dominant in the southern half of the site. At the interface of the Bronze Age and Hellenistic-Late Roman/Byzantine settlements, significant quantities of pottery slag as of a yet undetermined date may well indicate the presence of a ceramic industry in one or both periods. In general, however, the 2009 labor-intensive dog leash survey added little new information to our previous surveys in 2006 and 2007 that were conducted as pedestrian transects.

Both Dağılbaz Höyük and Dutlu Tarla are the most prominent sites in the İskenderun Plain during the Early Bronze (Dutlu and, to a lesser degree, Dağılbaz), Middle-Late Bronze/ Iron I (Dağılbaz) and Persian (Dağılbaz and probably Dutlu) periods. The size of the third-millennium settlement at Dutlu Tarla most likely reflects the early stages of the development of complex society in the İskenderun Plain. It is noteworthy that occupation during the second millennium BCE had shifted southwards from Dutlu Tarla to Dağılbaz Höyük. Relatively modest quantities of Hellenistic pottery were documented on both sites. During the Roman and Late Roman/Byzantine periods, settlement continued at Dutlu Tarla only.

Based on the survey results, Dağılbaz Höyük may have served as a fortress guarding the exit of the western branch of the Bahçedere that flows down from the Belen Pass above. The substantial remains of massive walls together with large quantities of Late Bronze pottery suggest to us that the site was the locale of a significant fortress, especially during the LBA. Based on the evidence documented at Dutlu Tarla and Dağılbaz Höyük, we propose that during the Early Bronze through Persian periods, the primary overland route connecting Syria and Asia Minor followed the Bahçedere, exiting at the fortress site of Dağılbaz Höyük and Early Bronze center of Dutlu Tarla (Fig. 10). This would explain the prominence of these two sites in the İskenderun Plain during much of the third through first millennia BCE.

With the establishment of a new urban center at Alexandreia kat'Isson, most likely at the end of the 4th (or possibly early 3rd) century BCE, the importance

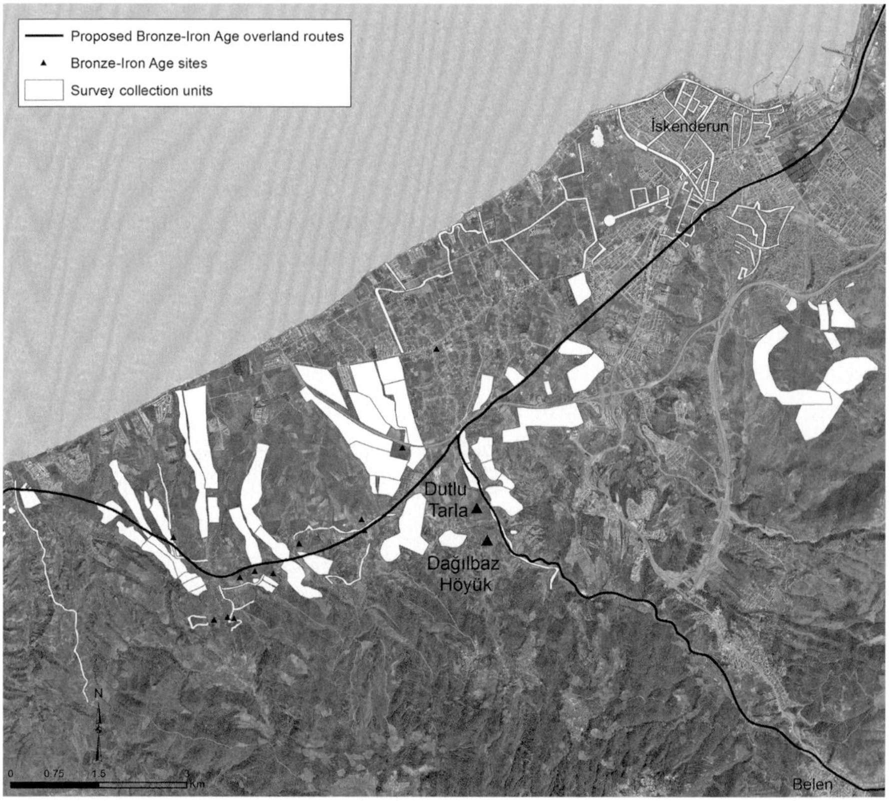

FIG. 10 Proposed Bronze-Iron Age and Persian-period overland routes. Satellite image provided by Digital Globe. Graphics by B. R. Olson. © Mopsos/BILAS Project.

of Dağılbaz Höyük and Dutlu Tarla and their hinterland subsides.[23] The resulting plethora of towns, villages, hamlets, quarries and various other features, including an aqueduct bringing water from Elmadağ (Hatay) to the city, in the vicinity of Alexandreia kat'Isson reflect its ascendance as the main population

23 Historical sources regarding the founding of Alexandreia kat'Isson are few. Jones (1971, 198–201) and Grainger (1990, 36–37, 108) argue that the city was founded by Seleucus I Nicator in honor of Alexander's victory at the Battle of Issus, though both note that no historical authority ascribes the foundation of the city to the king). The largely discredited Pseudo-Scymnus, the name given to an unknown author writing in classical Greek (Müller 1882, 1:235; Pseudo-Scymnus 923), attributes the founding of the city to Alexander the Great himself. The city began minting bronze coinage under Antiochus IV Epiphanes and autonomous bronze coinage in 163 BC (Head 1911, 716). See Cohen (2006, 73–76) for a recent discussion. Ceramic evidence from our survey indicates an early Hellenistic date for the initial settlement of Alexandreia kat'Isson.

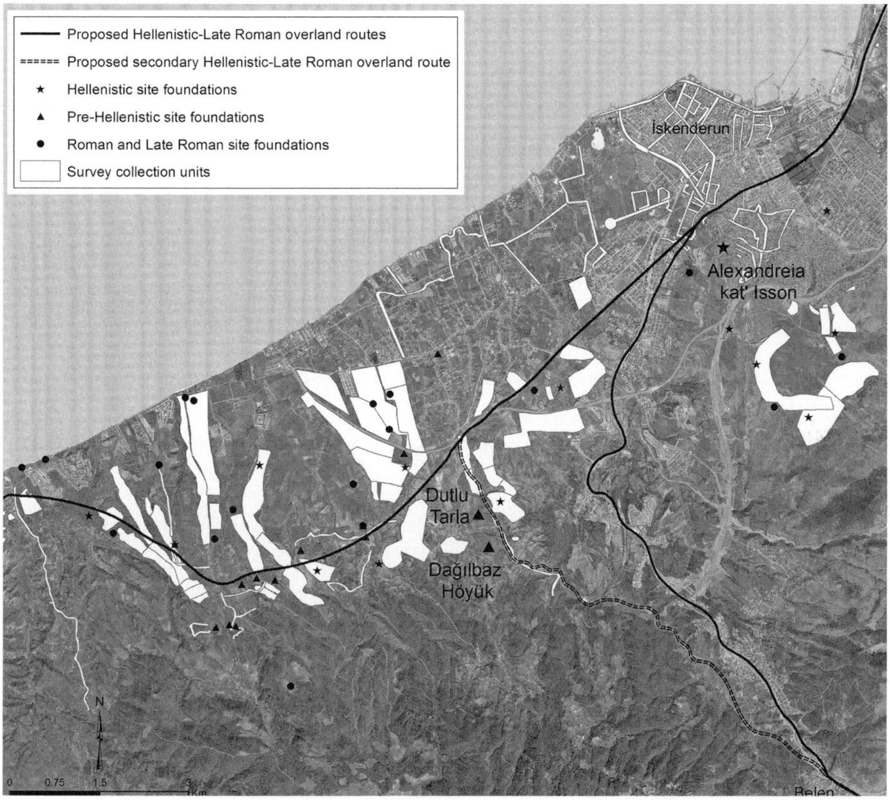

FIG 11 Proposed Hellenistic-Late Roman overland routes. Satellite image provided by Digital Globe. Graphics by B. R. Olson. © Mopsos/BILAS Project.

and urban center in the İskenderun plain. Based on these settlement patterns, we suggest that the main route connecting the Amuq Valley and İskenderun Plain via the Belen Pass shifts to the northeast, following a path parallel to the current highway connecting these two regions (FIG. 11). While the modern pass leads from Belen northwards to İskenderun along the crest of the Amanus foothills, the ancient route most likely followed the eastern branch of the Bahçedere. This hypothetical ancient route would have avoided the mountains with their woods and difficult passage choosing a more convenient way for Hellenistic traffic to the newly established city of Alexandreia kat'Isson.

REFERENCES

Aruz, J., K. Benzel and J.M. Evans, eds., *Beyond Babylon: Art, Trade, and Diplomacy in the Second Millennium BC.* New York: Metropolitan Museum of Art/New Haven, CT, 2008.

Badre, L., *Les figurines anthropomorphes en terre cuite à l'âge du bronze en Syrie*. Bibliothèque archéologique et historique 103. Paris: Geuthner, 1980.

Braidwood, R. J. and L. S. Braidwood, *The Earlier Assemblages, Phases A-J.* Vol. 1 of *Excavations in the Plain of Antioch.* Oriental Institute Publications 61. Chicago: University of Chicago Press, 1960.

Chammas, P., *Alexandrette.* Alexandrette: Imp. Al-Jihad, 1931.

———. "Une tournée archéologique dans l'Amanus." *Revue Archéologique Syrienne* 3 (1933): 6–18.

Cohen, G. M., *The Hellenistic Settlements in Syria, the Red Sea Basin, and North Africa.* Berkeley: University of California Press, 2006.

D'Alfonso, L. and A. E. Killebrew, "A New Anatolian Hieroglyphic Seal Impression from Dağılbaz Höyük, Bay of İskenderun, Turkey." *Near Eastern Archaeology* 74 (2011): 113–115.

Gates, M.-H., "Potmarks at Kinet Höyük and the Hittite Ceramic Industry" in *La Cilicie: espaces et pouvoirs locaux (2e millénaire av. J.-C.–4e siècle ap. J.-C.; actes de la table ronde internationale d'Istanbul, 2–5 novembre 1999*, ed. É. Jean, M. Dinçol and S. Durugönül,, 137–158. Paris: De Boccard, 2001.

Gjerstad, E., "Cilician Studies." *Revue Archéologique* (1934): 155–203.

Goldman, H., ed. *The Hellenistic and Roman Periods.* Vol. 1 of *Excavations at Gözlü Kule, Tarsus.* Princeton: Princeton University Press, 1950.

———. ed., *From the Neolithic through the Bronze Age.* Vol. 2 of *Excavations at Gözlü Kule, Tarsus.* Princeton: Princeton University Press, 1956.

Gough, M., "Augusta Ciliciae." *Anatolian Studies* 6 (1956): 165–177.

Grainger, J.D., *The Cities of Seleukid Syria.* Oxford: Clarendon Press, 1990.

Hartmann, M., "Das Liwa Haleb (Aleppo) und ein Teil des Liwa Dschebel Bereket." *Zeitschrift der Gesellschaft für Erdkunde zu Berlin* 29 (1894): 142–188 , 475–550.

Head, B.V., *Historia Numorum: A Manual of Greek Numismatics.* 2nd ed. Oxford: Clarendon Press, 1911.

Heinz, M., *Tell Atchana, Alalakh: die Schichten VII-XVII.* Alter Orient und Altes Testament 41. Kevelaer: Butzon & Bercker, 1992.

Hellenkemper, H. and F. Hild, *Neue Forschungen in Kilikien.* Veröffentlichungen der Kommission für die Tabula Imperii Byzantini 4. Wien: Österreichische Akademie der Wissenschaften, 1986.

Hild, F. and H. Hellenkemper, *Kilikien und Isaurien.* Tabula Imperii Byzantini 5. Wien: Österreichische Akademie der Wissenschaften, 1990.

Jones, A.H.M., *The Cities of the Eastern Roman Provinces.* 2nd. ed., revised by M. Avi-Yonah. Oxford: Clarendon Press, 1971.

Killebrew, A. E., "Summary of the 2009 Cilicia Survey (İskenderun Bay Region)." *Araştırma Sonuçları Toplantısı* 28 (2011): 39–46.

Killebrew, A. E. and G. Lehmann, "Summary of the 2008 Cilicia Survey (İskenderun Bay Region)." *Araştırma Sonuçları Toplantısı* 27 (2010): 319–338.

Killebrew, A. E., G. Lehmann and M.-H. Gates, "Summary of the 2007 Cilicia Survey (İskenderun Bay Region)." *Araştırma Sonuçları Toplantısı* 26 (2009): 227–238.

Lehmann, G., "Aegean-Style Pottery in Syria and Lebanon during Iron Age I" in *The Philistines and Other 'Sea Peoples' in Text and Archaeology*, ed. A. E. Killebrew and G. Lehmann, 265–328. Society of Biblical Literature Archaeology and Biblical Studies 15. Atlanta: Society of Biblical Literature, 2013.

Lehmann, G., A. E. Killebrew and M.-H. Gates, "Summary of the 2006 Cilicia Survey (İskenderun Bay Region)" in *Araştırma Sonuçları Toplantısı* 25 (2008): 171–188.

Lehmann, G., A. E. Killebrew, M.-H. Gates and B. Halpern, "The Mopsos Project: The 2004 Season of Archaeological Survey in the Bay of İskenderun, Eastern Cilicia." *Araştırma Sonuçları Toplantısı* 23 (2006): 79–88.

Müller, K., *Geographi Graeci Minores*. 2 vols. Paris: Firmin-Didot, 1882.

Özgen, İ. and M.-H. Gates, "Report on the Bilkent University Archaeological Survey in Cilicia and the Northern Hatay: August 1991" in *Araştırma Sonuçları Toplantısı* 10 (1993): 387–394.

Pruß, A., *Die Amuq-Terrakotten: Untersuchungen zu den Terrakotta-Figuren des 2. und 1. Jahrtausends v. Chr. aus den Grabungen des Oriental Institute Chicago in der Amuq-Ebene*. Turnhout: Brepols, 2010.

Seton-Williams, M. V., "Cilician Survey." *Anatolian Studies* 4 (1954): 121–174.

Steadman, S., "Prehistoric Sites on the Cilician Coastal Plain: Chalcolithic and Early Bronze Age Pottery from the 1991 Bilkent University Survey." *Anatolian Studies* 44 (1994): 85–103.

Tobin, J., *Black Cilicia: A Study of the Plain of Issus During the Roman and Late Roman Periods*. BAR International Series 1275. Oxford: British Archaeological Reports, 2004.

Woolley, C.L., *Alalakh: An Account of the Excavations at Tell Atchana in the Hatay, 1937–1949*. Reports of the Research Committee of the Society of Antiquaries of London 18. Oxford Society of Antiquaries, 1955.

Yener, K.A., ed., *Tell Atchana, Ancient Alalakh. Volume 1. 2003–2004 Excavation Seasons*. İstanbul: Koç University Press, 2010.

La cornaline dans les sources paléo-assyriennes

Cécile Michel[1]

Abstract

La cornaline, une pierre semi-précieuse originaire de la vallée de l'Indus, figure parmi les marchandises exportées par les Assyriens en Anatolie centrale au 19e siècle av. J.-C. Attestée sous forme de perles et éléments de parure dans les textes, d'une valeur inférieure au lapis-lazuli, elle était achetée par les hommes et les femmes à Aššur, et négociée à Kaneš selon les mêmes conditions que les autres marchandises importées. Les découvertes d'objets en cornaline dans les tombes des marchands assyriens d'Aššur et de Kaneš font écho aux données textuelles et permettent d'en préciser certains usages.

Les caravanes assyriennes affrétées par les marchands d'Aššur au 19e siècle av. J.-C. transportaient principalement des étoffes et de l'étain destinés à l'exportation vers l'Asie Mineure ; d'autres produits et matières premières étaient parfois ajoutés aux chargements, en moindre quantités. Parmi les plus précieux figuraient le fer, le lapis-lazuli et plus rarement la cornaline.

Lapis-lazuli et cornaline, toutes deux originaires de l'Est, représentaient les pierres semi-précieuses les plus appréciées par les habitants de l'ancienne Mésopotamie. Dans les incantations relatives à la naissance comparant la femme en travail à un bateau chargé de produits exotiques, le lapis-lazuli, de couleur bleue sombre, préfigurait le garçon, tandis que la cornaline, de couleur sanguine annonçait la fille à venir.[2] Après avoir, il y a une douzaine d'années, dédié à Klaas Veenhof un article sur le lapis-lazuli dans les données textuelles et archéologiques paléo-assyriennes,[3] il m'est particulièrement agréable, aujourd'hui, d'offrir cette note sur la cornaline à Marie-Henriette Gates, amie très chère, grande spécialiste de l'archéologie anatolienne, qui, dans les années 1980, a montré avec brio la voie du dialogue entre textes, images et données archéologiques.[4]

1 CNRS, ArScAn-HAROC, Maison de l'Archéologie et de l'Ethnologie, Nanterre.

2 Cohen 1976, 136, l. 18–21.

3 Michel 2001.

4 Nous devons entre autres à Marie-Henriette Gates les synthèses sur l'archéologie turque (« Archaeology in Turkey ») parues régulièrement dans l'*American Journal of Archaeology*, dans les années 1990 à 2005 ; voir également la synthèse Gates 2011.

Le lapis-lazuli apparaît régulièrement dans les transactions des Assyriens en Anatolie centrale, et nombre d'objets exhumés à Kaneš et dans quelques tombes de marchands d'Aššur sont faits de lapis-lazuli ou comportent un élément taillé dans cette pierre. La cornaline est plus rare ; néanmoins, une petite vingtaine de textes permettent de définir entre autres sa provenance, son prix et son usage, et ces données textuelles peuvent être comparées avec les quelques éléments de parure et objets en cornaline découverts à Aššur et à Kaneš.

1 Identification de la cornaline

1.1 Cornaline et agate, des pierres voisines

La cornaline, tout comme l'agate, est une variété de calcédoine, un terme qui désigne des quartz micro-cristallisés. Son nom vient du latin, *corneus* « corne » ou encore *cornus* « (fruit du) cornouiller ».[5] Pierre translucide variant du jaune au rouge, elle obtient sa couleur rouge-orangé grâce à un traitement thermique[6] ; elle est principalement utilisée en bijouterie. Elle a été régulièrement confondue avec certaines variétés d'agates, même si la cornaline présente une couleur unie contrairement à l'agate qui apparaît souvent finement zonée (c'est-à-dire avec une superposition de couches de couleurs légèrement différentes). De fait, ces pierres présentent les mêmes caractéristiques dans leur formule chimique (SiO2), ce sont des pierres dures (6–7 sur l'échelle de Mohs) et leur densité (masse volumique) est environ de 2,6. La distinction parfois difficile entre cornaline et agate a amené quelques spécialistes comme M.-L. Inizan à utiliser le terme « cornaline » pour désigner toute une série de pierres semblables[7] : « [La cornaline] est une variété microfibreuse de silice comme toutes les calcédoines, nous utiliserons le terme cornaline par commodité, même si dans bien des cas,

Dans Gates 1988, elle propose une étude croisée des différentes sources (textes, images, artefacts) sur des sujets aussi variés que la céramique, les ossements de faune, le métal ou l'architecture. Dans Gates 1989, elle s'intéresse à l'art et aux artisans de Mari, toujours dans une perspective interdisciplinaire.

5 Cohen 1976, 135–140. La série *abnu šikinšu*, « la pierre dont l'apparence est... », compare la cornaline au fruit du lyciet (*eddetum*), STT 108:5. *cf.* également Schuster-Brandis 2008, 413–415. La couleur rouge de la cornaline rappelle le cycle féminin, *cf.* André-Salvini 1999.

6 Roux 2000, 27–28.

7 Inizan 1999, 128. Les publications archéologiques montrent l'hésitation de leurs auteurs sur l'identification de la pierre dans laquelle un objet a été taillé. Par exemple, la petite tête de suidé exhumée en 1995 à Kültepe est, dans une même publication, tantôt définie comme étant en cornaline (Özgüç 2003, 230, no. 237 « Carnelian, a pink translucent stone head of a boar of Level Ib »), tantôt en agate (Özgüç 2003, 231, no.4 « As for the agate head of a boar », etc.).

il s'agit d'agate, de sardoine, d'onyx, etc., leur origine et leur travail sont à peu près identiques pour toutes. »

1.2 Les attestations de cornaline

La cornaline, na_4-gug en sumérien, est désignée par le terme *sāmtum* en akkadien, identifiée ainsi par sa couleur caractéristique, rouge, *sāmum;*[8] les sources paléo-assyriennes utilisent à parts quasiment égales les deux mots sumérien et akkadien, sans raison particulière.[9] L'usage du mot akkadien a parfois prêté à confusion. En effet, le terme *sāmtum* correspond également au féminin de l'adjectif qualificatif « rouge » qui peut désigner la laine teinte en rouge[10] : « de la laine teinte en rouge est disponible » ou encore « 80 talents (de laine) blanche, 20 talents (de laine) rouge ».

Liste lexicale paléo-assyrienne découverte en 1968, en deux fragments, dans une maison de la ville basse de Kaneš datée du niveau Ib (18e siècle), Kt t/k 76+79, mentionne au revers la cornaline parmi environ une quarantaine de pierres, après une brève liste de métaux (or, fer natif, étain, cuivre, bronze).[11] La liste des pierres couvre deux colonnes et commence par quelques gemmes semi-précieuses[12] : « pierre [...], lapis-lazuli, cornaline, cristal de roche? [...] ».

8 Michel 1999, 405. À Mari, le mot sumérien na_4-su_{13}-a « pierre rouge » est également employé pour désigner la cornaline, *cf.* Arkhipov 2012, 36–37.

9 na_4-gug : AKT 2, 30:42 ; BIN 6, 89:4, 16 ; CCT 4, 18a:4 ; CCT 4, 40a:5, 24 ; ICK 2, 321:10; Kt t/k 76+79:12 ; Kt 93/k 196:7; Kt 94/k 1746:4, 12; Kt j/k 97: 44; TC 3, 178:7 ; TTC 2:5. *sāmtum* : AKT 5, 52:37 ; AKT 6a, 144:22; AKT 6a, 145:38 ; BIN 6, 179:3' ; CCT 3, 29:28 ; Kt a/k 611:13 ; Kt 88/k 292:6 ; Kt 94/k 1471:8.

10 CCT 4, 27 :1'–2', síg!hi-a *sà-am-tum$_8$-ma, i-ba-ší-ma* ; CCT 4, 47a:30–31, 80 gú, *pá-ṣí-tum*: 20 gú *sà-am-tum*. Pour des textiles et vêtements rouges, *sāmum, cf.* BIN 4, 162:4; KTS2, 35:30 ; TC 1, 43:24, 27 ; Michel & Veenhof 2010, 234, 252.

11 Hecker 1993, 286–290, pl. 47–48 ; Michel 2008, 349.

12 Kt t/k 76+79:rev. v10–14, na_4 x z[a x], na_4-za-[gìn], na_4-g[ug], na_4-du_8-[šu-a], n[a_4 ...]. Pour l'identification possible de la pierre na_4-du-šu-a, *duhšum*, avec le cristal de roche, *cf.* Michel 1999, 405, contra Schuster-Brandis 2008, 407–409 et Steinkeller 2006, qui proposent de l'identifier au chlorite. L'usage de cette pierre dans les textes de Mari ne convient pas pour le chlorite, *cf.* Arkhipov 2012, 33–34. Selon Durand 2009, 153–154, la laine *d/tuhšum* ne serait pas nécessairement à relier à la couleur de cette pierre. L'ordre donné dans cette liste diffère de celui de ur_5-ra XVI (MSL 10, 5–16), qui consacre 456 lignes aux pierres, dans la mesure où, dans ce texte, la pierre na_4-du-šu-a apparaît avant les autres. Sur la colonne vi de Kt t/k 76+79 figurent d'autres pierres semi-précieuses, comme le *ziganšarrum*, et des pierres plus ordinaires comme la pierre de meule (na_4–ur_5).

2 L'origine de la cornaline

2.1 La cornaline, une pierre semi-précieuse de la vallée de l'Indus

Les principaux gisements de cornaline se trouvent en Inde. Son exploitation remonte sans doute au 7e millénaire en Asie Centrale ; elle était importée au Proche-Orient, via le Golfe arabo-persique, dès le 5e millénaire av. J.-C. [13] Pierre dure, qui se taille comme le silex, la cornaline était souvent importée sous la forme de perles en provenance de la vallée de l'Indus à partir de la seconde moitié du 3e millénaire et arrivait en Mésopotamie via Ur, où les perles étaient parfois inscrites. [14] En Mésopotamie, des ateliers de fabrication de perles de petite taille en cornaline ont été découverts à proximité de Larsa, datant du début du 3e millénaire. [15] À Tello, l'antique Girsu, des tombes de la seconde moitié du 3e millénaire ont produit plus de 600 perles dont une centaine en cornaline. [16] Cet ensemble comporte principalement de petites perles cylindriques ou en forme de disque, grossièrement réalisées, un groupe de perles de types variés, biconiques, à facettes et présentant d'autres formes, ne dépassant pas les 3 cm, et huit longues perles harappéennes d'environ 8 cm de long. Si les premières ont vraisemblament été réalisées en Mésopotamie, peut-être à Larsa, les dernières ont été importées finies depuis la vallée de l'Indus.

Parallèlement, le travail de la pierre est attesté en Afghanistan (Kandahar) pour la fin du 4e millénaire, puis en Iran du nord-est ; par conséquent la cornaline était aussi importée en Mésopotamie, avec le lapis-lazuli et l'étain, à travers le plateau iranien. [17]

Les perles découvertes dans les tombes paléo-assyriennes d'Aššur furent, pour une part, importées depuis l'Afghanistan, et pour l'autre part, réalisées dans la vallée de l'Indus par des spécialistes harappéens. En effet, la tombe d'Aššur n°37 contenait entre autres quatre perles en cornaline gravées, semblables à celles découvertes en nombre dans les sites de Mésopotamie du sud, mais qui sont rares dans le nord mésopotamien. [18]

2.2 Provenance de la cornaline dans les textes

Les sources écrites paléo-assyriennes montrent très nettement que la cornaline était importée depuis l'est, vraisemblablement avec l'étain et le lapis-lazuli ; cer-

---

13 Roux 2000, 27–28, 31.

14 Inizan 1999, 127. Voir par exemple la perle en cornaline dédiée par Šulgi à la déesse Ningal et découverte à Suse. Pour les perles inscrites, voir en dernier lieu Abrahami 2008 et Abrahami 2014.

15 Chevalier, Inizan & Tixier 1982.

16 Inizan 1993.

17 Inizan 1999, 127.

18 Aruz 1995, 50–51; l'une de ces perles avec décor guilloché aurait toutefois un parallèle à Tell Asmar daté du début du 2e millénaire, *cf.* ci-dessous section 4.1.

taines pièces ont pu toutefois être apportées à Aššur depuis le sud babylonien. Elle était achetée à Aššur, en même temps que les étoffes, l'étain et les ânes pour le transport.[19] La cornaline est fréquemment associée à des transports d'étain et d'étoffes à destination de l'Anatolie. Un convoi de presque 700 textiles et 600 kg d'étain chargés sur 34 ânes noirs, transportait également des clous, de l'huile fine, de la cornaline, des pierres fines (*zigašarrum*), des fibules en bronze, du safran et du cèdre.[20] En plus de l'étain et des étoffes, cette caravane transportait donc vers Kaneš divers produits de luxe. De même, un memorandum fait état d'un transport de près de 300 étoffes et 200 kg d'étain chargés sur 15 ânes noirs auxquels ont été ajoutés les biens suivants : cornaline, pierres fines (*zigašarrum*), cuivre, vieilles faucilles et huile, le tout confié à Aššur-malik, vraisemblablement à Kaneš ; la provenance de ces produits n'est toutefois pas explicite.[21] La cornaline subissait le même sort que les autres marchandises en route et pouvait être retenue au passage de l'Euphrate : « J'apprends que ton étain et la cornaline se trouvent à Hahhum dans la maison d'Iddin-Aššur, fils de Dadīya ».[22] En d'autres occasions, les pierres étaient transportées par des voyageurs, indépendamment des convois d'étain et d'étoffes.[23]

3 Le commerce de la cornaline

3.1 Formes sous la cornaline est négociée

La forme sous laquelle la cornaline intervient dans les transactions est rarement précisée. Un document inédit fait toutefois état d'un lourd bloc de pierre et d'une pièce allongée:[24] « (Ilī-wēdāku t'apporte 1 mine d'argent à notre sceau) pour

19 Kt 88/k 292 (L.G. Gökçek, *Archivum Anatolicum* 8/1, 61) achat d'étoffes et d'étain à Aššur, ainsi que de l'huile, de la cornaline, des ânes. TTC 2 mentionne l'envoi de cornaline avec de l'étain.

20 AKT 6a, 144 et le texte parallèle AKT 6a 145.

21 TC 3, 178.

22 CCT 4, 18a: 3–5 (lettre d'Imdīlum à Puzur-Aššur, Michel 2001, n° 203), *a-ša-me-ma* an-na-*kà*, na_4-gug *i-na, Ha-hi-im* é *I-dì-A*-šùr dumu *Da-ì-a i-ba-ší.*

23 La lettre BIN 6, 179, 3' dont l'incipit est cassé, mentionne l'envoi de perles en lapis-lazuli et cornaline par Asānum, ainsi que des boucles d'oreilles, *cf.* ci-dessous note 24.

24 Kt 94/k 1471:6–14 (lettre inédite d'Aššur-Šamšī et Dadaya à Alāhum, transcription de M. T. Larsen), 10 gín : *hu-sà-ru-um*, sig_5 *wa-at-ra-am le-qé-a-am, ší-tí* kù-babbar : *sà-am-tum, mì-iš-lúm* : *kà-bu-tum, mì-iš-lúm* : *a-ra-ak-tum, lu ra-*bi_4*-a-at, ku-nu-uk-ma, a-na* : Il_5*-we-da-ak, dí-in-ma*. Ce passage est cité par K. R. Veenhof, AKT 5, 163. Notons que le texte mentionne un peu plus loin du lapis-lazuli et de l'agate rubannée quantifiés au poids. Abrahami 2014, 148, n. 5, mentionne l'existence de blocs (*takassu*) de pierres semi-précieuses à tailler.

prendre 10 sicles de lapis-lazuli d'excellente qualité, (et) avec le reste de l'argent, de la cornaline pour moitié en pierre lourde (et) pour moitié en une pièce longue qui soit grande, scelle-(le tout) et remets-le à Ilī-wēdāku. » L'expression « pierre lourde » n'est pas claire ; s'agit-il d'un bloc suffisamment important pour y tailler un objet ? D'autre part, la description d'une « pièce longue » fait penser aux perles allongées taillées par les joalliers harappéens ; la question se pose toutefois sur l'état de cette pierre, était-elle déjà taillée ou non ? Un autre texte renvoie plus explicitement au commerce de perles en pierres semi-précieuses, sans toutefois préciser la forme de ces dernières : « quatre perles de lapis-lazuli, deux de cornaline ».[25]

Hormis le bloc de pierre dont on ne connaît pas la forme, les autres attestations renverraient plutôt à l'usage de la cornaline pour des éléments de parure. Les archives royales de Mari contemporaines confirment cet emploi de la cornaline.[26]

3.2 Quantités citées

Toutes les autres occurrences renvoient vraisemblablement à un ou plusieurs blocs de pierre dont le poids est parfois donné. On trouve des quantités de cornaline assez variables selon les textes, allant de 90 g à un peu plus de 15 kg, ce qui est assez exceptionnel. Le poid le plus élevé de cornaline mentionné est la propriété commune de trois marchands (ci-dessous note 28) ; il est deux fois plus important que le poids de lapis-lazuli le plus élevé attesté dans la documentation paléo-assyrienne.[27] Si l'on retire les deux poids les plus élevés, la cornaline est négociée avec un poids moyen d'environ 1 mine, soit 500 g.

---

25 BIN 6, 179:2'–3', [*ar*]-*bé-et zi-mì-zi*, [*ša* n]a$_4$-za-gìn : *ší-na* : *ša sà-am-tim*. Noter l'écriture en toutes lettres des chiffres. Ce texte est cité par Dercksen 2004, 25. Deux textes, qui ne sont pas commerciaux, font état d'objets en cornaline dont on ne sait s'ils existaient réellement. L'incantation contre un chien mentionne des pots en cornaline ; Kt a/k 611:12–13, [*kàr-pá-tì*]-*ki-na*, *ša sà-am-tim*. L'autre référence se trouve dans la Légende de Sargon (d'Akkad) Kt j/k 97:44–47, *i-na wa-ṣa-i-a* : *ša* na$_4$-gug, *ù* na$_4$-za-gìn : *qá-nu-a-am, lu ar-ku-ús-ma* : *a-na ma-tim, lu ú-za-iz*, « Lors de mon départ, je nouai un roseau de cornaline et lapis-lazuli et je le distribuais au pays ».

26 Michel 1999, 408–409, évoque des colliers faits de perles en pierres semi-précieuses (cornaline, agate, cristal de roche, lapis-lazuli) alternant avec des perles cannelées en or, ainsi que des fibules avec une tête décorée d'un lapis-lazuli ou d'une cornaline enchâssés. Les textes de Mari attestent en effet de perles de formes variées : ARMT 21, 223:35, 44, 52 ; ARMT 21, 246:7 ; M. 12255:2 ; Arkhipov 2012, 490:6'-7', 12' ; des incrustations en cornaline et lapis-lazuli sur divers bijoux et objets de luxe en or ou en fer (ARMT 24, 141:5' ; ARMT 24, 290+:2 ; ARMT 31, 187:6' ; ARMT 31, 232:9' ; M. 5291+:8 ; M. 6495+:ii13'M. 8515:10' ; M. 8647:5 ; M. 9013+:8) et de la pierre brute (ARMT 21, 118:7 ; ARMT 21, 223:48 ; M. 10759:29). Les textes en M. cités dans cette note sont édités dans Arkhipov 2012 = ARMT 32.

27 Kt 94/k 757:1–2 (transcription M. T. Larsen), *i-na* 16 5/6 *ma-na hu-sà-ri-im, ša ik-ri-bi ša A*-šùr, « 16 5/6 mines de lapis-lazuli appartenant au dieu Aššur ».

poids de cornaline	texte
30 5/6 mines	AKT 5, 52:37–38
6 mines	BIN 6, 89:3–5
3 mines	Kt 93/k 196:7
1 mine 55 sicles et 3 1/6 sicles	TTC 2:4–5
2/3 mine 2 1/3 sicles	CCT 3 29:28
1/2 mine 2 1/3 sicles	Kt 92/k 176:23
1/3 mine 2 sicles	AKT 6a 144:21–22// AKT 6a 145:38
11 sicles	ICK 2, 321:10

3.3 Prix

Divers montant d'argent ont été dépensés pour l'achat de cornaline, mais la quantité et la forme – taillée ou non – de la pierre obtenue demeurent généralement inconnues : il peut s'agir de perles vendues à l'unité ou d'un bloc de pierre. Les montants d'argent versés pour de la cornaline, quelque que soit son état, sont les suivants :

prix	achat	texte
1 1/3 mine d'argent fin	cornaline	Kt 94/k 1746:3–4 [28]
15 sicles d'argent	cornaline et *zigašarrum*	TC 3, 178:7–8
5 mines 5 sicles d'argent	30 5/6 mines de cornaline	AKT 5, 52:37–38 [29]

Ce dernier texte permet de calculer le prix d'achat de la cornaline, sans doute sous forme brute, à Aššur, à savoir à peu près 6 sicles de cornaline pour 1 sicle d'argent. La cornaline était donc meilleur marché que le lapis-lazuli ; celui-ci valait un peu moins de 2 sicles de lapis-lazuli pour 1 sicle d'argent, tandis qu'à Kaneš, il se négociait deux à trois fois le prix de l'argent. [30] On peut donc supposer une plus-value également importante pour la vente de cornaline en Anatolie.

3.4 Transactions sur la cornaline

Les textes témoignent surtout de l'achat de cornaline à Aššur, sans véritablement de précisions quand aux circonstances de cet achat ou sur l'identité des vendeurs. [31]

---

28 Kt 94/k 1746:3–4, (lecture M. T. Larsen), 1 1/3 *ma-na* kù-babbar *ṣa-ru-p*[*á-am*], *ší-im* na_4-gug[ti]-*k*[*à*]...*ku-nu-ki-a Du-du na-áš-a-*[*kum*].

29 AKT 5, 52:37–38, 30 5/6 ⸢*ma-na*⸣ *sà-am-tám*[(sic)] *ša ba-ri-ni*, 5 *ma-na* 5! (6) gín kù-babbar ⸢*it*⸣-*ba-al*, « 30 5/6 mines de cornaline, notre propriété conjointe, a coûté 5 mines 5! sicles d'argent » ; *cf.* le commentaire à ce texte p. 163. Les trois propriétaires de cette pierre sont Bēlum-bāni, Zagal'u et Adad-bāni.

30 Michel 2001 ; Dercksen 2004, 19.

31 Textes témoignant directement ou non de l'achat de cornaline à Aššur : AKT 5, 52 ; AKT 6a, 144 ; AKT 6a, 145 ; BIN 6, 179 ; ICK 2, 321 ; Kt 88/k 292 ; Kt 93/k 196 ; TC 3, 178.

J. G. Dercksen a supposé que la cornaline était vendue à l'Hôtel de Ville, mais aucun texte n'y fait allusion.[32] La pierre était achetée par des marchands assyriens, mais les femmes pouvaient également en acquérir.[33] La pierre fine était ensuite acheminée vers l'Anatolie avec l'étain, les étoffes et quelques autres marchandises pour y être vendue.

La vente de cornaline à Kaneš est attestée par deux lettres – dont l'une très fragmentaire – expédiées à Puzur-Aššur par Iddin-Aššur. Celui-ci explique avoir pris contact avec Adad-rabi à Kaneš pour une transaction secrète concernant la vente de cornaline, de lapis-lazuli et d'étoffes, mais ce dernier a refusé de s'en charger. Lapis-lazuli et cornaline doivent donc êtres déposés à crédit auprès d'agents-*tamkārum* pour lesquels Puzur-Aššur doit préciser l'identité.[34] La cornaline était donc négociée en Anatolie selon les mêmes techniques commerciales que les autres marchandises importées depuis Aššur.

4. Les usages de la cornaline : données archéologiques

Les textes apportent finalement très peu d'information sur l'usage de la cornaline à Aššur et Kaneš. Les quelques perles mentionnées étaient vraisemblablement montées sur fil pour faire des colliers. Le port de ces colliers avait bien sûr un but esthétique, mais aussi magique. Chaque pierre avait des vertus particulières[35] ; montées sur un collier, les pierres permettaient de se protéger contre certaines maladies ou démons (Lamaštu, par exemple), ou elles aidaient à la guérison.

4.1 La cornaline dans les tombes paléo-assyriennes d'Aššur

Quelques riches tombes d'Aššur datées de la période paléo-assyrienne contenaient des perles en cornaline, toutefois celles-ci semblent avoir été beaucoup plus rares que les perles en lapis-lazuli ou en agate à en croire les publications archéologiques. La tombe n°37 (= Haller 1954, n°20), simple trou quadrangulaire creusé à même le sol, recelait néanmoins plusieurs colliers constitués entre autres de perles en cornaline. Ces perles présentent des formes assez variées : sphérique, lentoïde, el-

32 Dercksen 2004, 25.

33 TTC 2:5–6, 3 1/6 gín na$_4$-gug, *a-ha-ma ša Ša-at-A-šùr*, « en outre, 3 1/6 sicles de cornaline provenant de Šāt-Aššur ».

34 CCT 4, 40a:24–28 = Michel 2001, no. 196, *a-na šu-mì* na$_4$-gug, *ù hu-sá*$^!$*-ri-im ša ta-áš-pu-ra-ni, um-ma a-ta-ma i-ṣé-er*, dam-gàr^{ri} *i-dí : šu-mì a-wi-li, wa-dí-a-ma lá-dí-in*. Voir aussi le texte fragmentaire BIN 6 89 :3–5, 6 *ma-na*, na$_4$-gu[g] *ù*, 2 *ma-na* [*h*]*u-sá-ru*.

35 Pour les vertues bénéfiques des pierres semi-précieuses selon le mythe du Lugale, *cf.* van Dijk 1983, 120–122, l. 531–545 ; pour les usages magiques et médicaux des pierres, *cf.* Schuster-Brandis 2008.

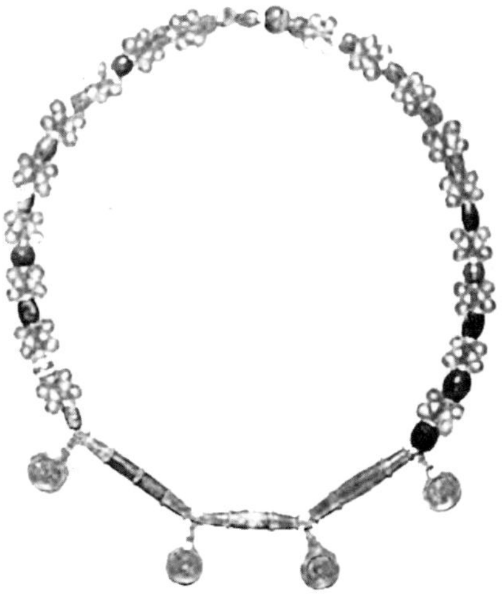

FIG. 1 Tour de cou exhumé dans la tombe 37 d'Aššur. Ass 20504g, h, u, x. Début du 2e millénaire. Photo : Harper *et al.* 1995, pl. 5, n°27.

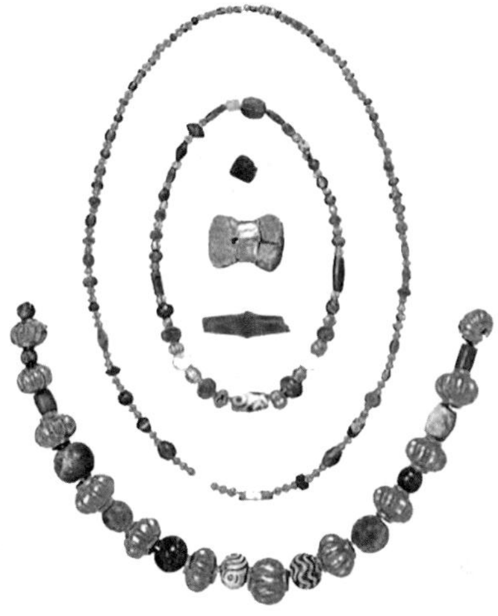

FIG. 2 Colliers et perles exhumés dans la tombe 37 d'Aššur. Ass 20504e, o, t, w, z sont en cornaline ou comportent des perles en cornaline. Début du 2e millénaire. Photo : Harper *et al.* 1995, pl. 6, depuis le bas n°30, 29, 28, 32b, 31, 32a.

liptique allongée, en forme de date et biconique.[36] Un tour du cou comportait deux perles allongées en cornaline encapuchonnées d'or, l'une avec un anneau d'or en son centre, ainsi qu'une douzaine de petites perles sphériques en cornaline (FIG. 1).[37]

De petites perles sphériques en cornaline figurent dans deux autres parures de cou (n°28 et 29), qui comportent également des perles biconiques à facettes (n°28). Quatre perles gravées ont été insérées dans ces différents colliers (n°28 et 30). Les dessins apparaissent en blanc car ils ont été obtenus à haute température avec l'utilisation d'une solution alkaline. Trois d'en elles sont sphériques et présentent des lignes ondulées et fond guilloché, la quatrième a la forme d'un barillet et son décor présente des points dans des cercles insérés dans un filet (FIG. 2).[38] La tombe contenait également une longue perle en cornaline, avec un bourrelet central, polie uniformément, de longueur L = 3,5 cm (n°32b).[39] Enfin, une perle en cornaline enfilée sur un anneau en or figurait également dans les parures de la tombe 37 (FIG. 3).

36 Aruz 1995, 50–51 et figure 14 pour la forme des perles.

37 Ass 20504g et Ass 20504t *cf.* Haller 1954, 10, pl. 10 et Hockmann 2010, 12, 111–112.

38 Ass 20504o, w ; Wartke 1995, 53, n°28 et 30.

39 Ass 20504t *cf.* Haller 1954, 10, pl. 10 et Hockmann 2010, 12, 111–112.

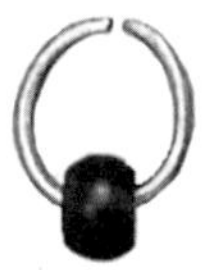

FIG. 3 Ass 20504aa, anneau en or (D = 1,5 cm) avec perle en cornaline (D = 0,9 cm) exhumé dans la tombe 37 d'Aššur. Début du 2e millénaire.Photo : Harper *et al.* 1995, pl. 7, n°37.

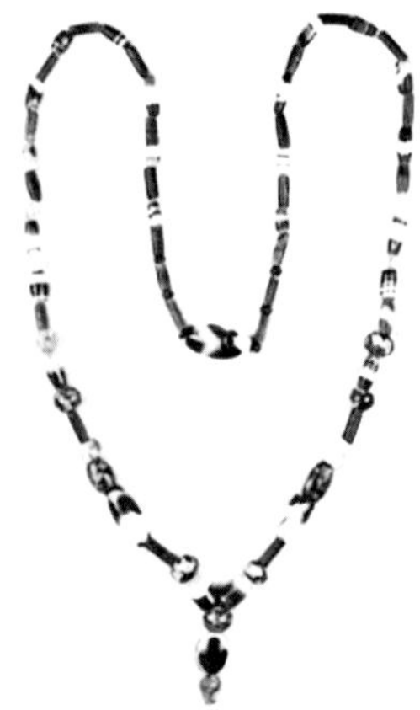

FIG. 4 Ass 12660o, tombe 13. Photo : Jakob-Rost *et al.* 1992, 186, n° 123.

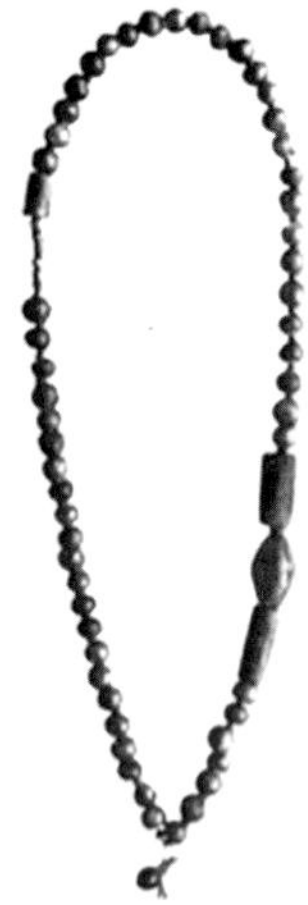

FIG. 5 Collier en or, cornaline et lapis-lazuli, Bronze ancien IIIc. Photo : Özgüç 1986a, pl. 75, 2, reproduite avec l'autorisation de F. Kulakoğlu.

La tombe 13 (anciennement n°35) comportait un collier fait de perles allongées en agate rubannée, cornaline et lapis-lazuli ; les 24 perles en cornaline sont de forme cylindrique (FIG. 4).[40]

Enfin, dans la tombe 34 (anciennement n°107) figuraient trois perles allongées en cornaline avec une perle en améthyste.[41]

4.2 Les objets en cornaline découverts à Kültepe

Les objets en cornaline découverts sur le site de Kültepe sont principalement des éléments de parure et plus particulièrement des perles datant des Bronze ancien et moyen, et une tête de suidé.

---

40 Ass 12660o, *cf.* Haller 1954, 112–113 et Hockmann 2010, 102–103. Pour une photo en couleurs de ce collier, *cf.* Jakob-Rost *et al.* 1992, 186, n°123.

41 Ass. 19796a, b, *cf.* Hockmann 2010, 109.

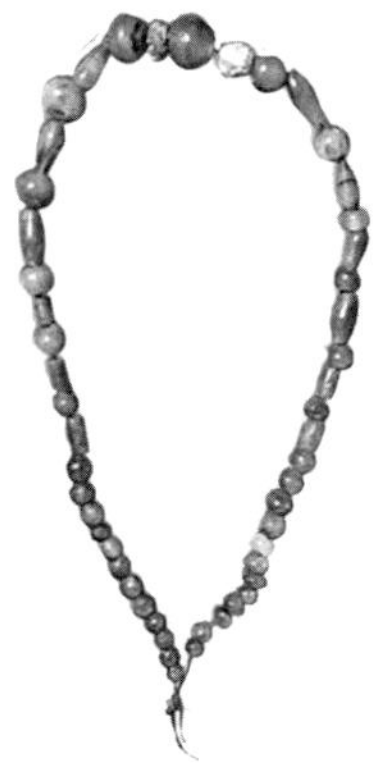

FIG. 6 Kt 85/k 112, collier en cornaline et fritte, ville basse, niveau II. Photo : Özgüç 2003, 257, n°288, reproduite avec l'autorisation de F. Kulakoğlu.

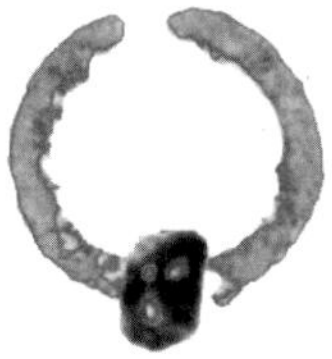

FIG. 7 Kt 84/k 159, anneau en bronze et perle en cornaline, ville basse, niveau II. Photo : Özgüç 1986a, pl. H.8, reproduite avec l'autorisation de F. Kulakoğlu.

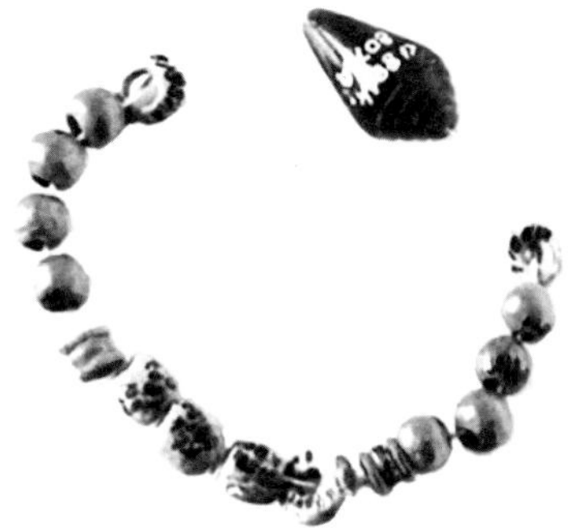

FIG. 8 Kt 88/k 806, collier en or, fritte et cornaline, ville basse, niveau Ib. Photo : Kulakoğlu & Kangal 2010, n°371, reproduite avec l'autorisation de F. Kulakoğlu.

4.2.1 Les perles

Dans une tombe exhumée sur la citadelle et datant du Bronze ancien IIIc (niveau 13) les archéologues ont découvert un collier composé de 71 petites perles annulaires en or séparant 55 perles sphériques en cornaline, une perle biconique en cornaline et 3 perles cylindriques en lapis-lazuli ; ces perles attestent de l'existence, déjà dans la deuxième moitié du 3e millénaire, d'importation de cornaline et lapis-lazuli en Anatolie depuis l'Est (FIG. 5).[42]

Dans la ville basse, des tombes contenaient également des parures de cou. Une tombe exhumée en 1985 et datant du niveau II (19e siècle) recelait un collier fait de 3 perles en fritte et 49 perles en cornaline, dont 37 perles sphériques de tailles variables, 5 perles cylindriques, 5 perles en forme de goutte et 2 perles biconiques (FIG. 6).[43]

Une autre tombe découverte la même année contenait une perle en cornaline enchâssée sur un anneau en bronze d'un diamètre de 1,8 cm (FIG. 7). Il s'agit d'une pièce unique pour Kültepe, mais similaire à l'anneau d'or découvert dans la tombe d'Aššur (*cf.* ci-dessus).

42 Özgüç 1986b, 44, fig. 3.41.

43 Kt 85/k 112 (Kayseri 85/3271), Özgüç 1986a, 37, pl. 74.6, 75.1.

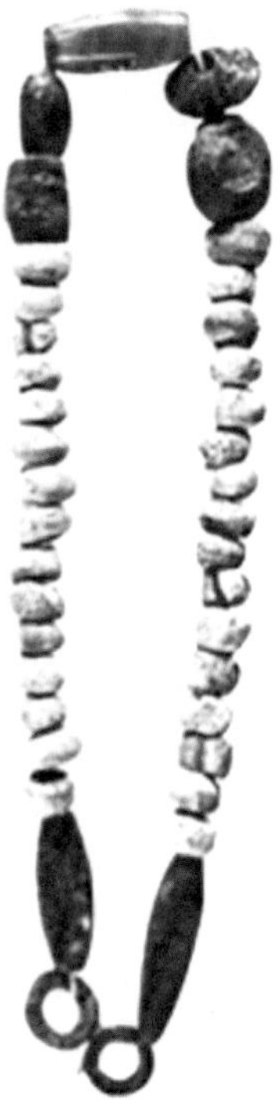

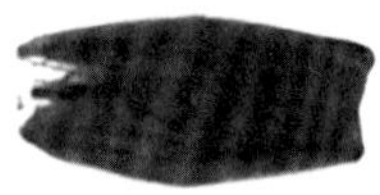

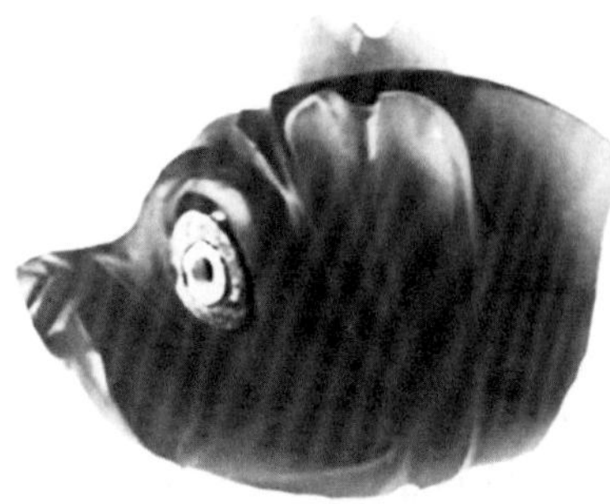

FIG. 9 Kt 83/k 52, collier en fritte, stéatite, or et cornaline, ville basse, niveau Ib. Photo : Özgüç 1986a, 36, pl. 74.2, reproduite avec l'autorisation de F. Kulakoğlu.

FIG. 10 Kt a/k 11339, perle en cornaline de 2,8 cm de long, ville balle, niveau Ib. Photo : Özgüç 1986a, pl. 74.8, reproduite avec l'autorisation de F. Kulakoğlu.

FIG. 11 Kt 95/k 110, tête de cochon en cornaline de 5,5 × 4,3 × 4 cm dans ses dimensions les plus larges. Ville basse, niveau Ib. Photo : Kulakoğlu & Kangal 2010, 253, n°203, reproduite avec l'autorisation de F. Kulakoğlu.

Des découvertes similaires ont été faites dans les tombes du niveau Ib. Parmi celles-ci, un collier (ou un bracelet) fait de 10 perles d'or et 6 perles en fritte, comporte une grosse perle en cornaline biconique, l'un des côtés étant taillé en cercles concentriques (FIG. 8).[44] Les dimensions de cette perle de longueur L = 8 cm et de diamètre sur sa partie la plus large D = 2,3 cm permettent d'en calculer sa masse, sachant qu'elle se compose de deux cônes, l'un d'une longueur L/3 et l'autre d'une

44 Özgüç 2003, 257, n° 287.

longueur 2L/3. Son volume (V) peut être estimé à 11 cm^3 et, sachant que la densité de la cornaline est de 2,6 g/cm^3, sa masse (M) serait légèrement inférieure à 30 g.[45]

Une femme inhumée dans une grande jarre portait un collier composé de 32 perles en fritte, 6 en stéatite, deux anneaux d'or une perle oblongue en cornaline (FIG. 9).

L'une des tombes en ruines exhumées en 1948 contenait une perle en cornaline de taille importante (FIG. 10).

4.2.2 Une tête de suidé

L'objet en cornaline le plus spectaculaire découvert à Kültepe, taillé dans un bloc de pierre rose translucide, est une petite tête de suidé exhumée en 1995 dans le niveau Ib de la ville basse ; malheureusement, le contexte précis de la découverte demeure inconnu. La tête présente un trou important sur l'arrière et deux petits trous en diagonale sur le sommet et la base ; elle devait être fixée en guise d'ornement sur un objet en bois ou en métal, comme un bâton ou un sceptre. Les yeux étaient incrustés de lapis-lazuli, l'iris étant en coquillage blanc.[46] Le groin est protubérant et les oreilles dressées : l'ensemble témoigne d'un fin travail d'artiste (FIG. 11). Cette pièce n'a pas de parallèle connu en Asie Mineure ; selon les archéologues, elle a été importée déjà manufacturée depuis l'Est.

On peut considérer que cette tête de suidé s'inscrit dans un cylindre de longeur hauteur H = 5,5 cm et de diamètre D = 4,3 cm, soit un rayon R = 2,15 cm. Comme la pièce ne rempli pas complètement le cylindre, on prendra comme mesure R = 1,75 cm de rayon. Ses mensurations permettent d'estimer son volume (V) à environ 53 cm^3, et sa masse (M) à un peu moins de 140 g.

*

La cornaline, plus rare que le lapis-lazuli dans les archives paléo-assyriennes, intervient toutefois de manière récurrente dans les transactions des marchands assyriens sous forme de bloc de pierre ou de perles; elle est davantage attestée que la pierre *pappardilum* qui s'apparenterait à l'agate rubannée. La cornaline figure en bonne place dans les parures exhumées dans les tombes d'Aššur et de Kaneš datées du début du 2e millénaire av. J.-C.

---

45 Le volume du cône est $V = \pi/3 \times r^2 l$ et sa masse $M = \rho V$, ρ étant la masse volumique ou densité. Le calcul ne tient pas compte du vide central – de volume négligeable – de la perle. A titre de comparaison, le poids en cristal de roche (densité 2,65 g/cm^3) Kt r/k 124 (Kulakoğlu & Kangal 2010, 319, n°385), de forme elliptique allongée et dont les dimensions sont à peu près de moitié par rapport à celles de la perle (L = 4,1 cm, R = 0,8 cm en sa partie la plus large), pèse 14,5 g.

46 Kt 95/k 110 publiée par Özgüç 1998, 252–254, 6ab ; Özgüç 2003, 230–232, n°237.

Cette pierre, originaire de l'Indus et de l'Asie centrale, circulait en quantités similaires au lapis-lazuli entre Aššur et l'Anatolie,[47] mais elle était meilleur marché. Les poids des plus gros objets taillés dans de la cornaline et découverts à Kaneš – une perle et une tête de suidé – correspondent aux poids les plus petits de pierre attestés dans les textes, respectivement moins de 4 sicles et 1/3 mine. Ces objets ont vraisemblablement été importés en Asie Mineure déjà manufacturés.

La cornaline était principalement utilisée pour tailler des perles, enfilées sur un fil, pour réaliser des colliers aux vertus magiques comme en temoigne le Lugale, ou encore la série *abnu šikinšu*, qui mentionne différentes variétés de cornaline[48] ; lapis-lazuli et cornaline étaient régulièrement employés pour confectionner des amulettes en Mésopotamie. On peut imaginer que la petite tête de cochon découverte en 1995 à Kültepe, quel que soit l'objet sur lequel elle était montée, avait une valeur symbolique particulière.

---

47 Michel 2001, 347, relève des quantités exceptionnelles de 12 et 30 mines de lapislazuli, sinon les quantités de pierre commercialisées s'échelonnent entre 1 sicle et 5 mines.

48 Schuster-Brandis 2008, 413–415.

BIBLIOGRAPHIE

Abrahami, Ph., « A propos d'une perle inédite : un élément de la parure-subi de Ninisina? » *Revue d'Assyriologie* 102 (2008): 39–48.

———. « Matériaux et produits précieux dans l'univers littéraire : symbole, poésie, mythologie. Les inscriptions cunéiformes sur objets en pierre fine » in *Les produits de luxe au Proche-Orient ancien, aux âges du Bronze et du Fer (3500–330 av. J.-C.)*, éd. par M. Casanova et M. Feldman, 147–156. Paris: Travaux de la Maison René-Ginouvès 19, 2014.

André-Salvini, B., « L'idéologie des pierres en Mésopotamie » in *Cornaline et autres pierres précieuses. La Méditerranée, de l'Antiquité à l'Islam*, éd. par A. Caubet, 373–400. Paris : La Documentation Française, 1999.

Arkhipov, I., *Le vocabulaire de la métallurgie et la nomenclature des objets en métal dans les textes de Mari*. Paris : ARMT 32 2012.

Aruz, J., « Grave 20 Beads » in *Assyrian origins : discoveries at Ashur on the Tigris: Antiquities in the Vorderasiatisches Museum, Berlin*, éd. par P. O. Harper, E. Klengel-Brandt et J. Aruz, 50–52. New York : Metropolitan Museum of Art, 1995.

Caubet, A., (éd.) *Cornaline et autres pierres précieuses. La Méditerranée, de l'Antiquité à l'Islam*. Paris : La Documentation Française, 1999.

Chevalier, J., M.-L. Inizan et J. Tixier, « Une technique de perforation par percussion de perles en cornaline (Larsa, Iraq). » *Paléorient* 8 (1982) : 55–65.

Cohen, M. E., « Texts from the Andrews University Archaeological Museum. » *Revue d'Assyriologie* 70 (1976) : 129–144.

Dercksen, J. G., *Old Assyrian Institutions*. Leyde : MOS Studies 4, PIHANS 198, 2004.

Durand, J.-M., *La nomenclature des habits et des textiles dans les textes de Mari*. Paris : ARMT 30, 2009.

Gates, M.-H., « Dialogues between Ancient Near Eastern Texts and the Archaeological Record: Test Cases from Bronze Age Syria. » *Bulletin of the American Schools of Oriental Research* 270 (1988) : 63–91.

———. « Artisans and Art in Old Babylonian Mari » in *Investigating Artistic Environments in the Ancient Near East*, éd. par A. C. Gunter, 29–37. Washington : University of Wisconsin Press, 1989.

———. « Southern and Southeastern Anatolia in the Late Bronze Age » in *The Oxford Handbook of Ancient Anatolia (8000 - 323 BCE)*, éd. par S. R. Steadman et G. McMahon, 393–412. Oxford : Oxford University Press, 2011.

Haller, A., *Die Gräber und Grüfte von Assur*. WVDOG 65. Berlin, 1954.

Harper, P. O., Klengel-Brandt, E., & Aruz, J. (éd.), *Assyrian origins : Discoveries at Ashur on the Tigris : Antiquities in the Vorderasiatisches Museum, Berlin*. New York: Metropolitan Museum of Art, 1995.

Hecker, K., « Schultexte von Kültepe » in *Aspects of Art and Iconography: Anatolia and its Neighbors. Studies in Honour of Nimet Özgüç*, éd. par M. J. Mellink, E. Porada et T. Özgüç : 281–291. Ankara : Türk Tarih Kurumu Basimevi, 1993.

Hockmann, D., *Gräber und Grüfte in Assur I, Von der zweiten Hälfte des 3. bis zur Mitte des 2. Jahrtausends v. Chr.* WVDOG 129. Wiesbaden: Harrassowitz Verlag, 2010.

Inizan, M.-L., « At the Dawn of Trade, Cornelian from India to Mesopotamia in the Third Millennium : The Example of Tello » in *South Asian Archaeology 1991, proceedings of the Eleventh International Conference of the Association of South Asia Archaeologists in Western Europe held in Berlin 1–5 July 1991*, éd. par A. J. Gail & G. J. R. Mevissen, 121–134. Stuttgart : F. Steiner, 1993.

———. « La cornaline de l'Indus et la voie du Golfe au IIIe millénaire. » in *Cornaline et autres pierres précieuses. La Méditerranée, de l'Antiquité à l'Islam*, éd. par Caubet, 125–138. Paris : La Documentation Française, 1999.

Jakob-Rost, L., Klengel-Brandt, E., Marzahn, J., Wartke, R.-B., *Das Vorderasiatische Museum*, Berlin : Verlag Philipp von Zabern, 1992.

Kulakoğlu, F. & Kangal, S., (éd.) *Anatolia's Prologue. Kültepe Kanesh Karum, Assyrians in Istanbul*, Kayseri Metropolitan Municipality Cultural Publication 78. İstanbul: Avrupa Kültür Başkenti, 2010.

Michel, C., « Les joyaux des rois de Mari » in *Cornaline et autres pierres précieuses. La Méditerranée, de l'Antiquité à l'Islam*, éd. par Caubet, 401–432. Paris : La Documentation Française, 1999.

———. « Le lapis-lazuli des Assyriens au début du IIe millénaire av. J.-C » in *K.R. Veenhof Anniversary Volume*, éd. par W. H. van Soldt, J. G. Dercksen, N. J. Kouwenberg & Th. J. Krispijn, 341–359. Leyde, 2001. (http://halshs.archives-ouvertes.fr/halshs-00350330)

———. « Ecrire et compter chez les marchands assyriens du début du IIe millénaire av. J.-C » in *Muhibbe Darga Armağanı*, éd. par T. Tarhan, A. Tibet & E. Konyar, 345–364. İstanbul : Sadberk Hanım Müzesi, 2008. (http://halshs.archives-ouvertes.fr/halshs-00443900)

Michel, C. & Veenhof, K. R., « The Textiles traded by the Assyrians in Anatolia (19th–18th Centuries BC) » in *Textile Terminologies in the Ancient Near East and Mediterranean from the Third to the First millennia BC*, éd. Par C. Michel & M.-L. Nosch, Ancient Textiles Series 8 : 209–269. Oxford : Oxbow Books, 2010.

Özgüç, T., *Kültepe-Kaniš II, New Researches at the Trading Center of the Ancient Near East.* Ankara : Türk Tarih Kurumu Yayınlarından V/41, 1986 (a).

———. « New Observations on the Relationship of Kültepe with Southeast Anatolia and North Syria during the Third Millennium BC » in *Ancient Anatolia. Aspects of Change and Cultural Develpment. Essays in Honor of Machteld J. Mellink*, éd. par J. V. Canby, E. Porada, B. S. Ridgway & T. Stech, 31–47. Madison : University of Wisconsin Press, 1986 (b).

———. « Boar-shaped Cult vessels and funeral objects at Kaniš. » *Altorientalische Forschungen* 25 (1998) : 247–256.

———. *Kültepe Kaniš/Neša. The Earliest International Trade Center and the Oldest Capital City of the Hittites.* Istanbul: The Middle Eastern Culture Center in Japan, 2003.

Roux, V. (éd.), *Cornaline de l'Inde. Des pratiques techniques de Cambay aux techno-systèmes de l'Indus.* Paris : Maison des Sciences de l'Homme, 2000.

Schuster-Brandis, A., *Steine als Schutz- und Heilmittel. Untersuchung zu ihrer Verwendung in der Beschwörungskunst Mesopotamiens im 1. Jt. V. Chr.* AOAT 46. Münster, 2008.

Steinkeller, P., « New Light on Marhashi and its Contacts with Makkan and Babylonia. » *Journal of Magan Studies* 1 (2006) : 2–7.

van Dijk, J. *LUGAL UD ME-LÁM-bi NIR-ĜÁL.* Leyde : Brill, 1983.

Wartke, R.-B., « Trade and Exchange : The Old Assyrian Period. Necklace beads (28–30) » in *Assyrian origins : discoveries at Ashur on the Tigris : Antiquities in the Vorderasiatisches Museum, Berlin*, éd. Par Harper, P. O., Klengel-Brandt, E., & Aruz, J., 44–47, 52–53. New York : Metropolitan Museum of Art, 1995.

Facing Muwattalli:
Some Thoughts on the Visibility and Function of the Rock Reliefs at Sirkeli Höyük, Cilicia

Ekin Kozal[1] — *Mirko Novák*[2]

Abstract

This article is an attempt to examine the functionality and the visibility of the Hittite rock reliefs at Sirkeli Höyük in its urban context, the rural landscape and network of roads arriving at the site. Two reliefs have been discovered so far. One of them can securely be dated, since the inscription refers to Muwattalli (II). The other one was mutilated in antiquity, and the identification of this Hittite king (Muršili III ?) is part of the discussion. Cup-like depressions, which are located on the reliefs, are also taken into consideration here. With the following thoughts and remarks on the function of these Sirkeli reliefs, we would like to honour Marie-Henriette and Charles Gates, two outstanding scholars in the field of Cilician archaeology, to whom we owe many important contributions. We hope that they will enjoy our small presentation, and we are looking forward to many future discussions, as fruitful as all the past ones.

Introduction

The function of Hittite open-air landscape monuments and rock reliefs is much disputed and still unresolved.[3] It seems clear that there is no monocausal explanation for their existence since there are remarkable differences between those reliefs that marked natural springs (Eflatun Pınar, Fraktin), those situated at important overland thoroughfares and passes through mountains (Hanyeri, İmamkulu), and those connected with monumental architectural structures (Gavur Kalesi) and urban settlements (Sirkeli Höyük).

---

1 E. Kozal, Çanakkale Onsekiz Mart University, Faculty of Sciences and Arts, Department of Archaeology, Çanakkale/ TURKEY, e-mail: ekozal08@gmail.com.

2 M. Novák, Universität Bern, Institut für Archäologische Wissenschaften, Abteilung für Vorderasiatische Archäologie, Bern/SWITZERLAND, e-mail: miroslav.novak@iaw.unibe.ch.
We thank Dr. Johanna Tudeau (Bern) for improving the English manuscript.

3 Glatz and Plourde 2011.

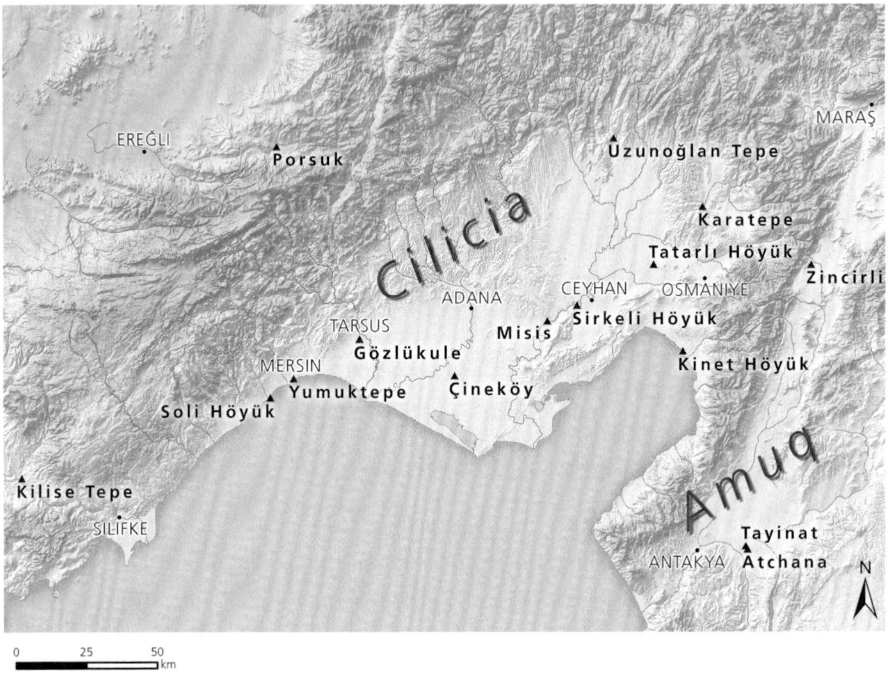

FIG. 1 Cilicia (© Susanne Rutishauser, IAW Bern)

The two Hittite rock reliefs located at Sirkeli Höyük are of some importance, especially because the one depicting Muwattalli II (*ca.* 1290–1272 BCE)[4] is the earliest relief securely attributed to a king.[5] The relief of Muwattalli II was first examined and published by Hans Gustav Güterbock during the campaign of John Garstang in 1936–1937, which was a part of the Neilson Expedition to Cilicia.[6] At that time the Ceyhan River flowed directly next to the rock outcrop on which the relief is carved. A photograph showing Güterbock on a ladder placed in the water gives an impressive view on the situation.[7] Güterbock published a second short note on the relief in 1997.[8] During later Sirkeli Höyük campaigns, which were directed by Barthel Hrouda (1992–1996) and Horst Ehringhaus (1997), a small earthen platform was filled up to enable the visitors to walk up to the reliefs. In 2015, with the generosity of Alemdar Öztürk, the mayor of Ceyhan, the

4 On the history of Muwattalli II see Klengel 1999, 202–218.

5 A new examination of the inscription will be published by David Hawkins soon. We thank him for giving us access to his manuscript.

6 Garstang 1937.

7 Güterbock in Garstang 1937, 66–68; Hrouda 1997a, pl. 5:3.

8 Güterbock in Hrouda 1997a, 104.

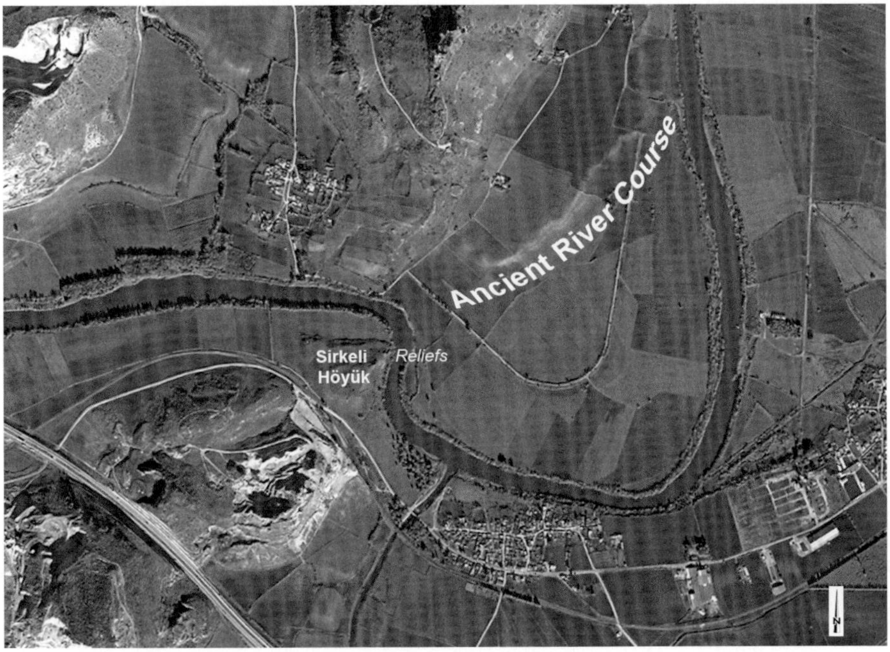

FIG. 2 Satellite image with traces of the ancient river course

Swiss-Turkish mission built a wooden platform here for visitors. During Hrouda's 1994 campaign, a second relief was discovered by Ehringhaus, only a few meters away from the Muwattalli relief. It had been chiselled out in antiquity.[9] This relief definitely represented a Hittite figure, displaying an identical but mirrored image of the Muwattalli relief.

The present paper deals with the ancient landscape around Sirkeli Höyük and the Late Bronze Age (LBA) structures at the site. The aim is to analyse the location, the visibility and the functionality of these two reliefs and of further potentially planned reliefs.

Location of Sirkeli Höyük and the Reliefs

Sirkeli Höyük, which is one of the largest settlement mounds in Plain Cilicia, is situated on the left bank of the Ceyhan River (ancient *Puruna* and *Pyramos*) right on the pass where the river breaks through the Misis Mountains and at the interface of Yukarıova (Ceyhan Ovası) and Çukurova (FIG. 1, FIG. 2). The site lies on the important thoroughfare from Syria to Central Anatolia, passing through

9 Ehringhaus 1995a; Ehringhaus 1995b; Hrouda 1997a, pl. 7.

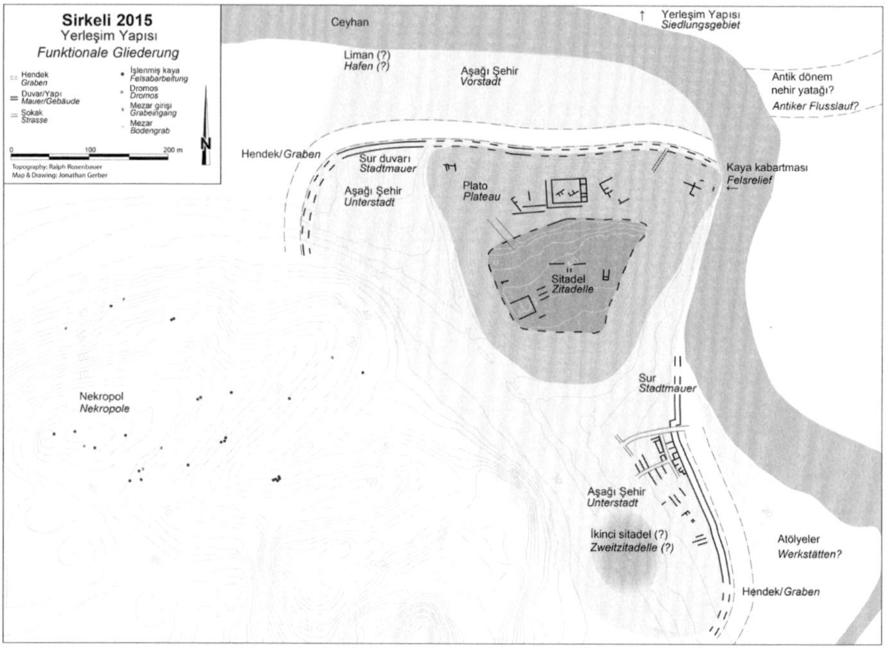

FIG. 3 Reconstructed city plan of Sirkeli (© Jonathan Gerber, IAW Bern)

the Cilician Plain via the Amanus and Syrian Gates in the east and the Cilician Gates and the Göksu Valley in the West. The modern highway, the old road and the railway still pass by the mound along this ancient route. Moreover, the site is situated *ca.* 40 km upstream from the coast on as side road linking the potential harbours at Karataş and Yumurtalık to Central Anatolia via Kozan, Feke and the Gezbel pass. The location of the site is understood to have preserved its importance also in later and modern ages.

The settlement is composed of: i) an 8 ha citadel mound, subdivided by elevation and fortification into a lower plateau and a higher inner citadel; ii) a southeastern and southern "Lower Town" of an additional minimum area of 12 ha; and iii) an extramural workshop areas to its north and east (FIG. 3). There is a suburb on the opposite side of the river to the north and a necropolis on a natural hill to the southwest. A smaller secondary mound lies to the south of the main mound and has been severely destroyed by road and railway constructions and recent mining activities. However, it was located *intramuros*, thus forming a kind of second elevated citadel.

With a size of over 20 ha *intramuros*, with the additional suburbs, workshop areas and a necropolis, the ancient settlement was one of the largest Bronze and Iron Age towns of Plain Cilicia. In the Bronze Age it first belonged to the kingdom and later to the Hittite province of Kizzuwatna, and in the Iron Age it was a city that was a part of the kingdom Hiyawa/Kawa, which later became the Assyrian province of Que. The city is not identified yet, but there are good reasons to believe that Tatarlı Höyük and Sirkeli Höyük, which are the two largest settlements in Yukarıova (the eastern part of Plain Cilicia), should be identified with the important cult towns of Lawazantiya/Lusanda and Kummanni/Kisuatni respectively.[10] If this is true, than Sirkeli Höyük / Kummanni was of religious importance both for the people of Kizzuwatna and the Hittite Empire.

The Images and their Identifications

Two imperial Hittite rock reliefs were carved into the natural rock outcrop that forms the eastern flank of the main citadel mound at the northeastern corner of the mound. The relief of Muwattalli II is one of the few Hittite reliefs that can be dated precisely (Fig. 4, Fig. 5). The inscription behind the head of the relief mentions not only the name of Muwattalli but also that of his father: "Muwattalli, Great King, the Hero, son of Muršili, Great King, the Hero". The king is depicted with his long robe and *kalmuš* in his left hand. His right arm is bent, with the elbow at the level of the waist and the closed hand pointing upwards. There is a round skullcap on his head, and he wears pointed shoes.[11] This depiction is comparable with the Sun God image from Chamber B at the Südburg in Boğazköy (with the exception of the winged sun disc),[12] as well as with the two depictions of Tudḫaliya at Yazılıkaya – one in Chamber A[13] showing him alone, and the other in Chamber B under the protection of Sarruma (*Umarmungsszene*).[14]

The second relief lies some 14 m north of Muwattalli's image (Fig. 6). In between, the rock face is stepped, forming different niches for each relief. Despite the fact that the second relief was mutilated in antiquity, the figure can be reconstructed according to the remaining traces. The figure wears the same garment and shows the same gesture as Muwattalli, but mirrored, thus looking to the right. Both figures bear their inscriptions on the back of their heads, although the inscription of the second relief was damaged in the past.

Due to the very careful way in which the relief has been chiselled out, leaving no possibility to identify the depicted figure, an act of pure vandalism can be

10 Forlanini 2013.

11 Ehringhaus 2005, 95–99, fig. 175; see also Kohlmeyer 1983, 95–101, and Glatz and Plourde 2011, 45–46.

12 Neve 1993, 63–80, figs. 211–212.

13 Seeher 2011, 82–83, figs. 86–88.

14 Seeher 2011, 110, figs. 112–120.

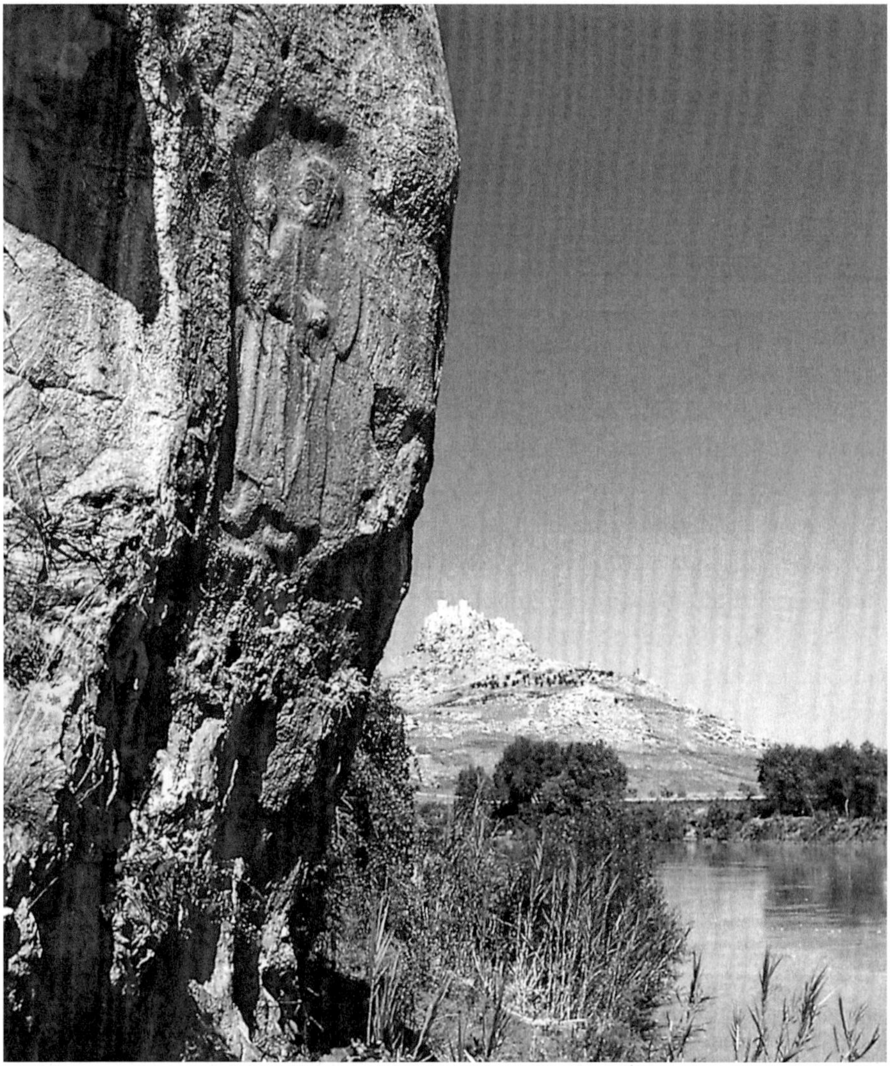

FIG. 4 Muwattalli's relief (© Horst Ehringhaus)

excluded. Dating the destruction to the times of Byzantine iconoclasm or Islamic fundamentalism can also be excluded since the nearby Muwattalli relief has remained untouched. This hints to a deliberate destruction by people who not only would have known very well to whom the images were dedicated but also respected Muwattalli, all the while subjecting the other figure to a *damnatio memoriae.*

It seems therefore likely to us that the second relief was representing one of Muwattalli's two sons, either Urḫi-Teššup, also known as Great King Muršili III, or Kurunta, who claimed the title of Great King and later became the ruler

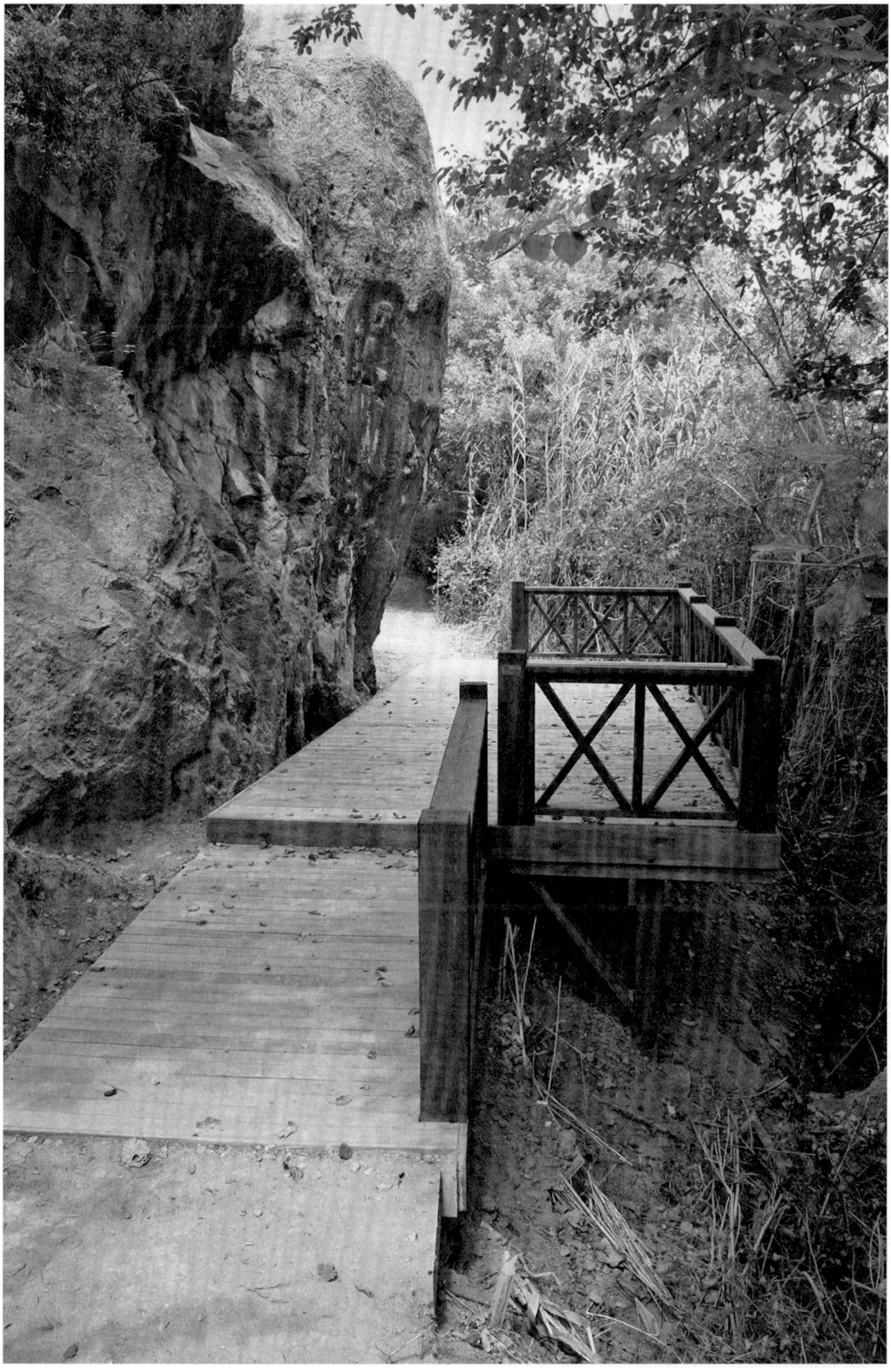

FIG. 5 Muwattalli's relief with the newly established platform (© Alexander Ahrens, IAW Bern)

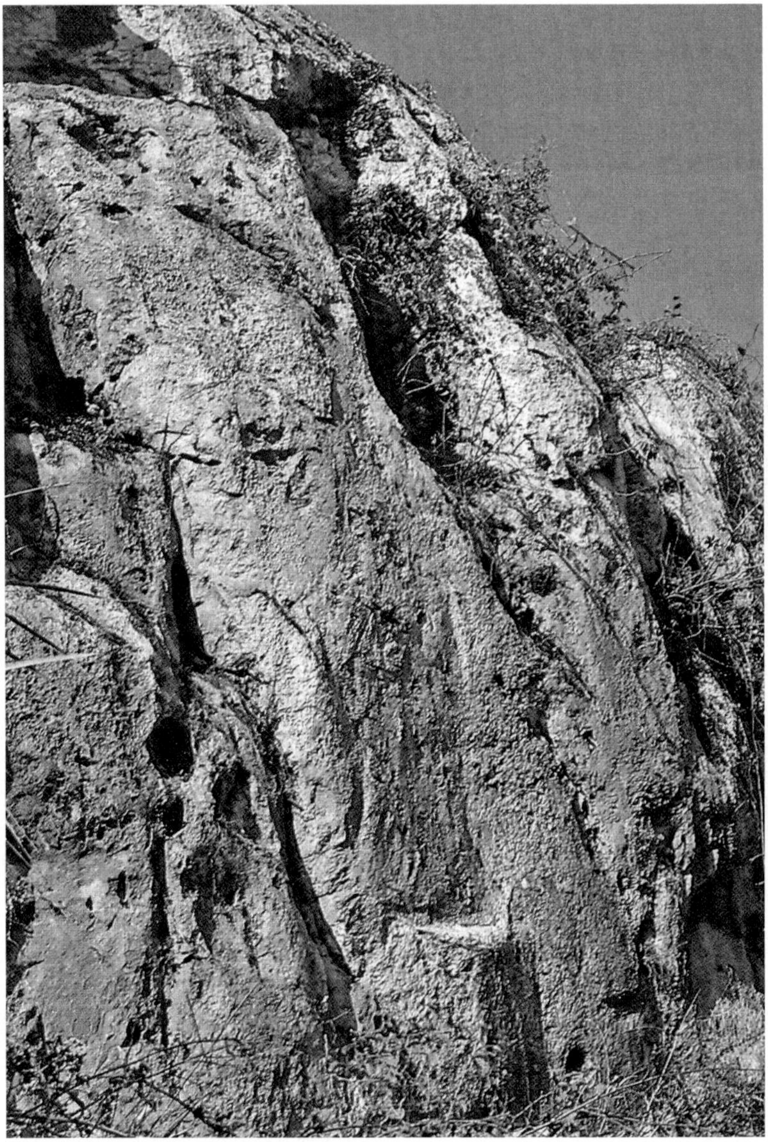

FIG. 6 Mutilated second relief (© Horst Ehringhaus)

of Tarḫuntašša. We prefer to identify the person on this second relief of Sirkeli Höyük as Urḫi-Teššup, since he, unlike his brother, underwent an official *damnatio memoriae* in Hatti after the *coup d'état* by his uncle Hattušili II ("III"). Urḫi-Teššup became the king of Hatti after the death of his father and gained the throne name Muršili. He moved the capital back from his father's residence in Tarḫuntašša to Hattuša, where he stayed seven years on the throne, before he lost power to his

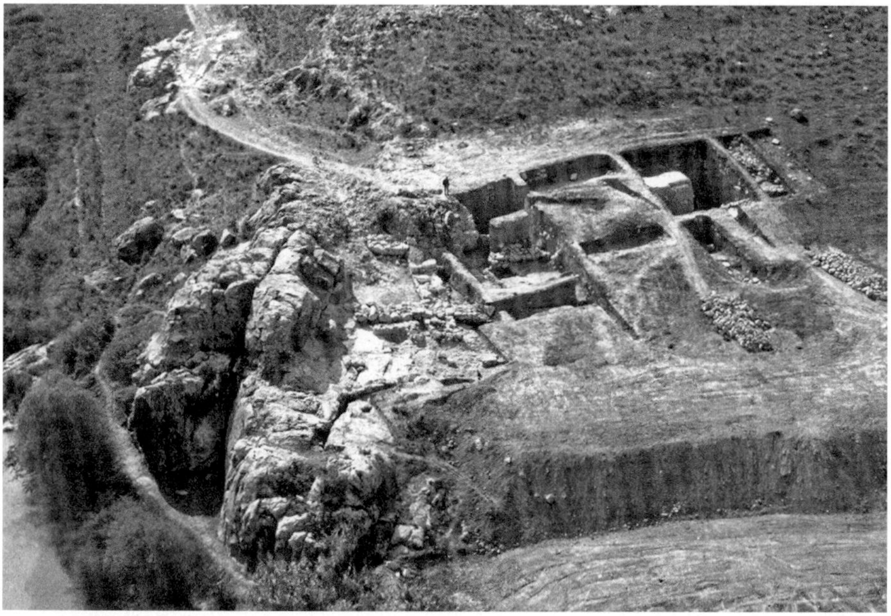

FIG. 7 Photo showing the Steingebäude, seen from the North with the relief rock on the left side (© Horst Ehringhaus)

uncle. He had to live in exile in several places in the Levant and finally in Egypt.[15] During the time of Hattušili II/III, he was mentioned exclusively with his Hurrian birth name Urḫi-Teššup (especially in Hattušili's apology), which hints at an attempt to disregard his time as king. It can be assumed that the erased relief at Sirkeli depicted Muršili III rather than Kurunta and was destroyed at Hattušili's order. In this case, the father and the son would have been portrayed next to each other. They would be wearing the same garments but facing different directions: Muwattalli's face is turned to the south whereas Muršili (?) faces the north, so they are looking in different directions and don't face each other.

A third relief was planned half way between the two reliefs. The face of the rock had already been prepared and smoothed out. A square field can still be easily discerned today. However, for uncertain reasons, this relief was never executed.

The *Steingebäude* and 'Shallow Cups'

The *Steingebäude* is a building excavated by B. Hrouda and H. Ehringhaus in 1996 and 1997 (FIG. 7). It is situated on top of the same rock outcrop that bears the reliefs

15 Klengel 1999, 218–235.

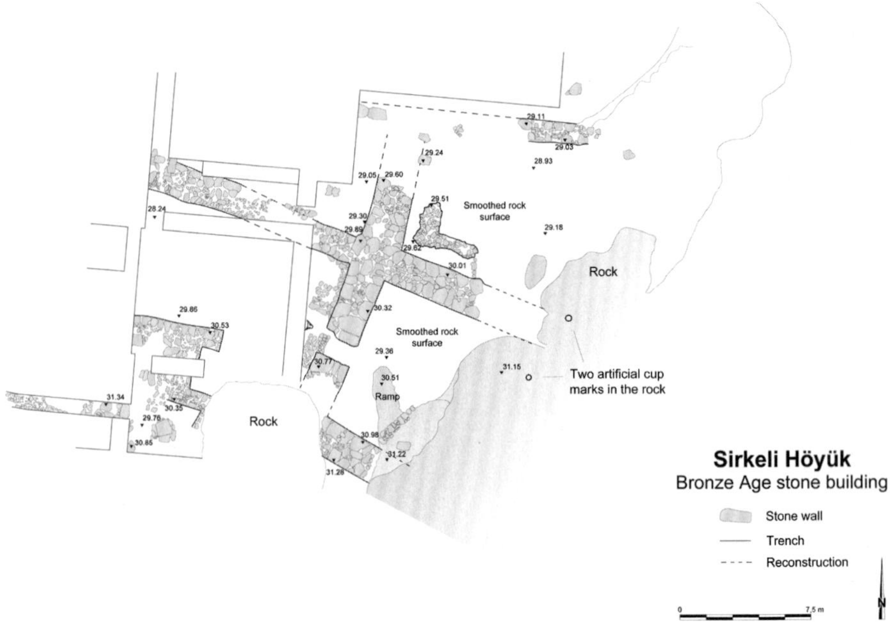

FIG. 8 Plan of the *Steingebäude* on top of the relief rock (© Gabriele Elsen-Novák and Jonathan Gerber, IAW Bern)

on its eastern flank and runs alongside the eastern edge of the citadel mound. Actually, the Chalcolithic and Early Bronze Age (EBA) settlement of Sirkeli Höyük was founded in the western shade of this rock and eventually grew in elevation during the more than three and a half millennia of occupation. This continuous settlement growth led to the rock being almost completely covered up, with only the easternmost outcrop 'breaking out' of the urban landscape and forming the very prominent and steep edge of the citadel towards the river plain.

The top surface of the rock was thoroughly smoothed out in its northwestern part, forming the ground and the floor of the *Steingebäude* (FIG. 8). To the south and east of this area the rock rises untreated to a higher level, that is, up to its sharp edge towards the east with the relief face.

Only one room of the building is preserved completely, whereas the architecture adjacent to the north is eroded and the rooms to the west are not yet excavated. A clear classification of the architecture is therefore only possible to a limited degree. However, it is clear that the building was set into an ankle of the rock, which was used not only as a floor but also as boundary on two sides. The room is thus partly defined by artificial walls and partly by natural settings, a type of architecture well-known from Central Anatolia during the Hittite period. The main room was flanked by at least one room to the west and another one to the north.

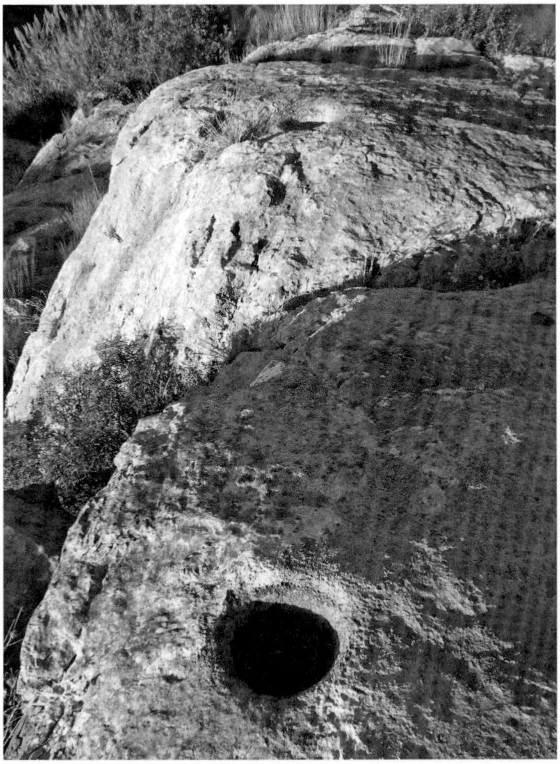

FIG. 9 Photo showing the Shallow Cups over the two reliefs

Access was possible through the west room. The foundations of the extremely thick walls of the main room are made of gigantic stones, resting immediately on the rock. The walls are 2 m thick and preserved to a height of about 75 cm. Whether they consisted exclusively of stones, which are not *in situ* any more, or were made of mud brick in the upper parts cannot be determined with certainty. Due to the debris discovered during the excavations, the latter alternative seems more likely, however. The mud brick superstructure may have vanished as a result of the melting of the mud bricks. The east side of the room and parts of its south side are defined by the higher parts of the rock. The broad entrance to this room is situated on the west wall. A zebu bull's head was found to the west of this doorway.[16] The only installation inside the room was a ramp cut out of the natural bedrock in the northern and lower part and artificially built by stones in its southern and higher part. This ramp was presumably the substructure of a staircase, perhaps consisting of wooden stairs that would not have been preserved. It facilitated access from the room up to the top of the higher parts of the outcrop close to the eastern edge. On this upper level two more interesting features have been discovered: the

16 Ehringhaus in Hrouda 1997a, 109–115.

so-called 'shallow cups' (Fig. 9). Such cup-like depressions, also designated as cup marks, are frequently associated not only with statues and tombs but also with Hittite rock reliefs. This connection is by no means a coincidence. For example, at Fraktin two of these cup-like depressions are situated on the rock above the two reliefs.[17] At Sirkeli, one depression measures 32 cm in diameter and 20 cm in depth, and the other 26 cm in diameter and 15 cm in depth.[18] The function of these depressions has already been discussed extensively, and so an elaborate repetition is not necessary here. David Ussishkin convincingly argued that they were used in cultic activities, namely for libation.[19] According to Charles Burney, these cup-like depressions are more specifically related to the ancestor cult, as they represent the cultic ditch in the reflection of the netherworld.[20] The ancestor cult was practised by both the gods and the kings.

A third depression has been detected at Sirkeli on another rock some 100 m south of the Muwattalli relief (Fig. 10). Nowadays the top of the rock is on ground level and therefore its clearly smoothed straight east face is deeply covered under the earth. If we expect a relief under each 'shallow cup,' then the face of this rock has to be revealed through excavation.

However, the special function of the *Steingebäude* is clear from the monumentality not of its rooms but of its walls, made of gigantic stones, as well as due to the zebu bull's head, which might have been fixed originally at the lintel and surely had a symbolic meaning. Moreover, its integration with the same rock with the reliefs and the 'shallow cups' indicates a special purpose. All these elements form an extraordinary ensemble. We will come to this later.

Late Bronze Age Settlement and Landscape[21]

The investigation and reconstruction of the urban development of the site embraced in its ancient landscape through its occupational history is one of the main goals of the recent project.[22] In this respect, settlement size, structure, and layout, as well as fortifications and large buildings, are examined. Besides excavation and intensive archaeological survey at the site, geophysical survey (geomagnetic, geoelectric tomography, ground-penetrating radar) and high-resolution satellite imagery have been applied. These studies yielded information not only about

17 Ussishkin 1975, 85–86, figs. 2–3.

18 Ussishkin 1975, 86–89, figs. 4–6.

19 Ussishkin 1975.

20 Burney 2004, 19–21.

21 See also Kozal 2013.

22 Kozal and Novák 2013.

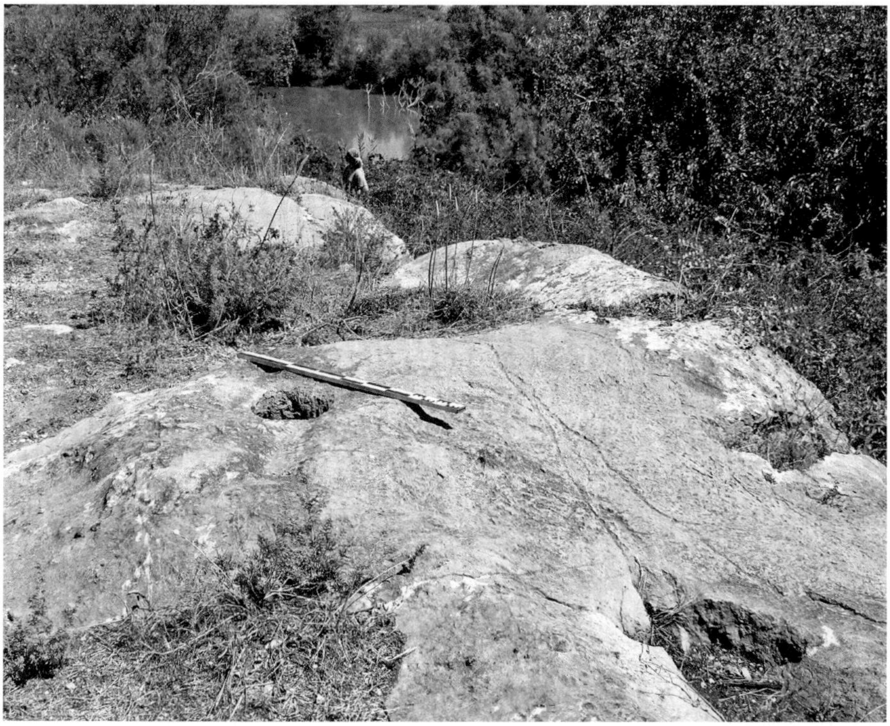

FIG. 10 Third 'shallow cup' south of the other two (© Laura Simons, IAW Bern)

unexcavated architectural remains, but also ancient riverbeds. Excavation of four sectors (A, C, D, and F) has been oriented accordingly to test the findings of satellite imagery and geophysical prospection. Sector A is located in the north-western corner and Sector C in the middle of the plateau. Sector D is situated on the southwest side of the citadel at its highest point. Sector F, which is in the southeastern lower town, was discovered recently by the geophysical investigations and followed by excavations.

In Sector A a large substantial building is still being excavated since 2006. The preliminary results show that the building was occupied from LB II into Iron II, succeeded by domestic architecture. In Sector C no LBA levels have been reached until now. In the neighbouring trenches of Hrouda however, LBA material has been revealed, thus providing evidence for the occupation of the whole plateau in that period.

Inside the fortified upper citadel, several trenches were excavated by Hrouda. Recent excavations have focused on a huge square building discovered by geophysical prospection in the southwestern fringe, labelled Sector D. Here a similar sequence to Sector A has been revealed, dating from the LBA to Iron Age III. Here we are dealing with a large building on the summit of the citadel, presumably a public building. Hrouda's excavation in the nearby Area 6 also yielded another neighbouring LBA building with stone foundations.

All these remains point to the urban nature of the LBA settlement. The ceramics reflect a Central Anatolian character, providing evidence for a strong Hittite impact.

Similar LBA material has also been collected during the survey of the northern suburb and the western Lower Town. The area north of the mound is nowadays a crop field that is cultivated regularly, making large-scale excavations impossible. However, a test trench opened in this field (Sector B) close to the northern border of the mound has revealed the upper phase of the fortification wall at a depth of *ca.* 3 m under river sediments. The materials on the topsoil in this area could have been washed down from the mound. However, this small test trench must not be representative of the complete area. Geophysical prospection has detected a canal-like structure *ca.* 30 m wide north of the fortification, running parallel to the north side of the mound. This is probably a ditch that runs around the fortification of the citadel. The strip between this ditch and the Ceyhan River was obviously used as a workshop area: defective pottery fragments were found during the survey, exactly at the spot where a kiln was detected through geophysical prospection. This evidence testifies to a link between the material on the surface and the geophysical findings under the earth. The material on the surface can thus be taken into consideration when questioning the dating of the northern lower town.

In contrast with the northern area, the southeastern Lower Town was not ploughed and therefore yielded a very limited amount of material. LBA pottery was not found on the surface. A dense settlement surrounded by a double fortification wall with a gate was found during geophysical prospection. Sector F was opened at the location where the gate was detected. The upper phases of the inner fortification wall with adjacent domestic architecture were recovered. They date from the Iron Age. Lower levels have not yet been reached, and it is therefore not yet possible to determine the initial occupation of the southeastern lower town. However, we can at least present here a feature of topography which was important in the Iron Age and which might have been projected by the earlier LBA architecture. The entrance to the Iron Age Lower Town from the southeast must have been through the southeastern gate that is detected both by geophysical prospection and in excavations. Today, the Ceyhan River runs directly east of the gate, thus blocking the entrance. This suggests that the river had a different course in earlier times.

Satellite imagery shows that the Ceyhan River changed its course east of Sirkeli Höyük several times (Fig. 2). It can be detected that the current bend is a more recent development of the preceding southward shift of the river's course. This was already observed by Ludwig Masch (Munich) in a geological survey connected with

Hrouda's investigations,[23] and it is also confirmed by the observations from 1997 to 2006 when an island on the river just opposite the Muwattalli relief disappeared due to the abandonment of the northern branch of the river. Although we cannot date the clearly visible ancient courses and the shifts of the river, we may assume that the course of the ancient river during the occupation of Sirkeli Höyük ran far to the north of the recent bend and approached the mound directly from the east. Contrary to the situation today, it would not have run parallel to the eastern fringe of the mound and the rock outcrop with the reliefs. This would mean the ancient thoroughfare coming from the Amanus Gates and continuing towards Adana and later to the Cilician Gates passed by Sirkeli Höyük on its northern side and not, as is the case today, on its southern side. It makes much more sense to have the identified city gate on the one side and the northern plateau—the lower and presumably also more 'public' part of the citadel—on the other side. Access to both the Lower Town and the citadel would thus have been arranged from the north.

These reconstructions have implications regarding the visibility of the reliefs. Today the river prevents a good view of the reliefs. But a person entering the LBA town coming from the east, that means from Syria, would have encountered the reliefs instantly. There is no evidence that the reliefs were hidden inside the fortifications as has been assumed for other reliefs like Gavur Kalesi.[24] In other words, the reliefs must have been not only directly visible to people entering the town from the east but must have also dominated the landscape towards the eastern gate.

Interpretation

To sum up the results so far: the ancient road may have approached the ancient city of Sirkeli Höyük exactly at the level of the reliefs, making them well visible to everybody reaching the city from the east along the "Cilician transverse highway"[25] from Syria. There were at least two reliefs. A third one can be suggested due to the existence of a third shallow cup. In addition, one more relief had been planned but was never executed. The *Steingebäude* and the area of the shallow cups were both visible as well and were seemingly hovering over the royal images. The prominent rock face at the northeastern edge of the citadel with the reliefs and the building was therefore a clear marker of the importance of the city and its relationship to the Great King Muwattalli.

The reliefs, the *Steingebäude*, and the shallow cups are components of the same ensemble, with clearly interrelated functions. Although we do not have any

23 Masch in Hrouda 1997, 133.

24 Kühne 2001.

25 Forlanini 2013, 3.

written evidence for its interpretation, we do have some hints: the ornate of King Muwattalli is identical with that of the Sun God in Hittite iconography. This could indicate a deification of the king even though the figure is not wearing a horned cap. Hittite kings were deified only after their death, which was described as "becoming a god."[26] However, as shown by Burney, the shallow cups seem to belong to the ancestor cult,[27] which would also place the reliefs and the *Steingebäude* in this context. Other reliefs of Hittite kings displaying either similar or comparable god-related iconographies and connections with shallow cups could then also be considered in the context of the ancestor cult. This has been suggested for Yazılıkaya and cannot be excluded for Fraktin.

Theo van den Hout following H. Otten raised the idea that the NA4*ḫegur*SAG.UŠ of Muwattalli II, mentioned in the treaty between Kurunta and Tudḫaliya III ("IV") on the Bronze Tablet from Hattuša, might have been located in Sirkeli, in connection with the relief.[28] This building was a memorial for the deceased, and thereby deified, Great King. In the treaty, Kurunta was guaranteed access to the memorial which lay outside his territory. If van den Hout's idea turns out to be correct, then our *Steingebäude* might be identified with the NA4*ḫegur*SAG.UŠ of Muwattalli II. But why then in Sirkeli? Could it be that Muwattalli died on his way back from Syria to his capital Tarḫuntašša? He must have passed by Sirkeli, taking the "Cilician transversal highway" to reach his residence located somewhere in Rough Cilicia or in the southern Konya Plain, localizing to the northwest of Cilicia. This would also fit well with the proposed identification of Sirkeli Höyük with the cult town of Kummanni.

This is a very attractive interpretation indeed, especially for the excavators of Sirkeli Höyük! However, as likely as it might appear, nothing has been proven yet, and there is a strong argument against it: the second mutilated relief shows clearly an identical iconography. Whether our identification of this image with Urḫi-Teššup or that of Hrouda and Ehringhaus with Kurunta is correct, the persons in question were alive when the image was carved. An ancestor cult would then be most unlikely.

We cannot provide definitive answers to the issues treated here yet, but we do hope that further research at Sirkeli Höyük will lead to more arguments in favour or against our interpretation of the ensemble.

26 Haas 2000, 53.

27 Burney 2004, 19–21.

28 Van den Hout 2002, 89–90; Balza and Mora 2011, 221-222.

REFERENCES

Balza, M. E. and C. Mora, "And I built this Everlasting Peak for him. The Two Scribal Traditions on the Hittites and the NA4*ḫekur* SAG.UŠ." *Altorientalische Forschungen* 38/2 (2011), 213-225.

Bryce, T., *Letters of the Great Kings of the Ancient Near East*, London: Routledge, 2003.

Burney, C., *Historical Dictionary of the Hittites*. Oxford: Scarecrow Press, 2004.

Ehringhaus, H., "Hethitisches Felsrelief der Grossreichszeit entdeckt." *Antike Welt* 26/1 (1995a): 66.

———. "Ein neues hethitisches Felsrelief am Sirkeli Höyük in der Çukurova." *Antike Welt* 26/2 (1995b): 118–119.

———. "Vorläufiger Bericht über die Ausgrabung auf dem Sirkeli Höyük, Provinz Adana / Türkei im Jahre 1997." *Istanbuler Mitteilungen* 49 (1999a): 83–140.

———. "Grabungen am Sirkeli Höyük 1997." *Kazı Sonuçları Toplantısı* 20 (1999b): 383–397.

———. "Kurunta als hethitischer Großkönig. Das großreichszeitliche Felsrelief von Hatip (Türkei)." *Antike Welt* 32/5 (2001): 515–520.

———. *Götter, Herrscher, Inschriften. Die Felsreliefs der hethitischen Großreichszeit in der Türkei*. Mainz: Zaberns Bildbände der Archäologie, 2005.

Forlanini, M., "How to Infer Ancient Roads and Intineraries from Heterogenous Hittite Texts: The Case of the Cilician (Kizzuwatnean) Road System." *KASKAL* 10 (2013): 1–34.

Garstang, J., "Explorations in Cilicia. The Neilson Expedition: Preliminary Report I." *Liverpool Annals of Archaeology and Anthropology* 24 (1937): 52–64.

Glatz, C. and A.M. Plourde, "Landscape Monuments and Political Competition in Late Bronze Age Anatolia: An Investigation of Costly Signaling Theory." *BASOR* 361 (2011): 33–66.

Haas, V., "Hethitische Bestattungsbräuche." *Altorientalische Forschungen* 27/1 (2000): 52–67.

Hrouda, B., "Vorläufiger Bericht über die Ausgrabungsergebnisse auf dem Sirkeli Höyük/ Südtürkei von 1992–1996" *Istanbuler Mitteilungen* 47 (1997a): 91–150.

———. "Damnatio memoriae? Neue Beobachtungen am Relief Nr. 2 bei Sirkeli/Türkei", *Antike Welt* 28/6 (1997b): 471–474.

Klengel, H., *Geschichte des Hethitischen Reiches*. Handbuch der Orientalistik I/34. Leiden: Brill, 1999.

Kohlmeyer, K., "Felsbilder der hethitischen Großreichszeit." *Acta Praehistorica et Archaeologica* 15 (1983): 7–135.

Kozal, E., "Exploring Sirkeli Höyük in the Late Bronze Age and its Interregional Connections" in *Across the Border: Late Bronze-Iron Age Relations between Syria and Anatolia, Proceedings of a Symposium held at the Research Center of Anatolian Studies, Koç University, Istanbul May 31–June 1, 2010*. Ancient Near Eastern Studies Supplement 42, ed. by K.A. Yener, 213–224. Leiden: Brill, 2013.

Kozal, E. and M. Novák, "Sirkeli Höyük. A Bronze and Iron Age Urban Settlement in Plain Cilicia" in *Anatolian Metal* VI. Der Anschnitt Beiheft 25, ed. by Ü. Yalçın, 229–238. Bochum: Deutsches Bergbau-Museum Publications, 2013.

Kühne, H., "Gavur Kalesi. Ein Ort der Ahnenverehrung?" in *Kulturgeschichten. Altorientalische Studien für Volkert Haas zum 65. Geburtstag*, ed. by Th. Richter, D. Prechel and J. Klinger, 227–243. Saarbrücken: Saarbrücken Dr. und Verlag, 2001.

Ussishkin, D., "Hollows, Cup-Marks and Hittite Stone Monuments." *Anatolian Studies* 25 (1995): 85–103.

van den Hout, Th., "Tombs and Memorials: The (Divine) Stone-House and Hegur Reconsidered" in *Recent Developments in Hittite Archaeology and History. Papers in Memory of Hans G. Güterbock*, ed. by K.A. Yener and H.A. Hoffner, 73–91. Winona Lake: Eisenbrauns, 2002.

Early and Middle Bronze Age Cylinder Seal Impressions from Salat Tepe

A. Tuba Ökse[1]

Abstract

The excavations conducted ias part of the Ilısu Dam salvage project at Salat Tepe brought out six architectural levels dating from the latest two centuries of the third millennium until the middle of the second millennium BC. A few cylinder seals and impressions of cylinder seals on vessels were found in the Middle Bronze Age (MBA) levels (Levels 4–2). The Upper Tigris region is separated from the Jezira by the Mardin Mountains, and from the Middle Euphrates by the Karacadağ Massive; however, a considerable amount of archaeological material point to strong cultural connections. The cylinder seals and impressions at Salat Tepe and at other sites in the vicinity determine a peripheral workshop of the Syrian glyptic style in the Upper Tigris region. Although neither cuneiform texts nor impressions on clay are found, the presence of cylinder seals in these sites point to the existence of an administrative structure of a socio-economic system during the Early and Middle Bronze Ages.

Introduction

Salat Tepe is one of the multi-period sites excavated as part of the salvage project for the Upper Tigris region that will be flooded by the Ilısu Dam. The site is *ca.* 90 km to the east of Diyarbakır, situated on the eastern bank of the Salat River. Salvage excavations revealed a whole sequence from the Chalcolithic to the medieval period.[2] The site was inhabited from the 6th millennium BC onwards and abandoned after Level 7 (EB I-IIA).

The mound summit was reoccupied in the Late Akkad Period in Level 6 (EB IVA). The post-Akkad period is represented by Level 5, dating to the last two centuries of the 3rd millennium BC (EB IVB).[3] In the beginning of the 2nd mil-

---

1 Department of Archaeology, Kocaeli University, Umuttepe Yerleşkesi 41380 Kocaeli, Turkey.

2 Ökse 2009; 2012.

3 For the EBA phasing, see Matthews 1997, 35.

lennium BC, the buildings of Level 5 were reused; the mound summit was levelled and enlarged with mud fills as substrata for new buildings (Level 4, MB I) and the mound summit was occupied by a weak architecture in Level 3 (MB II).

The mound summit was reorganized towards the end of the eighteenth century BC. The architectural remains of the preceding architecture were levelled and an extended flat substratum for a new settlement had been established by thick mud fills. Level 2 is dated to the 17th and early 16th centuries BC.[4] (MB III). Following the destruction of this settlement, Level 1 was established in the Mitanni Period.

In the Middle Assyrian period the mound was once again abandoned. The mound summit housed in the Iron Age nomadic communities living in pit houses and in the medieval period those living in tents and simple huts. The mound became a graveyard in modern times.

A total of five cylinder seals and eight impressions on potsherds found in reliable contexts and in secondary deposits of the EBA and MBA levels represent several styles dating from the beginning of the 3rd to the earlier half of the 2nd millennium BC.

Geometric Style with Hatched Design

The Cylinder Seal (Fig. 1) was found in a wash layer covering Level 7. The seal is carved with three horizontal zigzag rows and small triangles filling the spaces on the top and bottom. A similar decoration appears on a cylinder seal found in the EBA contexts of Kenantepe.[5] Identical seals are also attested in a wide region stretching from the Levant[6] to the Zagros Mountains during the EB II-IV. Similar decorations on impressions are found near the western extension of the *Kleinen Anten-Tempel* at Tell Chuera[7] and in the EB III-IV contexts of Ebla;[8] the original seals are dated to the Jemdet Nasr period.

One of the impressions (Fig. 2) was found in the fill on a floor in Level 5 and the other impression (Fig. 3) in a fill on a floor in Level 7. Both impressions are on chaff-tempered Coarse Ware potsherds. The preserved parts of both impressions are hachured by three short diagonal line clusters, each asloping to the left and to the right one after another, forming a zigzag pattern. The triangular spaces between these diagonal line boundaries are all hachured each by four horizontal lines. Impressions of the same style with broadly carved

4 Ökse and Görmüş 2006, 141–142.

5 Parker *et al.* 2000, 629, 639–640, fig. 8B.

6 Lapp 1989, 2, no. 2828.

7 Moortgat and Moortgat-Correns 1976, 58, fig. 21 a-b.

8 Mazzoni 1993, 412, fig. 7.

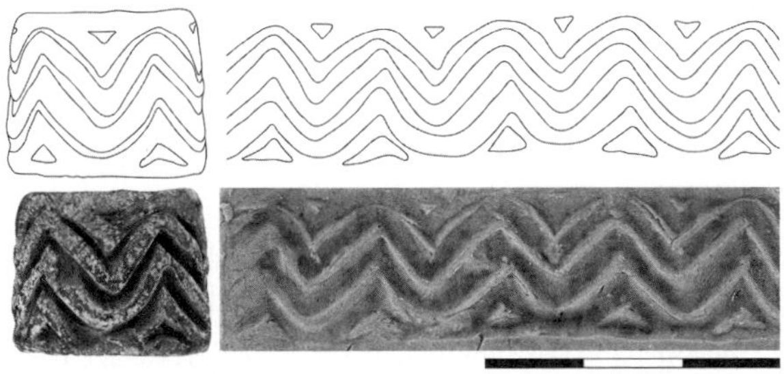

FIG. 1 Cylinder Seal J12/0029/X/01

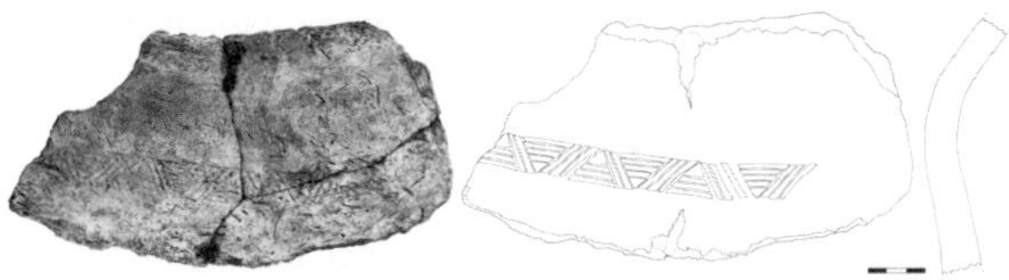

FIG. 2 Impression K12/0164/S/01

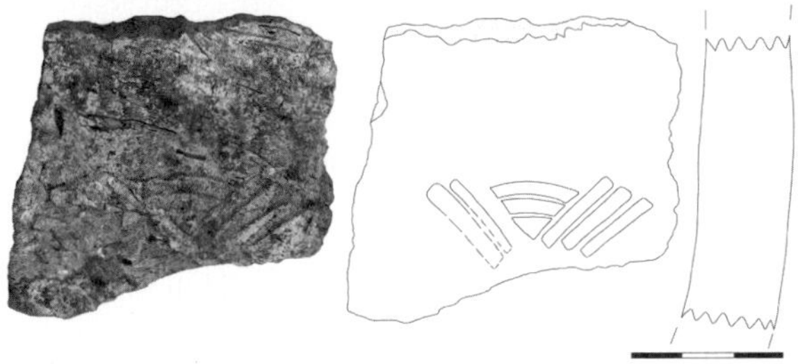

FIG. 3 Impression K13/0256/S/03

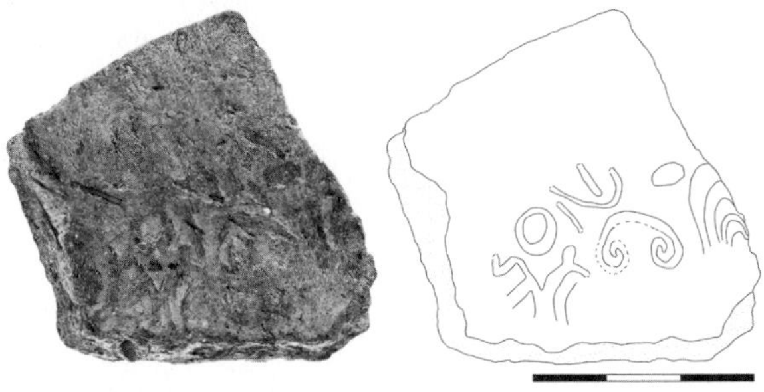

FIG. 4 Impression K13/0253/S/04

geometric design consisting of zigzag patterns and chevrons appear already in the Late Chalcolithic period in the Upper (Arslantepe VI B),[9] the Middle Euphrates region (Hassek Höyük EB I)[10] and the Upper Habur region (Tell Leilan IIIa).[11] This group became more common in the early 3rd millennium contexts

9 Palmieri 1981, fig. 10:1.

10 Behm-Blancke 1981, 25, pl. 11:5–6.

11 McCarthy 2011, 298, Type 1.

of Southern [12] and Northern Mesopotamia; [13] in Early Jezirah 0–3. [14] The scene of another impression (FIG. 4) on a monochrome sherd found in the mud fill in Level 5 is composed by concentric arches, similar to several examples of the Jemdet Nasr-ED I geometric style. [15]

In the second half of the 3rd millennium BC seals and sealings of the geometric style were further in use. Several examples are uncovered in the Khabur region, [16] the Middle Euphrates region [17] and in Western Syria. [18] This style is called "Peripheral Jamdet Nasr style" [19] or the "Piedmont Style." [20] These seals had also been used for decorating vessels in Northern Syria and Northern Mesopotamia throughout the EBA. [21]

---

12 Frankfort 1955, pl. 8:52, 12:99, 13:114, 16:154, 21:217, 35:357, 76:827, 81:862; Wiseman 1962, pl. 11d, 12b-d, h, 29d; Buchanan 1981, 81, 86, 89, no. 228–230; Collon 1987, 14–15, 20–23, fig. 11, 41, 50; Moortgat 1988, 8, pl. 9:52, VA 5965. For cylinder seals at Jemdet Nasr see: Matthews 2002, fig. 6.5–7, pl. 18; at Fara see: Martin 1988, 21, 68, 228–231, no. 44–87; at Ur see: Legrain 1936, pl. 7; Legrain 1951, 11, pl. 2, no. 35, pl. 3, no. 36, 38; at Khafaja see: Frankfort 1955, pl. 22, no. 228; at Tell Agrab see: *ibid.* pl. 76, no. 827.

13 For the Upper Euphrates region see: Hauptmann 1974, pl. 80:1–2; Hauptmann 1982, pl. 26:2; Hauptmann 2000, 421, abb. 2:1; Frangipane and Palmieri 1988, 296; Sagona 1994, 9, 110, fig. 69:6; for the Upper Euphrates region see: Sertok and Ergeç 1999, 94, 107, şek. 12; Ökse 2006, fig. 1–3, for the Upper Khabur region see: Mallowan 1937, pl. 12:2; Mallowan 1947, 72, 134, pl. 21: 7–8; Ingholt 1940, pl. 15:1–2; Moortgat and Moortgat-Correns 1976, 57–58, fig. 21; Matthews 1997, 130, pl. 10:58, 32:403–404; Muchaev and Merpert 1998, 505, fig. 8.1; Akkermans and Schwartz 2003, 216, fig. 7.4; for the Middle Khabur region see: Porada 1948, 7, pl. 7: 33, 39, 42, 50; Teissier 1984, no. 311 (3100–2900 BC).

14 McCarthy 2011, Tab. 1, Type 1, 5.

15 Teissier 1984, no. 43 (3100–2900 BC); Collon 1987, fig. 42, Period IIa; Valdés Pereiro 1999, 121, 126, fig. 3b (Level V: EB II)

16 Sagona 1994, 9; Matthews 1997, 75, 172, pl. 32: 405–415. For Tell Brak ED IIIa to the Ur III contexts see: *ibid.* pl. 32, 33: 421, 425–428, 35: 465–466; for Abu Hureyra EB III levels see: *ibid.* pl. 39: 525; for the Ninevite-V period of the Middle Habur see: Fortin 1988, fig. 10.

17 For Gre Virike Period II (EB III-IV) see: Ökse 2006, fig. 1–3; for Oylum Höyük see: Özgen *et al.* 1997, abb. 27.1; for Tell Halawa B Level 1 see: Lüth 1989, 108–109, abb. 69:6; for Tall Bi'a see: Strommenger and Kohlmeyer 1998, pl. 76: 16; for Tell el-'Abd' EB III levels see: Finkbeiner 1995, 69, abb. 8; for Tell Selenkahiye ED I-II levels see: Van Loon 2001, pl. 12.6 a-d, 12.13b; for Tall Munbaqa see: Werner 2004, 1–4.

18 For the parallels at Hama K see: Ingholt 1940, pl. 6:7, 15:1–2; for Amuq G see: Braidwood and Braidwood 1960, 331, fig. 254.1.

19 Amiet 1973, 217, fig. 1; Buchanan 1981, 74.

20 Akkermans and Schwartz 2003, 216; McCarthy 2011, 290. Other terms are used for different geographical regions: Parayre (1994: 557, fig. 28.1) defines the ED I seals of this group in the Diyala region as "Brocade style", and Mazzoni (1989: 34, fig. 10) uses the term "popular style" for Ebla seals.

21 Czichon 2004, 5–8.

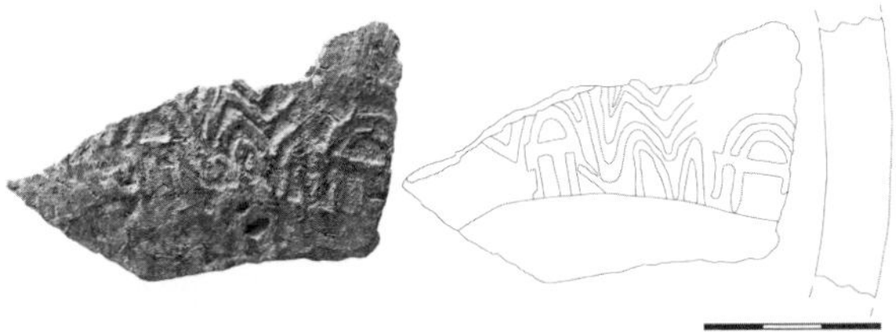

FIG. 5 Impression K13/0172/S/02

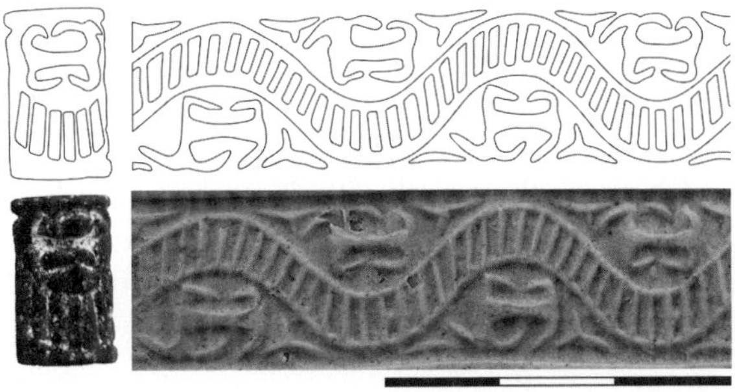

FIG. 6 Cylinder Seal L12/0261/X/05

Geometric Style with Architectural Design

The preserved part of the impression (FIG. 5) found in the mud fill covering Level 7 is composed of two domed buildings separated by two elongated arcs roofed by three zigzag lines. The quadrangular buildings seem to have a buttressed façade of three units, and the domes are both represented by two concentric arcs. Scenes with concentric elements are depicted on several seals in the Jemdet Nasr period.[22] Buildings with a zigzag fill on the top are depicted on Fara seals from Level 5 dating to EB II,[23] further domed structures filled with diagonal lines are depicted on seals from Tell Brak[24] and those with horizontal hatchings are found at Ur.[25]

Geometric Style with Scematic Animal Figures

The scene on the cylinder seal (FIG. 6) found in Level 4 is organized by a wavy band filled with vertical hatching. The semicircular spaces at the upper and lower edges are filled with a recumbent goat flanked by two eagles. The goat is depicted

22 Pittman 1994, fig. 17, no. 16:6.

23 Martin 1988, 21, 233, no. 100 (Level 5). For further doomed structures depicted on seals from Fara, see: *ibid.* 232, no. 95.

24 Akkermans and Schwartz 2003, 216, fig. 7.4.

25 Legrain 1936, 2, 32–33, pl. 17: 333–344, pl. 18: 345–350, pl. 40.

in a linear style. The front legs turned backwards, the hind legs facing forward, the tail raised upright, and the head in profile are shown with simple lines; and the horns with a curved line. The eagles are given in three short lines depicting stretched wings and the body.

Combinations of geometric design together with schematic figures appear in the Early Jezirah 1–2 contexts in the Upper Habur region.[26] Hatched waves are found on seals dating from the turn of the fourth to the 3rd millennium BC onwards including the Early Dynastic period in Mesopotamia.[27] However, instead of stylized goats, eagles are depicted on these seals.[28] Goats are occasionally depicted alongside hatched zigzags and arches.[29] The goats are carved in a schematic linear style resembling the style on seals of the Jemdet Nasr period (3100 BC).[30] Several goats resemble the schematic depiction on the Salat seal.[31] A more detailed version of the stylized sitting goats is found at Alalakh[32] and in the ED I style group at Fara.[33]

Stick-Figure Style

On a cylinder Seal (Fig. 7) found in a pit probably used in Level 3, the scene is bordered by a vertical band filled with three cross-signs on a vertical line. The scene consists of a human figure and a goat depicted with simple lines associated with drillings. The figure sits on a stool with one arm stretched out forward the head and the knees are formed by simple drilled dots. In front of this figure is the image of a caprid , rotated 90° to the right, facing the top. Its head is depicted by a simple drilled dot and the horns by a pair of arch-shaped lines; forks in the horns are indicated by three short lines.

The linar style fits well with the local "Stick-Figure" design dating to EJZ 2–3, contemporary with the Ninevite V assemblages of the Upper Habur region and

26 Tell Leilan IIIb-d, see: McCarthy 2011, 298, Type 3.

27 Pittman 1994, fig. 3, 10b. A similar hatched wave is also depicted on a seal dating to ED III period; see: Frankfort 1939, pl. XIVa.

28 For a Fara seal from the ED I period see: Martin 1988, 237, Nr. 130; for an ED III seal in the Diyala region see. Frankfort 1955, pl. 37, no. 384, pl. 39, no. 416; for an ED III seal from Ur see: Legrain 1951, pl. 2, no. 35, pl. 3, no. 36, 38; Collon 1987, fig. 94, Period IIe.

29 Pittman 1994, fig. 12, 2:15, 7:8.

30 Moortgat 1988, pl. 4:21, VA 11048.

31 Pittman 1994, fig. 18, no. 21:16; for similar seals from Samsat Höyük see: Özkan and Öztan 2009, 483, 487, fig. 16.

32 Collon 1982, no. 57, 74.

33 Martin 1988, 243, no. 194.

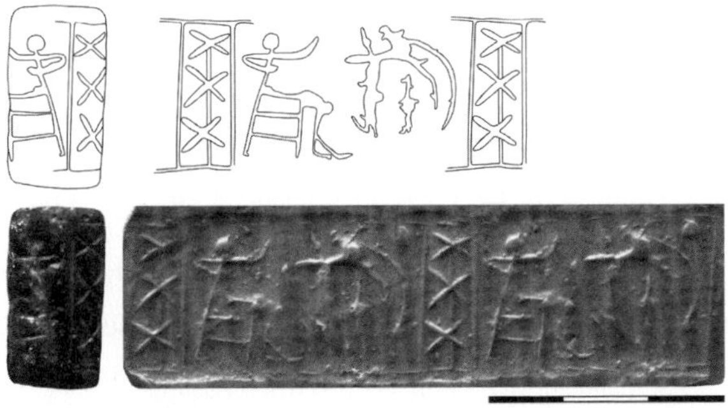

FIG. 7 Cylinder Seal K14/0230/X/02

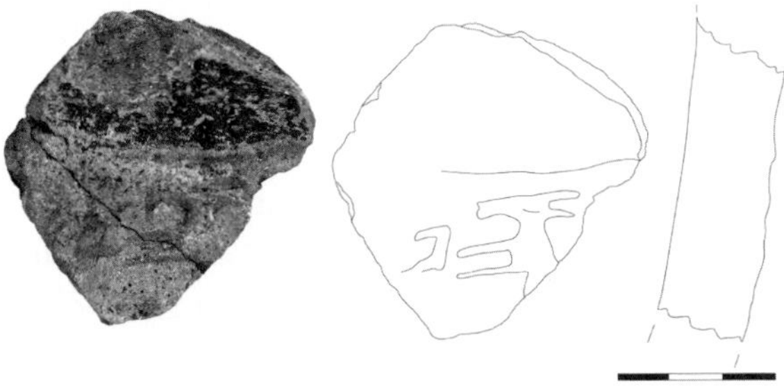

FIG. 8 Impression L11/0154/S/02

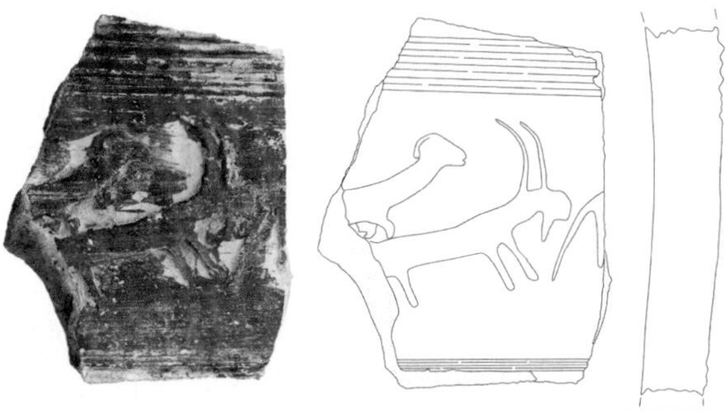

FIG. 9 Impression K13/0115/S/01

with ED I (*ca.* 2700 BC); this style is represented at Tell Brak, Tell Chuera and Abu Hujaira.[34] Standing human figures with outstretched hands and animal figures facing the top at right angles, on an impression from Tell Chuera[35] and those from Alalakh[36] are parallel to the Salat Tepe seal. Seals and sealings with a similar style are also known from several Mesopotamian sites.[37] Similarly stylized goat figures

34 McCarthy 2011, 290, 298, Type 4; for seals from Tell Brak see: Oates 2001, 122; for seals from Tell Chuera see: Moortgat-Correns 1995, pl. 13b.

35 Orthmann *et al.* 1986, 55–56, abb. 34. The impression is found at Tell Chuera level 2a, Gebäude B, Hof 6.

36 Collon 1982, no. 97.

37 Amiet 1961, no. 965–968.

on impressions at Khafaja are defined as "ED I style."[38] An impression of this style is dated to early ED IIIb at Abu Salabikh,[39] and similar schematic figures appear further in the Akkad and Ur-III periods,[40] although the composition scheme differs.

Local Figured Style

The local figured style is represented by several impressions on potsherds. On the preserved parts of two impressions animal scenes are depicted. One of these (Fig. 8) is on a vessel of the Red-Brown Wash Ware found in the mud fill used for levelling the mound summit in Level 4. The preserved part of the scene contains two roughly shaped goats facing to eachother. The figures are carved in a linear style resembling the schematic style depicted on seals dated from the Uruk IV/VI-Jemdet Nasr transition to the Mesilim Period;[41] same type of a goat head is seen on the impression on a jar stop from the early ED IIIb Ash-Tip at Abu Salabikh.[42]

The other impression (Fig. 9) is on a vessel of the Red-Brown Wash Ware found in a fill to the west of wall K13/021/D in Level 2. The preserved part of the scene contains a roughly shaped ram and a goat facing right. The position of the ram resembles those of a flock of small cattle on the meadow. Similar scenes appear on the bullae dating to the transition to the Mesilim period in Ur,[43] on the ED I seals in Fara.[44] These impressions resemble the *einheimisch-nordsyrischen* style of the 3rd millennium BC at Tell Chuera.[45] An impression found at Abu Salabikh, the Ash-Tip[46] and the "piedmont Ninevite V" impressions on pottery from the ED IIIb contexts at Tell Brak[47] determine the existence of this group further in the late ED III and Akkadian period.

38 Frankfort 1955, pl. 24, no. 243. A seal from an ED III context Khafaja (*ibid* no. 369) is seggested to earlier in date (*ca.* 2700–2300 BC), see: Orthmann *et al.* 1986, 52; Collon 1987, fig. 59, Period IIb-c.

39 Martin and Matthews 1993, fig. 2.57. The impression is on a jar stop from the Ash-Tip.

40 Moortgat 1988, 21, pl. 25:178, VA 3176.

41 For the seals dating to the Jemdet Nasr period (3100 BC) see: Moortgat 1988, 5–6, pl. 2:7–8, VA 10540, 10543, 3889; for the seals dating to the transition to the Mesilim period see: *ibid.* pl. 11:65, 67, VA 684; for those dating to the Mesilim Period see: *ibid.* 9, pl. 12:71, VA 2061.

42 Martin and Matthews 1993, fig. 2.88.

43 For the bullae found in levels SIS 4 and 5 below the Royal Graves of Ur see: Moortgat 1988, 9, pl. A, 3; Legrain 1936, pl. 48, no. 287; for seals contemporary with the latest examples of the Jemdet Nasr style see: Moortgat 1988, 8.

44 Martin 1988, 239, no. 150–151.

45 Orthmann 1995, 37, fig. 14.

46 Martin and Matthews 1993, fig. 2.11.

47 Oates 2001, 127–128, fig. 156–157.

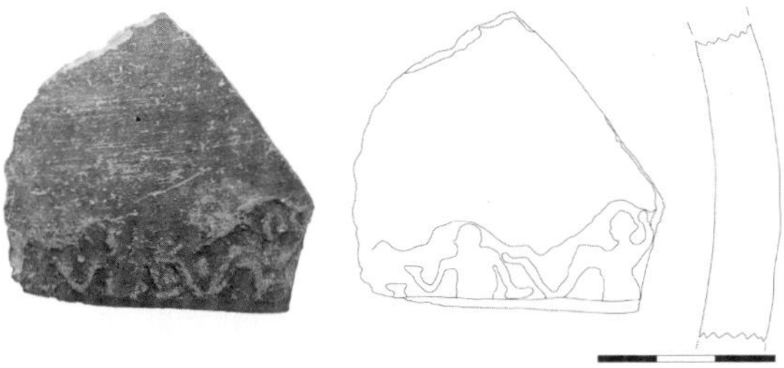

FIG. 10 Impression K13/0099/S/01

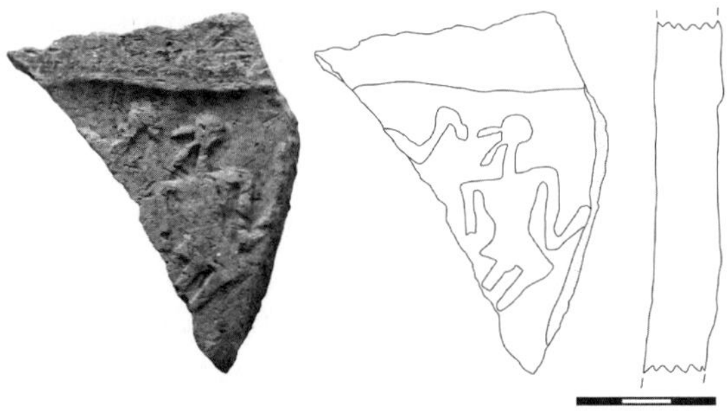

FIG. 11 Impression K14/0238/P/01

On the preserved parts of two more impressions, human figures are depicted. On the upper part of the rolling of the impression (FIG. 10) on a Red-Brown Wash Ware sherd found in the debris of Level 2, two persons with arms outstretched to both sides are depicted. The figures, facing left, hold conical bowls in both hands, with arms bent at the elbows. The bodies are roughly shaped with wide shoulders and thin waists. No remarkable details are present remarkable either on the faces or the bodies. Another impression (FIG. 11), on a Coarse Ware sherd with chaff temper found under a wall in Level 3, shows a person again with arms stretched out to both sides. Both arms are bent by the elbows but the hands are not preserved in the rolling. The body is roughly shaped with a long narrow neck and wide shoulders without any details. The head is formed by a small circle with two projecting parts attached to the left side. The head and long neck of a second person is preserved to the left of the first.

Similar impressions are found also on the Red-Brown Wash Ware assemblages from the late 3rd - early 2nd millennium BC contexts at Kenantepe,[48] located *ca.* 20 km to the west of Salat Tepe. Similarly depicted shepherd figures are seen on cylinder seals dating to the turn from the Uruk IV/VI period to the Jemdet Nasr period and the Jemdet Nasr period (3100 BC).[49] The human figures resemble the

48 Swartz Dodd 2012, 218–219, fig. 3A.

49 Moortgat 1988, 4, 8, pl. 1:4, VA 7234, pl. 7:40, VA 10544.

ED I style at Fara [50] and those from Alalah, [51] and the *einheimisch-nordsyrischen* style of the 3rd millennium BC at Tell Chuera. [52] The shape of the upper part of the human bodies on a cylinder seal found at Selenkahiye [53] and the "Syrian ritual" seal type from Tell Brak, [54] both dated to the late ED also resemble those depicted on the Salat impressions.

Figurative seals with similar shapes named the "broad relief style" [55] or the *rustikaler Stil*[56] appear from the Late Chalcolithic period onwards including the EB II in the Upper Euphrates region. [57] In the Balikh region these examples are known as the peripheral Late Uruk style, [58] and in the Middle Euphrates region this group is attested at several settlements throughout the 3rd millennium BC. [59] The schematic caprid and human figures of the "brocade style" [60] or "common style" [61] of Northwestern Syria appears in the EB I and continues until the end of the ED III period. [62] Parayre [63] defines this as "Syro-Palestinian EB IV glyptic", Buchanan [64] calls it the "Peripheral Early Dynastic style" and Amiet [65] refers to them as "cylindres prédynastiques schèmatiques." In Northern Mesopotamia and adjacent regions seals carved in this style appearing in the EJZ 1 contexts

---

50 Martin 1988, 240, no. 159.

51 Collon 1982, no. 5.

52 Orthmann 1995, 37, fig. 14.

53 Van Loon 1979, 103, fig. 11.

54 Oates 2001, 122–123, fig. 145b.

55 Frangipane and Palmieri 1988, 424, fig. 70:17.

56 Behm-Blancke 1993, 253, fig. 2:1.

57 Frangipane 1993, 194, fig. 2.2. For Arslantepe VI A (EB IA), see. Collon 1987, 14, fig. 11; Ferioli and Fiandra 1988, fig. 67: 1–4, 69: 11, 70: 17; A. Palmieri (1981, 118) defines the Arslantepe VIA group as forrunners of the Arslantepe VIB (EB IB) glyptic. For Han İbrahim Şah VIII (EB II) see: Ertem 1988, pl. 62: 1–2, and for the EB I pit at Hassek Höyük see: Behm-Blancke 1981, 25, pl. 11: 4.

58 Hammam et-Turkman, see: Van Loon 1983, 3, fig. 5.

59 Kurban Höyük V, Hassek Höyük, Lidar Höyük IIa1, see: Matthews 1997, 183; Van Loon 2001, pl. 12.12–13a; Gre Virike II, see: Ökse 2006, fig. 4–5; Jerablus Tahtani, see: Peltenburg et al 1995, 70; Tell Selenkahiye, see: Van Loon 2001, pl. 12.11 a-b; Umm el-Marra, see: Schwartz *et al.* 2003, 329, fig. 4.

60 Mazzoni 1984, 34; Mazzoni 1993, 406, 410–411, fig. 6; Mazzoni 2000, fig. 4.4,5.

61 Collon 1987, 20–23, 113, fig. 62–66, Period IId; Finkbeiner 1995, 71, fig. 9.

62 For Hama J 5, see: Ingholt 1940, pl. 14:3; see also Collon 1987, 152, fig. 678; for Ras Shamra see: Courtois 1962, fig. 21: H. B. Teissier (1984, 190–193) classifies similar seals as "Syrian Seals from 2900–2200 BC."

63 Parayre 1990, 557–558.

64 Buchanan 1981, 21, 137, no. 51, 361.

65 Amiet 1961, 33.

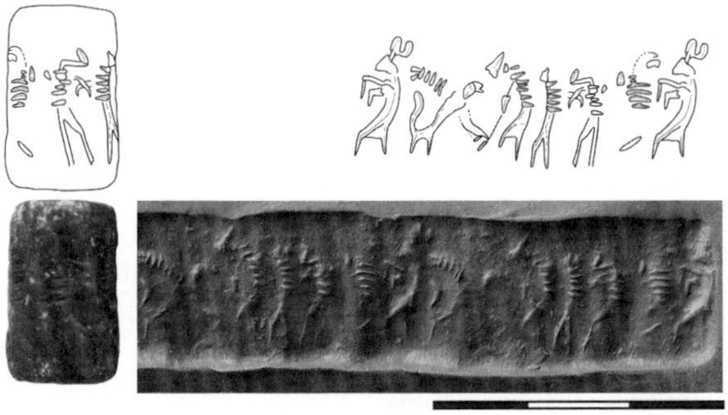

FIG. 12 Cylinder Seal L12/0165/X/01

are defined as regional/local styles[66] with parallels in the Early Dynastic style of Southern Mesopotamia. Similar impressions dating to the ED IIIa are found on jars in several sites of the Upper Habur region.[67]

Early Dynastic Style

A cylinder seal (FIG. 12) found in the debris covering the southern part of the main entrance of the central courtyard of Level 2 suffered abrasion. The scene consists of seven animals standing on their hindquarters: Two rampant lions crossing eachother, three lions facing left, and a hybrid-lion in combat. The lions' manes are depicted by five short horizontal lines. The upper parts of their hindquarters are depicted in a more voluminous fashion compared with the thinner lower parts. The S-shaped tails are raised and the open mouths indicate roaring.

Similar combat scenes with animals standing on their hindquarters are common in the mid-late 3rd millennium BC (ED II-III) in Mesopotamia.[68] The schematic and thin bodies resemble the figures depicted on seals dating to the ED II[69] and from the mid/late 3rd millennium BC contexts at Tell Brak.[70] The position and the mane resemble the ED II style at Fara,[71] which Boehmer defines as "Gruppe 5:

66 Akkermans and Schwartz 2003, 216; A. P.; McCarthy 2011, 289.

67 For Tell Muh Kabīr see: Meijer 1986, fig. 9; for Tell Leilan III see: Parayre 1990, 556–558, fig. 28:4, and for Tell Brak see: Matthews 1991, 148–152, fig. 2.13–14; Matthews 1997, pl. 38: 502–503. The impressions found at Tell Chuera is defined as products of local seal carvers, and named the "Chuera-style". See: Moortgat and Moortgat-Correns 1976, 58; fig. 22; see also Moortgat and Correns 1988, fig. 7, 18; Orthmann 1990, 36, fig. 34, 35:4; Matthews 1997, 145, 172.

68 Teissier 1984, no. 56–57 (2750–2500 BC); Orthmann 1975, 229–230, fig. 42a.

69 Frankfort 1939, pl. Xc; 1955, no. 320 and 554; Karg 1999, pl. 6:11, 7:4, 8:2, 8:6, 10:1, 10:8, 10:12; Moortgat 1988, 10–11, pl. D, 1; pl. 14:81, VA 3962, 15:90–91, VA 10394, 3421; Collon 1987, fig. 79, Period IIe (ED III).

70 Akkermans and Schwartz 2003, 242, fig. 8.7 b.

71 Martin 1988, 260, no. 364.

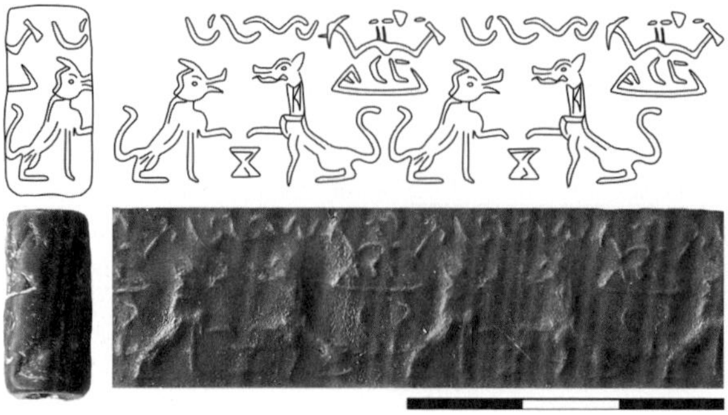

Fig. 13 Cylinder Seal L13/0079/X/01

sumero-akkadische."[72] On an impression found in a building dating to the Mesilim period (early ED II) at Tell Chuera[73] both the lions' manes and the goats' fell are depicted similarly to those on the Salat Tepe seal. Similar scenes dating to the ED III period are found on an impression from the Ash-Tip at Abu Salabikh,[74] on a seal from Alalah,[75] Khafajah, and Tell Agrab.[76] Similar positions and hatching to indicate manes appear in the Royal Graves of Ur from the EB III and Sargonid periods[77] as well as from the Early Akkadian contexts (Area SS, Room 18) from Tell Brak.[78]

Provincial Old Syrian Style

The main scene on a cylinder seal (Fig. 13)[79] found within the mud brick collapse of Level 2 consists of two lion figures at the bottom, facing to each other at both sides of a footed bowl, probably an altar. The lions are depicted as sitting on their hind legs with one front leg placed on the altar situated between them. The shoulders and rumps of the lions are depicted in a voluminous fashion with the use of a drill. The manes and the muscles are emphasized by curved lines. The S-shaped tails are raised and the open mouths indicate roaring. The scene is bordered at the top by a guilloche in the form of two strings twisted over each other, broken by a seated human figure positioned over the tails of the lions. The figure sits on a platform aligned with the heads of the lions. The bottom of the platform is formed by a straight line, and the upper surface is convex. The human figure is also incised

72 Boehmer 1965, 8, 10, pl. 3:27.

73 Moortgat and Moortgat-Correns 1976, 47, 50, fig. 19 a-b.

74 Martin and Matthews 1993, fig. 2.26.

75 Collon 1982, no. 4.

76 Frankfort 1955, pl. 39, no. 419: Khafaja, pl. 50, no. 515.

77 Legrain 1951, pl. 6, no. 86: pl. 13 (EB III) and no. 172 (Sargonid Grave 159).

78 Oates 2001, 130–131, fig. 162, 197:9.

79 Ökse and Görmüş 2006, 170, fig. 15.

with simple lines, has big eyes and the hair is indicated with large bored circles. The arms, bent at the elbows, are stretched out to both sides. The figure holds in the left hand a tool resembling a double hook, and in the right hand a hand-axe.

The human figure is depicted in a linear style similar to those on some Syrian seals with Hurrian influence.[80] The figure holds a tool and an axe, similar to those from Alalakh VII[81] dating to the late 18th and late 17th centuries BC. Parallels to lion figures sitting face to face with similar tails are known from the Old Syrian Style Groups I[82] and II.[83] Parallels to the horizontal lines across the lions' necks are known from the First Syrian Group[84] such as those from Alalakh VI, and the heads resemble those in Alalakh XIII. Moortgat[85] defines a similar scene as a Syrian style with Hurrian influence. Otto classifies similar scenes as "Stielgruppe 1" of the Old Syrian glyptic style, extending in a region from Cilicia to the western part of the Upper Habur region in the 19th–18th centuries BC.[86] Guilloche is used on the seals of the Old Babylonian Simple Style[87] and is characteristic for the early phase of the Old Syrian Style Group I dating to the 17th–19th centuries BC.[88] as well as of the Group II dating to 1600–1350 BC.[89] A similar design is known from Alalakh VIII-VII seals dating to late 18th to early 17th and to the 15th centuries BC[90] as well as from Alalakh IV from the 14th–13th centuries BC.[91] Figures on a line or a platform on the upper half of the scene is known from the Old Babylonian seals[92] and Old Syrian glyptic Group I.[93] The Salat Tepe cylinder might be a product of a provincial workshop of the Syrian Style, such as those at Kenan Tepe.[94]

80 Moortgat 1988, no. 542.

81 Collon 1975, pl. XX, 15, XV, 14, XXIV, 31.

82 Porada 1948, 118, no. 926; Buchanan 1966, pl. 56, no. 886; Collon 1982, 3, 36, no. 4, pl. 38, no. 7; see also Collon 1987, no. 210–211, Period IVf.

83 Porada 1948, 124–125, no. 945, 980; Contenau 1922, pl. XXVI, 185, 187, 189.

84 Porada 1948, 118, no. 921.

85 Moortgat 1988, no. 535.

86 Otto 2000, 35, 110, 117, 279, pl. 2:15: Stilgruppe 1a (Buchanan 1981, no. 1253), pl. 7:84: Stilgruppe 1d (Teissier 1984) and for other parallels see pl. 11:137: "Stilgruppe" 2b (Carchemish Hofstil); Teissier 1984, no. 552 (1850–1720 BC), 561 (1850–1800 BC). A. Otto dates the "frühklassisce" stil to 1830–1790 BC and the "hochklassisce" to 1795–1760 BC.

87 Buchanan 1981, 315, no. 850.

88 Buchanan 1966, 165, pl. 55, no. 855, 858, 863–864; Porada 1948, 118, no. 926.

89 Buchanan 1966, 123, no. 980.

90 Collon 1975, 4, 44, 50–51, pl. L-LI, no. 112.

91 Collon 1975, 169, 193–194.

92 Buchanan 1981, 316, no. 851.

93 Porada 1948, 118, no. 926; Buchanan 1966, pl. 56, no. 855.

94 Parker and Swartz Dodd 2003, 66, fig. 15.

Conclusion

The cylinder seals and impressions of cylinder seals on vessels found in the Early and MBA levels of Salat Tepe, one of the sites excavated within the salvage project of the Ilısu Dam, demonstrate strong cultural connections of the Upper Tigris region with Northern Mesopotamia.

The Geometric Group of the Jemdet Nasr Piedmont style is diagnostic for the period from *ca.* 3100 BC to the beginning of the later phase of the Ninevite-V period, the Early Jezirah 0–3 in the Habur region. This style is represented by two cylinder seals and three impressions at Salat Tepe. One of the seals (Fig. 1) and two impressions (Fig. 3, Fig. 5) of this group are found in contexts dating to EB I at Salat Tepe, contemporary with the presence of this style in Mesopotamia. Moreover, the impressed vessels belong to a handmade chaff-tempered ware produced in the Late Chalcolithic and EB I. Thus, both the stratigraphical positions and the stylistic analyses date these pieces to the early centuries of the 3rd millennium BC. Although one impression (Fig. 2) was found in a fill of a level dating to the later two centuries of the 3rd millennium BC, it seems to have been deposited with the material used for infilling the previous architecture creating substrata for new buildings.

One cylinder seal with a hatched wave design and stylistic animal figures (Fig. 6) is found in a later context dating to the earlier two centuries of the 2nd millennium BC; however, its parallels are mostly dated to the earlier half of the 3rd millennium BC. Thus, the existence of the Salat seal in a later context might determine a longer lifetime for this style in these northern regions. One cylinder Seal (Fig. 7) found in a pit probably used in Level 3 is carved in the Stick-Figure Style dating to the Early Jezirah 2–3, contemporary with the Ninevite-V assemblages in the Habur region. On the other hand, Salat Tepe was abandoned in this period, and Level 3 was inhabited in the MB II. Thus, the seal might have been brought to the site at a later period.

The second group of impressions found in the MBA contexts of Salat Tepe resembles the Peripheral Early Dynastic Style of Northern Mesopotamia. Three of these impressions (Fig. 8, Fig. 10) are on Red-Brown Wash Ware sherds of the EB IV-MBA assemblages of the local production in the Upper Tigris region, and the other two (Fig. 4, Fig. 11) on monochrome sherds. The stylitic parallels of the animal and human figures imprinted on these sherds are dated to a period from the Late Chalcolithic to the end of the ED period. The stratigraphical positions and the ware groups are obviously later than the stylistic parallels, so, the EBA regional styles might have been used in the Upper Tigris region further in a period including the earlier two centuries of the 2nd millennium BC.

Of the Salat Tepe seals, two found in the debris of Level 2 have suffered abrasion. The debris is dated to the 17th century BC; however, both seals are carved in earlier styles. One of these is a product of the Early Dynastic style of Mesopotamia (Fig. 12), and Salat Tepe was abandoned in the Early Dynastic period, so, this seal might have been secondarily brought to the site in the MBA, and might have been used as an amulet or bead. The other seal (Fig. 13) is a product of the Provincial Old Syrian Style Group I dating to the 19th–17th centuries BC, contemporary with Level 2. This piece might be a product of a provincial workshop, such as those at Kenan Tepe.

Although neither cuneiform texts nor impressions on clay are found at Salat Tepe, the presence of cylinder seals in these sites point to the existence of an administrative structure as part of a socio-economic system during the Bronze Age. On the other hand, two of the cylinder seals (Fig. 12, Fig. 13) which were damaged by abrasions might have been used secondarily as amulets.

Catalogue

Cylinder Seal J12/0029/X/01 (Fig. 1): Baked clay. Height 16 mm; diameter 19.5–19.8 mm; width of perforation 4.2 mm; depth of carving 2.2. Found in a wash layer covering Level 7 dating to EB I. Geometric Style with Hatched Design. EB I-II.

Impression K12/0164/S/01 (Fig. 2): From a handmade chaff-tempered potsherd in the fill on the south-western part of floor K12/101/T in Level 5 dating to EB IVB. Geometric Style with Hatched Design. EB I-II.

Impression K13/0256/S/03 (Fig. 3): From a handmade chaff-tempered potsherd in the fill to the north of hearth K13/107/F in Level 7 dating to EB I. Geometric Style with Hatched Design. EB I-II.

Impression K13/0253/S/04 (Fig. 4): From a monochrome sherd in the mud fill to the southwest of wall K13/106/D in Level 5 dating to EB IVB. Geometric Style with Hatched Design. EB I-II.

Impression K13/0172/S/02 (Fig. 5): From a handmade vessel with pale brown burnished slip in the mud fill covering Level 7 dating to EB I. Geometric Style with Architectural Design. EB I-II.

Cylinder Seal L12/0261/X/05 (Fig. 6): Serpentine. Height, 14 mm; diameter 8 mm width of perforation 4 mm. Found in Room L12/080/M in Level 4 dating to MB I. Geometric Style with Scematic Animal Figures. EB I-II.

Cylinder Seal K14/0230/X/02 (Fig. 7): Serpentine. Height, 22 mm; diameter 12 mm; width of perforation 2 mm. Found in Pit K14/125/Ç probably used in Level 3 dating to MB II. Stick Figure Style. EB II-IV.

Impression L11/0154/S/02 (Fig. 8): From a Red-Brown Wash Ware sherd in the mud fill levelling the mound summit in Level 4 dating to MB I. Local Figured Style. EB II-IV.

Impression K13/0115/S/01 (Fig. 9): Found on a Red-Brown Wash Ware sherd in a fill to the west of wall K13/021/D in Level 2 dating to MB III; Local Figured Style; date: EB II-IV.

Impression K13/0099/S/01 (Fig. 10): Found on a vessel of the Red-Brown Wash Ware sherd in the debris of Level 2 dating to MB III; Local Figured Style; date: EB II-IV.

Impression K14/0238/P/01 (Fig. 11): Found on a chaff-tempered coarse sherd under wall K14/120/D in Level 3 dating to MB II; Local Figured Style; date: EB II-IV.

Cylinder Seal L12/0165/X/01 (Fig. 12): Serpentine; height 17.50 mm; diameter 11.50 mm; width of perforation 3.3 mm; found in the debris of the main entrance of the central courtyard of Level 2 dating to MB III; Early Dynastic Style; date: EB II-III.

Cylinder Seal L13/0079/X/01 (Fig. 13): Serpentine; height 16.85 mm; diameter 8.69 mm; width of perforation 2.54 mm; found in the mud brick fill of the central courtyard of Level 2 dating to MB III; Provincial Old Syrian Style Group I; date: MB II-III (1900–1600 BC).

REFERENCES

Akkermans, P. M. M. G. and G. M. Schwartz, *The Archaeology of Syria from Complex Hunter-Gatherers to Early Urban Societies (ca. 16,000–300 BC)*. Cambridge : Cambridge University Press, 2003.

Amiet, P., *La glyptique mésopotamienne archaïque.* Paris: Editions du Centre National de la Recherche Scientifique, 1961.

———. "Aperçu préliminaire sur la glyptique archaïque d'Arslantepe." *Origini* 7 (1973): 217–224.

Behm-Blancke, M., "Hassek Höyük. Vorläufiger Bericht über die Ausgrabungen der Jahre 1978–1980." *Istanbuler Mitteilungen* 31 (1981): 5–30.

———. "Glyptische Traditionen beiderseits des Ost-Taurus in ausgehenden 4. und frühen 3. Jahrtausend v. Chr" in *Between the Rivers and over the Mountains: Archaeologica Anatolica et Mesopotamica. Alba Palmieri Dedicata,* ed. by M. Frangipane, H. Hauptmann, M. Liverani, P. Matthiae, M. Mellink, 247–259. Roma: Università di Roma "La Sapienza," 1993.

Boehmer, R. M., *Die Entwicklung der Glyptik während der Akkad-Zeit.* Berlin: De Gruyter, 1965.

Braidwood, R. J. and L. S. Braidwood, *Excavations in the Plain of Antioch I: The Earlier Assemblages, Phases A-J* (Oriental Institute Publications 61). Chicago: University of Chicago Press, 1960.

Buchanan, B., *Catalogue of Ancient Near Eastern Seals in the Ashmolean Museum I: Cylinder Seals of Babylonia and Assyria.* Oxford: The Clarendon Press, 1966.

———. *Early Near Eastern Seals in the Yale Babylonian Collection.* New Haven – London: Yale University Press, 1981.

Collon, D., *The Seal Impressions from Tell Atchana/Alalakh.* Alter Orient und Altes Testament 27. Neukirchen-Vluyn: Neukirchener Verlag, 1975.

———. *The Alalakh Cylinder Seals: A New Catalogue of the Actual Seals Excavated by Sir Leonard Woolley at Tell Atchana and from Neighbouring Sites on the Syrian-Turkish Border.* British Archaeologial Reports, International Series 132. Oxford: Archaeopress, 1982.

———. *First Impressions: Cylinder Seals in the Ancient Near East.* London: British Museum Publications, 1987.

Contenau, G., *La Glyptique Syro-Hittite.* Bibliothèque archéologique et historique du Service des Antiquités de Syrie, t. II. Paris: Paul Geuthner, 1922.

Courtois, J.C., "Contribution à l'étude des Civilisations du Bronze Ancien à Ras Shamra-Ugarit (Sondages 1959)." *Ugaritica* 4 (1962): 415–475.

Czichon, R. M., "Echter und nachgeahmter Rollstempeldekor" in *Tall Munbāqa-Ekalte III: Die Glyptik* (Wissenschaftliche Veröffentlichungen der Deutschen Orient-Gesellschaft 108), ed. by P. Werner, 5–8. Saarbrücken: Saarbrücker Verlag, 2004.

Ertem, H., "Han İbrahim Şah Excavations, 1971" in *Keban Project 1971 Activities*, 59–69. Ankara: Orta Doğu Teknik Üniversitesi Keban Projesi Yayınları, 1974.

Ferioli, P. and E. Fiandra, "Clay Sealings from Arslantepe VI A: Administration and Bureaucracy." *Origini* 12/2 (1988): 455–509.

Finkbeiner, U., "Tell el-Abd." *Damaszener Mitteilungen* 8 (1995): 51–83.

Fortin, M., "Rapport préliminaire sur la première campagne de fouilles à Tell Atij, sur le moyen Khabour." *Syria* 55 (1988): 139–171.

Frangipane, M., "New Groups of Clay-Sealings From the 4th Millennium Levels of Arslantepe-Malatya" in *Aspects of Art and Iconography: Anatolia and Its Neighbours. Studies in Honor of Nimet Özgüç*, ed. by M. J. Mellink, E. Porada and T. Özgüç, 191–200. Ankara: Türk Tarih Kurumu Basımevi, 1993.

Frangipane, M. and A. Palmieri, "A Protourban Center of the Late Uruk Period." *Origini* 12/2 (1988): 287–454.

Frankfort, H., *Cylinder Seals A Documentary Essay on the Art and Religion of the Ancient Near East*. London: Macmillan, 1939.

———. *Stratified Cylinder Seals from the Diyala Region*. Oriental Institute Publications 72. Chicago: The University of Chicago Press, 1955.

Hauptmann, H., "Die Grabungen auf dem Norşun Tepe 1971" in *Keban Project 1971 Activities*, 71–107. Ankara: Orta Doğu Teknik Üniversitesi Keban Projesi Yayınları, 1974.

———. "Die Grabungen auf dem Norşun Tepe, 1974" in *Keban Project 1974–1975 Activities*, 15–70. Ankara: Orta Doğu Teknik Üniversitesi Keban Projesi Yayınları, 1982.

———. "Zur Chronologie des 3. Jahrtausends v. Chr. am Oberen Euphrat aufgrund der Stratigraphie des Norşuntepe" in *Chronologies des pays du Caucase et de L'Euphrate aux IVe-IIIe Millenaires,* ed. by C. Marro and H. Hauptmann, 419–448. Paris: Institut Français d'Études Anatoliennes d'Istanbul-De Boccard, 2000.

Ingholt, H., *Rapport préliminaire sur sept campagnes de fouilles à Hama en Syrie* (*1932–38*). Kopenhagen: Ejnar Munksgaard, 1940.

Karg, N., "Gre Dimse 1998: Preliminary Report" in *Salvage Project of the Archaeological Heritage of the Ilısu and Carchemish Dam Reservoirs Activities in 1999*, ed. by N. Tuna and J. Öztürk, 237–296. Ankara: Orta Doğu Teknik Üniversitesi, 1999.

Lapp, N. L., "Cylinder Seals and Impressions of the Third Millennium BC from the Dead Sea Plain." *Bulletin of the American Schools of Oriental Research* 273 (1989): 1–15.

Legrain, L., *Ur-Excavations III: Archaic Seal Impressions*. New York-London: Trustees of British Museum-University of Pennsylvania, 1936.

———. *Ur-Excavations X: Seal Cylinders*. New York-London: Trustees of British Museum-University of Pennsylvania, 1951.

Lüth, F., "Tell Halawa B" in *Halawa 1980–1986* (SBA 52), ed. by W. Orthmann, 85–109. Bonn: R. Habelt, 1989.

Mallowan, M. E. L., "Excavations at Brak and Chagar Bazar." *Iraq* 9 (1937): 1–259.

———. "Excavations at Tall Chagar Bazar and an Archaeological Survey of the Habur Region, Second Campaign, 1936." *Iraq* 4 (1947): 91–150.

Martin, H. P., *Fara: A Reconstruction of the Ancient Mesopotamian City of Shurrupak*. Birmingham: Chris Martin, 1988.

Martin, H. P. and R. J. Matthews, "Seals and Sealings" in *The 6G Ash-Tip and its Contents: Cultic and Administrative Discard from the Temple? Abu Salabikh Excavations 4,* ed. by A. Green, 23–81. Melksham: British School of Archaeology in Iraq, 1993.

Matthews, D. M., "Tell Brak 1990: The Glyptic." *Iraq* 53 (1991): 147–157.

———. *The Early Glyptic of Tell Brak: Cylinder Seals of Third Millennium Syria*. Orbis Biblicus et Orientalis 15, Series Archaeologica. Fribourg-Göttingen: University Press of Fribourg-Vadenhoeck & Ruprecht, 1997.

———. *Secrets of the Dark Mound: Jemdet Nasr 1926–1928*. Iraq Archaeological Reports 6. Wiltshire: British School of Archaeology in Iraq, 2002.

Mazzoni, S., "Seal Impressions on Jars from Ebla in EB IA-B." *Akkadica* 37 (1984): 18–44.

———. "Cylinder Seal Impressions on Jars at Ebla: New Evidence" in *Aspects of Art and Iconography: Anatolia and Its Neighbours. Studies in Honor of Nimet Özgüç*, ed. by M. J. Mellink, E. Porada and T. Özgüç, 399–414. Ankara: Türk Tarih Kurumu Basımevi, 1993.

———. "From the Late Chalcolithic to Early Bronze I in North-West Syria" in *Chronologies des pays du Caucase et de L'Euphrate aux IVe-IIIe Millenaires,* ed. by C. Marro and H. Hauptmann, 97–114 (Varia Anatolica 11). Paris: Institut Français d'Études Anatoliennes d'Istanbul-De Boccard, 2000.

McCarthy, A. P., "Glyptic" in *Jezirah. Associated Regional Chronologies of the Ancient Near East I,* ed. by M. Lebeau, 287–300. Turnhout: Brepols, 2011.

Meijer, D. J. W., *A Survey in Northeastern Syria*. Leiden: Nederlands Instituut voor her Nabije Oosten, 1986.

Moortgat, A., *Vorderasiatische Rollsiegel: Ein Beitrag zur Geschichte der Steinschneidekunst.* Berlin: Gebr. Mann Verlag, 1988.

Moortgat, A. and U. Moortgat-Correns, *Tell Chuera in Nordost-Syrien: Vorläufiger Bericht über die Siebente Grabungskampagne 1974.* Schriften der Max Freiherr von Oppenheim-Stiftung 9. Berlin: Gebr. Mann Verlag, 1976.

Moortgat-Correns, U., *Tell Chuera in Nordost-Syrien: Vorläufiger Bericht über die neunte und zehnte Grabungskampagne, 1982 und 1983.* Berlin: Gebr. Mann Verlag, 1988.

———. "Die Unveröffentlichen Rollsiegel vom Tell Chuera aus der Grabung 1955" in *Studies for Ancient Near Eastern Studies in Memoriam İ. Metin Akyurt and Bahattin Devam,* ed. by A. Erkanal, H. Erkanal, H. Hüryılmaz and A. T. Ökse, 221–222. İstanbul: Arkeoloji ve Sanat Yayınları, 1995.

Muchaev, R. M. and N. Y. Merpert, "Tell Hazna I-The Most Ancient Cult Centre in North-East Syria" in *Light on Top of the Black Hill. Studies Presented to Halet Çambel*, ed. by G. Arsebük, M. J. Mellink and W. Schirmer, 499–514. İstanbul: Ege Yayınları, 1998.

Oates, J., "The Evidence of the Sealings" in *Excavations at Tell Brak 2: Nagar in the Third Millennium BC*, ed. by D. Oates, J. Oates and H. McDonald, 121–150. Oxford: British School of Archaeology in Iraq, 2001.

Ökse, A. T., "Gre Virike'de Bulunan Silindir Mühür ve Kaplar Üzerindeki Silindir Mühür Baskıları" in *Cultural Reflections. Studies in Honor of Hayat Erkanal*, ed. by A. Erkanal-Öktü, E. Özgen S. Günel and E. Sifil, 546–551. İstanbul: Homer Kitabevi, 2006.

———. "Salat Tepe Orta Tunç Çağı Seramiklerinin Stratigrafik Dağılımı ve Tarihlendirilmesi" in *I. ODTÜ Arkeometri Çalıştayı. Türkiye Arkeolojisinde Seramik ve Arkeometrik Çalışmalar*, ed. by A. Özer and A. G. Türkmenoğlu, 50–60. Ankara: Orta Doğu Teknik Üniversitesi, 2009.

———. "Salat Tepe Stratigrafisine göre Yukarı Dicle Havzası Kronolojisi." *Ege Üniversitesi Edebiyat Fakültesi Arkeoloji Dergisi* 17:1–29 (2012).

Ökse, A. T. and A. Görmüş, "Excavations at Salat Tepe in The Upper Tigris Region: Stratigraphical Sequence and Preliminary Results of the 2005–2006 Seasons." *Akkadica* 127/2 (2006): 119–149.

Orthmann, W., *Tell Chuera: Ausgrabungen der Max Freiherr von Oppenheim-Stiftung in Nordost-Syrien*. Bonn: R. Habelt, 1990.

———. *Der Alte Orient*. Propyläen Kunstgeschichte 14. Berlin: Propyläen Verlag, 1975.

———. "Die Grabungen am Steinbau 1" in *Ausgrabungen in Tell Chuera in Nordost-Syrien I: Vorbericht über die Grabungskampagnen 1986 bis 1992*, ed. by W. Orthmann, 17–72. Saarbrücken: Saarbrücker Druckerei und Verlag, 1995.

Orthmann, W., H. Klein and F. Lüth, *Tell Chuera in Nordost-Syrien 1982–1983: Vorläufiger Bericht über die 9. und 10. Grabungskampagne*. Schriften der Max Freiherr von Oppenheim-Stiftung 12. Berlin: Gebr. Mann Verlag, 1986.

Otto, A., *"Die Entstehung und Entwicklung der Klassisch-Syrischen Glyptik"* Untersuchungen zur Assyriologie und vorderasiatischen Archäologie 8. Berlin-New York: De Gruyter, 2000.

Özgen, E., B. Helwing and H. Tekin, "Vorläufiger Bericht über die Ausgrabungen auf dem Oylum Höyük." *Istanbuler Mitteilungen* 47 (1997): 39–90.

Özkan, S. and A. Öztan, "Samsat Höyük Kalkolitik ve Eski Tunç Çağı Mühürleri" in *Studies in Honour of Altan Çilingiroğlu: A Life Dedicated to Urartu on the Shores of the Upper Sea*, ed. by H. Sağlamtimur, E. Abay, A. Uü. Erdem, A. Batmaz, F. Dedeoğlu, M. Erdalkıran, M. B. Baştürk, E. Konakçı, 479–488. İstanbul: Arkeoloji ve Sanat Yayınları, 2009.

Palmieri, A., "Excavations at Arslantepe (Malatya)." *Anatolian Studies* 31 (1981): 101–119.

Parayre, D., "Seals and Seal Impressions From Tell Leilan 1985." *American Journal of Archaeology* 94 (1990): 556–567.

Parker, J. B., A. Creekmore, E. Moseman and R. Sasaki, "The Upper Tigris Archaeological Research Project (UTARP). A Preliminary Report from the Year 2000 Excavations at Kenan Tepe" in *Salvage Project of the Archaeological Heritage of the Ilısu and Carchemish Dam Reservoirs, Activities in 2000,* ed. by N. Tuna and J. Velibeyoğlu, 613–643. Ankara: Orta Doğu Teknik Üniversitesi, 2002.

Parker, J. B. and L. Swartz Dodd, "The Early Second Millennium Ceramic Assemblage from Kenan Tepe, Southeastern Turkey. A Preliminary Assessment." *Anatolian Studies* 53 (2003): 33–69.

Peltenburg, E., S. Campbell, P. Croft, D. Lunt, M. A. Murray and M. E. Watt (eds.), "Jerablus-Tahtani, Syria, 1992–4: Preliminary Report." *Levant* 27 (1995): 1–28.

Pittman, H., *The Glazed Steatite Glyptic Style. The Structure and Function of an Image System in the Administration of Protoliterate Mesopotamia*. Berliner Beiträge zum Vorderen Orient 16. Berlin: Dietrich Reimer Verlag, 1994.

Porada, E., *Corpus of Ancient Near Eastern Seals in North American Collections: The Collection of the Pierpont Morgan Library*. The Bollingen Series 14. Washington: The Bollingen Foundation, 1948.

Sagona, A. G., *The Aşvan Sites 3: The Early Bronze Age*. Monograph 18. Ankara: The British Institute of Archaeology at Ankara, 1994.

Schwartz, G. M., H. H. Curvers, S. Dunham and B. Stuart, "A Third Millennium BC Elite Tomb and Other New Evidence from Tell Umm el-Marra, Syria." *American Journal of Archaeology* 107 (2003): 325–361.

Sertok, K. and R. Ergeç, "A New EBA Cemetery. Excavations near the Birecik Dam, SE Turkey. Preliminary Report (1997–98)." *Anatolica* 25 (1999): 87–107.

Strommenger, E. and K. Kohlmeyer, *Tall Bi'a-Tuttul I: Die altorientalischen Bestattungen*. Saarbrücken: Saarbrücker Druckerei und Verlag, 1998.

Swartz Dodd, L., "Filling a Niche: Settlement Expansion and Innovation in the Upper Tigris River Valley during the Middle Bronze Age" in *Looking North: The Socioeconomic Dynamics of the Northern Mesopotamian and Anatolian Regions during the Late Third and Early Second Millennium BC*, ed. by N. Laneri, P. Pfälzner and S. Valentini, 213–228. Wiesbaden: Harrassowitz Verlag, 2012.

Teissier, B., *Ancient Near Eastern Seals from the Marcopoli Collection*. Berkeley-Los Angeles-London: University of California Press, 1984.

Valdés Pereiro, C., "Tell Qara Quzaq: A Summary of the First Results" in *Archaeology of the Upper Syrian Euphrates: The Tishrin Dam Area*, Aula Orientalis-Supplementa, ed. by G. Del Olmo Lete and J.-L. Montero Fenollós, 117–127. Barcelona: AUSA, 1999.

Van Loon, M., "1974 and 1975 Preliminary Results of the Excavations at Selenkahiye Near Meskene, Syria" in *Archeological Reports from the Tabqa Dam Project: Euphrates Valley, Syria*, The Annual of the American Schools of Oriental Research 44, 97–112. American Schools of Oriental Research: Cambridge U.S.A., 1979.

———. "Hammâm et-Turkmân on the Balikh: First Results of the University of Amsterdam's 1982 Excavation." *Akkadica* 35 (1983): 1–23.

———. *Selenkahiye: Final Report on the University of Chicago and University of Amsterdam Excavations in the Tabqa Reservoir, Northern Syria, 1967–1975.* Leiden: Nederlands Instituut voor her Nabije Oosten, 2001.

Werner, P., *Tall Munbaqa-Ekalte III: Die Glyptik.* Wissenschaftliche Veröffentlichungen der Deutschen Orient-Gesellschaft 108. Saarbrücken: Saarbrücker Verlag, 2004.

Wiseman, D. J., *Catalogue of the Western Asiatic Seals in the British Museum I: Cylinder Seals, Uruk-Early Dynastic Periods.* London: The Trustees of the British Museum, 1962.

Revisiting the Issue of Late Bronze II Drab Ware with Potmarks

Remzi Yağcı[1]

Abstract

Potmarked vessels excavated in many LBA contexts have led to various interpretations about the probable functions of these potmarks. One of the most remarkable suggestions is to explain the presence of these potmarks as evidence of political and socio-economic affiliations of a given region in the Hittite period. This paper aims to re-assess the function of these potmarks by focusing on pottery assemblages of Soli Höyük dated to the 15th and 14th centuries BC in order to provide a better perception of administration and control of trade in the Hittite province of Kizzuwatna.

Many excavation reports focusing on the Late Bronze Age (LBA) contexts and related publications abound in pottery on which there are incised potmarks. Although these potmarks are frequently noted, they have not been subjected to thorough examination until recently.[2] The literature on potmarks has primarily tried to comment upon the vessels and the location of the marks in order to explain their possible function(s) and their linguistic significance.[3] Recent research has, on the other hand, underlined the importance of the marks as a source of information for political and socio-economic affiliations of the period.[4] In this paper,[5] which places special emphasis on Soli Höyük, by studying and re-assessing why, how and where the vessels were marked, I aim to reach a better understanding of the administration and control of trade in the Hittite controlled province of Kizzuwatna. I dedicate this article to Marie-Henriette Gates and Charles Gates for their invaluable contribution to Anatolian archaeology and their devotion to teaching Archaeology. I think that this article will mean more to Marie-Henriette who has pioneered research on Anatolian potmarks.

1 Dokuz Eylül University, Faculty of Letters, Department of Museology, Tınaztepe Campus, Buca, İzmir.

2 Glatz 2012.

3 Mielke 2006.

4 Gates 2001.

5 This paper was originally presented at the 6th International Congress on the Archaeology of the Ancient Near East in London, in April 2010.

A brief look at recent publications reveals a number of comprehensive studies on the subject. For instance Hirschfeld [6] and Lindblom [7] investigated the significance of these marks in Cypriot-Mycenaean pottery, while Mielke [8] and Gates studied them in Hittite or Hittite-controlled territory. Mielke associated these marks with Luwian hieroglyphs whereas Gates discussed these potmarks in a wider perspective and suggested that these potmarks were "indices for wide-scale government enterprise revealing the complex relationships between the center and the periphery." [9] More recently Glatz underlined that there are "clear regional differences in contemporary traditions that are indicative of different communities of practice rather than a centrally homogenized production organization." [10] Remarkably, she also highlighted that these marks were frequently used in earlier periods, for instance in Arslantepe, with fewer signs of centralized authority. [11]

The mass-produced drab ware was the most dominant pottery type of LB II period. Within Hittite controlled territory and economy, drab ware is represented by a monochrome fabric produced in a limited range of shapes and it was widely distributed. The most common forms of drab ware were plates, platters, and craters supplemented by less frequent juglets, pitchers and flasks. Frequently, drab ware vessels were incised with different potmarks consisting of lines, cuts, wedges, ovals etc. before firing. The incised potmarks on the shoulder, base or body of the mass-produced monochrome drab wares were common both at the center (i.e. Boğazköy, Maşat Höyük, Kuşaklı, Alacahöyük, Gordion, Korucutepe) and in the peripheries (i.e. in Kilise Tepe, Soli, Yumuktepe, Tarsus and Kinet Höyük) during the LB II (15th and 13th centuries) in Anatolia. [12]

Different Interpretations

As stated, these potmarks have been interpreted in different ways. Interpretations include a wide range of possibilities as regards "the future owner, consumer, and recipient or alternatively, place the storage location, contents or intended purpose of the contents of marked vessels within a state-controlled environment." [13] Firstly, potmarks were seen as a sign of a professional potter or potter's workshop. Since

6 Hirschfield 1992, 315–319; Hirschfield 1993, 311–318; Hirschfield 2008,1–2.

7 Lindblom 2007, 1–2.

8 Mielke 2006, 153–154.

9 Gates 2001.

10 Glatz 2012.

11 Glatz 2012, 3

12 *Cf.* Gates 2001, 138; Glatz 2012, 6, fig. 1

13 Glatz 2012, 6.

the demand for pottery production necessitates cooperative labor in a precise routine, potters might use these marks to signal individual production.[14] The large numbers of potmarks in the mass-produced LB II Anatolian drab ware assemblage may show that the potters in the Hittite Period used to mark their own products in shared or multiple work facilities where payment—in any form—was apportioned individually. In brief, the potmarks were seen as indicators of potter's workshops.

Secondly, in a wider framework, the potmarks were regarded as indicators of a large scale industry with specific standards that may change locally. As recent research straightforwardly puts forward the application of single potmarks and a standardized ceramic industry with local mass-production were common to the eastern Mediterranean states of the LBA, from Mycenaean Greece to Cyprus, the Levant and Egypt.[15]

Thirdly, these marks were interpreted as an indicator of controlled enterprise in the Hittite empire. According to the textual evidence, there were similar kinds of markings on other commodity types such as metal ingots and herded animals.[16] The assumption that these marks were associated with Luwian Hieroglyphs i.e., reading the marks as Luwian logograms such as King (REX L. 14)[17] and City (URBS L. 225) seem to strengthen the presence of central economic control. Mielke studied the Kuşaklı pottery repertoire by re-discussing the views of Müller-Karpe, Gates and Glatz.[18] Mielke distinguishes two main types of potmarks in Kuşaklı.[19] In the first group, there are potmarks that may be read as Luwian hieroglyphs and he refers to three logograms (the King (L.14), City (L. 225) and Happiness/Health (L. 370). Mielke claims that there are other potmarks that cannot be read or interpreted as script and suggests that supra-regional and more detailed research is needed for more concrete conclusions. However, these potmarks that cannot be classified as script, he suggests, may refer to the type of pottery or the quantity they contain. More interestingly, Mielke highlights the relationship with some vessel shapes and some marks.[20]

Gates, on the other hand, refuses the association between the potmarks and script and highlights other functions of the potmarks. Gates' hypothesis claims that prefiring potmarks are diagnostic of a centralized economy through which the Hittite state sought to bring even distant regions under effective administra-

14 Hirschfield 1992, 315–319; Hirschfield 1993, 311–318; Hirschfield 2008,1–2.

15 Hirschfield 2008; Gates 2001, 140.

16 Gates 2001, 141.

17 Gates 2001, 141.

18 Mielke 2006, 151–155.

19 Mielke 2006, 151–155.

20 Mielke 2006, 151–155.

tive control.[21] More recently, Glatz in her detailed study compares findspots for vessels, location of potmarks, associations of marks with vessel forms as well as distribution patterns of potmark motifs and relative motif diversity and points out the existence of regional differences rather than evidence of a standardized and centralized system.[22] Under the light shed by those abovementioned views on LBA drab ware with potmarks, if the assemblage of Soli is revisited, it may provide insights into some of these problematic and open-ended interpretations.

Context

Soli Pompeiopolis excavations 11 km west of Mersin provide useful contextualized material to revisit the issue of potmarks through the pottery sherds with incised potmarks. According to written sources Soli must have been located on the border between Tarhuntassa and Kizzuwatna in the 2nd millennium BC.[23] Soli possibly was a very important harbor city for both land and maritime commercial activity in the Kizzuwatna-Hittite territory. Archaeologically, the ceramic repertoire of the Hittite Imperial period mainly consists of Red Lustrous Wheel-made (or its local production red burnished) ware,[24] painted pottery with cross-hatching decoration,[25] White Slip II pottery[26] and mass produced "drab ware" of which some with potmarks were found, revealing the position of Soli both as a part of centralized and/or local economy and as an active port located on an international trade route. There are several suggestions on the possible toponymy of Soli in the 2nd millennium BC, T. Bryce claims that Soli may be identified with Ura[27] attested in the Hittite texts during LBA. Ellipra and Egara (İngirā)[28] are other possibilities.

Pottery with potmarks in Soli Höyük is found within an official context and is closely associated with the surrounding fortification walls[29] that are partly unearthed (Fig. 1). The most prominent evidence related to the fortification wall system is the fact that a bulla *(m)u-wa-zi* (Fig. 2),[30] a grain jar (Fig. 3) containing

21 Gates 2001,137–138.

22 Glatz 2012, 34–35.

23 As it was Cilicia Aspera and Cilicia Campestris or Pedias in the Classical Period.

24 Jean 2006, 325–327.

25 Yağcı 2010.

26 Yağcı 2003.

27 Bryce 2009, 662.

28 Yağcı 2001, 161; Yağcı 2007, 798; Forlanini 2013, 3–4.

29 Lorenz and Schrakamp 2011, 146; for detailed bibliography see note 90.

30 Yağcı 2007, 800, n. 21.

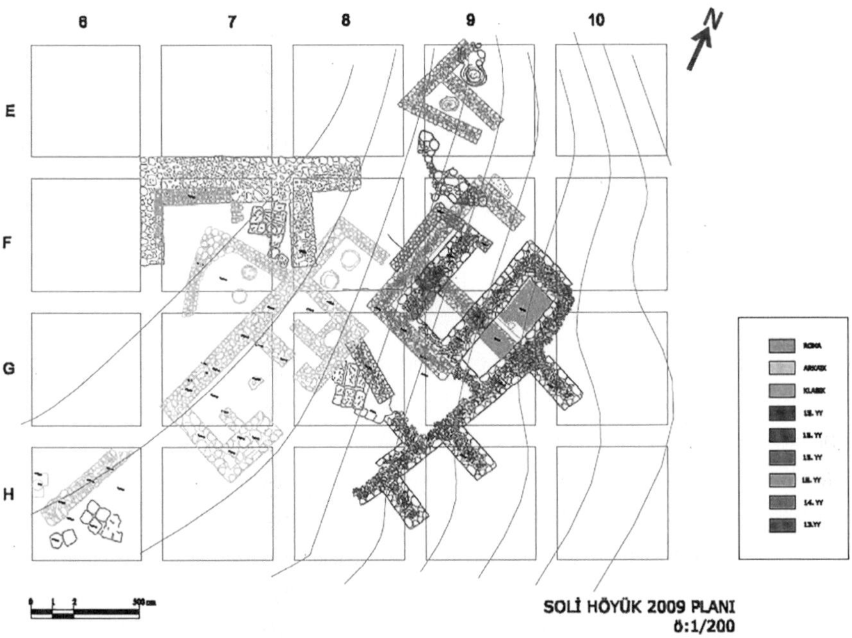

FIG. 1 Plan of Soli Höyük Fortification Walls

carbonized barley (*Hordaeum vulgare*)[31]seeds according to C14 analysis[32] and a plate with a potmark (FIG. 4) within an ash layer were found just behind the fortification walls in the east of the mound (FIG. 5).[33] Barley was among the most frequent grains that were stored in these facilities both for official and domestic purposes.[34] In the Hittite texts, apart from being an animal feed, barley was cited

31 Excavation in Soli Pompeiopolis (2009) provided further carbonized grains. The majority of the grains were barley *Hordeum vulgare* (150 grains), a relatively low number of emmer wheat *Triticum dicoccum* (50 grains) and lentils *Lens culinaris* (16 grains). Although there is scant archaeological evidence on the type of grains (alimenta), we know that barley and emmer wheat were among the most common type of grains in the Hittite world. Barley seeds were unearthed in the temple contexts in Kuşaklı and Maşat Höyük, see Hoffner 2001, 201–203. ŠE in the Hittite texts is equivalent to barley, *Hordeum vulgare*, see Ertem 1974, 4–6. In many Bronze Age societies, barley and different species of wheat formed also the basis of cereal production due to guaranteed minimum harvest even in hardest weather and geographical conditions. Dörfler *et al.* 2011, 106.

32 See footnote 28

33 In Hittite cities, storerooms were closely connected to defense systems and the most typical example of this connection is seen in Boğazköy where the storeroom is directly located at the back of the postern wall. Dörfler *et al.* 2011, fig. 4.

34 Hoffner 2001, 202–203, fig.1, ZÍZ (bread wheat) and ŠE are more frequently used than *šeppit* (einkorn) and KANĀSU (emmer).

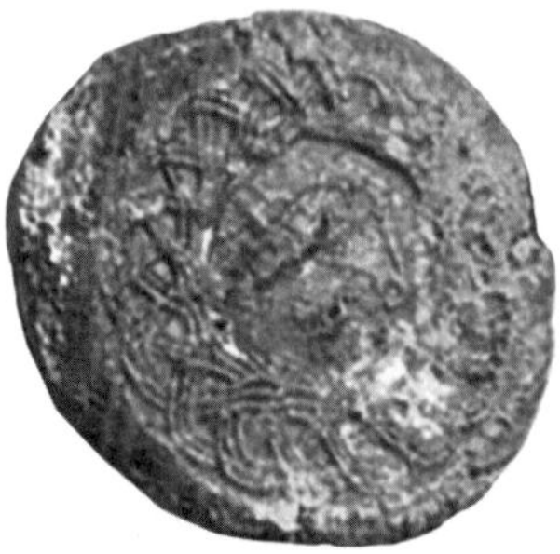

FIG. 2 Muwazi bulla

as soldiers' provision which was measured in *PARISU* and distributed to soldiers together with wheat during military campaigns.[35] According to law, barley was cheaper than wheat and 1 *PARISU* was equivalent to ¼ silver shekel.[36]

According to published material, the findspots of pottery with potmarks are rather sporadic. Most of the marks come from habitation areas. Official and religious contexts and burial sites are other spots where pottery with potmarks were frequently excavated. In Korucutepe, potmarks are associated with the Phase I fortification system and the summit of the mound.[37] In this context, there is a close parallelism with Korucutepe since Soli Höyük's assemblage is also found in a context related with the fortification wall system.

The casemate fortification on the slopes of Soli Höyük dates back to the 15th century BC. Foundations and the walls of buildings from the Hittite Imperial Period (14th and 13th centuries), were also unearthed. The 1.35 m wide wall on the eastern slope of the mound is located at the level 13.91 m and is fortified by casemates as casemate rooms are built in. Mudbricks used for the construction of casemates were manufactured in standardized sizes (18x13 cm 9.10 cm wide). Chronologically, the casemate walls of Soli Höyük are in close parallelism with Yumuktepe walls,[38] Boğazköy uppercity walls and Yerkapı Büyükkaya North walls.[39]

35 Hoffner 2009, 83, 164–165. The texts from Tapikka/Maşat Höyük, demonstrate a reorganization and reconstitution of territories and the letters reveal that groups up to twenty-two persons were supervised by a DUGUD-officer and they were provided with barley rations of two *sūtu* per person

36 Ertem 1974, 4–6.

37 Glatz 2012, 12.

38 2 Sigma calibrated result (%95 probabilty): Cal. BC 1440 to 1380. According to the report provided by Beta Analytic Radiocarbon Dating Laboratory. *cf.* Jean 2006, 326; Manuelli 2009, 257.

39 Naumann 1971, 255, 310–311, figs. 327, 328. Mielke 2011, 178; Lorenz and Schrakamp 2011, 146, for a detailed bibliography see note 90. The earliest casemate walls and rooms in Anatolia are unearthed in Kizzuwatna again, in Yumuktepe in the Chalcholitic period (level XVI) and the most developed version in Tarsus in the EBA. Naumann 1971, fig. 305–307. J. Garstang suggests that casemate rooms are connected to

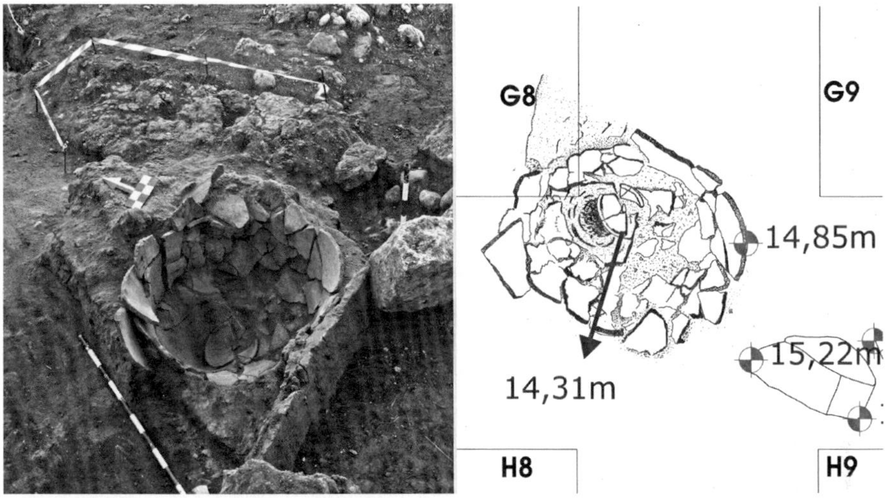

FIG. 3 The grain jar and the plate with potmark

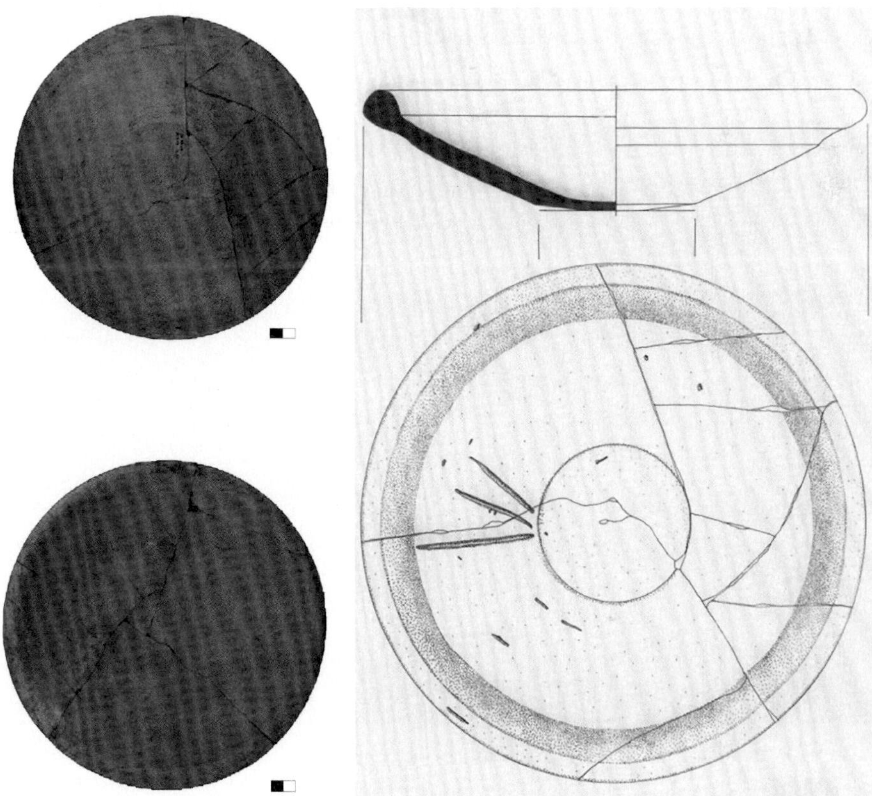

FIG. 4 Plate with potmark

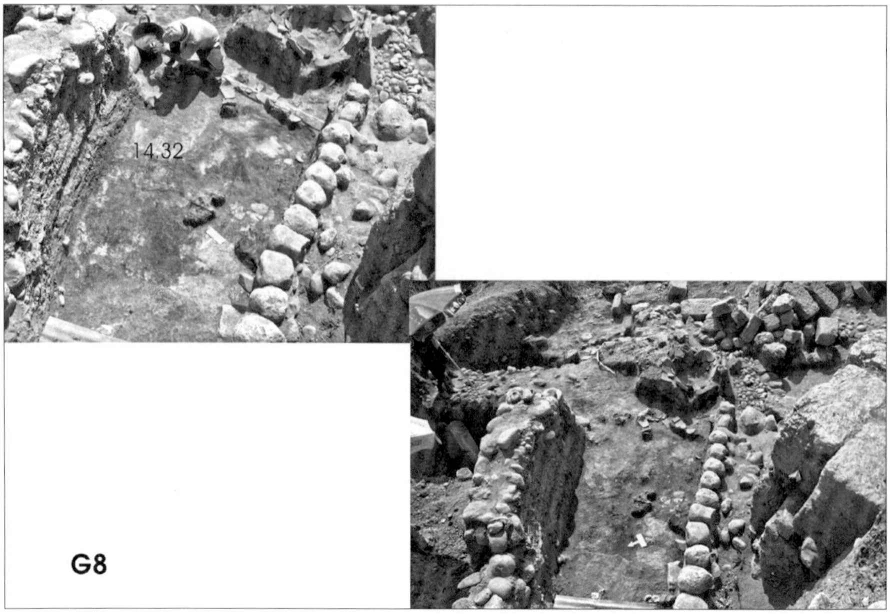

Fig. 5 Ash layer adjoining the fortification wall and the grain jar

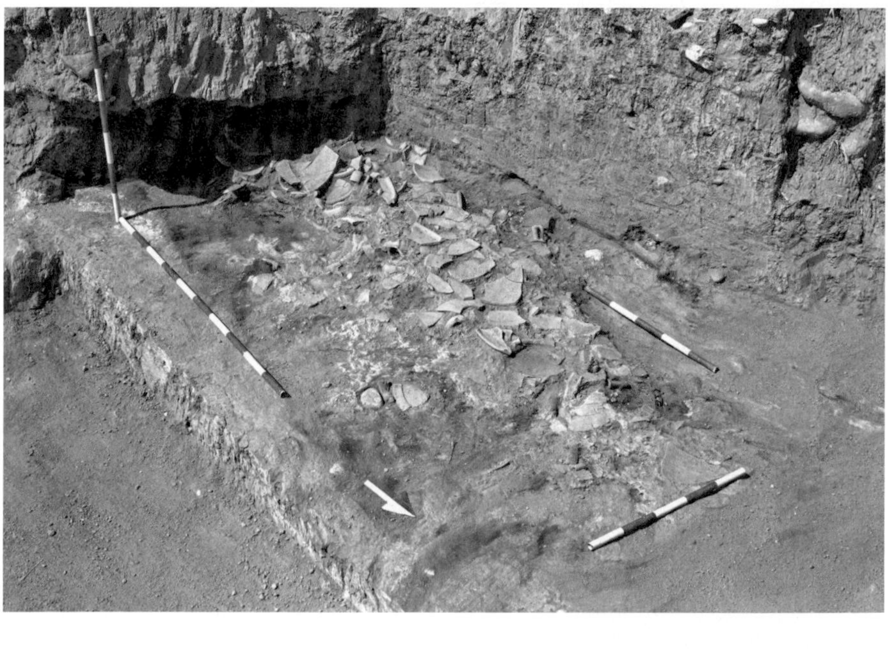

Fig. 6 Pottery assemblage dated to 15th century in the debris

Casemate rooms—from the Chalcholithic Period to the Hittite Period—seem to be related to storerooms and grain jars. The barley jar and the plate excavated near the casemate wall in Soli Höyük point to a functional relationship.

These rooms in the Hittite Period were not used for residential purposes rather they were used as storerooms for both food and ammunition. The grain jar and a number of monochrome plate with a potmark were found in a burnt layer in Soli Höyük. This context is closely related to the casemate rooms and thus the wall.

The plate with the potmark within the grain jar may be seen as an indicator of the fact that the measurement system and control mechanisms decided upon the border treaties between the Hittites and Kizzuwatna were stil valid. In other words, the walls of Soli and Yumuktepe are indicative of the border treaties between the Hittites and Kizzuwatna. In these treaties, all kinds of measurement were standardized and the issues of defense were decided.[40] It is evident that these issues were elaborated carefully.

The architectural remains demonstrate that Soli was among these cities that were fortified in the 15th century BC.[41] The remains reveal that the walls were destroyed by a devastating fire and were no longer in use in the 14th century and the rectangular buildings with big kilns and workshops were built on those walls.[42]

In Cilicia, the context in which pottery with incised potmarks were frequently unearthed is dated to the 15th century BC. Similar to other Hittite centers in Cilicia, at Soli Höyük these drab ware vessels began to be used in from the Middle Hittite Period. As is stated, Soli in the 15th century was surrounded by city walls and the sherds are found scattered within and/or under the ash layer. Garstang, suggests that the ceramic evidence that is closely related to fortification walls reveals that the Hittite cultural sphere has begun in the level VII in Yumuktepe east of Soli.[43] A large number of pottery with or without potmarks have been found

married soldiers by taking into account the fact that hearths, cooking pots and grain jars are excavated together within these contexts. Garstang 1953, 249–250.

40 For instance, the treaty between Sunassura, the King of Kizzuwatna and Suppiluliuma (1350–1320 BC.) or Tuthalia I/II (1450–1420 BC), the king of the Hittites states that: "Toward the sea *Lamiya* belongs to the *Sun* (and) *Pitura* belongs to *Sunassura;* They will measure out of the territory together and divide (it). The *Sun* will not fortify *Lamiya*. *Aruna* belongs to the *Sun*. Toward *Pitura they will measure out the territory and divide (it) themselves*. The *Sun* must not fortify *Aruna*." Goetze, 1940, 51.

41 There is no proof that Soli was still fortified in the 14th and 12th centuries.

42 Yağcı 2009 , figs. 2, 3, 6

43 Garstang dates this period to the 15th century BC and identifies the presence of early Hittite ceramic in relation to the agreement between Isputahsu, the king of Kizzuwatna and Telipinu, the Hittite king and he claims that the Yumuktepe walls were built during Telipinu's reign. Garstang 1953, 237-238. The fortification walls in Soli (if they were still used) and Yumuktepe show us that these cities were strategically important for both kingdoms since they were fortified.

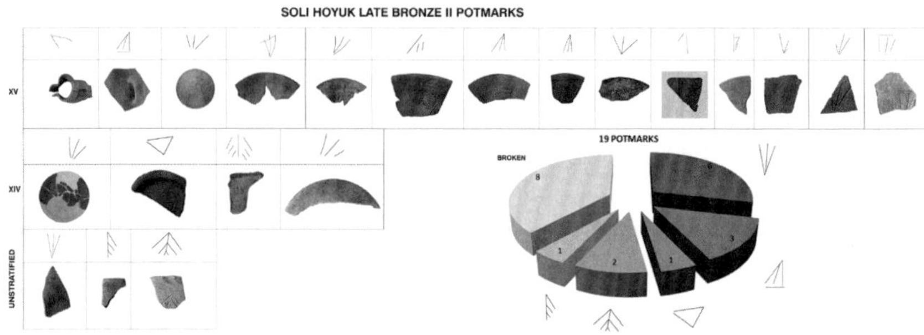

FIG. 7 Soli Höyük Late Bronze II potmarks

within the burnt layer of the 15th century. Their find spot adjoining the casemate rooms suggests that they have a governmental or official function related to the fortification walls. They might be used to distribute grains or provisions to soldiers. Especially, the grain jar with barley remains is important to reassess the function of the pottery with potmarks. We can assume by looking at the poor quantity of barley in the grain jar that the city had withstood for a long period before it had fallen into fire and destruction. We are able to date the fire layer thanks to C14 analysis and a HH bulla (*(m)u-wa-zi*) dated to the 15th century BC. The C14 analysis of barley grains founded in grain jar adjoining the fortification walls that were located at the center of Gridsquares G8, G9, H8 and H9 enables us to date the context to the 15th century BC. The grains identified as barley (*Hordeum vulgare*) were dated to 1440–1380 BC through double calibration procedures. These finds help us give a more or less precise date for the context.

Soli Assemblage

Having discussed different interpretations of potmarks and the archaeological contexts in which potmarked vessels have been found, it is essential to look at the Soli assemblage as a whole and reach at some conclusions on probable functions of these potmarks. At Soli Höyük, a total of twenty one drab ware sherds incised with potmarks have been unearthed together with a wide ceramic repertoire (FIG. 7). Most of these sherds (14 sherds) were found within the fire layer dated to the 14th century BC. Four sherds were unearthed in the 15th century and three of the sherds with potmarks were recorded in unstratified spots.

SOLI Chronology & Assemblage	Typology[44]	Spatial Distribution	Probable Explanation	Pottery Type
XV1	Type 2-simple chevrons	Alacahöyük, Hattusa, Tarsus, İmikuşağı	Different professions denoting administrative categories, ration distribution	Closed form (XV1)
XV2, 4, 14	Type 10c-triangles	Alacahöyük, Maşathöyük, Korucutepe	Luwian Hieroglyph for king or an associated symbol for royalty, connection with royal store houses and distribution systems	Closed form handle (XV2), open form (XV 4, 14)
XV 3,5, 6, 7, 8, 9, 10(?),11(?), 12, 13 XIV 1, 4, Unstratified I	Type 3-chevrons with one parallel line in one side	Kinet Höyük Tarsus	Profession (?), ration distribution	Open form (XV3, 5–10, 12, 13) (fig.9) Open form (XIV 1,4), Open ware (Unstratified1)
XIV 3, Unstratified 2,3	Type 6- tree or twig motifs	Hattusa(?) Alacahöyük Tarsus	Unknown	Closed form, handle (XIV 3), Open form (Unstratified 2, 3)
XIV 2	Type 10a-triangles	Gordion, Mersin-Kinet Höyük, Korucutepe	Luwian Hieroglyph for health and luck	Base- closed form (XIV2)

Table 1

Table 1 shows the distribution of potmarks from the Soli assemblage. Most of the four types, namely Type 2 (one example), Type 3 (thirteen examples), Type 6 (three examples), Type 10 (four examples), are seen on nineteen sherds with potmarks

44 Typology after Glatz 2012, fig. 2

from Soli Höyük. Most of them are body sherds (18) and there are two handles (2) and a base (1). Only one marked sherd belongs to painted pottery (XV 6) while all the others are monochrome drab ware.

Type 2, simple chevrons, is represented by a single sherd, from the body of a closed ware. Type 10 (both 10a and 10c), triangles, is one of the best known motifs, potmark usually associated with the Luwian hieroglyph for "king" (REX) (L. 14),[45] or luck and health (BONUM/SANITAS?) (L. 370) and generally accepted to indicate a connection with royal storehouses and distribution systems. Type 10 is represented by four examples in the Soli assemblage. Three bear dissected triangles whereas the other one bears a simple triangle (FIG. 8). Type 6, tree or twig motifs, is represented by three examples, one dated to the 14th century and two unstratified sherds. It is one of the rare motifs for marked pottery in the Hittite geography and it is remarkable to find them among the Soli examples in Cilicia.

Type 3, chevrons with one parallel line in one side, according to Glatz' typology is the most frequent potmark and is represented by thirteen samples in the Soli Assemblage. This type seems to be closely related to Cilicia according to present publications and strengthens Gates' suggestion as indicating the existence of a local standard production as is the case with Kinet Höyük and Tarsus pottery with potmarks.[46] The plate found in the grain jar bears also a Type 3 potmark and is a medium sized example of this primarily Cilician pattern and mode of production. The context in which the plate is found, i.e., the grain jar just behind the fortification walls is highly important as it suggests a possible function of the plate and the potmark on it. The plate weighs 952 gr. together with the weight of the jar in which it was found. This plate might well be used as a scale while distributing ration allowance to officials/soldiers as a part of widespread and/or local system of measurement. Moreover, the typology of potmarks and the profile and shape of related pottery may be compared to the examples of Kinet Höyük as evidence of a locally produced standard pottery with potmarks in different sizes, which were probably used for measurement in a mostly regional level.[47]

In the Soli assemblage, most of the sherds (18 sherds) are from open and shallow vessels (most probably plates) and only three sherds belong to medium to large sized closed vessels. Two of them are handles and the third one is a base on which the motif of a triangle is clearly visible. The open vessels are generally marked below the rim and the lower vessel body. This seems to strengthen the argument that there is a tendency to mark open vessels in Cilician centers. If we persist in our hypothesis of the existence of a local measurement, distribution and

45 Mielke 2006, 153, fig. 145.

46 Glatz 2012, 22.

47 Gates 2001, fig. 8, 1–3 and fig. 9.

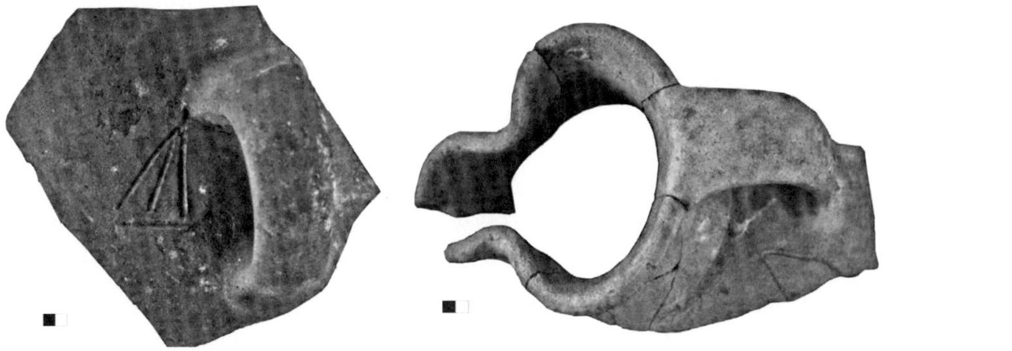

Fig. 8 Closed forms (Type 10c and Type 2)

mass production system, the closed vessels might be used to measure liquids and the potmarks on the vessels (Type 2, Type 6, Type 10) may refer to the volume or the content of the container.

Table 1 also provides information on the correlations of potmarks between different centers. Although there is a clear prevalence of Type 3 and a high level similarity with Tarsus and Kinet Höyük, Korucutepe has also a connection to Soli both in terms of the findspots and type of potmarks (Type 10). The analysis also reveals low level connections with other Hittite centers such as Alacahöyük, Maşathöyük, Hattuša, etc.[48]

Within this framework, if we revisit the twenty one potmarks from Soli Höyük, we firstly see that these are mostly in the common shape of Type 3 (13) and Type 2 (1) and as is demonstrated in Table 1, they are probably a reference to different professions denoting administrative categories or to ration distribution. I suggest that these potmarks refer to the capacity of the container depending on whether it is a closed or open vessel. The open and shallow vessels might be used to measure grains while the closed vessels were used for liquids. A similar function may also be valid for Type 10 potmarks. The triangle shape was mostly incised on open vessels in Cilicia, however, the examples of Soli seem to add a different dimension to the discussion since here we see that Type 10 (both 10a and 10c) potmarks were incised both on open and closed vessels. At the first sight, these drab ware vessels may look rather simple to reveal a connection to royal/central authority. However, a holistic look at the Soli examples suggests that these vessels may be manufactured to fit to standards adopted by the King or a local authority especially if we focus on the appearance of Type 3 potmarks as is seen in the

48 *Cf.* C. Glatz 2012, fig. 2.

plate found within the barley jar and those in Type 10 which are associated with the King or a royal storehouse and distribution system. These marks most likely reflect a wide-spread industry conforming locally to standards set elsewhere; most probably by the central authority and/or a local authority related to the state.

Only a limited number of pottery bears potmarks and this strengthens the view that these marks had a specific function. Since each and every vessel is not incised with potmarks, this practice was not surely coincidental. For instance, in Kinet Höyük, only 10–15% of vessels are marked.[49] The fact that all the drab ware vessels were not marked seems to complicate to interpret these potmarks as mere signs since this interpretation remains partial and narrow under given circumstances. Although these marks have been widely accepted to signify pottery workshop or the potter in accordance with functional and traditional usages, our case provides promising insights about further uses of these marks and pottery vessels bearing them. Overall, all these factors together with the analysis of the marked pottery in Soli may indicate one or several means of organizing local standardized production in the Hittite-Kizzuwatna region.

49 M-H.Gates, Potmarks and the Late Bronze Pottery, pp.137–138, 143.

REFERENCES

Bryce, T., *The Routledge Handbook of the Peoples and Places of Ancient Western Asia*, New York: Routledge, 2009.

Dörfler, W., C. Herking, R. Neef, R. Pasternak, A. von den Driesch, "Environment and Economy in Hittite Anatolia" in *Insights into Hittite History and Archaeology*, ed. by H. Genz and D.P. Mielke, 99–124. Leuven: Peeters, 2011.

Ertem, H. *Boğazköy Metinlerine Göre Hititler Devri Anadolusu'nun Florası*, Ankara: Türk Tarih Kurumu, 1974.

Forlanini, M., "How to Infer Ancient Roads and Itineraries from Heterogeneus Hittite Texts: The Case of The Cilician (Kizzuwatnean) Road System." *KASKAL* 10 (2013): 13–34.

Garstang, J., *Prehistoric Mersin, Yumuktepe in Southern Turkey*, Oxford: Clarendon Press, 1953.

Gates, M-H., "Potmarks and the Late Bronze Pottery Industry" in *La Cilicie – espaces et pouvoirs locaux IIe millénaire av. J.-C. – IVe siècle ap. J.-C.*, ed. by É. Jean et al. 137–157. Paris: De Boccard, 2001.

Genz H. and Mielke, D.P. (eds.), *Insights into Hittite History and Archaeology*, Colloquia Antiqua 2. Leuven: Peeters, 2011.

Glatz, C., "Bearing the Marks of Control: Reassessing Pot Marks in Late Bronze Age Anatolia." *American Journal of Archaeology* 116 (2012): 5–38.

Goetze, A., *Kizzuwatna and the Problem of Hittite Geography*. Yale Oriental Series Researches 22. New Haven: Yale University Press, 1940.

Hirschfield, N., "Cypriot Marks on Mycenaean Pottery" in *Mykenaika*, ed. by J.P. Olivier, *Bulletin de Correspondance Hellénique*, CH Supplement 25, 315–319. Paris, 1992.

———. "How and Why Potmarks Matter." *Near Eastern Archaeology* 71, (2008): 1–2.

———. "Incised Marks (Post-Firing) on Aegean wares" in *Wace and Blegen. Pottery as Evidence for Trade in the Aegean Bronze Age 1939–1989*, ed. by C. Zerner *et al.* 311–318. Amsterdam: J.C. Gieben, 1993.

Hoffner H. A. Jr., "Alimenta Revisited" in *Akten des IV. internationalen Kongresses für Hethitologie, Würzburg, 4.-8. Oktober 1999*, ed. by G. Wilhelm, 199–212. Wiesbaden: Harrassowitz Verlag, 2001.

———. *Writings from the Ancient World Letters from the Hittite Kingdom*. Atlanta: Society of Biblical Literature, 2009.

Jean É. *et al.* (eds.), *La Cilicie – espaces et pouvoirs locaux IIe millénaire av. J.-C. – IVe siècle ap. J.-C.*, Varia Anatolica XIII. Paris: De Boccard, 2001.

———. "The Hittites at Mersin-Yumuktepe: Old Problems and New Directions" in *Structuring and Dating in Hittite Archaeology*, ed. by D.P. Mielke, U.-D. Schoop, J. Seeher, 311–332. İstanbul: Ege Yayınları, 2006.

Lindblom, M., "Book Review, N. Hirschfeld, Marks and Makers: Appearance, Distribution and the Function of Middle and Late Helladic Manufacturers' Mark on

Aeginetan Pottery." *American Journal of Archaeology Online Book Reviews*, January (2007): 1–2.

Lorenz, J., I. Schrakamp, "Hittite Military and Warfare" in *Insight into Hittite History and Archaeology*, Colloquia Antiqua 2, ed. by H. Genz and D. P. Mielke, 125–152. Leuven: Peeters, 2011.

Manuelli, F., "Local Imitations and Foreign Imported Goods. Some Problems and New Questions on Red Lustrous Wheel-Made Ware in the Light of the New Excavations of the Southern Step Trench at Yumuktepe/Mersin." *Altorientalische Forschungen* 36 (2009): 251–267.

Mielke, D.P., *Die Keramik vom Westhang. Kuşaklı – Sarissa*. Rahden: VML Vlg Marie Leidof, 2006

———. "Hittite Cities: Looking for a Concept" in *Insights into Hittite History and Archaeology*, Colloquia Antiqua 2, ed. by H. Genz and D. P. Mielke, 153–194. Leuven: Peeters, 2011.

Naumann, R., *Architektur Kleinasiens von ihren Anfangen bis zum Ende der hethitischen Zeit*. Tübingen: Wasmuth, 1971.

Wilhelm, G. (ed.), *Akten des IV. Internationalen Kongresses für Hethitologie, Würzburg, 4.-8. Oktober 1999*. Wiesbaden: Harrassowitz Verlag, 2001.

Yağcı, R., "The Importance of Soli in the Archaeology of Cilicia in the Second Millennium BC" in *La Cilicie – espaces et pouvoirs locaux IIe millénaire av. J.-C. – IVe siècle ap. J.-C.*, Varia Anatolica XIII, ed. by É. Jean *et al.* 159–165. Paris: De Boccard, 2001.

———. "The Stratigraphy of Cyprus WSII and Mycenaean Cups in Soli Höyük Excavations" in *Identifying Changes the Transition from Bronze to Iron Ages in Anatolia and its Neighbouring Regions*, ed. by B. Fischer, H. Genz, É. Jean, K. Köroğlu, 93–106. İstanbul: Türk Eskiçağ Bilimleri Enstitüsü Yayınları, 2003.

———. "Hittites at Soli." *Studi Micenei ed Egeo-Anatolici* XLIX, I (2007): 797–814.

———. "Soli/Pompeiopolis Antik Liman Kenti 2007 Kazıları" 30. *Kazı Sonuçları Toplantısı* 3 (2009): 465–474.

———. "Pottery with Hatched Decoration at Soli Höyük in Late Bronze Age" in *Acts of the VIIth International Congress of Hittitology* II, ed. by A. Süel, 971–987. Ankara: Anıt Matbaa, 2010.

———. "Revisiting the Issue of Late Bronze II Drab Ware with Potmarks" International Congress on Archaeology of the Near East, London, April 2010 (unpublished paper).

———. "Kizzuwatna in the Bronze Age and in Later Periods: Continuity and/or Discontinuity" in *Nostoi: Indigenous Culture, Migration and Integration in Aegean Islands and Western Anatolia during the Late Bronze and Early Iron Age, March 2011 International Symposium held at Koç University*, ed. by Ç. Maner, K. Kopanias, N. Stampolidis, 499–515. İstanbul: Koç University Press, 2015.

Secondary Smelting:
The Analysis of Three Copper-Based Samples from Kinet Höyük

K. Aslıhan Yener — Gonca Dardeniz [1]

It is both an honor and pleasure to have been invited to contribute an article to a Festschrift for Marie-Henriette Carre Gates and Charles Gates: a pleasure because it is gratifying to have the opportunity to pay tribute to two scholars who played such important roles in the early stages of my (Yener's) career; and an honor because of their eminence as archaeologists of such extensive backgrounds. In the course of distinguished careers, Professors Gates touched on many aspects of the LBA and Classical periods in general and in particular, the Hatay region and Syro-Anatolia. While our contribution does not address Charles' particular expertise, we will address the results of metal samples taken from Marie-Henriette's domain, Late Bronze I (hereafter, LBI) Kinet Höyük; the excavation where both husband and wife have devoted several decades of research.

Abstract

Three LBI copper-based samples from the site of Kinet Höyük in Hatay, Turkey were analyzed in 2013 at KUYTAM (Koç University Surface Technologies Center) and ARHA Laboratories at Koç University, İstanbul. As part of the urban tier of an Anatolian production model for producing bronze, a secondary lowland processing practice was identified at the site. During the preliminary metallographic examination using a polarizing light microscope, an arsenical copper metal prill was discovered embedded within a slag matrix in ingot sample (KT 11421c). The second sample taken from the same ingot (KT 11421d) contained lead, copper and tin. The third sample (KT 127491) was a relatively pure copper slag. This paper reports the results of these analyses.

1 Department of Archaeology and History of Art, Koç University, Rumelifeneri Yolu, 34450 Sarıyer, İstanbul, Tukey.
This study was carried out at Koç University Laboratories (KUYTAM) in İstanbul, Turkey. We thank Marie-Henriette Carre-Gates for permission to publish this material.

Introduction

The highland production model defined for Anatolia is one that involves the two-tiered production of metal artifacts.[2] The first tier entails the mining and smelting operations in the metalliferously rich ore deposits and forests, usually located in the mountains. The second tier comprises the lowland urban centers where the processed ores, either in the form of ingots or semi-processed materials are then refined, re-smelted, alloyed and cast into the idiosyncratic metal corpus of each site. Recent research in ancient metallurgy and its sources have led to a better understanding about cultural relations especially during the formative periods of metal technology and state formation in Anatolia. Once metal became locked into a cultural system as an indicator of wealth, disparities in access to labor and resources influenced how individuals operated within and between communities of producers and consumers. These relations often linked distant groups together into cooperative agreements, yet to be determined for Kinet Höyük. Therefore, metal technologies are strategically placed in complex networks and institutions of production, exchange, and consumption that effectively unite disparate highland resource areas and agricultural lowlands—in effect, a multi-tiered production model.[3] The analytic results of these copper-based metal fragments have important ramifications in illuminating the practices of bronze production in the early second millennium BC.

Context and Methodology

Over the course of several decades, Marie-Henriette Carre-Gates and Charles Gates have provided us with a fine-grained understanding of the dynamic human landscape of coastal Hatay of which Kinet Höyük is part. With their team of archaeologists, specialists and students, their intensive exploration and excavations in the region around Dörtyol have revealed a kaleidoscope of changing shorelines and river courses, a cultural sequence going back at least 7,000 years and encroaching absorption into the Hittite empire.[4] The western slope excavations during the 1999 season at Kinet Höyük yielded copper-based fragments from local Period 15 tentatively dated to the LBI. On a visit to the site on November 5th 2000, Yener received for analysis two fragments, labeled KT 11421c and 11421d respectively. Preliminary notes taken at the site indicate that KT 11421 was possibly an ingot weighing 1.18 kg and found in room 135 (Locus 541). Samples KT 11421c and KT 11421d were taken from different parts of this ingot. The other sample, KT 127491, was found in room 159 adjacent to room 135, and dated to the middle of Period 15 (Period 15B).

2 Yener 2000.

3 Yener *et al.*, 2015; Lehner and Yener 2014, 165–174.

4 Gates 1999, 77–111; Gates 2006, 293–309.

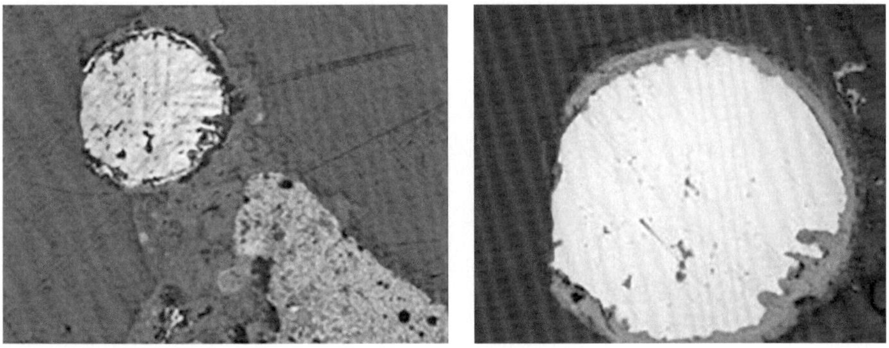

FIG. 1 5x magnified optical microscope image of KT 11421c (left), 10x magnified image of the sample (right).

The artifact analyses presented here began ten years ago at the Oriental Institute of the University of Chicago metallurgy laboratory (polished cross sections and polarizing light microscopy) by Yener, and continued at the newly established KUYTAM and ARHA Laboratories at Koç Universtiy, with the participation of Dardeniz in 2013. These instrumental analyses utilized a Scanning Electron Microscope (SEM-EDX) for composition and imaging. The three samples (KT 11421c, KT 11421d and KT 127491) had been embedded in epoxy resin and subsequently ground and polished at the Oriental Institute. At Koç University the samples were examined with the aid of an Olympus BX51 optical microscope (OM) and Zeiss Ultra Plus Scanning Electron Microscope (SEM). Semi-quantitative analyses were done using the SEM-EDX connected to a Zeiss Ultra Plus attachment. Cell^A software used for OM and Quantax software was used to evaluate the SEM-EDX data.

KT 11421c revealed a copper prill which was observed in a 10x image taken by the optical microscope (FIG. 1). Subsequent semi-quantitative analyses of the prill by SEM-EDX showed copper as a major element together with carbon and oxygen. Analytical measurements by SEM-EDX indicated 79.64% copper in the sample (FIG. 2). A heterogeneous structure (FIG. 3A) was observed in the sample and its colors change from black to gray and white (FIG. 1 (left) and FIG. 3A). Its micro structure shows a diversity of globules and cubic dendrites.

The interpretation of the metallographic images suggested that this fragment was a product of alloying with the bronze prill entrapped inside the matrix. Arsenic content in the prill (FIG. 3B-C) yielded high values of up to 9.19% with semi-quantitative analysis. It is obvious that the metal prill is an arsenical bronze, but the exact trace levels (ppm) of the arsenic should be confirmed by ICP-MS. Further processing would necessitate grinding and extracting the entrapped bronze prills from the slag matrix in order to cast a bronze artifact.

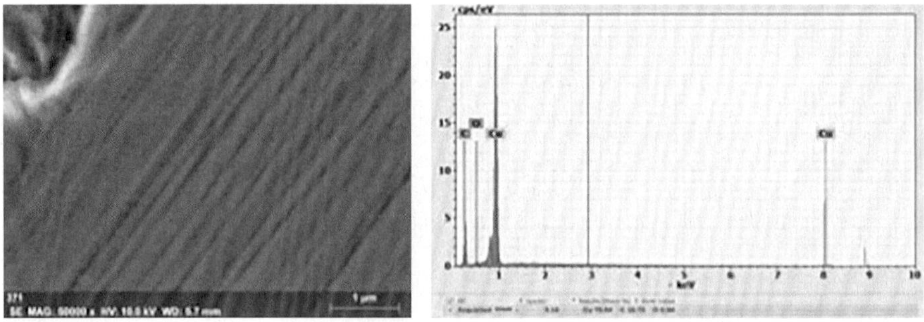

FIG. 2 SEM image (left) and EDX graphic (right) of sample KT 11421c. Magnification, working distance and semi-quantitative elemental compositions are indicated below image.

Examination of sample KT 11421d from the same ingot indicated a heterogeneous content. SEM-EDX analyses confirmed the presence of tin and lead together with copper. EDX results of the flat surface (FIG. 4B) yielded 60.38% copper and 5.53% tin (FIG. 4C). Furthermore light gray whitish granules around the flat grain indicate a 31.72% lead in the sample (FIG. 4D). Generally lead facilitates casting by lowering melting temperatures, however, such high amounts would not be considered good bronze, making it too soft. Whether this sample was the product of re-smelting (refining), re-melting scrap metal containing tin and arsenic or alloying using a tin-arsenic ore is a research question beyond the scope of these investigations.

Sample KT 12749 labeled "Cu industrial sample" was determined to be copper slag (FIG. 5). Semi-quantitative measurements on the light gray surfaces determined that the sample contained copper (77.78wt%), carbon (13.97 wt%), and oxygen (8.25 wt%) (FIG. 6A). The slag matrix was composed of iron and silicate, which is a characteristic copper slag matrix.

Conclusions

The examination of three copper-based fragments has illuminated an urban tier of a highland production model for Anatolia first proposed in 2000.[5] Semi-quantitative analyses (SEM-EDX) of the first ingot fragment (KT 11421c) determined the presence of an arsenical bronze prill entrapped in an ingot. Another sample from the other side of the ingot (KT 11421d) was determined to contain tin and substantial amounts of lead, suggesting a very heterogeneous product as an ingot.

5 Yener 2000.

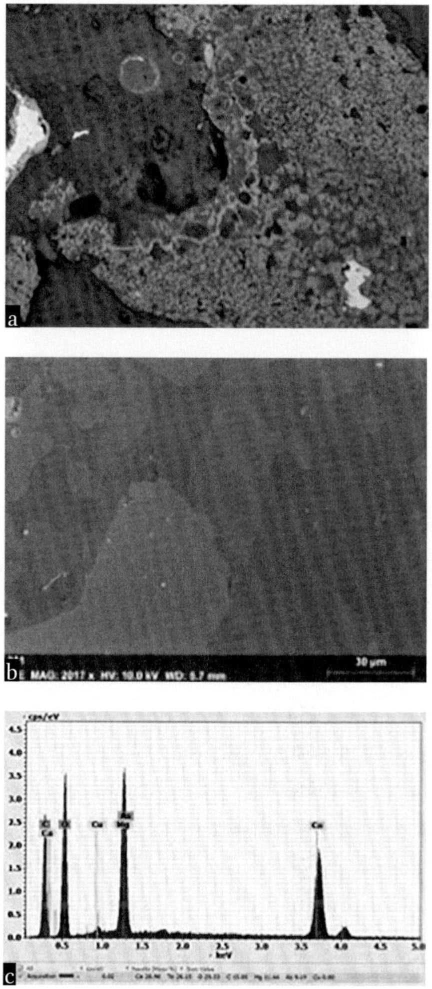

FIG. 3 (a) 10x magnified image of KT 11421c. (b) SEM image of KT 11421c. Measurement details are in the legend. (c) KT 11421(c) SEM-EDX graph showing composition. Note arsenic and copper peaks.

Sample (KT 12749) was determined to be copper slag found inside a crucible, a residue of alloying (or re-smelting) copper.

On a site-based level the analyses indicated the presence of a secondary production of bronze during LBI Kinet Höyük. The find places of the ingot samples containing the prill as well as the crucible within proximity of each other suggests a crafting quarter in this sector of the site. Secondary processing involved the refining and resmelting of copper and alloying materials obtained from the "primary processing" tier elsewhere, usually near the mines. As part of a highland production model for Anatolia,[6] the nearby Taurus and Amanus Mountains would be good candidates as a source where the ores would be pro-

6 Lehner and Yener 2014, 165–174.

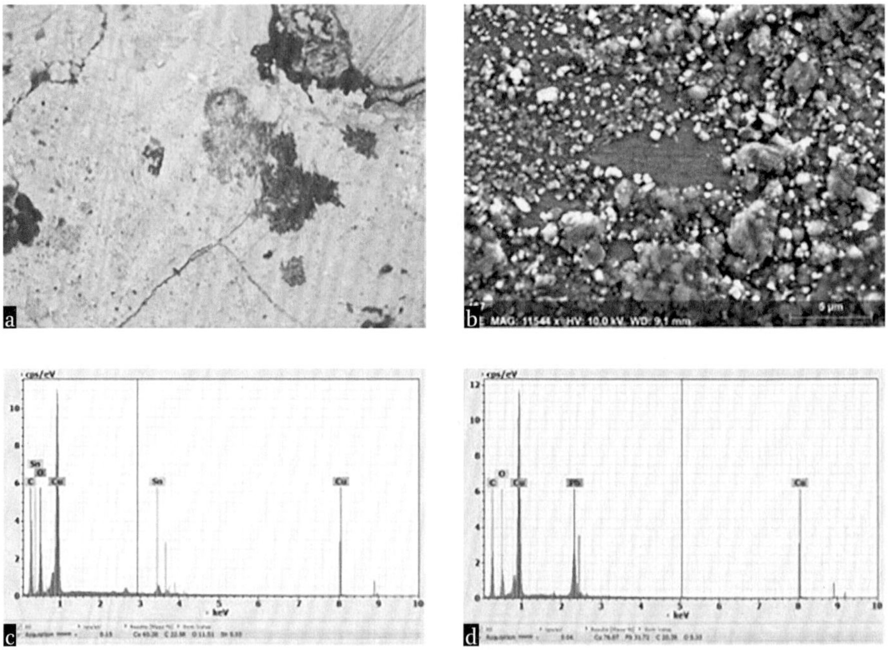

FIG. 4 (a) 10x magnified optical microscope image of KT 11421d. (b) SEM image of KT 11421d. (c) SEM-EDX graph of KT 11421d indicating presence of Sn and Cu. (d) KT 11421d SEM-EDX graph of KT 11421d indicating presence of Pb and Cu.

cessed in the first tier of production and then transported to lowland urban centers such as Kinet Höyük.

However, sourcing the location of the copper, tin, lead and arsenic mines is a topic that would necessitate further analysis. Certainly lead isotope ratios would reveal the lead ore deposits exploited, given the high levels of lead in one of the samples. Lead ores are part of the massive argentiferous lead-zinc-copper deposits of the Taurus Mountain range[7] within the vicinity of the site. Tin sources have been fully substantiated in Turkey both at Kestel Mine in the Taurus Mountains,[8] and recently at Hisarcık near the Erciyes volcano in Kayseri.[9] Intriguingly, the tin deposits of Hisarcık contain high levels of arsenic ore (yazganite). Given the fact that the Kinet ingot sample contains both tin and arsenic as do contemporary bronzes at Alalakh and Tarsus,[10] two processing possibilities present themselves.

7 Yener *et al.* 1991, 541–577.

8 Yener 2000.

9 Sarp and Cerný 2005, 367–374; Yazgan 2005, 135–138; Yener *et al.* 2015.

10 Özbal 2006, 303–313; Yener 2000.

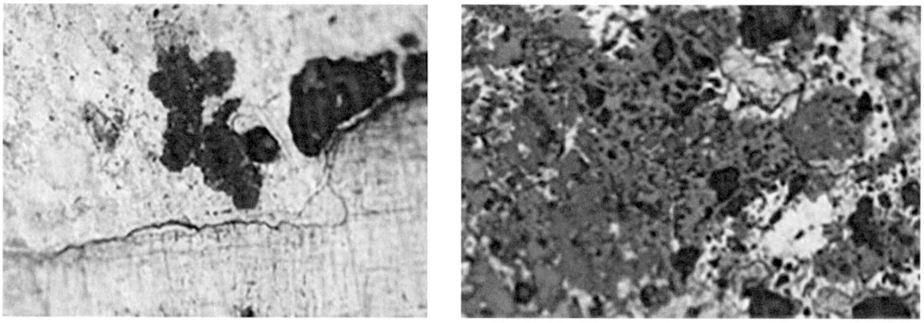

FIG. 5 10x optical microscope images of sample KT 12749 from different perspectives showing heterogeneity of the sample.

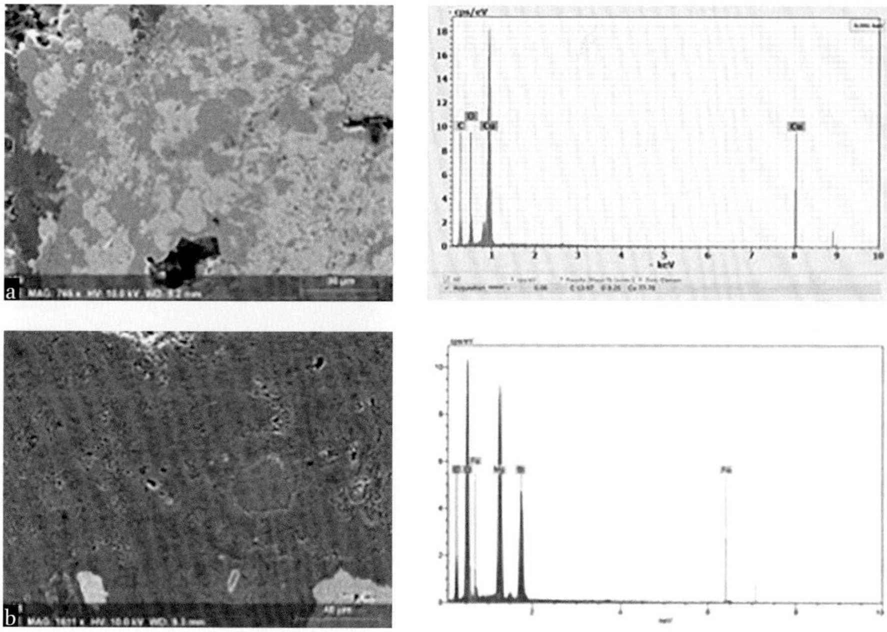

FIG. 6 (a) KT12749 SEM image (left) and EDX graph (right) showing Cu, C and O in the light gray microstructures. (b) KT12749 SEM image (left) and EDX graph (right) showing the composition of the slag matrix.

One would be re-melting scrap metal, or more likely, the use of the heterogeneous arsenic-tin ores of Hisarcık mines in operation during Kinet's occupation.

REFERENCES

Gates, M.-H., "Kinet Höyük (Hatay, Turkey) and MB Levantine Chronology." *Akkadica* 120 (1999): 77–111.

———. "Dating the Hittite Levels at Kinet Höyük: a Revised Chronology" in *Structuring and Dating in Hittite Archaeology. BYZAS* 4, ed. by D. P. Mielke, J. Seeher and U. D. Schoop, 293–309. Istanbul: Ege Yayınları, 2006.

Lehner, W. and K.A. Yener, "Organization and Specialization of Early Mining and Metal Technologies in Anatolia" in *Archaeometallurgy in Global Perspective: Methods and Synthesis* ed. by B. W. Roberts and C. P. Thornton, 165–174. New York: Springer, 2014.

Özbal, H., "Tell Atchana Metal Buluntularının Kimyasal Analizi." *Arkeometri Sonuçları Toplantısı* 21 (2006): 303–313.

Sarp, H. and R. Cerny, "Yazganite, NaFe3+2 (Mg,Mn) (As04) 3.H20, a New Mineral: Its Description and Crystal Structure." *European Journal of Mineralogy* 17 (2005): 367–374.

Yazgan, E., "Cassiterite (tin) Mineralization Related with Erciyes Volcanic Activities and the Mode of Formation of the Magnetite-cassiterite-yazganite-tridymite Paragenesis." *58th Geological Congress of Turkey, 11–17 April 2005 abstracts,* 135–138. Ankara 2005.

Yener, K.A., *The Domestication of Metals: The Rise of Complex Metal Industries in Anatolia (c. 4500–2000 BC)*. Leiden: Brill, 2000.

———. "The Small Finds" in *Tell Atchana, Ancient Alalakh. Volume 1. 2003–2004 Excavation Seasons*, ed. by K. A. Yener, 102–107. Istanbul: Koç University Press, 2010.

Yener, K.A. , F. Kulakoğlu, E. Yazgan, R. Kontani, Y. S. Hayakawa, J. W. Lehner, G. Dardeniz, G. Öztürk, M. Johnson, E. Kaptan and A. Hacar, "New Tin Mines and Production Sites near Kültepe, Ancient Kanesh in Turkey: A Third Millennium BC Highland Production Model." *Antiquity* 89 (2015): 596–612.

Yener, K.A., E.V. Sayre, E. Joel, H. Özbal, I.L. Barnes and R.H. Brill, "Stable Lead Isotope Studies of Central Taurus Ore Sources and Related Artifacts from Eastern Mediterranean Chalcolithic and Bronze Age Sites." *Journal of Archaeological Science* 18 (1991): 541–577.

Çine-Tepecik Yerleşmesine Ait Figürlü Miken Seramiği

Sevinç Günel[1]

Abstract

Tepecik is located to the south of Menderes, on the plain that is crossed by Çine River. In the stratigraphical definition of the mound, the late phase of Level II belongs to the Late Bronze Age (LBA) settlement, Level II 1. This Level yields a fortified settlement plan. Besides local pottery in this settlement, another important ware group consists of Mycenaean painted vessels. The shapes, as well as the decorative motifs, correspond to the Mycenaean painted pottery tradition, which had a wide distribution not only in Greece and the Aegean Islands, but also in the West Anatolian coastal region. Among the Mycenaean pottery, figured examples with depictions of birds, fish, deer, as well as warriors on deep bowls and krater fragments belong to the 'pictorial style' in Mycenaean pottery development. These examples reflect certain scenes on figure painted Tepecik Mycenaean vessels and are similar to decoration on ceramic development of Late Helladic IIIB-Helladic IIIC (LH IIIB-LH IIIC) early and middle phases.

Batı Anadolu'da gerçekleşen yeni arkeolojik kazı ve araştırmalar, bölgenin tarihöncesi ve tarihi dönemlerinin detaylı ve yeni bir bakış açısıyla ele alınmasını sağlamıştır. Bu araştırmalar, Batı Anadolu'nun sınırlı bilgilere dayalı erken dönem kültürel yapısının çok daha zengin bir birikime sahip olduğunu ortaya koymaktadır. Son araştırmaların verdiği neticeler, bölgede yerel bir kültürel yapının yanı sıra bölgelerarası ilişkilerin yoğunluğuna işaret etmektedir. Batıda Ege deniziyle, doğuda ise, Anadolu'nun iç bölgeleriyle bağlantıları sağlayan derin vadiler, Tunç Çağları ve tarihöncesi dönemlere ait yerleşmelerin yayılım alanında ve yerleşim biçimlerinde önemli bir rol oynamıştır. Batı Anadolu Bölgesine ait kültürel şekillenme, MÖ 2. binyıla uzanan zaman dizininde çevre kültürlerle ilişkileri öne çıkaran boyutlarıyla takip edilmektedir. MÖ 2. binyıl, Anadolu'da Hititlerin siyasi konumu ve buna paralel olarak geniş bir coğrafyada politik güce sahip olan Hitit İmparatorluğu ile gelişimini sürdürdüğü bir süreçtir. Bu kültürel gelişime paralel olarak, Batı Anadolu'da, Hititlerin varlığı ve etkisi, arkeolojik veriler ve

1 Hacettepe Üniversitesi, Arkeoloji Bölümü, 06800, Beytepe, Ankara.

filolojik kaynaklarla anlaşılmaktadır. Bu dönemde, Batı Anadolu'da siyasi güçler ve politik olaylarla ilgili yeterli bir tanımlama yapılamasa da, Hititlerin bu bölgeye ilgisi, yazılı metinlerden öğrenilmektedir. Bu bilgiler Batı Anadolu'daki ülkelerin/toprakların ve bazı siyasi güçlerin tanınmasını sağlamıştır.[2] Öte yandan Batı Anadolu'da, öne çıkan diğer bir kültürel etkileşimi Ege dünyasından tanınan Miken kanıtları göstermektedir. MÖ 2. binyılın ortalarından son evresine değin takip edilen Miken kültürünün yansımaları ise, bölgelerarası bağlantılara somut arkeolojik verileriyle ışık tutmaktadır. Bu kanıtlar, Ege ve Doğu Akdeniz bölgelerinde, Batı Anadolu'yu da içine alan bir kültürel birlikteliği ortaya koymakta ve aynı zamanda kronolojinin oturtulmasına katkı sağlamaktadır.

MÖ 2. binyıl kültür tarihi, Batı Anadolu'nun kıyı şeridi ve kıyı şeridinden içerde İç Batı Anadolu'da yer alan yerleşim birimlerine ait kültür kalıntılarıyla tanımlanmakta ve belli bir kronolojik ayrımı vermektedir.[3] Aydın ili, Çine ilçesi, Karakollar köyü sınırlarında yer alan Çine-Tepecik, Menderes ve güneyinin MÖ 2. binyıl yerleşim modelinin ve kronolojik gelişiminin anlaşılmasını sağlayan yeni bir merkezdir. Tepecik, Menderes'in güneyinde, Çine Çayı'nın uzandığı ovada kesintisiz bir yerleşim sürecini yansıtmaktadır.[4] Höyüğün stratigrafik ayrımında, II. 2. kültür tabakası, Orta Tunç Çağı (OTÇ) yerleşmesini; II. 1 kültür tabakası ise, savunma sistemine sahip Geç Tunç Çağı (GTÇ) yerleşim planını vermektedir (Res. 1). GTÇ yerleşmesinde, höyüğün batısında sura ait 55 metrelik uzantı takip edilmiştir. Sur duvarı, 2.20 m kalınlığında ve 6.32 m boyutlarında kare planlı kulelerle destekli bir planı gösterir. Surla çevrili yerleşmede, özellikle depolamaya yönelik yapılar ve pithosların yerleştirildiği geniş bir alana yayılan taş platform, kentin idari sisteminde ekonomi faktörünü ve dönemin ekonomik gücünü ortaya koymaktadır.

Depolamayla ilgili bu yapılardan biri, sura ait kule yapılarından biriyle bağlantılıdır. Savunma sisteminin güneybatı uzantısında birinci kuleyle bağlantılı olan bu yapı, 3.50 m uzunluğunda ve yaklaşık 2.00 m genişliğinde dikdörtgen planlıdır (Res. 1; Yapı 1). Söz konusu bu yapının kuzeyi, kulenin 1.30 m kalınlığını veren güney duvarına, batısı, sur duvarına dayanmaktadır. Yapının güney ve doğusu ise, 0.45–0.50 m kalınlığında, ufak taşların oluşturduğu bir duvar örgüsüyle sınırlanmıştır. Bu alandaki mevcut mimari kalıntılara göre, bu yapı kulenin güneydoğu köşesinde yaptığı çıkıntıya uygun olarak inşa edilmiş olmalıdır. Yapı içinde, yanmış ağaç izleri ile kerpiç kalıntıları arasında iç içe yerleştirilmiş kaplar *in situ* ele geçmiştir. Bu kaplar arasında, Batı Anadolu'nun yerli seramik örneklerinin yanı sıra Miken kültürünün

---

2 Forrer 1926; Garstang 1943; Garstang ve Gurney 1959; Heinhold-Krahmer 1977; Hawkins 1998; Ünal 2003; Strobel 2008.

3 Günel baskıda.

4 Günel 2008, 130–139.

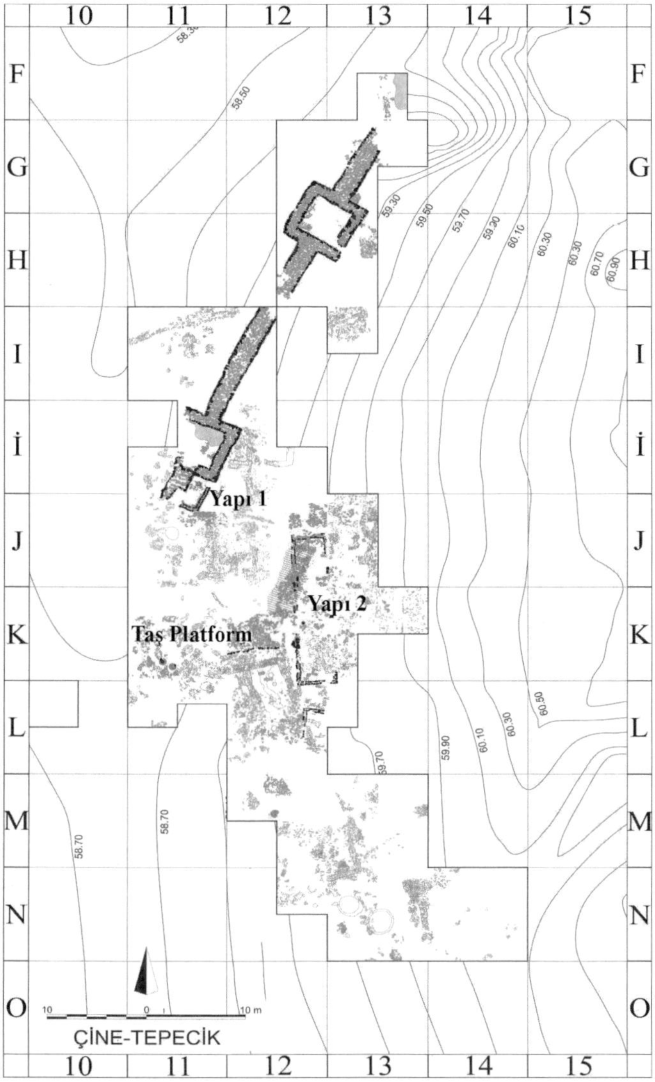

Res. 0

seramik geleneğinden tanınan boya bezeli kaplar yer almaktadır.[5] Miken seramik grubuna ait üzengi kulplu kaplar, ithal ve yerli üretim olmak üzere form ve özellikle kaplar üzerine uygulanan motifleri açısından Geç Hellas III B2 (GH III B2) ve Geç Hellas III C (GH III C) erken-orta evrelerinin özelliklerini taşımaktadır.[6] Surla bağlantılı olan bu mimarinin işlevine ilişkin olarak gerek yapının boyutları ve gerekse kapların buluntu durumu, depolamaya yönelik bir kullanıma işaret etmektedir.

5 Günel 2010, 25–49.

6 Günel 2010, 30–39.

Surla bağlantılı bu yapılaşmanın doğusunda daha büyük boyutta ikinci bir yapı ise, dikdörtgen planlı olup, 16.50 m uzunluğunda ve 4.50 m genişliğindedir (Res. 1; Yapı 2). Yapıda, çok sayıdaki pithos parçalarının buluntu durumu, pithosların yapı içinde belli bir düzende yerleştirildiğini göstermektedir. Özellikle *in situ* durumda olan pithos diplerinin konumlarından, pithosların yapının batı duvarı boyunca kuzey-güney doğrultusunda yerleştirildiği anlaşılmaktadır. Bu pithoslardan biri, yapının güney kesiminde sağlam durumda ve *in situ* ele geçmiştir.[7] Üzeri düzgün bir kapak taşı ile kapatılmış olan ve depolama amaçlı kullanım gören bu pithoslar, Yapı 2'nin 'depo/magazin' olarak tanımlanmasını desteklemiştir. Bu yapı içinde, pithosların yanı sıra farklı malzeme-teknik özelliklere sahip ve aynı zamanda form açısından çeşitlilik gösteren kaplar yer almaktadır. Bu kapların önemli bir grubunu, Miken boya bezeli kaplar oluşturur. Bu kaplar arasında, özellikle derin kase ve krater parçalarında kuş, balık, geyik ve bunun yanı sıra savaşçı tasvirlerin de işlendiği figürlü örnekler *Pictorial style* olarak tanımlanan seramik geleneğine aittir.[8] Tepecik'te arkeolojik verilerin yanı sıra bölgenin tarihi coğrafyası açısından anlamlı olan mühür baskıları ise, bu yapıya aittir.[9] Hitit İmparatorluk dönemine tarihlenen mühür baskıları, GTÇ yerleşmesinin kronolojik ayrımında seramik buluntularıyla paralel bir dönemi temsil etmektedir. Tepecik mühür baskıları, kültür tabakası belli olan bir arkeolojik kontekste, depo yapısında bulunmuştur. Hiyeroglif kitabe içeren bu mühürler, yüksek kaliteli bir işlenişe sahip olup, Hititlerin çekirdek bölgesiyle karşılaştırılabilecek niteliktedir. Ayrıca her iki mühür baskısı da kitabeye yönelik bilgilerin yanı sıra Tepecik merkezinin bulunduğu coğrafyada siyasi ve ticari anlamda bir güce sahip olduğuna işaret etmektedir. Mühür baskılarının yanı sıra depolama amaçlı pithoslar, kentin idari sistemi içinde belli bir ekonomik faktörün işlediğini ortaya koymaktadır. Bu sistemi, Yapı 2'nin hemen batısında yer alan ve ufak taşlardan oluşan bir alan desteklemektedir (Res.0; Taş Platform). Bu platformda, gövdenin yarısına kadar toprağa gömülü iri boyuttaki pithoslar, ufak taşlarla çevrelenmiş bir depolama sisteminin uygulandığını göstermiştir. Buna göre, gerek depo yapıları (Yapı 1 ve Yapı 2) ve gerekse taş platformun oluşturduğu alandaki iri boyuttaki pithoslar, kente ait ürünlerin belli bir sisteme dayalı depolandığını ve ekonomik anlamda bir organizasyona gidildiğini ortaya koymaktadır. Bu alanın hemen güney yönünde uzanan mimari, daha çok dikdörtgen plan veren yapı kalıntılarıyla yerleşmenin güney ve güneybatı yönünde genişlediğini göstermiştir. Bu alanda, bir arada olmak üzere çok sayıda ağırlıklara rastlanmıştır.

7 Günel 2011, 3–4.

8 Tepecik II 1 kültür katına ait yerleşmeden ele geçen Miken boya bezeli ve figürlü seramiğe ait bir grup eserle ilgili yayın: Günel 2015, 607–626. Magazin yapısına ait savaşçı ve av sahneli iki kraterle ilgili yayın çalışması: Günel ve Herbordt 2014, 4–8.

9 Günel ve Herbordt 2010, 9, fig. 4–6. İlgili yayında, mühür baskısına ait çizimler, Ch. Müller-Hazenbos ve S. Herbordt'a aittir. Aynı yapıya ait ikinci mühür baskısı ile ilgili yayın; Günel, S ve S. Herbordt 2014, 8–11.

Bu ağırlıklardan bir grubu, kaba nitelikte ve iyi pişirilmemiş olup 'makara' biçimindedir. Benzer örnekler, Ege ve Doğu Akdeniz'e uzanan coğrafyada özellikle GH III C döneminde daha belirgin bir yoğunlukta görülmektedir.[10] Bir arada ele geçen diğer grup ise, pişmiş toprak piramit biçimli ağırlıklardır. Farklı tiplerde ve çok sayıda olmak üzere bir arada ele geçen ağırlıklar, bu alanda atölye/atölyelerin varlığına işaret eden ip uçlarıdır. Mimari kalıntıların oluşturduğu bu yerleşim planında, II.1 kültür tabakasına ait bir grup figürlü Miken seramiği, bölgelerarası bağlantılara ve kronolojik ayrıma katkı sağlamaktadır.

Miken Figürlü Seramik Buluntuları

Geç Tunç Çağı yerleşmesinde mimariyle bağlantılı ve aynı zamanda bu yapıların çevresindeki alanlardan ele geçen seramik buluntuları arasında Miken figürlü kaplara ait parçalar, bu süsleme anlayışının detaylarını ortaya koymaktadır. Bu örneklerden biri, krater tipi kaba ait bir parçadır (Kat. 1, Res. 2-3). Bu kap parçasında, gövdede yatay bantlar arasında yer alan ana sahnede, insan figürü tasvir edilmiştir. Figür, kısmen korunmuş olup, 5.03 cm uzunluğa sahiptir. Söz konusu figür, üçgen görünüme sahip üst gövde, oldukça ince bir bel ve belden aşağısı tekrar üçgen görünüm veren giysisiyle gösterilmiştir. Figürün dirsek hizasından kıvrılan sağ kolu, yukarıya doğru kalkmış durumda işlenmiştir. Sol kolu ise, aşağıya doğru olup, elinde olasılıkla silahı/mızrağı ile betimlenmiştir. Öte yandan figürün beli hizasında ve arkasına gelecek şekilde yatay bir uzantı görülmekte ve olasılıkla sırık görünümlü bu uzantıda asılı olan torbasını taşımaktadır. Ayrıca figürün bel hizasında torbasına destek olan yatay sırıkla bağlantılı saçak görünümlü çizgiler, giysisinin arkasında ve etek hizasında üç çizgi halinde gösterilmiştir. Figürün ayaklarına yakın yerde kısmen korunmuş kuşa ait olduğu anlaşılan ayaklar ise, ana sahnede bir kuş tasvirinin yer aldığını göstermektedir. Söz konusu figürün önünde ise, kırık olması nedeniyle anlaşılamamakla birlikte, bir hayvan figürünün işlendiği düşünülmektedir.

Ege dünyasında, Miken figürlü seramik geleneğinde işlenen ana konulardan biri av sahnesidir. Miken kraterlerinde, av sahnesinde avcı ve ona eşlik eden birden fazla köpek ve aynı zamanda aynı sahnede yer alan kuşlar, söz konusu bu resimsel anlatımı tamamlamaktadır. Buna göre, Tepecik figürlü kap parçasında yer alan figürle karşılaştırılabilecek örnekler, burada bir avcının tasvir edildiğini göstermiştir. Bu kapsamda, Phthiotis-Kalapodi'de bir kraterde avcı, omuzlarına dayadığı sırıkla benzer tipte torba taşımakta ve aynı zamanda Tepecik örneğinde olduğu gibi, figürün arakasında saçak görünümü veren çizgiler yer almaktadır.[11]

10 Rahmstorf 2003; 2005; 2008.

11 Crouwel 2006, 18, fig. 7.

Tepecik figürlü kaplar arasında en yaygın görülen kuşlardır. Tepecik Miken seramiğinde, kuş tasvirleri, işleniş açısından detaylarda farklılık göstermekte ve bu yönüyle oldukça zengin bir grup oluşturmaktadır. Kuş tasvirlerinin daha çok kabın ağız kenarının alt hizasında işlenmiş örneklerine rastlanmaktadır. Bu tipe giren bir örnek, dışa kalınlaştırılmış ağız kenarlı bir kasede görülmektedir (Kat. 2; Res. 4-5). Kasenin ağız kenarını çevreleyen zikzak bezemenin altında, kuş betimlenmiştir. Kuş tasvirinde baş ve kanat kısmen korunmuş olmasına rağmen, gövdeden ayrı işlenmiş kanatların duruş biçimi, hareket anında/uçar pozisyonda olduğuna işaret etmektedir. Kanatlar birbirine paralel çizgi taramadan oluşmaktadır.

Benzer bir örnek, diğer bir kabın dışa kalınlaştırılmış ağız kenarının hemen alt hizasında, görülmektedir (Kat. 3; Res. 6-7). Bu kaba ait kuş tasvirinde, baş ve gaga işlenişi, son derece zarif boyun kısmıyla tamamlanmaktadır. Bu kuş tasvirinde de kanatların durumu, kuşun hareket anında/uçar konumda olduğunu göstermektedir. Gövde, yarım daire oluşturan kalın bantlarla gösterilmiş, kanatlar ise, yine birbirine paralel ince çizgilerle verilmiştir. Tepecik kuş figürlü diğer kaplar arasında, burada söz edilen gövde işlenişine sahip benzer örneklere rastlanmaktadır (Res. 1). Kuş tasvirinin ön kısmında ise, dikey ve birbirine paralel işlenmiş çizgilerden oluşan bir sınırlama görülmektedir (Furumark Motif 75:11). Bu çizgilerin oluşturduğu paneller arasında ana figür işlenmiştir (Res. 1). Bu tasvir tarzı, GH III B-C evrelerinde ana motif/sahnede görülmektedir.[12] Benzer bir uygulama, Rhodes-Ialysos buluntuları arasında görülmektedir.[13] Kuşun gövde işlenişinde iç içe yarım daireler ve kanatların çizgi tarama halinde verildiği örneklere, Kos-Seraglio kraterlerinde görmek mümkündür.[14] Ayrıca her iki örneğe ait kanat işlenişi (Kat. 2–3), Argolis-Midea'da Miken figürlü bir kapta görülmektedir.[15]

Kaplar üzerinde kuşların hareket anında/uçar konumda tasvir edildiklerini gösteren diğer bir örnekte, kanatların yanı sıra ayakların duruşu da bu hareketliliği yansıtmaktadır (Kat. 4; Res. 8). Kratere ait bu parçada, kuşun gövdesinin ön kısmı, çevresinin noktalarla sınırlandığı yarım daire şeklinde verilmekte, kuyruk kısmına doğru ise, çizgi taramayla tamamlanmaktadır. Gövdede yer alan noktalarla sınırlandırılmış yarım daire motifi (FM 43: i), Miken motifleri arasında GH III B - GH III C evrelerinin karakteristik motifleri arasında yer almaktadır.[16] Miken kaplarında genelde ana sahnenin yanı sıra görülen bu motif, söz konusu bu örnekte, kuşun gövdesine uyarlanmış bir süsleme anlayışıyla gösterilmiştir. Bu da seramik sanatçısının figürlerle motifler arasındaki kombinasyonda ortaya koy-

12 Furumark 1941, 414.

13 Benzi 1992, 107.

14 Crouwel 2006, 21, fig. 17.

15 Demakopoulou 2006, 41, fig. 26.

16 Furumark 1941, 345.

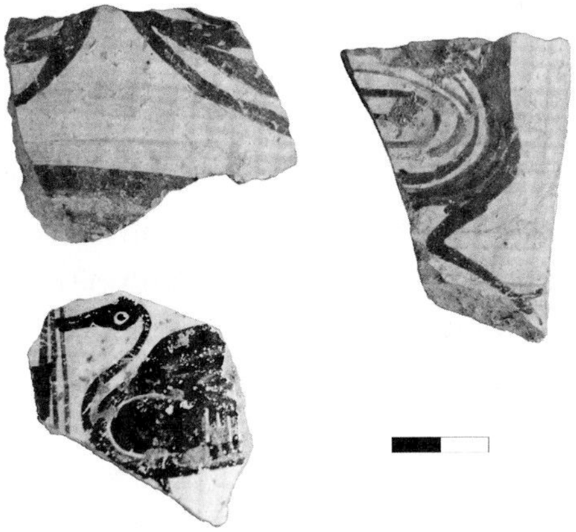

Res. 1

duğu bir zenginliği göstermektedir. Kuş betimlemesinin hemen önünde ise, yine Miken motiflerinden çok iyi bilinen çevresi noktalarla sınırlanmış daire motifi yer almaktadır. Böylece sanatçı gerek kuş tasvirinde gerekse motif olarak popüler olan süslemeyi aynı kap üzerine uygulamıştır. Daire motifi de, GH III B - GH III C evrelerinin motifleri arasında görülmekte ve paralel bir kronolojiyi vermektedir. Daire içinde 'artı' işareti görünümde çizgiler, Miken süsleme geleneğinde farklı tipte yer almaktadır (FM 17; FM 26; FM 41). Nokta ya da çizgi taramayla verilmiş daire motifleri, GH III C orta evresinde ana sahnede yer alarak motif zenginliğini ortaya koymaktadır.[17] Kuş tasvirinde gövde işlenişi açısından yakın bir örnek, Kos-Seraglio'da bir krater üzerinde yer almakta ve GH III C orta evresine paralel bir kronolojiye oturtulmaktadır.[18]

Kratere ait olduğu düşünülen diğer bir gövde parçasında, kuş tasviri detaylarda farklılık gösteren bir işlenişle görülmektedir (Kat. 5; Res. 9-10). Yatay bir bant bezeme ve bu bant bezemeyle bağlantılı üçgen motiflerin oluşturduğu süsleme, olasılıkla kabın ağız kenarını çevrelemektedir. Üçgen motif, iç içe çizgilerden oluşmakta ve dış çevresi ise, çizgi taramayla sınırlanmaktadır. Üçgen motifin yer aldığı tasvir bandında, kuşun kanatları yine gövdeden ayrı olarak işlenmiştir. Ancak yukarıda ele alınan örneklerden farklı olarak kanatlar, çizgi taramayla verilmemiş olup tamamen boyalıdır. Gövdesi ise, birbirine paralel çizgi taramalarla şekillendirilmiştir. Öte yandan zarif bir boyun işlenişi, gözlerin nokta olarak gösterilmesi gibi özellikleriyle diğer kuş betimlemeleriyle benzerlik göstermektedir. Kap üzerinde kuşların, üçgen motifler arasına gelecek şekilde sıra halinde birbirini takip ettiği düşünülmektedir.

Kaplarda kuşların sıra halinde işlendiğini, bir krater üzerinde görmek mümkündür. Bu örnekte, kuşlar dışa kalınlaştırılmış ağız kenarının alt hizasında bir-

17 Mountjoy 1999, 1068, fig. 438: 268.

18 Mountjoy 1999, 1106, fig. 452:101.

birini takip edecek şekilde yer almaktadır (Kat. 6; Res. 11-12). Kuşların kanatları ve ayakların işleniş biçimi, yine hareket anında/uçar pozisyonundadır. Kuşların kanatları tamamen boyalı, gövde ise, çizgi taramayla verilmiştir. Kuyruklar ise, birer kalın çizgiyle gösterilmiştir. Öte yandan kuşların baş, gaga biçimi ve boyun kısımları diğer örneklerde olduğu gibi, zarif bir işlenişi yansıtmaktadır. Kuşların sıra halinde resmedildiği bir diğer örnek, bu tarz süsleme geleneğinin etkin olduğunu göstermektedir (Kat. 7; Res. 13-14). Kratere ait dışa kalınlaştırılmış ağız kenarında, yer alan kuşlar birbirini takip edecek düzende yerleştirilmiş olmalıdır. Mevcut korunan parçada, kuşların kanatları diğer kuş betimlemelerinde olduğu gibi gövdeden ayrıdır. Kanatlar tamamen boyanmıştır. Gövde ise, çizgi tarama ile belirginleştirilmiştir. Bu açıdan yukarıda ele alınan örneklere ait (Kat. 5–6) kuş betimlemeleriyle benzer bir tasvir anlayışını yansıtmaktadır. Ayrıca kanatların konumu ve ayakların duruşu, hareket anını göstermiştir. Kuşların tasvir edildiği bu alan, bir bantla sınırlanmıştır. Kuş tasvirleri, kırmızı yüzey üzerine bej/beyaz renktedir. Böylece görsel açıdan daha dikkat çekici bir görünüm kazanmıştır. Kuş tasvirlerin yer aldığı ana sahne, yarım dairelerin oluşturduğu yatay bant bezeme ile sınırlanmaktadır (FM 42: 4). Bu bezemeye, Tepecik Miken boya bezeli gruba ait diğer kaplar üzerinde de rastlanmaktadır.[19]

Tepecik figürlü Miken kapları arasında bu örnekler, kuş tasvirlerinin oldukça popüler bir süsleme olarak yer aldığını göstermiştir. Kaplar üzerinde, kuşların özellikle kanatlarında ve gövde işlenişiyle ilgili detaylarda farklılıkları görmek mümkündür. Bu çeşitliliği, Miken seramik grubunda hamur yapısı, hamur rengi, yüzey işlenişi ve boya bezeme rengi de göstermektedir.

Değerlendirme

Batı Anadolu'nun Ege dünyasıyla olan kültürel ilişkilerinde Tepecik'te ele geçen Miken seramiği, GH III B-C dönemlerini kapsayan bir kronolojiyi vermiştir. Ege'nin Geç Tunç Çağı'na bakıldığında, Ege ve Doğu Akdeniz'de ticaret ağının en etkin olarak gerçekleştiği dönemler (GH III A- GH III B) Miken saraylarının ekonomik anlamda en güçlü ve etkin olduğu süreci ortaya koymaktadır. Saray dönemi sonrası, GH III B sonu ve GH III C, sarayların tahribatıyla politik anlamda bir güç kaybı ve buna bağlı bir tutarsızlık dönemine uzanmaktadır. Bu süreç, Ege ve Doğu Akdeniz'i kapsayan ticaret sisteminde seramik üretimindeki yenilikleriyle, diğer materyallerin yanında yerini almıştır.[20] Bu değişim, özellikle GH III C dönemi mimarisinde, ölü gömme geleneğinde, ticari bağlantılarında ve aynı zamanda seramik üretiminde bölgesel ve yerel kültürel bir anlayışın oluşmasıyla

19 Günel 2010, 38–39, fig. 21, 24, tab. 1: 11–12.

20 Shelton 2010, 145; Burns 2010, 297.

takip edilmektedir.[21] Saray sisteminin kırılmasıyla (GH III B2/GH III C erken) Ege dünyasında politik değişim ve ekonomik faktörler, Miken seramik geleneğinde görülen farklılaşmayla takip edilmektedir.[22] Ege ve Doğu Akdeniz'i içeren bu kültürel yapıda, GH III B2/GH III C erken ve orta evrelerine ait seramik geleneğinde belli motifler öne çıkmaktadır. Söz konusu dönemin süsleme anlayışında, yarım daire motifinin farklı kaplar üzerinde uygulanan en popüler süsleme arasında yer aldığı görülür.[23] Bu motifler, iç içe yarım daireler, içi boyalı yarım daireler ya da dışı noktalarla sınırlanmış iç içe çizgilerin oluşturduğu yarım daireler olmak üzere çeşitlilik göstermektedir (FM 43). Bu bezeme stili, Çine-Tepecik II 1 kültür tabakasına ait yerleşmede kase, krater ve üzengi kulplu kaplarda en yaygın uygulanan motiflerdir.[24] Miken boya bezeli seramikte söz konusu bu motiflerin yanı sıra özellikle kaselerde uygulanan dalga bezekler (FM 53) ve ayrıca krater gibi derin kaplar üzerinde görülen dama tahtası da (FM 56) yaygın görülmekte ve paralel bir kronolojiyi vermektedir.[25]

Öte yandan Ege'de derin kaseler ve kraterler üzerine uygulanan figürlü süsleme geleneğine (*Pictorial Style*) GH III B2 evresinde rastlanmaktadır.[26] Ege'de GH III B2 evresi, Miken kraterlerinde kuş, keçi, boğa ve araba sahnelerinin resimsel bir anlatımla işlendiği *Pictorial Style* grubunda görülür.[27] Bu gelenek, GH III C erken evresinden itibaren ise, politik değişime paralel olarak bölgesel bezeme stilleriyle gelişimini sürdürmüştür.[28] Yunanistan'da figürlü tasvirler, büyük boyutlu kaplarda, kraterlerde ya da derin kaselerde uygulanmaya devam etmiştir. Bu kaplar arasında kraterler, Yunanistan ve adalarda geniş bir yayılım alanına sahiptir.[29] Doğu Ege adalarında ve Batı Anadolu'da figürlü seramik geleneğini, Geç Hellas III C orta evresine değin takip etmek mümkündür.[30] GH III C erken ve orta evrelerine ait figürlerde ve motiflerde zengin bir süsleme anlayışı görülmektedir. Ege dünyasında kuş betimlemelerinde detaylarda görülen farklılıklar, bu zenginliği yansıtmaktadır.[31] Figürlü kaplarda kuşlar ve balıklar ya friz halinde ya da keçi,

---

21 Shelton 2010, 146.

22 Jung 2010, 174, tab. 13.1.

23 Furumark 1941, 340–348.

24 Günel 2010, fig. 16–22, tab. 4.

25 Günel 2010, 13–15, 32–39, fig. 8–23, tab. 4.

26 Mountjoy 1999, 35.

27 Mountjoy 1999, 35.

28 Vermeule 1964, 206–210; Mountjoy 1999, 44, 50; Crouwel 2006, 15–22; Crouwel 2007, 73–82.

29 Mountjoy 1999, 44.

30 Mountjoy 1999, 50; Crouwel 2007, 73–82.

31 Furumark 1941, 250–255, FM 7.

at ve geyik gibi hayvanlarla bir arada resmedilmiştir.[32] Miken seramiğindeki bu zenginlik, Ege'de kültürel anlamda tekrar bir canlanmayı ifade etmekte ve ayrıca Doğu Akdeniz'e uzanan geniş coğrafyada bölgelerarası ilişkilerin yoğunluğunu ortaya koymaktadır.[33] Miken seramiğinin kronolojik gelişiminde, GH III C evresine ait Miken kraterlerinde konu olarak silahlarıyla birlikte işlenmiş figürlerin yer aldığı askeri bir konu ya da hayvanlarla birlikte resmedilmiş bir avcı öne çıkmaktadır.[34] Kraterlerdeki bu resimsel anlatımlarda gerek figürlerin işlenişi gerekse ana sahnede yer alan motifler bölgesel etkileri yansıtır.[35] Benzer sahneleri ve bölgesel etkiyi, Tepecik'te yerli Miken kraterleri de ortaya koymaktadır. Tepecik'te bu iki ana konunun yanı sıra diğer Miken kaplarında da farklı stilde işlenmiş kuş tasvirleri, balık ve aynı zamanda geyik, keçi tasvirlerinin işlendiği zengin bir grup bulunmaktadır. Tepecik derin kase ya da kraterleri üzerinde uygulanan bu figüratif betimlemeler, Miken seramik geleneğiyle paralel bir kronolojiyi ve tasvir anlayışını yansıtmaktadır.

Bu değerlendirmeler kapsamında, Tepecik Geç Tunç Çağı yerleşmesine ait Miken seramiği, GH III B ve GH III C erken ve orta evrelerinin malzemesini oluşturmakta ve en yakın paralellerine Yunanistan ve Doğu Ege adalarında rastlanmaktadır. Ayrıca Ege ve Doğu Akdeniz'de, GH III C dönemi Miken seramik gelişiminde yerli üretimlerin artması, adalara uzanan bir göç dalgasının göstergesi olarak açıklanmaktadır.[36] Bu kronolojik gelişimde, Tepecik figürlü derin kase ve kraterleri, GH III B2-GH III C erken/orta evrelerinin süsleme geleneğini yansıtmaktadır. Tepecik Miken seramiğinde yerli üretim kapların sayıca belirgin bir yoğunlukta olması da, Ege'de gerçekleşen bu hareketlilikle bağlantılı olmalıdır. Buna göre, Tepecik, bölgelerarası ilişkilerin varlığına ışık tutmasının yanı sıra Miken kültürel etkisinin kıyı şeridinden içerde, Çine bölgesine değin takip edilebileceğini ortaya koyan bir merkez olarak bölge arkeolojisinde yerini almaktadır.

---

32 Slenczka 1974, 73–75, pl. 25–31, 39; Crouwel 2006, fig. 16; Mountjoy 1999, 922, fig. 376; 1073, fig. 438, 267; 1106, 452, 101; Güntner 2000, 85–127, 261–288, pl. 38–59; Vlachopoulos 2003, 221, fig. 4: b.

33 Doğu Akdeniz Bölgesi'nde, Kıbrıs – Enkomi Miken figürlü kaplar arasında kuş tasvirleri için Bkz.: Vermeule / Karageorghis 1982, 204, 208, fig. V.61-V.72, VI. 29-VI. 39; Güney Anadolu – Tarsus Miken seramiği; Mountjoy 2006, 118–120, fig. 8.

34 Crouwel 2006, 16.

35 Crouwel 2006, 20.

36 Rutter 2010, 420.

Katalog

Kat. 1 , Res. 2–3
Env. No: 10/29
Cinsi: krater parçası
Bul. Yeri: açma: M/12; plankare: I-V/a-e; derinlik: 58.10 m
Tarihlendirme: tabaka: II 1; dönem: GTÇ
Hamur: Orta nitelikte; hamur rengi: kırmızı (2.5 YR 5/6- red)
Astar: içte: kırmızı (5 YR 5/6-yellowish red); dışta: bej (10 YR 7/3–7/4- very pale brown)
Boya Bezeme: içte: kırmızı (5 YR 5/6- yellowish red) dışta: kırmızı/ kırmızımsı-kahverengi (5 YR 5/3-reddish brown; 5 YR 5/4- reddish brown; 5 YR 5/6-yellowish red)
Ölçüler: kor. yük. 12.99 cm; kor. gen. 7.03 cm ; cidar kal 1.32 cm.

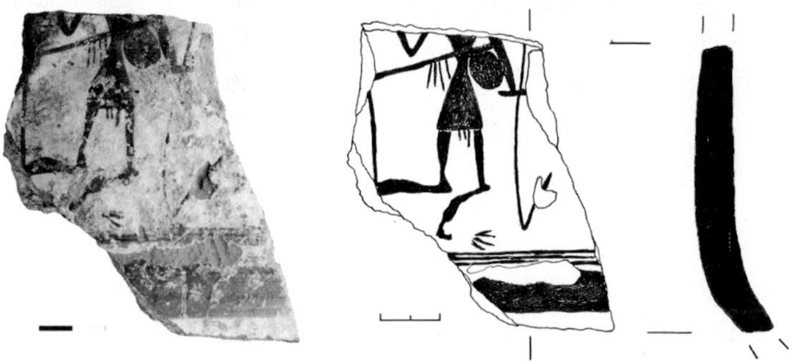

Kat. 2, Res. 4–5
Env. No: 13/95
Cinsi: kase parçası
Bul. Yeri: açma: M/11; plankare: V/g; derinlik: 57.37 m
Tarihlendirme: tabaka: II 1; dönem: GTÇ
Hamur: Orta nitelikte; hamur rengi: kırmızı/kiremit kırmızı (5 YR 5/6-yellowish red)
Astar: Bej (10 YR 8/3- very pale brown)
Boya Bezeme: içte: kırmızı (2.5 YR 5/6-red); dışta: kırmızı (2.5 YR 5/6-red)
Ölçüler: ağız çapı 15.04 cm; kor. yük. 3.63 cm; kor. gen. 2.95 cm; cidar kal. 0.42–0.51 cm

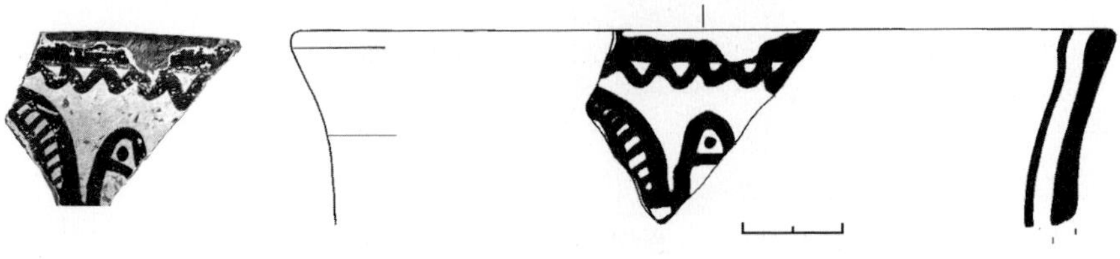

Kat. 3, Res. 6–7
Env. No: 11/71
Cinsi: kase parçası
Bul. Yeri: açma: L/12 ; plankare: VIII-X/d-i; derinlik: 58.05–57.96 m
Tarihlendirme: tabaka: II 1; dönem: GTÇ
Hamur: Orta nitelikte; hamur rengi: kırmızı (5 YR 4/4-reddish brown)
Astar: içte: gri (5 YR 4/1-dark gray); dışta: bej (10 YR 7/3-very pale brown)
Boya Bezeme: içte: kırmızı (5 YR 6/6-reddish yellow); dışta: kırmızı (5 YR 5/6-yellowish red)
Ölçüler: ağız çapı 16.02 cm; kor. yük. 7.64 cm; kor. gen. 6.45 cm; cidar kal.0.99 cm

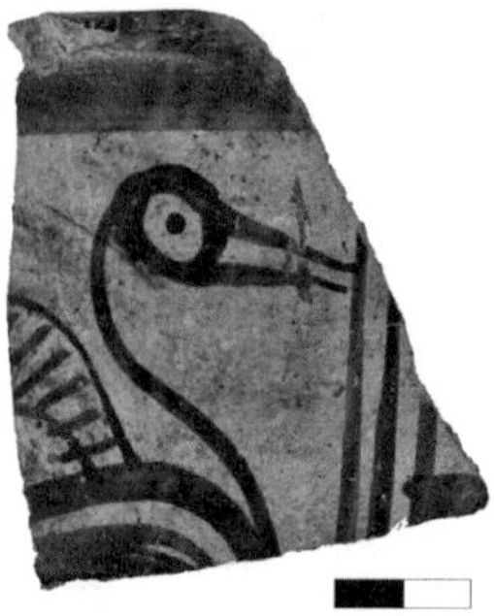

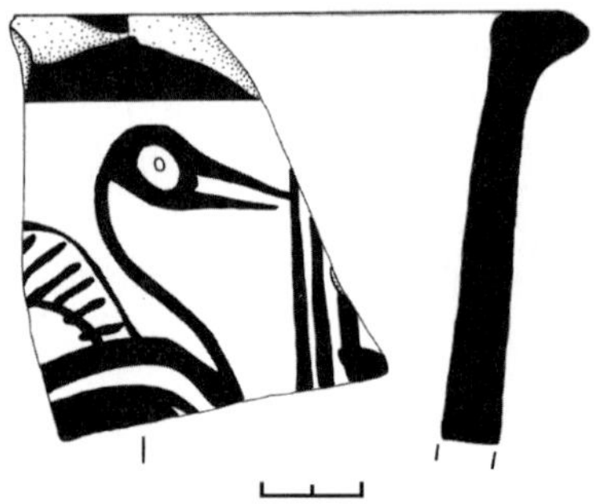

Kat. 4 , Res. 8
Env. No: 13/99
Cinsi: krater parçası
Bul. Yeri: açma: K/12 ; plankare: I-VI/f-i ; Derinlik: 57.66
Tarihlendirme: tabaka: II 1; dönem: GTÇ
Hamur: Orta nitelikte; hamur rengi: kırmızı (5 YR 4/4-reddish brown)
Astar: içte: kırmızımsı-devetüyü (5 YR 6/6-reddish yellow); dışta: Bej (10 YR 7/3-very pale brown)
Boya Bezeme: kırmızı (5 YR 5/6-yellowish red)
Ölçüler: kor. yük.: 6.03 cm; kor. gen. 7.01 cm; cidar kal.: 0.72 m

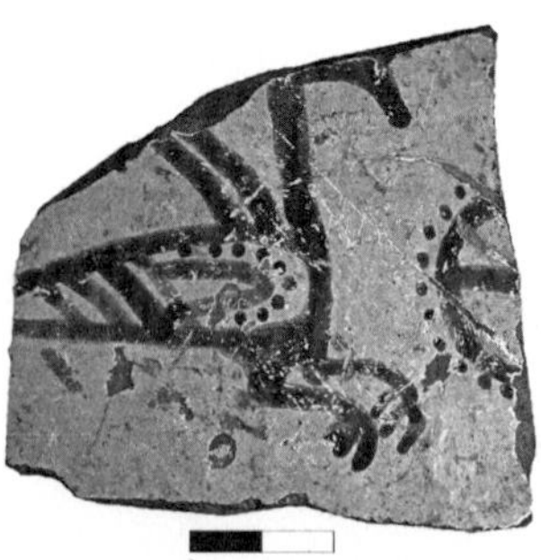

Kat. 5 , Res. 9–10
Env. No: 13/08
Cinsi: krater parçası
Bul. Yeri: açma: L/13; plankare: VI-X/a-c; derinlik: 58.31–58.20 m
Tarihlendirme: tabaka: II 1; dönem: GTÇ
Hamur: Orta nitelikte; hamur rengi: kırmızı (2.5 YR 5/6-red)
Astar: içte: kırmızı (2.5 YR 5/6-red); dışta: bej/krem (10 YR 8/3-very pale brown)
Boya Bezeme: dışta: kırmızı (2.5 YR 5/8-red)
Ölçüler: kor. yük. 6.68 cm; kor. gen. 12.69 cm; cidar kal.0.81 cm

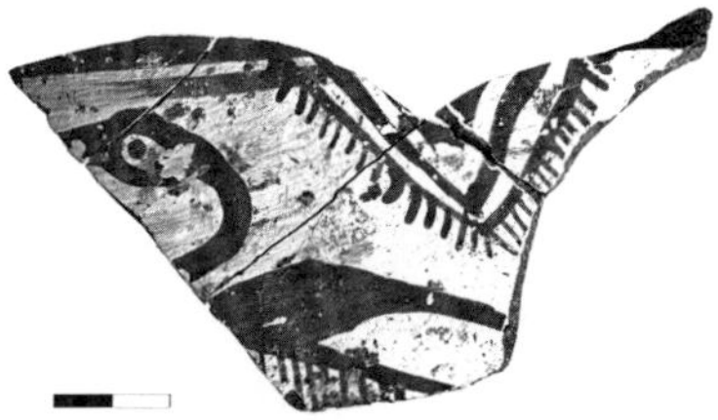

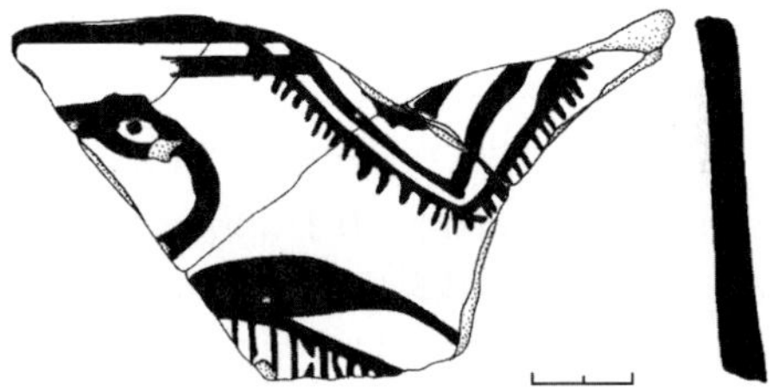

Kat. 6 , Res. 11–12
Env. No: 13/66
Cinsi: kase parçası
Bul. Yeri: açma: M/11 ; plankare: I-V/a-e; derinlik: 57.10–57.05 m
Tarihlendirme: tabaka: II 1; dönem: GTÇ
Hamur: Orta nitelikte; hamur rengi: devetüyü (2.5 YR 5/6-reddish brown)
Astar: içte: devetüyü (2.5 YR 5/6-reddish brown); dışta: bej/krem (10 YR 7/4-pale brown)
Boya Bezeme: içte: koyu siyahımsı- kahverengi (10 YR 3/2- very dark grayish brown); dışta: koyu kahverengi (10 YR 4/2- dark grayish brown; 10 YR 4/3-brown)
Ölçüler: ağız çapı 27.03 cm; kor. yük. 5.28 cm; kor. gen. 9.92 cm; cidar kal.0.93 cm

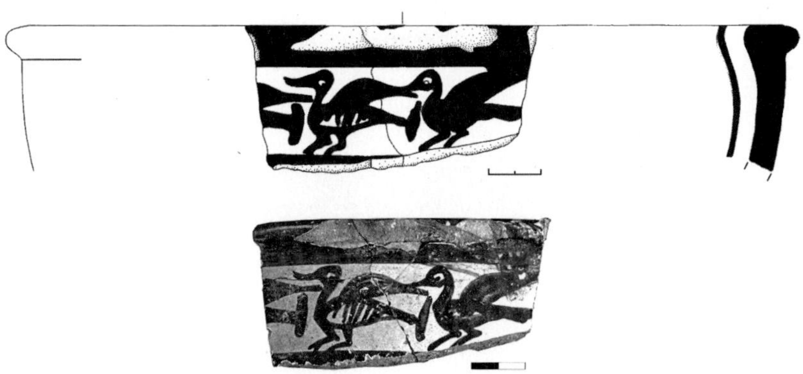

Kat. 7 , Res. 13–14

Env. No: 09/10

Cinsi: Krater parçası

Bul. Yeri: açma: K/12 ; plankare: I-V/f-i ; derinlik: 58.23–58.14 m

Tarihlendirme: tabaka: II 1; dönem: GTÇ

Hamur: Orta nitelikte; hamur rengi: kırmızı (5 YR 5/6-yellowish red); özü gri (5 YR 5/1-gray)

Astar: içte: gri (10 YR 4/1-dark gary); dışta: bej (10 YR 8/3-very pale brown)

Boya Bezeme: dışta: kırmızı (5 YR 5/6-yellowish red; 2.5 YR 5/8-red; bej (10 YR 8/3-very pale brown)

Ölçüler: ağız çapı 30.01 cm; kor. yük. 6.54 cm; ağız çapı 27.02 cm; cidar kal. 0.95 cm

Cinsi: krater parçası

Bul. Yeri: açma: L/13; plankare: VI-X/a-c; derinlik: 58.31–58.20 m

Tarihlendirme: tabaka: II 1; dönem: GTÇ

Hamur: Orta nitelikte; hamur rengi: kırmızı (2.5 YR 5/6-red)

Astar: içte: kırmızı (2.5 YR 5/6-red); dışta: bej/krem (10 YR 8/3-very pale brown)

Boya Bezeme: dışta: kırmızı (2.5 YR 5/8-red)

Ölçüler: kor. yük. 6.68 cm; kor. gen. 12.69 cm; cidar kal.0.81 cm

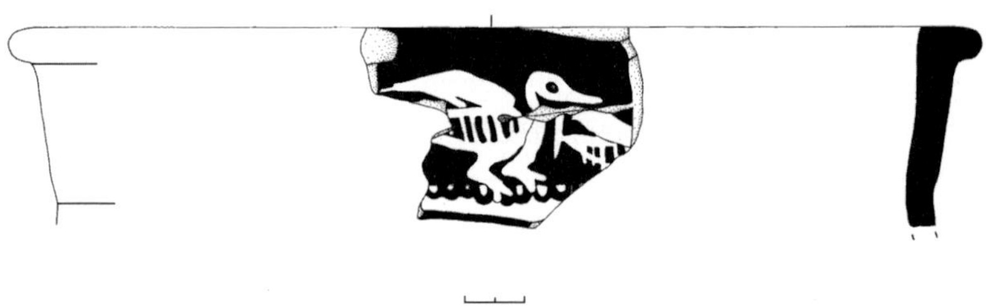

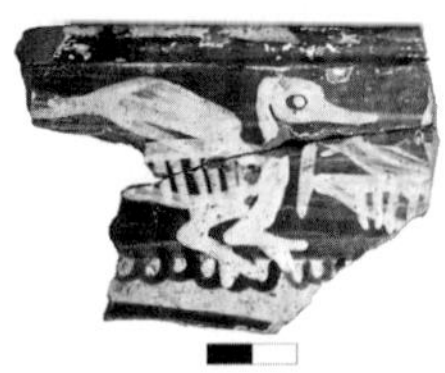

KAYNAKÇA

Benzi, M., *Rodi e la civiltá Micenea*. Rome: Gruppo Editoriale Internazionale, 1992.

Burns, B.E., "Trade" in *The Oxford Handbook of the Bronze Age Aegean (ca. 3000–1000 BC)*, ed. by E. H. Cline, 291–304. Oxford: Oxford University Press, 2010.

Crouwel, J.H., "Late Mycenaean Pictorial Pottery a Brief Review" in *Pictorial Pursuits. Figurative Painting on Mycenaean and Geometric Pottery*, ed. by E. Rystedt and B. Wells, 15–22. Stockholm: Svenska Institutet i Athen, 2006.

———. "Pictorial Pottery of LH III C Middle and its Antecedents" in *LH III C Chronology and Synchronisms II LH III C Middle*, ed. by S. Deger -Jalkotzy and M. Zavadil, 77–88. Vienna: Verlag der Österreichschen Akademie der Wissenschaften, 2007.

Demakopoulou, K., "Mycenaean Pictorial Pottery from Midea" in *Pictorial Pursuits. Figurative painting on Mycenaean and Geometric Pottery*, ed. by E. Rystedt and B. Wells, 31–43. Stockholm: Svenska Institutet i Athen, 2006.

Forrer, E., *Forschungen*. Band 1, Heft 1. Berlin 1926.

Furumark, A., *The Mycenaean Pottery. Analysis and Classification*. Stockholm: Kungl, 1941.

Garstang, J., "Hittite Military Roads in Asia Minor. A Study in Imperial Strategy with a Map." *American Journal of Archaeology* 47 (1943): 35–62.

Garstang, J. and O. R Gurney, *The Geography of the Hittite Empire*. London: British Institute of Archaeology at Ankara, 1959.

Günel, S., "Çine-Tepecik Kazıları ve Bölge Arkeolojisine Katkıları" in *Batı Anadolu ve Doğu Akdeniz Geç Tunç Çağı Kültürleri Üzerine Yeni Araştırmalar*, ed. by A. Erkanal-Öktü, S. Günel and U. Deniz, 129–139. Ankara: Hacettepe Üniversitesi Yayınları, 2008.

———. "Mycenaean Cultural Impact on the Çine (Marsyas) Plain Southwest Anatolia: the Evidence from Çine-Tepecik." *Anatolian Studies* 60 (2010): 25–49.

———. "Çine-Tepecik Geç Tunç Çağı Yerleşmesi." *Türk Eskiçağ Bilimleri Enstitüsü. Haberler* 32 (2011): 1–8.

———. "Çine-Tepecik: New Contributions on Late Bronze Age Cultures in Western Anatolia" in *NOSTOI Indigenous Culture, Migration+Integration in the Aegean Islands+Western Anatolia during the Late Bronze+Early Iron Age*, ed. by N. Chr. Stampolidis, Ç. Maner and K. Kopanias, 607–626. Istanbul: Koç University Press, 2015.

———. forthcoming. "Contributions on the Cultures of Western Anatolia in the Second Millennium BC" in *The Geography and Landscape of the Hittites*, ed. by L. Ullmann and M. Weeden. Leiden: Brill.

Günel, S. and S. Herbordt, "Ein hethitischer Siegelabdruck aus Çine-Tepecik." *Archäologischer Anzeiger* 1 (2010): 1–11.

———. "Mykenische Kraterfragmente mit figürlichen Darstellungen und ein Siegelabdruck eines hethitischen Prinzen aus der spätbronzezeitlichen Siedlung von Çine-Tepecik." *Archäologischer Anzeiger* 1 (2014): 1–14.

Güntner, W., *Figürlich bemalte mykenische Keramik aus Tiryns, Tiryns XII,* Mainz am Rhein: Von Zabern, 2000.

Hawkins, J.D., "Tarkasnawa King of Mira. 'Tarkondemos', Boğazköy Sealings and Karabel." *Anatolian Studies* 48 (1998): 1–31.

Heinhold-Krahmer, S., *Arzawa. Untersuchungen zu seiner Geschichte nach den hethitischen Quellen.* Texte der Hethiter 8. Heidelberg: Carl Winter Universitätsverlag, 1977.

Jung, R., "End of the Bronze Age" in *The Oxford Handbook of the Bronze Age Aegean* (*ca. 3000–1000 BC*), ed. by E. H. Cline, 171–184. Oxford: Oxford University Press, 2010.

Mountjoy, P.A., *Regional Mycenaean Decorated Pottery.* Berlin: Vermeule, 1999.

———. "Mycenaean Pictorial Pottery from Anatolia in the Transitional LH IIIB2- LH IIIC Early and the LH IIIC Phases" in *Pictorial Pursuits. Figurative Painting on Mycenaean and Geometric Pottery,* ed. by E. Rystedtand B Wells, 107–121. Stockholm: Svenska Institutet i Athen, 2006.

Rahmstorf, L., "Clay Spools from Tiryns and Other Contemporary Sites. An Indication of Foreign Influence in LH IIIC?" in *2nd International Interdisciplinary Colloquium. The Periphery of the Mycenaean World, 26–30 September 1999, Lamia,* ed. by N. Kyparissi-Apostolika and M. Papakonstantinou, 397–415. Lamia, 2003.

———. "Ethnicity and Changes in Weaving Technology in Cyprus and the Eastern Mediterranean in the 12th Century BC" in *Cyprus: Religion and Society from the Late Bronze Age to the End of the Archaic Period. Proceedings of an International Symposium on Cypriote Archaeology, Erlangen, 23–24 July 2004,* ed. by V. Karageorghis, H. Matthäus and S. Rogge, 143–169. Möhnesee: Bibliopolis, 2005.

———. *Kleinfunde aus Tiryns. Terrakotta, Stein, Bein und Glas/Fayence, vornehmlich der Spätbronzezeit, Tiryns XVI.* Mainz am Rhein: Von Zabern, 2008.

Rutter, J.B., "Mycenaean Pottery" in *The Oxford Handbook of the Bronze Age Aegean* (*ca. 3000 1000 BC*), ed. by E. H. Cline, 412– 429. Oxford: Oxford University Press, 2010.

Shelton, K., "Mainland Greece" in *The Oxford Handook of the Bronze Age Aegean* (*ca. 3000–1000 BC*), ed. by E. H. Cline, 139–148. Oxford: Oxford University Press, 2010.

Slenczka, E., *Figürlich bemalte mykenische Keramik aus Tiryns, Tiryns VII.* Mainz am Rhein: Phillip von Zabern, 1974.

Strobel, K., "Neues zur Geographie und Geschichte des Alten Anatolien. Eine Einführung mit Beiträgen zur Hethitischen Geographie des westlichen Anatolien" in *New Perspectives on the Historical Geography and Topography of Anatolia in the II and I Millennium BC, Eothen* 16, ed. by K. Strobel, 9–16. Florence: Logisma Editore, 2008.

Ünal, A., *Hititler Devrinde Anadolu.* İstanbul: Arkeoloji ve Sanat Yayınları, 2003.

Vermeule, E., *Greece in the Bronze Age.* Chicago: University of Chicago Press, 1964.

Vermeule, E. and V. Karageorghis, *Mycenaean Pictorial Vase Painting.* Cambridge, MA: Harvard University Press, 1982.

Vlachopoulos, A., "The Late Helladic III C 'Grotta Phase' of Naxos. Its Synchronisms in the Aegean and Its Non-Synchronisms in the Cyclades" in *LH III C Chronology and Synchronisms. Proceedings of the International Workshop Held at the Austrian Academy of Sciences at Vienna*, ed. by S. Deger-Jalkotzy and M. Zavadil, 217–234. Vienna: Österreichische Akademie der Wissenschaften, 2003.

PART 4

Iron Age

The Performance of Neo-Assyrian Prophecy in the Temple: an Archaeological-Textual Approach

Selim F. Adalı[1] — *Erkan Akbulut*[2]

It is a great privilege and pleasure to write for this volume prepared in honour of Marie-Henriette and Charles Gates. This contribution investigates a topic that confirms their emphasis on the need to interpret both the textual and the archaeological record.

Abstract

The present contribution investigates the prophetic performance that took place in Ešarra, the temple of Aššur. This is a detailed study of cuneiform tablet K 2401 (= State Archives of Assyria [SAA] 9 3) which records prophecies in the temple. The temple's architectural context also contributes to a better understanding of the setting, the socio-political standing and even some of the wording of the prophecies. Such prophecies were sponsored by the Assyrian Empire as part of its mission to control its subjects.

Judaism, Christianity, and Islam are religions that have preserved prophetic traditions to our day. There were, however, other older traditions in the ancient Near East. The two main corpora of cuneiform texts concerning ancient Near Eastern prophecy are the Old Babylonian texts from Mari during the reign of Zimri-Lim

---

1 Department of History, Ankara Social Sciences University, Hükümet Meydanı No.2, Ankara 06030, Turkey.

2 The Skirball Department of Hebrew and Judaic Studies, New York University.
Selim F. Adalı would like to acknowledge the benefit of the Senior Fellowship awarded to me by Koç University's Research Center for Anatolian Civilizations when concluding the present contribution. Both authors would also like to acknowledge Bilkent University Library. We would also like to thank the editors of the present volume for accepting our paper, as well as Yağmur Heffron and Tevfik Emre Şerifoğlu for providing us with very helpful feedback. Responsibility for any possible error in this paper belongs to the authors alone. This paper was completed before the availability of Ponchia 2014.

(1775–1762 BC) and the Neo-Assyrian texts from Nineveh during the reigns of Esarhaddon (680–669 BC) and Assurbanipal (668–631/627? BC.).[3] Neo-Assyrian prophetic texts include oracle collections, letters and various other texts with quotations of or references to prophecy or prophets.[4] Prophecies/oracles can be defined as divine messages in the form of first-person speech, uttered and recited by human transmitter(s).[5] This paper applies a combined archaeological and textual approach to certain Neo-Assyrian prophecies performed in Ešarra, the temple of Aššur. This is because the architectural context of the temple helps better understand the content of the prophecies performed. A brief discussion of some of the broader implications of this interpretation for the social and political context of Neo-Assyrian prophecy will conclude our study.

The cuneiform tablet K 2401 (= SAA 9 3) is an oracle collection which records certain prophecies delivered within Ešarra, the temple of the national god Aššur in the ancient city of Aššur (modern Qalʿat Šerqāṭ).[6]

The content of SAA 9 3 is divided into two parts and five sections. All sections are divided by a single line, except the double ruling between the third and fourth sections. The first part consists of the first three sections, separated by the double ruling from the second part, which consists of sections four and five.

If recording more than one oracle from different settings, the Neo-Assyrian oracle collections delineate each oracle with a single line.[7] The double line in SAA 9 3 seems to make a further distinction. Weippert proposed that the double line separates Aššur's *šulmu* prophecies in the first part from the *abutu* ("word") of Ištar of Arbela in the second part.[8] Prophecies labelled as *šulmu* ("well-being") in the Neo-Assyrian texts are prophecies which express good tidings for whom they are addressed.

3 Nissinen 2003; Stökl 2012, 29–34.

4 Collected in Nissinen 2003, 101–177; Stökl 2012, 104–109, with further references.

5 Nissinen 2003, 1–2; *cf.* Stökl 2012, 7–11. Negotiating a more precise definition for prophecy is beyond the scope of the present paper. For our purposes, the terms 'prophecy' and 'oracle' are used interchangeably, while noting that otherwise both terms may be viewed within wider semantic ranges.

6 For the editions of K 2401, see Parpola 1997, 22–27 (= SAA 9 3); Nissinen 2003, 118–124, with further references. We thank the Trustees of the British Museum for the photographs of K 2401, available online to the public. The transliteration of SAA 9 3 confirms Parpola's edition unless otherwise stated. Parpola's collations and philological readings have received positive reviews (*cf.* Postgate 2002), despite objections to his views on Assyrian religion (Frahm 2000/01, Lambert 2001/02, among others). For the name of Ešarra ("House of the Universe"), see George 1993, 145, 1035.

7 K 4310 (= SAA 9 1) also has a double line, but the preceding section is mostly destroyed and the final three lines preserve merely a few words; the purpose of the double line is unclear.

8 Weippert 2002, 16.

Part One, Section One (SAA 9 3.1)	Introduces participants of the ceremony; *šulmu* in fragmented context
Part One, Section Two (SAA 9 3.2)	Aššur's *šulmu* oracle before the 'Lord of the Courtyard'
Part One, Section Three (SAA 9 3.3)	Aššur's *šulmu* oracle before the 'Image'
Part Two, Section Four (SAA 9 3.4)	Word of Ištar of Arbela (*abat Issār ša Arbail*), by a designated *raggimu*[9]
Part Two, Section Five (SAA 9 3.5)	Word of Ištar of Arbela (*abat Issār ša Arbail*), by a designated *raggimu*

In the first part, there are short descriptions of where the *šulmu*-oracles were delivered (SAA 9 3 ii 8–9; ii 26). They can be regarded as postscripts, with subsidiary information about the rituals and the setting.[10] The double line served to distinguish between the oracles of Aššur and Ištar of Arbela, respectively. It may be that the oracles of these two deities referred to two different occassions collected on one tablet. According to this view, the double line (instead of the usual single line mentioned above) is delineating two different texts on one tablet.[11]

The exact function of the double ruling is unclear, since SAA 9 3 mentions only one prophet, despite recording different divine messages, bearing in mind that the established practice, as seen in the other Neo-Assyrian oracle collections, was to register the prophet of every recorded oracle.[12] On the other hand, scribes could insert a double ruling even when they continued the same text and indicated no new divide.[13] In another Neo-Assyrian prophetic text, Bayâ spoke consecutively

9 *Raggimu* is a unique Neo-Assyrian term for someone who performs prophecy. Its etymology and significance is discussed further below in the conclusion.

10 There is a similar situation in SAA 9 1 v 26–36 (with an extra 8[?] lines destroyed) where an oracle (not preserved) was accompanied by certain descriptions of the goddess Ištar of Arbela. De Jong (2007, 173) notices that the unit has a description of the activities of Ištar of Arbela and the text is broken even before the description ends. The text says that the goddess went out to the "steppe" (EDIN) and sent a *šulmu*, a message of well-being. An oracle followed this description and was recorded and delineated in the same manner as all the previous eight units in SAA 9 1, as well as in the subsequent oracle. SAA 9 1 v 26f. was designed to contain an oracle. It is therefore possible to have a record of an oracle with other information as conceived by the scribe and the *Sitz im Leben*.

11 Lambert 2001/02, 209; Villard 2001, 80.

12 Parpola 1997, lxiii-lxiv. Parpola restores the name of the prophet in SAA 9 3 iv 31 as [*Lā-dāgil-i*]*li*. The text only has [... DIN]GIR, according to Parpola's collation. The trace of this sign is hard to see, but the identification cannot be excluded; *cf.* Stökl 2012, 112, 212.

13 E.g. Heeßel 2007, 44–50, 164–165: text 11 (where the single and double rulings function in the same way).

in the name of Bēl Marduk, Ištar of Arbela, and Nabû.[14] Scholars disagree as to why,[15] but the point here is that such a change in deities could potentially occur in other texts. Did the *raggimu* of SAA 9 3 consecutively prophesy in the name of Aššur and Ištar of Arbela? Regretably, the final subscript of SAA 9 3 is not completely intact. The name of the *raggimu* is missing. If the name is to be restored as [Lā-dāgil-il]i as proposed by Parpola, then a Lā-dāgil-ili from Arbela is indeed known.[16] He may have travelled to Aššur for the ceremony in Ešarra,[17] but he may have prophesied in Arbela. The alternative tentative hypothesis is that he or another prophet(ess) participated in two separate rituals.[18] The postscript in SAA 9 3 consists of more than his name and the designation *raggimu* (iv 31–35). The extra line may have had more information about him or his circumstances.

Aššur's *šulmu* messages are recorded as oracles alongside those of Ištar of Arbela, regardless of whether or not the two parts of SAA 9 3 are concerned with the same ceremony. The second part of SAA 9 3 has a ritual setting, as well as the *raggimu* delivering prophecy. For the purposes of this paper, we will not take sides on this debate. Rather, we will focus on the first part of SAA 9 3 and Aššur's *šulmu*-oracles delivered in Ešarra, because this is where we get the information relating to their archaeological setting.

The literary and retrospective features of Aššur's oracles, along with the mention of rituals in SAA 9 3, may raise questions about the origin and character of these oracles.[19] The use of the term *šulmu* in other Neo-Assyrian prophecies, however, helps see that they are oracles. In SAA 9 1 v 26, *šulmu* (DI-*mu*) *ana Aššūr-aḫu-iddina* ("*šulmu* to Esarhaddon") refers to the *šulmu*-oracle that has come to the king from Ištar of Arbela, referred to in the same text as *šulmu ana mūrīšá* "(an oracle of) well-being to her calf (i.e. Esarhaddon)" (v 29).[20] Here is an oracle named *šulmu*, indicating good tidings. SAA 9 2 i 33′ has [*š*]*ul-me*, restored by Parpola. This refers again to the well-being of Esarhaddon. Another oracle in the

14 SAA 9 1 ii 16′–40′.

15 Parpola (1997, xvii-xx) proposed that the two deities were considered identical. Frahm (2000/01, 228) argued against this and states that there are other visions involving more than one deity (ARM 26 208). Kwasman (2001, 228) argued each deity in Bayâ's oracle represented a stage in Esarhaddon's life. For Lambert (2001/02, 209), the Mesopotamian prophet could speak in the name of a succession of deities, however unusual that may seem today.

16 SAA 9 1 vi 31–32; SAA 9 2:28′; *cf.* Parpola 1997, l.

17 There are cases whereby a prophet's/prophetess' place of origin did not coincide with the place where s/he delivered the prophecy. For example, a prophetess from Arbela spoke in Nineveh (SAA 9 9); *cf.* Toorn 2000, 73.

18 *Cf.* Stökl 2012, 140, n. 68.

19 Villard 2001, 80; Pongratz-Leisten 1999, 77, 267, 272; de Jong 2007, 173–174, 185–186.

20 Parpola 1997, 10.

same text bids the king to send out two burnt offerings to the presence of the gods of Esaggil so that they will announce, says Lā-dāgil-ili to the king, "your well-being (*šulmu*)" (SAA 9 2 ii 27′). The *šulmu* of Esarhaddon announced before the presence of the god Aššur in Ešarra is, we argue, a similar type of oracle of well-being. SAA 9 3.1 is too fragmented to infer further details about this, but most probably the *šulmu* oracle here, called the "introductory oracle" by Nissinen, is an oracle from Aššur, as are the next two in the first part of SAA 9 3.[21]

Prophetic Performance in Ešarra

The first section in SAA 9 3 introduces a ceremony which the god "Aššur has arranged in Ešarra" ([... *ina*] E2.ŠAR2.RA ^{d}*Aš-šur is-sa-kan*; i 14).[22] Parpola reads *isinnu* in the gap before the name of Ešarra in this line.[23] Postgate proposes the Neo-Assyrian form of the word, *sinnu* ('festival'). He suggests that a wordplay links i 14 with iv 28, rendering iv 28b-30 as *ina* UGU *sin-ni-šú-nu* [*a-na* ^{GIŠ}]*za-qi-ba-a-ni* [*as*]*-sa-kan-šú-nu* "for their festival I will put them on stakes."[24] The wordplay, in our view, indicates that the gathering in i 14 was also on the occasion of a festival of a similar kind, one of the implications being that festivals legitimated royal rule (or rebels may participate in festivals assuming a false ruler).[25] The prophecies in SAA 9 3 allude to the early years of Esarhaddon (*c.* 681–679 BC), i.e. the king's civil war victory. The mention of the treaty/loyalty oaths (*adê*) and the ritual descriptions in SAA 9 3 are seen as linked with and/or embedded into the king's coronation

21 Nissinen 2000, 251–252. The third person references to Aššur do not prevent them from being words from this god; *cf.* SAA 9 9:3–7, r.1–3 as noted by Nissinen 2000, 252, n. 62.

22 The festival is placed in Aššur, i.e. "Inner City"; SAA 9 3 i 15.

23 Note that in the second part of SAA 9 3, Ištar of Arbela also says: "I organized a [fest] ival" ([x x x *sin*]–*nu a-sa-kan*); SAA 9 3 iv 6. We take [x x x *sin*]–*nu* instead of [x x x *i-sin*]–*nu*, see Postgate's (2002, 313) proposal to read the Neo-Assyrian form *sinnu* in place of *isinnu* in SAA 9 3 iv 28. This must be separated from 'Aššur's festival' (*i-sin-ni* AN.ŠÁR) held at the *akītu* chapel of Aššur; Parpola 1997, 22:i 14.

24 Postgate 2002, 313. The drop in the initial vowel is examplified by Postgate with Neo-Assyrian *killu* for *ikkillu* (SAA 9 3 ii 14; *cf.* SAA 9 5:3). One can add Neo-Assyrian *garinnu* for *agarinnu* "mother" (SAA 9 3 i 24; *cf.* Parpola 1997, 23: i 24).

25 The information at hand does not help settle if the two parts of SAA 9 3 are referring to the same festival or separate ones. Ištar of Arbela's festival is also referred to as a 'banquet' (*qarītu*; SAA 9 3 iii 26). For a *qarītu*-festival of Ištar of Arbela, as well as of other deities, see Menzel 1981, 21–22. Most pertinent documents concern the *qarītu*-festival of Ištar of Arbela, but it is not clear if this was a regular festival. One letter (SAA 13 147: 11) assumes a *qarītu*-festival of Ištar of Arbela in Arbela, whereas there was also a functioning cult of the same goddess in Aššur (Menzel 1981, 81). A text (VAT 8767, 1–5) found in Aššur mentions offerings made for a *qarītu*-festival of the same goddess; Menzel 1981, 22.

rituals.[26] Pongratz-Leisten proposes that all of the oracle collections (SAA 9 1–3; SAA 9 4 is too fragmentary to comment on) represent an abbreviated version of the narrative of Esarhaddon's rise to the throne, written long after the events to support the appointment of Assurbanipal as heir.[27] SAA 9 3 lacks a date, and the proposed dates are tentative.[28]

The "festival" (*sinnu*) in SAA 9 3 refers merely to a festival organized in the name of Aššur. This is not to dismiss the historical background of the prophecies or the dating proposals. Rather, SAA 9 3 records the prophecies without regard to a specific event. The prophecies allude only broadly to past events. SAA 9 3 records oracles delivered during a festival by Aššur, a festival affirming the king. The ritual descriptions of the sprinkling of oil, making sacrifices and the burning of incense are very general and can be associated with any festival.

This first section of SAA 9 3 is very fragmented. Their location is not clear. Esarhaddon is mentioned several times.[29] Besides him, certain persons arrive (*illakūni*; i 22), and (other?) persons burn incense(?) (*išarrupū*; i 23). The persons (or divine statues? in line 22) cannot be identified. The role of the *raggimu* here is not clear, as explained above. Extant is a reference to "his mother" (*ga-ri-ni-šu*).[30] Parpola notes *garinnu* "mother" as a word referring to Esarhaddon's mother Naqi'a/Zakûtu.[31] Naqi'a is mentioned in other texts of Neo-Assyrian prophecy, referred to as the "mother of the king."[32] What is known about her role in ritual processions,

---

26 Parpola 1997, lxviii-lxx; Nissinen 2000, 251; Nissinen 2003, 101; Toorn 2000, 77; Villard 2001, 79; Weippert 2002, 18. The precise meaning and etymology behind *adê* remains unclear. We retain the translation "oaths" because oath-taking was a major component of what constitutes the *adê*. We assume, however, a wider semantics for "oath" in accordance with the fact that oath-taking was part of a process whereby the divine realm assigned as 'destiny' certain obligations of the subjects of the empire, as will be discussed below and as discussed by Lauinger (2013), who additionally suggests that *adê* can be translated as 'duty, destiny' since the practice of *adê* has more contexts than the taking of oaths. We prefer to stay with the translation "oaths" also because the social context of the *adê* and the Tablet of Destinites (discussed further below) remains to be better understood (e.g., how is destiny understood in terms of duty as opposed to oaths?), and the precise etymological relation of *adê* with the homophonous word *adû* ("work assignment, duty") is not clear, since the pertinent data is from late in the Neo-Assyrian period. This needs to be addressed elsewhere.

27 Pongratz-Leisten (forthcoming). Pongratz-Leisten will publish an updated version of her proposal in her upcoming book on religion and ideology in Assyria.

28 *Cf.* de Jong 2007, 250.

29 For this section, SAA 9 3 i 11, 12, 16, 21; also *cf.* SAA 9 3 ii 34, iii 15, 17, iv 13, 14.

30 SAA 9 3 i 24.

31 Parpola 1997, 23: i 24.

32 AMA.LUGAL, SAA 9 1 v 13; AMA.MAN, SAA 9 2 i 13′. These prophecies assume Naqi'a's support for Esarhaddon during his exile; Nissinen 1998, 22–24. SAA 9 5:4 has a text break in the first line. The name of the addressee is lost. Perhaps this

rites, temple offerings, and other such activities, resembles the role of the king.[33] For the 'Zakûtu-Treaty' (SAA 2 8, an *adê* ("oath")-text), Naqi'a took the place of the king and made the Assyrians swear loyalty to her grandson Assurbanipal.[34] She may be present in SAA 9 3, involved in another *adê*-document (discussed below) concerning the king. The 'sons of Assyria' also attend to listen to the oracles and the oaths read out.[35] Assyrian royal correspondance and other texts give the impression that these Assyrians participating in temple rituals were part of the political and religious elite.[36] Preserved in this section is the pronouncement of *šulmu* to the universe, Ešarra, and Esarhaddon:[37]

9 [DI-*mu a*]-*na* AN-*e u* KI-*tim*[38]
10 [DI-*m*]*u*$^{!}$ *a-na* É.ŠÁR.RA
11 [DI-*mu*] ⌈*a*⌉-*na* ^{m}*Aš-šur*-PAB.AŠ MAN KUR *Aš-šur*
12–13 [*šul-m*]*u* šá ^{m}*Aš-šur*-PAB.AŠ [*iš-kun*]-*u*$^{!}$-*ni*$^{!}$ *ina* UGU GÌR.II *lil-lik*

9 Good tidings (*šulmu*) to Heaven and Earth!
10 Good tidings (*šulmu*) to Ešarra!
10–11 Good tidings (*šulmu*) to Esarhaddon king of Assyria!
12–13 May the good tidings (*šulmu*) of Esarhaddon reach before *his* feet!

Parpola translates lines 12–13 as "[May the well-b]eing which Esarhaddon [has established] *gain footing*!"[39] Building on Parpola's reading [*šul-m*]*u*, we propose that "the feet," written in logograms (GÌR.II), may be assuming a third person

is a reference to Naqi'a, in part due to a later expression using feminine suffixes indicating an address to a female figure; Parpola 1997, 34. These feminine suffixes, however, may refer to a goddess, perhaps Ištar of Arbela, called to mediate for and protect Esarhaddon; de Jong 2007, 174, n. 121.

33 Discussed in Svärd 2012, 109–110. For Naqi'a's significance in general, see Svärd 2012, 106–116, et passim. Svärd's dissertation is due as a State Archives of Assyria Studies volume.

34 Discussed in Svärd 2012, 113–116, with a discussion of the nature of the political power associated with Naqi'a; *cf.* Melville 1999; Melville 2004, 53–57.

35 DUMU.MEŠ KUR *Aš-šur* (SAA 9 3 i 27).

36 Whether people of private individuals or lower classes had access to parts of the temple is not known; Menzel 1981, 297. Future excavations and research could investigate this possibility with a systematic archaeological perspective.

37 SAA 9 3 i 9–13.

38 Instead of KI.TIM (= *kaqquru*), clearly also much used, we propose KI-*tim*, standing for *erṣetim* in the cosmic sense in the traditional expression *šamê u erṣetim* "heaven and earth"; *cf.* CAD E s.v. *erṣetu*, 308–310 with many examples.

39 Parpola 1997, 22.

ending not written out. If so, this reference may be to the feet of Aššur, in reference to the god being the organizer of the festival and news of the king's well-being reaching him symbolically. If correct, Aššur "hears" the good news on line 13, and line 14 refers to him organizing a festival, as discussed above. Additionally, line 20, broken, states: "in front of Aššur" (IGI ᵈ*Aš-šur*). This may be a reference to the statue of Aššur, as the god is the festival organizer. On certain occassions, Aššur could travel in his temple.[40] Even if the statue is mentioned in line 13,[41] it cannot be excluded that the statue had already exited the cultroom during this specific part of the ritual.

The second and third *šulmu*-oracles have legible postscripts indicating where they were delivered. The second *šulmu* was delivered in one of Ešarra's courtyards: "This is the *šulmu* before Bēl-Tarbaṣi and the gods" (*an-ni-u šul-mu ša ina* IGI ᵈEN. TÙR *ina* IGI DINGIR.MEŠ-*ni šá-ki-nu-u-ni*; SAA 9 3 ii 8–9). The god Bēl-Tarbaṣi (ᵈEN.TÙR, 'Lord of the Courtyard') was one of Ešarra's gatekeepers (ᵈÌ.DU8.MEŠ É.ŠÁR.RA) listed in the *Götteraddressbuch* of Aššur.[42] We are unable to precisely identify his gate in the textual and archaeological record. Since he is a gatekeeper, the *šulmu* delivered before him was delivered before a gate. In any case, this *šulmu* oracle was delivered in front of this statue and the gods of the courtyard.[43] The second element of Bēl-Tarbaṣi's name is *tarbaṣu* ("courtyard"). This word does not indicate one specific courtyard, but Driel posits that it may refer to the annexe on the southeastern front of Ešarra, i.e. the *Ostanbau*.[44]

The *Ostanbau* was built under Sennacherib and directly connected with Aššur's cultroom.[45] W. Andrae conceived the *Ostanbau* as enclosed by walls and with limited access to the cultroom and to the paved processional way. The plan drawn by Andrae has gained acceptance, despite the current state of the remains,[46]

---

40 Driel 1969, 143.

41 *Cf.* Weippert 2002, 17.

42 T149:45, 48 (in Menzel 1981). Parpola (1997, 23:ii 8f) quotes the *Götteraddressbuch* and also notes SAA 1 76 r.6 according to which an *adê*-ceremony took place in one of the courtyards of Ešarra. In SAA 1 76, the governor of the Aššur province, Ṭab-ṣilli-Ešarra, informed Sargon II that the 'treaty/oaths tablet of Gurdî' was brought by the Palace Superintendent (LÚ *šá* IGI.É.GAL) for ceremonies in the temple as soon as Gurdî's emissaries arrived. Gurdî was an Anatolian vassal king (of Tunna or Atuna?) of the the Tabal region; *cf.* Fuchs (1994, 411–412).

43 *Cf.* Parpola 1997, lxiv; Nissinen 2000, 252.

44 Driel 1969, 45, 105.

45 For the construction under Sennacherib and the identification of Aššur's cultroom, see Driel 1969, 21–24 and 37 respectively.

46 The denudation of the soil made it very difficult for the excavators to draw an adequate plan of Ešarra, especially for the Neo-Assyrian period; Driel 1969, 32. For a critical appraisal of the problems, see especially Galter 1984.

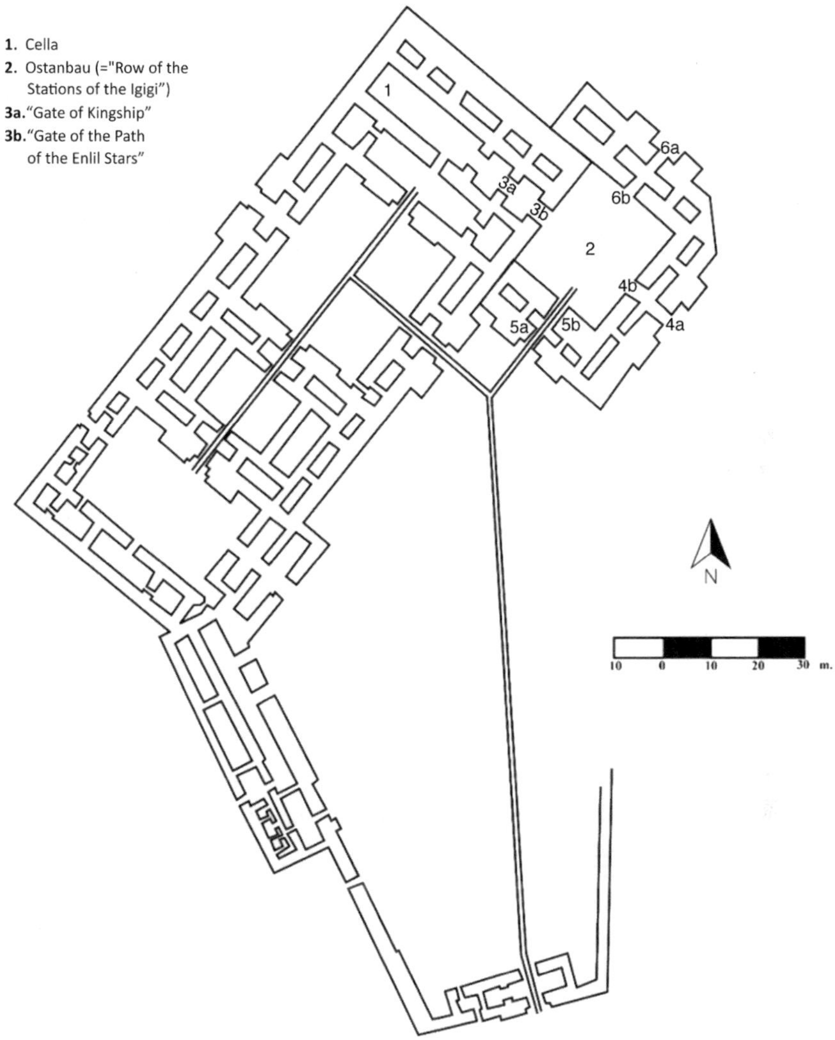

FIG. 1 Ground plan of Ešarra.

partly because it does allow for sufficient entrances, accounting for the new gates named in the texts (see FIG. 1).[47]

Sennacherib built the *Ostanbau* to provide the temple with a courtyard of the divine assembly with Aššur as the king.[48] The *Götteraddressbuch* of Aššur

47 Huxley 2000, 109–110. For the plan, see Haller and Andrae 1955, 51; *cf.* Stępniowski 2003, 244. The temple's ground plan provided in this paper (fig. 1) follows Andrae's plan. For the names of the gates, see George 1992, 182–183, 191–195.

48 Huxley 2000, 119, following George 1989, 119; *cf.* George 1992, 286–291 on the significance of the "dais of destinies" in the Babylonian context.

gives the "Gate of the Dais of Destinies" as the inner gate of the "Gate of the Wagon Star."[49] During the time of the Neo-Assyrian Sargonid dynasty in Ešarra, the "dais of destinies" (*parak šīmāti*) was the shrine which contained the throne occupied by the king of the gods. King Aššur fixed the fates of the universe.[50] The courtyard of the *Ostanbau* is recognized as the "Row of the Stations of the Igigi" (*kisalli sidir manzāz* ᵈ*Igīgī*).[51] The *Ostanbau* appears to be a courtyard where the divine assembly meet under Aššur and the gods.

What about Bēl-Tarbaṣi? Among the gatekeepers associated with Bēl-Tarbaṣi in the *Götteraddressbuch* is "Ninurta of the stable" (ᵈMAŠ *ubusāti*).[52] A text of Sargon II (ND 1120: 19, 22) refers to a "house of the stable" (*bīt ubusāti*) of Ninurta.[53] After Sennacherib's reconstruction, the "house of the stable" is under the god Mandanu, mentioned in the ritual BM 121206 ix 39'. This god is not in the *Götteraddressbuch* which names Bēl-Tarbaṣi alongside "Ninurta of the stable."[54] By the time of the ritual BM 121206, Ninurta was in another chapel named "house of the king" (*bīt šarri*).[55] The "house of the king" and the "house of the stable" were both near the *šaḫūru*-house (*bīt šaḫūri*), all probably corresponding to various chambers adjacent to Aššur's cultroom and in connection with the *Ostanbau*.[56] Driel notices that the "house of the stable" is mentioned together with what may be restored as [...KÁ *kam*]-*su* ᵈ*Igīgī* "Bent are the Igigi Gate" in BM 121206 ix 41–42.[57] This gate is the southwestern outer gate of the *Ostanbau* courtyard. Bēl-Tarbaṣi, as a gatekeeper, must have been guarding one of the gates of the *Ostanbau*. We suggest that it was one of the inner gates because SAA 9 3 (ii 8–9) assumes Bēl-Tarbaṣi is present alongside the gods in the courtyard. The postscript states that the *šulmu* was delivered before Bēl-Tarbaṣi and not Aššur. This means, in our view, that the participants of the ritual in SAA 9 3 were oriented in a way that differed from the next *šulmu*, delivered before the *ṣulmu* ("image").

49 George 1992, 182–183, 194.

50 George 1989, 119.

51 Driel 1969, 45; George 1989, 199. One could translate *manzāzu* as "pedestal." Translating it as "station" appeals to the use of the term *manzāzu* in astrological texts for the station of a star or planet; Huxley 2000, 110, *passim*.

52 Due to damages, the full list of fellow gatekeepers eludes us; *cf.* Menzel 1981, T149:45–47. The other gatekeepers we can read are ᵈKAL.KAL, ᵈPIRIG.MEŠ, ᵈUR.MAḪ.MEŠ, ᵈ*En-pi*, and ᵈMU.DINGIR.KUR.

53 Quoted and discussed in Driel 1969, 38.

54 Driel 1969, 38–39.

55 Driel 1969, 38.

56 For details, see Driel 1969, 38–39.

57 Driel 1969, 39.

A tablet (Ass. 3916) discovered at Aššur contains an account of Esarhaddon's restorations in Ešarra. It begins with the cella (*atmanu*).[58] Next is the "dais of destinies" wherein the god Aššur has taken up residence, and this is the dais where "they (the gods) decree the fate of heaven and earth" (*ši-mat* AN-*e u* KI-*tim i-ši-mu*).[59] It may be assumed that the dais was in the cultroom,[60] linking the description of the dais with the previous account of the cella. Alternatively, the description of the dais may be tied with the subsequent description of the gates of the *Ostanbau*.[61] The gates in the *Ostanbau* were chosen in reference to the throne of Aššur and the dais of destinies.[62] Esarhaddon's text assumes that the dais was in a place where Aššur is seated on the throne while the fates are decreed. The gods are also present in the throne room. This does not mean that the gods dwelled there. Each god had its own chapel or cultroom and came from their own rooms for ceremonies. For example, a letter responds to a royal query about the attendance of the gods in an *adê*-ceremony, stating that Nabû(?) will not leave his room until a particular day.[63] If the gods came to the space of the throneroom from their own residences, one may assume that their king Aššur also had his private chamber. This may correspond to the cultroom, where the king offered food to Aššur in certain other rituals.[64]

The preserved parts of SAA 9 3 do not mention the "dais of destinies," but since the fates are decided there during the time of Esarhaddon, the presence of the dais may be assumed in SAA 9 3. SAA 9 3 states that the gods are present and records the announcement of the good news (*šulmu*) not only for king Esarhaddon but also for Ešarra and "*heaven and earth*" (just as with Esarhaddon's text [Ass. 3916]).[65] It may be puzzling that there was a *šulmu* delivered before a Bēl-Tarbaṣi (Lord of the Courtyard) when the god Aššur was enthroned in the same courtyard. Bēl-Tarbaṣi, as a gatekeeper, was near one of the *Ostanbau* gates, perhaps the "Bent are the Igigi

58 RINAP (The Royal Inscriptions of the Neo-Assyrian Period) 4 60 22b′–25′.

59 RINAP 4 60 26′–27a′.

60 Driel 1969, 37.

61 For Esarhaddon's claim to refurnish these gates; RINAP 4 60 29b′–33a′. The preceding description of the dais contains references to the 'images' of Esarhaddon and Assurbanipal; *cf.* fn. 68.

62 Huxley 2000, 110.

63 SAA 13 32. This short letter not fully preserved. The full nature of the ceremony assumed in the communication cannot be discerned. The part mentioning Nabû is damaged, and the reading of the divine name is not certain.

64 E.g. Driel 1969, 142.

65 It is unfortunate that the first section of SAA 9 3 is not well preserved. It may have contained relevant information about the dais; note the presence of Aššur (IGI ^{d}*Aš-šur*; i 20).

Gate" or its inner gate.[66] We surmise that the delivery of the oracle before this god was not due to his status but served to orient the reader by pointing to a part of the courtyard. After the oracle was delivered facing the gate guarded by Bēl-Tarbaṣi and the gods, recognizing the gods around the same space, the next oracle was delivered towards the "image" (*ṣalmu*). The final *šulmu*-oracle in SAA 9 3 is the "*šulmu* before the 'image'" (*šul-mu šá ina* IGI *ṣa-al-me*).[67] This 'image' refers most probably to that of Aššur.[68] The god would have been enthroned on the dais of destinies. It will be recalled that the "Gate of the Dais of Destinies" was the inner gate of the "Wagon Star Gate"; the Wagon Star remains visible in the night sky throughout the year, and is associated with the king of the gods in Babylonian tradition, whereas Enlil's dais was the Wagon Star.[69] Aššur, the king of gods, on the dais of destinies in Ešarra (*cf.* Esarhaddon's text discussed above), was enthroned somewhere near one of the gates not occupied by Bēl-Tarbaṣi. The dais of destinies itself may have been close to the "Gate of the Dais of Destinies," named after the dais itself.[70]

This situation also explains a connection between the two *šulmu*-oracles, since the latter, i.e. the one before the image, begins with *annūrig* ("now"). The adverb *annūrig* regularly occurs in letters, usually initiating a new temporal phase in the progression of the same message.[71] In SAA 9 3, initiating the final oracle with *annūrig* ("now") connects the oracle with the previous one delivered towards

66 One is still tempted to say Bēl-Tarbaṣi stood by the outer gate, but SAA 9 3 ii 8–9 is clear that Bēl-Tarbaṣi and the gods shared the same space, and the gods were not outside the *Ostanbau* during the ritual.

67 SAA 9 3 ii 26.

68 E.g. Parpola 1997, 24:ii 26; Weippert 2002, 16–17. Esarhaddon's text (RINAP 4 60 28′–29′) indicates that the king had, at some stage, built an image (*ṣalmu*) of himself and of his heir Assurbanipal on the same dais of destinies upon which Aššur was entroned. In SAA 9 3, the rendering *ṣa-al-me* could also represent 'images' (*ṣalmē*). There is a possibility that the reference was to the images of the god Aššur, the king and the crown prince on the dais. This would mean dating SAA 9 3 to a later period of Esarhaddon's reign and already Pongratz-Leisten (forthcoming) has argued that SAA 9 3 and the other oracle collections represented Esarhaddon's rise to power in order to legitimate Assurbanipal as the successor. Such a dating, however, is still open to discussion and until further evidence, we will presume the reference is to Aššur alone. But see also the discussion by Dalley (1986, 99) that *ṣalmu* was a divine symbol on which loyalty oaths were sworn.

69 Huxley 2000, 118–119. Sennacherib had built the *Ostanbau* as part of the Assyrian policy to emulate the Babylonian cult of Marduk. The gate named after the dais of destinies commemorates the presence of the dais in Ešarra; George 1989, 119.

70 The dais may have also been somehow connected with the "Gate of Kingship," as well as the "Wagon Star Gate." The specifics remain unclear. The symbolism of the gates assumed the throne of Aššur and the Gate of Kingship in the northern sky; Huxley 2000, 113.

71 E.g. SAA 1 1:7; SAA 10 30:5; SAA 10 315:13.

the gate where Bēl-Tarbaṣi stood, whereas the final *šulmu*-oracle was directed, in a matter of moments changing orientation, saying *annūrig*, towards the image on the dais of destinies in the courtyard, where Aššur was enthroned. There was a procession towards the statue of Aššur in the throneroom,[72] but our analysis indicates that all the rituals recorded in SAA 9 3 (perhaps even the fragmented account in the first section) took place in the *Ostanbau*. The individuals present in the ceremony listening to the prophecies are addressed as the 'sons of Assyria'.[73] They are referred to when the oracle is delivered before the gate kept by Bēl-Tarbaṣi.

Arguably, one can also see impact of the *Ostanbau* settting with the wording of the oracles. A few remarks are made here to demonstrate this specific point.[74] Aššur's *šulmu*-message before Bēl-Tarbaṣi and the gods begins with a general proclamation of the king's triumph against his enemies (SAA 9 3 i 28–34), "from sunset to sunrise, from sunrise to sunset" ([*issu rab*]*ā Šamši* [*adi napā*]*ḫ Šamši* [*issu napā*]*ḫ Šamši* [*adi rab*]*ā Šamši*; [i 31–34]). The sun's path, and Šamaš's daily 'sunrise' and 'sunset,' comprised important parts of the symbolism of the *Ostanbau* gates.[75] The oracle is therefore in accord with this symbolism while expressing the greatness of the Assyrian Empire under divine support, using it to praise the king with the attributes of Šamaš.[76] The allusions to temple symbolism are selective and were adapted to the genre of the oracles, recalling also how allusions creatively adopt from Mesosopotamian literature.[77]

Aššur's *šulmu*-message before the "image" presents us with another case of the courtyard's influence. Aššur boasts of hurling down fire from the "great gate of heaven" (KÁ.GAL AN-*e*) against traitors.[78] The Gate of Anu, known from various types of Assyrian texts, including literary texts such as Nergal and Ereškigal and the Adapa Epic, was the first gate reached from earth, at the peak of heaven, leading

72 But not into the cultroom; *cf.* Nissinen 2000, 252–253. It is not clear if the final phase of the procession was the temple terrace. This relies on a difficult reading in the second part of SAA 9 3, *ina* UGU [*tam-l*]*e-e ḫi-*⌜*ir*⌝*-ṣ*[*u*! x x x] (iii 2). Parpola (1997, 25:iii 2) mentions a terrace (*tamliu*) located outside the gate that leads into the cella of Aššur. The other problem is the unclarity as to whether the two parts of SAA 9 3 relate to the same ceremony, as discussed above.

73 "Listen, O Assyrians!" ([*si-ta-am*]*-me* DUMU.MEŠ KUR *Aš*-šur); SAA 9 3 i 27.

74 A full exploration of this will require further study. The descriptions mentioned are also recognized from other Assyrian texts and even from standard formulae.

75 Huxley 2000, 116, 124–125, passim. The symbolism is also appreciated after seeing the background for the sculptured figures of protective mythological beings (e.g., the scorpion-men) adorning the gates.

76 Further to the point, the king is said to shine as bright as the sun (SAA 9 3 ii 7).

77 The prophetic allusions to Mesopotamian literature are discussed in Halton 2009.

78 SAA 9 3 ii 15–17.

into the presence of the gods in their celestial courtyard.[79] The symbolism of the *Ostanbau* assumes Aššur, as the king of the gods, to be on his celestial throne.[80] Seeing all of Esarhaddon's enemies, be they foreign or traitors from within, Aššur's punishment is expressed in celestial terms from his throne in his cosmic palace, interacting with the cosmological symbolism of the *Ostanbau*.[81]

The *šulmu*-oracles are followed by the rather enigmatic "oaths tablet of Aššur" (*ṭuppi adê ša Aššūr*; SAA 9 3 ii 27–32) provided within a ritual context:

ii 27 *ṭup-pi a-de-e an-ni-u* šá d*Aš-šur*
ii 28 *ina* UGU *ḫa-'u-u-ti ina* IGI LUGAL *e-rab*
ii 29 Ì.DÙG.GA *i-za-az-ri-qu*
ii 30 UDU.SISKUR.MEŠ *ep-pu-šú*
ii 31 ŠEM.ḪI.A *il-lu-ku*
ii 32 *ina* IGI LUGAL *i-sa-as-si-u*

ii 27–28 The oaths tablet of Aššur enters the king's presence on a cushion.
ii 29–31 Fragrant oil is sprinkled, sacrifices are made, incense is burnt,
ii 32 They read it out in the king's presence

The identification of *ṭuppi adê anniu ša Aššūr* is problematic, and a full treatment of the relevant scholarly literature requires a separate study. Some brief observations will be offered here. The 'oaths tablet of Aššur' may be a reference to Aššur's oracles so far discussed.[82] Or it may be a separate document, perhaps the standard Assyrian loyalty oaths between the king and his subjects, mainly on the grounds that the previous messages were already named as *šulmu*, and other Assyrian texts

79 For details, see Horowitz 1998, 59, 65, 250, 266–267. For other aspects of the "gate of heaven" in SAA 9 3, see Parpola 1997, 24: ii 15f.

80 Huxley 2000, 111–113.

81 For a study of celestial divine punishment in Assyrian prophecy from a different philological and comparative angle; see Stökl 2013. Stökl raises a range of issues that need to be discussed further, demonstrating the depth of the topic.

82 Weippert 1981, 79, 92. Parpola (1987, 181) proposes, based on the oracles, that it referred to the god's promises to the king; *cf.* Parpola 1997, xix-xx. Ishida (1977, 114–116) offered that the first part of SAA 9 3 concerned a treaty between Aššur and the king, whereas the second part referred to a vassal treaty established by Ištar of Arbela (*cf.* Weippert 2002, 18). On Ishida's point about a reference to a treaty between god and king, see fn. 107. The self-binding nature of Aššur's oracles (*cf.* Parpola 1987, 181) may be upheld by itself, without necessarily associating them with the 'oaths tablet of Aššur,' from an etic view that analyses how the god is bound by his decrees. Pongratz-Leisten (forthcoming) provides a similar approach for the god's seal for Esarhaddon's succession treaty.

do not clearly attest to oaths taken by Aššur.[83] Pongratz-Leisten places the 'oaths tablet of Aššur' as part of the ritual context quoted above, noting that the ritual descriptions employ the present tense, whereas the oracles employ the preterite and perfect tenses, further supporting the view that *ṭuppi adê anniu ša Aššūr* does not refer to the oracles.[84] Considering that SAA 9 3 emphasizes the rise of Esarhaddon and the fate of the rebels, Pongratz-Leisten finds it more likely that the oaths in question where the very important standard loyalty oaths imposed on subjects.[85]

Pongratz-Leisten proposes that the construction *ṭuppi adê anniu ša Aššūr* should be interpreted as "Diese *adê*-Tafel [geschworen] bei Aššur" and not as the "Bund des Aššur (mit dem König)," noting labels such as *māmīt ša* DN or *nīš ilāni.*[86] One can find references to *adê māmīt ša ilāni* ("*adê* of the oath/curse of the great gods"), *adê ilāni rabûti* ("oath of the great gods"), *māmīt ša* ^{d}*Aššūr* ("oath/curse of Aššur"), *nīš ilāni* (oath sworn by the gods) and *adê nīš ilāni* (an *adê* with oath sworn by the gods).[87] These cases assume treaties or loyalty oaths backed by the gods as divine witnesses, who have guaranteed punishment for the violators of the *adê* agreement when the oath takers seal in their divine names.[88]

We agree with Pongratz-Leisten's view that the delivery of the oracles was followed by an *adê* ceremony, briefly described in the above quoted section of

---

83 For these and other arguments raised, see Pongratz-Leisten 1999, 78–80; Pongratz-Leisten (forthcoming); Weeks 2004, 48–49. The entire question has also been considered in relation to the study of the formation and transmission of Deuteronomy and the covenant in Biblical tradition, since similar phraseology and other features can be found in Deuteronomy and Esarhaddon's succession treaty containing loyalty oaths; *cf.* Steymans 1995, 284–312; Otto 1999 (chapter two); Levinson 2009; Mack 2011; *cf.* Radner 2006, 374–375. SAA 9 3 is also important for these inquiries because it testifies to loyalty oaths being administered in temple contexts and shows that, like Deuteronomy, treaty was connected with temple, something that can also be inferred for the Syria-Palestine region due to the copy of Esarhaddon's treaty found in Tell Tayinat in a temple setting; Levinson 2012, 55–56.

84 Pongratz-Leisten 1999, 78. The use of the demonstrative *anniu* is also found with the standard Assyrian loyalty oaths; SAA 2 6:283, 291, 397, 555A, 612A, as discussed in Pongratz-Leisten 1999, 80.

85 *Ibid.* 1999, 78–80.

86 *Ibid.* 1999, 80. DN stands for "divine name."

87 CAD A I s.v. *adû* A, 131. The words *nīš* (lit. "life") and *māmītu* are synonymous words for oaths but with different uses. The word *māmītu* (oath; curse [as a consequence of a broken oath]) is more of a second millennium word when compared with *adû*; CAD N II s.v. *nīšu* A, 290–291; CAD M I s.v. *māmītu*. The use of the word *adû* for oath terminology begins in the early first millennium BC; Radner 2006, with further references.

88 For the divine witnesses in the Neo-Assyrian period, see Parpola and Watanabe 1988, xxxvii.

SAA 9 3.[89] SAA 9 3 explicitly states that they "read out aloud" (*isassiū* [from *sasû*]; SAA 9 3 ii 32) the *ṭuppi adê ša Aššūr* in front of the king. The readers ("they") are in the plural.[90] This is not said for the delivery of the *šulmu*-oracles, which were instead "established" (the verb *šakānu,* which has a very wide semantic range). These readers of the oaths may have been different from the deliver(ers) of the oracles. In any case, the use of the impersonal verbs here indicate that the scribe of SAA 9 3 wants to emphasize the 'oaths tablet of Aššur' and the rituals associated with its recitation. We think that SAA 9 3 concerns the Assyrian loyalty oaths. Esarhaddon's treaty of loyalty oaths (SAA 2 6) is a good example for the type of text in mind.[91] It is a very long document (due to detailed stipulations, curses, etc.) and could not have been reproduced in the space reserved for recording oracles in SAA 9 3.

Esarhaddon's succession treaty was a text of loyalty oaths sworn by subordinates throughout the Assyrian Empire (672 BC), recognizing and upholding Assurbanipal as the heir. Samples of these loyalty oaths are known from Nimrud.[92] The oath-takers in this case were rulers of countries on the Median and Zagros frontiers of the Assyrian Empire and their people.[93] Fragments of the same text have been found in Aššur, and they also correspond to various lines of the text known from Nimrud.[94] A recent discovery at Tell Tayinat (Unqi) has revealed a text

89 Pongratz-Leisten 1999, 80. Pongratz-Leisten (forthcoming) connects this oath ceremony with Esarhaddon's policy of ensuring the succession of Assurbanipal.

90 For the verb *sasû* as "to read out, to recite" for this context, the semantic range of the verb needs to be taken into consideration, *cf.* CAD Š II s.v. *šasû*, 146, 151–152, 162–163. Clearly, the readers did not keep the reading to themselves during the ceremony. Reading out loud was the expected mode of reading in public. For example, St. Augustine (AD 354–430) remarks on Bishop Ambrose's habit of reading silently instead of reading out aloud. It was unexpected; *Confessions* (VI.3).

91 Given the uncertainties with the dating of SAA 9 3, the *adê*-document mentioned may be referring to something before Esarhaddon's succession oaths but similarly imposed. Alternatively, and if Pongratz-Leisten's late dating (*cf.* fn. 27) holds, SAA 9 3 may concern Esarhaddon's succession treaty.

92 Wiseman 1958. More recently with additional fragments; Watanabe 1987; SAA 2 6. For the date, see Fales 2012, 135–136.

93 Ḫumbareš of Naḫšimarti, Bur-Dadi of Karzitali, Ḫatarna of Sikris, Larkutla of Mazauma, Ramataya of Urakazabanu, Tunî of Ellipi and a ruler of Izaya whose name is not preserved; Parpola and Watanabe 1988, xxx. Liverani (1995) alternatively proposes that these were Medians serving in Assyria. The reference to people of those lands (SAA 2 6:3–10) and their title, EN.URU (*bēl āli*; "city ruler" [SAA 2 6:3]), is more likely a term for the ruler of a region with settlements; *cf.* Fales 2012, 144–145.

94 VAT 11543 corresponds to lines 229–236; Parpola and Watanabe 1988, xlviii. VAT 12374 and VAT 9424 correspond to lines 54–62 and 509–516, respectively; Frahm 2009, 135–136. The provenance of all three fragments remains unknown.

(manuscript T) "almost identical" with that in Nimrud, only that the oath-takers are now the "governor" (*bēl pāḫiti*) of the province Kullania and all its peoples.[95]

Esarhaddon's succession treaty is called the "oath of Esarhaddon" (*adê ša Aššūr-aḫu-iddina*) and has the three seals of Aššur.[96] The act of sealing the "oaths tablet" (*ṭuppi adê*) elevated it to the status of the "tablet of destinies" (*ṭuppi šīmāti*).[97] In other words, such documents can be considered the earthly counterparts of the theological concept of destinies being fixed in the divine assembly. By sealing them, Aššur is determining his vassals' destinies.[98] Aššur seals the destinies of gods and men with the Seal of Destinies.[99] George argues that the document ratified by Aššur's seals is, on the mythological plane, the tablet of destinies.[100]

It would be inconceivable that the oaths tablet recited during the rituals in SAA 9 3 lacked the seal of Aššur. The description of the "oaths tablet of Aššur" (*ṭuppi adê ša Aššūr*) emphasized the ownership of the god. In fact, the recent text found at Tell Tayinat restores the expression "this *adê*, tablet of Aššur king of the gods and of the gods" (*a-de-e an-ni-e ṭup-pi Aš-šur* MAN ⌜DINGIR⌝.MEŠ *u* DINGIR.⌜MEŠ⌝).[101] We read from Ass. 3916 that Aššur and the gods decreed the fates (as discussed above), and SAA 9 3 mentions the gods along with Aššur during the delivery of the oracles concerning the fate of the king as well as "heaven and earth" (also discussed above). It is tempting to argue that the *adê*-document in SAA 9 3 could have been the same as the one for which copies exist for oath takers from the Median countries, Kullania and possibly other Assyrian dominions awaiting

---

95 For details and the text, see Lauinger 2012.

96 SAA 2 6:i-iii; Lauinger 2012, 91:i-iii. For the three divine seals, see Watanabe 1985.

97 Lauinger 2012, 87. To our knowledge, no monument showing the "tablet of destinies" has yet been discovered; *cf.* George 1986, 138.

98 George 1986, 140–141. George also draws attention to the fact that the oath tablets at Nimrud (Kalhu) were found in rooms adjoining the temple of Nabû in that city and discusses the possibility that the temples of Nabû in Kalhu and Aššur prepared and stored state documents; George 1986, 141; Fales 2012, 137.

99 According to the seal inscription; Watanabe 1985, 380–381; Lauinger 2013, 109–110.

100 George 1986, 140–141. Lauinger (2013, 109–115) builds on this with a scenario as to how vassals interacted with the temples of Nabû, and proposes that the transformation of the *ṭuppi adê* to a 'tablet of destinies' is connected with its use in the *akītu*-ceremonies associated with the temples of Nabû, and this way the oath-takers' obligations become their destinities.

101 Lauinger 2012, 98: T v 64. SAA 2 6:400–401 expresses this slightly differently, with [EN? *ṭup*]*-pi a-de-e an-ni-i* [^{d}*Aš-šur*] MAN DINGIR.MEŠ *u* DINGIR.MEŠ "this oath tablet of [Aššur] the king of the gods and of the gods". The restoration of "Aššur" proposed by Parpola and Watanabe is confirmed. De Jong (2007, 411n211) has also noticed the significance of this expression for understanding the *adê*-document in SAA 9 3, arguing similarly to Pongratz-Leisten that it is an oath tablet sworn and guarded by Aššur.

discovery, but because the dating of SAA 9 3 remains unclear (*cf.* fn. 91), this cannot be said with full certainty. In any case, the Tell Tayinat discovery further supports the view that the Nimrud copies are to be seen as part of a wider socio-political structure within the Assyrian Empire.[102] We note that the Nimrud copies were found in the throne room of Ezida, the temple of Nabû.[103] The Tell Tayinat text was found in the inner sanctum of Building XVI, a Neo-Assyrian temple.[104] This encourages us to view the *adê*-documents as belonging within a temple and a ritual setting. In this case, Esarhaddon's *adê* had become a god-like entity, venerated in public viewings.[105] The *adê*-document mentioned in SAA 9 3 was performed amidst prophecies with the King of the Gods residing, and therefore a similar transformation of the document must have taken place.[106]

The *adê*-documents existed prior to the time Esarhaddon, and functioned in such ways that it is not always possible to refer to them as oaths imposed on subjects. At times they may be referred to as types of treaties.[107] The exact nature of the *adê*-document in SAA 9 3 is unknown, except that it involved oaths binding the Assyrians participating in the ceremony, either by loyalty oaths or by a vassal treaty.[108] The type of loyalty oath in mind can also be examplified with a reference to those sworn by the vassal Gurdî. SAA 1 76 refers to an *adê*-ceremony during the time of Sargon II, held at a temple courtyard (TÙR *ša* É.DINGIR; r. 6), probably in

---

102 Watanabe (1987, 1–5) had argued before the discovery of the text at Tell Tayinat that the Nimrud copies were part of a wider socio-political structure. The exact nature of the system awaits further discussion, as well as future discoveries; *cf.* Fales 2012.

103 Parpola and Watanabe 1988, xixx.

104 Lauinger 2012, 90.

105 Fales 2012, 153–153.

106 This expands upon Lauinger's (2013, 112–113) comment that the recitation of the *adê*-document during the ritual of SAA 9 3 connects somehow with the transformation of the tablet into the divine realm. The entire ritual, with Aššur's *šulmu* oracles, becomes a full experience of divine presence for the participants.

107 Parpola and Watanabe 1988, xv-xxv; Radner 2006. SAA 3 33:19′ mentions how the Assyrian king (Sargon II?) did not keep the oaths (*adê*) of the king of the gods (i.e. Aššur) and was slain. The context is not clear. Ishida (1977, 116) notes it as a possible treaty between Aššur and the king, if not a literary designation of the king's commitment to his god. There are also cases where *adê* refers not to representatives of territorial-political units, but to individual members of the elite; Fales 2012, 139–142; Lauinger 2013, 103–105.

108 On the Assyrians as members of the elite taking oaths, see Radner 2006, 360–363. The Neo-Assyrian oaths in the seventh century BC covered a wider range of government and palace representatives and potentially all subjects of the Empire; Fales 2012, 135–136. Fales notes the possibility that SAA 9 3 referred to SAA 2 4, an *adê* document that may relate to the accession of Esarhaddon; Fales 2012, 135, n 16. Problems discussed above concerning the dating of SAA 9 3 mean that there is no definite answer here.

Ešarra.[109] If current estimates are accurate and the *Ostanbau* was built during the time of Sennacherib,[110] then the courtyard in question was probably elsewhere. In any case, the governor of the Aššur province, Ṭab-ṣilli-Ešarra, informed the king that the 'oaths tablet of Gurdî' (*ṭuppi adê ša Gurdî*) was brought by the Palace Superintendent (LÚ *šá* IGI.É.GAL) for ceremonies in the temple as soon as Gurdî's emissaries arrived. Gurdî was a king (of Tunna or Atuna?) from Anatolia's Tabal region.[111] His emissaries took the oaths on his behalf, and arguably on behalf of the people of their country. The temple did not keep the tablets.[112] Rather, the oaths tablet was returned after the ceremonies. The Palace Superintendent made sure of this.[113] SAA 9 3 (ii 27–32) emphasized that the 'oaths tablet of Aššur' was brought into the ceremony. Perhaps they were also returned to the temple of Nabû.

Conclusion

We studied one case where prophetic activity was joined with rituals and the recital of the oaths in Ešarra. Exploring them *vis-à-vis* their *Ostanbau* setting has provided some new insights. Can we gain further insights about Neo-Assyrian prophecy from the material remains?

In SAA 9 3, certain individuals named the 'sons of Assyria' (how many were present is unknown) participated in a public event in the temple. Public events provide the state with the space and opportunity to exercise control and hegemony.[114] The political organization of the Assyrian Empire sought to incorporate diverse areas and peoples into their system of exploitation for the Assyrian heartland.[115] An archaeological approach may draw the interpreter to look for clues as to the ways in which the Empire may have used the material facilities available to them.

The *Ostanbau* courtyard housed the prophetic performance alongside ritual. This communicated, in comprehensible language, the will of the gods to legitimize the deeds of the king, the loyalty oaths regulating the commitments of their subjects and the might of the kingdom to punish rebels.[116] The *Ostanbau* could

109 *Cf.* Parpola 1997, 23:ii 8f.

110 Esarhaddon's text (Ass. 3916) ascribes the work for the *Ostanbau* to his ancestors and not specifically to his father Sennacherib; RINAP 4 60 27′. Such statements may be regarded as too typical and general; *cf.* George 1989, 119.

111 Fuchs 1994, 411–412.

112 Were they stored in the palace and/or the temple of Nabû? *Cf.* fn. 98.

113 SAA 1 76:r. 8–12.

114 Smith 2011, 421.

115 Parker 2011, 359

116 This is never to reduce ritual and prophecy to politics. There are multiple aspects to this topic, worthy of several other studies.

accommodate up to nearly one thousand individuals (with an area of approximately 600m^2, based on the published ground plan). Did they use this potential? Haller and Andrae did point out that the mudbrick paving floor of the *Ostanbau* was repaired several times during its lifetime.[117] This would suggest an intense use of the entire courtyard. Since the *Ostanbau* only provided access into the sacred cella as a walkway, too much human traffic therein is not normally expected. The extensive use of space in the courtyard, however, may indicate a possible function as a gathering area for ritual activity, such as the prophetic performances discussed in the present study. Future archaeological surveys can help clarify and expand upon this specific point, amongst others. The texts usually will not inform us about the attendance and may even give the impression that a limited number of individuals, like emissaries of a vassal king, attended a given ceremony. Nor do we usually know the regularity of the festivals and other rituals organized. Were they regarded as rare events with great significance? Or were they used regularly to engage the elite and the subjects?

The terms *raggimu* and *raggintu*, used for prophet or prophetesses respectively, are exclusively Neo-Assyrian,[118] and are based on the verb *ragāmu* "to shout, to call, to proclaim, etc." This verb is applicable to the act of proclaiming the divine message and oracles in public.[119] The *Sitz im Leben* of Neo-Assyrian prophecy is mostly unknown. Based on anthropological, Biblical and Old Babylonian parallels, Neo-Assyrian prophecy can be considered as having a public aspect.[120] There is a passage according to which the prophets could address a very large group of people. We do not know the number of the 'sons of Assyria' in SAA 9 3, but Ištar of Arbela does, through a prophetess and in another oracle, speak "to the cro[wd] (*a-na ma-a'-*[*du-ti*]; SAA 9 2 ii 34').[121] How much of a crowd? Were prophets "speakers to the masses" (*cf.* Parpola 1997, xlv)? Or how do we posit a more limited crowd? In other words, is there a way to detail some ways the prophets had public access? If, for the sake of argument, temples were the main venue for state sponsored prophecy during the Neo-Assyrian period, then we know that temples dominated the urban Mesopotamian landscape[122] and varied in size. This may also mean that prophecy was widespread also thanks to the fact that it was attached to the performance of rituals

117 Haller and Andrae 1955, 70–71.

118 The words *raggimu* and *raggintu* are based on the form *parris*, a Neo-Assyrian variant of the G participle form of the verb *ragāmu*, with the doubling of the second radical and the shortening of the preceding vowel; Parpola 1997, CII, n. 212; *cf.* Stökl 2012, 111.

119 *Cf.* Parpola 1997, CIII, n. 217; *cf.* CAD R s.v. *ragāmu,* 62–63.

120 Stökl 2012, 112.

121 The oracle entry in SAA 9 2 iii 18' merely indicates that the prophetess is from Kalhu, but this does not even prove her location during the oracle.

122 *Cf.* George 1993.

in temples. Looking at the archaeological data with an eye for ritual spaces can also potentially inform us about prophecy (assuming equal attention given to the texts).

Does this mean that the oracles were part of the cult? Mār-Issār mentions that he heard a prophetess (*raggintu*) "had prophesied" (*tartugum*) "before" (*pānāt*) the cultic work for the substitute king ritual in Akkad. He then assures the king that the apotropaic rituals were successful.[123] The oracles are quoted to support this view and were probably delivered in different contexts.[124] The same prophetess also "spoke to him" (*taq-ṭi-ba-áš-šu*), i.e. Damqî, in the council of the land (*ina* UKKIN *ša* KUR).[125] The authorities must have arranged this, because Damqî was the designated substitute king and under constant watch. On the other hand, this prophetic address was public.[126] Mār-Issār reports that the "Akkadians" (*Akkadû'a*), and Babylonian administrators and representatives (*šatammāni qēpāni ša māt Akkadî*), were afraid (*iptalḫū*). This claim, be it true or not, touches upon the great fear of persecution if a rebellion began. The obligation to report words of treason in the succesion treaty of Esarhaddon (SAA 2 6) mentions the *raggimu*-prophets and the *maḫḫû*-ecstatics among the potential speakers of evil words.[127]

SAA 13 37 states that a *raggintu* prophesied in the temple ([*ina*] ⸢É⸣.DINGIR *tart*[*u*]*gum*).[128] Afterwards, there is a dispute between her and Adad-aḫu-iddina, a temple administrator who did not want to turn over the "throne" (^{GIŠ}GU.ZA), a cultic item. It was mentioned in the oracle of the *raggintu*.[129] In another text, Ištar of Arbela served oath takers with bread and water, symbolizing their return to their cities and provinces where they will eat, drink, and keep their oaths.[130] The items were symbols used for the specific wording of oracles. SAA 13 144 reports sacrifices, and that a prophetess "prophesied" (*tartugu*[*m*]). The mention of the prophecy alongside the sacrifices implies their connection.

123 SAA 10 352:22–r.6.

124 How long "before" the rituals were the oracles delivered? This is hard to say also because the perfect tense in "she prophesied" (*tartugum*) is more aspectual than temporal, as is expected in Semitic languages. The oracles quoted address Damqî as "king." Mār-Issār quotes the oracles to assure Esarhaddon that this person was the right choice for the substitute king in the ritual; *cf.* Nissinen 1998, 73–77.

125 SAA 10 352:e.23–25, r. 1–2.

126 Parpola 1997, xlv.

127 SAA 2 6:116–117.

128 SAA 13 37:9–10.

129 The oracle is not well preserved, but the first words are: [GIŠ]GU.ZA TA É.[DIN]GIR "[The t]hrone from the te[mp]le ..."; SAA 13 37:11.

130 SAA 9 3 iii 2–6. The reference to the cities and the provinces implies that the oath takers were subjects introduced in the gap between columns ii and iii; Weeks 2004, 49. The gods called to the oaths on ii 35–36 were probably witnesses and divine council members.

The peculiar public role of the prophets and prophetesses in the temple cult may explain at least in part the emergence of the unique Neo-Assyrian terms *raggimu* and *raggintu*. Their prophesying in the temple or in relation to a ritual often takes the verb *ragāmu* as the examples above indicate. An aspect of "prophesying" in the Assyrian Empire meant, we propose, a sort of prophetic public address and performance in temple setting, associated with rituals and complementing them. This complementary character seems to indicate that sometime in Assyrian history, taking the period of Esarhaddon as the *terminus ante quem*, there emerged a class of prophets called the *raggimu/raggintu*, performing in temples and rituals, voicing the royal agenda.

REFERENCES

Dalley, S., "The God Ṣalmu and the Winged Disk." *Iraq* 48 (1986): 85–101.

Fales, M. F., "After Ta'yinat: The New Status of Esarhaddon's Adê for Assyrian Political History." *Revue d'Assyriologie* 106 (2012): 133–158

Frahm, E., *Keilschrifttexte aus Assur literarischen Inhalts III: Historische und historisch-literarische Texte* (*Historical and Historical-Literary Texts from Assur*). Wiesbaden: Harrossowitz Verlag, 2009.

———. "Wie 'christlich' war die assyrische Religion? Anmerkungen zu Simo Parpolas Edition der assyrischen Prophetien." *Die Welt des Orient* 31 (2000/2001): 31–45.

Fuchs, A., *Die Inschriften Sargons II aus Khorsabad*. Göttingen: Cuvillier Verlag, 1994.

Galter, H., "Die Bautätigkeit Sanheribs am Aššurtempel." *Orientalia* 53 (1984): 433–441.

George, A., "Sennacherib and the Tablet of Destinies." *Iraq* 48 (1986): 133–146.

———. "Review of Simo Parpola 'The Correspondence of Sargon II, Part I: Letters from Assyria and the West.'" *Bulletin of the School of Oriental and African Studies* 52 (1989): 118–120.

———. *Babylonian Topographical Texts*. Leuven: Peeters, 1992.

———. *House Most High: The Temples of Ancient Mesopotamia*. Winona Lake: Eisenbrauns, 1993.

Haller, A. and W. Andrae, *Die Heiligtümer des Gottes Assur und der Sin-*Šamaš*-Tempel in Assur.* Mit Beiträgen van W. Andrae Berlin, 1955.

Halton, C., "Allusions to the Stream of Tradition in Neo-Assyrian Oracles." *Ancient Near Eastern Studies* 46 (2009): 50–61.

Heeßel, N. P., *Divinatorische Texte I: Terrestrische, teratologische, physiognomische und oneiromantische Omina*. Wiesbaden: Harrossowitz Verlag, 2007.

Horowitz, W. *Mesopotamian Cosmic Geography*. Winona Lake: Eisenbrauns, 1998.

Huxley, M., "The Gates and Guardians in Sennacherib's Addition to the Temple of Assur." *Iraq* 62 (2000): 109–137.

Ishida, T. *The Royal Dynasties in Ancient Israel: A Study on the Formation and Development of Royal-Dynastic Ideology*. Berlin: De Gruyter, 1977.

Jong, M. J. de. *Isaiah among the Ancient Near Eastern Prophets: A Comparative Study of the Earliest Stages of the Isaiah Tradition and the Neo-Assyrian Prophecies*. Leiden: Brill, 2007.

Kwasman, T., "Review of Assyrian Prophecies by Simo Parpola." *The Jewish Quarterly Review, New Series* 92 (2001): 227–232.

Lambert, W. G., "Review of Simo Parpola. Assyrian Prophecies. Helsinki. 1997. State Archives of Assyria 9." *Archiv für Orientforschung* 48/49 (2001/2002): 208–211.

Lauinger, J., "Esarhaddon's Succession Treaty at Tell Tayinat: Text and Commentary." *Journal of Cuneiform Studies* 64 (2012): 87–123.

———. "The Neo-Assyrian *adê*: Treaty, Oath or Something Else?" *Zeitschrift für Altorientalische und Biblische Rechtsgeschichte* 19 (2013): 99–115.

Levinson, B. M., "The Neo-Assyrian Origins of the Canon Formula in Deuteronomy 13:1" in *Scriptural Exegesis: The Shapes of Culture and the Religious Imagination. Essays in Honour of Michael Fishbane*, ed. by D. A. Green and L. Lieber, 25–45. Oxford: Oxford University Press, 2009.

———. "Die neuassyrischen Ursprünge der Kanonformel in Deuteronomium 13,1" in *Viele Wege zu dem Einen: Historische Bibelkritik—Die Vitalität der Glaubensüberlieferung in der Moderne*, ed. by S. Beyerle, A. Graupner and U. Rüterswörden, 23–59. Neukirchen-Vluyn: Neukirchener Verlagsgesellschaft, 2012.

Liverani, M., "The Medes at Esarhaddon's Court." *Journal of Cuneiform Studies* 47 (1995): 57–62.

Mack, R., *Neo-Assyrian Prophecy and the Hebrew Bible: Nahum, Habakkuk, and Zephaniah*. Piscataway: Gorgias Press, 2011.

Melville, S. C., *The Role of Naqia/Zakutu in Sargonid Politics*. Helsinki: Neo-Assyrian Text Corpus Project, 1999.

———. "Neo-Assyrian Royal Women and Male Identity: Status as a Social Tool." *Journal of the American Oriental Society* 124 (2004): 37–57.

Menzel, B., *Assyrische Tempel. Untersuchungen zu Kult, Administration und Personal*. Rome: Biblical Institute Press, 1981.

Nissinen, M., *References to Prophecy in Neo-Assyrian Sources*. Helsinki: Neo-Assyrian Text Corpus Project, 1998.

———. "Spoken, Written, Quoted, and Invented: Orality and Writtenness in Ancient Near Eastern Prophecy" in *Writings and Speech in Israelite and Ancient Near Eastern Prophecy*, ed. by E. B. Zvi and M. H. Floyd, 235–271. Atlanta: Society of Biblical Literature, 2000.

———. *Prophets and Prophecy in the Ancient Near East*. Atlanta: Society of Biblical Literature, 2003.

Otto, E., *Das Deuteronomium: Politische Theologie und Rechtsreform in Juda und Assyrien*. Berlin: De Gruyter, 1999.

Parker, B. J., "The Construction and Performance of Kingship in the Neo-Assyrian Empire." *Journal of Anthropological Research* 67 (2011): 357–386.

Parpola, S., "Neo-Assyrian Treaties from the Royal Archives of Nineveh." *Journal of Cuneiform Studies* 39/2 (1987b): 161–189.

———. *Assyrian Prophecies*. Helsinki: University of Helsinki Press, 1997.

Parpola, S. and K. Watanabe, *Neo-Assyrian Treaties and Loyalty Oaths*. Helsinki: University of Helsinki Press, 1988.

Ponchia, S., "The Neo-Assyrian Adê Protocol and the Administration of the Empire" in *From Source to History: Studies on Ancient Near Eastern Worlds and Beyond.* Dedicated to Giovanni Battista Lanfranchi on the Occasion of His 65th Birthday on June 23, 2014, ed by S. Gaspa *et al.*, 501–525. Münster: Ugarit-Verlag, 2014.

Pongratz-Leisten, B., *Herrschaftswissen in Mesopotamien. Formen der Kommunikation zwischen Gott und König im 2. und 1. Jahrtausend v.Chr.* Helsinki: University of Helsinki Press, 1999.

———. "'The Writing of the God' and the Textualization of the Neo-Assyrian Prophecy" in *Spotlights on Jewish Prophecy: Functions of Prophecy in Jewish Scriptures and Beyond*, ed. by A. Lange and B. H. Reynolds III. Göttingen, forthcoming.

Postgate, J. N., "Review: Simo Parpola. Assyrian Prophecies. (State Archives of Assyria, vol IX). Helsinki University Press. Helsinki. 1997." *Journal of Semitic Studies* 47 (2002): 312–313.

Radner, K., "Assyrische ṭuppi adê als Vorbild für Deuteronomium 28, 20–44?" in *Die deuteronomistischen Geschichtswerke: Redaktions- und religionsgeschichtliche Perspektiven zur 'Deuteronomismus'—Diskussion in Tora und Vorderen Propheten*, ed. by M. Witte *et al.*, 351–378. Berlin: De Gruyter, 2006.

Smith, A., "Archaeologies of Sovereignty." *Annual Review of Anthropology* 40 (2011): 415–432.

Stępniowski, F.M., "The Temples in Aššur. An Overview of the Sacral Architecture of the 'Holy City'." *Revista sobre Oriente Próximo y Egipto en la antigüedad* 6 (2003): 233–244.

Steymans, H.U., *Deuteronomium 28 und die adê zur Thronfolgeregelung Asarhaddons: Segen und Fluch im Alten Orient und in Israel*. Göttingen: Vandenhoeck & Ruprecht, 1995.

Stökl, J., *Prophecy in the Ancient Near East: A Philological and Sociological Comparison*. Leiden: Brill, 2012.

———. "'I Have Rained Stones and Fiery Glow on Their Heads!' Celestial and Meteorological Prophecy in the Neo-Assyrian Empire" in *'Thus Speaks Ishtar of Arbela': Prophecy in Israel, Assyria, and Egypt in the Neo-Assyrian Period*, ed. by R. P. Gordon *et al.*, 239–251. Winona Lake: Eisenbrauns, 2013.

Svärd, S., *Power and Women in the Neo-Assyrian Palaces*. PhD Dissertation, University of Helsinki. Helsinki, 2012.

van der Toorn, K., "Mesopotamian Prophecy between Immanence and Transcendence: A Comparison of Old Babylonian and Neo-Assyrian Prophecy" in *Prophecy in its Ancient Near Eastern Context. Mesopotamian, Biblical and Arabian Perspectives*, ed. by M. Nissinen, 71–87. Atlanta: Society of Biblical Literature, 2000.

van Driel G., *The Cult of Aššur*. Studia Semitica Neerlandica 13. Assen, 1969.

Villard, P., "Les prophéties à l'époque néo-assyrienne" in *Prophètes et rois: Bible et Proche-Orient*, ed. by A. Lemaire, 55–84. Paris: Persee, 2001.

Watanabe, K., "Die Siegelung der 'Vasallenvertrage Asarhaddons' durch den Gott Aššur." *Baghdader Mitteilungen* 16 (1985): 377–392.

———. *Die adê-Vereidigung anlässlich der Thronfolgeregelung Asarhaddons*. Berlin: Mann Verlag, 1987.

Weeks, N., *Admonitions and Curse: The Ancient Near Eastern Treaty/Covenant Form as a Problem in Intercultural Relationships*. New York 2004.

Weippert, M., "Assyrische Prophetien de Zeit Asarhaddons und Assurbanipals" in *Assyrian Royal Inscriptions: New Horizons in Literary, Ideological, and Historical Analysis. Papers of a Symposium Held in Cetona (Siena), June 26–28, 1980*, ed. by F. M. Fales, 71–115. Rome: Istituto per l'Oriente, 1981.

———. "'König, fürchte dich nicht!' Assyrische Prophetie im 7. Jahrhundert v. Chr." *Orientalia* 71 (2002): 1–54.

Wiseman, D. J., "The Vassal-Treaties of Esarhaddon." *Iraq* 20 (1958): 1–99.

Lycia and the Hatay: Understanding Communication between Coast and Interior

Tamar Hodos[1]

Abstract

The Iron Age of Anatolia's Mediterranean coastline was a period of transformation, especially during the first half of the first millennium BCE. During this time there is increasing evidence of material similarities, especially in ceramic styles, which has given rise to arguments for an Iron Age Mediterraneanisation. The interactions that promoted these common styles were remarkably diverse, however. Comparing and contrasting the coastal region of the Hatay, in the northeastern corner of the Mediterranean, with Lycia's upland zone, in the southwestern landmass of Anatolia, this contribution examines the phenomenon of the development of common ceramic styles amid different networks of engagement. It assesses the complexity of the balance between shared and divergent practices and the mechanisms that underpin the social and cultural developments of the Mediterranean's Iron Age as seen along its Anatolian shores.

Preface

I first met Marie-Henriette in July 1993, when I came to Turkey to participate in Kinet Höyük's initial two-month excavation season. I had just completed the first year of my doctorate and had limited fieldwork experience under my belt. Little did I realise then how that one summer would shape both my professional and personal lives. Kinet was meant to be a five-year project. I stayed for a decade, and the project continued for another decade afterwards. During those summers, I learned not only the skills of excavation, survey, post-excavation analysis and interpretation, but I also witnessed first hand a model of professionalism in challenging circumstances. The physical environment was relentless. In addition to the extreme heat and humidity, early seasons also included vicious mosquitoes, oversized cockroaches, erratic water and electricity supplies (in combination with

1 Department of Archaeology and Anthropology, University of Bristol, 43 Woodland Road, Bristol BS8 1UU, United Kingdom.

one another during the 1993 seasons), and livestock invasions of the various dig house residences. These particular aspects of adventure came to an end in the late 1990s, when the permanent dig house was constructed and the municipality commenced its programme to keep the mosquito population in check by belching diesel fumes over the district every few weeks. Living communally in close quarters every summer had its own understandable challenges, regardless of abode. Nevertheless, every member of the project was always equally valued: our views were listened to, our concerns respected, our requests considered (and usually honoured). Professionally, we were given opportunities to explore our own interests and pursue our developing specialisms. Externally, the project was famous for its genuine welcome: every traveller who made the effort to visit us received outstanding hospitality from the moment of arrival with the warmest *hoşgeldiniz* to the time of departure and the *su gibi git, su gibi dön*. I have carried this model of efficient, effective project management, team building and heartfelt welcome with me to my own subsequent field projects. In addition, I have gained much personally from the wisdom of both Marie-Henriette and Charlie in the over two decades that I have had the privilege and honour to call them friends.

There is also a serendipitous symmetry between my fieldwork career in Turkey and that of Marie-Henriette, as well as an underlying unity. While Marie-Henriette may be best known for her work at Kinet Höyük, she began her fieldwork in Turkey in the Elmalı region of Lycia, working under the direction of Machteld Mellink, her undergraduate Bryn Mawr College professor and mentor. Twenty years after Marie-Henriette graduated from Bryn Mawr, I completed my own undergraduate degree at the same institution. My first field experience in Turkey was at Kinet, where I worked actively from 1993 until 2003. In 2007, I commenced my own field project in Turkey, this time in the Seki plain in Lycia, the upland plateau adjacent to Elmalı. Thus, it seems a fitting tribute to Marie-Henriette to look at these two regions we have in common.

The Iron Age Along Anatolia's Mediterranean Shores

The Mediterranean's Iron Age was a period of transformation, especially during the first centuries of the first millennium BCE. During this time along the lands that circumscribe the sea, we see increasing evidence of material similarities, especially in ceramic styles. This has given rise to arguments for an Iron Age Mediterraneanisation as a kind of global Mediterranean.[2] This notion derives from contemporary processes of globalisation, a concept that refers to our recognition of the world as a coherently bounded place. This one-placeness does not reflect a

2 E.g., Morris 2003; Hodos 2009.

unified culture or world society, however. Rather, the sense of unity is generated by sets of shared practices that are used by those interacting at the global level, and which thereby transcend cultural or national practices. At the same time, these common traits also generate a sharper delineation of the boundaries between those groups involved with one another at the global level. This reinforcement of cultural heterogeneities is one of the paradoxes of globalisation processes.

During the Mediterranean's Iron Age, we see a number of common features develop, notably and most obviously with regard to ceramic forms. In particular, it is Greek ceramic shapes and decorative motifs that gain popularity around the Mediterranean. This process begins in earnest during the eighth century BCE, and explodes during the seventh and sixth centuries BCE.[3] The widespread use of Greek pottery, and imitations of its styles, at this time is one of the factors that creates the sense of one-placeness we associate with Mediterraneanisation. This does not mean, however, that these styles were used in the same way or had the same social meanings in different contexts, nor that the social, economic, political or cultural networks that brought these wares to these various regions were similar. Closer analysis of the patterns of import and imitation in the ceramic assemblages of two regions along Anatolia's Mediterranean shores, the Hatay and Lycia, and even within two sites, Kinet Höyük in the Hatay, and Çaltılar Höyük in Lycia, between the eighth and sixth centuries BCE will enable us to assess the complexity of the balance between shared and divergent practices and to explore the mechanisms that underpin this phenomenon of broadly shared ceramic taste.

The Hatay and Lycia

The Turkish regions of the Hatay and Lycia are modern delineations related to contemporary politics. The political situation during the Iron Age was much more ambiguous and flexible than it is today, especially from the eighth century BCE onwards. In the eastern Mediterranean, this is the era of the Neo-Hittite states. The lower Orontes Valley is identified politically as Unqi, with its seat at Tell Tayinat. The coastal strip that circumscribes the İskenderun Gulf, where Kinet has its commanding views around the entire bay, seems to have been part of Que, whose capital city was at Karatepe. In terms of material culture, however, Kinet has more in common with settlements in the Amuq than those further west,[4] reminding us of the complexities and differences between social and political identities.

The significance of this littoral zone should not be underestimated. It represents the end of the shortest caravan route between Mesopotamia and the

3 Hodos forthcoming.

4 Hodos 2006, 48.

Mediterranean. The Orontes River itself was the primary natural route from the northeastern corner of the Mediterranean to the interior of Syria and on to not only Mesopotamia but also the Anatolian highlands, Syro-Palestine and further Levantine regions. Therefore, it should not be surprising that this is where the most intensive importation of Greek pottery to the Near East can be found, a trade that begins with regularity during the eighth century BCE.[5] Kinet, while engaging in trade, may have also played a strategic role in protecting the gulf, and thus perhaps the Orontes itself, from seaborne menaces from the west, given its centred location at the head of the bay; it surely controlled the coastal strip that lay between the two access points down to the sea from the Amanus mountains, at Arslanlı Bel to the west and Belen to the east.

In southwestern Anatolia at this time, the politics were somewhat different. According to ancient literary sources, the coastal zone may be affiliated with Lycians, but the upland zones are associated with Milyans in and around the Elmalı plain, and Kabalians in the area extending from the Seki plateau up to Burdur and Gölhisar. How they distinguished themselves from one another in name and material culture remains uncertain, however.[6] The Elmalı basin was accessed from the coast near Finike, in eastern Lycia, while contact between the Elmalı and Seki plains was via the mountains. Although the precise routes of antiquity are uncertain, ceramic evidence from the two basins suggests communication and exchange with one another. The Seki plateau itself is accessed from the coast via the Xanthos River. The route of the river played a vital role in connecting the southwestern coastal zone of Lycia with the inland kingdoms of Anatolia. An Ottoman bridge, Roman inscription, and Hellenistic watchtower along the course of the Xanthos River in the Seki basin attest the long-lived importance of the Seki route between the interior zones of Anatolia and the sea. Today, the highway between Fethiye and Antalya across the mountains follows the same route. A blade from Çaltılar Höyük of Nenezi Dağ obsidian, worked in a manner that recalls Bronze Age Aegean techniques, illustrates the longevity of this route as a conduit (and consumer) between inland and coastal regions.

Kinet Höyük and Çaltılar Höyük

Kinet Höyük was first investigated by Marie-Henriette Gates as part of her 1991 regional survey of the northern Hatay and Cilicia.[7] Fieldwork at the site itself commenced the following year and continued until 2012, when the project celebrated

5 Hodos 2008.

6 Hodos 2015, 93–95.

7 Gates and Özgen 1993.

its twentieth birthday and final season. The primary fieldwork methodology was excavation. This consisted of a series of strategically placed trenches of various sizes in locations on top, around the edges and down the sides of the mound to generate a holistic understanding of the various periods of occupation. In addition, trenches were opened in the lower terraces and fields surrounding the mound, revealing that during certain periods of the settlement's life, its residents lived beyond the mound itself. Survey work conducted in and around the site included various geomorphological surveys and a topographical survey, which established that the mound covers an area of 3.3 ha and is 26 m high.

The site is famous for, amongst other things, its extremely well-stratified Iron Age contexts, although its periods of occupation extend from the Neolithic to the middle of the first century BCE, with a brief reoccupation between the twelfth and fourteenth centuries CE. It is, in fact, one of few sites in Anatolia, and the eastern Mediterranean in general, with excellent stratigraphy for the Iron Age. Although the final publication of its Iron Age strata is still being prepared, preliminary reports give an indication of the nature of its Iron Age assemblage.[8] For the purposes of this particular contribution, the periods of particular interest are its eighth, seventh and sixth century BCE contexts. Monumental structures on stone foundations and with plastered walls characterise the site during the ninth and first half of the eighth centuries BCE. During the second half of the eighth century BCE, a sudden and dramatic change took place. Buildings were reconstructed along new orientations, with different techniques and less precise finishes (jogs and niches in the walls; occasional absence of stone foundations). The ceramic assemblage included Assyrian wares and a corresponding substantial drop in local painted outputs (down to 5%, when they had previously comprised 30%). Even the diet of the community changed, with a marked disinterest in fish, despite the site's coastal setting, and in contrast to previous and subsequent periods. Collectively, these have been interpreted as a period of Neo-Assyrian occupation with settlement by an inland group. Some time after the beginning of the seventh century BCE, this population left. After a brief break in occupation, the site was reconstructed, and there appears to have been an emphasis on domestic and industrial workings, with modest multi-roomed buildings situated adjacent to cobbled areas, hearths and ovens across the excavated settlement areas. Kilns associated with both the late ninth/early eighth century BCE and late seventh century BCE were excavated at the eastern side of the site. Collectively, strata pertaining to these periods are preserved to a depth of over 2 m.[9]

8 In addition to the annual reports published by M-H. Gates in *Kazı Sonuçları Toplantısı*, see also C. Gates 2006; 2010; Hodos 1999; 2000; 2006, 25–88; Hodos *et al.* 2005.

9 Hodos 2008, 66.

Çaltılar Höyük was first recorded in 1988 as part of the Balboura Survey, directed by Jim Coulton, University of Oxford, UK. The mound covers an area of 3 ha and is thus slightly smaller in area than Kinet's höyük, yet it is only 12m high at its highest point. The site has never been excavated. Instead, a series of intensive surveys was conducted by the Çaltılar Archaeological Project between 2008 and 2010.[10] This included a topographic survey, rapid reconnaissance survey, and intensive collection survey, as well as magnetometer and electrical resistance tomography surveys to detect sub-surface features without excavation. Material culture pertaining to the site's occupation history was gathered through the intensive collection survey. This involved a systematic total collection of all visible artefacts from a series of 5 m x 5 m squares from across all visible areas of occupation, the extent of which had been established by the rapid reconnaissance survey. Over the two collection seasons, *c.* 33,000 sherds and nearly 1,000 other artefacts (flint, blades, querns, slag, and occasionally a shotgun cartridge case and a donkey shoe) were recorded.

Ceramic evidence indicates occupation from the Chalcolithic period until the middle of the sixth century BCE. Like Kinet, it is clear that the physical extent of occupation fluctuated between periods. This was especially apparent in areas to the immediate north and south of the mound, where the fields were rich in pottery (alluvium overlies the eastern and western extents of occupation). The Iron Age material from these areas was considerably worn, suggesting long-term exposure and natural movement down the slopes of the mound; this contrasts noticeably with the Chalcolithic and Bronze Age material retrieved from the same squares, which showed little comparable erosion evidence. This suggests that the settlement extended beyond the contours of the mound in periods prior to the first millennium BCE. Without stratified contexts, there is a limit to what we can say about the settlement itself. Proportions of sherds by period, for instance, are of limited value since the most recent periods of occupation are likely to be the most represented in a surface collection. Indeed, ceramics dated to the Iron Age represent 75% of all the sherds (and 62% by weight). We also lack good contextual information that might indicate how various areas of the site were used. Nevertheless, despite the fact that our evidence is drawn only from surface collection, a number of important observations from the collected assemblage have enabled several signficant interpretations to be suggested about the nature of the site and its residents.

10 Momigliano *et al.* 2011.

Ceramic Consumption Patterns

Consumption and demand are not direct consequences of production and distribution, as simple or automatic responses to the availability of goods. Instead, they are culturally, temporally, socially, and even politically specific, although this does not mean that they are unrelated to production and distribution matters. Amphoras and wine drinking vessels seem to have been the primary commodity of many ships during the Iron Age, or at least of those ships that never reached their destinations. Ships carried single-origin or multi-origin cargoes, and it is clear that both cabotage and redistribution networks operated. Our earliest post-Bronze Age evidence dates to the eighth century BCE, with the Tanit and Elissa wrecks near Ashkelon, both of which carried Phoenician amphoras bound for Egypt or the western Mediterranean. Evidence for mixed cargoes exists from the seventh century BCE, with examples such as the Kekova wreck, with its assemblage of southeast Aegean, Corinthian, and Cypro-Levantine amphoras.[11] The more substantial evidence from over the course of the sixth century BCE confirms that ships regularly carried wares of mixed (e.g. Giglio; Gela; Pointe Lequin 1A) and single origins (e.g. Ecueil de Miet, Grand Ribaud F).

From even before the eighth century BCE, Kinet's ceramic repertoire belonged to a Cypro-Cilician milieu, much like its regional neighbour Tarsus. Its painted products include Cypro-Cilician geometric, bichrome, black-on-red, white slip, red slip, and burnished wares, which together represent nearly a third of the total ceramic assemblage of the ninth and eighth centuries BCE. During the seventh century BCE, its potters adhered to the Cypro-Cilician tradition, but supplemented their decorated output with the introduction of Wave Line styles, associated with East Greece, during the later part of the seventh century BCE. Between the last quarter of the seventh century BCE and the end of the sixth century BCE, Wave Line wares came to dominate the painted repertoire and to represent a substantial proportion of the entire assemblage. Banded bowls and so-called Ionian bowls also became popular forms for Kinet's workshops. Kinet craftsmen also produced some figural and non-figural vessels in so-called orientalising styles, in imitation of East Greek and Corinthian workshops.[12]

Imported pottery includes Greek geometric wares, such as Euboean pendent semi-circle skyphoi, and Cypriot Bichrome, examples of both dating particularly to the second half of the eighth century BCE. Assyrian palace ware and related imports characterise imports of the late eighth and early seventh centuries; no Greek wares were imported during this phase.[13] East Greek bird bowls represent

11 Hodos 2009, 224 with references.

12 C. Gates 2006, 369; 2010, 44.

13 Gunnar Lehmann, personal comment. I am extremely grateful to Gunnar for shar-

the main foreign wares during the first half of the seventh century BCE, while a few examples of figural and non-figural decorated classes, such as Wild Goat jars and Ripe Corinthian juglets, were imported during the later seventh century BCE. A so-called 'Sidonian' bottle belongs to the sixth century BCE.[14] No Chian or Fikellura wares have been found; Attic Black Figure (and later Red Figure) appears rarely. Attic SOS and East Greek transport amphoras (including a one-handled example from Miletus) illustrate the bulk import habits between the second half of the seventh and sixth centuries BCE (although very few of the imported transport vessels, if any, can be assigned clearly to the sixth century[15]). Levantine wares include basket-handled amphoras and glazed earthenware vessels during the seventh century.

Çaltılar's ceramic output is harder to characterise, for there are no well-published Iron Age strata from neighbouring sites with which to compare its local outputs. Most Iron Age contexts in modern Lycia and its neighbouring regions come from sporadic soundings at major Graeco-Roman city-states; Iron Age material collected from surveys, such as the Balboura Survey, are unstratified. Sites that have been more widely excavated have not yet been published, such as Hacımusalar. Our parallels are therefore often drawn from sites further away, such as Clazomenai or Kilise Tepe. Nevertheless, their plain and decorated products enable us to offer some general dating and understanding of Çaltılar's own assemblage. The site's painted outputs include banded and geometric motifs, in increasing complexity and more precise execution, over the course of the ninth to sixth centuries BCE. Mixing and pouring shapes, with a variety of rim shapes and sizes, complement a range of drinking vessels. There are also storage and cooking wares, although precise dating of these is difficult in the absence of stratified contexts or published parallels from well-stratified neighbouring sites.

Study suggests that there is a number of Iron Age imports from as early as the ninth century until the middle of the sixth century BCE. The majority of these come

---

ing with me his current assessment of Kinet's Iron Age ceramic periodisation, including the site's import patterns.

14 This particular vessel form exemplifies the complexities of globalisation. The 'Sidonian' bottle is a shape of Phoenician origin that was known in Aegean and central Mediterranean contexts, and probably produced widely. For instance, Culican (1975), regards them as imitations of Phoenician examples and made by a variety of workshops. S. Morris (1995, 136, n. 149) views the Theran examples as material cultural support for the presence of Phoenicians on Thera. The Kinet example has a Greek letter on it that was inscribed prior to firing. This suggests that the vessel was manufactured in a Greek-speaking environment. So does this make it a Greek product, or a transplanted Phoenician object (and if so, then how are we to address its Levantine origin?), neither, both, or something new? Further discussion, especially about the roles and natures of hybridisation within globalisation processes, lies beyond the scope of the present contribution.

15 Gunnar Lehmann, personal comment.

from western Anatolia. This includes several micaceous fabrics associated with East Greek outputs of the eighth and seventh centuries BCE, decorated with banded and wave line motifs. There is also a notable collection of Southwestern Anatolian ware that consists of several visually distinctive, petrographically discrete sub-groups. This may indicate more than one production centre, or, rather, that Çaltılar imported wares from more than one producer. Black-on-red plates and flasks that have been recovered are more likely to come from Rhodes or the Anatolian mainland itself, rather than the eastern Mediterranean, judging by their petrography. Several Phrygian pieces were also recovered, including an example of a large, closed vessel of the ornate brown-on-buff style, known at Gordion during the late eighth and early seventh centuries BCE, and possibly a discrete group of burnished grey ware open and closed vessels (research is ongoing to determine if this group is, indeed, of Phrygian origin; Phrygian influence in Lycia at this time makes the kingdom a plausible candidate). A small number of Greek sherds were also found, including Protocorinthian open vessels (plates or kotylai) and a possible Euboean closed vessel. Several bird bowls were also recovered, indicative of seventh century BCE contact with the western Anatolian littoral and islands, as is a Chian chalice bowl fragment with cable motif. Slightly later imports include a piece of Lydian marbled ware open form (sixth century BCE output). Although several Attic black glazed body sherds were retrieved, no Attic Black Figure pieces were collected from the mound surface (and nor was Attic Red Figure, although the site was no longer occupied by its floruit). Other classes are harder to pin down, such as a fine ware red fabric group with a grey core (open and closed forms), which originates probably in central-western Anatolia. Several figural and banded vessels can be associated with a temporal horizon between the seventh and early-mid sixth centuries BCE, but their places of manufacture cannot yet be identified; they are likely to be in western Anatolia, however. Some depict animal motifs (ears, a hoof, or polychrome feathers) that relate to outputs such as Wild Goat and similar ones, while others are monochrome and bichrome banded table wares common during the seventh and sixth centuries BCE. There is no evidence of material from further east, such as the Levant or Cyprus.

Similarities and Differences

Quantitative comparisons between the two sites are pointless, as the nature of the data collection is completely different for each. The imported wares identified at Çaltılar are, presumably, only a fraction of what lies under the ground still. That already there is evidence for imports from Greece, Lydia, Phrygia and around western Anatolia is suggestive of the site's connections with both Anataolia and the Aegean during this period. More cannot be said, however, until evidence from under the surface becomes obtainable. Equally, Kinet's Iron Age assemblage comes from predominantly the northeast and southwest edges of the settlement. Iron Age strata were never excavated in the areas in the centre of the top of the settlement. Nevertheless, with these limitations in mind, observations about both assemblages, and comparisons between them, can be made fruitfully.

It is surprising that Kinet, with its harbours, does not have more imports. The community was engaged regionally, especially with Cyprus and the nearby Levant, and more widely with the Aegean, with stylistic influence moving from one to the other over the course of the eighth to sixth centuries BCE. Given the proximity of Cyprus, a direct relationship between Kinet and Cyprus is assumed. The precise nature of the site's links with the Aegean has not been explored either, although they are presumed to be commercial rather than of a settlement nature.[16] The limited number of imports in comparison with local production in imitation of those imported styles must be probed. As noted above, the Cypro-Cilician painted output accounts for nearly a third of the entire ceramic assemblage of the ninth and eighth centuries BCE, while it has been estimated that 40% of the total ceramic assemblage during the seventh and sixth centuries BCE is in imitation of painted Aegean styles.[17] The presence of a major trading site at Al Mina during this time in contrast with the limited number of imports in each phase at Kinet suggests multiple networks of commerce and communication in this littoral zone. More specifically, the networks that connected Kinet with Cyprus, and then the Aegean, seem to have been separate from the routes between those regions and Al Mina, which served as a major port. Perhaps ships were more willing to sail for an additional hour or two to reach this regional emporium, at the mouth of the Orontes River, bypassing a neighbouring harbour like Kinet.

If Kinet were involved in trade in a substantial way, we would expect to see either direct evidence of warehouses, such as at Al Mina, or a substantial percentage of imported goods, such as we see at emporia elsewhere in the Mediterranean at this time (e.g., Naukratis and various emporia in France[18]). No warehouse structures have been identified at Kinet during these Iron Age periods, and Kinet does not appear to have been a vast consumer of imported material. One might then question whether the business of trade really was a core activity during this time. A consideration of the geographic networks of connection may also support such a doubt. The river that ran alongside the site originates in the Amanus Mountains, but there is no evidence that its course provided a route over and across the mountains, which are surprisingly high. Furthermore, the site's central location

16 C. Gates 2006, 369.

17 C. Gates 2010, 44.

18 Naukratis: e.g., Möller 2001; France: e.g., Dietler 2010, 148–155. See also Demetriou 2013.

within the bay and its notable elevation—it is the only geographical feature in an otherwise extraordinarily flat landscape—lend it a particularly valuable strategic position to keep an eye over the comings and goings through the northeastern corner of the Mediterranean by both land (between the two passes from the Amanus mountains discussed above) and by sea. Trade, such as it was during this period, may have been a byproduct, or secondary industry. Yet the fashions of the era did not pass Kinet by. Rather, it was actively engaged with wider fashions, tastes and habits. Initially this was expressed through preference for Cypro-Cilician styles and may reflect a shared system of taste, and perhaps values, with the site's Cypriot and Cilician neighbours. During the seventh and sixth centuries BCE, as East Greek table wares began to dominate regional markets, Kinet's talented potters and painters copied the styles that were so in fashion, but perhaps slightly harder to access directly precisely because ships did not offload their cargoes on a regular basis at Kinet's port. Nevertheless, Kinet was a full participant in the global Mediterranean of the Archaic period, producing ceramic styles that were expressions of the sense of one-placeness we see in the wider Mediterranean at this time. A strong network of importation is not necessary to enable a settlement to be globally connected; other networks, such as those that revolve around social values and understandings, may play a stronger role.

It is equally surprising that Çaltılar has as many imports as it does, given its location in a modest upland plateau that seems to be neither a gateway nor a major production centre. It is only alongside a transit route, rather than at a significant physical feature of such a route, like a confluence of roads or rivers, or a natural point of transition between landscape types. The site's import pattern, therefore, may be indicative of the site's function, and this may relate to the single clear architectural feature identified by the sub-surface surveys. An archaeological feature was noticed in the northern sector of the site, rather than one pertaining to the modern farming terraces that otherwise mark the surface of the mound. The magnetometry results outlined a structure of 10 x 20 m in size. The electrical resistance tomography survey indicated that this was made of stone, and that its walls are extant from just below the current ground level to a depth of 2.5 m. Given that the latest occupation at the site, judging by the ceramic assemblage, is the middle of the sixth century BCE, it is most likely that this construction relates to that era (seventh-sixth centuries BCE). Stone buildings of such dimensions at this time are usually identified as a temple or fortification. One example is the Inner Defence Platform at Old Smyrna, which is believed to have served as a fortress during the eighth and seventh centuries BCE, although votive evidence suggests it might have been a contemporary temple, and this part of the site evolved into the city's main cult area by the sixth century BCE. The majority of the later seventh and sixth century BCE ceramics from Çaltılar is dining wares, including various cup forms, mixing shapes, and serving vessels (including so-called fruit stands). As feasting and drinking are often associated with cultic activities, it is possible that such activities may have taken place in and around the structure itself. The quantity and variety of imported pottery between the eighth and sixth centuries BCE retrieved just from the surface and not from excavated contexts were surprising. That many of these seem to be large, ornately decorated, and presumably expensive, high status vessels suggests that the site was something significant during this time, perhaps serving as a sanctuary, not just for the community itself but more regionally. The imported vessels may represent dedications or be related to ritual observance by visitors. Thus, Çaltılar, too, participated in the global Mediterranean world of the seventh and sixth centuries BCE, its residents and/or visitors replete with the latest ceramic fashions, especially those originating in the East Greek/west Anatolian world.

A Global Mediterranean

Kinet residents strongly favoured wave-line and so-called Ionian bowls, while the inhabitants of Çaltılar preferred other decorated forms (figural; geometric; banded wares), yet the general repertoire of import origins between the two sites is comparable, as, indeed, it is often in the Mediterranean at this time because of widespread usage of common types, some of which were undoubtedly mass produced.[19] In both cases, despite the proximity of Greeks resident in both regions,[20] there is little evidence that the Greeks themselves played a direct role in shaping tastes at either site. Indeed, given the mixed nature of many cargoes, and evidence for cabotage networks of exchange, the geographic or ethnic origins of ship owners or crew are less exclusive to questions of trade in general than once thought. The point is that direct trade does not seem to form a substantial core of either site's activities. The popularity of Greek wares at these two sites, and elsewhere at this time, instead reflects the pervasion of shared practices that we associate with the level of global connectivity in globalising processes. Shared practices are not the same as identical ones, however. One of the features of globalisation, and one that is often misunderstood, is that engagement at the global level does not necessarily involve identical activity or belief, but rather represents common understanding;

19 Dupont 2010. Increasingly, studies are revealing that such wares were also often locally produced rather than widely imported. For example, for Kinet itself: Songu 1997; Hodos *et al.* 2005, 80–81. For Çaltılar: Momigliano *et al.* 2011, 94–97; Hodos 2015, 108–111.

20 Greeks in Cilicia are reputed to be at Soloi, Nagidos and Kelenderis, according to ancient literary sources; archaeologists have often argued for Greeks at Tarsus and Al Mina, as well. See C. Gates 2006, 369 with references. Greeks in Lycia are at Phaselis: Hansen and Nielsen 2004, 1140–1141.

nevertheless, the practices are particular to each participating community. The widespread use of similar styles may reveal broadly shared values pertaining to the social contexts of the use of such types. The use of East Greek wares at both sites suggests that in general these were desirable commodities; that they were objects in demand derives precisely from commonly held notions of social status display, even if each site exhibits features of that display in a locally-specific, locally-appropriate manner.

Political matters in each region may not have played a significant role in long-term tastes. Kinet's Iron Age period is marked by a brief Neo-Assyrian phase. While this particular period is notable for its site-wide differences, the continuities evident between the periods before and after this phase are surprising. Architecturally, the site is rebuilt in traditional techniques. Ceramic-wise, Cypro-Cilician outputs are resumed, although initially supplemented with, and then supplanted by, the new Aegean style of Wave Line ware and the so-called Ionian bowls, while the residents themselves returned to their fish-eating ways. Political changes may have had some disruption, but daily life patterns sustained for far longer. Çaltılar seems to have been similarly unbothered by major political issues during the eighth and seventh centuries BCE, perhaps being too far away from the power centres of Phrygia and Lydia, although their influence and activities may have encouraged Çaltılar's links with inland zones and interior Anatolia. Persian activity in the sixth century BCE almost certainly put an end to the site's existence, however, as the abandonment of the site, judging by its ceramic evidence, corresponds with literary records of Harpagus's conquest of Lycia in the middle of the century.

The networks of connectivity, whether for political, economic or cultural purposes, were very different for each site. For Kinet, sea links must have been vital, but not necessarily long-distance ones. It would have been perfectly possible to bypass the Gulf of İskenderun altogether moving in a westerly direction from somewhere like Al Mina, especially if one wanted to go considerably west and to do so quickly.[21] Kinet was more likely part of a cabotage network, with smaller crafts hugging the coast as they moved along from port to port. Equally, Çaltılar would not have been easy to reach from the coast, given the steepness of the mountains to reach the Seki basin, whether one follows a riverine or road route.

Despite these differences, the ceramic import and production patterns at these two sites during the Iron Age demonstrate that both communities were active participants in the wider Mediterranean world. They were not passively taking what they could get, but they made active choices about what to procure and produce. Political developments may have impacted upon availability, temporarily or longer-term, perhaps encouraging the development of new links, and

21 Oflaz 2006, 10, fig. 1–5.

opening up new influences. The common taste for Greek ceramic styles, however, especially during the seventh and sixth centuries BCE, represents shared practices. These were tempered by local needs and interests, though, with Kinet favouring especially Wave-Line vessels and Ionian bowls, and Çaltılar preferring a wider variety of banded table wares. This exemplifies the balance between practices in common at a global level and differences that define a region or community. Both Kinet and Çaltılar were just as much a part of the global Mediterranean as the Greeks themselves.

REFERENCES

Culican, W., "Sidonian bottles." *Levant* 7 (1975): 145–150.

Demetriou, D., *Negotiating Identity in the Ancient Mediterranean: the Archaic and Classical Greek Multiethnic Emporia*. Cambridge: Cambridge University Press, 2013.

Dietler, M., *Archaeologies of Colonialism. Consumption, Entanglement, and Violence in Ancient Mediterranean France*. Berkeley: University of California Press, 2010.

Dupont, P., "The Contribution of Archeometric Results to our Understanding of Archaic East-Greek Trade" in *Archaic Greek Culture: History, Archaeology, Art and Museology: Proceedings of the International Round-Table Conference, June 2005, St-Petersburg, Russia*, ed. by Sergey Solovyov, 37–40. Oxford: Archaeopress, 2010.

Gates, C., "Orientalizing and Archaic East Greek Pottery Types from Kinet Höyük (Cilicia)" in *Hayat Erkanal'a Armağan: Kültürlerin Yansıması/Studies in Honor of Hayat Erkanal: Cultural Reflections*, ed. by Armağan Erkanal-Öktü, 368–372. İstanbul: Homer Kitabevi, 2006.

———. "Greeks in the East: A View from Cilicia" in Sergey Solovyov, ed. *Archaic Greek Culture: History, Archaeology, Art and Museology. Proceedings of the International Round-Table Conference, June 2005, St-Petersburg, Russia*. 41–45. Oxford: Archaeopress, 2010.

Gates, M.H. and İ. Özgen, "Report on the Bilkent University Archaeological Survey in Cilicia and the Northern Hatay (1991)." *Araştırma Sonuçları Toplantısı* 10 (1993): 387–394.

Hansen, M. H. and T. H. Nielsen (eds.), *An Inventory of Archaic and Classical Poleis*. Oxford: Oxford University Press, 2004.

Hodos, T., "Kinet Höyük and Al Mina: New Views on Old Relationships" in *Periplous: Festschrift to Professor Sir John Boardman*, ed. by G. Tsetskhladze, A. M. Snodgrass and A. J. N.W. Prag, 145–152. London: Thames and Hudson, 1999.

———. "Kinet Höyük and Pan-Mediterranean Exchange" in *The Sea in Antiquity*, ed. by R. Brock, T. Cornell, S. Hodkinson, and G. J. Oliver, 25–37. Oxford: British Archaeological Reports, 2000.

———. *Local Responses to Colonization in the Iron Age Mediterranean*. London: Routledge, 2006.

———. "Relative Ceramic Densities in the North-Eastern Mediterranean." *Olba* 16 (2008): 57–72.

———. "Colonial Engagements in the Global Mediterranean Iron Age." *Cambridge Archaeological Journal* 19.2 (2009): 221–241.

———. "Lycia and Classical Archaeology: the Changing Nature of Archaeology in Turkey" in *Classical Archaeology in Context: Theory and Practice in Excavation in the Greek World*, ed. by C. Antonaccio and D. Haggis, 87–118. Berlin: De Gruyter, 2015.

———. forthcoming. "Greeks and Cultural Development in the Pre-Roman Mediterranean" in *A Companion to Greeks Across the Ancient World*, ed. by F. De Angelis. Oxford: Wiley-Blackwell.

Hodos, T., C. Knappett and V. Kilikoglou, "Middle and Late Iron Age Painted Ceramics from Kinet Höyük: Macro, Micro and Elemental Analyses." *Anatolian Studies* 55 (2005): 61–87.

Möller, A., *Naukratis. Trade in Archaic Greece*. Oxford: Oxford University Press, 2001.

Momigliano, N., A. Greaves, T. Hodos, B. Aksoy, A. Brown, M. Kibiroğlu and T. Carter, "Settlement History and Material Culture in Southwest Turkey: Report on the 2008–2010 Survey at Çaltılar Höyük." *Anatolian Studies* 61 (2011): 61–121.

Morris, I., "Mediterraneanization." *Mediterranean Historical Review* 18.2 (2003): 30–55.

Morris, S., *Daedalos and the Origins of Greek Art*. Princeton: Princeton University Press, 1995.

Oflaz, S. A., *Taxonomy and Distribution of the Benthic Foraminifera in the Gulf of Iskenderun, Eastern Mediterranean*. Unpublished MSc dissertation, Middle East Technical University, 2006.

Songu, F., *Wave-Line Pottery from the Late Iron Age Levels of Kinet Höyük*. Unpublished MA dissertation, Bilkent University, 1997.

Ritual Landscapes and Cultural Identities in Ionia: Evidence from the Rural Cult Places of Klazomenai

Elif Koparal[1]

To MH&C Gates for the splendid days I've spent in Kinet, where I found friendship, wisdom and inspiration.

Abstract

Cult was one of the essential components of *polis*, and each *polis* has created its identity through rituals. The cult places on the frontiers of the Ionian *poleis* and the sanctuaries located within the asty provided a network of communication that maintained the order and solidarity of Ionian societies. Archaeological evidence about the cults of Klazomenai and related rituals are scanty, and architectural remains are highly arbitrary and unsuitable for locating a sanctuary within the *asty*. Yet the systematical archaeological surveys conducted at its *khora* documented rural sanctuaries on the territorial borders with its neighbors Teos and Erythrae. All of those places situated at prominent locations such as caves, hilltops and promontories have been used prior to the emergence of *poleis* around the eighth century BC. Although they may have functioned as a shelter or a numinous place before the first millennium BC, they were integrated into the network that designated territorial borders, together with forts, tumuli and border markers, as well as the natural frontiers. This article presents those cult places located around the *khora* of Klazomenai and discusses their function as landmarks for defining the borders, and also how they were inherited and integrated into the ritual landscape formed during the formation of the *polis*.

Theoretical Framework

Archaeology has long sought to comprehend the social dynamics of past societies through the remains of cultic and ritual activities. Merritt,[2] quoting Jung,[3] wrote

---

1 Hitit Üniversitesi Fen Edebiyat Fakültesi Arkeoloji Bölümü, Çorum.

2 Merritt 2008.

3 Jung 1965, 144, 300–302.

he felt it was tragic that modern people lacked a mythical dimension in their lives, and emphasized the importance of developing a symbolic perspective.[4] Cauvin[5] suggested that the "psycho-cultural" revolution which took place at the beginning of the Neolithic should be perceived as an intellectual transformation leading to the "symbolic construction of community."[6] Organized ritual activities have frequently been correlated with sedentary communities, but recent evidence clearly shows that the symbolic construction of communities took place prior to the social transformation of communities during the Neolithic period.[7] Therefore we can speak of symbolic landscapes and ritual networks, constructed one over another through a very long time, much longer than previously thought. Landscapes are dynamic not only in a geomorphological sense, but also in terms of the way they were perceived by people. In fact, even if features of the geographical landscape may not have changed, the way they were perceived may well have.[8] Landscapes and places are not static entities, and in this sense, time can be seen as the hidden fourth dimension.[9] Yet, paradoxically, natural places such as mountains, caves and promontories preserve their positions as cult places for long periods of time despite the dramatic shifts in political and social contexts.[10] This may be explained by the ultimate needs and aspirations of human beings, which remain unaltered regardless of time and place[11] and yield to repeating symbolism.

Archaeological perspectives have frequently revealed the gaps between the ancient mind and today's way of thinking. In the context of cult archaeology, the gap is created by the concept of secularism. From the Age of Enlightenment to recent times, the modern world excluded religion from social and political formation practices. It was generally not accepted as an organizing element of modern societies. However, secularism is a synthetic concept that emerged in recent centuries, and it is naive to think that the modern world is lacking "deities" and the symbolism that created cultural landscapes. Before the Age of Enlightenment, politics could hardly be divorced from religion, and the palimpsests of the past landscape are still visible components of modern landscapes.

For any ancient society, religion was the essential component of the state and policies were employed through the veins of cult and ritual. Rituals are variously

---

4 Jung, 1976, 286.

5 Cauvin 2000.

6 Watkins 2008.

7 Schmidt 2010.

8 Bradley 2000, 33.

9 Tilley 2004, 12.

10 Bradley 2000, 155.

11 Nash and Children, 2008.

described as "determined modes of action,"[12] "stereotyped patterns of action,"[13] or "performances of more or less invariant sequences of formal acts and utterances not encoded by the performers."[14] The practice of rituals is personal and social to the same degree. It is a way of communication that provides information about the performers and a situation that serves to maintain the order and the solidarity of a group, in order to disguise inequalities and help deal with anxieties.[15] Archaeologically it is not possible to recognize a sacred place unless a ritual was practiced there, since ritual is the only tangible component of cultic practices.

Accordingly, religion was the organizing element of the Greek *polis*, upon which its identity was founded. Sanctuaries were not only monumental buildings constructed within urban centers, but were also situated at natural places in their rural territories. Such cult places, whether adorned with a building or not, had a long history as numinous settings, and there is a high tendency to identify such places with a political function, such as sanctifying a frontier.[16] The formation of the state and emergence of the *polis* are mostly linked with the concept of a sanctified border, although the use of landmarks and morphological features for demarcating the borders was probably in use long before.[17] The continuity and rupture in the use of these places for cultic activity complicate the issue of employing rural sanctuaries for territorial demarcations. It may be deceptive because at least some of these cult places were already in use in prehistoric times.

De Polignac, who classified sanctuaries in terms of their geographical reference to the urban center, emphasized the use of cult places as landmarks and explained how they articulated the territories of urban centers.[18] His work grouped sanctuaries as urban or extra-urban, and by such spatial grouping, his work attempted to demonstrate the *polis* as a composition of urban center and *khora*. According to De Polignac, the political function of those cult places situated at the fringes of the territories was to integrate the rural land into the *polis* as well as marking a frontier that divided one territory from another.[19] This bipolar model suggests that the control of the countryside was asserted by implanting extramural sanctuaries. In the socio-political context, these sanctuaries might have functioned as places of mediation and exchange between different groups, presumably Greeks

12 Durkheim 1915, 36.

13 Burkert 1979, 34.

14 Rappoport 1979, 175.

15 Shanks and Tilley 1992, 129–154.

16 Sourvinou-Inwood 1993, 10.

17 Hall 2014, 88.

18 De Polignac 1995.

19 De Polignac 1995, 33–41.

and indigenous communities.[20] Vallet has also made a similar classification that categorizes sanctuaries no more than 1 km from the city as sub-urban and those further away, up to 40 km, as extra-urban.[21] Such terminology provides us with the knowledge about the geographical location of the sanctuary in reference to one of the urban centers. However, it may be misleading regarding the function of these cult places as common places for more than one society. On the other hand, such a division has also been criticized on the grounds that political power was not supposed to be linked to the notion of the city as an urban center, but rather with the political body, regardless of where its members resided.[22]

Most of the sanctuaries placed at the borders of khorai were marking a topographic feature or geographical unit. Most of them were located in eccentric positions that marked the outer limits of the land available for agriculture. Particularly caves and groves on mountains and promontories were common settings for cult places. Perhaps mountains are the most obvious sacred spots in nature, being visible from afar and evoking a sense of proximity to the gods.[23] Promontories with temples are also a common feature of the ritual landscapes at various parts of the Greek *koine*.[24] The distribution of promontory sanctuaries follows two principles: one is that of the harbor sanctuary providing a safe cove for sailors, and the other that of a geographical position linked with trade routes.[25] Caves, as natural features, were multifunctional. They were used as shelter, water source, mine, quarry, dump, animal pen, execution place or even for the disposal of bodies (Thucydides. I, 134; Pausanias IV, 184 f), as well as cult places. The sanctity of groves is also a common phenomenon in the Greek context, but it may be difficult to find any of these well-preserved with cultic features, since groves are the most likely to be destroyed or vanish with time amongst other land features.

The position of cult places at eccentric parts of the landscape cannot be explained solely by the isolation of the believers in nature. Such parts of the territory, hardly accessible and sparsely inhabited, were shared by different social groups.[26] The notion of frontiers might have been crucial due to the heavy demand for land, particularly during the formation phase of *poleis*. It was necessary for societies to strengthen their control over space to guarantee the exploitation of natural

20 Edlund 1987, 41.

21 Vallet 1968, 67–142.

22 Polinskaya 2006, 79.

23 Rutkowski 1986, 200–201, 247.

24 Semple 1927, 353–386.

25 Edlund 1987, 48.

26 De Polignac 1995, 33.

sources, which is also crucial for the control of routes and for defending the land.[27] There are some good examples that represent the function of sanctuaries as border marks between different *poleis*. On the island of Rhodes, the Zeus Atabyrios sanctuary, located on the highest point of the border zone, separates Ialysos, Lindos and Kamiros. Artemis Limnatis is on the border between Messenia and Lacedaemon, and both shared possession of the cult.[28] Other examples are Heraion at Argolis, which lay between Argos, Mycenae and Tyrins; and, Aphrodision between Lato and Olonte on Crete. Some examples are known to have been shared by two communities, such as Artemis Hymnia by Orchomenos and Mantinea in Boeotia, and Artemis Hemerasia by Pheneos and Cleitor in Arcadia.

The appropriation of a cult site marked the boundary of the relevant territory and formed the basic step for unifying the components of a society into a single entity, which is the *polis*.[29] The network of sanctuaries placed at the rural area around the urban center articulated the territory of *poleis*. Construction of such a network might have been a conscious response to the political and social needs of newly emerging states. The land possessed by the cult sites was used for agricultural activities, which also contributed to the pastoral economy. The close environs of cult places might have been left as neutral zones, uncultivated. The Eleusinian land between Attica and Megara is a well known example of this phenomenon.[30]

Here the archaeological case on rural cult places is presented from the perspective of an Ionian *polis*, Klazomenai. I will argue that the rural cult places around Klazomenai were multi-functional in a socio-political sense. They may have articulated the territory and provided control of pastoral land and trade routes, as well as being places for the establishment of Ionian identity. The archaeological context of rural cult places may offer ground to debate issues of cultural continuity and the establishment of national identity in Ionian lands. Archaeological evidence clearly reveals the use of cult places long before the supposed date of Ionian migrations. In fact, the integration of local cults into Ionian ritual landscapes is a common phenomenon and was followed clearly at central large sanctuaries.[31] Such evidence from rural cult places has significant potential to contribute to cult archaeology in Ionia to explain the process of cultural and political transformations during the *polis* formation and the establishment of Ionian identity.

---

27 Pausanias IV.41; De Polignac 1995, 33–59.

28 McInerney 2006, 50.

29 De Polignac 1994, 33–59.

30 McInerney 2006, 52.

31 Archaeological evidence is present for the occupation of Ephesus well before the supposed period of Ionian migration; Büyükkolancı 2000.

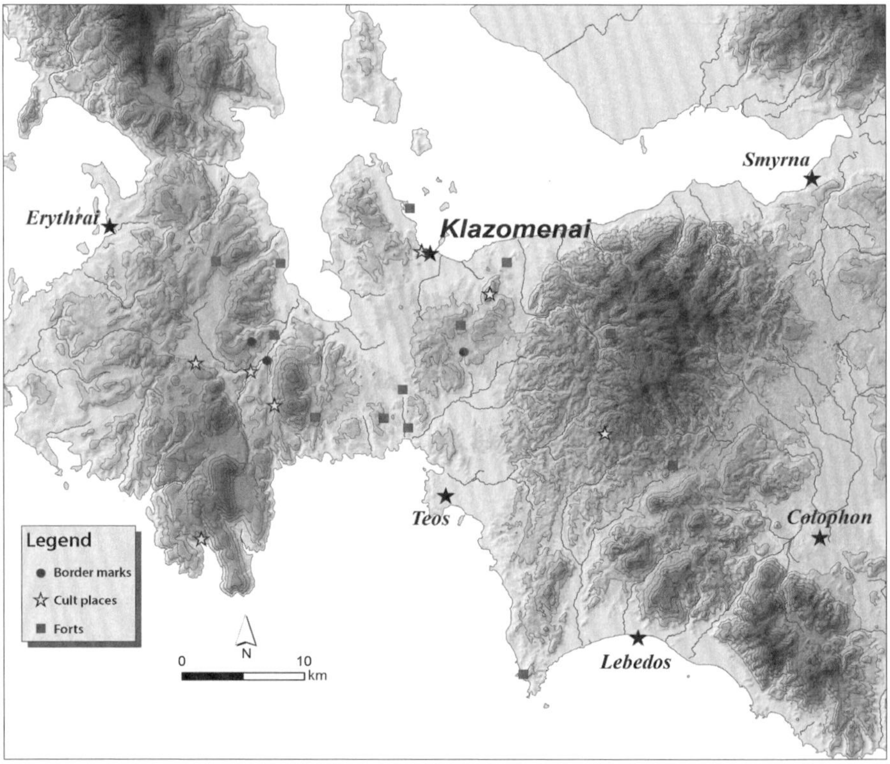

Fig. 1 Topographic map showing the distribution of cult places, border marks, forts and tumuli in Klazomenian *khora*.

Rural Cult Places in the Klazomenian *Khora*

Systematic archaeological surveys conducted in the territory of Klazomenai aimed to define the settlement patterns in the region and attempted to explain the social, political and environmental dynamics that caused the shifts. Even though mapping sites and labeling each period in terms of layers may be regarded as somewhat artificial and analytical only in a basic sense, these methods do present us with a perspective for understanding the dynamics of cultural and political landscapes and networks. Klazomenai is today located at Urla-İskele in the İzmir region on the western coast of Anatolia. The Klazomenai Survey mapped sites with various functions, as well as the distribution of forts, border marks, tumuli and cult places marking the borders of its territory (Fig. 1). The placement of these sites almost perfectly overlapped with natural frontiers created by mountains encircling the Urla basin, a geographical unit which formed the core of the Klazomenian *khora*.[32]

32 For further information on Klazomenian *khora* see: Koparal 2013.

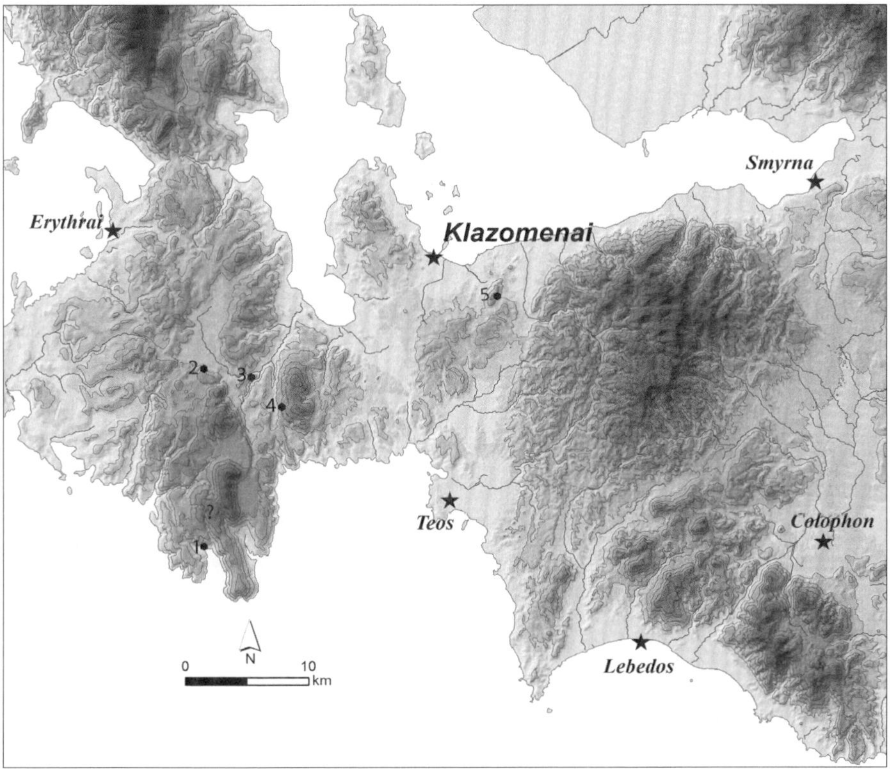

FIG. 2 Topographic map showing the distribution of cult places (1.Cılga; 2.Köytepe; 3.Kazankaya; 4.Söğüt; 5.Inkaya, ?.Korykos).

Currently, six cult places have been documented by the archaeological surveys around Klazomenai (FIG. 2). Epigraphic evidence for the cults of Klazomenai is rare and fragmentary. Yet, a few inscriptions, as well as coin iconography, do refer to the presence of cults dedicated to certain deities. Fragmentary inscriptions found around Klazomenai reveal the presence of cults dedicated to Hermes,[33] Athena Polias,[34] Zeus Tropaiophoros,[35] Zeus Soter and Herakles.[36] The coin iconography

33 Engelmann and Merkelbach 1972–1973; Jeffrey 1951, 345, no. 63; Simon 1986, 64–65.

34 Simon 1986, 64–65. The Archaic temple located on Karantina island was identified as a shrine dedicated to Athena Polias by Oikonomos. Simon associated the Archaic deposit that included some Archaic figurines with an inscription found nearby referring to the cult of Athena Polias.

35 Woodward 1926–1927, 117, no 1; Simon 1986, 64.

36 Engelmann and Merkelbach 1972–1973, no. 518–519; Simon 1986, 64–65.

depicts Kybele,[37] Hermes,[38] Zeus,[39] Apollo,[40] Athena,[41] and Artemis Ephesia.[42] Yet it is not possible to make a conclusive identification of deities associated with the individual cult places. Those sanctuaries located at remarkable natural settings are likely to fall into disputed territories between the *poleis* of Erythrae, Teos, Smyrna, and Klazomenai.

Cılga is a sheltered cove situated on the southwestern coast of the Urla-Çeşme peninsula, and it is not easily accessible from land. The cave, located at the tip of the promontory situated to the west of the cove, functioned as a cult place with a height of 150 m above present sea level. The site was first documented by H. Erkanal.[43] It is likely that the area was disputed between Erythrae, Teos and Klazomenai. The coves situated on the highly indented southwestern coast like Kokar, Cılga and Düverlik were probably shelters for sailors and pirates and remained as isolated places. The cave has a very narrow entrance opening into a front gallery preceding a second gallery 16 m long. There are three more galleries connected to this one, and the total length of the cave is approximately 40 m. In the front gallery, there is a 2 m high debris filled with terracotta figurines presumably depicting Hecate, although this is not confirmed by epigraphic evidence. Intriguingly, Hecate was associated with crossroads, entrance ways, and moonlight. Therefore, perhaps symbolically, her presence indicated the crossroads between the *poleis*, as well as showing the way to sailors with her torches. It is known that a Sybille from Erythrai who migrated to Cumae served Hecate.[44] The deposit of figurines also included pottery sherds dating to the Archaic and Classical periods.[45]

Köytepe is a hilltop site overlooking the Barbaros plain situated to the west of Klazomenaian territory at the Uzunkuyu-Zeytinler region. The hilltop is densely covered with maquis and pine trees, and for this reason the surface visibility is low almost year around at the site. Despite low surface visibility, some well-preserved surface material (FIG. 3–4) revealed the long-term use of the site beginning with the Neolithic period. The northern portion of the hill was destroyed during the motorway construction. There are remains of a building on the western part of the hill, where a foundation wall of 15 m extending in a north-south direction and

37 Simon 1986, 64–65; BMC Ionia 32 (no. 123–123), 33 (no. 128), 35 (no. 136).

38 Simon 1986; BMC Ionia 28 (no. 98, 100–101).

39 Simon 1986; BMC Ionia 27 (no. 87–91); 29 (no. 105–106).

40 Simon 1986; BMC Ionia 17–31 (no. 46–47).

41 Simon 1986; BMC Ionia 21–26 (no. 32–45, 51–86).

42 Simon 1986

43 Erkanal 1995.

44 Akalın 2008.

45 Erkanal 1995.

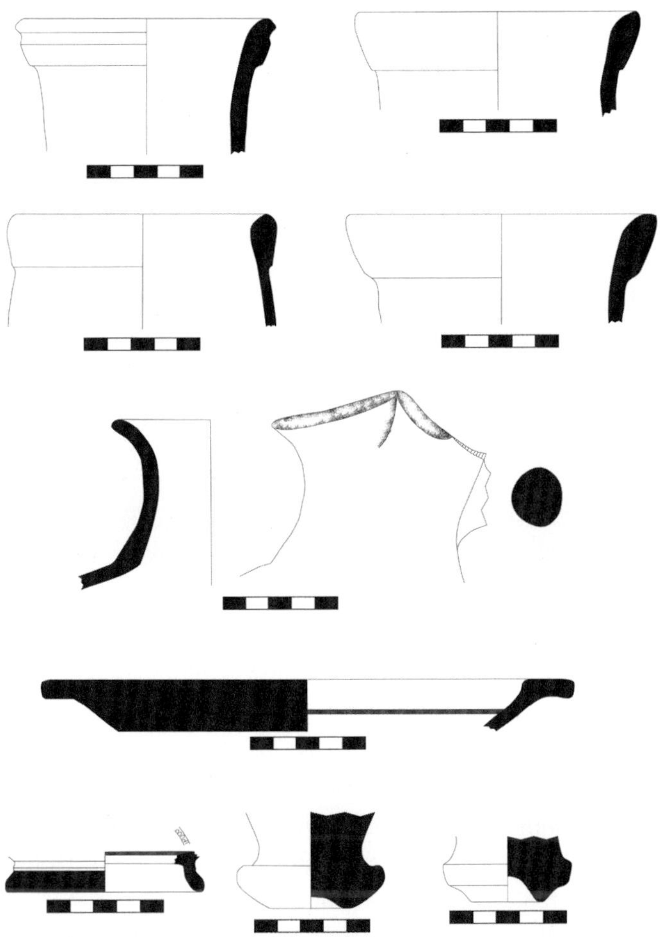

FIG. 3 Drawings of selected surface material from Köytepe.

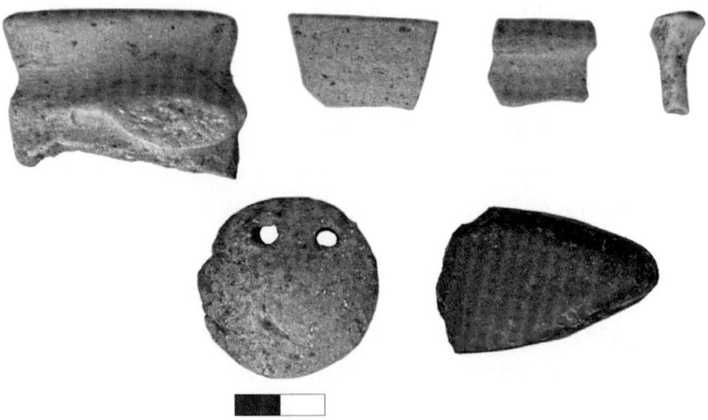

FIG. 4 Photo of selected surface material from Köytepe, including a stone axe fragment.

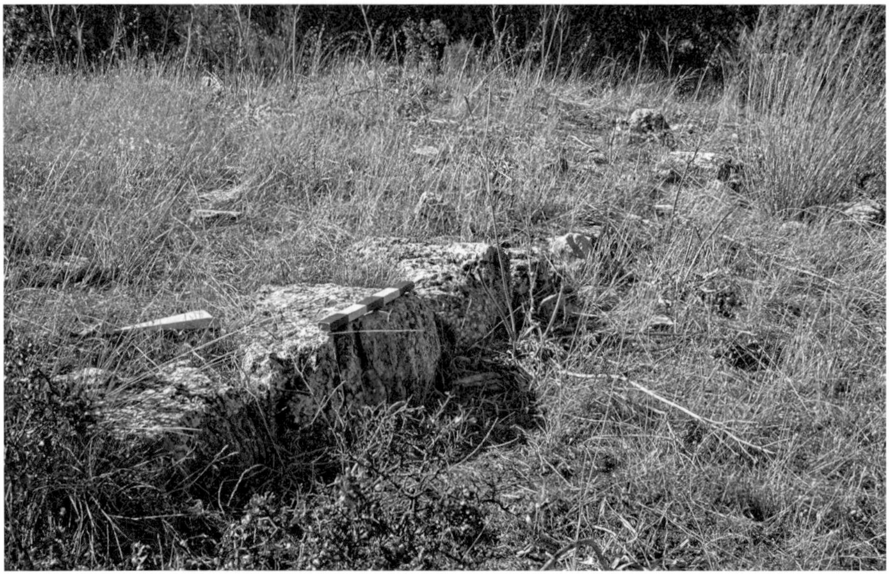

Fig. 5 Photo of wall foundation at Köytepe.

a 5 m foundation wall extending in a east-west direction are preserved (Fig. 5). The walls are built of huge cut-stone blocks without any mortar, and their width reaches 0.9 m. The use of dry wall technique suggests an early date of the building, before the Late Roman period. The portable stone cult altar dating to the Archaic period and a fragment of an architectural relief (Fig. 6) also dating to the Archaic period provide significant evidence related to the dating and the function of the building. An inscription found at Zeytinler near Pyrge (probably the village of Birgi) mentions the border of a sanctuary dedicated to Zeus Olympios.[46] On the basis of archaeological and epigraphic evidence, Köytepe should be regarded as a plausible candidate for the setting of the Zeus Olympios temple. Not far from the building, a disturbed pithos burial was found on top of the hill. The burial, enclosed by a wall of 0.4 m, is associated with a trefoil rimmed oinochoe and a pithos whose mouth faced north. The mostly burned fragmentary human bones were scattered around, probably pulled out of the pithos by smugglers. The oinochoe, which might be a burial gift, dates to the end of the fourth century BC.

Kazankaya is situated on an outcrop rock that stands as a landmark on the main route from Urla to Çeşme (Fig. 7). There is a cistern cut into the rock on the top of it, with a diameter of 0.5 m diameter and a depth of 1.5 m. There are also remains of the foundations of dry walls extending in a north-south direction around

46 Simon 1986, 64; Engelmann and Merkelbach 1972–1973, no. 231.

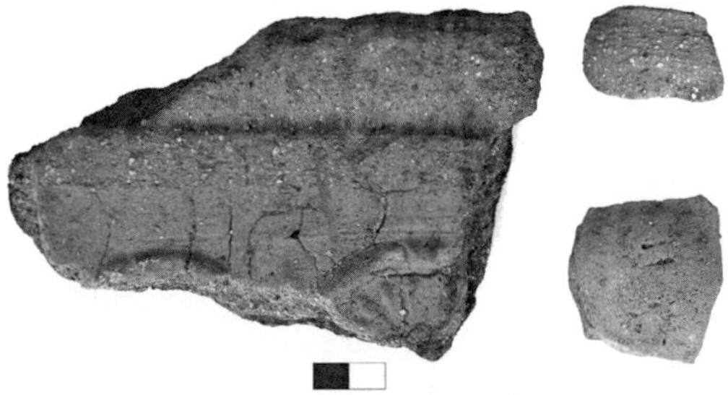

FIG. 6 Photo of architectural relief from Köytepe.

the rock. Surface materials consist of non-diagnostic body sherds and are few in number. Despite the lack of sufficient evidence, the location and natural setting of the site fits the scheme of the ritual network around Klazomenai.

Söğüt is a natural cave located to the southwest of Klazomenian territory, in a 350 m wide valley extending in a north-south direction leading to Kokar Cove on the southern coast to the east of Cılga. The valley is located within the mountainous mass that presumably set the frontier between Erythrae and Klazomenai. A colluvium plain lies in front of the small cave (FIG. 8) and is today inhabited seasonally by lumberjack families. The valley consists of a geographic unit where almost ten settlements, whose sizes range between 0.5–5 ha, are distributed. The surface pottery collected in that area roughly indicates a settlement history from the Geometric period to the Late Ottoman era. However, few prehistoric sherds were found around the cave, which might have functioned as a cult place for a long period of time. The findings clearly indicate the use of the cave as early as the Early Bronze Age, perhaps even before.[47] The cave has an entrance 11.5 m wide and 20 meters high. Inside the cave, a throne is carved on the wall with a cross on top of it (FIG. 9). Due to the cross, it would not be far from reality to suggest the use of the cave as a sanctuary during the Christian period, most probably for the Virgin Mary. It seems likely that the original reliefs carved on the wall were modified during the Christian era. Below the cross there is a rock cut seat protruding from the cave wall that resembles a throne, and perhaps the original figure was a seated female, most probably Kybele. This place is highly likely to be the sanctuary consecrated to the games of Alexander, which is described by Strabo as being situated to the north of Khalkideis at Khersonessos Isthmus (XIV.1.31).

Korykos (shown with a question mark in FIG. 2) is solely known from textual sources as the setting of a sanctuary, where rituals were practiced for Kybele.[48] Pausanias mentions seer women who lived in rocky places and grottos and were well respected by society (X.12). Korykos is named Kırandağ today, and it is part

47 Meriç *et al.* 2012, 42.

48 Akalın 2008.

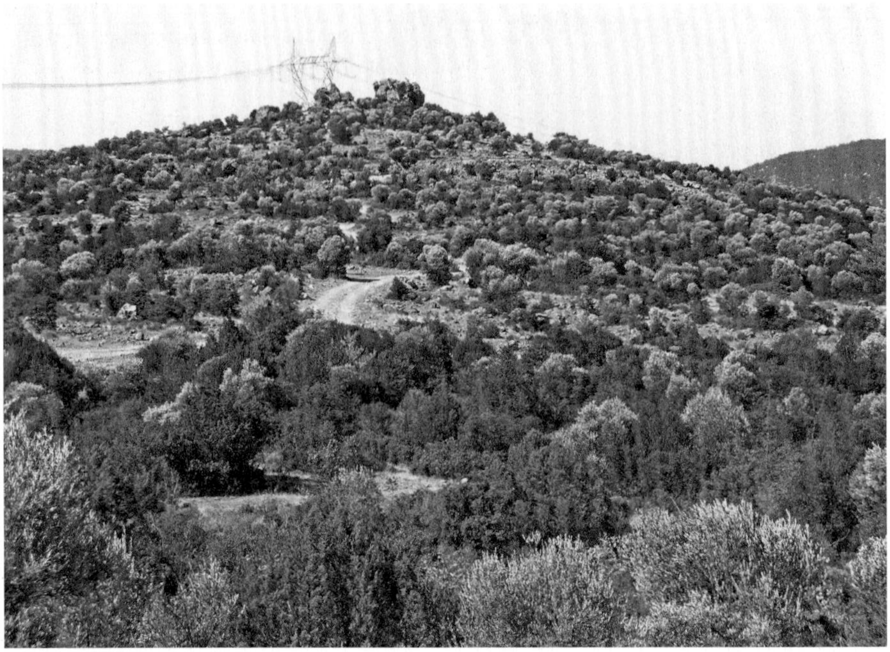

Fig. 7 View of Kazankaya.

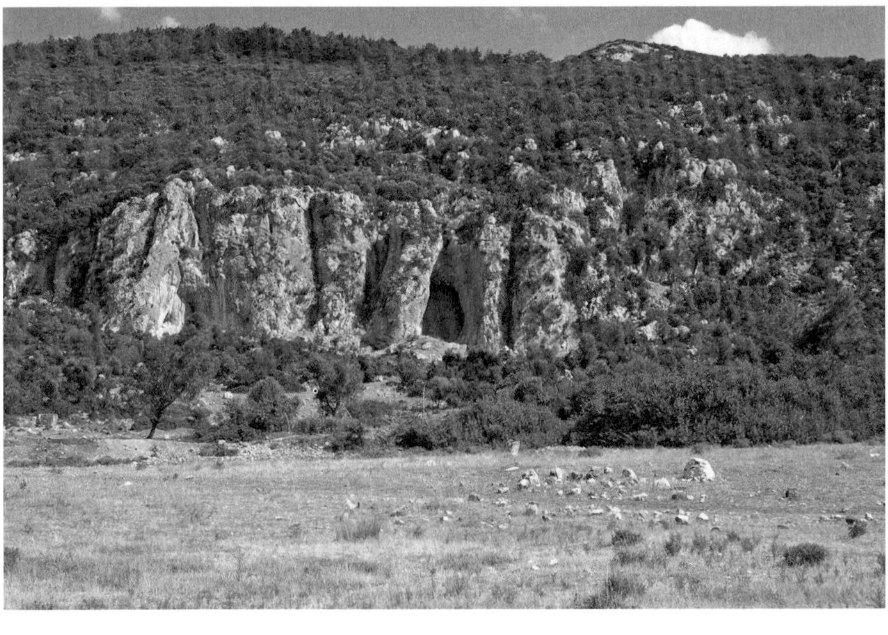

Fig. 8 View of Söğüt cave.

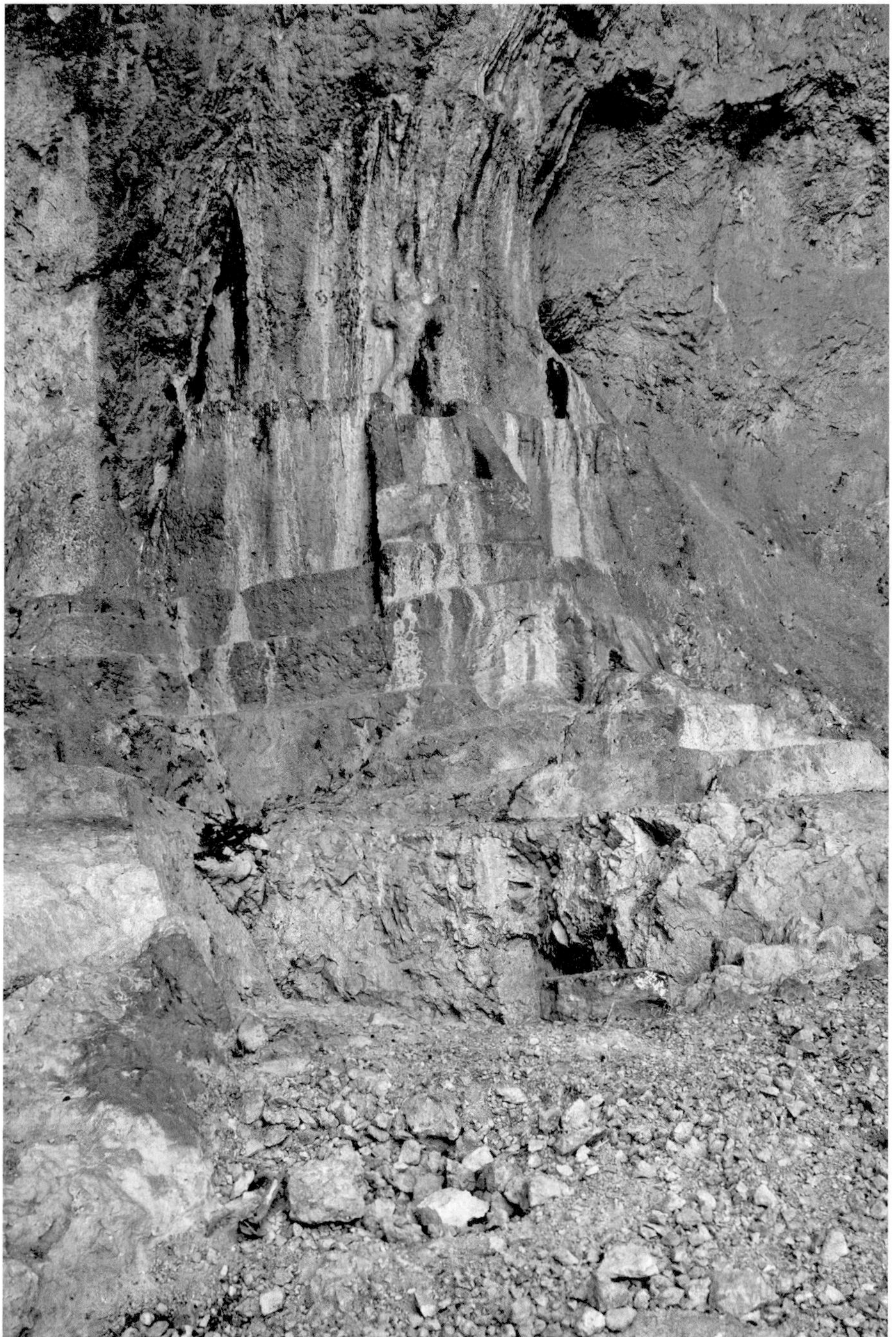

Fig. 9 View of Söğüt cave, relief on wall.

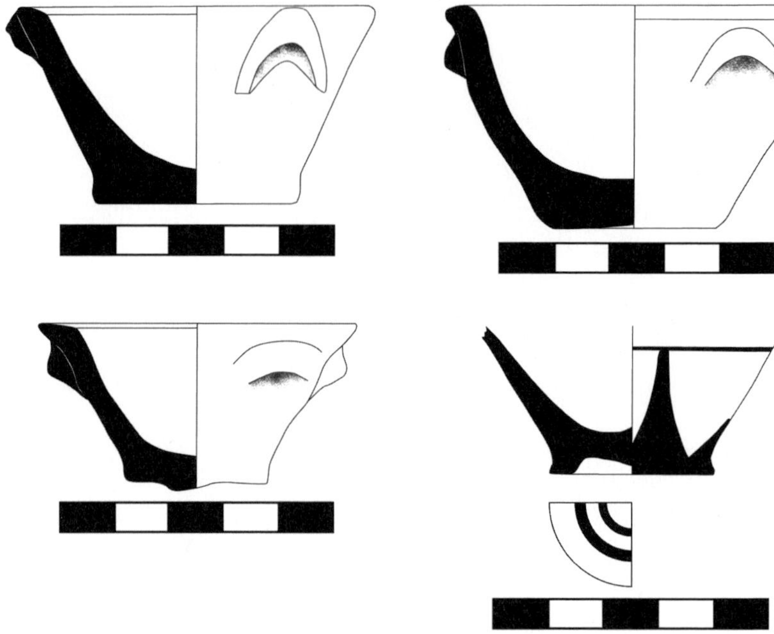

Fig. 10 Drawing of selected votive cups from Inkaya cave.

of the mountainous mass that sets the natural frontier between the territories of Klazomenai and Erythrae. The setting of the sanctuary dedicated to Kybele is not localized precisely yet. It might not be so far from Söğüt.

The İnkaya Cave is situated on the summit of Kocadağ on the western tip of a mountain range that defines a natural frontier between Teos and Klazomenai. The total length of the cave is about 200 m and reaches a depth of 30 m. The pottery sherds found on the floor of the cave suggest the long-term use of the cave. Perhaps the cave was used primarily as a shelter and subsequently turned into a sanctuary. The large quantity of sherds, which date to the prehistoric period, includes small votive cups (Fig. 10) and Geometric-Early Archaic bowls (Fig. 11) and continue into the Ottoman era. Such continuity in the use of the place marks its function as a numinous place.[49]

There are also two more sanctuaries which are known to us from literary sources, but which have not yet been located. Strabo[50] mentions a temple dedicated to Apollon Gryneus mentioned by Servius[51] near Smyrna where hot springs

49 Atalay 1987.

50 XIV.I.36.

51 Aenid 4.345; Simon 1986, 64–65.

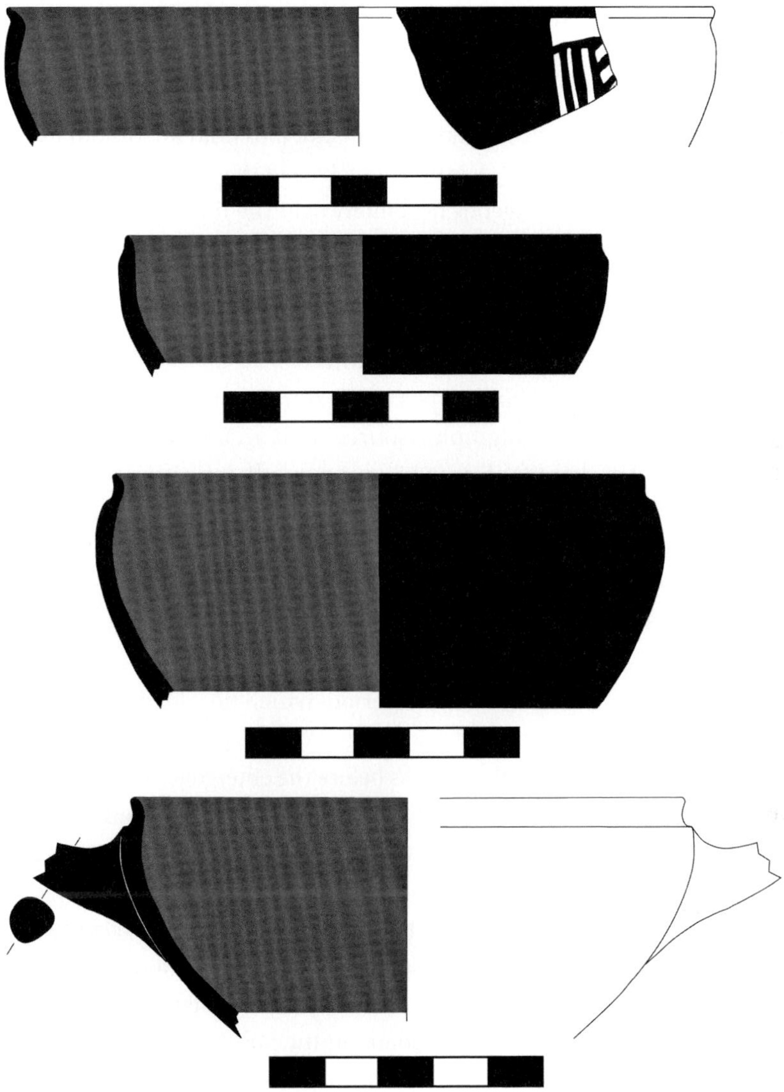

FIG. 11 Drawing of selected bowls from Inkaya cave.

were present. The setting or any associated remains are not yet identified, but it might have been a place near Balçova or İnciraltı. The other one is mentioned by Diodoros, who refers to Klazomenians having consulted Pythia of the Delphi Apollon about a dispute which arose after the death of Tachos, who had founded a city near the sea. The dispute, between Kyme and Klazomenai, was over the hegemony of Leukai, where a shrine dedicated to Apollon was located. Pythia decided that the shrine should belong to the *polis* that offered the first sacrifice in Leukai, and each side should start from their own city. Kyme, being much closer to the targeted destination assumed itself advantageous. However, the Klazomenians forestalled them in performing the sacrifice by choosing a lot from their own citizens to found a city near Leukai. They decided to hold an annual festival to bear its name, Prophthaseia.[52] All this took place in the fourth century BC when Klazomenai used its advantageous hegemony over the northern sea through the islands and extended its borders towards the north.[53]

Conclusion

The evidence for the ritual landscapes of Klazomenai is scanty in comparison with other *poleis* in Ionia. Epigraphic sources and archaeological evidence are seldom integrated and are far from presenting a full definition of the religious structure of the *polis*. Therefore, the archaeological evidence from the rural cult places around Klazomenai is significant in shedding light on this issue. Although it was not possible to identify to whom these sanctuaries were dedicated, some suggestions could nevertheless be made, as discussed above. The rural sanctuaries undoubtedly marked the territorial borders of Klazomenai at different stages, but in particular during the Early Archaic period, which heralded state formation. However, all sanctuaries were used prior to the Archaic period and most probably were elements of different ritual networks before the emergence of *poleis*. Therefore the network of these cult places might have formed with the emergence of *poleis* for the articulation of the territory, but their cultural and cultic functions in terms of bringing together different societies was most probably inherited.

The Early Archaic period is widely accepted as a revolutionary time when Greek communities went through a socio-cultural transformation[54] and constructed a collective identity. It is beyond doubt that rituals were significant actors during the formation of *poleis* together with economic and political aspects. Archaeological evidence both from the mainland and the territory reveal that the early Archaic

52 Diodoros, 15.18.1–2.

53 The Klazomenians claimed a peraea near the mouth of Hermos after 385 BC (Diodorus 15.18.3), probably due to lack of sufficient grain. The name of the settlement is not mentioned in the texts, but it is likely to have synoceised with Leukai. The source of the grain might have been in the close environs such as Smyrna, Phocaea or even Khios, but not the Black Sea or Egypt (Aristotle, *Oeconomica*, II.16.1348b). In the late 380's Klazomenai was at war with Kyme over the recently founded city of Leukai (Diodorus 15.18.1–2), and the silver and gold coins bearing Apollon/swan are assumed to to have been minted for the mercenaries employed by Klazomenai. This assumption is fairly based on the fact that this type of coin was minted very briefly and never repeated according to Meadows 2009, 253; Kinns 1989, 183–193.

54 Finley 1954.

period was a time of state formation and institutionalization for Klazomenai as well.[55] The defensive networks were formed around its territory either by the use of earlier forts or by constructing new forts and watch posts.[56] Tumuli and border markers were other components of the newly formed political landscape around the Klazomenian territory. Yet the ritual landscape was clearly inherited from previous inhabitants, who expressed their symbolic perception on the landscape before the supposed arrival of the Ionians. However, as there are different forms of rupture and continuity in the use of these cult places, "continuity" by itself cannot be regarded as the most significant parameter related to the formation of ritual landscapes.[57] Regardless of whether they were used by prehistoric communities or not, there was a revival during the early Archaic period as indicated by the quantity and the dating of the pottery. However, the pre-existence of a ritual landscape, presumably with minor alterations, generates several questions about the construction of cultural identity in Ionia. It seems likely that the Ionian identity may have been represented by the continuity of a long-existing heritage[58] rather than a simple takeover into which previous cultural aspects dissolved. Continuing archaeological surveys around the *khorai* of Klazomenai and Teos can potentially discover new cult places, but the spatial pattern is likely to remain without any major alterations. The cult places marked certain topographic features such as caves, coves, and hilltops which were prominent features of the natural landscape.

55 Ersoy 2013; Koparal 2009, 57–79.

56 Koparal 2013.

57 De Polignac 1994, 9.

58 Antonaccio 1994, 86.

REFERENCES

Akalın, A. G., "Traces of Mother Goddess in Erythri." *Asia Minor Studien* 66 (2008): 1–7.

Antonaccio, C. M., "Placing the Past: The Bronze Age in the Cultic Topography of Early Greece" in *Placing the Gods: Sanctuaries and Sacred Space in Ancient Greece*, ed. by S. Alcock and R. Osborne, 79–105. Oxford: Clarendon Press, 1994.

Arnason, J. P., "Exploring the Greek Needle's Eye: Civilizational and Political Transformations" in *The Greek Polis and the Invention of Democracy: A Politico-cultural Transformation and Its Interpretations*, ed. by J. P Arnason, K. A. Raaflaub and P. Wagner, 21–46. Chichester: Wiley-Blackwell, 2013.

Atalay, E. Ö., "İzmir ve Aydın Yörelerinde Mağara Araştırmaları." *V. Araştırma Sonuçları Toplantısı Cilt* 2 (1987): 297–321.

Bammer, A. and U. Muss, "Ein frühes Quellheilingtum am Ayasolukhügel in Ephesos." *Anatolia Antiqua* 15 (2007): 95–101.

Barclay V. H. and R. S. Poole, eds., British Museum Catalogue of the Greek Coins of Ionia: London 1892.

Bradley, R., *An Archaeology of Natural Places*. London: Routledge, 2000.

Burkert, W., *Structure and History in Greek Mythology and Ritual. Sather Classical Lectures 47.* Berkeley: University of California Press, 1979.

Büyükkolancı, M., "Excavations on Ayasuluk Hill in Selçuk, Turkey" in *Die Ägäis und das Westliche Mittelmeer: Beziehungen und Wechselwirkung 8. bis 5. Jhdt. v. Chr. Akten des Symposions, Vienna, 24. bis 27. März 1999*, ed. by F. Krizinger, 39–43. Vienna: Österreichische Akademie der Wissenschaften, 2000.

Cauvin, J., *The Birth of Gods and the Origins of Agriculture*. Cambridge: Cambridge University Press, 2000.

De Polignac, F., *Cults, Territory and the Origins of the Greek City-State*. Tr. by J. Lloyd. Chicago: University of Chicago Press, 1995.

———. "Mediation, Competition and Sovereignty: The Evolution of Rural Sanctuaries in Geometric Greece" in *Placing the Gods: Sanctuaries and Sacred Space in Ancient Greece*, ed. by S. Alcock and R. Osborne, 3–19. Oxford: Clarendon Press, 1994.

Durkheim, E., *The Elemental Forms of the Religious Life*, tr. by J. W. Swain. London: Allen Lane and the Penguin Press, 1915.

Edlund, I. E. M., *The Gods and the Place: the Location and the Function of Sanctuaries in the Countryside of Etruria and Magna Graecia (700–400 BC) (Skrifter Utgivna Av Institutet I Rom, Acta Instituti Romani Regni Sueciae, 4°, XLIII)*. Stockholm: Skrifter utgivna av Svenska Institute i Rom, 1987.

Engelmann, H. and R. Merkelbach, *Die Inschriften von Erythrai und Klazomenai I*. Bonn 1972–1973.

Erkanal, H., "İki Koy Mağara ve Foklar." *Atlas* 27 (1995).

Ersoy, Y.E., "Klazomenai'de Tunç Çağı'ndan Arkaik Dönem Sonuna Kadar Yerleşim Düzenleri ve Değişimleri: Siyasal, Sosyal ve Çevresel Etkiler" in *Yerleşim Sistemleri ve Mekan Analizi*, ed. by Ö. Çevik and B. Erdoğu, 257–280. İstanbul: Ege Yayınları, 2013.

Finley, M.I., *The World of Odysseus.* New York: NYRB Classics, 1954.

Hall, J.M., *A History of the Archaic Greek World, ca.1200–479 BCE.* Chichester: Wiley-Blackwell, 2014.

Herda, A., "Apollon Delphinios-Apollon Didymeus: Zwei Geschichter eines milessischen Gottes und ihr Bezug zur Kolonisation Milets in archaischer Zeit" in *Kulturkontakte: Apollon in Milet/Didyma, Histria, Myus, Naukratis und auf Zypern*, ed. by R. Bol *et al.*, 13–86. Rahden 2008.

Jeffrey, L.H., *The Local Scripts of Archaic Greece. A Study of the Origin of the Greek Alphabet and Its Development from the Eight to the Fifth Centuries BC.* Oxford: Oxford University Press, 1961.

Jung, C.G., *Memories, Dreams, Reflections*, ed. by A. Jaffe, tr. by R. Winston and C. Winston. New York: Vintage, 1965.

———. *The Collected Works of C.G. Jung Vol. 18.* ed. by H. Read *et al.* Princeton: Princeton University Press, 1976.

Kinns, P., "Ionia: The Pattern of Coinage During the Last Century of the Persian Empire." *Revue des etudes Anciennes* (1989): 183–193.

Koparal, E., "Border Forts of Klazomenai: Cinderesi Fortification" in *Zurück zum Gegenstand: Festschrift für Andreas E. Furtwängler* (*ZAKSSchriften 16*), ed. by R. Einicke *et al.*, 501–507. Langenweißbach: Beier & Beran Verlag, 2009.

———. "Land Use and Agricultural Potential in Klazomenian *Khora*" in *Settlement Archaeology Series IV, 12–13 May 2011, Ankara*. Symposium Proceedings IV, ed. B. Erciyas, 125–145. İstanbul 2013.

———. "Grek Polisi İmgesi ve Değişen Gerçekler: Klazomenai Örneği" in *Yerleşim Sistemleri ve Mekan Analizi*, ed. by Ö Çevik and B. Erdoğu, 57–79. İstanbul: Ege Yayınları, 2013.

MacSweeney, N., *Foundation Myths and Politics in Ancient Ionia*. Cambridge: Cambridge University Press, 2013.

McInerney, J., "On the Border: Sacred Land and the Margins of the Community" in *City, Countryside, and the Spatial Organization of Value in Classical Antiquity*, ed. by R. M. Rosen and I. Sluiter, 35–59. Leiden: Brill, 2006.

Meadows, A. R., "The Hellenistic Silver Coinage of Klazomenai" in *Ancient History, Numismatics and Epigraphy in the Mediterrenean World. Studies in Memory of Clemens E. Bosch and Sabahat Atlan and in Honour of Nezahat Baydur*, ed. by O. Tekin, 247–262. İstanbul: Ege Yayınları, 2009.

Meriç, A. G., K. Öz and A. Uhri., "Urla Söğüt Kutsal Alanı Seramik Buluntularının Değerlendirilmesi." *Dokuz Eylül* Üniversitesi *Edebiyat Fakültesi Dergisi* 1/1 (2012): 40–54.

Merritt, D. L., "Sacred Landscapes, Sacred Seasons: A Jungian Ecopsychological Perspective" in *The Archaeology of Semiotics and the Social Order of Things* (*BAR In-*

ternational Series 1833), ed. by G. Nash and G. Children, 153–170. Oxford: British Archaeological Reports, 2008.

Nash, G. and G. Children, *The Archaeology of Semiotics and the Social Order of Things* (*BAR International Series 1833*). Oxford: British Archaeological Reports, 2008.

Polinskaya, I., "Lack of Boundaries, Absence of Oppositions: the City-Countryside Continuum of a Greek Pantheon" in *City, Countryside and the Spatial Organisation of Value in Classical Antiquity* (*Mnemosyne Supplementum vol. 279*), ed. by R. M. Rosen and I. Sluiter, 61–92. Leiden: Brill, 2006.

Rappoport, R. A., *Ecology Meaning and Religion*. Richmond: North Atlantic Books, 1979.

Rutkowski, B., *The Cult Places on the Aegean*. New Haven: Yale University Press, 1986.

Schmidt, K., "Göbekli Tepe, the Stone Age Sanctuaries: New Results of Ongoing Excavations with a Special Focus on Sculptures and High Reliefs." *Documenta Praehistorica* 37 (2010): 239–256.

Semple, E., "The Templed Promontories of the Ancient Mediterranean", *The Geographical Review* 17 (1927): 353–386.

Shanks, M. and C. Tilley, "Ideology, Symbolic Power and Ritual Communication: a Reinterpretation of Neolithic Mortuary Practices" in *Symbolic and Structural Archaeology*, ed. by I. Hodder, 129–154. Cambridge: Cambridge University Press, 1982.

Simon, C. G., *The Archaic Votive Offerings and Cults of Ionia*. PhD Thesis, University of California, 1986.

Sourvinou-Inwood, C., "Early Sanctuaries, the Eighth Century and Ritual Space: Fragments of Discourse" in *Greek Sanctuaries; New Approaches*, ed. by N. Marinatos and R. Hagg, 1–17. London: Routledge, 1993.

Tilley, C., *The Materiality of Stone: Explorations in Landscape Phenomenology*. New York: Bloomsbury Academic, 2004.

Vallet, G., "La Cité et son territoire dans les colonies grecques d'occident" in *La Citta e il suo territorio. Atti del VII Convegno di Studi Sulla Magna Grecia, Taranto 8–12 Ottobre 1967*, 67–142. Naples: ISAMG, 1968.

Watkins, T., "Ordering Time and Space: Creating a Cultural World" in *Proceedings of the 5th International Congress on the Archaeology of the Ancient Near East, Madrid, April 3–8 2006/ Madrid, 3 a 8 abril de 2006, Actas del V Congreso Internacional de Arquelogía del Oriente Próximo Antiquo, Vol. III*, ed. by J. M. Cordoba *et al.*, 647–659. Madrid 2008.

Woodward, A. M., "Some Notebooks of Sir William Gell." *Annual of the British School at Athens* 28 (1926–1927): 107–127.

Eighth Century BCE Mortaria at Kinet Höyük

Gunnar Lehmann[1]

It is a great pleasure to dedicate these lines to Marie-Henriette and Charles Gates, good friends and exemplary scholars. Being invited by them to study the Iron Age pottery from Kinet Höyük, I am happy to have the opportunity to present some preliminary results of these studies, focusing on the earliest appearance of ceramic mortaria in the Levant during the Iron Age.

Abstract

The paper discusses eighth century BCE mortaria made of clay found in Kinet Höyük and other sites in the Levant. Such mortaria were apparently imported to the Levant during the late eighth century BCE. During the Assyrian period the import of mortaria may have been interrupted and resumed only in the mid-seventh century BCE.

Introduction

After E. Stern's study of the "Material Culture of the Land of the Bible in the Persian Period",[2] the archaeological community became more conscious about a specific type of ceramics usually called "mortaria". These vessels are often associated with the Persian (or Achaemenid) period. Mortaria made of clay are, however, much older. The first examples of ceramic mortaria appear in the eastern Mediterranean as early as the eighth century BCE. During the seventh century BCE, mortaria became more frequent and were found in large quantities in Cilicia, Syria, Phoenicia and Palestine. Later types of mortaria made of clay remained in use throughout the Achaemenid, Hellenistic and Roman periods. This paper deals with the earliest ceramic mortaria found at Kinet Höyük that were produced in the eighth century BCE.

Mortaria are shallow wide bowls with a thick wall and rim. They often show traces of heavy use inside, where they are extremely worn. A number of studies

1 Department of Bible, Archaeology and Ancient Near Eastern Studies, Ben-Gurion University, P.O.B. 653, Beer Sheva 84105, Israel.

2 Stern 1982.

focused over the last two decades on these vessels discussing questions related to their typology, function, distribution and chronology.[3] Villing concluded convincingly that mortaria were most probably used as grinding bowls.[4] Figurines and drawings from Greece dating to the fifth and fourth centuries BCE show mortaria being used in that way.[5] It is, however, unclear, what was processed in these bowls and whether the mortaria in the eastern Mediterranean were all used for the same purpose throughout the centuries of their occurrence.

New evidence for the earliest ceramic mortaria, dating to the eighth century BCE, was recently found at Kinet Höyük. The site is located in the northeastern corner of the Mediterranean, on the east side of the Gulf of İskenderun (Hatay province, Turkey). Excavations were conducted between 1992 and 2012 under the direction of one of our honorees, Marie-Henriette Gates of Bilkent University, Ankara. The eighth century BCE mortaria found during the excavations at Kinet Höyük not only provide additional evidence for early ceramic mortaria, but they also help to understand previously published mortaria from Cilicia that were found at Tarsus and Mersin.

The mortaria presented here were found in Kinet Höyük Periods 8 and 9. Period 9 dates to the eighth century BCE and represents a local Cilician settlement with a material culture that developed out of the earlier Iron Age presence at the site. Period 8 represents a somewhat intrusive material culture that is associated with the Assyrian presence in the Levant. Period 8 dates to the late eighth and early seventh century BCE. In this paper it is argued that the eighth century BCE mortaria were especially typical for the Cilician local settlement of Period 9 and foreign to the Assyrian style material culture of Period 8.

Among the structures of Period 9 at Kinet Höyük, a major building stands out on the western parts of the mound, which has distinctive features with mud-brick walls of *ca.* 1 m width. The building was destroyed in a conflagration. Parts of the building were coated with a thick plaster that turned bright pink and rock-hard as a result of the conflagration.[6] This appearance contributed to nicknaming the building "Pink Palace."

The material used for the mudbrick walls is unparalleled at Kinet: a compact mixture of gravel, soil and sherds, but no vegetal temper. Thick plaster served to preserve the mud-bricks. The plastered floor level of the largest room (5.5 m wide) was lower than those to its north and south, suggesting that it occupied the center

3 Lehmann 1996; Salles 1985; Sapin 1998; Spataro and Villing 2009; Villing 2009; Villing 2006; Villing and Pemberton 2010; Zukerman and Ben-Shlomo 2011.

4 Villing 2006, 34; Zukerman and Ben-Shlomo 2011, 88.

5 Villing 2006, 34, fig. 14; Villing and Pemberton 2010, figs. 26–30.

6 Gates 2004, 407.

of the building, which is preserved here for a total length of 14.35 m. Finally, the building had been carefully cleaned out before the destruction due to a fire. It was later razed to an even height (0.90 m for the central room) in preparation for the Period 8 constructions.[7]

Most of the ceramics found in association with the "Pink Palace" were not found in the building itself but had been dumped immediately outside its north-eastern end, where they were found in a pit and spilled out on the ground around it. There were no traces of fire in the pit or the area around it, and the absence of animal bones or any other trash shows that the pit was not used for garbage disposal, but instead to bury a discrete collection of items.[8] The same practice was used to clean out a large Period 9 building on the mound's eastern side excavated in Operation A in 1998, where broken but near-complete jars of similar types had been packed into two pits set just outside its entrance.

The pit in front of the "Pink Palace" contained five or six storage jars, two torpedo amphoras, a two-handled amphora of "Aegean" type, fragmentary red-slipped bowls and the rims of two Geometric cups from the Greek Mainland. One of the jars bears a complete, nine-letter Phoenician inscription, written just below its collar rim before firing. It may state: "To Sarmakaddanis," a name with Luwian or Hurrian elements.[9] Context and imported Greek pottery would date it to the second half of the eighth century BCE. According to André Lemaire, who proposes this still preliminary reading, the jar would provide a rare example of an eighth century Phoenician cursive inscription. For Kinet Höyük itself, this discovery provides the site with its first onomastic reference. It also underscores the status of the west slope sector in this period, attests to the use of the Phoenician alphabet here and connects the name of its owner back to an indigenous Bronze Age tradition.[10]

After Period 9 was destroyed and leveled, the area was filled in to provide a new building ground for the construction of Period 8, dated to the Assyrian period. The material culture of this stratum has an intrusive character that is apparent from its distinctive architecture. Its builders made no effort to continue with the previous local building customs. Layout and construction techniques of architectural remains in Operation EH demonstrate the break with the previous architectural traditions: different wall orientation; walls with jogs and shallow niches (apparently structural); foundations of varying heights casually put together with stones of all sizes and shapes, from small cobbles to roughly squared blocks;

7 Gates 2004, 407-408.

8 Gates 2004, 408.

9 Gates 2004.

10 Gates 2004, 408.

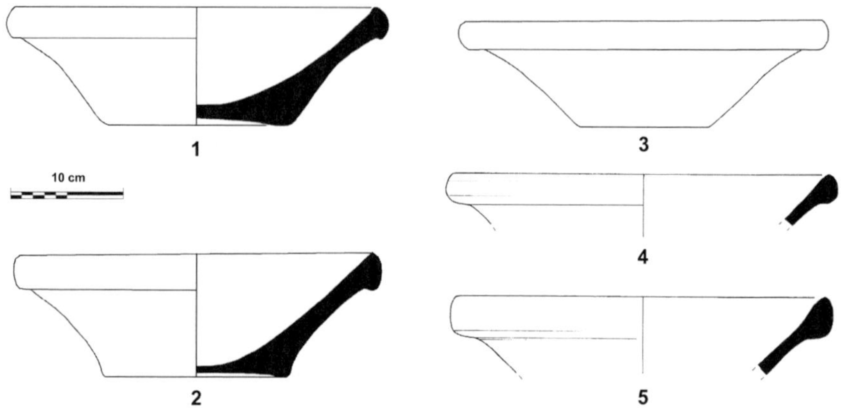

FIG. 1

1 Kinet Höyük KT 17503-03.
2 Mersin Level IV, Barnett 1939-40, Pl. 52:1.
3 Tell Jemmeh Building D Room M, Duncan 1930, 7X.
4 Qubur el-Walaydah Stratum 2-6.
5 Qubur el-Walaydah Stratum 2-6.

large square bricks typical for Assyrian buildings; cobbled pavements, and pisé ovens of a new, unprecedented design.[11] The intrusive character of the material culture of Period 8 is also evident in the faunal sample from this phase, with its unusual number of equid bones and the near-absence of marine products.[12]

The pottery also presents discontinuity with the preceding tradition: the assemblage includes thick-walled and chaff-tempered vessels, rib-rimmed bowls and fine white plates and a majority of plain wares, in shapes paralleled by the eighth-century Neo-Assyrian repertoire.[13]

The ceramic mortaria found in these levels include:

Period 9

KT 17224, Locus 366, Lot 866, Operation EH 2003, Period 9 Early. Found in sediments under the "Pink Palace" at elevation levels top 19.19–22 m, bottom 18.88 m.

KT 17359, Locus 342, Lot 817, Operation EH 2003, Period 9 Late. Floor level of Period 9 Late with pottery from the destruction level of Period 9.

KT 17375, Locus 342, Lot 824, Operation EH 2003, Period 9 Late. On the

11 Gates 2004, 406-407.

12 Gates 2004, 407.

13 Gates 2003, 285.

floor level of Period 9 Late. Context like KT 17359.
17503–03 (Fig. 1.1), Locus 342, Lot 825, Period 9 Late. On the floor level of Period 9 Late. Context like KT 17359.
KT 17554, Locus 355, Lot 833, Operation EH 2003, Period 9 Late. On the floor level of Period 9 Late.

Period 8
KT 16013 Locus 278, Lot 634, Operation EH 2002, Period 8 Late. Room between W280 and W251 with floor level at *ca.* 19.88 m.
KT 16015, Locus 290, Lot 635, Operation EH 2002, Period 8 Early. Debris of Period 8 Early under the floor level of Period 8 Late.
KT 16950, Locus 339, Lot 809, Operation EH 2003, Period 8 Early. Excavated in 1998 season Op. F as Locus 52. The pit cuts into the large public building of Period 9 at the West Slope nicknamed the "Pink Palace". Adjacent to wall 320. The pit may contain earlier material from Period 9.
KT 17018, Locus 311, Lot 750, Operation EH 2002, Period 8 Early. Found during the removal of wall W311 of Period 8 Early.

Only one fragment was found in the later phase of Period 8, where it is an isolated find. The three remaining fragments all come from very early contexts in Period 8. One fragment (KT 17018) was probably found in the fill dumped to prepare the buildings of Period 8. This fill contained material from Period 9. The pit in which KT 16950 was found is cutting into levels of Period 9 and may contain material of this earlier stratum. Thus, two of the four mortaria dated to Period 8 may in fact originate in Period 9. If this understanding is correct, the evidence suggests that ceramic mortaria are typically associated with Period 9 and are rare as isolated finds in Period 8.

As all these mortaria are typologically very similar, it appears to be sufficient in this preliminary report to illustrate only one of these vessels here (Fig. 1.1). The vessels have thick walls between 1.5–3 cm. They are wide and shallow, KT 17503–03 has a diameter of 34 cm and a height of 10 cm. They have a wide form, and their straight walls open at an angle of about 40 degrees. The rims are folded and thick. They are not triangular or overhanging as many of the later mortaria rims in the mid seventh century BCE. Often, around the edge of the base are finger imprints. The fabric is distinctive with a light yellowish surface and a bright orange fabric inside.

A very close parallel was found in the Kekova Adası shipwreck.[14] Another early mortarium was found aboard the Phoenician shipwreck Elissa in the deep waters west of Ashkelon.[15]

14 Greene *et al.* 2013, fig. 11.

15 Ballard *et al.* 2002, fig. 9:3.

More parallels come from eighth century BCE contexts in Israel: Ashdod Stratum VIII,[16] Stratum VII[17] and Stratum VI-VII.[18] While the vessel forms at Ashdod are very similar to the examples at Kinet Höyük, the rims are somewhat different.

Closer parallels from southwest Israel were found at Tell Jemmeh in Building D Room M (Iron Age IIB) (FIG. 1.3)[19] and in eighth century BCE levels at Qubur el-Walaydah (FIG. 1.4-5).

In Phoenician contexts, a mortarium was found in Beirut in the "Level of Abandonment,"[20] another one comes from Horvat Rosh Zayit Building 306[21] and one from Tyre Stratum III.[22] The fragment of a mortarium at Tell Keisan Stratum 5[23] was found in a level with eighth and seventh century BCE material; it cannot be dated safely to the eighth century BCE.

Some of the earliest mortaria on Cyprus were found at Salamis Tomb 79[24] and are dated to about the middle of the eighth century.[25]

In the light of the evidence at Kinet Höyük and the parallels listed here, I would like to reevaluate the evidence at Mersin and Tarsus. The evidence from Mersin is difficult to assess. I have dealt with the stratigraphy in more detail elsewhere.[26] The mortarium from Mersin is marked as being from Level IV (FIG. 1.2).[27] This level contains "mostly [...] material of the eighth century BC."[28] The comparisons of the rather few published examples of pottery from that level with the ceramics from Kinet Höyük generally confirm this date. However, the publications of Mersin are not detailed enough to understand the stratigraphy in the necessary depth. In any case, the form of the mortarium found at Mersin is quite similar to the ones excavated from Kinet Höyük Period 9.

The largest number of early mortaria predating the seventh century BCE were

16 Dothan 1971, fig. 50:1.

17 Dothan 1971, fig. 53:8; Dothan and Freedman 1967, fig. 40:11; Dothan and Porath 1982, fig. 19:14.

18 Dothan and Freedman 1967, fig. 41:11.

19 Duncan 1930, 7X.

20 Badre 1997.

21 Gal and Alexandre 2000, fig. VII.11:19.

22 Bikai 1978, pl. 9:19.

23 Briend and Humbert 1980, pl. 45:5.

24 Karageorghis 1973–1974: 116.

25 According to Coldstream 1979, 266–267.

26 Lehmann 1996, 166–170, 310–312.

27 Barnett 1939–1940: 107, pl. 52:1.

28 Barnett 1939–1940: 98.

found at Tarsus.[29] These vessels need a special revision, as the stratigraphy of the site was considered to be particularly problematic due to contextual disturbances, and the chronological homogeneity of the ceramic assemblages was questioned.[30] A careful examination of the stratigraphy at Tarsus suggests that although there are disturbances and contaminations, most of the evidence can still be used in the discussion about the earliest appearance of mortaria in the Levant. It is impossible to discuss the stratigraphy of the Iron Age levels at Tarsus here in full detail. However, the importance of the evidence demands proper treatment. In a critique of the stratigraphy at Tarsus, Boardman has demonstrated that the period of Assyrian domination is in fact the last phase of the "Middle Iron Age" levels.[31] Ironically, the phase called by the excavators "Assyrian" is in fact post-Assyrian (or terminal-Assyrian) and should be dated to the middle or early second half of the seventh century BCE. The cuneiform tablets found in this context should also be dated to the same period.[32] One of the tablets from Tarsus was erroneously dated to 636 BCE by Goetze,[33] as was demonstrated by Dalley.[34]

Tarsus Stratigraphy

Goldman/Hanfmann[35]	Boardman[36]
"Assyrian Period"	Second half of the seventh century BCE
Middle Iron Age ca. 14.60 – 14.10–30 m	Late eighth and first half of the seventh century BCE (Assyrian)
Middle Iron Age ca. 15.00 – 14.70 m	Eight century BCE

Early mortaria found at the site are discussed in the volume *Tarsus III*,[37] where Hanfmann published a number of vessels that belong typologically among the eighth century BCE examples of ceramic mortaria from sites discussed above. These were noted by him in strata of the Early and the Middle Iron Age, as well as in the Assyrian period. Mortaria found in later levels of the seventh century BCE that are typologically not related to the Kinet Höyük mortaria of Period 9 are not discussed in this paper.

29 Hanfmann 1963.

30 Zukerman and Ben-Shlomo 2011, 90–91.

31 Boardman 1965.

32 Boardman 1965.

33 Goetze 1939, 16, no. 9.

34 Dalley 1999.

35 Goldman 1963, Hanfmann 1963.

36 Boardman 1965.

37 Hanfmann 1963, 71, 75, 90–91.

Mortaria reported from levels of the Early Iron Age at Tarsus are:
297 15.70–16.10 m[38]
298 Jw 14.60 m and below[39] (in fact Middle Iron Age, see below)
299 Jsw above 15.10 m floor[40] (in fact Middle Iron Age)
300 K 14.82[41] (in fact Middle Iron Age)

Mortaria reported from levels of the Middle Iron Age at Tarsus:
921 intrusion starting at 15.00 m[42] (type different from Kinet)
922 Jo Pottery Deposit at floor level 15.03 m[43] (same type as Kinet)
923 Destruction Level, Tarsus: Destruction Level[44] (same type as Kinet)
924 N floor level at 14.30 m[45] (type different from Kinet, this level is in fact late seventh century BCE)

Vessels listed as mortaria[46] that I do not consider to be true mortaria:
925 Oven 5a[47]
926 Street fill at 15.50 m[48]
927 South of Oven 5[49]
928 Oven 5, upper fill[50]
929 Oven 5[51]
930 Destruction Level[52]

Two mortaria are reported from levels of the "Assyrian Period" at Tarsus; in fact both vessels come from levels of the late seventh century BCE.[53]

38 Hanfmann 1963, fig. 119.
39 Hanfmann 1963, fig. 119.
40 Hanfmann 1963, fig. 119.
41 Hanfmann 1963, fig. 64.
42 Hanfmann 1963, fig. 132.
43 Hanfmann 1963, fig. 79.
44 Hanfmann 1963, fig. 132.
45 Hanfmann 1963, fig. 79.
46 Hanfmann 1963, 233–234.
47 Hanfmann 1963, fig. 132.
48 Hanfmann 1963, fig. 132.
49 Hanfmann 1963, fig. 132.
50 Hanfmann 1963, fig. 132.
51 Hanfmann 1963, fig. 132.
52 Hanfmann 1963, fig. 132.
53 Boardman 1965.

1152 Xc to 13.95 m, Tarsus Assyrian[54] (different from Kinet)
1153 Y, to 13.93 m (not illustrated)

The early dating of four mortaria to Early Iron Age levels at Tarsus is problematic. The Early Iron Age levels contain material predating the Cypriot Geometric III period. They should, thus, date to the late eleventh through early ninth centuries BCE at the latest. This date appears to be extremely early for the appearance of mortaria. A close look at the stratigraphic context of the mortaria assigned to the Early Iron Age levels demonstrates that these vessels should in fact be assigned to later levels. The necessary stratigraphic information for the following discussion can be found in *Tarsus III*.[55] Tarsus number 297 was found at 15.70–16.10 m. This would associate number 297 with levels of the Late Bronze Age or the transition from the Late Bronze Age to the Iron Age at the latest. This is such an extreme exception that the stratigraphic context of the sherd may be an intrusion.

Number 298 was found in unit Jw at "floor level 14.60 m and below".[56] The floor at 14.60 m was dated to the Middle Iron Age.

Number 299 was found in room Jsw above a floor at 15.10 m.[57] As the sherd was found *above* the floor at 15.10 m, it was close to the preserved top of the collapsed Early Iron Age walls. It may have been deposited after the abandonment of the Early Iron Age level in the debris of that level. This could have happened during the leveling of the Early Iron Age level and the construction of the foundations of the Middle Iron Age room Jsw with its first floor at 14.70 m.

Number 300 was found in room K on a floor at 14.82 m. This floor belongs to the Middle Iron Age level: the first Early Iron Age floor beneath lies at 15.30 m, half a meter below.[58]

All four mortaria assigned to the Early Iron Age levels may have originated in the Middle Iron Age. One of them was found on a Middle Iron Age floor, two probably in Middle Iron Age foundations and one in Late Bronze Age levels, apparently in an intrusion. Against this evidence, I suggest associating the beginning of mortaria at Tarsus with the earliest levels of the Middle Iron Age.

Among the mortaria recorded in Middle Iron Age levels, number 921 was found in a pit that was dug from floor level at 15.00 m that can be dated to the Middle Iron Age. Number 922 was part of the Jo Pottery Deposit on the earliest Middle Iron Age floor level at 15.03 m. Number 923 comes from the "Destruction

54 Hanfmann 1963, fig. 137.

55 Goldman 1963, 3–5, 19–21, 92–97 and the associated architectural plans.

56 Hanfmann 1963, 187.

57 Hanfmann 1963, 187.

58 Hanfmann 1963, 187.

Level." Boardman has interpreted the "Destruction Level" as make-up fill at the end of the Assyrian phase of the first half of the seventh century BCE in preparation for the building of the stratum dated to the second half of the seventh century BCE.[59] The fill of the "Destruction Level" contained numerous sherds from the late eighth century BCE. Number 924 appears to be a find from a floor level of the second half of the seventh century BCE.

As already pointed out, the so-called "Assyrian Period" at Tarsus should accordingly be re-dated to the early second half of the seventh century BCE. Mortaria numbers 1152–1153 found in the "Assyrian Period" level thus date, in fact, to this time.

To summarize, at Tarsus, mortaria were in use during the Middle Iron Age in the eighth century BCE; in the Assyrian period, there is no evidence for mortaria, which re-appear only in the second half of the seventh century BCE.

The evidence discussed here indicates that most of the earliest ceramic mortaria appeared in pre-Assyrian levels of the eighth century BCE. When they were found in Assyrian period levels, they seem to be out of context or are isolated finds representing an exception. In this way, they resemble Aegean pottery, which is extremely rare in the Assyrian period and which almost disappeared from the region.[60]

The few Aegean imports to the northern Levant were found almost exclusively at Al Mina and Tarsus. The ceramics at these two sites include exports of the last Euboean Late Geometric styles to the eastern Mediterranean. More representative for the end of the eighth and the first half of the seventh century BCE is Early and Middle Proto-Corinthian pottery (some of which are in fact Euboean imitations), as well as the now increasingly dominant East Greek styles. Al Mina Ware, apparently a Cypriot production inspired by Aegean pottery, occurred also in levels of the Assyrian period at Al Mina and Tarsus.

The lack of imports and a preference for unpainted pottery at most sites during the Assyrian period are apparent also in the reduced number of Cypriot and local Cypro-Cilician painted outputs, which at Kinet Höyük drop to 5% in the Assyrian Period 8, when they had previously comprised 30% of the ceramics in Period 9. The evidence suggests that the import of mortaria was drastically reduced in the Levant during the Assyrian period. Zukerman and Ben-Shlomo have recently reaffirmed that ceramic mortaria were apparently originally produced on Cyprus.[61] While there is increasing evidence for an early appearance of mortaria during the eighth century BCE in the Levant, this type of vessel almost disappeared during the period

59 Boardman 1965.

60 Fantalkin 2008; Vacek 2012; Waldbaum 1994.

61 Zukerman and Ben-Shlomo 2011, with references.

of Assyrian dominance in the Levant and reappeared in substantial quantities only during the second half of the seventh century BCE with new types that are clearly distinguishable from earlier eighth century BCE forms. The reappearance of mortaria together with Greek and Cypriot imports is apparently associated with the dominance of the Egyptian 26th Dynasty in the Levant.

The restriction of imports from the Aegean and Cyprus may have been a well-considered decision of the Assyrian empire. Whether this was due to ideological reasons [62] or rather as a result of strict Assyrian control of the Mediterranean trade remains to be discussed. The Assyrians were a continental power, unable to control the seas. Greeks are mentioned in a few Assyrian references as pirates and seafarers, appearing from out of the unknown, from the "midst of the sea" (*qabli tâmti*). [63] Assyrian control of Mediterranean trade was restricted to the coast of the Levant and Cilicia. Repeated conflicts with the Phoenician cities and the establishment of governmental *kāru*-trading posts reflect Assyrian land-based attempts to gain control over the activities in the Mediterranean. [64]

In this context, a royal 'store-house' was established at Ahta, probably Al Mina Stratum 7. [65] There was no trading station at Tarsus, and the Greek imports during the Assyrian period there are probably due to direct contacts with nearby Greek settlements. This does not necessarily mean that Tarsus was a Greek colony itself, although Greeks may have been one component of the population of Cilicia. [66] In contrast to Al Mina and Tarsus, our preliminary analysis indicates that there were no Greek imports at Kinet Höyük Period 8 during the Assyrian period. The fact that mortaria from Cyprus disappeared during this period as well provides further evidence for severe restrictions of maritime interaction during the Assyrian period in the Levant in general and the harbor of Kinet Höyük in particular.

62 Fantalkin 2008, 208–219.

63 Lang and Rollinger 2010; Rollinger 2001.

64 Elat 1978; Na'aman 1979.

65 Zadok 1996.

66 Bing 1969; Bing 1971; King 1910; Desideri and Jasink 1990; Gander 2012; Helm 1980; Jasink 1989; Schmitz 2009.

REFERENCES

Badre, L., "Bey 003 Preliminary Report: Excavations of the American University of Beirut Museum 1993–1996 [at Beirut]." BAAL *Bulletin d'Archéologie et d'Architecture Libanaises* 2 (1997): 6–94.

Ballard, R.D., Stager, L.E., Master, D., Yoerger, D., Mindell, D., Whitcomb, L.L., Singh, H. and Piechota, D., "Iron Age Shipwrecks in Deep Water off Ashkelon, Israel." *American Journal of Archaeology* 106.1 (2002): 151–168.

Barnett, R.D., "Explorations at Mersin: 1938–1939: The Greek Pottery." *Annals of Archaeology and Anthropology* 26 (1939–1940): 98–130.

Bikai, P.M., *The Pottery of Tyre*. Warminster: Aris and Phillips, 1978.

Bing, J.D., *A History of Cilicia during the Assyrian Period*. Unpublished Ph.D. Thesis, Indiana University, Bloomington, Ind. 1969.

———. Tarsus "A Forgotten Colony of Lindos." *Journal of Near Eastern Studies* 30 (1971): 99–109.

Boardman, J., Tarsus, "Al Mina and Greek Chronology." *Journal of Hellenic Studies* 85 (1965): 5 15.

Briend, J. and J.-P. Humbert, J.P., *Tell Keisan (1971–1976): Une cité phénicienne en Galilée*, Orbis Biblicus et Orientalis, Series Archaeologica, 1. Freiburg (Switzerland) and Göttingen: Freiburg Universitätsverlag and Vandenhoeck & Ruprecht 1980.

Coldstream, J.N., "Geometric Skyphoi in Cyprus." *Report of the Department of Antiquities of Cyprus* (1979): 255–269.

Dalley, S., "Sennacherib and Tarsus." *Anatolian Studies* 49 (1999): 73–80.

Desideri, P. and A. M. Jasink, *Cilicia: Dall'eta di Kizzuwatna alla conquista macedone.* Torino: Casa Editrice le Lettere, 1990.

Dothan, M. and D. N. Freedman, *Ashdod I: The First Season of Excavations 1962.* 'Atiqot 7. Jerusalem, 1967.

Dothan, M., *Ashdod II-III: The Second and Third Seasons of Excavations 1963, 1965.* 'Atiqot 9–10. Jerusalem: Department of Antiquities and Museums, 1971.

Dothan, M. and Y. Porath, *Ashdod IV: Excavation of Area M: The Fortifications of the Lower City*, 'Atiqot 15. Jerusalem: Department of Antiquities and Museums, 1982.

Duncan, J.G., *Corpus of Dated Palestinian Pottery: Including Pottery of Gerar and Beth-Pelet, and Beads of Beth-Pelet*. London: British School of Archaeology in Egypt, University College. 1930.

Elat, M., "The Economic Relations of the Neo-Assyrian Empire with Egypt." *Journal of the American Oriental Society* 98 (1978): 20–34.

Fantalkin, A., *Contacts Between the Greek World and the Southern Levant during the Seventh-Sixth Centuries BCE*. Unpublished Ph. D. Thesis Tel Aviv University, 2008 (Hebrew).

Gal, Z. and Y. Alexandre, *Horbat Rosh Zayit: An Iron Age Storage Fort and Village*, Israel Antiquities Authority, Reports 8. Jerusalem, 2000.

Gander, M., „Ahhiyawa - Hiyawa - Que: Gibt es Evidenz für die Anwesenheit von Griechen in Kilikien am Übergang von der Bronze- zur Eisenzeit?" *Studi Micenei ed Egeo-Anatolici* 54 (2012): 281–309.

Gates, M.-H., "2001 Season at Kinet Höyük (Yeşil-Dörtyol, Hatay)." *Kazı Sonuçları Toplantısı* 24.1 (2003): 283–298.

———. "2002 Season at Kinet Höyük (Yeşil-Dörtyol, Hatay)." *Kazı Sonuçları Toplantısı* 25.1 (2004): 405–416.

Goetze, A., "Cuneiform Inscriptions from Tarsus." *Journal of the American Oriental Society* 59.1 (1939): 1–16.

Goldman, H. ed., *Excavations at Gözlü Kule, Tarsus: Vol. III: The Iron Age*. Princeton: Princeton University Press, 1963.

Greene, E.S., Leidwanger, J. and H.A. Özdaş, "Expanding Contacts and Collapsing Distances in Early Cypro-Archaic Trade: Three Case Studies of Shipwrecks off the Turkish Coast" in *The Transport Amphorae and Trade of Cyprus*, ed. by M.L. Lawall and J. Lund, 21–34. Aarhus: Aarhus University Press, 2013.

Hanfmann, G.M.A., "The Iron Age Pottery of Tarsus" in *Excavations at Gözlü Kule: Tarsus III: The Iron Age*, ed. by H. Goldman, 18–332. Princeton: Princeton University Press, 1963.

Helm, P.R., *'Greeks' in the Neo-Assyrian Levant and 'Assyria' in Early Greek Writers*. Ph.D. University of Pennsylvania 1980 DissAbstr 41: 1168-A 8018554, 1980.

Jasink, A.M., "I Greci in Cilicia nel periodo neo-assiro." *Mesopotamia* 24 (1989): 117–128.

Karageorghis, V., *Excavations in the Necropolis of Salamis*, Volume III, Salamis 5. Nicosia: Department of Antiquities, Cyprus, 1973–1974.

King, L.W., "Sennacherib and the Ionians." *Journal of Hellenic Studies* 30 (1910): 327–335.

Lang, M. and R. Rollinger „Im Herzen der Meere und in der Mitte des Meeres: Das Buch Ezechiel und die in assyrischer Zeit fassbaren Vorstellungen von den Grenzen der Welt" in *Interkulturalität in der Alten Welt: Vorderasien, Hellas, Ägypten und die vielfältigen Ebenen des Kontakts,* ed. by Rollinger, R, Gufler, B., Lang, M. and Madreiter, I., 207–264. Wiesbaden: Harrassowitz Verlag, 2010.

Lehmann, G. *Untersuchungen zur späten Eisenzeit in Syrien und Libanon: Stratigraphie und Keramikformen zwischen ca. 720 bis 300 v.Chr.*, Altertumskunde des Vorderen Orients 5. Münster: Ugarit Verlag, 1996.

Na'aman, N., "The Brook of Egypt and Assyrian Policy on the Border of Egypt." *Tel Aviv* 6 (1979) 68–90.

Rollinger, R., "The Ancient Greeks and the Impact of the Ancient Near East: Textual Evidence and Historical Perspective (*ca.* 750–650 BC)" in *Mythology and Mythologies: Methodological Approaches to Intercultural Influences: Proceedings of the Second Annual Symposium of the Assyrian and Babylonian Intellectual Heritage Project. Held in Paris, France, October 4–7, 1999*, ed. by R.M. Whiting, Melammu Symposia 2, 233–264. Helsinki: Neo-Assyrian Text Corpus Project, 2001.

Salles, J.-F., "Cuvettes et 'mortiers' du Levant au 1er millénaire avant J.-C" in *De l'Indus aux Balkans: Recueil à la mémoire de Jean Deshayes*, ed. by J.-L. Huot, M. Yon and Y. Calvet, 199–212. Paris: Editions Recherche sur les Civilisations, 1985.

Sapin, J., "'Mortaria': Un lot inédit de Tell Keisan: Essai d'interprétation fonctionnelle." *Transeuphratene* 16 (1998): 87–120.

Schmitz, P.C., "Archaic Greek Names in a Neo-Assyrian Cuneiform Tablet from Tarsus." *Journal of Cuneiform Studies* 61 (2009): 127–131.

Spataro, M. and A. Villing, "Scientific Investigation of Pottery Grinding Bowls in the Archaic and Classical Eastern Mediterranean." *British Museum Technical Research Bulletin* 3 (2009): 89–100.

Stern, E., *Material Culture of the Land of the Bible in the Persian Period 538–332 BC.* Warminster: Aris & Phillips 1982.

Vacek, A., *Greek and Related Pottery from Al Mina: A Case Study of Production, Consumption and Distribution of Greek Pottery in the Eastern Mediterranean from the 9th to the End of the 7th Century BC*. Unpublished D. Phil. Thesis, University of Oxford, School of Archaeology, Merton College, 2012.

Villing, A., "'Drab Bowls' for Apollo: The Mortaria of Naukratis and Exchange in the Archaic Eastern Mediterranean" in *Naukratis: Greek Diversity in Egypt: Studies on East Greek Pottery and Exchange in the Eastern Mediterranean*, ed. by A. Villing and U. Schlotzhauer, 31–46. London: British Museum Press, 2006.

———. "The Daily Grind of Ancient Greece: Mortars and Mortaria between Symbol and Reality" in *Shapes and Uses of Greek Vases (7th–4th centuries BC)*, ed. by A. Tsingarida, 319–333. Brussels: CReA-Patrimoine, 2009.

Villing, A. and E.G. Pemberton, "Mortaria from Ancient Corinth: Form and Function." *Hesperia* 79 (2010): 555–638.

Waldbaum, J.C., "Early Greek Contacts with the Southern Levant, *ca.* 1000–600 BC: The Eastern Perspective." *Bulletin of the American Schools of Oriental Research* 293 (1994): 53–66.

Zadok, R., "Geographical and Onomastic Remarks on H. Tadmor, 'The Inscriptions of Tiglath-pileser III, King of Assyria'." *Nouvelles Assyriologiques Brèves et Utilitaires* 1 (1996): 11–13.

Zukerman, A. and D. Ben-Shlomo, "Mortaria as a Foreign Element in the Material Culture of the Southern Levant during the 8th–7th Century BCE." *Palestine Exploration Quarterly* 143.2 (2011): 87–105.

Greek and Native Contact in Transcaucasian Iberia

Jacques Morin[1]

Introduction

This paper will attempt to correlate the information offered by Classical and Georgian Medieval sources about Iberia, within the Caspian watershed to the east of Colchis, with what is known in the field, to verify whether the literary sources and the archaeological record match. A further question will be to examine the nature and form of the contacts with Greek civilisation and cultural norms within a long-term historical perspective, extending from the sixth century BC to the Late Roman period. The investigated area is limited to the valley stretching between the Caucasus Mountains to the north and the Trialeti range to the south, along the middle reaches of the Mtkvari River (the Kyros of ancient sources), i.e. the heartland of the Ancient Iberian kingdom, as well as its mountainous marches to the north and south, including the upper course of the river where the author has excavated.

The presence of Greeks and elements of their material culture in the territory of Colchis, present-day Western Georgia, is well attested during Antiquity, since at least three Ionian settlements mentioned in Classical sources were established along the easternmost coast of the Black Sea at Dioskourias, partially submerged offshore of present day Sokhumi, Gyenos further to the south near the town of Ochamchire, and Phasis, on an isthmus between the mouth of the eponymous river (the modern Rioni) and a coastal lake (the present day Paliostomi). The foundation date of none of the towns can be ascertained archaeologically because,

---

1 Department of Archaeology, Faculty of Humanities and Letters, Bilkent Universtiy, 06800 Ankara, Turkey.

I wish to extend my thanks to the editors of this Festschrift for their invitation to contribute to celebrate two esteemed colleagues. The project from which this paper derives was funded by the *Social Sciences and Humanities Research Council of Canada* and was conducted in collaboration with the team of Dr. Vakhtang Licheli, then from the *Archaeological Research Centre of the Georgian Academy of Sciences*, Tbilisi, but now at Tbilisi State University, between 1993 and 1998. This paper is a revised and considerably expanded version of a talk delivered at the 100th Meeting of the *Archaeological Institute of America*, held in Washington in December 1998. The presence of the author in Washington was made possible by a faculty grant of Bilkent University, Ankara. I warmly thank all institutions and people who made this project possible. All photographs and drawings by the author.

for the most part, the sites are inaccessible.[2] In addition, archaeological research has revealed traces of other Hellenic establishments in Colchis, unknown to the ancient chroniclers or ignored by them, near the coast[3] as well as native settlements where evidence of contacts with the Greeks has been found further inland (see map, Fig. 1).[4]

Such evidence demonstrates the penetration of Greek culture in Colchis, both along the coast and far in its hinterland. A process of acculturation can be reconstituted in general terms, at Pichvnari-Kobuleti in the mixed Colchian-Greek necropolis[5] at Vani and perhaps Sairkhe. It appears quite clearly that adoption by locals of Greek cultural norms occurred only after a long period of close contact between Greeks and the élite among Colchian populations.

The Central Iberian Evidence for Contact

Can similar phenomena be documented in Iberia? Given the geographical extent of the penetration of Greek cultural elements in Colchis, especially the presence of Classical finds in graves at and near Sairkhe, one would expect to find equivalent

2 For an overview of Greek finds in Georgia see Licheli 2007, 1083–133. The earliest Greek material in Colchis, however, dates back to the late seventh and early sixth centuries BC (see Lordkipanidze 1991, 129–130; Kacharava 1997, 137–146).

3 *Eshera*, 10 km northwest of *Dioskurias* (see Lordkipanidze *op. cit.*, 126, 138 and Tsetskhladze 1998, 22–25), a settlement as yet unpublished, near the town of *Tsikhisdziri* (Kacharava *op. cit.*), on the coast north of *Batumi*, an important necropolis of the fifth-fourth century BC a short distance from the latter at *Kobuleti-Pitchvnari* where abundant finds of Attic red-figure vessels in graves suggest a Greek presence (Lordkipanidze *op. cit.*, 130; Kacharava *op. cit.*, 140–141) (fig. 1), as well as *Bathys Limen* within today's Batumi, and at the nearby Batumi fort (Kacharava *op. cit.*; Vickers 1998, 15; Vickers M. and A. Kakhidze 1999, 11–12; Vickers M. and A. Kakhidze 2000, 13–14.

4 Most notably the remarkable site of Vani, probably ancient *Surium/Suris* that offers a clear picture of the acculturation of a local élite, presenting a wealth in Greek- (and Persian-) style decorative and monumental arts, fragments of Greek inscriptions, numerous imports, representations of Greek divinities and perhaps, by extension, of Greek cults, since Greek gods are named in one inscription, and cut-stone architecture, notably a distinctly Hellenic-style system of fortifications (Lordkipanidze *op. cit.*, 138–145; Lordkipanidze 1991, 151–195; Tsetskhladze *op. cit.*, 114–158). *Vani* lies, furthermore, at the convergence of two routes towards the Colchian hinterland and Iberia (see Licheli 1997, 147–153.) For instance, in addition, at the site of Sairkhe near the eastern issue of one branch of the *Sarapana* pass were excavated several wealthy burials containing Greek pottery, a stone-built circuit wall, and several carved stone architectural elements perhaps in Greek and—certainly—in Persian style, on the basis of which a Doric style temple has been theoretically reconstituted (Nadiradze 1990, 213–222; Tsetskhladze *op. cit.*, 153–154, fig. 57; see Braund 1994, 130 on the problems of this reconstruction.

5 Vickers and Kakhidze 1999; Vickers M. and A. Kakhidze 1999, 11.

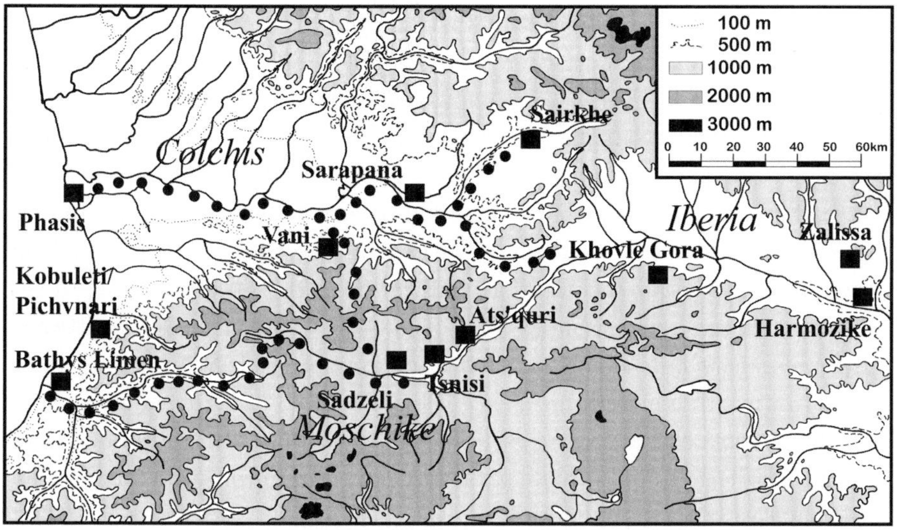

FIG. 1 Map of Colchis, Iberia and Moschike. Dotted line = pathways from the coast; squares = sites mentioned in the text

materials also in Iberia. No major topographical obstacle prevents communication between Sairkhe and the Iberian hinterland, located a short distance from the site, beyond the watershed. Furthermore, several mentions in the Classical sources and the Georgian Medieval traditions suggest that the impact of Greek culture also spread eastwards into Iberia. Can the archaeological record reflect such claims?

Colchis and Iberia are separated by the massif of the Moschic mountains which runs roughly along a south-west north-east axis about 100 km inland of the Black Sea coastal area, linking the Greater Caucasus to the north with the eastern Anatolian plateau to the south. This range, today called the Surami Ridge in Georgia, culminates at slightly more than 3000 m above sea-level. In spite of its appearance as a formidable barrier, it is segmented by numerous river valleys, which allow passage towards the hinterland by way of several relatively low passes between the highest peaks. Although at first glance on a map, and no doubt from the perspective of a newcomer arriving from the Black Sea coast, the massif may appear impenetrable, in reality it offers several adequate, although steep at places and lengthy, pathways between the two regions.

Hard evidence in support of each case described below is far from abundant, but contact between the Black Sea and Caspian watersheds can be documented along four axes at this latitude (FIG. 1), all leading more or less directly towards the course of the Kyros. The northernmost of these paths follows the course of the Phasis River up to the Sarapana pass, then down again into the Caspian watershed and leads directly to the central Iberian plain, exiting the mountains near the modern town of Khashuri where it connects with the Kyros River. According to Strabo (11.2.17) the Phasis was navigable up to Sarapana, from where a road, which could accommodate the circulation of wagons, led to Iberia on the Caspian watershed. The trip from Sarapana to Iberia lasted four days. The prominence of this road in Strabo suggests that it should have constituted the main communication axis between the two regions.[6] Little evidence has been published from various locations within the pass that confirms the text of Strabo. But since it has been the main communication axis throughout later Georgian history, as attested by the presence of forts along its course, it seems improbable to dismiss it simply on the grounds that material evidence is insufficient.[7] It is true, however, that certain segments of the pass are very difficult to negotiate. In addition, one has to consider whether the alternate paths offer any advantages over it in terms of speed and ease of access to Iberia.

A second pathway runs along the Phasis up to the site of Vani where it bifurcates south towards Sulori to reach a low pass in the mountains and then descends towards the modern village of Sadzeli, west of Akhaltsikhe. On the outskirts of Sadzeli can be recognised a large pre-Christian settlement, from which one can easily reach the Kyros. V. Licheli,[8] on the basis of the length of the journey, shorter than through the Sarapana pass, and the discovery of Greek pottery at Ats'quri on the Kyros about 25 km downriver from Sadzeli (see *infra*, 485–488), has suggested that this pathway should be considered the preferable axis for the diffusion of Greek material towards Iberia. The lack of material evidence from the path itself between Vani and Sadzeli, however, leaves open any question of precedence.

A third path follows the Adjaritskhali river, which empties into the Black Sea near Batumi, up into the mountains towards yet another low pass and continues downhill on to Sadzeli. This possible route-way has never been surveyed, but its potential should not be dismissed out of hand because it provides the shortest possible route across the mountains and appears easy because it involves travelling along only one river before scaling one mountainous ridge.[9]

The idea that a southern itinerary through Sadzeli is shorter than the one through the Sarapana pass needs careful investigation, which to my knowledge has never been attempted. It is true that reaching the course of the Kyros at Akha-

---

6 Braund *op. cit.*, 40–41 has expressed doubts on the accuracy of Strabo's account and the actual existence of the road before the Sassanid period.

7 Few regional surveys have been conducted in the area, which might fill out a map; our view of the record is forcibly skewed towards remains clearly visible on the surface.

8 Licheli *op. cit.*, 148, 151.

9 The fourth pathway along the Chorokhi River leads to Armenia.

ltsikhe, about 5 km distant from Sadzeli, starting either at Vani or at the mouth of the Adjaritskhali River would take less time than walking (or driving a cart) through the Sarapana pass to Khashuri, but if one adds the distance between Sadzeli and the Iberian issue of the Sarapana pass, then the trip would certainly prove as long, for there are more than 70 km between Akhaltsikhe on the Mtkvari and Khashuri, a sizeable portion of which passes through very rough relief. The difficulties of the terrain are such that I seriously doubt anyone could cover such a distance in less than three days by foot; the trip would take somewhat less time downriver by boat, since the river is navigable with a light craft. From the perspective of length of voyage and ease of access, the alternate itineraries offer no substantial advantages or evident disadvantage over the Sarapana pass; it all depends on destination.

Given the lack of proper surveys along the potential routes linking Colchis and Iberia, it would be imprudent to exclude any line of communication between the two areas, since relative advantages can be demonstrated for all of them. All routes may have been used concurrently. The northern route via the Sarapana pass must have been the preferred way towards the core area of Iberia, since it is mentioned by Strabo as a road leading to it, and since it provides reasonably direct access.[10] Making this the only path along which people and material transited to the interior, on such basis, would overemphasize our reliance on one literary—albeit well informed—source at the expense of the potential offered by the topography. It might suggest that the Iberian kingdom, at least at the time of Strabo, was sufficiently powerful to direct traffic along a preferred axis and to redistribute imports within its territory from the capital or a point within the core of the kingdom, an unlikely feat of centralisation. Furthermore, nothing in the known archaeological record suggests that Iberia controlled extensive territories along the upper reaches of the Kyros Valley, either during Hellenistic or Early Roman times;[11] Strabo's assertion (11.2.18) that Iberia controlled the middle part of the Moschic lands may be accurate, but his geographical characterisation of the area is too general for us to pinpoint the actual location and extent of the area he meant.

The path taken by Greeks or Romans and the material they carried towards the interior cannot be proven, short of discovering discarded cargo along the way, but the position of each route offers potential for hypotheses. The town sites of Phasis, Tsikhisdziri, Pichvnari-Kobuleti and Bathys Limen lie at the Black Sea end of these axes; they are thus of prime importance as the centres from which people and objects began their journey to the interior. The town of Phasis was clearly the most important centre on the coast, by virtue perhaps of its central position vis-à-

10 *Contra* Braund *op. cit.*, 40–41.

11 *Contra* Lordkipanidze 1991, 157.

vis its Colchian neighbours, as well as its location on the most important river of the region, and the focal point for exchanges associated with the river Phasis. We should not underestimate, however, the importance of the lesser known southern establishments, since the Adjaritskhali Valley offers the shortest access to the Caspian watershed, leading towards both Iberia and to the northernmost portions of Armenia. One may tentatively suggest that the two Phasis to Iberia route-ways were used primarily by people and cargo which reached Colchis from the north, while the Adjaritskhali to Iberia and Chorokhi to Armenia (plus Iberia?) itineraries were favoured for materials shipped along the southern Black Sea shore. Ultimate destination must also have influenced the choice of pathways, with the core area of Iberia favouring a northern itinerary and the upper reaches of the Kyros—the present day Samtskhe-Javakheti and adjacent areas, Ancient Moschike—and Armenia favouring a southern road.

Strabo in his description of Iberia presents the picture of widespread influence from Classical civilisation, stating (11.3.1) that the Iberians lived in urbanised settings with several of the amenities of Classical life: orderly planned towns and markets, houses covered with tiled roofs. He also mentions the presence of sanctuaries to Greek divinities or heroes (Phryxos, Leukothea, Jason) throughout the countryside (11.2.17)—including the Moschic Mountains. The local historical tradition also presents many hints of Graeco-Roman influence, several of them evidently spurious, such as the conquest of the Caucasus by Alexander[12] deriving from the late Alexander Romance. It suggests, nevertheless, the existence of close relations between Iberia and the Hellenistic, Roman and Byzantine states and institutions. It also mentions that Greek gods had been worshipped at various locales in the kingdom—Aphrodite, near Mtskheta, for instance, as well as Artemis and Apollo at Sosangeti-Atsqueri.[13]

The first contacts of Greeks with the hinterland of Moschike[14] can be recognised archaeologically as early as the late sixth century BC. The nature of the contacts between the Archaic period and early Hellenistic times remains unknown, whether direct or indirect, involving trade or some other form of exchange. The paucity of material finds, however, does not offer much ground to reconstruct elaborate or continuous relations. The earliest Greek finds in the territory of Iberia proper consist of a fragment from a Black-Figure vessel at Khovle Gora and one

12 *Kartlis Tskhovreba*, 17–18.

13 *Kartlis Tskhovreba*, 58 and see Thomson 1996 on the lateness of the tradition.

14 I separate out in this section *Iberia* proper along the middle course of the Mtkvari River (the ancient Kyros) from *Moschic* lands along the upper course of the *Mtkvari* for two reasons. First, Strabo (11.2.18) seems to make some distinction between the two regions, which the archaeological data might reflect. Then, to allow a more detailed description of the finds made at *Ats'quri*.

handle from a fikellura amphora discovered at Avlebi, in East Georgia [15]; later finds are almost as sparse and also involve only a handful of sherds from Inner Kartli—i.e. the core of the later Iberian kingdom. [16] Such paltry results most probably indicate that contacts were at best episodic and may very well have consisted in chance occurrences. It is also evident that only objects changed hands, for during the fifth and fourth centuries BC no signs of borrowing, neither in building techniques nor in cultural behaviour can be detected anywhere. The only possible exception to this situation in the entire hinterland remains the site of Sairkhe (see above, n. 4), liminal to Iberia and possibly Colchian. If the Doric temple hypothesis were confirmed, the building would stand in stark contrast to the neighbouring landscape, where no such elaborate Greek-inspired structure has been uncovered, for, in fact, the evidence in Iberia points overwhelmingly in the opposite direction at this time: towards Persia and Persian culture. [17] The situation shifts during the 3rd century BC with the recession of Persian power and the rise of the Seleucid kingdom replacing it.

Relations with Greek culture from then on assume a somewhat more concrete aspect, when viewed from their material perspective; they continue developing from this point on throughout the Roman period. The new context can be recognised in Iberia by the appearance of new forms of architecture and the use of new types of materials typical of Greek building methods. The most remarkable features are the use of cut stone in architecture and of tiling for roofs, forms and materials found relatively often along the Iberian plain and in particular around the capital of the kingdom, Harmozike, but almost totally absent from the outlying mountainous areas framing it. Several examples are well known, dating from the second century BC to the third century AD. It is not necessary in this format to provide an exhaustive list, but the most important include: a large complex on the acropolis of Mtskheta, the capital of Iberia (at the place called Armazischevi or Armaztsikhe), a Roman type bath, and nearby several cut-stone tombs with gabled and tiled roofs; at Sarkine, 10 km upriver from Mtscketa, are reported cut-stone architecture and roof tiles, as well as terra-cotta statuettes representing Dionysos; at Dsalisi (ancient Zalissa) was excavated a monumental complex including a

15 See Licheli *op. cit.,* 147 and Kacharava *op. cit.,* 138.

16 Licheli *op. cit.,* 150.

17 A vast body of literature and abundant finds, notably in architecture, attest to the importance of the Achaemenid Empire in shaping the local culture, particularly its religion. This is shown by the presence of Persian type buildings, notably fire temples, and decorative arts at several locations in the countryside (see Gagoshidze 1996, 125–136; Kimiashvili and Narimanishvili 1995–1996, 309–318; Knauß 1999, 81–114). As well, one issue of the Journal *Ancient Civilizations from Scythia to Siberia* (13, 2007) is devoted to this question. This phenomenon is manifest also in Strabo's description of the Iberians, who are said to dress like the Medes and the Armenians (11.3.3).

large bathhouse and mosaic-paved halls, one mosaic representing the marriage of Dionysos and Ariadne.[18]

From the Hellenistic period down into Roman times, we also notice the appearance of coins in some graves, a feature foreign to local custom but well known from the Classical world. Such occurrences are relatively rare proportionately to the total number of graves but are distributed widely throughout Iberia: the cemetery at Samadlo, near Harmozike, has produced many examples—both Roman and Parthian types—dated between the first and third centuries AD.[19] They constitute, perhaps, the only sure sign that Graeco-Roman customs had started to have an impact on the beliefs of the local population, for the remainder of the cultural complex shows little signs of Hellenic beliefs. How such beliefs were transmitted is unknown.

Finally, one type of evidence is not mentioned in the Classical sources but must be covered: the epigraphical texts which exist in small numbers both in Greek and in a local version of Aramaic, especially in the neighbourhood of the capital. Most of the inscriptions consist of public documents or epitaphs inscribed on stone—and not bronze as in Colchis—and all are dated to Roman times. One, a Flavian building inscription, is clearly a Roman document, since it uses the Roman dating system in identifying Vespasian and his two sons. It most probably was erected by the Roman engineers who designed and built Harmozike's fortifications; it demonstrates eloquently that by the end of the first century AD, the two regimes had grown very close, essentially that Rome considered Iberia as an ally.[20]

But what is the significance of the truly local documents? In the first place, they are not very numerous, many are epitaphs, some appear on objects of every day usage they are written either in Greek or are bilingual (Greek and Aramaic). Braund[21] has suggested they show that during the period of the Roman Empire, Greek had become the main language of the Iberian élite. This would imply that the process of acculturation had modified the local culture to such an extent that the leaders of society had abandoned their own language. There are signs of acculturation represented by the élite structures mentioned previously (bathhouses, mosaics, terra-cotta Greek gods). The flimsy material evidence, however, cannot support such a conclusion. The absence of inscriptions in the local language (or languages) does not constitute proof that the king and his entourage did not conduct their business in their native tongue. Most of the known inscriptions mention either a king, a queen, a *pitiax* or some other high official. It may, therefore, be

18 See in particular an extensive discussion in Lordkipanidze *op. cit.,* 156–176.

19 See Braund *op. cit.,* 208.

20 Braund *op. cit.,* 227–230.

21 Braund *op. cit.*, 212–215.

more prudent to consider the presence of Greek and Aramaic within the political context of the times more as symbols of political realities and allegiance than of personal culture. Since Iberia was an ally of Rome, the prevalence of the use of Greek, the diplomatic language of that Empire in the east, by the local authorities may simply indicate where their loyalties lay, and such documents may have been erected primarily for Roman—and Parthian/Sassanid—envoys to see and read as political messages; if the intended audience had been the local populace, then local languages might have been used instead.

Samtskhe and Ats'quri

I now turn to an area in South Georgia, bordering on Iberia: Samtskhe, where contacts with the Black Sea coast show a distinctly different profile. According to most scholars this region was part of the Moschic lands, inhabited by the Moschoi, seemingly different ethnically from the Iberians, if one is to trust Strabo (11.3.17 & 18). The Georgian toponym Samtskhe itself—and its Russian equivalent of Mescheti—is believed to derive from the ancient term.[22] Modern Samtskhe, however, is not co-terminous with the ancient region of Moschike, for it stretches only over a very limited segment of the area along the upper course of the Mtkvari.

Samtskhe is a rough mountainous country, with limited amounts of flat arable lands. These are restricted to scattered stretches on the bottom of the river valley since, for a sizable portion of its course between Borjomi and Akhaltsikhe, the Mtkvari flows through a steep-sided gorge. The valley widens considerably further north to constitute the heartland of Iberia proper. Water is abundant as the river system demonstrates, and it must also have been so in Antiquity, so that the entire region should have been thickly wooded, as the lesser accessible parts of the landscape still are today. The relief is very harsh, and although vegetation today is green and lush, most of the landscape is better adapted to animal husbandry than to intensive agriculture. It must have been relatively poor in Antiquity, as it remains today, and capable of sustaining only a limited population.

The region appears to have been marginal throughout all of Antiquity, both geopolitically due to its location between larger and more powerful neighbours (Colchis, Iberia, Armenia, the Parthian and Seleucid Empires), and economically because of the rugged nature of its terrain. Political control must have proven difficult at any period, as Strabo's portrayal suggests (11.2.18). The importance of the region relates essentially to the hypotheses that it constituted a buffer zone between, sometimes, rival states, and that the valley itself was one of the main communication arteries between them. As a communication axis, it should pro-

22 Lordkipanidze 1996, 141–153.

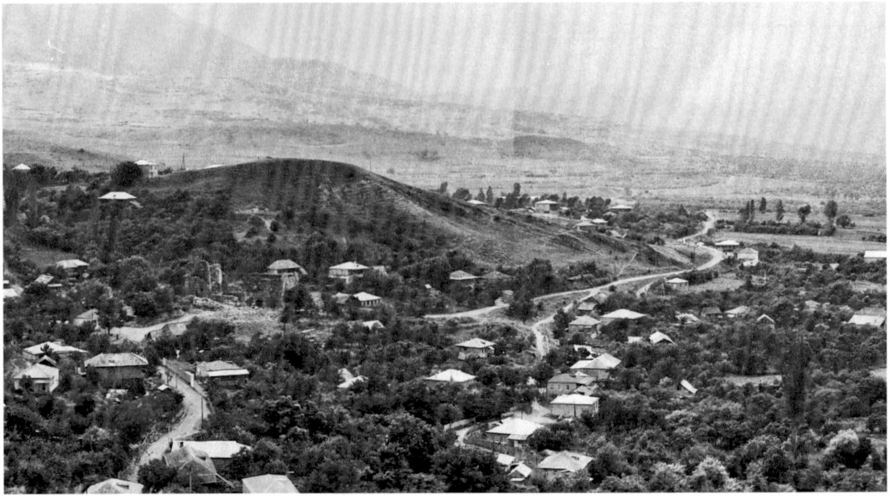

FIG. 2 The valley of the Mtvari river at Ats'quri, looking south

vide, therefore, fertile ground for contact between local inhabitants and their neighbours, including the Greeks of the Black Sea coast.

Few sites have been explored extensively in the region, so that it is difficult to develop a proper perspective encompassing the nature of society, its level of development and its integration to any regional political unit. A great deal is known of the archaeology of the Medieval period because of the great visibility of remains of that date. Exploration of Antiquity, on the other hand, had provided much less fruitful, producing only very modest material, most of which are chance finds. This situation is attributable, essentially, to thick post-Medieval colluvium covering the remains of Antiquity. Discovery depends mostly upon the vagaries of natural erosion. Small portions of two sites of relevant date have been excavated: Ats'quri, a settlement within which graves are dispersed, dating from the sixth century BC to at least the first century AD, and Tsnisi, a necropolis of the third and second century BC, with an associated settlement presumed to lie under the modern village but still unlocated. A third settlement is known from surface material only: Sadzeli. Information collected at the excavated sites suggests, nevertheless, a village-based society. The finds demonstrate neither urban developments, nor the trappings of a distinct entrenched élite: all houses consist of simple one or two room structures, all graves contain modest amounts of offerings and fine ceramics, metal objects and jewellery are extremely rare, as are imported materials. It appears as if, in spite of the presence of several developed states around this area, the region was never properly integrated into any state structure or, although under nominal control, the population remained untouched by social development therein. This contrasts

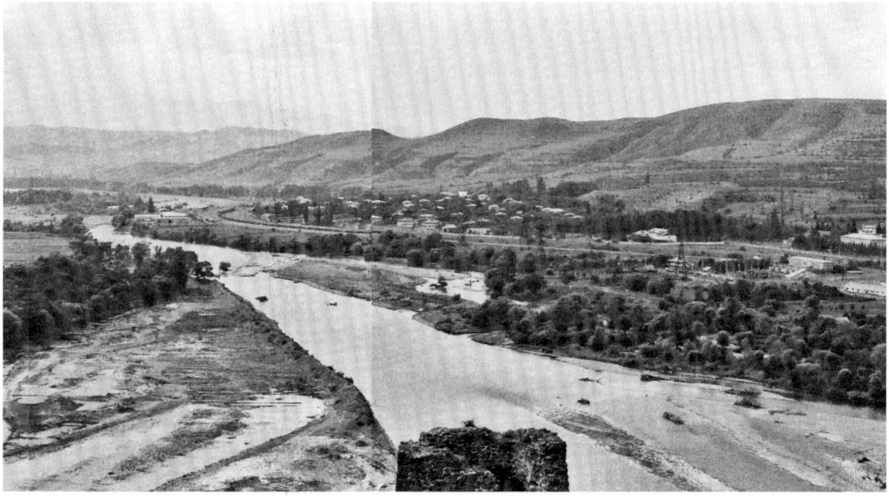

with the ancient sources. Herodotus (3.94) mentions that the Moschoi were part of the 21st satrapy along with the Tibareni, Macrones, Mosynoichoi and Mares during Achaemenid times, but by the time of Strabo (11.2.18), control of the area appears to have been divided vaguely from north to south between the Colchians, Iberians and Armenians. At some point in Medieval times, the area was integrated to the Georgian kingdom, as is evidenced by architecture and a few Georgian inscriptions.

The site of Ats'quri is located on the upper course of the Mtkvari, about halfway between the towns of Akhaltsikhe and Borjomi, at the head of a small plain (Fig. 2), closely ringed by steep hills on the shore where the ancient village was located. The valley extends more widely on the shore facing the settlement, but no ancient site is known there. Today Ats'quri stands as a modest farming village of about 2.000 inhabitants, with settlement extending on both shores of the river; it presents, however, clear signs of a much more prominent past with a sheer rock bastion crowned by an extensive fortified complex, which controlled communications along the valley, and a cathedral of a scale comparable to the largest in Georgia; both date to Medieval times. The site of pre-Christian Antiquity extends exclusively along the south-western shore of the Mtkvari, while the Christian agglomeration moved across the river to take advantage of the protection afforded by the fortress. The result of this move is that few traces of Medieval habitation remain above the levels of Antiquity, simplifying the stratigraphy. The objective of our investigations, begun there in 1993, was to study the impact of Greek culture on the local populations in Antiquity; we concentrated our efforts on the earlier phase of the site's occupation.

It would be tempting to assume that Ats'quri was the main regional settlement in Antiquity, because it benefits from a sizable arable area and extends over at least 5 ha, but lack of information on the other establishments prevents us from concluding this. In fact, Sadzeli is perhaps better located to exploit a dominant position, since it sits near the junction of two pathways leading from the Black Sea across the mountains and would afford communications both downriver to Iberia and upriver to Armenia. Unfortunately, apart from a brief examination of its surface, it has never been studied in any detail.

Less than 1% of the surface of Ats'quri was excavated. The excavations demonstrate, nevertheless, that the site was inhabited continuously from at least the sixth century BC,[23] and that it spread almost from its foundation over the entire surface of the later settlement, since material of this date can be found throughout the site. No houses of early date have been excavated, so that the record for that period is limited to scattered sherds. Faint remains under one house suggest that the location of some early habitations were reused at later times, perhaps as an economical measure, for several of the known houses were semi-subterranean, dug-out from the slopes of low hills with their floors as low as 1.50 m below ground level and with thick walls above ground. This is not a sign of poverty or primitiveness, but a logical adaptation to the local climate, which can be bitterly cold and with thick snow accumulation in winter. As far as the limited stratigraphical information allows a date, the excavated houses belong to the fourth and third centuries BC. Few complete plans are available, but the best preserved house consists of one large, irregular, rectangular room (about 5 x 6.5 m) with a hearth platform in one corner and a narrower room to the side with an oven (Plate 2). At least one and possibly two clay-lined pits were dug in front of the house. The walls are made of fieldstones, and their inner surface was plastered with clay, as was the floor. No traces of any roofing were found *in situ*, but some disarticulated burned remains, perhaps from another house nearby, point towards a timber and clay structure. Fragments of houses fitting this description have been found in two excavated areas; in both cases the overall pattern shows a high building density with only narrow passageways between individual buildings (1–1.5 m wide) and a courtyard in front of some.

Houses of the type just described are known elsewhere in Georgia, particularly in Iberia, where exact parallels of somewhat earlier date can be found.[24] They stand in stark contrast, however, with what Strabo (11.3.1) writes of Iberian architecture and town planning. While we cannot exclude that a marketplace existed in the unexcavated portion of Ats'quri, the likelihood that one will ever be found is very low indeed, for not one single feature of Strabo's description can apply at this site.

23 Recent work has pushed the initial occupation date of the site to the Bronze Age (see Licheli 2007, 55–66.)

24 See Abramishvili *et al.* 1986, 45–51 and Apakidze 1978, 109–119.

There are no signs of a street grid; for instance, in the excavated areas only one possible area paved with small stones near the shore of the river could be a street. Not a single element from any monumental urban structure has ever been found at the site, and no carved or cut stone of appropriate date on the southwest shore of the river has ever been unearthed by anyone in the village. In one area, the fragmentary remains appear to be roughly aligned, which might suggest some form of grid, but the free spaces between the houses are mere trodden earth paths. The houses do not fit into any Hellenic pattern: plans, building techniques, and materials all follow local customs; not one single fragment of tile has been found anywhere in the settlement of Antiquity. Consequently, although many of these elements can be observed in Iberia proper, the phenomenon did not spread beyond the core area of the kingdom, where they were adopted perhaps only by the élite. Strabo's urban description cannot be recognised in the finds of this region. The distinction he makes (Strabo 11.3.3) between the Iberians of the plains and the mountaineers to the north of the country appears to apply to this region also.

The archaeological record, however, is not entirely bare, since small quantities of imported Greek material have been collected in excavation, mostly ceramics but also a number of glass paste beads and a small blue frit scarab. The totals, although very small compared to numbers in Colchis, suggest that large-scale excavation might be very productive. The earliest finds consist of three fragments of sixth century BC East-Greek banded ware, one from a drinking cup, a sherd from the shoulder of a small container and another small painted sherd, all perhaps to be associated with the service of wine (Fig. 3.1–2, Fig. 4). A slightly larger number of sherds of the fifth and fourth centuries, but still only a handful—no more than 20 examples *in toto*—have also been collected, all of them black-glazed pottery, save for one fragment of a palmette cup. Athenian products appear to dominate the assemblage (Fig. 3.3–6, Fig. 5). Hellenistic pottery has also been found, in slightly lesser quantities than the Classical. Most of this material was reduced to very small fragments, very few of which join. Most appear to belong to open vessels—cups and plates—associated with the service of wine in the Hellenic world. The Hellenistic banded ware, by contrast, consists only of closed shapes. Finally, our collection includes a number of transport amphora sherds, all very small non-joining fragments, so it is not possible to reconstruct any shapes, or establish dates and provenances. None of the handles were stamped. No recognisably Roman pottery was collected on the site. The presence of Greek pottery forms does not appear to have influenced the local craft, unless one considers the introduction of ring bases in Hellenistic times as a form of influence.

All in all, the excavations at Ats'quri have produced about 60 imported Greek sherds, including the amphorae. This may appear insignificant at first glance, except that it constitutes one of the largest collections of Greek pottery in all of the

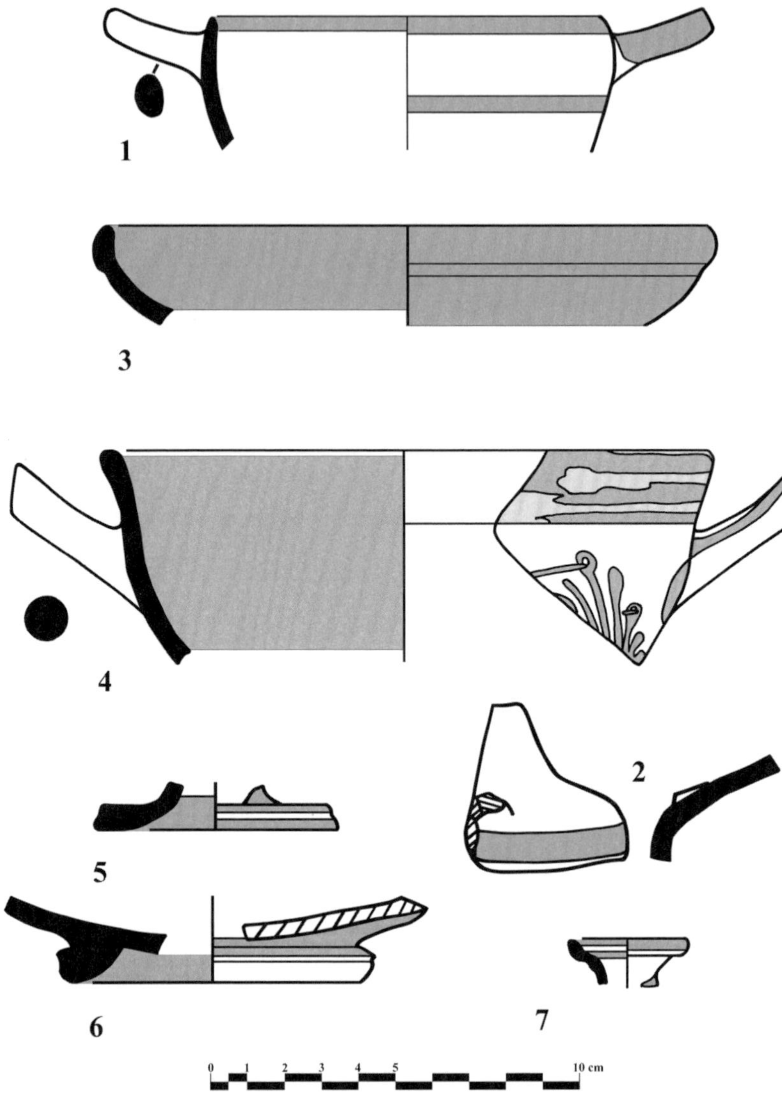

FIG. 3 Greek pottery from Ats'quri (1 & 2 Archaic; 3-6 Classical; 7 Hellenistic)

Transcaucasus, resulting from a very limited excavation (less than 500 m^2 *in toto*). All areas of the site and almost all deposits have produced the odd Greek sherd (about one Greek sherd per 1000), but almost two thirds were collected from one single deposit, where they amounted to 0.5% of all material. All appear to have been the result of discard following domestic use. None has been found in graves, and most are represented by very small non-joining fragments, an indication that

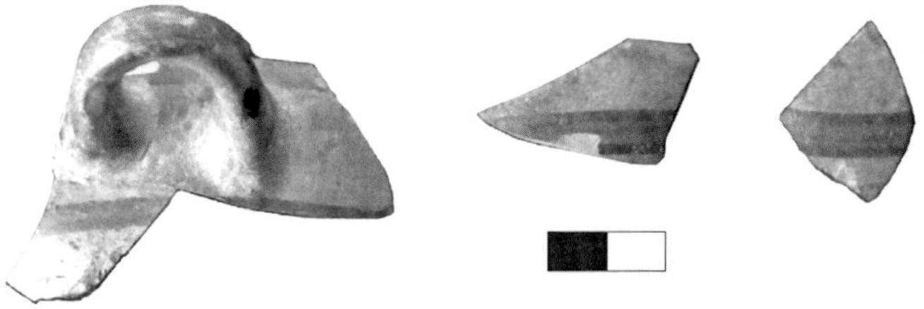

FIG. 4 Archaic Greek Pottery from Ats'quri.

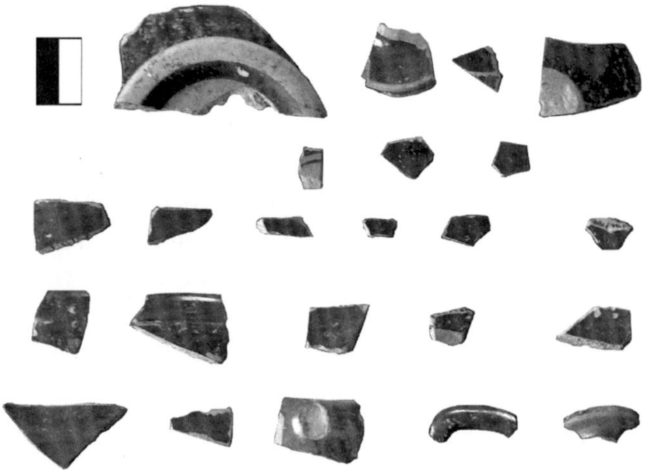

FIG. 5 Classical and Hellenistic Black-Glazed Pottery from Ats'quri.

they were exposed to the elements after discard and thus dispersed. Some might, nevertheless, have been deposited in graves disturbed later in Antiquity—for which we possess evidence—and one indication to that effect is that the deposit where most of the Greek sherds were found also contained a considerable quantity of glass beads, which would be in place in graves; however, no human bones were collected with them. The only excavated fifth or fourth century grave did not contain imported material. Given the very limited scope of the excavation, it is not possible to draw conclusions as to the intra-site distribution of this pottery, much less to infer any preferential distribution within the local social groupings. The apparently skewed distribution might constitute an artefact of a very restricted sample.

The deposition of coins in graves, already noted in Iberia, is also present at Ats'quri. Only one grave produced a coin. It contained the skeleton of a tall male (nearly 1.90 m in height) in a contracted position laid on his right side, with his face turned to the southeast. The grave appears wholly unremarkable, apart from the height of the individual, and displays the same scarcity of funerary goods noticed in other graves on the site: one jug, a meat offering, a few glass-paste and carnelian beads, and the silver coin of Polemon II, which provides a good date. The exact placement of the coin—in either the mouth or the hand of the deceased—could not be ascertained, for it was found while sifting the earth collected around the skeleton.

It is generally assumed that coins are a sign of acculturation in these parts, but the fact that we possess only one at Ats'quri weakens this hypothesis and begs for more than a blanket interpretation. Other graves with coins are known from the region; several are reported at Tsnisi about 20 km south of Atsquri, still unpublished but of Hellenistic date,[25] and one at Satkhe[26] far to the south of Akhalkalaki, also of Hellenistic date. The later date and provenance of the Ats'quri coin itself may allow a different perspective on the process of acculturation at the site in that it can link our individual with known history. Polemon had extended his realm to include Colchis (Strabo, 11.2.18), which his widow maintained. The mountain route-ways discussed earlier attest by themselves to some form of contact between the coast and the valley of the Kyros, as do the Greek imports. Could it be that the region also fell to Polemon, or was allied with him? One of the outlets for young men in a relatively poor region, such as this one, may have been, like today, to join an army. Could it be that we have here the remains of one man who joined Polemon's army as a mercenary and came back home at the end of his service, having adopted some Greek beliefs during his army years? This, of course, cannot be proven.

Strabo (11.2.17) mentions the presence in the Moschic Mountains of a sanctuary to Leukothea associated with an oracle of Phryxos. One must seriously doubt that Greek divinities and heroes were worshipped in the area, since no physical evidence can be adduced to prove their presence. What we may have in Strabo's text, however, is the assimilation of local divinities by the Greeks to their own religious tradition. If there really was an oracle in the area, it would have inevitably attracted the attention of the local Greeks, who might have consulted it, rather than travelling long distances to traditional Hellenic oracular shrines. We should be able, therefore, to identify traces of their passage by offerings they left at the sanctuary and other objects along the way.

The sanctuary has never been located and, consequently, several hypotheses have been advanced as to its location. The subject is discussed by Braund[27] who states that it must be located somewhere along the Kyros, in the region bound by Borjomi and Akhaltsikhe. He favours a location associated with water springs,

25 This information was provided by V. Licheli, who has worked in this region for more than 30 years.

26 See Pearce *et al.* 1993, 17–20.

27 Braund *op. cit.,* 149; see also Braund 2000, map 88, B-3.

given the nature of Leukothea, perhaps near Borjomi or Abastumani, famous today for their mineral springs. Ats'quri constitutes one of the potential other locations of the sanctuary. Its case can be argued on the basis of the Georgian Medieval sources, which, although reflecting a considerably distorted view of the pagan divinities, reveal functional features similar to those hinted at in the Classical tradition.

Ats'quri during Medieval times was the location of a see, whose ruined cathedral can still be observed within the village on the northeast shore of the river, the core of the Medieval settlement. Reused architectural elements provide evidence for an earlier church at the same spot. It is associated with a legend stating that the apostle Andrew visited the town, identified in the chronicles as Atsqueri, formerly known as Sosangeti, while on a mission of evangelisation.[28]

Excavation within the cathedral has revealed no sign of any cult building or deposit dated to pre-Christian times at that location, and finds demonstrate that the earliest activity there occurred during Medieval times. The location of the present cathedral cannot correspond to that of the sanctuary of Leukothea. If such a sanctuary ever existed in association with Atsquri, it must have been located across the river, where the pre-Christian settlement is located. The local sedimentary history and built up conditions have prevented the identification of any building or deposit commensurate with the text of Strabo. The most that can be said is that the relatively large quantity of Greek material—from a local perspective—might be notionally linked to either the stay at Ats'quri of Greek consultants of the oracle, or to their passage through the site on their way to the sanctuary. The presence of Greek pottery and other imported materials could then be explained as offerings at the sanctuary or as gifts left in exchange for various services (shelter, guidance, safe passage, etc).

To sum up the regional evidence, it is clear that whatever contacts existed between the inhabitants of the region and the Greeks—and later Romans—of the coast produced only superficial effects on the culture of the Moschoi, limited to a few individuals. This could be due to the very marginal nature of the region and its weak links to the more firmly established élite structures of the neighbouring areas where true states emerged, as if the local leaders did not feel the need or did not have the resources to match their neighbours.

28 Thomson, *op. cit.*, 355–359, provides a text of the legend. I have argued elsewhere (Morin 2009) that this legend constitutes a clear attempt to foster the idea that the Christian church in Georgia was founded by an apostle and should be understood in the light of the Medieval politics of prestige surrounding the apostolicity of churches. It finds a parallel in the story of the same Andrew introducing the Christian cult and founding churches in Constantinople. Artemis and Apollo may reflect the Christianization of the Medieval and later Georgian tradition of Dali, goddess of the wild and the hunt and her hero son Amirani.

Conclusions

How can we consider the nature of the contacts discussed above within a long-term historical perspective? Relationships between the coast and the hinterland can be divided in three phases and their nature linked both to political and social developments in Iberia and among its neighbours.

First, from Archaic times to the Early Hellenistic period, there is no recognisable state organisation in Iberia, save perhaps for some form of Persian domination, as is suggested by the recent finds at Gumbati in Eastern Georgia,[29] and relationships involve small Greek *poleis* with local groups. During this period, contacts were merely episodic and materials changed hands and were carried back and forth. There is no visible impact on the Iberian hinterland. This may be related to the fact that Iberia was then a relatively unorganised society and that its élite relied on the Persians for bestowal of status.[30]

Second, from Hellenistic to Roman times, the newly formed Iberian kingdom figures in relationships linked to the power politics of major empires, first between itself and the Seleucid kingdom, and later with Rome and their Parthian adversaries. It seems at this point that the contacts are slightly more intensive; there are political relations, perhaps even treaties. In Iberia itself, the emerging, and then dominant, élite, chiefly but not only the rulers, adopt some of the trappings of urbanised Hellenistic, then Roman, life. As a result, urban life spreads throughout the kingdom, at least in the core area of Iberia. There is also slight penetration of Greek ideas, as is shown by the coins found in some graves; through what agency this occurs is not understood. Any impact is felt mostly in the core area of the kingdom, while marginal areas remain relatively unaffected.

Third, from late Roman times onwards, a new phenomenon causes realignment in local culture: the adoption of Christianity by the Iberians. This is the period when Greek culture had its most profound impact, as is exemplified by the myth of the temple of Artemis at Sosangeti-Atsqueri, as well as by the integration of considerable Hellenic materials in the local historical traditions (e.g. the Romance of Alexander) and the adoption of Greek church nomenclature. Historically, this is also a period when Iberia enters into alliances with Christian states in opposition to first Mazdeist, then Muslim Persia and eventually the Ottomans.

29 See Furtwängler 1995, 177–111; Furtwängler and Knauß 1996, 363–381; *idem* 1997, 353–387.

30 I have suggested this is the case in Morin 2004, 108–119.

REFERENCES

Abramishvili, R.M., M.R. Abramishvili, T.R. Vashakidze, N.I. Giguashvili, I.B. Sultanishvili and G.F. Chocovani, "Arkheologicheskiye Raskopi v Tbilisi (Archaeological Work in Tbilisi)." *Polebie Arkheologicheskiye Isledovaniya* (*Journal of Archaeological Research*), (1986): 45–51.

Apakidze, *Mtskheta* II. Tbilisi: Metsniereva, 1978.

Braund, D., *Georgia in Antiquity, a History of Colchis and Tanscaucasian Iberia 550BC-AD 562*. Oxford: Oxford University Press, 1994.

Braund, D. and R.J. Talbert (ed.), *The Barrington Atlas of the Greek and Roman World*. Princeton: Princeton University Press, 2000.

Furtwängler, A.E., "Gumbati, archäologische Expedition in Kachetien 1994 1. Vorbericht." *Eurasia Antiqua* 1 (1995): 177–111;

Furtwängler, A.E. and F.S. Knauß, "Gumbati, archäologische Expedition in Kachetien 1995 2. Vorbericht." *Eurasia Antiqua* 2 (1996): 363–381

———. "Gumbati, archäologische Expedition in Kachetien 1996 3. Vorbericht." *Eurasia Antiqua* 3 (1997): 353–387.

Gagoshidze, I., "The Achaemenid Influence in Iberia." *Boreas* 19 (1996): 125–136.

Kacharava, D., "The Graeco-Kolkhian Trade Connection in the 7th–4th Century BC" in *Proceedings of the First International Conference on the Archaeology and History of the Black Sea* , ed. by J. M. Fossey, 137–146. Amsterdam: Gieben, 1997.

Kimiashvili, K. & G. Narimanishvili, "A Group of Iberian Fire Temples (4th Cent. BC-2nd Cent. AD)." *Archäologische Mitteilungen aus Iran und Turan* 28 (1995–1996): 309–318.

Knauß, F.S., "Achämeniden in Transkaukasien" in *Fenster zur Forschung* ed. by S. Lausberg and K. Oekentorp, 81–114. Münster: Museumvorträge der Museen der Westfälischen Wilhelms-Universität, 1999.

Licheli, V., "Black Glazed Pottery in Transcaucasia: its Diffusion Rout" in *Proceedings of the First International Conference on the Archaeology and History of the Black Sea* , ed. by J. M. Fossey, 147–153. Amsterdam: Gieben, 1997.

———. "Hellenism and Ancient Georgia" in *Ancient Greek Colonies in the Black Sea 2,* BAR International Series 1675, ed. by D. V. Grammenos and E. K. Petropoulos, 1083–1133. Oxford: Archaeopress, 2007.

———. "Oriental Innovations in Samtskhe (Southern Georgia) in the 1st Millennium BC." *Ancient Civilizations from Scythia to Siberia*, 13 (2007): 55–66.

Lordkipanidze, O., *Archäologie in Georgien von den Altsteinzeit zum Mittlealter* VCH *Acta Humaniora*. Weinheim: VHC Verlagsgesselschaft, 1991.

———. "Vani an Ancient City of Colchis." *Greek, Roman and Byzantine Studies* 32 (1991): 151–195.

———. *Das alte Georgien* (*Kolchis und Iberien*) *in Strabons Geographie, neue Scholien*. Amsterdam: Hakkert, 1996.

Morin, J., "Long-term Cross-Cultural Relations and State-Formation in Transcaucasian Iberia, An *Annaliste* Perspective." *Ancient Near Eastern Studies* 41 (2004): 108–119.

———. "Mythmaking and Acculturation in the South Caucasus—Artemis and Apollo at Ats'quri" in *Zurück zum Gegenstand Festschrift für Andreas E. Furtwängler*, ed. by R. Einicke et alii, 423–431. Langenweißbach: Beier & Beran, 2009.

Nadiradze, D., "Le site archéologique de Saïrké" in *Le Pont-Euxin vu par les Grecs,* ed. by O. Lordkipanidze and P. Lévêque, 213–222. Paris: Annales littéraires de l'université de Besançon, 1990.

Pearce, J., E.A. Carson, P.L. Kohl and C. Edens, "International Program for Research in the Caucasus: Field Seasons 1990 and 1991." *Archaeological News* 18 (1993): 17–20.

Thomson, R.W., *Rewriting Caucasian History, The Mediaeval Armenian Adaptation of the Georgian Chronicles.* Oxford: Oxford University Press, 1996.

Tsetskhladze, G.R., *Die Griechen in der Kolchis*. Amsterdam: Hakkert, 1998.

Vickers, M., "Pichvnari." *Anatolian Archaeology* 4 (1998): 15.

Vickers M. & A. Kakhidze, "Pichvnari, Ajarian AR, Georgia 1999." *Anatolian Archaeology* 5 (1999): 11–12.

———. "Pichvnari, Ajarian AR, Georgia 1999." *Anatolian Archaeology* 5 (1999): 11.

———. "Pichvnari, Ajarian AR, Georgia 2000." *Anatolian Archaeology* 6 (2000): 13–14.

Women and Music in Ancient Anatolia: The Iconographic Evidence

Tuna Şare[1]

To my dear professors, Marie-Henriette and Charles Gates, whose music turned the scholarship of the art and archaeology of Turkey into a festivity. It was an honor to be your student. You will always be our Muses.

Abstract

This article examines the imagery of female musicians in ancient Anatolia. It is a preliminary investigation of a topic which has never been dealt with in detail in previous scholarship. Through depictions on a variety of objects, this study explores and offers some provisional thoughts on the semantic value of female musicians and their socio-religious associations within Anatolian civilizations from the Bronze Age to the Classical period. Among questions sought to be answered are: in what kind of contexts did the female musicians (singers, dancers, instrument players) appear? With what type of musical instruments were female musicians associated? What do these associations imply? And what was the status of a female musician?

The overall review in this study reveals the continuous existence of female musicians active in cult ritual, in weddings, and in funerals specific to each Anatolian civilization, a tradition still in practice in rural villages of Asia Minor. The musical

---

1 Department of Art History, Çanakkale Onsekiz Mart University, Terzioğlu Campus, 17100 Çanakkale, Turkey.

While this article was in press, the conference "Representations of Musicians in the Coroplastic Art of the Ancient World: Iconography, Ritual Contexts and Functions" organized by Angela Bellia and Clemente Marconi at the Institute of Fine Arts brought more insight to the topic. Especially two presentations, one by Doğan-Gürbüzer on the male and female terracotta figurines with stringed instruments from the Sanctuary of Apollo Clarios from Claros in Ionia and another by Holzman on the seventh century tortoise shell lyres from Gordion are important in relation to this essay's topic. The proceedings of this conference are yet to be published.

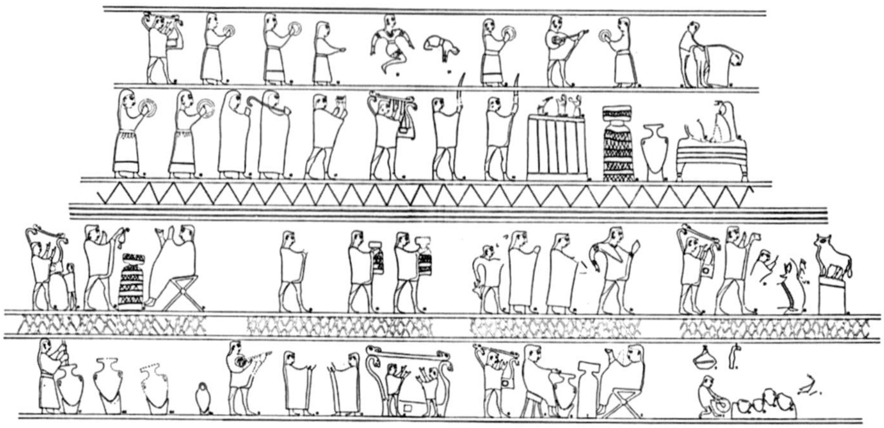

FIG. 1 Drawing of the reliefs of İnandık Vase, after Dinçol 1999, 5.

instruments mostly associated with women in Hittite iconography are percussion instruments (membranophones and idiophones), usually used in cult practices. Professional female musicians appear playing all sorts of musical instruments, including stringed, wind and percussion (chordophones, aerophones, membranophones and idiophones, respectively) in courtly wedding ceremonies of the Urartian culture. From sixth century BCE[2] onwards, professional female dancers and musicians playing stringed and wind instruments seem to have continuously performed in cultic performances, in funereal and nuptial ceremonies and in courtly activities of the rich in Western Anatolia. Finds from the Hellespontine tombs of the Late Classical period imply that the knowledge of professional musical training and poetry seem to have become an indicator of an elite identity for women. Key pieces in the discussion are Hittite relief vessels, from the sites of İnandıktepe and Hüseyindede, an Urartian belt from the Sadberk Hanım Museum in İstanbul, the Polyxena Sarcophagus and Late Classical terracotta figurines from ancient Assos. The classification of the musical instruments in the discussion is based on the Hornbostel and Sachs system.[3]

2 Hereafter all dates are BCE unless indicated otherwise.

3 According to the Hornbostel and Sachs's (1914) classification, the instrument producing sound through an instrument itself vibrating is an idiophone; an instrument producing sound through a column of air is an aerophone; an instrument producing sound by way of vibrating a stretched membrane is a membranophone; and an instrument producing sound by way of vibrating strings is a chordophone. Different terminologies used in previous studies of ancient musical instruments cause confusion and inconsistency. See Celasin and Beşiroğlu 2006 for the investigation of this methodological problem, especially for Hittite musical culture.

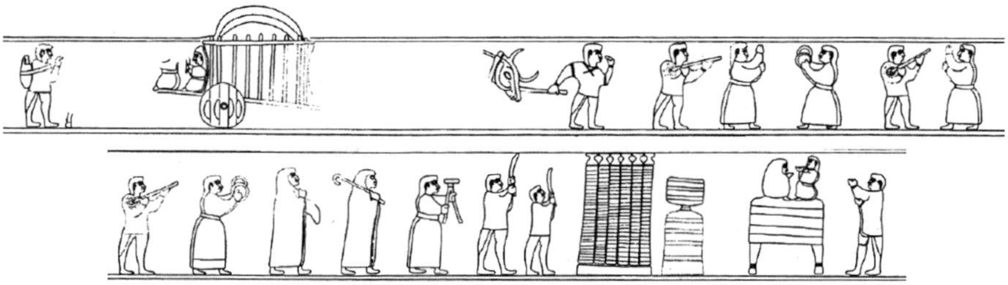

FIG. 2 Drawing of the reliefs on the first two registers of the Hüseyindede Vase I, after Yıldırım 2008, figs. 5.1 and 6.1.

The Imagery of Female Musicians in Hittite Art

The importance of music and dance in Hittite culture is perhaps best attested in the representations on the relief vases of Early Hittite art.[4] Dancers, singers, and early musicians playing a variety of instruments, including the lute, lyre, cymbals, and flutes, often along with acrobats, decorate the registers of relief vases. On vases from Alişar, Eskiyapar, Boğazköy, Bitik, İnandıktepe, Kabaklı, and Hüseyindede, musicians appear as part of courtly ritual ceremonies.[5] Perhaps, the best preserved and most complete of all these vases comes from İnandıktepe.[6] The İnandık Vase, 86 cm in height and 50 cm in width, dates to the 17th century and displays representations of ritual ceremonies in low relief on four superimposed registers surrounding the body and the neck of the vase (FIG. 1). The top register, which depicts a procession of musicians and dancers leading to the scene of a couple's ritual intercourse, includes four female musicians. Unlike the lyre- and lute-playing men on the same register, all of these females (clad in long and belted dresses) are shown as playing the large clash-cymbals in their upraised hands. The procession in the second register starts with two more female cymbal players, dressed similarly to the female musicians of the above register, except for their belts with fringes hanging down. In the fourth (bottom) register, two female dancers face each other and dance with their upraised hands to the music of a male lutanist and two male harpists.

A similar relief vase, both in size and overall decoration, discovered at Hüseyindede Tepesi also includes female musicians in a lively procession decorating its registers

4 Musicians and dancers are described in several Hittite texts, and they also appear in Hittite glyptic art. For examples of musicians on Hittite stamp seals, see Boehmer and Güterbock 1987, 104, pl. XXXVII/ 301; see also Alp 1999, 4. For a discussion of Hittite texts with references to musicians and musical instruments see Alp 1999, 2–13, 50–60; Güterbock 1995, 57–72; De Martino 1995.

5 Alp 1999, 1–19.

6 Özgüç 1988.

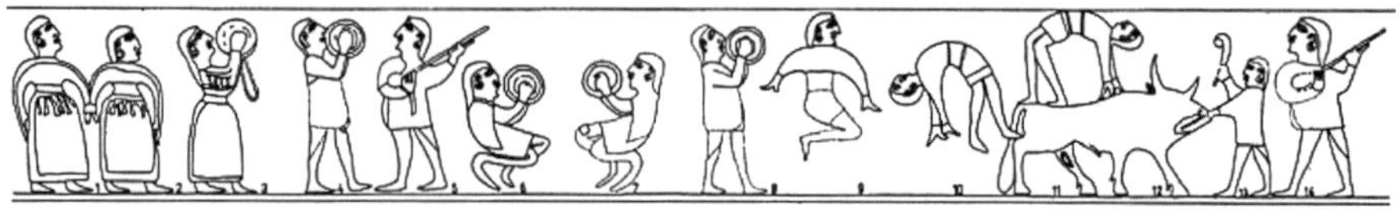

FIG. 3 Drawing of the reliefs on Hüseyindede Vase II, after Yıldırım 2008, fig. 6.9.

(FIG. 2).[7] The ceremonial procession on the top register contains three female dancers, dancing to the music of male lutanists with their arms raised high. One of the dancers also plays her cymbals in her upraised hands. Both discs of the clash-cymbal pair can be seen, since the far disc is depicted as lifted higher up. One more female cymbal-player appears as part of the procession on the second register. Another vase of the mid 17th century found in a temple, again at Hüseyindede, contains only one relief band around the neck of the vase (FIG. 3). Among the 13 human figures in a procession with a bull-leaping scene, two females in long dresses with fringed belts hold each other's hand. Unlike the profile view of the other members of the procession, the bodies of the two women are shown frontally, possibly to signify their role as dancers performing a group dance to the rhythm provided by the female cymbalist in front of them. The female cymbalist's uplifted head and slightly open mouth indicate that she is also singing. The fabric hanging down from her cymbals is probably a secure-band used to hold the cymbals together. The fringes hanging down from the belt of the dancers may have also produced a rhythmic sound as they danced. The other performers on the relief band, including cymbalists, lutanists and acrobats, are all male.

Cymbal-players of both genders also appear in processional scenes of the vases from Bitik, Alişar, Boğazköy, and Kabaklı.[8] The majority of the cymbal-players in these representations are female. Possibly referred to as *galgalturi-* in Hittite cuneiform texts, the cymbals are made of iron, bronze, and copper and are produced in pairs.[9] Early examples of metal cymbals were discovered from Levels II and Ib of Kültepe-Kaneš, an Assyrian trade colony of the 18th century.[10] Though they seem to

7 For Hüseyindede vases, see Sipahi 2000; Yıldırım 2000a; 2000b; 2001; 2002; 2005; 2008.

8 Yıldırım 2002, 597.

9 Güterbock 1995, 57; Alp 1999, 10; Bittel 1968; Dinçol 1999, 50–51; Yıldırım 2002, 597. De Martino (1995, 2662), considering the information that they are produced in pairs, defines *galgalturi-* as castanets and *ḫuḫupal-* as the cymbal. Yet, as the representations on Hittite relief vases show, *galgalturi-* were also produced and used as clashing pairs.

10 Earlier than the Kaneš examples, are the cymbals found along with castanets and sistra in the royal tombs of Horoztepe dating from the end of the 3rd millennium. The skeletons in these tombs are too damaged to know whether these instruments come from male or female tombs: see Özgüç and Akok 1958. For Kaneš cymbals, see Alp 1999, 10; Dinçol 1999, 49; Yıldırım 2002, 597. Dinçol and Yıldırım also note

be slightly smaller than the sizes indicated by vase imagery, these cymbals provide a better observation of what cymbals looked like in real life. They are smooth on the outside and curved inwards at the edges with a bulbous protrusion in the middle. The holes in the middle of the bulbous form possibly allowed tying a string to attach them to the hands of the players and also the cymbals to each other.

Musicians and dancers also appear on the orthostat reliefs with royal processional scenes of Neo-Hittite art, including the well-known examples from Karatepe, Zincirli, and Carchemish, though there is no known example of a female musician in these representations.[11]

As this brief review of the female musicians in representational Hittite art shows, female musicians either dance, sing or play the cymbals in ceremonial processions. The inclusion of the so-called "bed scenes" of a couple sitting on top of what appears to be a bed, as on the second registers of the İnandıktepe and Hüseyindede Vases, and the scene of a man unveiling (?) a woman on the Bitik Vase,[12] have led scholars to argue that these processions on Hittite vases are festive ceremonies for a sacred marriage of the king and the queen or the god and the goddess.[13] Whether for a royal or a divine couple, the common consensus among scholars is that these ceremonies are related to Hittite festivals which celebrated fertility and reproduction.[14] Discovery of these vases in cult centers prove their function as ritual objects. If we accept that the artists who decorated the vases reflected the societal attitudes and actual practice, the representations on the vases mimic the ritual acts of the participants. Thus, female musicians seem to have acted as singers, cymbal-players, and dancers in these ceremonies.

It is interesting to note that there are no wind instruments (aerophones) in these representations. Also, stringed instruments (chordophones) like lutes and lyres, which require more technical training to play, always appear in the hands of male musicians, while the cymbals, an essentially rhythmic percussion instrument (idiophone), are mostly exclusive to women. Indeed, despite the existence of different designations for professional musicians and non-professional musicians of both genders, the terms used in the Hittite texts for professional musicians are predominantly in the masculine form.[15]

---

the continuous use of these cymbals in Anatolia during the Old Hittite Period and Phrygian Period through examples from archaeological discoveries.

11 Alp 1999, 30–36.

12 Özgüç 1957.

13 Yıldırım (2008, 844) provides a review of different scholarly interpretations. Also contributing to the interpretation of these ceremonies as related to marriage is the inclusion of carriages (carrying the dowry of the bride, or cult objects?) on the celebrative scenes on the vases from Hüseyindede, Boğazköy, and Alişar.

14 Alp 1999, 24; Yıldırım 2008, 844–845.

15 De Martino 1995, 2663.

Reinforcing the rhythm, which is already inherent in the melody of the songs, percussion instruments are often seen as supportive, not forming part of the music in their own right.[16] They are associated with ecstatic worship, which involves transitional stages in ritual activities usually performed by females, as is well-known from the cult of Cybele and Dionysus in the ancient Greek world (see below).[17] Indeed, one can infer from the Hittite texts that alongside professional singers and musicians employed as temple personnel, other priests or priestesses played instruments like tambourines that are apparently considered as within the technical competence of non-professionals and had magical properties in ritual.[18] The cymbal-players on the Hittite relief vases must have been priestesses as such.

As for the dancers and singers, Hittite texts also imply a distinction between professional performers and those who dance and sing only during a cult ritual. Most of the priestesses represented on the vases must have belonged to the second category. Yet, there are also specific references to "some women and girls" required for special kinds of dances during special occasions, suggesting the existence of professional females performing.[19] Also professional were the exclusively female chorus of lamenters performing in funerary rituals, named "*taptara-* women" in the texts.[20]

As can be inferred from the Hittite laws and official letters preserved on the cuneiform archives from Boğazköy-Hattuša, the capital of Hittites, the role of women in Hittite society was mostly bound to the domestic sphere. Although female members of the royal family, such as Queen Puduhepa, exercised considerable independent power, an ordinary woman depended mostly on her husband.[21] Outside of their home, women could be employed in the medical sector or as agricultural workers, as cooks, millers, weavers, innkeepers, cellar keepers, musicians, singers and dancers, the last three mostly as part of temple personnel.[22] Yet, as Hoffner notes in his study of Hittite law codes, a ratio of wages paid to men and women for comparable tasks was roughly two to one.[23]

Thus, female musicians, dancers, and singers depicted on the Hittite vases seem to be priestesses working for the temple in rituals. Although they appear

16 Landels 1999, 81; West 1994, 122.

17 Burkert 1985, 102; West 1994, 124. As Bundrick (106–116) notes, the most frequently depicted musical instruments in Dionysiac scenes on Athenian vases are percussion instruments: *cymbala* (cymbals), *krotola* (clappers), and *tympana* (shallow drums).

18 De Martino 1995, 2664.

19 De Martino 1995, 2666.

20 Rutherford 2008.

21 Hoffner 1995, 567–568.

22 Imparati 1995, 579.

23 Hoffner 1995, 567.

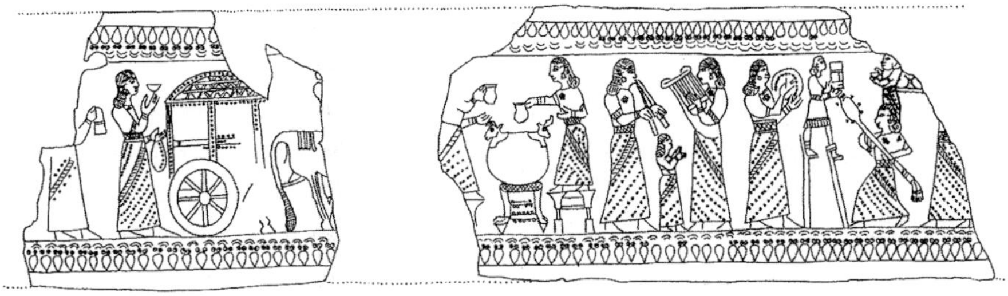

FIG. 4 Drawing of the Urartian belt from Sadberk Hanım Museum, after Anlağan 1998, 61, drawings 1-2.

singing and dancing side by side with males, the only musical instrument they play are cymbals, suggesting that male musicians received a more professional musical training than the females.

The Imagery of Female Musicians in Urartian Art

Unlike the Hittite examples, almost all known representations of musicians in Urartian art are females, implying a gender-specific role of the profession in certain festivities of Urartian culture. Urartian texts do not provide much evidence about music and dance, but musicians appear cast on a group of Urartian bronze belts with dates ranging from the late eighth to early sixth centuries. The smaller size of these belts and the representations of processions with female gift bearers, musicians, dancers and acrobats, compared to the larger sized belts with hunt and battle scenes, indicate that they belonged to females.[24] The short length and traces of usage further indicate that these belts were used by young females in their lifetime and buried with them in their tombs.[25]

Providing the most extensive imagery of female musicians is perhaps the belt now in the Sadberk Hanım Museum (FIG. 4).[26] Dated to the late eighth-early seventh century, the fragmentary belt displays a procession of females. On the far left are the two gift bearers, walking towards the right, behind an elaborately decorated cart pulled possibly by oxen. Following this is a libation scene with two females pouring liquid into a large cauldron with bull protomes on its neck. Next comes the procession of female musicians: a musician playing the double flute, a small girl clapping hands and possibly singing, a lyre-player, another musician

24 Kellner 1991, 142–160; Seidl 2004, 133–150.

25 Seidl 2012, 163.

26 Anlağan 1998.

playing a single frame drum (a tambourine), a smaller figure walking on sticks while playing a xylophone-like instrument, a dancing figure with a long rattling instrument (see below for the discussion of the latter two instruments), and finally another small figure balanced on the shoulders of the rattling woman playing possibly a metal bowl by striking a small stick on it. All of the females are clad in long-sleeved dresses belted at the waist.

There are several different interpretations as regards the meaning of the celebrative processions depicted on these belts. Miyashita's view is that the scenes refer to events in the afterlives of the deceased women, but this can be dismissed since the belts were used before death.[27] By pointing out the existence of central elderly women on some belts, Seidl and Ziffer suggest that the scenes refer to the banqueting at the court of the queen, where old women taught young girls courtly activities.[28] This latter interpretation is an appealing one. Yet, these elderly authoritative females could also refer to the mothers of a bride and groom, in charge of the arrangements for wedding festivities. Indeed, as Belli proposes, the scenes on these belts more likely depict nuptial ceremonies for aristocratic families. Used briefly during a woman's lifetime, the belts might have been given as wedding presents to the brides and buried along with them after their death.[29] In fact, silver and gold bridal belts are still part of traditional wedding costumes in the eastern part of Anatolia. Furthermore, the celebrative preparations, which include a variety of 'womanly' tasks, such as cooking and loom weaving, as can be seen within the processions on some belts, could easily be associated with wedding preparations and related ritual activities, rather than courtly teachings of a female banquet as Seidl suggests.[30] The most common actors of the processions on these belts are the gift bearers and the musicians, indicating the festive character of the occasion depicted, thus implying once more that these festivities are for a specific event. As acts of bravery such as hunting and battling are representative of aristocratic male identity, marriage and wedding ceremonies represent the most important occasions shaping a woman's gender identity in many ancient cultures.[31] Thus, the scenes on Urartian belts of both genders provide a perfect comparison for the expected gender roles within Urartian culture.

27 Miyashita 1983.

28 Seidl 2012; Ziffer 2002.

29 Indeed, the existence of decorative carts pulled by oxen within the processions in some of the scenes could refer to the dowry of the bride, see Belli 2007, 103, figs. 15–16.

30 Seidl 2013, 163.

31 See for examples, Oakley and Sinos 1993 and Blundell 1995 (especially 86) for marriages and weddings in ancient Greece.

The female musicians shown on at least seventeen Urartian bronze belts[32] appear singing; dancing, either with bent knees, twisted bodies, or clapping upraised hands; playing the single-framed hand drums, round or rectangular in shape, usually with jingling metal discs attached to the outer rims; playing metal bowls with sticks; playing castanets, or playing the lyre and the double flute. One obscure instrument on the scenes resembles a xylophone with two parallel sidepieces connected by wooden pegs with strips in between, possibly producing sound when the strings were struck. It can be seen in the hands of the small figure (gender is not certain) walking on sticks (Fig. 4).[33] Another instrument with an oval top and a long stick extending down, defined as a long-necked lute by Belli, is perhaps a rattling standard top as Seidl suggests (see the second figure on the right on Fig. 4).[34] Seidl rightly points out that in all of the known representations of this instrument, strings are missing, there are metal discs attached to the top of the circular part and, unlike the lutes, the long neck of the instrument is situated below the circular part, not above.[35]

The above review of the Urartian belts shows that although the majority are rhythmic percussion instruments, female musicians appear playing a variety of instruments that belong to the families of idiophones, membraphones, aerophones, and chordophones, the latter two certainly requiring professional training. This variety might suggest the existence of an aristocratic school of musicians in which females were trained. The dancing of the females also looks more professional, with agitated movements, when compared to the dancers on Hittite vases. One example shows the dancer with a completely twisted body wearing a special (possibly sound-producing) high headdress.[36] The depictions on the belts reveal a joyful feminine world of musicians, dancers, and singers performing within an elite community, as a unique aspect of Urartian society. As Belli also notes, as an exclusively female profession in the Urartian period, the traditions of female musicians and dancers performing in celebrations and singers lamenting in funerals still continue in the villages of Eastern Anatolia.[37]

32 Belli (2004) lists 16 Urartian belts with depictions of female musicians. Seidl's article (2012, fig. 1) includes another elaborate example in the Munich Archäologische Staatssammlung.

33 See Seidl 2012, 165 for the discussion.

34 Belli 2004, 89.

35 Seidl 2012, 165.

36 Seidl 2012, fig. 2h.

37 Belli 2004, 96.

Female Musicians of Lydia and Phrygia

Despite the lack of extensive literary and archaeological evidence from Phrygia itself, the power of music in Phrygian culture, especially in relation to the cult of Phrygian Cybele, is well attested in Greek literature and artistic representations. These Greek sources refer to the extensive use of the Phrygian flute, the tympanum, and the cymbals, creating an ecstatic music for the encircling dances of women for the Phrygian goddess.[38] The late fifth century poet Diogenes, for example, states,

> [The Phrygian women who] with their tympana and the whirling of the resounding brass and the clashing of the cymbals in their hands roar out the wise and the healing music of the gods.[39]

Starting with the introduction of the cult of Cybele into Greek religion in the late sixth century, the followers of the goddess appear playing the *tympana*, castanets, and the *auloi* (double-flutes) on Greek vases.[40] Greek Cybele herself always holds a tympanum in her left hand as her main attribute in Greek representations, indicating the significance of the ecstatic music in her cult.[41] She acquires this attribute, however, only in Greek imagery. Her main attributes on the sixth century representations from Phrygia itself are an animal of prey (usually a bird) and a phiale, which she holds in both hands.[42] The only known image of Cybele from Phrygia that includes musicians is the so-called Boğazköy Cybele: the large sixth century statue shows the goddess standing with two smaller-sized male musicians, an *aulos*-player and a *kithara* player, on either side (Fig. 5). Interestingly, as Roller points out, these instruments, the *kithara* and the *aulos*, have nothing to do with the percussion instruments that create unrestrained ecstatic music associated with the cult of Cybele and her followers in Greco-Roman sources.[43] Thus, the Boğazköy statue shows us that the music in the Cybele cult in Phrygia incorporated *kithara* and *aulos*, and possibly other musical instruments, played by musicians of different genders in cult ritual.

Sixth century funerary reliefs from Lycia offer a few depictions of musicians, specifically *kithara*-players, performing in public festivities next to wrestlers.[44]

38 Among the other Greek sources on the music of Cybele: Euripides Bacchae 55–63, 124–134; Euripides Helen 1308, 1347; Strabo 10.3.15–17; Catullus 63. 22–26. See Roller 1999, 151–161 for a broader discussion.

39 Diogenes *Athenaios* 1.2. Also see Roller 1999, 151, n. 24.

40 See for example, Roller 1999, 152, fig. 43.

41 See the discussion in Roller 1999, 136–138, fig. 41.

42 See for example, the Cybele relief from Gordion in Akurgal 1961, 98, fig. 62

43 Roller 1999, 110.

44 See the *kithara*-players on the famous Wrestler relief from Xanthos and the reliefs of the Pillar Tomb I from Isinda. Draycott 2007a, 109–110, figs. 3–4.

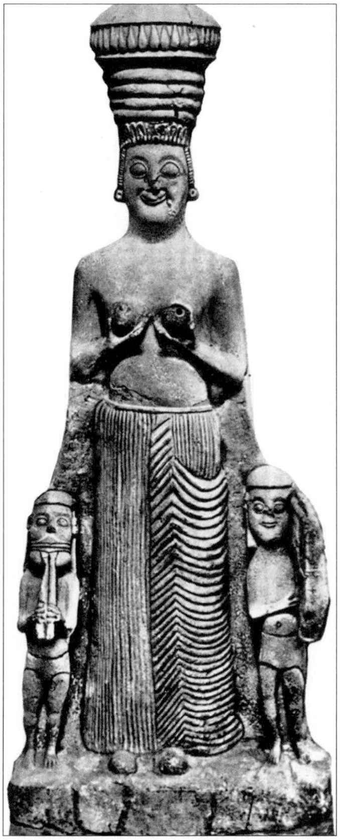

FIG. 5 Boğazköy Cybele, photo after Akurgal 1961, 91, fig. 55.

Musicians also appear on the later fifth and fourth century Lycian art.[45] Yet, in all of the extant examples the musicians are male. Furthermore, there is not any extensive literary evidence to enlighten musical practices in Lycia.

There are no musical representations found at Lydian Sardis so far.[46] Yet, the influence of Lydian music on Greek culture is well attested in literature and art.[47] The harp, for example, which appears in Greek imagery of the early fifth century, is believed to have been introduced into Greek culture from Lydia.[48] Similarly, another stringed instrument, the *barbitos*, which appears in Greek iconography in the sixth century, and is often linked with Eastern Greek poets like Sappho, Alkaios, Anakreon, seems to have come to Greek musical culture through Lydian

45 See, for example, the trumpet-players in the procession of Perikle on the west frieze of the Heroon of Perikle at Limyra, Şare 2013, 62, figs. 7–9.

46 Franklin 2007, 197.

47 Franklin 2007, 196–200.

48 West 1994, 349; Bundrick 2005, 30.

contacts.[49] Not only the specific instruments but also the so-called "Lydian mode" and the so-called "Phrygian mode" in Greek music seem to have their origins in Asia Minor.[50]

Greek literature also hints at a more independent social status for the women of Western Anatolia, compared to Greek women in the sixth and fifth centuries. When comparing Lydian and Greek social customs, Heredotus, for example, mentions working class Lydian girls, who raise their own dowry through prostitution until they get married (I. 193).[51] Heredotus' note is nothing more than an outsider's perception of Lydian culture, but representations of local women on Achaemenid period art found within the cultural periphery of former Lydian lands indeed implies different status and roles for women.[52] On several Achaemenid period funerary stelai and frescoes women appear side by side with their husbands in banquets being entertained by musicians and being served by male and female servants, whereas in contemporary Attic art, citizen women are mostly shown confined to women's quarters with only female servants. Furthermore, Athenian wives are never shown as reclining or sitting with men in banquet scenes, the task being reserved for *hetariai* performing in symposiastic banquets.[53] Based on this comparison, then, one can envision the possible existence of Lydian females working as professional musicians and singers. Yet, it is still hard to identify with certainty on which occasions the female musicians of Lydia performed and what kind of instruments they used. Not from Sardis, but close to the Lydian land, we know of female poetic social groups like that of Sappho in Mytilene, whose meetings included musical performances

49 Franklin 2007, 197; West 1994, 336; Bundrick (2005, 22) notes that unlike the harp, which was continuously used in Greek imagery after the fifth century, the imagery of *barbitos* disappears after the fifth century, as does the instrument itself in Greek musical culture.

50 West 1994, 331, 358.

51 Heredotus (I, 173) also says that Lycians were matrilineal, taking their mother's name rather than their father's.

52 The role and status of women in Western Anatolia during the sixth and fifth centuries have not been dealt with in detail in the scholarship. The only focus on this issue thus far has been Draycott's talk at the Annual Meeting of the AIA in 2007. Through her investigation of the representations of women in funerary art of Western Anatolia, Draycott suggests that there were more relaxed marital relations and more potential for female roles of power in the region when compared to mainland Greece, see Draycott 2007c.

53 Draycott (2007c) points out that the female enthronement scenes on some of these funerary stelai suggest greater female authority than that suggested by the otherwise similar mistress and maid images of Attic funerary art. She also stresses the emphasis on the "nuptial couple" motif on the funerary banquet scenes, which come closer to the same motif in Etruscan art.

accompanying the poems, including wedding songs and hymns.[54] Considering the interplay between Anatolian and Greek culture in early sixth century Western Anatolia, one can consider the likelihood of the existence of similar groups within the cultural periphery of the Lydian empire.[55] Another aspect of Greek musical culture, choruses of young females and dancers performing in rituals, and female singers lamenting in funerals might have also continued in the cities of Western Anatolia under Lydian and under Achaemenid political control after 546.[56] Indeed, on a late sixth century fragmentary column drum from Cyme, a young female cult participant is shown frontally holding hands with two other frontally shown figures, possibly to indicate that she is performing in a ring dance.[57]

Despite the lack of imagery of female musicians and dancers in sixth century Lydia and Phrygia, Hellespontine Phrygia provides rich visual evidence. The so-called Polyxena Sarcophagus discovered in a tumulus in Gümüşçay in the Troad region includes female dancers and musicians in its extensive sculptural program (FIG. 6). The product of a Greek workshop and dated to between 500–490 on stylistic grounds, it is the earliest stone sarcophagus with figural reliefs ever to be found in Asia Minor.[58] Its frieze includes the representation of the brutal sacrifice of Polyxena by the tomb of Achilles and mourning Trojan women on one side (Side A); and a processional festivity with gift bearers, musicians, and dancers on the other long side (Side C). The two short sides depict a mourning scene including Polyxena's mother, Hecuba, under a barren tree (Side B) and an indoor scene with females seated on a *kline* (Side D).

Side C contains 17 figures involved in a celebration with gifts, music and dances. The protagonist of the frieze is a large veiled female seated on an elaborate throne with a flower in her hand. From the right, two women approach her, one with a bowl of eggs and a mirror and the other with alabastra in both hands. On the left, four more women approach the girl from behind. The one on the far left holds a *chelys* lyre with a plectrum attached to the end of a cord in one hand and an egg in the other hand,[59] the

54 See Blundell (1995, 82–92) for the extant fragmentary poems of Sappho. As Blundell notes, it is not certain whether Sappho's poems were performed in a small community restricted to females or for the general public.

55 For the amalgamation of Greek and Lydian customs in the sixth century BCE, see for example Rein 1997.

56 See Calame (1997) for choruses of young females and Stears (2008) for female lamenters in ancient Greece.

57 For the relief of the column drum from Cyme, see Akurgal 1961, 257, fig. 220.

58 For the detailed discussions of the Polyxena Sarcophagus see Sevinç 1996; Steuernagel 1998; Reinsberg 2001; Draycott 2007b; Ateşlier and Öncü 2004; Rose 2013. Here, I preferred to use Rose's dating of the sarcophagus (Rose 2013, 100).

59 The cords, which were typically used to attach the plectrum to the lyre to keep it being lost, are commonly represented on Athenian vases with images of *chelys* lyres, see Bundrick 2005, 18.

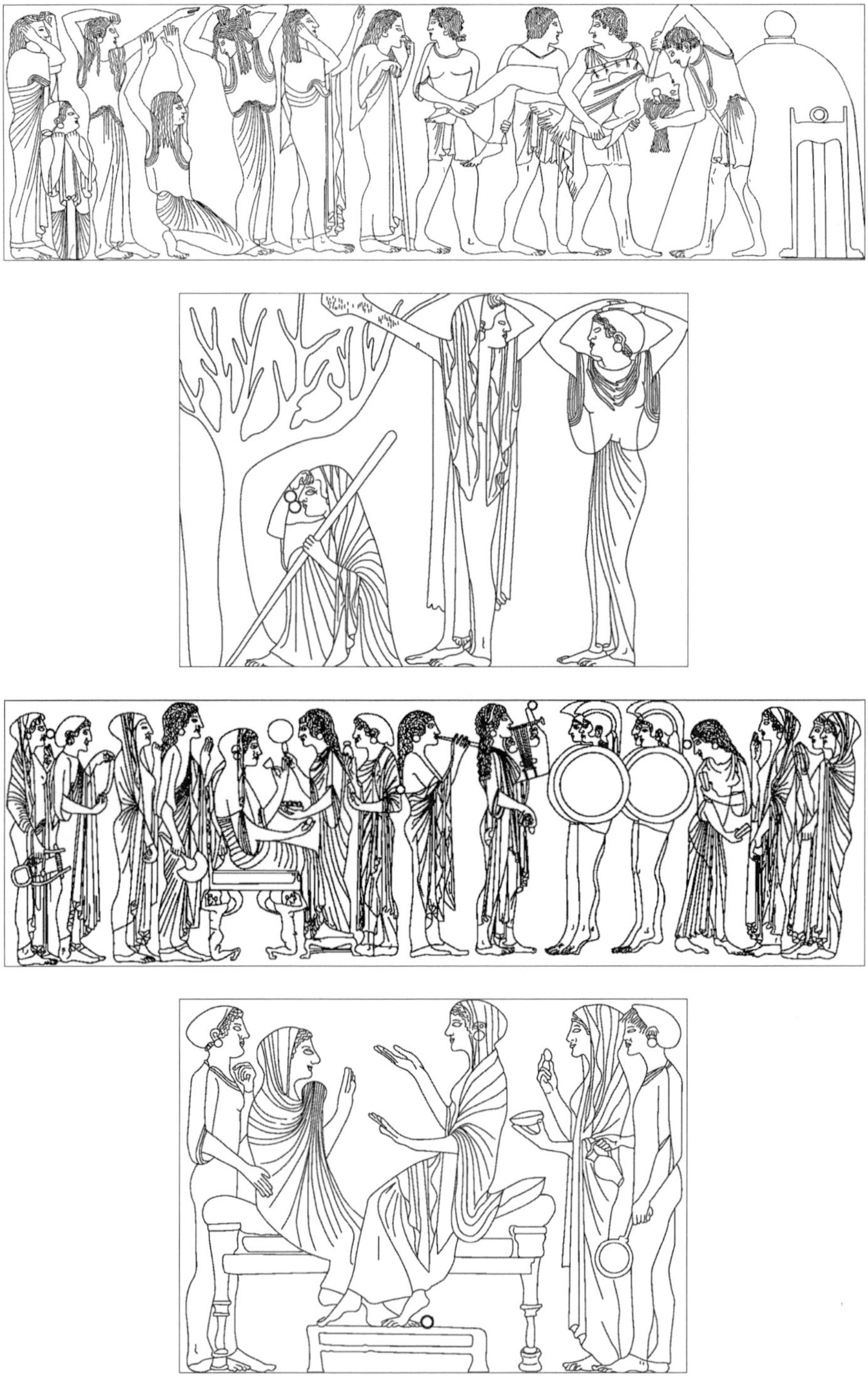

Fig. 6 Drawings of the reliefs of the Polyxena Sarcophagus, after Draycott 2007, pl. 50. Side A, Side B. Opposite Side C and Side D

second carries a fillet, the third is without an offering, and the fourth holds a fan. On the right side of the frieze, the composition becomes more energetic with four armed (Pyrrhic) dancers, dancing on tiptoes to the music played by a female *aulos*-player and a *kithara*-player, who holds the *kithara* against her left shoulder and a plectrum (attached to the *kithara* via a long cord hanging down) in the right hand.[60] One other woman with a twisted body dances to the rhythms of the castanets she plays in her hands. Three more women on the right end of the frieze watch the dance scene.

Despite the obvious mythological references, namely the sacrifice of Polyxena on Side A and Hecuba in mourning on Side B, proposed identifications of the indoor scene on Side D, two females seated on a *kline*, and a processional celebration with musicians on Side C have remained controversial. Most scholars have preferred to interpret the depictions on Sides C and D as funerary rituals (a funerary procession and a funerary banquet, respectively).[61] Others, however, have suggested that they refer to courtly celebrations in a women's quarter, possibly a wedding ceremony.[62] Indeed, the central females seated on a throne on Side C and on a *kline* (next to a larger female figure) on Side D seem to represent a court bride receiving gifts and being entertained (Side C) and being prepared for her passage of life in an indoor initiation ceremony (Side D).[63] An overall look at the iconography of the

60 Because she is the tallest and she wears a fillet, Rose (2013, 90) suggests that the *kithara*-player is presumably the band-leader.

61 Sevinç 1994, 260; Steuernagel 1998, 171. Rose (2013, 89–95) interprets Sides C and D as celebrations, but a funerary one celebrating the life of the deceased.

62 Draycott (2007b, 119) considers the scene as a courtly celebration, not specifically a funerary one. Ateşlier and Öncü (2004, 59–61) argue that the scene depicts the wedding of Polyxena and Achilles in the underworld. Reinsberg (2001) and Şare (2006) also argue for a representation of a wedding ceremony.

63 Rose disagrees with the wedding ceremony interpretation for Sides C and D by pointing out that the ceremony lacks the common gifts presented to the brides on wedding scenes on Greek vases such as kalathoi, lekanai, and jewelry chests. Stressing the use of eggs, common funerary offerings in Greek, Etruscan, and Anatolian iconography, Rose suggests that the ceremony is funereal (see Rose 2013, 94). Yet, the presence of eggs as offerings to the bride might have also functioned as a fertility offering to the bride to be. Within the general iconographical program, the offering of eggs on Sides C and D might have been used as a provision for eternal energy and life in the underworld for the unmarried girl, with the frieze giving the message that "the funeral is taking place like a wedding"; in other words, she is 'marrying her death.' Both literary and archaeological evidence exists for such a conflation of death and marriage, especially for girls who died unmarried. The artists of the sarcophagus seem to have utilized the overlapping features of the nuptial and funereal practices well known in Greek culture to emphasize the heroism of the deceased. In both the wedding and the funeral the girl is ritually bathed, adorned and dressed by women. The deceased is covered, as the bride is covered with a veil. Both ceremonies involve a procession with music and dance. Thus, the girl, about to abandon her kin, is accompanied to her unknown dwelling (see Şare 2006 for a detailed discussion).

sarcophagus reveals a program combining the brutal death of a young girl with the courtly wedding of another.[64] The intentional conflation of death and marriage on the Polyxena sarcophagus suggests that the sarcophagus was initially produced for an unmarried aristocratic woman, whose tragic "marriage to death" has been associated with that of another heroine from mythology.[65]

Having interpreted the friezes of Sides C and D as bridal-funereal arrangements for a woman who perhaps never lived to see her marriage and whose status is elevated to that of a heroine, we can now turn back to the female musicians of Side C. As mentioned above, one of the women approaching the enthroned bride holds a *chelys* lyre with a plectrum attached to the lyre via a cord. The lyre as an offering, which is not played by the woman who carries it, might refer to the educated musical ability of the court bride herself, as the fan, mirrors, and the fillet held by other female maids might refer to her luxurious courtly status.[66] Indeed, starting with its earliest appearance in the early seventh century in Greek art, the lyre is associated with aristocratic education.[67] In Athenian art, apart from the Muses, the *chelys* lyre appears in the hands of mortal aristocratic women only in the second half of the fifth century, several decades after the Polyxena sarcophagus. Another stringed instrument shown played by a female on the sarcaphagus is the concert *kithara*. This kind of *kithara* is always associated with virtuoso performances of professional male musicians, namely *kitharodes*, in public contests in Greek culture. Mortal Greek women never appear playing the *kithara* in contemporary and slightly later Athenian art.[68] Dressed in a chiton and with a long mantle hanging down from her shoulder, the *aulos*-player of the frieze also departs from its Greek contemporaries since the *aulos* usually appears being played by divinities and immortal Muses or nude or semi-nude courtesans in the contexts of male symposia.[69]

64 See Şare 2006 for the detailed discussion of the conflation of death and marriage in the iconographical program of the Polyxena Sarcophagus.

65 Surprisingly, the looted sarcophagus contained only the bones of a middle-aged man. The abundant female iconography, however, suggests that the reliefs were intended for a female occupant. Unfinished details of the friezes, such as the drill holes and not yet carved body parts, especially on Side D, further indicate that the sarcophagus was intended for someone else, but it was reassigned for a man's use before it was finished. See Rose (2013, 97–100) for the relation between the patron and the iconography. A very recent shocking theory by Tim McNiven (2014) explains the confusing relationship between the female oriented iconography and the male occupant of the sarcophagus by suggesting that a transvestite eunuch priest of Cybele is buried inside.

66 Draycott 2007c, 105. Rose (2013, 90) suggests that the fillet being offered to the girl is possibly meant to represent a luxurious textile dyed in expensive Tyrian purple.

67 Bundrick 2005, 14.

68 Bundrick 2005, 18–26.

69 Bundrick 2005, 37–39.

The female dancer with castanets is one of the earliest that appears in the work of a Greek sculptor.[70] The twisted pose of her body to convey the art of dancing is unique. Steuernagel suggests that this posture indicates performance of an "ecstatic" dance.[71] Like the exaggerated poses of the mourners on Side A, the posture may indicate an Anatolian way of dancing or maybe a special dance like the *imeneos*, the dance of the marriage with a lot of twists and turns.[72] The gender of the Pyrrhic dancers on the frieze has been a controversial issue. Draycott and Reinsberg suggest that they are probably armed female dancers, since they are not nude but wear *perizomai* (shorts) and the shields they held in their hands obscure their bodies.[73] Draycott and Reinsberg also point out the existence of female Pyrrhic dancers who performed not in funerals but in celebrations like weddings in Greek art and literature.[74] Rose, on the other hand, by pointing out the hairstyle of the soldiers, which correspond to the male soldiers holding Polyxena on Side A, and also the tendency to depict males clothed rather than nude in the arts of Western Anatolia suggest that they are indeed male Pyrrhic dancers performing in a public funeral.[75] Whether they are armed males dancing to the music played by professional female musicians or male soldiers, they are part of a celebrative public event, directed, attended and performed by women. This is interesting in itself, since it shows the kind of power and entertainment afforded to an aristocratic woman in Hellespontine Phrygia, as opposed to the representations of more modest preparations for wedding festivities mostly restricted to the women quarters on Athenian vases.[76] The concert *kithara* played by a female musician and armed dancers (male or female) performing to a female audience are exceptionally unusual, since the instrument and the similar dancers (of male gender) appear in male-dominated public events in contemporary Greek art and culture.[77] Furthermore, a female *kithara* player and the association of an aristocratic girl with the ability to play a lyre are indicative of the professional musical

70 Even though the iconography of the sarcophagus has unique Anatolian features, the style is Greek, indicating that it is the product of Greek sculptors, see also Brian 2013, 101–103 on this.

71 Steuernagel, 1998, 172.

72 *Imeneos* was danced by the bride with her mother and friends in ancient Greek wedding ceremonies, see Lawler 1965.

73 Reinsberg 2001, 83–84; Draycott 2007b, 106.

74 Reinsberg 2001, 83–84; Draycott 2007b, 106. McNiven (2014) identifies the scene on Side C as a seated Kybele with attendants and the armed dancers as Coribantes of uncertain gender.

75 Rose 2013, 94.

76 Oakley and Sinos 1993.

77 See also Draycott 2007b, 106.

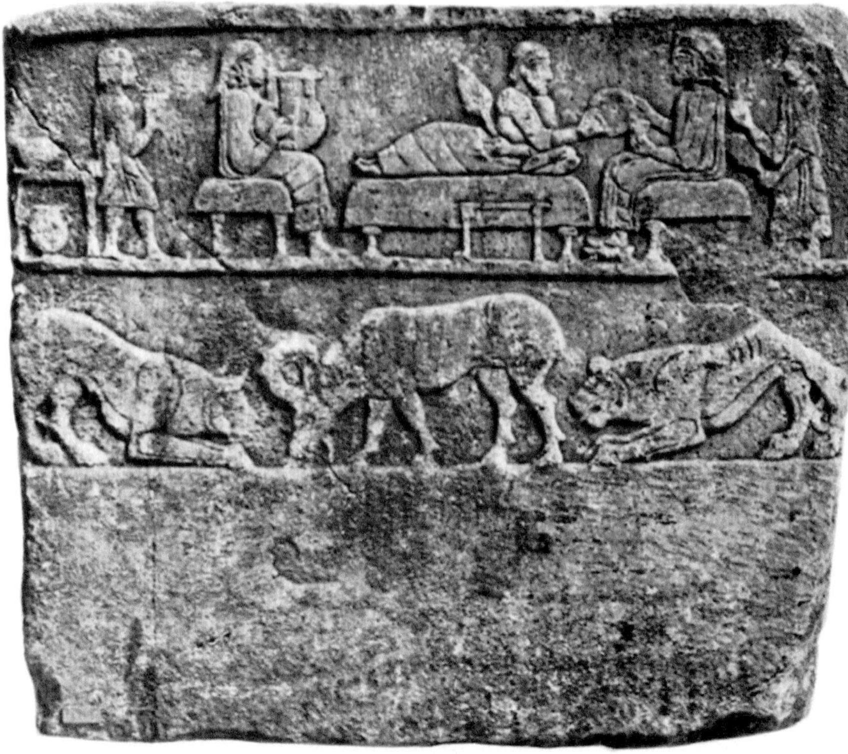

Fig. 7 Ödemiş relief, photo after Dentzer 1982, pl. 58, fig. 318.

education provided to females in Hellespontine Phrygia in the sixth and fifth centuries. The all-women music band and the dancers on the Polyxena sarcophagus are very unique with no parallel in Greek iconography, but with parallel imagery on earlier Urartian iconography.

The Imagery of Female Musicians in Western Anatolia in the Fifth and Fourth Centuries

Images of musicians continue to exist in the arts of Western Anatolia in the fifth and fourth centuries. The visual data from Achaemenid centers, such as funerary stelai from Daskyleion, indicate that the *kithara*- and *aulos*-players were part of courtly activities attended both by male and females. Because of the crude style of most of the extant examples, the gender of these musicians is uncertain.[78] Only on one fifth

78 See the musicians of the banquet scene on the top register of the Stele of Addā from Daskyleion, dated to around 450 BCE (Draycott 2007b, 290, cat. no. 17).

century stele from Ödemiş, now in the İzmir Archaeology Museum, a female *kithara*-player in a banquet scene is discernible (FIG. 7).[79] Unlike the standing servants, she appears clad in an elaborate dress, suggesting her higher social standing compared to the servants. She is one of the two women symmetrically placed as seated on each side of a reclining man, underscoring a similar high status for both women. As already mentioned above, the most popular motif on the Achaemenid reliefs of Western Anatolia, the funerary banquet or *Totenmahl* depictions, usually incorporate respectable female family members of a male protagonist seated next to him. Overall, the popular motif conveys the notion of a princely house with its members of both genders and their courtly activities.[80] Thus, the Ödemiş relief implies the possible existence of professional female musicians of high status performing in courtly and ritual activities to an audience of both genders in Western Anatolia.

The female musicians, especially dancers and *aulos*- and *kithara*-players, appear in the form of terracotta figurines in fourth century Asia Minor.[81] The most striking among these are a group of female musicians discovered in a late fourth century tomb of a woman at the Western Necropolis of Assos (FIG. 8A–B).[82] Found along with a variety of other types of figurines, vases and jewelry, the female group consists of a *kithara*-player, a female poet holding a scroll, an *aulos*-player, a rattle- (*krotolas*) player and a dancer by an altar. Apart from the dancer, who wears a long belted tunic and a bashlyk, and the nude *aulos*-player, all of the females are dressed in long chitons with mantles on top. Only the poet seems to have an additional tunic with long loose sleeves. All the seated figurines wear *sakkoi* covering their hair buns. Except the dancer, they are all shown as seated on chairs with their feet resting on footstools.

The dancer, with hands clasped over the tilted head as the body sways towards the altar, has several parallels in fourth century Greek mainland and Anatolian

79 The relief is often associated with the Kayster River Valley (see Altınoluk 2013, 78, fig. 136; Draycott 2007b, 305, cat. no. 29).

80 See Draycott, forthcoming, on the *Totenmahl* representations in late Archaic and Achaemenid Western Anatolia.

81 For the female musician type in terracotta in general, see Winter 1903, II, 138–142; most examples come from the third century tombs of Myrina and Tanagra. The known examples closest to Assos are two female *kithara* players slightly later in date: a later fourth century seated *kithara*-player from the so-called Dardanos Tumulus (not published yet) and another standing third century example from Ilion (Thompson 1963, 107, pl. xxvi, fig. 102), both in the collection of the Çanakkale Archaeology Museum.

82 See Şare and Arslan, 2015, for the detailed discussion of the tomb and the figurines. The analysis of the skeletons confirm that one woman and another adolescent of unknown gender were buried in this cist grave, the so called M4 tomb.

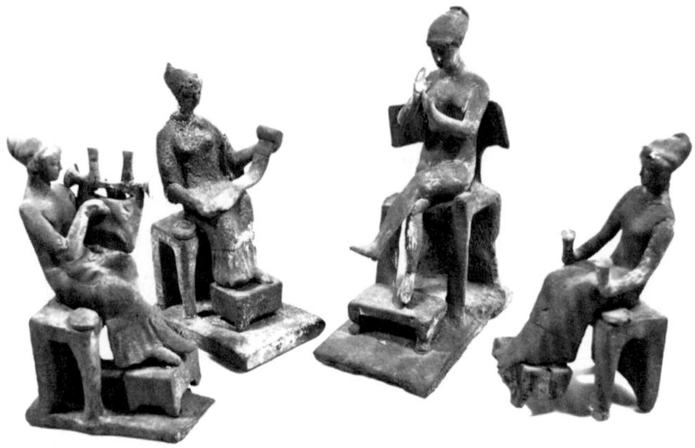

Fig. 8a Terracotta figurines of seated musicians from M4 Tomb, photo credit @ Assos Excavations.

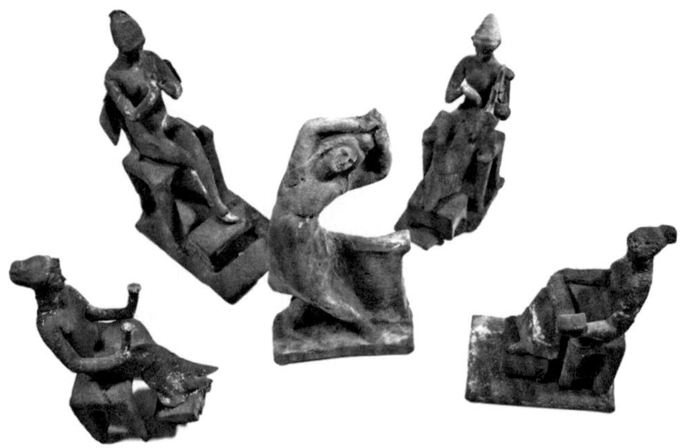

Fig. 8b Terracotta figurines of seated musicians and dancers from M4 Tomb, photo credit @ Assos Excavations.

iconography (Fig. 8b).[83] The type, known as the *oklasma* dancer, is often associated with female performers of the cult rituals of Dionysus and Cybele. As typical of fourth century male fashion in Anatolia, the figure is clad in 'oriental' dress—tight pants, knee-length tunic and bashlyk.[84] This dress is suggestive of male gender for the figure, but one should not rule out the existence of female cross-dressing in ritual activities. Indeed, we have discussed the possible female identity for the armed Pyrrhic dancers on the earlier Polyxena sarcophagus above.

At first glance, the cache of seated figurines is reminiscent of a group of Muses (Fig. 8a). Yet, there is no way of knowing whether these figurines refer to mortal

83 For the type in general see Winter 1903, II 158, figs. 1–8. See Thompson 1963, 100–102, pl. 23, no. 86 for a similar example of an *oklasma* dancer type from Ilion and the origin and the iconographic discussion of the type.

84 See Şare 2011 for Western Anatolian dress fashions in fourth century Western Anatolia.

or immortal women. If the figurines represent Muses, they provide evidence for the kinds of inspiration the female occupant of the tomb needed for her daily activities at Assos or activities that mourners hoped she would practice in the afterlife: reading poetry and playing the *kithara*, the *aulos*, and the rattles. If, on the other hand, they are mortal women, they reflect the social gatherings (usually for religious purposes) of high-class Assian women in the early fourth century. As mentioned earlier, such female social groups with musical performances accompanying the poems are well known from nearby Archaic Lesbos. In either case, the figurines hint at the intellectual environment of aristocratic women at Assos and indicate the existence of professionally trained female musical groups in fourth century Asia Minor.

In which contexts (private or public) these female musicians performed are hard to know. If it is indeed a female, the Assian dancer by the altar implies the involvement of female dancers in cult ritual. The rich gold jewelry, perfume bottles, the amount and the types of other figurines found in the same tomb suggest that the Assian woman tomb owner came from an economically high class. Thus, the figurines of female musicians in her possession reflect, once again, the social gatherings (usually for religious purposes) of aristocratic Assian women in the mid fourth century.

Similar to the group from Assos, gold diadems found in mid fourth-century Hellespontine tombs display cast images of female musicians reading scrolls and playing a variety of instruments, flanking the central figures of Dionysus and Ariadne.[85] Among these, the so-called Ilgardere diadem contains eight seated female musicians playing the harp, the *aulos*, the lyre and a lute-like instrument and two female poets, each of whom reads a poem from a scroll on opposite sides of the divine couple. Once crowning the head of a high-status woman, possibly the occupant of the tomb, the diadem reflects the significance of music and poetry in a woman's life and afterlife in the region. The actual discovery of *auloi* and *kithara* fragments from the late fourth century Hellespontine tombs suggests that female musicians like those on the earlier Polyxena sarcophagus continued to perform in courtly and cultic activities in this region.[86] Rose suggests that these are the instruments used in the musical performances of funerary ceremonies and buried along with the deceased in the tomb.[87] Yet, they might also be the belongings of the deceased aristocratic women who had received a sophisticated musical education.

85 For the Ilgardere diadem and contemporary parallels from the same region, see Körpe 2004.

86 For the fragments of an ivory *aulos* discovered at the Dedetepe tomb, see Rose 2013, 122. For the fragments of a stringed instrument discovered at Dardanos Tumulus, see Byrne 1993.

87 Rose 2013, 174.

The instruments might have been buried along with them as tribute to their elite status and also as their essential needs in the afterlife.[88]

Conclusion

Ancient depictions of musicians remind us of the variety of occasions and different social contexts in which music is played or deployed. Perhaps it is a cliché to point this out, but we sometimes take for granted the omnipresence of music in our lives today and forget about its omnipresence in the past as well, a past that is silent since music can only be heard in the present, in the moment it is being played. Thus, the depictions of musicians have the evocative power of bringing us back to that 'moment' in that past.

With the hope of shedding some light on past musical cultures, in my discussion of the imagery of female musicians in ancient Anatolia, I have tackled several intertwining issues, such as gender and social status, gender and music and musical education and status. Due to the limitations of the evidence, not every question is answered but with the examination of the specific imagery we have encountered both professional and non-professional female musicians, (singers, instrument players, and dancers) consistently active in cult ritual, funereal, and nuptial ceremonies. Hittite imagery indicates that priestesses in cultic festivities danced, sang, and played percussion instruments while stringed instruments were reserved for male priests, who probably obtained a more professional training. The representations on Urartian belts imply the existence of a professional group of female musicians playing a variety of instruments, dancing and singing in courtly nuptial festivities in the Urartian culture of Eastern Anatolia. The iconography of the Polyxena sarcophagus and Achaemenid-style stelai indicate that similar female musical bands and dancers continued to perform in nuptial, funereal, and cultic ceremonies in late sixth and fifth century Western Anatolia. Representations of these women not simply as low-class entertainers, but as essential members of the courtly ceremonies, and the range of instruments they appear playing suggest a high social status for them. Indeed, in the fourth century, the knowledge of literature and music, especially the ability to play stringed and wind instruments seem to have become an indicator of elite female identity in Western Anatolia.

88 Indeed, among the variety of goods for multiple burials found in the Dardanos Tumulus, the stringed instruments and the terracotta figurines of seated females playing the *kithara* seem to be contemporary.

REFERENCES

Akurgal, E., *Die Kunst Anatoliens von Homer bis Alexander.* Berlin: De Gruyter, 1961.

Alp, S. *Hititlerde Şarkı Müzik ve Dans.* Ankara: Kavaklıdere Kültür Yayınları, 1999.

Altınoluk, S., *Hypaipa. A Lydian City During the Roman Imperial Period.* İstanbul: Ege Yayınları, 2013.

Anlağan, T., "Sadberk Hanım Müzesi'ndeki Bir Urartu Kemeri Üzerine Gözlemler." *PALMET* II (1998): 51–60.

Ateşlier, S. and Öncü, E., "Gümüşçay Polyksena Lahiti Üzerine Yeni Gözlemler: Mimari ve İkonografik Açıdan Bakış." *Olba* 10 (2004): 45–87.

Belli, O., "Urartularda Kadın Müzisyen ve Dansçılar" in *Festschrift in Honor of Belkıs Dinçol and Ali Dinçol,* ed. by M. Alparslan and M. Doğan-Alparslan, 87–105. İstanbul: Ege Yayınları, 2007.

Bittel, K., "Cymbeln für Kybele" in *Festschrift fur Wasmuth zum 80 Geburtstag,* ed. by Kollegen und Autoren, 79–82. Tübingen, 1968.

Blundell, S. *Women in Ancient Greece.* Cambridge: Harvard University Press, 1995.

Boehmer, R. M. and Güterbock, H.G., "Glyptik aus den Stadtgebiet von Boğazköy, Grabungskampagnen 1931–1939, 1952–1978." *Boğazköy-Hattusa XIV.* Berlin, 1987.

Bryne, M., "The Dardanos Fragments and the 40° Angular Lyre" *The Galpin Society Journal* 46 (1993): 3–25.

Bundrick, S. *Music and Image in Classical Athens.* New York, 2005.

Burkert, W. *Greek Religion.* Cambridge, 1985.

Calame, C. *Choruses of Young Women in Ancient Greece: Their Morphology, Religious Role, and Social Functions.* Lanham, 1997.

Celasin, C. and Beşiroğlu, Ş., "Hitit Medeniyeti Müzik Kültürünün Analizinde Arkeolojik Verilerin Rolü" *İTÜ Dergisi-Sosyal Bilimler* 2 (2006.):35–46

De Martino, S., "Music, Dance and Processions in Hittite Anatolia" in *Civilizations of the Ancient Near East IV,* ed. by J.M. Sasson. 2661–2670. New York: Charles Scribner's Sons, 1995.

Dentzer, J.M., *Le motif du banquet couché dans le Proche-Orient et le monde grec du VIIe siècle avant J.-C.* Rome: Bibliothèque des écoles françaises d'Athène de de Rome, 1982.

Dinçol, B., *Eski Önasya ve Mısır'da Müzik.* Eskiçağ Bilimleri Enstitüsü Yayınları 11, İstanbul, 1999.

Draycott, C.M., "Dynastic definitions: Differentiating Status Claims in the Archaic Pillar Tomb Reliefs of Lyci" in *Anatolian Iron Ages* 6. *The Proceedings of the Sixth Anatolian Iron Ages Symposium,* Ancient Near Eastern Studies Supplement 20, ed. by A. Sagona and A. Çilingiroğlu, 103–134. Louvain: Peeters, 2007a.

———. *Images and Identities in the Funerary Arts of Anatolia, 600–450 BC: Phrygia, Hellespontine Phrygia, Lydia.* D. Phil. Thesis, University of Oxford, 2007b.

———. "Roles and Representations of Women in the Funerary Monuments of Archaic Period Western Anatolia." Paper presented at the *109th Annual Meeting of American Institute of Archaeology*, 2007c.

———. "Drinking to Death: The 'Totenmahl', drinking culture and funerary representation in late Archaic and Achaemenid Western Anatolia" in Proceedings of the Conference *Dining & Death: Interdisciplinary Perspectives on the 'Funerary Banquet' in Ancient Art, Burial and Belief*, ed. by C. M. Draycott. Oxford, forthcoming.

Franklin, J. C., "A Feast of Music": A Greco- Lydian Musical Movement on the Assyrian Periphary" in *Anatolian Interfaces: Hittites, Greeks and Their Neighbors,* ed. by B.J. Collins, M. Bachvarova./ I. Rutherford, 193–203. Oxford: Oxbow Books, 2007.

Güterbock, H.G., "Reflections on the Musical Instruments arkammi, galgalturi and huhupa in Hittite" in *Studio Historiae Ardens. Festschrift fur Ph. H.J. Houwink ten Cate,* ed. by Theo P.J. van den Hout and J. de Roos, 57–72. İstanbul: Nederlands Historisch-Archaeologisch Instituut te İstanbul, 1995.

Hoffner, H.A., "Legal and Social Institutions of Hittite Anatolia" in *Civilizations of the Ancient Near East I,* ed. by J.M. Sasson, K. Rubison, J. Baines, 555–569. New York: Charles Scribner's Sons, 1995.

Hornbostel, E. M. and Sachs C., "Systematik der Musikinstrumente: Ein Versuch" *Zeitschrift für Ethnologie* 46 (1914): 553- 590.

Imparati, F., "Private Life Among the Hittites" in *Civilizations of the Ancient Near East I,* ed. by J.M. Sasson, K. Rubison, J. Baines, 571–585. New York: Charles Scribner's Sons, 1995.

Kellner, H., *Urartu A Metalworking Center in the First Millennium BCE.* Tel Aviv, 1991.

Körpe, R., " A Gold Diadem from Ilgardere-Gelibolu" *Studia Troica* 14 (2004): 141–145.

Landels, J.G., *Music in Ancient Greece and Rome*. London and New York: Routledge, 1999.

Lawler, L.B., *The Dance in Ancient Greece*. Middletown: Wesleyan, 1965.

Mathiesen, T., *Apollo's Lyre: Greek Music and Music Theory in Antiquity and the Middle Ages.* Nebraska: ACLS Humanities, 1999.

McNiven, T., "Woman as Status Symbol? The Polyxena Sarcophagus and a Krater from Thrace." Paper presented at the *115th Annual Meeting of the American Institute of Archaeology*, 2014.

Miyashita, S., "La scène du banquet dans les ceintures urartéennes." *Bulletin of the Ancient Orient Museum* 5: 299–318. 1983

Oakley, J and Sinos, R., *The Wedding in Ancient Athens*. Wisconsin: University of Wisconsin Press, 1993.

Özgüç, T., "The Bitik Vase." *Ankara Üniversitesi, Dil ve Tarih-Coğrafya Fakültesi Dergisi* XVI/1–2 (1957): 1–18.

———. *Kültepe-Kanis II, Eski Yakındoğu'nun Ticaret Merkezinde Yeni Araştırmalar.* Ankara: Türk Tarih Kurumu Yayınları, 1986.

———. *İnandıktepe. Eski Hitit Çağında Önemli bir Kült Merkezi.* Ankara: Türk Tarih Kurumu Yayınları, 1988.

Özgüç, T. and M. Akok, *Horoztepe.* Ankara, 1958.

Redmond, L., *When the Drummers Were Women: A Spiritual History of Rhythm.* New York: Three Rivers Press, 1997.

Rein, M.J., " 'Anatolianism' and the Costume of the East Greek Korai." *American Journal of Archaeology* 96 (abstract), 1992.

Reinsberg, C., "Der Polyxena-Sarkophag in Çanakkale." *Olba* 4 (2001): 70–99.

Roller, L.E., *In Search of God the Mother: The Cult of Anatolian Cybele.* Berkeley: UNiversity of California Press, 1999.

Rose, B., *The Archaeology of Greek and Roman Troy.* Cambridge: Cambridge University Press, 2013.

Rosenzweig, R., *Worshipping Aphrodite: Art and Cult in Classical Athens.* Ann Arbor: University of Michigan Press, 2004.

Rutherford, I., "When you go to the Maedow....'": The Lament of the Taptara-Women in the Hittite Sallis Wastais Ritual" in *Lament: Studies in the Ancient Mediterranean and Beyond,* ed. by A. Suter, 55–70. Oxford: Oxford University Press, 2008.

Şare, T., "'*Marriage to Death' on the Polyxena Sarcophagus.*" MA Thesis, Rutgers University, 2006.

———. *Dress and Identity in the Arts of Anatolia: The Seventh through Fourth Centuries BCE.* PhD thesis, Rutgers University, 2010.

Şare, T. and N.A. Aslan, *Terracotta Treasure from Assos.* İstanbul: Ege Yayınları, 2015.

Seidl, U., *Bronzekunst Urartus.* Mainz: Verlag Philipp von Zabern in Wissenschaftliche Buchgesellschaft, 2004.

———. "Rattling and Clapping Urartian Girls: Idiophones in Urartu" in *Archaeology of Armenia in Regional Context,* ed. by P. Avetisyan and A. Bobokhyan, 163–170. Yerevan: Academy of Sciences Press, 2012.

Sevinç, N., "A New Sarcophagus of Polyxena from the Salvage Excavations at Gümüsçay." *Studia Troica* 6 (1996): 251–264

Sipahi, T., "Eine altethitische Reliefvase von Hüseyindede Tepesi." *Istanbuller Mitteilungen* 50 (2000.): 61–81.

Stears, K., "Death Becomes Her: Gender and Athenian Death Ritual" in *Lament: Studies in the Ancient Mediterranean and Beyond,* ed. by A. Suter, 139–156. Oxford: Oxford University Press, 2008.

Steuernagel, D., "Ein spätarchaischer Sarkophage aus Gümüşçay im Museum von Çanakkale. Ikonographsiche Beobachtungen" in *Archäologische Studien in Kontaktzonen der Antiken Welt,* ed. by R. Rolle, K. Schmidt, 165–177. Göttingen, 1998.

Thompson, D.B., *Troy: The Terracotta Figurines of the Hellenistic Period.* Princeton: Princeton University Press, 1963.

West, M. L. *Ancient Greek Music.* New York: Clarendon Press, 1994.

Winter, F., *Die Antiken Terrakotten*, Vol II. Stuttgart, 1903.

Yıldırım, T., "Yörüklü / Hüseyindede: Eine neue hethitische Siedlung im Südwesten von Çorum" *Istanbuller Mitteilungen* 50 (2000a): 41- 60.

———. "Music in Hüseyindede/Yörüklü: Some New Musical Scenes on the Second Hittite Relief." *Anadolu Araştırmaları* 16 (2000b): 591–560.

———. "Hüseyindede Kabartmalı Vazosunda Betimlenen Dans Eden Bir Hittitli" *Ankara Üniversitesi Dil ve Tarih Coğrafya Fakültesi Dergisi* 41 (2001.): 1–7.

———. "Hüseyindede Tepesi'nde Bulunan İkinci Kabartmalı Vazoya Ait Yeni Bir Müzisyen." *Ankara Üniversitesi Dil ve Tarih Coğrafya Fakültesi Dergisi* 42 (2002): 1–7.

———. "Hüseyindede Tepesinde Bulunan Yeni Bir Kült Vazosu", *V. Uluslararası Hititoloji Kongresi Bildirileri, Çorum 02–08 Eylül 2002,* 761–774. Ankara, 2005.

———. "New Scenes on the Second Relief Vase from Hüseyindede and their Interpretation in the Light of the Hittite Representative Art" in *Studi Micenei ed Egeo-Anatolici VI Congresso Internazionale di Ittitologia, Roma, 5–9 Settembre 2005,* ed. by. A. Archi and R. Francia, 837–850. Roma, 2008.

Ziffer, I., "Four Belts from the Land of Ararat and the Feast of the Women" in *Sex and Gender in the Ancient Near East* (CRRAI 47), ed. by S. Parpola and R. Whiting, 645–657. Helsinki: Neo-Assyrian Text Corpus Project, 2002.

A Seal from Toprakkale:
Selective Emulation of Assyrian Elements in Urartian Art

Tuğba Tanyeri-Erdemir[1]

It is a pleasure to dedicate this article to our professors Marie-Henriette and Charles Gates. From early on, they taught us how to look at things with focused attention and to analyze them rigorously.

Abstract

A cylinder seal with clear Assyrian affinities was excavated from the Urartian site of Toprakkale. Assyrian elements frequently occur in the art of the Urartian Kingdom, however the transmission of imagery is at times more intensified than others. During the seventh century BC there was a marked increase in the appearance of Assyrian influence in Urartian imperial art. I use the Toprakkale seal to explore whether or not it may have served as a model for the infiltration of Assyrian visual imagery into Urartian art and to analyze the selective emulation and strategic articulation of Assyrian iconographic and stylistic elements in the Urartian artistic repertoire of the seventh century BC.

In its heyday, the kingdom of Urartu controlled a large territory extending across eastern Turkey, northwestern Iran and Armenia between the ninth and sixth centuries BC. Throughout this time and across this geography, there is a considerable degree of uniformity in different forms of artistic production and a remarkable centralization of architectural production of the state. Most of what we categorize under Urartian art is state art, which is deeply embedded in state ideology and serves as part of a ruling strategy. In its royal art and ruling ideology, the Urartian Kingdom was inspired by its powerful southern neighbor, the Assyrian Empire.

---

1 Center for Science and Society Science and Technology Museum Middle East Technical University, Ankara 06531. Middle East Technical University, Ankara. I would like to thank Halil Demirdelen of the Museum of Anatolian Civilizations for his assistance in producing images of the Toprakkale seal, Dr. Marie-Henriette Gates and Prof. Altan Çilingiroğlu for allowing me to use images from Kinet Höyük and Ayanis, respectively.

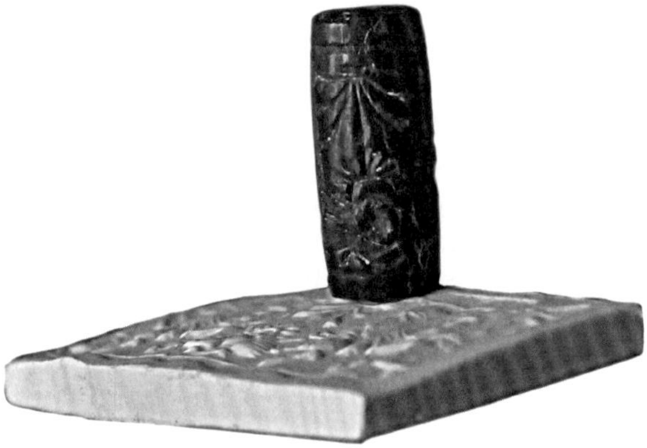

Fig. 1 The Toprakkale seal. Courtesy of Museum of Anatolian Civilizations, Ankara.

The written sources indicate that the contemporary and neighboring kingdoms of Urartu and Assyria frequently interacted, though mostly in conflict and not through peaceful coexistence.[2] The interactions between the two powers, even at times of hostility and warfare, appear to have inspired imitations in art.

Both kingdoms were also part of a larger Near Eastern cultural sphere which shared, among other things, a common visual vocabulary for the expression of kingly power and state art. Exposure and circulation of imagery across the Near East inspired different artistic traditions and enabled each to adapt and imitate ways of the others. As such, the transmission of stylistic and iconographic elements between various states and across this formidable geography is multi-directional and not necessarily contemporaneous.

We catch glimpses of interaction between Urartu and Assyria in the stylistic and iconographic elements inspired by Assyrian examples in Urartian art. The end product, namely the finished Urartian artefacts bearing similarities to Assyrian models, indicate that the Urartian artists were exposed to imagery created in the Assyrian artistic domain. The processes through which this exposure happens is still not well understood. In this paper, I present a cylinder-seal of Assyrian origin which was excavated from the seventh century Urartian site of Toprakkale. This particular seal, which has not been adequately published formerly, is an important artifact to consider in discussions of stylistic and iconographic sharing between Urartu and Assyria. I argue that the Toprakkale seal holds important clues to understand selective emulation and strategic articulation of Assyrian stylistic and iconographic elements into Urartian art of the seventh century BC.

2 See Radner 2011; Salvini 1995.

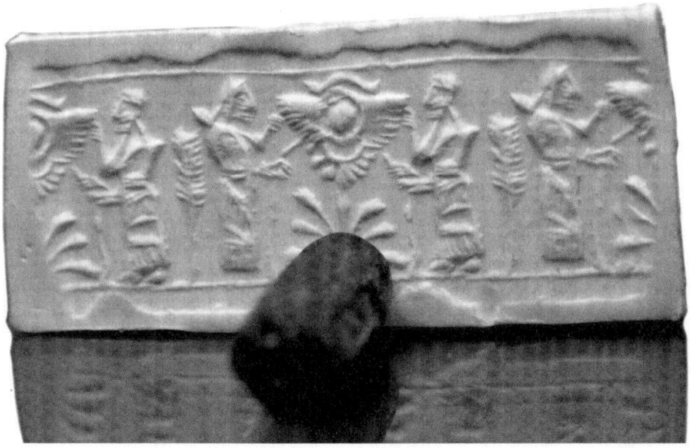

FIG. 2 Impression of the Toprakkale seal. Courtesy Museum of Anatolian Civilizations, Ankara.

The Toprakkale Seal

The cylinder seal of our investigation was excavated from Toprakkale, an Urartian imperial foundation of the seventh century BC, located to the west of Lake Van. It is in the collection of the Museum of Anatolian Civilizations in Ankara (inventory number: 152–4-64).[3] The Toprakkale seal (hereafter, TK seal) has been in the collection of the Museum of Anatolian Civilizations for over half a century, and I can attest to the fact that it has been on display for over a decade at least. Yet, the seal has not appeared in any publication except for a brief note in Ursula Seidl's analysis of the Toprakkale Throne.[4] Most of the Iron Age and Urartian seals from the collection of the Museum of Anatolian Civilizations, which have shared the

3 The Toprakkale Seal was excavated by Afif Erzen probably sometime during the 1959–1961 excavation seasons. Unfortunately, the inventory card at the Museum of Anatolian Civilizations contains no information about the exact location or the year of excavation of the artifact. The 1976 excavations by the same team focused mostly on preparing a topographic plan of the site, and in the publications, the excavator notes that there were only a few small finds encountered and very few pieces of pottery (Erzen 1977, 25). There is no mention of a cylinder seal in the list of small finds. Likewise, there is no mention of a cylinder seal in the publication of the 1977 season report (Erzen 1978, 6). Oktay Belli's short retrospective synopsis of the excavations conducted by İstanbul University under Erzen, however, notes that the temple and storage facilities were exceptionally rich in small finds, including over 1000 pieces of metal objects (Belli 2000, 227). The better published 1976 and 1977 seasons both note that there was little recovered in terms of small finds. It is highly possible that the seal was excavated in 1959–1961, but was never included in the items selected for the few primary publications of the site. Erzen's overview of the excavations does not mention this particular find (Erzen 1962). The excavations of 1959–1961 focused on two main areas: the Urartian temple which was excavated down to the foundation plaques (Erzen 1962, 395–408) and the southern end of the site (Erzen 1962, 408–414). The seal could have come from either location.

4 Seidl 1994, 83, Abb. 12. Seidl includes a sketch of the impression of the seal and mentions it as a possible indication of Assyrian influence in Toprakkale. Her sketch does not include an inventory number, nor any information on the size and formal qualities of the object.

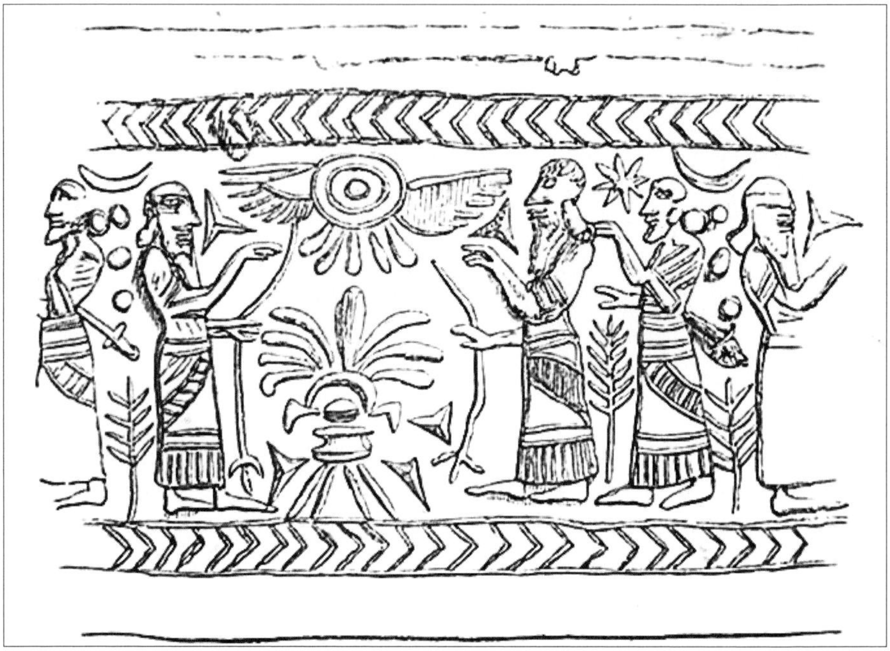

FIG. 3 Drawing of a cylinder seal excavated by Austin Henri Layard. After Layard 1853, pl. 69, fig. 45.

same display case with the TK seal in the last decade, have been published,[5] yet the TK seal was not included in those publications.

The TK seal is 2.9 cm high and 1.2 cm in diameter, carved out of a grained black stone, possibly steatite (FIG. 1). The picture-frame is bordered by straight lines above and below (FIG. 2). The composition shows two standing male figures flanking a central palmette placed on the ground. A winged solar-disc hovers above the palmette, and each male figure holds the streamers coming out of its wings. Streamers continue to the ground and terminate in front of the feet of each male figure. The solar disc has a carved round center, surrounded by a circular line, topped with a soft-curved arch, the ends of which curl up. Two flaring wings emerge out to the sides, and there is a semi-circular line below connecting the two wings. A series of tear-shaped feathers hang below this semi-circular line, forming the tail of the solar-disc. The central figure of the scene is a palmette. The palmette has no trunk and sits directly above the straight line defining the picture frame of the seal. Seven leaves radiate out of a single rectangular, horizontal dent. Two male figures flanking the palmette wear long fringed robes. Neither appears to

5 Çelikel 1987; Yağcı 1995.

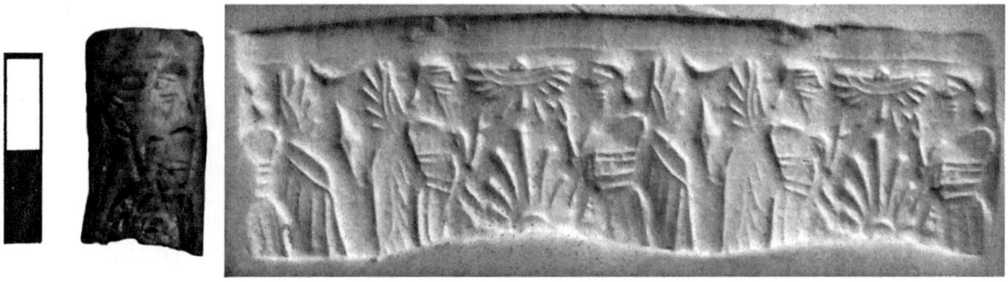

FIG. 4 Cylinder seal from Kinet Höyük. Courtesy Prof. Dr. Marie-Henriette Gates.

be bearded. The one to the left (on the seal impression) has a hairstyle that curls upwards above the shoulders. The poses of the figures are almost identical, each holding a streamer with one hand and extending their opposite arms to the wings of the solar-disc, as if supporting it. It is hard to see whether they are depicted as mirror images or one from the left and the other from the right. Between the backs of the two standing figures there is a single standing vertical feature, which appears to be a stylized tree with branches of short, slightly angled straight lines. If the cylindrical seal is cut diagonally in half, one line would go through the line formed by the central leaf of the palmette and the center of the circle of the sun-disc and the other though the straight vertical line formed by the stylized tree.

Assyrian Parallels and Artistic Inspirations in Urartu

The style and subject matter of the TK seal is very similar to Assyrian cylinder seals of the first millennium BC. The overall configuration and subject matter of the seal, two standing human figures flanking a central vertical element (sacred tree or a palmette) under a sun-disc, is commonly attested in the Assyrian glyptic repertoire with several variations. The closest parallel to the TK seal is a cylinder seal excavated by Austen Henry Layard (FIG. 3) from one of several sites he was working at in northern Mesopotamia in the mid 19th century.[6] Bordered on the top and bottom with a chevron motif, this seal shows three figures in long fringed garbs, depicted in a very similar fashion to the Toprakkale example. Two of the figures flank a central figure of a palmette placed on top of a triangular base, located beneath a sun-disc with wings flaring out of a concentric circular center. The third person stands behind the figure to the right, and there are two vertical trees with angled linear branches pointing up, first behind the second flanking figure to the right, and the other after the figure following him. The execution of

6 Included in Layard 1853; currently in the collections of the British Museum, BM WA 89347 (N 1068) published in Collon 2001, 94–95, no. 163, pl. XL, XLIII; 1987, 75–76, no. 340.

the sun-disc, the palmette and the two vertical stylized trees, as well as that of the male figures, is almost identical to the TK seal, with minor alterations. The most significant difference between the two is the addition of a third attendant to the scene. Another similar seal was excavated at Nineveh.[7] Although the Nineveh seal is not as well preserved as the one excavated by Layard, the configuration of the scene, with two attendants, sun-disc and palmette is parallel to the Toprakkale example. A partial cylinder seal excavated from Kinet Höyük dated to the eighth century BC (FIG. 4) displays similarities in style and composition: in this example, an abbreviated version of the sun-disc hovers above a palmette.[8] The most significant difference in the Kinet example is the fact that the two standing male figures are winged. The presence of a similar style seal on the Eastern Mediterranean coast indicates that this seal type was in circulation around the neighboring territories of Assyria.

In terms of its execution, the TK seal fits into the Neo-Assyrian linear-style.[9] These seals are not drilled, but cut into grained stones (such as serpentine), and thus the final designs look more linear than curved, with less plasticity and abbreviated details. The Assyrian linear-style seals were produced in the ninth and eighth centuries BC.[10]

The central theme of the TK seal is frequently illustrated in Neo-Assyrian glyptic repertoire both in the linear style on softer stones (serpentine and limestone)[11] but also in the drilled style, on hard and finely grained, sometimes semi-precious, stones such as quartz or carnelian. Multiple variations of the scene exist in examples of the latter kind as well: those that display a stylized sacred tree[12] and those with a deity coming out of the sun-disc.[13] The scene depicted on the TK seal showing a ritual with a sacred tree is loaded with symbolism, which is well attested across different cultures of the Near East. In Neo-Assyrian art, the discussions and analysis of the sun-disc[14] as well as the sacred tree[15] are extensive. Both symbols occur in a variety of configurations, sometimes in conjunction with each other, as we see in the example from Toprakkale, but also as separate images.

7 In the collections of the British Museum, BM WA 99407 (1904–10–9, 440) published in Collon 2001, 94, no. 162, pl. XIII.

8 Gates 2000, 197, fig. 8.

9 Porada 1948, 72–73, especially nos. 640–645; Collon 2001, 84.

10 Collon 1987, 75.

11 See Porada 1948, 72–73, especially nos. 640–645.

12 Collon 2001, 86–88, 92, nos. 151 and 159.

13 Collon 1987, 78–79, no. 345, 355; Lambert 1979, 24, no.67.

14 Collon 2001, 79–82; Goldman 1961.

15 Parpola 1993.

The theme of two figures flanking a central sacred tree has many examples also in Urartian glyptic, however none displays the exact configuration as this particular seal from Toprakkale. With a few exceptions, which I will discuss in the following pages, similar compositions in the Urartian glyptic repertoire show sacred trees in elaborate stylizations organized in geometric patterns, with multiple branches and tear-shaped leaves and almost always flanked by fantastic composite creatures.[16] Thus, the TK seal itself has its closest affinities amongst the Assyrian glyptic repertoire, and not the Urartian one.

Thus far, I illustrated that this particular seal excavated from the seventh century BC Urartian imperial site of Toprakkale is highly likely to be of Assyrian origin. The strong stylistic and iconographic affinities of the TK seal indicate that it was produced in the Assyrian realm, or by an artisan trained in the Assyrian glyptic production sometime in the ninth or eighth centuries BC. We do not know when and how it made its way into the Urartian realm, but because of its presence in an Urartian site, it can be regarded as a carrier of Assyrian stylistic and iconographic elements into Urartu. To test this, we need to identify and illustrate the similarities of the TK seal with the Urartian artistic repertoire. This will give us evidence whether or not the TK seal may have generated stylistic and iconographic inspirations in the art of Urartu.

Let us start with two Urartian examples that display both a close similarity in composition and individual elements. These are a cylinder seal impression on a bulla and a bronze helmet, both excavated from Ayanis and both dated to the seventh century BC, to the reign of the Urartian king Rusa II. The cylinder seal impression on a clay bulla excavated at Ayanis (Fig. 5) has a similar configuration to the TK seal, though with several adjustments.[17] The top border of the impression bears a cuneiform inscription, which identifies it "as the seal of x house".[18] The image depicted on this seal impression illustrates two pairs of standing figures dressed in long garbs and pointed high-helmets holding tall staffs in their hands. The pair to the left flanks what appears to be a large pithos-like vessel, indicated by a dotted line of small circles, which stands beneath a winged sun-disc; the second pair flanks a sacred tree. The sacred tree in this example has a tall trunk, reaching almost as high as the heads of the flanking figures. The leaves of the tree flare out of the top of the trunk in five fleshy leaves, very much like a palm tree. As

16 See, for instance, for Bastam: Seidl 1979, 137–140, A1, A2; for Ayanis: Abay 2001, 223–225, A1, figs. 1–3; for Karmir-Blur: Piotrovskii 1962, fig. 72.

17 Abay 2001, 329, fig. 7, A3.

18 The defining sign to identify this "house" could not be identified. Thus, the identity of this "house", whether it is a building or an institution, is not clear, as the cuneiform symbol before the word "house" had not been formerly attested elsewhere in the Urartian texts (Salvini 2001, 317, AY6).

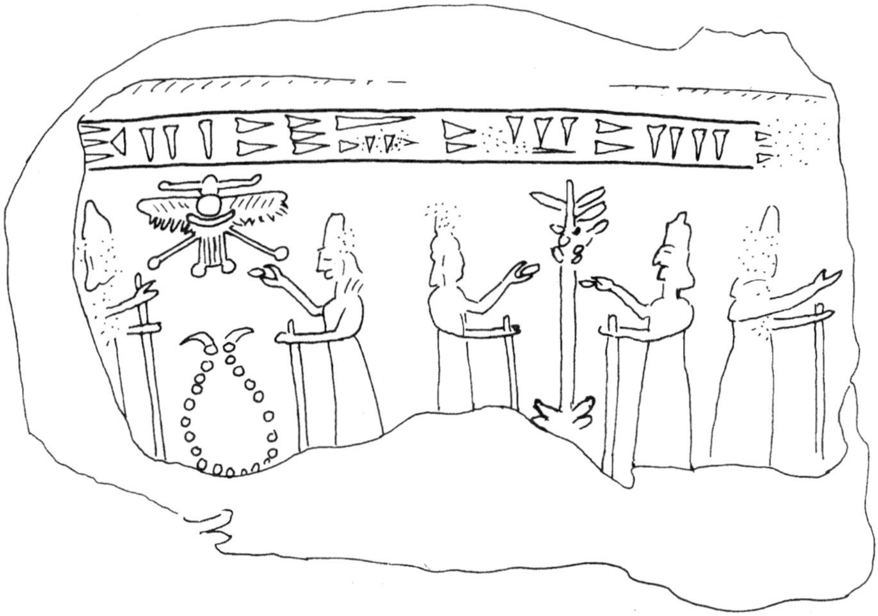

FIG. 5 Line drawing of the cylinder seal impression on a bulla from Ayanis (AY.135.90). After Salvini 2001, 317.

such, this particular representation is rather unusual in Urartian art, where sacred trees are commonly depicted either in a highly stylized manner, as elaborate trees with multiple branches coming out in symmetrical shapes terminating in tear-like leaves, or in some ritual scenes with down-turned branches without leaves. This particular sacred-tree is probably representing a palm tree, as Abay has noted.[19] Although this seal is not unique in its composition with figures flanking central objects, possibly engaged in ritual actions, some of the motifs represented are not common in the Urartian artistic repertoire. The palm tree, for instance, occurs only in one other object, namely the bronze helmet of Rusa II from Ayanis, with a similar depiction. Some other motifs, such as this particular depiction of the sun-disc with flaring wings or the pithos-like feature, appear in the art of the seventh century BC and not earlier.

The bronze helmet of Rusa II from Ayanis (FIG. 6) is a peculiar object in many respects.[20] It differs from earlier examples of Rusa II's forefathers dated to the eighth century BC not only in its overall design, but also in the choice of subject matter and style. The earlier imperial bronze helmets of Sarduri II and Argišti I

19 Abay 2001, 329.

20 Derin and Çilingiroğlu 2001, 164, fig. 13.

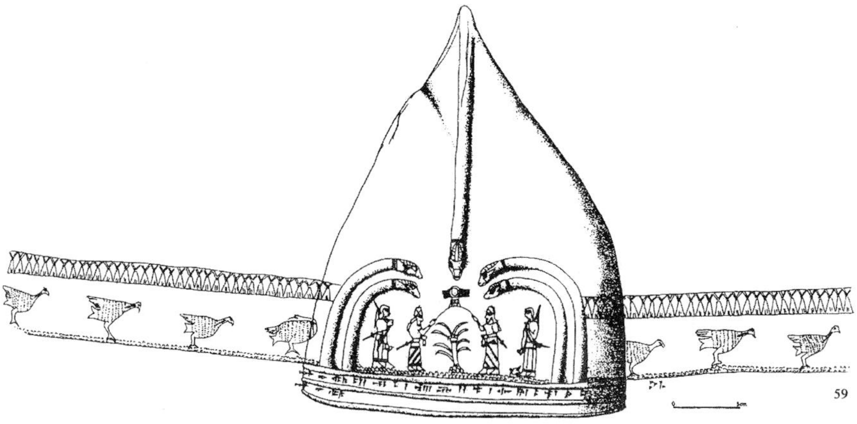

FIG. 6 Line drawing of the bronze helmet of Rusa II. After Çilingiroğlu and Derin 2001, 181, Fig.13, Catalogue number 59.

excavated from Karmir-Blur, for instance, have repetitive, formulaic, highly symmetrical depictions: 11 pairs of divine figures pollinating highly stylized sacred trees in the front of the helmet in two rows of five pairs and a single pair placed on top, framed by curved features terminating in lions' heads; repetitive depictions of chariots and warriors on their horses encircle the rest of the helmet in two rows.[21] Rusa II's helmet from Ayanis, in contrast, displays only a single, central representation framed in curved features terminating in goats' heads and a single row of repetitive, but not identical, images of fowl. Although this artifact is unique in many aspects, such as the very natural depiction of fowl, here we will focus on the central theme, which would have been placed right above the forehead of the wearer, in the most visible position.

The scene is organized in a symmetrical fashion, with a vertical center defined by thc sacred tree and a sun-disc hovering above it. On either side of the central element, two male figures are depicted. First, a pair of bearded figures dressed in long diagonally-fringed garb and high crowns and wearing swords at their belts is shown flanking a sacred tree, as they hold the streamers coming down from the winged sun-disc with their right hands and hold what appear to be small buckets in their left hands. Two other non-bearded figures in soldiers' attire, carrying bows on their shoulders and swords at their belts, stand behind each one of them. In terms of his pose, the fourth figure of the scene appears similar to the third figure depicted on the Assyrian seal excavated by Layard (FIG. 3; for references see n. 5 above). The sacred-tree is also unique in its depiction: it is planted on a heap of earth shown as

21 Seidl 2004, fig. 29 (Argišti I) fig. 30 (Sarduri II).

small circles on the ground and has a short trunk and flaring, large curved leaves coming out of the top and the sides. On top of the trunk, there are three small circles which appear to be the fruits of the tree. The depiction of the tree, in contrast to the earlier eighth century BC examples, is neither symmetrical nor stylized. Like the fowl encircling the helmet, the sacred tree in this scene is depicted naturally and somewhat unbalanced with uneven leaves. The sun-disc has two wings and a tail coming out of a central circle with two streamers coming down. As stated previously, the motif of a sacred tree flanked by figures is attested frequently in Urartian art.

What is new in the bronze helmet of Rusa II is the overall configuration under a sun-disc, with identifiable humans as members of the highest strata of society (possibly the king and the crown prince), and soldiers flanking a very naturally depicted palm tree. The absence of fantastic animals or divine figures and the natural depiction of the central tree figure are peculiar. As such, both the impression on the bulla, as well as the helmet of Ruse II from Ayanis, contrasts with earlier Urartian examples and bear strong resemblance to the formula of the Neo-Assyrian linear-style seals in general, and the TK seal in particular.

The appearance of the sun-disc in conjunction with a stylized palm tree is attested on the incised scene on the lid of a stone box from Karmir-Blur.[22] In this example, the central theme is flanked by two bird-headed winged genii. The sun-disc has a circular center, out of which wings and a tail spread out; two wiggly streamers come out to the sides and terminate in open claws. Like the TK seal, there is a line ending in volutes above the circular center, connecting the tops of two wings. The stylized tree in this example differs from most Urartian examples: the leaves of the tree are long, fleshy and slightly curved, depicted in two groups. The first, just above the ground, spreading out of a triangular-shaped trunk, appears to bear three circular fruits. The second set of leaves flare out of the elongated trunk, just below the sun-disc. Both the shape and structure of the leaves, as well as the round fruit, indicate that this is a highly-stylized palm tree.

Individual motifs of the TK seal appear frequently in seventh century Urartian art produced in different media. One of the most popular motifs is the sun-disc in the particular configuration as seen in the TK seal. This specific configuration with a circular center, two wings coming out of it and with streamers coming down at each end, sometimes topped with a straight line terminating in volutes, appears on a myriad of objects. The sun-disc was already a favored symbol of the Urartian art of the ninth century BC, especially attested on artifacts inscribed with king Išpuini's name.[23] The earlier representations show a deity coming out of the winged sun-disc. This particular configuration is attested on a bronze shield

22 Piotrovskii 1967, fig. 48.

23 Merhav 1991, figs. 27–30.

excavated from Yukarı Anzaf, which shows a number of deities depicted standing on their animals and with their attributes. The second deity is depicted as standing on a striding bull and emerges out of a winged sun-disc (Belli 1998, 33ff). The representation on this shield indicates that each deity was identified through their attributes, and thus the god coming out of a sun-disc is not a generic deity, but rather the representation of a particular deity of the Urartian pantheon.

The sun-disc motif of the seventh century, however, differs significantly from the earlier examples of the ninth century BC in the absence of the deity coming out of it. The seventh century representations are similar to the TK seal and appear frequently on artifacts dated to the reign of Rusa II. The motif is particularly popular in the glyptic repertoire.[24]

The sun-disc appears on art produced in different media. One of the most elaborate and finely crafted examples appears on a bronze furniture piece in the form of a lion's paw from Toprakkale.[25] This particular sun-disc was meticulously designed, showing an interest in the overall symmetry of the design, with each feather on the wings and the tail, the central circle, and the connection of the two wings depicted as a straight line ending in two small volutes and two straight streamers ending in claws cut into the bronze. These holes were once inlaid with colored stones. A small golden sun-disc from Ayanis bears similarities to these examples, however it differs stylistically in its execution and proportions, as the wings are shorter and the tail longer.[26] The broad distribution of this particular formulation of the winged sun-disc across a wide geography and the appearance of it on diverse media indicates that the motif was widely used and accepted into Urartian artistic culture.

The Urartian seal repertoire has examples showing narrative scenes involving actors (possibly the king himself or a high religious official, a priest) engaged in ritualistic actions around sacred trees. Those scenes display some variety and are not limited to images of two individuals flanking a central sacred tree. The richness of this data has allowed scholars to investigate the ritualistic function of such trees. Nevzat Çevik's study investigated the cosmological dimensions of sacred trees and ritual scenes in Urartian art, tying these to the archaeological record, and analyzing how such rituals may have been enacted.[27]

The appearance of male human figures, as opposed to fantastic creatures or repetitive formulaic representations, is yet another popular theme of the seventh

24 See for instance, for Karmir-Blur: Piotrovskii 1962, figs. 71, 72; for Ayanis: Abay 2001, figs. 7, 12, 16, 19, 21; for Bastam: Seidl 1979, 139, C1-C5, D1.

25 Seidl 1994, fig. 11.

26 Batmaz 2013, fig. 23.

27 Çevik 1999.

century BC Urartian art. These male human figures are dressed in garbs, and there are indications in their paraphernalia probably pointing to their status in society or offices. As such, they could be identified by the ancient audience. Although human forms can be found in the art of the earlier periods (for example, the warriors and charioteers on the helmets of Argišti I and Sarduri II from Karmir-Blur[28]) these are generic, repetitive, formulaic representations. In the seventh century, standing male figures engaged in various ritual activities start to appear in the glyptic art. Alina Ayvazian's study on ritual scenes in the Urartian seal repertoire includes several such representations, among them the aforementioned seal impression from Ayanis.[29] Ayvazian suggests that such images of an "individual in the process of the ritual action" are seen only on cylinder seals and not on stamp seals.[30]

The specific type of representations with a human involved in ritual action in the sacred-tree rituals occurs in the seventh century BC glyptic art.[31] The excavations at Ayanis provide us with archaeological evidence supporting that those rituals were indeed carried out in an area connected to the Temple grounds.[32] As such, the representations of the scene, like the bronze helmet and seal impression from Ayanis, depicting individual actors in actual actions, may have been popularized in the seventh century. In the art of the seventh century BC we can clearly see a different understanding and attitude towards representation of the ritual sphere. If such scenes from the art of the ninth and eighth centuries can be seen as alluding to deeply embedded, highly symbolic cosmological concepts, similar scenes in the art of the seventh century BC, by contrast, are more narrative and refer to actual actions of rituals. This is not to say that the earlier representations of the divine sphere with fantastic beings flanking sacred trees were abandoned (even in the seal repertoire). These more realistic depictions of standing human figures in ritual actions emerge in the seventh century BC, along with a continuation of the earlier compositions.

The palmette motif can be seen on several examples of Urartian art of the seventh century BC. It is not novel to the art of the seventh century BC, though attested rarely before the seventh century BC. The wall paintings in Erebuni, for instance, dated to the reign of Argišti I in the second quarter of the eighth century BC, illustrate a similar palmette.[33] The palmette is a popular motif across the Near East and appears in the art of several different cultures. Thus, the appearance of

28 Seidl 2004, fig. 29 (Argišti I), fig. 30 (Sarduri II).

29 Ayvazian 2004, 124, fig. 3.

30 Ayvazian 2004, 123.

31 See for instance a seal impression from Toprakkale: Batmaz 2013, fig. 17.

32 Batmaz 2013.

33 Azarpay 1967, 19–20, fig. 4.

the motif in Urartian art prior to the seventh century may have been inspired from a variety of sources.

What is new in the seventh century is the naturalistic representation of palm trees. Two examples in particular bear significant similarities to the TK seal in composition and selection of elements: the bronze helmet of Rusa II and the seal impression on a bulla from Ayanis (AY6). They both display naturalistically depicted palm trees. I tend to see them as similar concepts to the palmette, perhaps replacing the abbreviated 'palm tree' represented as a palmette. The reason why I think this way is the fact that the particular configuration of sun-disc together with a sacred-tree in Urartu has only limited examples, and in all three, the tree itself differs significantly from the Urartian stylized tree representations. These examples are Rusa II's helmet, the seal impression from Ayanis (AY6), and the Karmir-Blur box-lid. Thus, the juxtapositioning of the two elements strongly suggests that the inspiration for this type of representation may have come from the Neo-Assyrian repertoire, perhaps following the specific example of the TK seal. In all three examples, the sacred tree is not the highly stylized geometrically patterned trees, but in two clearly depicts a palm tree, and in third, a stylized palm tree. It is highly likely that these palm trees are replacements for the palmette.

Selective Emulation and Strategic Articulation of Assyrian Elements

The composition, individual elements and their particular configuration(s) on the TK seal appear frequently in Urartian art of the seventh century BC. Starting with its early kings of the ninth century BC, the Urartian Empire appears to have been inspired by the Assyrian Empire in its expressions of rulership, writing system,[34] and art from the ninth century BC onwards.[35] However, the influx of Assyrian influence in Urartu does not appear to have had a steady flow, but rather fluctuated thorugh time.

The timing and rate of cross-cultural artistic transmissions may depend on a variety of factors. As Irene Winter noted, "[i]n the case of Assyrian relations with the west, it seems evident that individual states had particular histories and individual Assyrian kings had specific personalities which governed the intensity of interaction on an artistic level."[36] This also seems to be the case for Urartu, that different Urartian kings had differing attitudes towards permitting or promoting artistic emulation. Assyrian stylistic and iconographic elements occur more prominently during the reigns of some kings than others. Although the infiltration of

34 Salvini 2006, 45.

35 Azarpay 1968, 7–15.

36 Winter 1982, 370.

Assyrian influence can be traced back to the ninth century BC, there seems to be a distinct and highlighted emphasis on the incorporation of Assyrian elements into Urartian artistic production of the seventh century BC, particularly during the reign of Rusa II. Seidl, for instance, noticed a strong Assyrian influence in her study of the Toprakkale throne.[37] Barnett made a similar observation in his investigation of material in the British Museum excavated from Toprakkale in the 19th century.[38] Likewise, Azarpay noted a similar trend of marked Assyrian influence in Urartian art of the seventh century BC.[39]

Did the TK seal serve as a model for the Assyrian-inspired imagery of the seventh century BC? There must have been a myriad of ways in antiquity through which Urartian artisans could be exposed to Assyrian art. Through trade, travel, and warfare, artifacts could travel. Especially small and durable items like cylinder seals would be highly mobile. Likewise, artisans working for Urartian kings could have been exposed to or perhaps even trained in other artistic traditions of the Near East. In our case, we have evidence of a seal, probably produced in Assyria some time between the ninth-eighth centuries BC and excavated from the seventh century Urartian imperial site of Toprakkale. We do not know how and when the TK seal made its way to Urartu or whether it was ever used by its Urartian owners in its intended function as a seal. The TK seal was probably one of many artifacts that endured a similar journey. It is precious for us, the researchers, because it not only survived but was also recovered archaeologically, from an Urartian imperial site of the seventh century BC. The presence of such an artifact at the site suggests that the image was available for Urartians. Furthermore, the presence of Assyrian stylistic and iconographic emulations in Urartian art of the seventh century BC, following the example of the TK seal, implies that the TK seal is a good candidate that could have served as a model for the transmission of imagery.

The imperial site of Toprakkale may have been a suitable locale for the initiation of Assyrian imagery into Urartu. The site is located near Lake Van, in the vicinity of perhaps the most emotionally charged Urartian site, namely Tušpa. Tušpa is commonly called the "capital" of the Urartian kingdom, though the exact meaning of the term is rarely discussed. Nevertheless, Tušpa was one of the pivotal centers of Urartu from the earliest days of the kingdom.[40] Assyrian records include numerous campaigns against Urartu, and some even claim to have reached and sacked Tušpa. Toprakkale is located on the slope of a mountain to the west of the site of Tušpa and overlooks Lake Van. Both sites are open for mobility routes

37 Seidl 1994.

38 Barnett 1950, 35–37.

39 Azarpay 1968, 63–65.

40 Tarhan 2011.

around Lake Van, though access between the Plain of Van and elsewhere would have been restricted by natural barriers. One route following the Hoşap Valley leading towards the east may have been the main access to the Lake Van Basin from Mesopotamia through the Urmia Basin.[41] Of the five major sites built by Rusa II in the seventh century BC, Toprakkale was the southernmost and closest in location to this southern route of communication with Mesopotamia.[42] As such, it would have been a likely outpost for Assyrian artifacts and concepts to enter the Urartian realm in the seventh century BC.

Even though Toprakkale was the first Urartian site ever excavated and has been investigated by a number of different teams of various nationalities over the span of a century, it is still one of the most enigmatic Urartian sites.[43] Unfortunately, the archaeological data at hand does not allow us to identify the architectural layout of the site and the spatial distribution of most artifacts. Nevertheless, the material culture generated from Toprakkale displays some of the strongest Assyrian influence in all of Urartian art. The Toprakkale Throne, for example, exhibits close affinities with Assyrian three and two-dimensional sculptural art.[44] It is likely that high quality, well crafted, elite objects of Assyrian origin would have been brought to imperial cities such as Toprakkale. Those artifacts may have inspired artisans working with various media. In the absence of identified workshops producing imperial art, such suggestions cannot be substantiated. However, the location and size of the site and the richness of finds bearing strong similarities to Assyrian models suggest that it may have served both as an entry hub and a place where experimentation with new emulated imagery may have taken place.

A survey of Urartian art of the seventh century BC indicates that the individual motifs, as well as their particular configurations as seen on the TK seal,

---

41 Zimansky 1985, 17–18.

42 The other seventh century BC sites founded by Rusa II are Adilcevaz on the western shore of Lake Van, Ayanis on the eastern shore of Lake Van, located to the north of Toprakkale, Karmir-Blur in Armenia and Bastam in northwestern Iran. See Zimansky 1995.

43 The site was initially excavated by the British Museum in 1879–1880 by H. Rassam, Emilius Clayton and Raynolds. Later it was extensively investigated and excavated by C.F. Lehmann-Haupt and W. Belck in 1898–1899, by I.A. Orbeli in 1911–1912, by N.Y. Marr in 1916 and by K. Lake in 1938. The Turkish excavations were directed by Afif Erzen in 1959–1961 and again in 1976 (Erzen 1977). Even though the excavations in the site have been numerous, the publications of those expeditions have been minimal, and thus our information about the site and the archaeological contexts of the finds still remains limited. The excavations conducted by independent teams were not necessarily carried out in a systematic manner, and with the existing information we cannot identify most of the architectural components of the site. To give one example, despite being investigated for over a century, there is not a proper and accurate plan of the site in the literature.

44 Seidl 1994.

appear on a variety of artifacts produced in various different kinds of media. Here it is important to note two factors.

First, this particular image was not copied verbatim. One needs to recognize this as a dual process: the Urartian artisans working for the central authority reproduced certain elements, while omitting others. The seal itself was not imitated as it is; in contrast, we see the infiltration of selected elements used on this seal into Urartian art. There is a pattern in the selection of those motifs and configurations. Some of them display similarities either in composition or in concept to Urartian art of earlier periods. As such, they were not alien for the ancient Urartian audience to a certain extent, but different enough to be distinct from earlier representations. Cosmologically meaningful, culturally embedded forms, perhaps reinterpreted through the adoption of new elements from Assyria, may have been one way of rejuvenating the art of the ruling ideology, without dramatically altering the status quo of artistic visual culture.

Second, these emulations are not restricted to Urartian glyptic, but were reproduced in other media. Production in each material type (bronze, stone, etc.) required trained artisans, who were working in independent groups employed by the state. The emergence of these Assyrian elements in the seventh century BC rather abruptly in different media (bronze armor, glyptic, stone) and across a wide geography (Toprakkale, Ayanis, Karmir-Blur) indicates that these were accepted by the central authority of the state and were perhaps promoted to be reproduced in various forms. This suggests that the reception of selected elements were conscious, and they were adapted fully into the Urartian corpus.

Conclusion

The Assyrian seal excavated from the Urartian site of Toprakkale offers us a chance to examine the transfer of iconographic and stylistic elements from one artistic culture of the ancient Near East to another. In this case we see the strategic integration of selected Assyrian stylistic and iconographic elements into the Urartian artistic repertoire of the seventh century BC. As Winter stated in relation to the development of a local style in Hasanlu after the Assyrian contact, "It is generally acknowledged that art objects embody cultural values, and serve as media for communication and information storage. Therefore, the adaptation of an art style and the molding of it into a local style is equally a function of the cultural process. In fact, the new style can be both a reflection of phenomena already existing at some level within the society and a mediating factor in reinforcing or integrating new social values on other levels."[45]

45 Winter 1977, 383.

What we observe in the Urartian case is a selective emulation and strategic articulation of Assyrian stylistic and iconographic elements. The ready availability of an image, on its own, does not imply that the image will be reproduced verbatim or imitated as it is. Rather, emulation takes place through a selective process which favors elements that have a level of familiarity for the recipient culture. Stylistically this refers to the symmetrical composition and particular configuration of elements. In terms of iconography, we see the integration of selected motifs into the Urartian repertoire of the seventh century BC. Elements depicted on the TK seal such as the solar-disc and the palmette, which can be linked to already existing motifs in the Urartian repertoire, were favored. In similar symmetrical compositions to the TK seal, the naturalistically depicted palm tree replaces the highly stylized sacred tree, although the sacred tree continued its use in other contexts. Likewise, the solar-disc can be related to the earlier motif of a deity coming out of a winged-disc; however in the particular depiction of the solar-disc of the seventh century BC reproduces the TK seal example closely. As such, the selective process of the recipient culture favored elements that could easily replace already existing cosmologically contextualized elements of the repertoire.

The Urartian art of the seventh century BC is considered to display a strong level of Assyrianization. In this article, I focused on a single Assyrian artifact excavated from an Urartian site and demonstrated the possible infiltration of some of the stylistic and iconographic elements into the Urartian art of the seventh century BC. The selective emulation of Assyrian elements in this period appears to be strategic in the reformulation of cosmologically meaningful, culturally embedded motifs. This could have been part of a larger artistic revival and imperial policy, in which already existing elements could convey new messages without a complete deviation of historically significant and familiar forms in artistic visual culture.

REFERENCES

Abay, E., "Seals and Sealings" in *Ayanis I: Ten Years' Excavations at Rusahinili Eiduru-kai 1989–1998*, ed. by A. Çilingiroğlu and M. Salvini, 321–353. Rome: Istituto per gli studi micenei ed egeo-anatolici CNR, 2001.

Ayvazian, A., *Urartian Glyptic: New Perspectives*. Unpublished PhD Thesis, Berkeley: University of California Press, 2006.

———. "Ritual Scenes in Urartian Glyptic." *Isimu* 7 (2004): 123–130.

Azarpay, G., *Urartian Art and Artifacts: A Chronological Study*. Los Angeles 1967.

Barnett, R., "The Excavations of the British Museum at Toprak Kale, near Van." *Iraq* 12 (1950): 1–43.

Batmaz, A., "A New Ceremonial Practice at Ayanis Fortress: The Urartian Sacred Tree Ritual on the Eastern Shore of Lake Van." *Journal of Near Eastern Studies* 72/1 (2013): 65–83.

Belli, O., *Anzaf Kaleleri ve Urartu Tanrıları*. İstanbul: Arkeoloji Sanat Yayınları, 1998.

———. "Urartu Krallığı'nın İkinci Başkenti Toprakkale (Rusahinili) Kazıları" in *Türkiye Arkeolojisi ve İstanbul Üniversitesi*, ed. by O. Belli, 223–227. Ankara: İstanbul Üniversitesi, 2000.

Çelikel, S., "Anadolu Medeniyetleri Müzesindeki Bir Grup Urartu Mührü." *Anadolu Medeniyetleri Müzesi 1987 Yıllığı* (1987): 68–79.

Çevik, N., "Hayat Ağacı'nın Urartu Kült Törenlerindeki Yeri ve Kullanım Biçimi." *Anadolu Araştırmaları* 15 (1999): 335–367.

Çilingiroğlu, A. and M. Salvini (eds.), *Ayanis I: Ten Years' Excavations at Rusahinili Eiduru-kai 1989–1998*, ed. by A. Çilingiroğlu and M. Salvini. Rome: Istituto per gli studi micenei ed egeo-anatolici CNR, 2001.

Collon, D., *First Impressions. Cylinder Seals in the Near East*. London: British Museum Publications, 1987.

———. *A Catalogue of Western Asiatic Seals in the British Museum. Cylinder Seals V. Neo Assyrian and Neo-Babylonian Periods*. London: British Museum Publications, 2001.

Derin, Z. and A. Çilingiroğlu, "Armour and Weapons" in *Ayanis I: Ten Years' Excavations at Rusahinili Eiduru-kai 1989–1998*, ed. by A. Çilingiroğlu and M. Salvini, 155–187. Rome: Istituto per gli studi micenei ed egeo-anatolici CNR, 2001.

Erzen, A., "Untersuchungen in der urartäischen Stadt Toprakkale bei Van in den Jahre 1959–1960." *Archäologischer Anzeiger* 2 (1962): 384–414.

———. "Çavuştepe Yukarı Kale ve Toprakkale 1976 Kazıları." *Anadolu Araştırmaları* 4–5 (1977): 1–59.

———. "Çavuştepe Yukarı Kale ve Toprakkale 1977 Çalışmaları." *Anadolu Araştırmaları* 6 (1979): 1–15.

Gates, M-H., "1998 Excavations at Kinet Höyük (Yeşil-Dörtyol, Hatay)." *Kazı Sonuçları Toplantısı* 21 (2000): 193–208.

Lambert, W.G., "Near Eastern Seals in the Gulbenkian Museum of Oriental Art, University of Durham." *Iraq* 41 (1979): 1–45.

Layard, A.H., *The Monuments of Nineveh From Drawings Made on the Spot*. Piscataway: Gorgias Press, 2004.

Merhav, R., "Chariot and Horse Fittings" in *Urartu: A Metalworking Center in the First Millennium BCE*, ed. by R. Merhav, 53–78. Tel Aviv: Sabinsky Press, 1991.

Parpola, S., "The Assyrian Tree of Life: Tracing the Origins of Jewish Monotheism and Greek Philosophy." *Journal of Near Eastern Studies* 52/3 (1993): 161–208.

Piotrovskii, B.B., *Iskusstvo Urartu VII-VI vv.* Leningrad 1962.

Porada, E., *Corpus of Ancient Near Eastern seals in North American Collections. The Collection of the Pierpoint Morgan Library*. New York 1948.

Radner, K., "Assyrians and Urartians" in *The Oxford Handbook of Ancient Anatolia*, ed. by S. R. Steadman and G. McMahon, 734–751. Oxford: Oxford University Press, 2011.

Salvini, M., *Geschichte und Kultur der Urartäer*. Darmstadt: Wissenschaftliche Buchgesellschaft, 1995.

———. "Inscriptions on Clay" in *Ayanis I: Ten Years' Excavations at Rusahinili Eiduru-kai 1989–1998*, ed. by A. Çilingiroğlu and M. Salvini, 279–319. Rome: Istituto per gli studi micenei ed egeo-anatolici CNR, 2001.

———. "An Overview of Urartian History" in *Urartu: Doğu'da Değişim-Transformation in the East*, ed. by K. Köroğlu and E. Konyar, 74–101. İstanbul: Yapı Kredi Yayınları, 2011.

Seidl, U., "Uraräische Glyptik" in *Bastam I: Ausgrabungen in den Urartäischen Analgen 1972–1975*, ed. by W. Kleiss, P. Calmeyer, S. Kroll, M. Salvini, U. Seidl and C. Strauss, 137–149. Berlin: Dietrich Reimer Verlag, 1979.

———. "Der Thron von Toprakkale. Ein neuer Rekonstruktionverscuh." *Archäologische Mitteilungen aus Iran* 27 (1994): 67–84.

———. *Bronzekunst Urartus*. Mainz am Rhein: Verlag Philipp von Zabern in Wissenschaftliche Buchgesellschaft, 2004.

Tanyeri-Erdemir, T. *Continuity, Change, and Innovation: Considering the Agency of Rusa II in the Production of the Imperial Art and Architecture of Urartu in the 7th Century BC*. Unpublished Ph.D. Thesis, Boston University, 2005.

Tarhan, T., "The Capital City Tushpa" in *Urartu: Doğu'da Değişim-Transformation in the East*, ed. by K. Köroğlu and E. Konyar, 288–337. İstanbul: Yapı Kredi Yayınları, 2011.

Winter, I., "Perspective on the Local Style of Hasanlu IVB: A Study in Receptivity" in *Mountains and Lowlands: Essays in the Archaeology of Mesopotamia*, ed. by L. D. Levine and T. C. Young, 371–386. Malibu: Undena Publications, 1977.

———. "Art as Evidence for Interaction: Relations Between the Assyrian Empire and North Syria" in *Mesopotamien und seine Nachbarn XXVe Rencontre Assyriologique Internationale (Berlin, 2–7 July 1978)*, ed. by H-J. Nissen and J. Renger, 355–382. Berlin: Dietrich Reimer Verlag, 1982.

Yağcı, R., "İnsan Başı ve Yumruk Biçimli Bir Grup Mühür ile Bir İğne." *Anadolu Medeniyetleri Müzesi Yıllığı 1995* (1996): 181–215.

Zimansky, P.E., *Ecology and Empire: Structure of the Urartian State.* Chicago: The Oriental Institute of the University of Chicago, 1985.

———. "An Urartian Ozymandias." *Biblical Archaeologist* 58/2 (1995): 94–100.

The Pottery of the Latest Iron IA Phase at Tell Tayinat, Amuq

Elif Ünlü[1]

As Director of the Kinet Höyük excavations, neighboring both the Amuq and Cilicia and tying the Syro-Anatolian world with the Mediterranean, Dr. Marie-Henriette Gates has been pivotal for our understanding of the ancient northeastern Mediterranean. Her intellectual and conceptual input into the workings of the Hittite potting tradition and its wider political impact is seminal. Her contributions to our comprehension of the Late Bronze-Iron Age transition in the region are also essential. Therefore, I write this with the hopes of relevance to her scholarship and to show my admiration for her work.

Abstract

The period spanning the end of the Bronze Age and the beginning of the Iron Age is one of the most discussed, yet still least understood, in the eastern Mediterranean. The material culture from different settlements indicate that this is a period both of instability and persistence, eventually taking different regions into their distinctive trajectories, each determined by a wide variety of variables, the combination of which is specific to each region. Tell Tayinat is located in the Amuq Plain at the important crossroads tying the Syro-Anatolian world with Cilicia and Central Anatolia, as well as to the maritime routes opening into the Mediterranean trade. The significance of this settlement for the region during the later Iron Age is apparent by the accumulation of new evidence from the recent excavations, along with data from the previous University of Chicago excavations.

Here pottery from the new excavations at Tell Tayinat is investigated analyzing the very last phase of the Iron IA Period (called Field Phase 3 by the excavators). Continuities and divergences from the earlier Iron IA phases are studied with the aim of understanding the reconfigurations of various networks operational during this period, and hence, elucidating at least some aspects of the formation of the later Neo-Hittite kingdom in the region.

1 Department of History, Boğaziçi University, Bebek, İstanbul, Turkey.
I would like to extend my deepest gratitude to Timothy P. Harrison, director of the Tayinat Archaeological Project, for allowing me to work on this material. The financial support of my research is provided by Boğaziçi University Scientific Research Fund nr. 8254.

Introduction

The mound of Tell Tayinat lies in the eastern half of the Amuq Plain close to the Orontes River (Fig. 1). The Amuq Plain, with the combination of a temperate climate, sufficient rainfall and a steady supply of fresh water from the Orontes (Asi) River, has been a fertile region for cash-crop agriculture, as well as for fruits and vegetables. The Amanos (Nur) Mountains form a barrier between the plain and the Mediterranean Sea, but also provide the occupants of the region a more diversified ecology. One of the main routes connecting northern Syria to the Mediterranean goes through this region, opening the greater Syro-Anatolian region to the eastern Mediterranean (Fig. 2). It also has relatively easy access to the Cilician Plain, which shares the northeastern corner of the Mediterranean with the Amuq Region. Within this geographical context, the Amuq Plain has been a conduit of goods, ideas, and peoples through the millennia of its uninterrupted occupation to the modern time.

Excavations on the mound of Tell Tayinat were first undertaken by the University of Chicago's Oriental Institute between 1935–1938 as part of the Syrian-Hittite Expedition project, followed by landmark publications establishing a sound chronological framework for the region. These excavations brought to light a strong Early Bronze and Iron Age occupation on the mound. After a period of archaeological inactivity in the region, recently several excavations were initiated on the plain, one of which is the Tayinat Archaeological Project (TAP). TAP started active excavations on the mound in 2004 headed by Professor Timothy P. Harrison under the auspices of the University of Toronto, Department of Near and Middle Eastern Civilizations. Due to the careful excavation and diligent record-keeping of the TAP team, a fine-tuned stratigraphy of the archaeological deposits has been emerging, enabling a detailed study of the settlement's material culture anchored to an intra-site phasing.

The Iron IA Period[2] remains at Tell Tayinat were first encountered in Field

2 This period corresponds to the early part of Amuq Phase N of the Syrian-Hittite Expedition (for Amuq periodization see Swift 1958, 58). In the eastern Mediterranean, various terms are used to designate the periods spanning the very end of the Late Bronze Age to the earlier phases of the Iron Age. This article uses the term Iron IA in accordance with the terminology preferred by the TAP team. For Anatolia, Iron IA would correspond to Late Bronze IIb (LB IIb) (see Goldman 1956, 64), for Cyprus, to Late Cypriot III (LC III), and for the Aegean, to Late Helladic IIIC (LH IIIC)/ Late Minoan IIIC (LM IIIC): this terminology emphasizes continuities present in this period. On the other hand, in the Levantine and Syrian regions it is denoted as the beginning of Iron I, emphasizing the discontinuities (see especially Mazzoni 2000). Conceptually this period should be regarded as a transition between the Late Bronze and Iron Age Periods to avoid the pitfalls and biases presented by the distinct narratives regarding both periods in the scholarship. It is the author's opinion that there is merit in studying the material culture of the very late phases of the Late Bronze Age and the early phases of the Early Iron Age together to fully understand the transformations and continuities taking place in the eastern Mediterranean during this unsettled period.

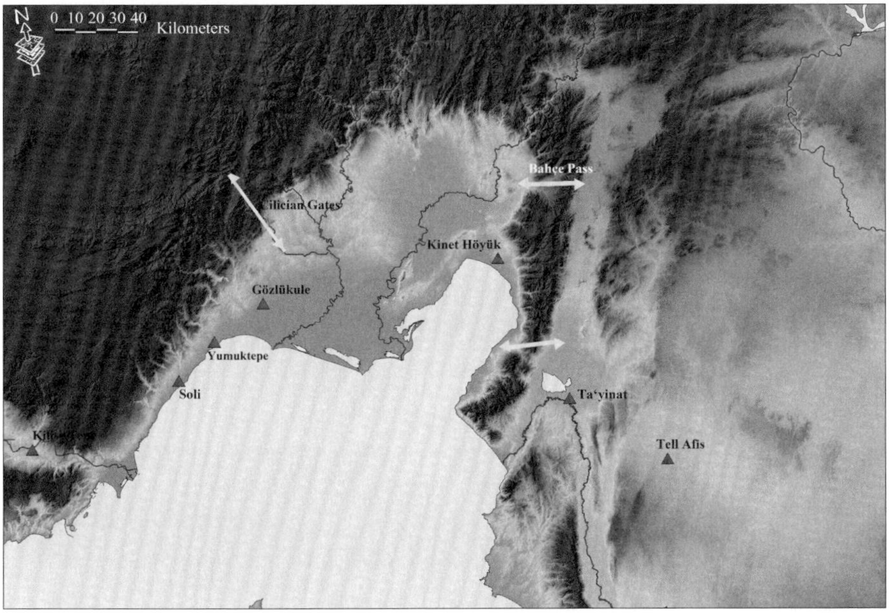

FIG. 1 Map of the region (by Stephen D. Batiuk)

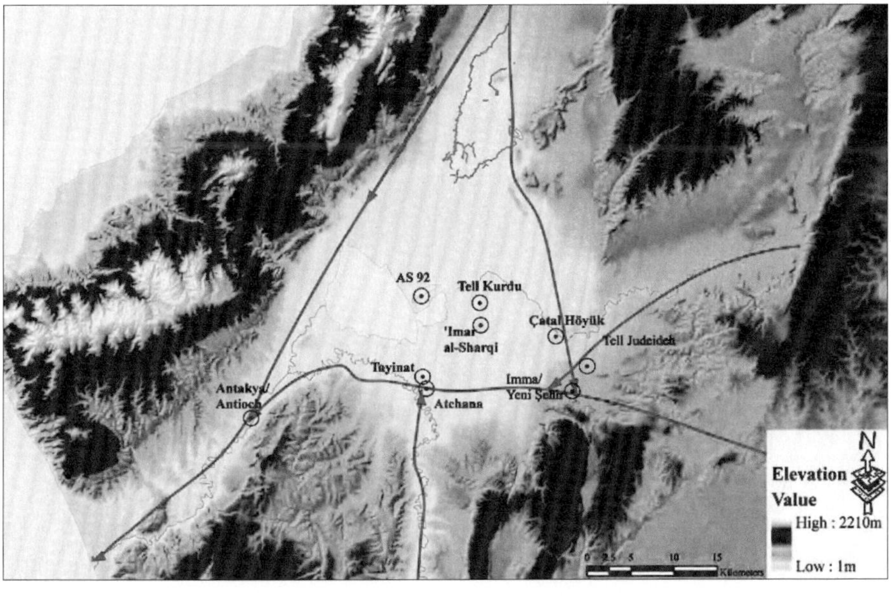

FIG. 2 Map of the Amuq Plain (by Stephen D. Batiuk)

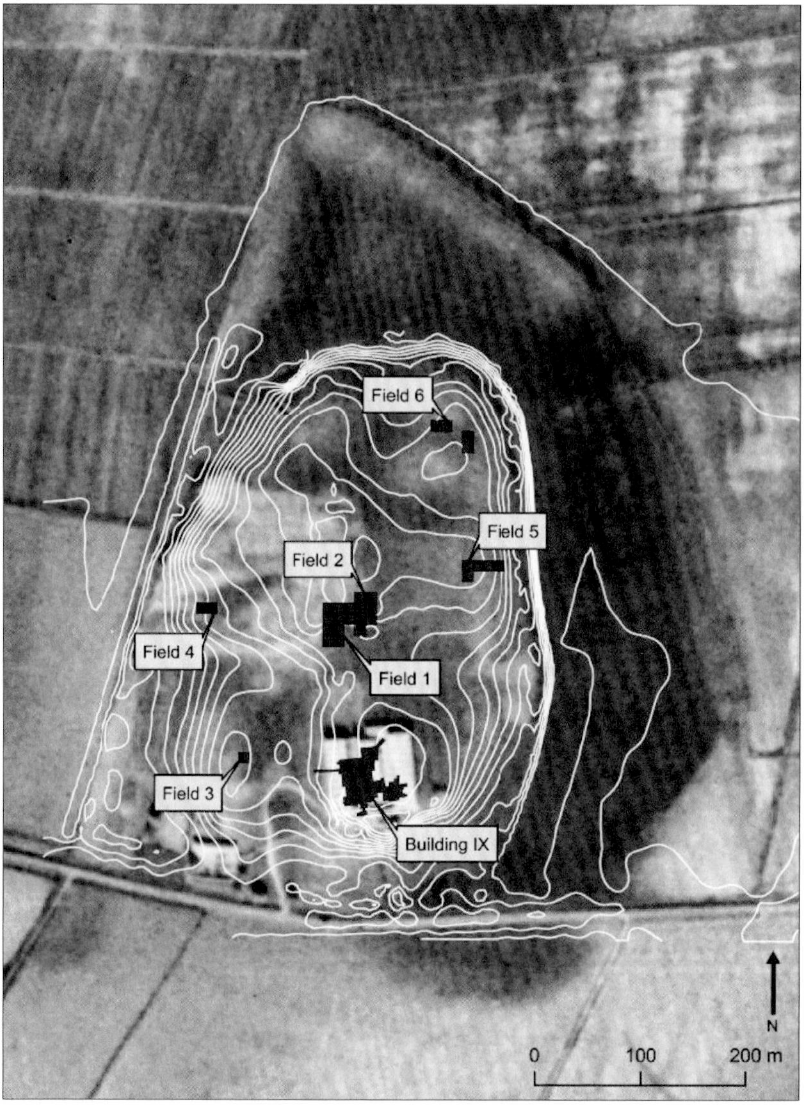

FIG. 3 The mound of Tell Tayinat (by Stephen D. Batiuk)

1 trenches G4 55 and G4 56 (FIG. 3), where the levels belonging to this period are separated into Field Phases 6–3 (hereafter, FP) by the excavators, the latter representing the latest the Iron IA phase on the mound.[3] This article focuses on the pottery of this very last phase of Iron IA Period on the mound, namely FP 3, which

3 Harrison *et al.*, forthcoming.

Trench G4 55									
Locus	Pail	Plain	Painted-NonLH IIIC	Cooking Pot-Shell	Cooking Pot-Lime	LH IIIC	Ir II*	Unidentified	Total**
18	23	6		3	1	2			12
36	68	17			1	5	2		25
36	78	3		7		3		1	14
36	80	14			1	5		1	21
36	83	22			1	4		1	28
36	84	15		5		6		1	27
36	91	17				6		1	24
36	94	10				6		1	17
36	95	35	1	12		11		1	60
36	100	14		6	1	4		1	26
36	101	6		1		1		1	9
36	115	7	1	6		6			20
72	120	4		2	1	5			12
	Total	170	2	42	6	64	2	9	295
	%	57.63	0.68	14.24	2.03	21.69	0.68	3.05	

* Ir II counts include both RSBW and Cypro-Cilician painted
** Intrusive Early Bronze sherds are excluded

TABLE 1 Percent counts of all diagnostic sherds from selected Field Phase 3 contexts

is mainly represented by pits in these trenches.[4] The material presented here comes largely from two pits, Loci 36 and 40. Even though not the ideal archaeological context, upon close investigation, the contents of these pits reveal a very homogeneous and internally consistent pottery assemblage that can be distinguished from both the earlier Iron IA phases and the later Iron II levels on the site.

Tayinat Field Phase 3 Pottery

The pottery of this 'enigmatic'[5] phase seems to be straddling the earlier phases with stronger Late Bronze Age (LBA) Anatolian and Aegean traditions and the later Iron II Period with its well-known pottery repertoire in the region. Counts taken from diagnostic sherds of selected pails reveal both the continuities and discontinuities from earlier Iron IA phases (TABLE 1). For example, during FP 3, Gray Ware and Anatolian Red Slipped Wares are not present anymore. The LH IIIC pottery, on the other hand, although fewer in numbers compared to the earlier phases, is still part of the assemblage during FP 3. It is noteworthy that, even though many of the shapes from FP 3 herald the later Iron II Period pottery, the Red Slipped and Burnished Ware (hereafter RSBW) amounts from these contexts are so small that they are statistically negligible.

The most common vessel type for this phase is the plate/shallow bowl (FIG. 4).[6] Vessels of this type are all wheelmade with medium fine to medium coarse purification levels of the clay. The pastes have grit and lime inclusions along with

4 Harrison *et al.*, forthcoming.

5 Designated so by the excavators, see Harrison *et al.*, forthcoming.

6 Because the plate/shallow bowl distinction is rather arbitrary, and they represent a similar food serving tradition, it is preferred here that they are not differentiated from one another.

very little mica. In a few cases there is chaff temper added. The color varies from pink to reddish yellow. In all cases, the surface treatment is restricted to simple smoothing. These vessels are well fired with hard biscuits and no dark cores. There are rare instances where the fabric of a typical plate/shallow bowl was additionally tempered with shell (Fig. 4.7). This is a novelty of FP 3. In earlier phases of Iron IA, shell tempered fabric is exclusively used in producing cooking pots (see below for more detail).

The shallow bowl/plate with a simple rim and a low pedestal base is the most typical shape within this category (Fig. 4.1–3, Fig. 4.7). The diameters vary in size from 19–44 cm within the selected sample, with the 28–32 cm range being the most common. This shape has good parallels in the later Iron II assemblage of the region.[7] Yet it is also not a new concept, as the plate/shallow bowl is the leading shape of the earlier Iron IA Period on the site[8] and in the region.[9] Therefore, here it does not represent a new eating custom; rather it is a simplification and standardization of the more elaborate and varied plate/shallow bowl shapes from earlier phases.[10] One consistent distinction is in the surface treatment: in the earlier phases, these vessels have rounded bases, which were left mostly untreated to the point that wheel-marks or scraping-marks towards the lower half of the body on the outside are visible.[11] This is in contrast to the carefully smoothed surface and the ring base of this shape.[12] One can consider these vessels as an intermediate stage tying the earlier Late Bronze Anatolian inspired tradition to the later Iron II tradition. Also plate/shallow bowl types with more elaborated rims, although fewer in numbers, are by no means discontinued in FP 3, still maintaining the earlier tradition during this phase (Fig. 4.4–6).

The painted plates/shallow bowls share common shapes with the plain ones and have the same fabric (Fig. 5). Decoration is mostly limited to wide bands ranging from red to dark brown on the outside just below the rim. Similar decoration also occurs in FP 4 (Fig. 7.2–3). The decoration of the rim with a single painted band is a typical Late Bronze Age characteristic in the region.[13]

7 For Tell Tayinat, see Osborne 2011, type 1A1, pl. 1.4; for Tell Qarqur, see Dornemann 2003, fig. 81.

8 Harrison *et al.*, forthcoming.

9 Venturi 2000b, 1718, see fig. 8.1–4 belonging to level 9a–8.

10 TP 6–5 plates/shallow bowls are in great conformity to the Hittite Monochrome Ware tradition (Harrison *et al.*, forthcoming).

11 Harrison *et al.*, forthcoming.

12 But it should be noted that ring bases on plates/shallow bowls seem to be present at Tell Atchana (Woolley 1955, plate CIX.3b).

13 For Tell Atchana, see Horowitz forthcoming, fig 9.1, 3; for Kinet Höyük, see Gates 2010, 73 *in passim*.

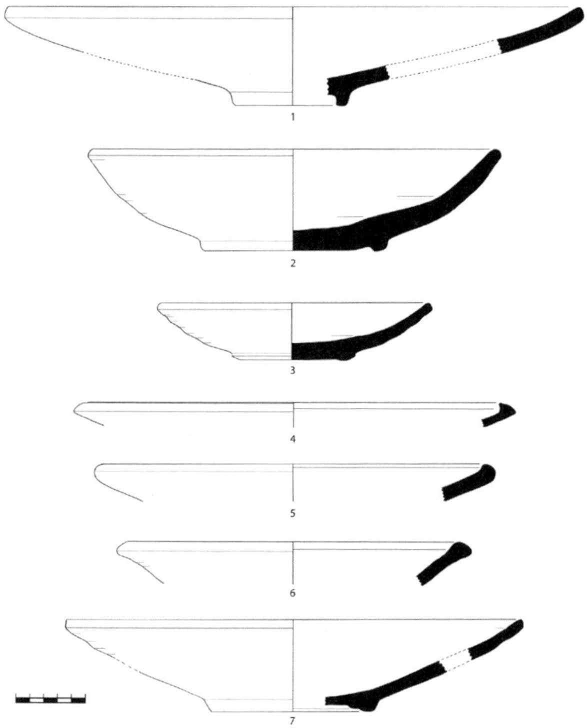

FIG. 4 Tell Tayinat FP 3 plain plates/shallow bowls

Brown Burnished vessels are a rare but consistently occurring type from the earliest phases of Iron IA (FIG. 6.1).[14] These vessels are self-slipped and medium burnished. Although macroscopically one cannot ascertain if they should be considered local, the distinctive yellowish brown color of the fabric and the surface are different from the common plain fabric. This ware type is also encountered in Tarsus LB IIb levels, as well as at the more easterly Cilician settlement of Kinet Höyük.[15] At this point it is not possible to link this ware type to the well-known RSBW tradition of the Iron II Period. The origin of the RSBW is a considerably discussed, yet still an unresolved, issue.[16] The red slipped plate/shallow bowl from Tayinat FP 4, which is not burnished but only smoothed, can

14 Represented by a shallow bowl in this case, but other vessel shapes are also present within the assemblage.

15 This ware was named "Brown Pattern Burnished Ware" at Kinet Höyük (Gates forthcoming, fig. 5.18).

16 An involved survey on the origin of RSBW is beyond the scope of this paper, but see Gates 2010, 72–75, where several issues (including associating this surface treatment ethnically with the Aramaeans) are succinctly surveyed. Here M.-H. Gates tentatively proposes that red slipped bowl examples from Kinet Period 12 may help tie this surface treatment to the Late Bronze Anatolian tradition. A red wash on plates is also attested in the Late Bronze levels of Tell Atchana, see Woolley 1955, 322.

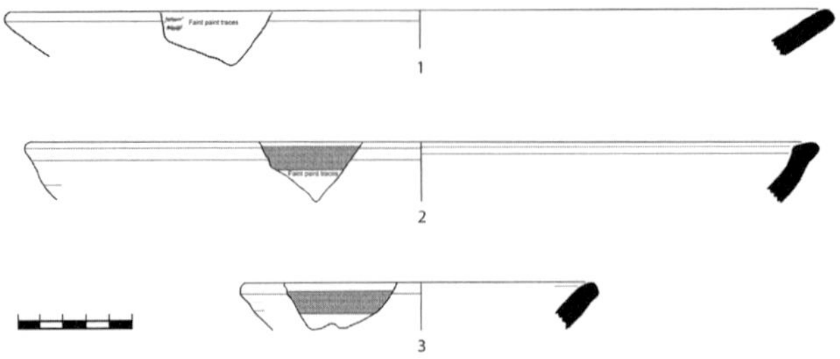

Fig. 5 Tell Tayinat FP 3 painted plates/shallow bowls

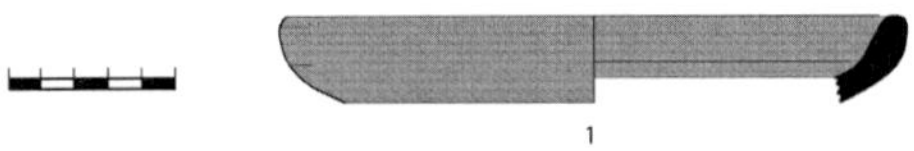

Fig. 6 Tell Tayinat FP 3 Brown Burnished Ware bowl

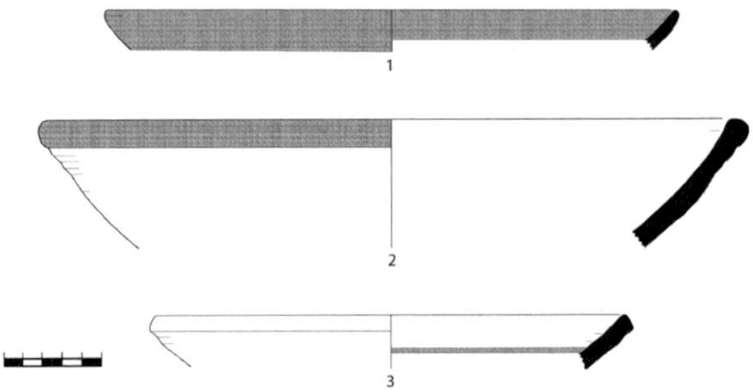

Fig. 7 Tell Tayinat FP 4 slipped or painted bowls

be considered an early RSBW form occurring here already in Iron IA (Fig. 7.1). But such examples at Tell Tayinat are few in number, and more stratigraphically secure data is needed to consider a linear development of the RSBW class from the local tradition as viable.

Another hallmark of the FP 3 repertoire is the bowl with a flaring rim and a smooth carination toward the base (Fig. 8.1–2). It is another shape that continues into the Iron II Period, but with a much sharper carination.[17] Their fabric is the same as the fabric of the plates/shallow bowls ranging from medium to medium fine purification levels. The color is also within the typical plain ware palette, but some of these deep bowls seem to have been fired at higher temperatures, as indicated by the completely oxidized, clinky, and very light colored fabric (Fig. 8.2). Their diameter varies from 11–25 cm, suggesting that these cups were used to serve a range of drinking portions. They are smoothed on the outside and inside

17 Osborne 2011, type 2C1, pl. 10; also at Tell Qarqur, see Dornemann 2003, 16–20, fig. 82.

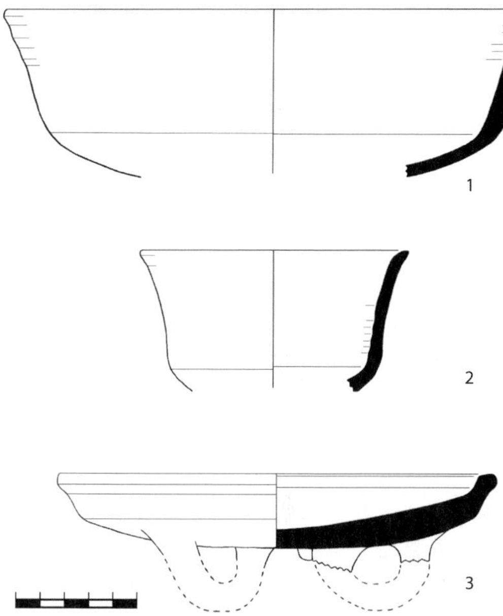

FIG. 8 Tell Tayinat FP 3 plain bowls and cups

until below the rim, and the rest of the interior is left untreated.[18] This shape may well be following an earlier LH IIIC tradition, with the important difference that these bowls do not seem to have handles.[19]

The tripod bowl (FIG. 8.3) is a type not encountered in the earlier phases of Iron IA. In FP 3 there are at least two examples (one not illustrated, but also has looped feet). They both come from the same pit deposition, which yielded large amounts of mendable pottery. Tripod bowls are encountered in Iron II levels in the region, but not generally with looped feet.[20] Tripod vessels with looped feet are encountered at the neighboring site of Tell Atchana from the earlier Bronze Age levels.[21] In fact, tripod vessels have been part of the Anatolian ceramic repertoire

18 This is a peculiar trait for a drinking cup.

19 This is the shallow angular bowl FS 295 tradition of LH IIIC. It is commonly encountered in the region: for Tarsus see Mountjoy 2005, 422, fig. 17.; for Tell Tayinat, see Janeway 2011, fig. 2.6, where it is further elaborated that at Tell Tayinat this version is less common and is encountered in FP 5, p. 175.

20 For Tell Tayinat, see Osborne 2011, type 2A4, pl. 6.12–14; for Al Mina Stratum 8, see Lehmann 2005, 6, fig. 3:4. Interestingly, a vessel identified as a lid (identified as such because the loops are of different sizes) from level IIc/d Kilise Tepe in Rough Cilicia could actually be a loop footed tripod bowl (Hansen and Postgate 2007, 357, 783, fig. 397.). But obviously also here it is an exotic shape.

21 See Woolley 1955, 332, 339, pl. CXXIV.161 (jar), 162 (bowl). 163 a–b are tripod footed bowls, but the feet are not looped. They are the most common type. Especially variant b was mostly covered with a red wash and burnished.

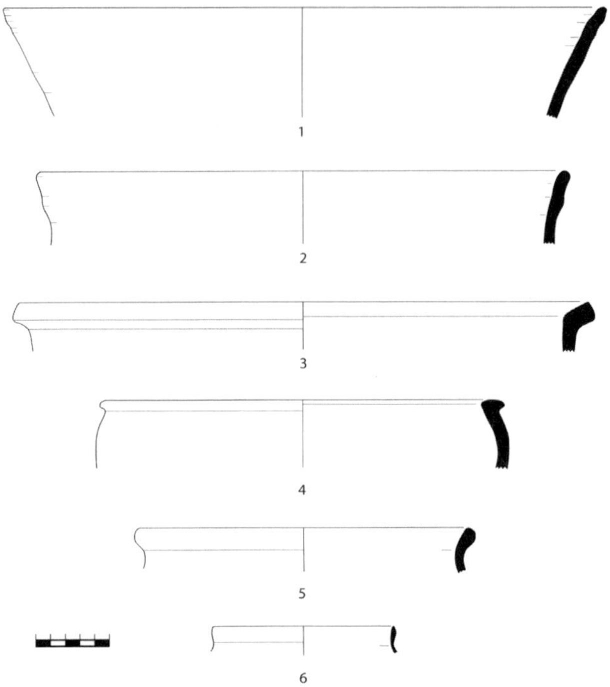

Fig. 9 Tell Tayinat FP 3 jars

since the Early Bronze Age.[22] So the tripod footed bowls from Tayinat FP 3 may represent a continuation of an earlier Bronze Age tradition strongly represented in Anatolia. One should note, however, that both of these tripod bowls are self-slipped and low to medium low burnished, an unusual surface treatment for the FP 3 phase at Tell Tayinat. Moreover, the fabric inclusions and color range from light reddish to yellow is somewhat off from the typical local plain ware fabric. Loop footed tripod vessels seem to be more at home in the southern Levant, found both on bowls and jars.[23] Therefore, considering the absence of this specific type of loop footed tripod vessels in Anatolia, it is very possible that these are imports from the southern Levant. Regardless of their origin, certainly these were not vessels of ordinary daily use, but rather for special, even maybe cultic, occasions.

The closed vessel repertoire at Tayinat FP 3 also shows a mixture of continuity from earlier phases along with some novelties. The jars with an everted rectangular rim (Fig. 9.3) or everted thickened out rim (Fig. 9.5–6) continue the LB II and

22 For Troy, see Blegen *et al.* 1951, 358, nr. 256, 277, 363; for Elmalı-Karataş, see Eslick 2009, pl. 67. KT 410; for Tarsus-Gözlükule, see Goldman 1956, 445, fig. 273.

23 Suggested to be a continuation of a LBA tradition in this region (see Harrison 2004, 24, 27; also see Shipton 1939, pl. 5.27, plain jar from stratum X) Good examples come from Megiddo VI levels: Harrison 2004, pl. 1.9 (painted bowl) and pl. 7.5–6 (painted jars).

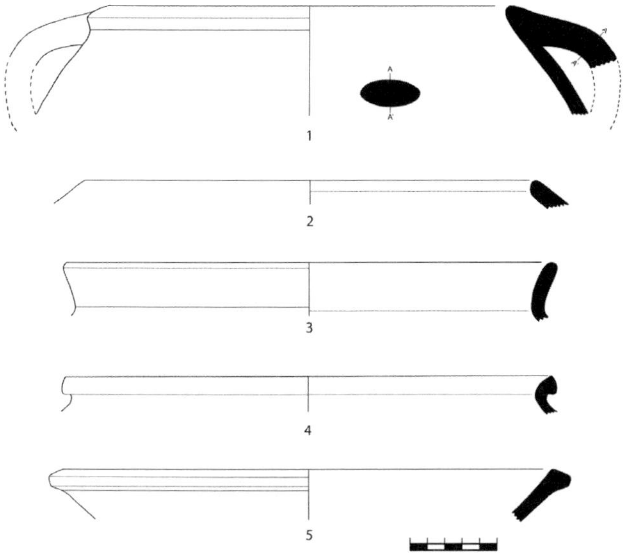

FIG. 10 Tell Tayinat FP 3 cooking pots

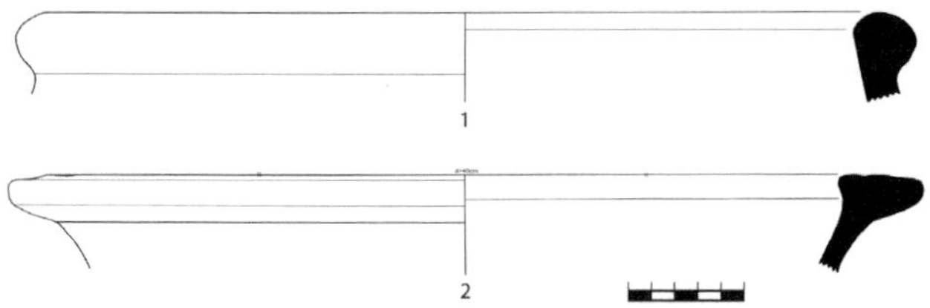

FIG. 11 Tell Tayinat FP 3 storage vessels

earlier Iron IA tradition.[24] On the other hand, jars with straight, strongly everted rims are common in FP 3 but are not present in earlier phases (FIG. 9.1–2). Another shape not encountered in earlier phases of Tell Tayinat are jars with globular bodies and horizontal pulled out rims (FIG. 9.4), though it finds somewhat distant parallels in the region.[25]

FP 3 cooking pots are predominantly made with a shell-tempered fabric (FIG. 10). The distinguishing feature of this fabric is the copious use of crushed shell along with lesser amounts of sand, lime, and chaff inclusions. This is a coarse fabric used in the production of large, closed vessels. These vessels are self-slipped and smoothed on the outside and on the inside until below the rim. Frequent mottling on their exterior surfaces ascertains their function for cooking.

24 For Tell Tayinat, see Harrison *et al*, forthcoming; for Tell Afis, see Venturi 2000b, fig. 5.9, 5.14; for Tarsus-Gözlükule, see Goldman 1956, fig. 389 O; for Mersin-Yumuktepe, see Sevin and Köroğlu 2004, fig. 7.13 (painted); for Lidar Höyük, see Müller 1999, figs. 5.1–2, 5.7.

25 For Kinet Höyük, see Gates, forthcoming, fig. 7.4; for Tell Afis, see Venturi 2000a, fig. 10.7 from the early part of Iron IA.

The use of crushed shell as temper for cooking pots has a long tradition in the northeastern Mediterranean from the LBA onward and continues to be used without significant changes to its paste recipe throughout the Iron IA Period,[26] continuing into the Iron II Period, but in a more restricted manner.[27] Some of the cooking pot shapes from FP 3 show continuity from the earlier phases, like the two-handled pot with a ridge running along the exterior of the rim (Fig. 10.1)[28] and the sharply rolled out rim but with the usual ridge (Fig. 10.4).[29] The hole-mouth cooking pot (Fig. 10.2), on the other hand, seems to be a later occurrence, perhaps in accordance with the general trend at simplification of the rims.[30] Here, it should be noted that in FP 3 (and even earlier in FP 4), the shapes within the shell tempered ware repertoire became more varied, and even shapes traditionally produced in plain fabric began to be produced in this ware type, albeit in very small numbers (Fig. 4.7). This perhaps indicates a less rigid demarcation of pottery and ware types based on their function and might signify a further breaking down of older production practices by this later Iron IA Period.

There is also a different type of cooking pot ware tempered with crushed lime. This occurs in very small amounts throughout all FPs. The shapes represented within this small group are also unusual, like the open plate/shallow bowl type presented here (Fig. 10.5).

Storage vessels have a coarse, mixed fabric, some having both lime and shell inclusions and some being further tempered with chaff. One of the most common traits of storage vessels from the Iron IA assemblage at Tell Tayinat is the thickened-out rim and inverted stance (Fig. 11.1). This type occurs in all FPs and the thickening out is at varying degrees of exaggeration. The pithos with both a thickened-in and thickened-out rim flattened horizontally[31] is another type that occurs through all phases, some of which are further grooved on top, like the one illustrated here (Fig. 11.2).[32]

26 Harrison *et al.* forthcoming.

27 Osborne 2011, pl. 24, types 8B1 and 8B2.

28 See Harrison *et al.*, forthcoming; Venturi 2000a, fig. 10.2 from level 9a.

29 See Venturi 2000b, fig. 5.18, from level 10–9c.

30 There is a variety of terminology used for this class of vessels, like "Cooking Pot à la Stéatite", "Band Handled Cooking Pot" etc., none of which acknowledge the strong LBA roots of the paste heavily tempered with shell. It is beyond the scope of this paper to go into the detail of these discussions. Suffice it to say that these shapes are very much at home within the general trends in shape development observed throughout the Iron IA Period at Tell Tayinat, and there is no need to look further afield for the origin of these pots.

31 This one has both lime and shell inclusions.

32 Such grooved tops on the rims are a very characteristic trait in LB II Tarsus-Gözlükule, see Goldman 1956, fig. 390 K-M.

Conclusion

The last phase of the Iron IA Period at Tell Tayinat displays mainly continuity, with some novelties not encountered in earlier phases. The most typical shapes continue the earlier Late Bronze practices, like the plate/shallow bowl tradition and the shell tempered cooking pot vessels. Some shapes seem to be inspired by the LH IIIC tradition present within the assemblage since FP 6.

However, this phase exhibits certain transformations, one of which is the general trend towards simplification of the formerly more elaborated rims. Moreover, the surface treatment is generally more careful, and some vessels (especially in the plate/shallow bowl category) are further decorated, ranging from simple painted bands to examples that are either partially or totally slipped in red. Some are also burnished.

It is clear that the Iron IA Period in the eastern Mediterranean was a synthesis of shifting networks, local and regional preferences, and changing demographics and played a significant role in forming the basis of the idiosyncratic cultures of the later Iron Age kingdoms in the region establishing themselves within the next few centuries. The growing historical and material evidence demonstrates that during the later Iron Age in the power vacuum created by the downfall of the Hittite Empire, the Amuq region contained an independent Neo-Hittite kingdom with epigraphic and stylistic affinities to the earlier LBA Hittite realm [33] (including continued use of Hieroglyphic Luwian). [34] This kingdom was then incorporated into the Neo-Assyrian Empire by Tiglath-pileser III, with Tell Tayinat as its provincial capital. [35] In the pottery assemblage of the Iron IA period at Tell Tayinat as well, we see continuation of the earlier Late Bronze traditions, while at the same time there is the intrusive new material with strong Aegean affinities. [36] The pottery of this latest phase of Iron IA demonstrates the process whereby different customs (new and old) started to be merged with each other and further simplified, yielding a more standardized material than before, which heralds the later Iron II pottery assemblage.

The residents of Tell Tayinat during the earlier phases of the Iron IA seem to have adopted a flexible strategy to include various practices into their repertoire, creating a new local syntax in response to the rapidly changing political, economic, and cultural conditions in the region. [37] During FP 3, a trend of standardization

33 The stratigraphic relationship between the Iron IA phase and the later Iron IC/II phases is not clear at Tell Tayinat (see Harrison 2009, 177).

34 See Harrison 2009, 187.

35 Harrison 2009, 175; Harrison and Osborne 2012, 125–126.

36 Harrison *et al.*, forthcoming; Janeway 2011.

37 For more detail on earlier phases see Harrison *et al.*, forthcoming.

and simplification can be observed, eliminating certain earlier traditions and introducing some novelties, which culminates in the well-known Iron II pottery repertoire of the region. This is a natural outcome, especially in environments of economic flexibility and social flux, whereby many distinct conventions coexisting for a while start to merge with each other. This, however, seems not to have occurred in a dichotomy of dominant and the fringe or old and the new, but rather smoothly taking on some aspects from certain practices and creating in the end a novel, regionally well-defined assemblage.

REFERENCES

Blegen, C. W., J. L. Caskey and M. Rawson, *Troy: Excavations Conducted by the University of Cincinnati, 1932–1938, Vol. 2. The Third, Fourth, and Fifth Settlements*. Princeton: Princeton University Press, 1951.

Dornemann, R.H, *Preliminary Excavation Reports and Other Archaeological Excavations. Tell Qarqur, Iron I Sites in the North-Central Highlands of Palestine*. Boston: The American Schools of Oriental Research, 2003.

Eslick, C., *Elmalı-Karataş V. The Early Bronze Age Pottery of Karataş: Habitation Deposits*. Oxford: Archaeopress, 2009.

Gates, M.-H., "Potters and Consumers in Cilicia and the Amuq during the 'Age of Transformations' (13th–10th centuries BC.)" in *Societies in Transition. Evolutionary Processes in the Northern Levant between Late Bronze Age II and Early Iron Age. Papers Presented on the Occasion of the 20th Anniversary of the New Excavations in Tell Afis, 15th November 2007*, ed. by F. Venturi, 65–81. Bologna: Clueb, 2010.

———. "From Late Bronze to Iron Age on Syria's Northwest Frontier: Cilicia and the Amuq" in *Percorsi di Archeologia Siriana: Celebrando 20 anni di archeologia a Tell Afis. Pisa, 27–28 November 2006*. Pisa, forthcoming.

Goldman, H., *Excavations at Gözlü Kule, Tarsus. From the Neolithic through the Bronze Age. Vol II*. Princeton: Princeton University Press, 1956.

Hansen, C. and J. N. Postgate, "Pottery from Level II" in *Excavations at Kilise Tepe, 1994–98: From Bronze Age to Byzantine in Western Cilicia*, ed. by J. N. Postgate, N. and D. Thomas, 343–370. Oxford: Oxbow Books, 2007.

Harrison, T.P., *Megiddo 3. Final Report on the Stratum VI Publications*. Chicago: The Oriental Institute of the University of Chicago, 2004.

———. "Neo-Hittites in the 'Land of Palistin'. Renewed Investigations at Tell Ta'yinat on the Plain of Antioch." *Near Eastern Archaeology* 72/4 (2009): 174–189.

Harrison, T. P. and J. F. Osborne, "Building XVI and the Neo-Assyrian Sacred Precinct at Tell Tayinat." *Journal of Cuneiform Studies* 64 (2012): 125–143.

Harrison, T.P., S. Batiuk, M. Capper, B. Janeway, D. Lipovitch, D. Lump, J. Roames, E. Ünlü and L. Welton, *Shifting Networks and Community Identity at Tell Tayinat in the Iron IA*. Forthcoming.

Horowitz, M.T., "The Evolution of Plain Ware Ceramics at the Regional Capital of Alalakh in the 2nd Millennium BC" in *Pots, Palaces and Politics: An International Workshop on the Evolution and Socio-Political Significance of Plain Ware Traditions in the 2nd millennium BC Near East and East Mediterranean*, ed. by C. Glatz. London, forthcoming.

Janeway, B., "Mycenaean Bowls at 12th/11th Century BC Tell Tayinat (Amuq Valley)" in *On Cooking Pots, Drinking Cups, Loomweights and Ethnicity in Bronze Age Cyprus and Neighbouring Regions. An International Archaeological Symposium Held in Nicosia*, ed. by V. Karageorghis and O. Kouka, 167–185. Nicosia, 2011.

Lehmann, G., "Al Mina and the East: A Report on Research in Progress" in *The Greeks in the East*, ed. by A. Villing, 61–92. London: British Museum Publications, 2005.

Mazzoni, S., "Syria and the Periodization of the Iron Age: A Cross-Cultural Perspective" in *Essays on Syria in the Iron Age*, ed. by G. Bunnens, 31–59. Ancient Near Eastern Studies Suppl. 7, Louvain, 2000.

Mountjoy, P.A., "The Mycenaean Pottery from the 1934–1939 Excavations at Tarsus" in *Field Seasons 2001–2003 of the Tarsus-Gözlükule Interdisciplinary Research Project*, ed. by A. Özyar, 83–134. İstanbul: Ege Yayınları, 2005.

———. "A Note on the Mixed Origins of Some Philistine Pottery." *Bulletin of the American Schools of Oriental Research* 359 (2010): 1–12.

Müller, U., "Die eisenzeitliche Stratigraphie von Lidar Höyük." *Anatolian Studies* 49 (1999): 123–131.

Osborne, J.F., *Spatial Analysis and Political Authority in the Iron Age Kingdom of Patina, Turkey*. Unpublished Ph.D. Thesis, Harvard University, 2011.

Sevin, V. and K. Köroğlu, "Late Bronze Age at Yumuktepe: New Evidence from Step-Trench South" in *Mersin-Yumuktepe: A Reappraisal*, ed. by I. Caneva and V. Sevin, 73–83. Lecce: Congedo, 2004.

Shipton, G.M., *Notes on the Megiddo Pottery of Strata VI-XX*. Chicago: University of Chicago Press, 1939.

Swift, G.F., *The Pottery of the 'Amuq, Phases K to O, and Its Historical Relationships*. Unpublished Ph.D. Thesis, University of Chicago, 1958.

Venturi, F., "Le Premier Age du Fer a Tell Afis et en Syrie Septentrionale" in *Essays on Syria in the Iron Age*, ed. by G. Bunnens, 505–536. Louvain, 2000a.

———. "Tell Afis et la "Dark Age" (les niveaux de la fin du Bronze récent II et de l'âge du Fer I)" in *First International Congress on the Archaeology of the Ancient Near East, May 18th–23rd 1998*, ed. by P. Matthiae, A. Enea, L. Peyronel and F. Pinnock, 1715–1730. Rome: Università degli studi di Roma "La Sapienza," 2000b.

Woolley, C.L., *Alalakh: An Account of the Excavations at Tell Atchana in the Hatay, 1937–1949*. Report of the Research Committee of the Society of Antiquaries of London 18. London: Society of Antiquaries, 1955.

PART 5

Hellenistic and Roman

Second-in-Rank Local Producers of Megarian Bowls in the Aegean and Elsewhere[1]

Jan Bouzek[2]

Charles and Marie-Henriette Gates were excellent hosts of the Black Sea Congress in Ankara in 2001 with their students from Bilkent University, and they have always been willing to help on other occasions, so it is my pleasure to support their students and contribute to a Festschrift dedicated to the couple.

Abstract

This article discusses the local production of Megarian bowls oriented toward a local market, which sometimes imitated the models of the main centres, but also brought interesting new combinations of motifs and new ideas. Though only with limited exports beyond their local areas, they contributed – similarly as the coroplasts did – to innovative facets of minor Hellenistic art.

The more profound study of Megarian bowls[3] started with an interest in iconography, notably in Homeric bowls,[4] and by analysing identical stamps and moulds.[5] The main production centres were identified by several scholars,[6] and their distribution was studied.[7] Megarian bowls had several main centres of production,

1 This paper was prepared in the frame of the project P 12 in the Faculty of Arts, Charles University, "History in Interdisciplinary Perspective".

2 Department of Archaeology and Museology, Faculty of Arts, Masaryk University, Arna Nováka 1/1, 602 00 Brno, Czech Republic.

3 See Courby 1922.

4 Hausmann 1959; Sinn 1979.

5 Especially Laumonier 1977; see Bouzek and Jansová 1974.

6 Ephesian workshops: De Luca 1984; Gassner 1997; also see Zabelina 1984; Bouzek 1990.

7 Bouzek 1990, 2006, 2007; Domăneanţu 2000.

of which first Athens,[8] and later the Ionian class,[9] identified as products from Ephesus,[10] led the way. Macedonia was a producer of Homeric bowls at Demetrias[11] and of simpler variations at Pella.[12] In Pergamon a more sophisticated variety with applied reliefs was invented.[13] These were the most important centres with most of their products destined for export,[14] while other workshops situated elsewhere exported less frequently. Kyme, Pergamon and Myrina had high quality workshops in contrast to inland sites,[15] but exceptions exist.

Corinth took a position between the two categories. It had excellent production until its destruction in 146 BC.[16] Its exports and impact were exerted notably in its earlier zone of interest, marked, for example, by its export of Red-Figured pottery. Corinthian bowls were found even in the eastern Adriatic and southwestern Balkans, where local workshops also imitated its style,[17] as did some potters in the Peloponnese, notably after they managed to escape from the destroyed city, as in Argos and Olympia,[18] where they reached a more sophisticated level.[19] Megarian bowls were produced in limited numbers probably even on the island of Aegina[20] and in Eretria,[21] while the Pylos cemetery yielded only Ionian imports.[22]

However, many local potters also produced their mainly less sophisticated imitations elsewhere. Pierre Dupont, in a brief contribution to the most recent Black Sea congress in Istanbul in 2009, mentioned clay analyses, which seem to show that local clay was probably used for some of the Megarian bowls similar to those from the main centres, but in the final publication[23] it was mentioned that

8 Rotroff 1982; Schwabacher 1941.

9 Laumonier 1977.

10 De Luca 1984; Gassner 1997; Krinzinger 2001; Rogl 2001; Dereboylu 2001; Günay-Tuluk 2001; Bouzek 2005.

11 Hausmann 1959; Sinn 1979.

12 Akamates 1993.

13 De Luca and Ziegenhaus 1968; Ziegenhaus and De Luca 1975; Hübner 1993.

14 Surveys by Domăneanţu 2000; Guldager Bilde 1993; Siebert 1977, 1980; Bouzek 2007; Lévêque and Morel 1987.

15 For Hierapolis in Phrygia see Semiraro 2003.

16 Edwards 1975, 1981.

17 Stobi: Anderson-Stojanović 1992; the Ohrid Region: Bitrakova-Grozdanova 2008; Croatia: Rusić 1999.

18 Hausmann 1996.

19 Siebert 1978.

20 Margreiter 1988; Smetana-Scherrer 1982.

21 Metzger 1969; Schmidt 2000.

22 Danadi 2004.

23 Dupont 2013.

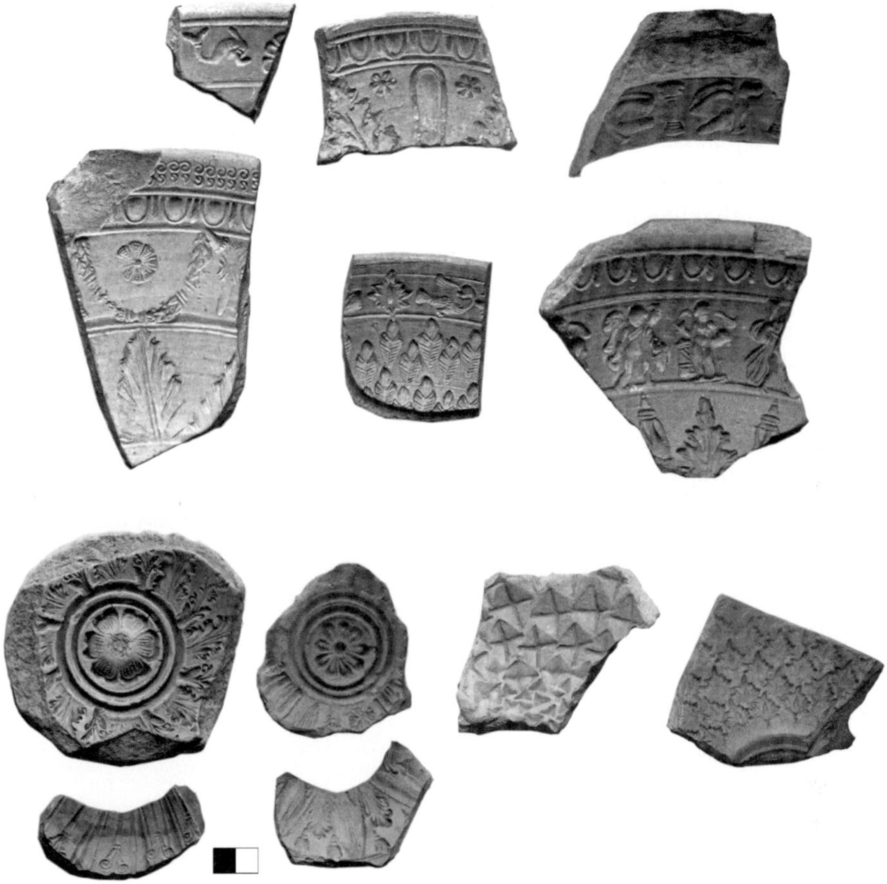

FIG. 1 Fragments of moulds from Kyme.

no local bowl were found among the finds from Histria. The study of taken-over patterns, starting with the Delos "Plagiaire" of Laumonier,[24] opened the discussion of the possibility of stamps being taken from the leading workshops to elsewhere. It is a challenge for the recent study of Hellenistic relief pottery to complete the picture of more specific local products.

A certain amount of locally made Megarian bowls were also produced at the minor Greek cities of the north Aegean. Besides Pella[25] and Demetrias with its Homeric class,[26] this was reflected by several small publications from Archailogikon

24 Laumonier 1977.

25 Akamates 1993.

26 Sinn 1979.

Deltion and Archaiologika Analekta ex Makedonias kai Thrakis, and by objects on display in the museums of Kavalla, Komotini, Maroneia, Thasos and elsewhere.[27] Where the Aegean islands are concerned, workshop debris from Hefaisteia on Lemnos was published,[28] and similar evidence came from Minoa on Amorgos,[29] while the Laumonier's "Plagiare" probably worked in Delos.

On the other hand, local centres in western Asia Minor, which mainly served local markets, existed notably in Kyme, where the new Italian excavations brought to light a much larger collection of moulds and bowls than previously published, and one of its products was found even at Histria;[30] the selection of moulds (Fig. 1) show well the inventiveness of the potters even in the 'second-in-rank' centres. The richness of inventions can also be seen at neighbouring Myrina.[31] Of another character are bowls from Milet,[32] Sardis[33] and Iassos,[34] while the Mayence set of moulds came from Ionia or Aeolis.[35] This does not mean that other ateliers did not produce Megarian bowls,[36] but it shows that their products are less well known and remain largely unpublished.[37]

In Tarsus,[38] Cyprus[39] and several centres in north Syria,[40] bowls of good quality were produced.[41] Further to the south, less sophisticated imitations appeared besides mainly Attic and Ephesian imports,[42] and a similar situation existed in Egypt and Cyrenaica.[43]

---

27 See Karadima 1997 and Rotroff 2010.

28 Massa 1990.

29 Pappa 2000.

30 Domăneanţu 2000, 112.

31 Courby 1922, pl. 10cd, pl. 11a.

32 Kossatz 1990.

33 Rotroff 1994.

34 Pierobon 1986; Pierobon and Benoit 1997.

35 Künzl 2002.

36 They did produce them, sometimes even with greater success, as seen at Samos; Tsakos 1994.

37 See Hellström 1965.

38 Goldman and Jones 1950.

39 Neuru 1991; Papuci-Wladyka 1995.

40 Antioch on the Orontes: Waagé 1948; Dura Europos: Cox 1949.

41 Less so from minor sites; Hama: Christensen and Johansen 1971; Tell Erfad: Boháč *et al.* 1997, 126, fig. 4; 1999.

42 For Beirut see Bouzek and Trefný 2002, 24–28, 102–105; for Savaria see Crowfoot and Kenyon 1957; Dor Rosenbaum and Heginbottom 1995a; 1995b; for Gezer see Gitin 1990.

43 Sha'arha-Amakim: Mlynarczyk 2000; Tell Anafa: Herbert 1997.

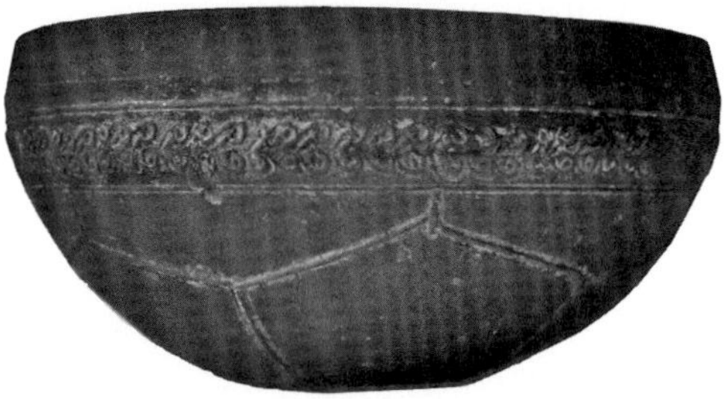

FIG. 2 Bowl with pentagonal patterns, no provenance, Charles University, Prague

As could be expected, in the wrecks and in *oppida* in southern France, Ephesian bowls prevail.[44] The Popilius workshop was successful in Campania; the last producer did not glaze his bowls but preferred the sharply cut relief,[45] as Demetrios from Panticapaeum did in the Black Sea[46] and as seen by the more modest Dacian imitations in the vicinity of Bucarest (FIG. 3). Several other workshops produced them in the Black Sea cities, notably in its northwestern corner,[47] but also in Messembria and perhaps even in Kabile, while among the finds from Apollonia and Mesembria, ones from the Attic and later Ephesian workshops took the leading position.[48]

The Kirbei bowls were probably made at Olbia, and many Black Sea cities had their own workshops.[49] The new study of bowls found in Romania, with the most notable ones being in the Constanţa, Bucureşti, Braila and Tulcea museums,[50] helped me recognize the situation. Many of the items from the Greek cities in the territory of Romania, that were studied more properly, are apparently products from local workshops in the area.[51]

The analysis of the samples from Histria[52] has shown that there were no local products among the materials from here, and at other places, *e.g.* Aegina,[53] the already made visual observations and the absence of good local clay seem to exclude such a possibility.

44 Benoit 1961.

45 See Puppo 1995; Hausmann 2004.

46 Bouzek 2007, 1232 with references.

47 Levi 1940; Bouzek 2007.

48 Bouzek 2007, 1231–1233, figs. 30–44, also see Čimbuleva 1969, 170–178, figs. 129, 150, 133–134

49 See Domăneanţu 2000, 119–122, 144–146; Guldager Bilde 1993, 201; Bouzek 2007, 1231–1233; 2012.

50 For which I am grateful to the keepers of the collections, and also for the kind invitation to a series of conferences in these cities, especially at Valeriu Sîrbu.

51 Bouzek 2012.

52 Dupont 2013.

53 Smetana-Scherer 1982; Margreiter 1988.

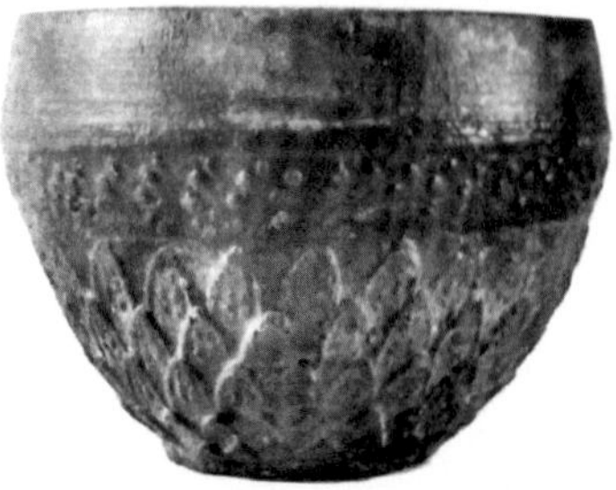

Fig. 3 Megarian bowl from near Kerch, mus. Pilsen

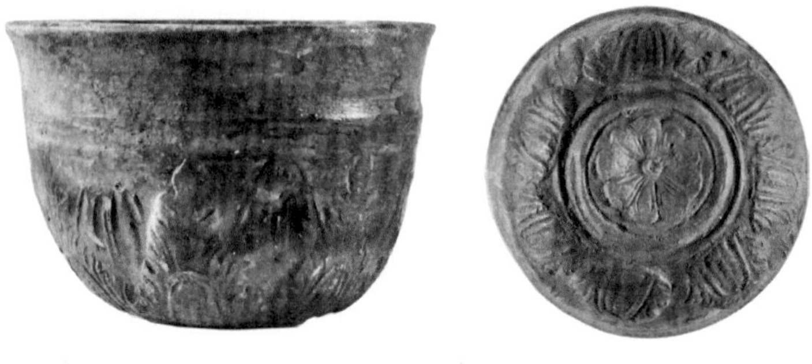

Fig. 4A-B Megarian bowl from near Kerch, mus. Pilsen

The Dacian bowls produced near Bucarest were half "barbarian,"[54] and the quality of the main exporting centres (first being Athens, later Ephesus, then Macedonia with Homeric bowls and in the first century especially Pergamon) was not reached by most of the local producers. This was also the case with some bowls I studied personally in the Chişinau Museum, and it applies also to the two bowls from Kerch in the Pilsen Museum. One with pine-cone decoration imitates Ephesian bowls, and a second example is of the class well represented in Olbia.[55] It should be noted, however, that some silver phalerae reputedly or certainly found in the eastern Balkans are closely similar in their decoration to the northwestern Pontic Megarian bowls, *e.g.* the three new phalerae in the Bojkov collection.[56] Clay bowls certainly imitated the much more expensive silver tableware. Some less sophisticated potters probably copied whole moulds or even bowls, as was usual in figural terracottas,[57] and perhaps even from silver bowls or from plaster models, as already supposed by Courby.[58]

54 Bouzek 1990, 68–69; Sirbu 2009; Petrova 2011; Varbanov 2012.

55 CVA Pilsen pl. 40; Bouzek 1990, pl. 14: 1–2, see figs. 4, 5a-b, 28.

56 Marazov 2011, nos. 185–187.

57 Muller 1997.

58 See Bouzek 2006.

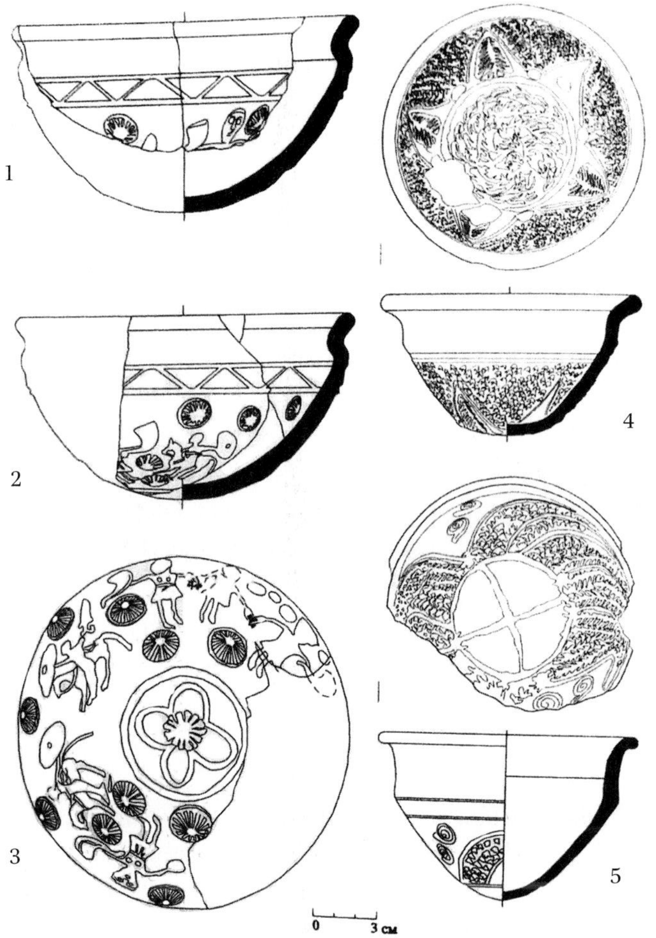

FIG. 5 Getic imitations of Megaran bows from Ruse northen Bulgaria, after Varbanov 2012.

To sum up, even if the main exporters, which were first Athens and later Ephesus and Pergamon, were the most important producers of Hellenistic relief pottery, nearly every Greek city in eastern Asia Minor, north Syria, Greece and around the Black Sea had some workshops, which produced for the local markets and were able to satisfy a large portion of local customers. However, in the eastern Balkans,[59] the Adriatic region, north Africa and southern France, hardly any local products have been detected until now.

59 Anderson-Stojanović 1992; Sokolovska 1986.

REFERENCES

Akamates, I., *Pelines metres aggeion apo ten Pella*. Athens 1993.

Anderson-Stojanović, V.R., *Stobi: The Hellenistic and Roman Pottery*. Princeton: Princeton University Press, 1992.

Benoit, F., *L'épave de Grand Congloué à Marseille*. Paris, 1961.

Bitrakova-Grozdanova, V., "Les bols à relief de la region d'Ohrid." *Archeološki otkritija na počvata na Makedonija* 18 (2008): 457–466.

Boháč, L., J. Bouzek and V. Grace, "Hellenistic and Roman finds from Bedřich Hrozný's excavations at Tell Erfad, Syria. I-II." *Eirene* 33 (1997): 122–157.

———. "III and Addenda." *Eirene* 35 (1999): 47–60.

Bouzek, J., *Studies of Greek Pottery in the Black Sea Area*. Prague: Charles University, 1990.

———. "Ephesier ausserhalb von Ephesus" in *Festschrift für Friedrich Krinzinger, Synergia Band II*, ed. by B. Brandt, V. Gassner and S. Ladstätter, 55–65. Vienna, 2005.

———. "Formen und Abformen" in *Mittel und Wege*, ed. by A. Doster, 11–22. Möhnesee: Bibliopolis, 2006.

———. "Greek Fine Pottery in the Black Sea Region" in *Ancient Greek Colonies in the Black Sea 2, Volume II*, ed. by D.V. Grammenos and E.K. Petropoulos, 1221–1262. Oxford: Archaeopress, 2007.

———. "Local production of Megarian bowls in the Black Sea and Thrace." *Studia Hercynia* 16/2 (2012): 43–48

Bouzek, J. and L. Jansová, "Megarian bowls" in *Anatolian Collection of Charles University, Kyme I*, ed. by J. Bouzek, 13–76. Prag: Charles University, 1974.

Bouzek, J. and M. Trefný, "Hellenistic Pottery in 'Czech excavations in Beirut, Martyrs' Square, 1996 (Bay 069, Sondage A, Part I." *Eirene* 38 (2002): 7–166.

Christensen, A.P. and Ch.F. Johansen, *Hama III,2, Les poteries hellénistiques et les terres sigillées orientales*, Copenhagen, 1971.

Crowfoot , J.W. and K.M. Kenyon, *The Objects from Samaria*. New Haven: Archaeological Institute of America, 1957.

Courby, F., *Les vases grecs à relief*. Paris, 1922.

Cox, D.H. *The Greek and Roman Pottery, Excavations at Dura Europos, Final Report IV,2*. New Haven 1949.

De Luca, G. and O. Ziegenhaus, *Das Asklepieion 2. Teil: Der nördliche Temenos-Bezirk und angrenzende Anlagen in hellenistischer und frührömischer Zeit, Altertümer aus Pergamon XI/2*. Berlin: De Gruyter, 1975.

De Luca, G., *Das Asklepieion 4. Teil. Via tecta und die Hallenstrasse, Die Funde, Altertümer von Pergamon XI,4*. Berlin: De Gruyter, 1984.

Dereboylu, E., "Weissgrundige Keramik und hellenistische Reliefbecher aus dem Hanghaus 2" in *Studien zur hellenistischen Keramik in Ephesos*, ed. by F. Krinzinger: 21–42. Vienna: Österreichisches Archäologisches Institut, 2001.

Domăneanţu, C., *Histria XI: Les bols hellénistiques à décor en relief.* Bucharest, 2000.

Dupont, P., "Les bols à reliefs hellénistiques d'Histria: données archéometriques préliminaires" in *The Bosporus Gateway between the Ancient Westand East 1st Millennium BC – 5th century AD,* ed. by G.R. Tsetskhladze, S. Atasoy, A. Avram, Ş. Dönmez and J. Hargrave 2013, 337–346. Oxford: British Archaeological Reports, 2013.

Edwards, G.R., *Corinth: Results of Excavations Conducted by the American School of Classical Studies at Athens. Volume VII Part III. Corinthian Pottery.* Princeton, 1975.

———. 1981: "Molded Relief Bowls." *Hesperia* 50 (1981): 189–210.

Gassner, V., *Das Südtor der Tetragonos-Agora: Keramik und Kleinfunde, Forschungen in Ephesos XIII/1/1.* Vienna: Österreichisches Archäologisches Institut, 1997

Gitin, S., *Gezer III (Biblical Archaeology III).* Jerusalem: Nelson Glueck School of Biblical Archaeology, 1990.

Goldman, H. and F.F. Jones, *Excavations at Gözlü Kule, Tarsus I: The Hellenistic and Roman Periods.* Princeton: Princeton University Press, 1950.

Guldager Bilde, P., "Mouldmade Bowls" in *Centre and Periphery in the Hellenistic World, Studies in Hellenistic Civilisation 4,* ed. by P.Bilde, 192–209. Aarhus: Aarhus University Press, 1993.

Günay-Tuluk, G., "Hellenistische Reliefbecher im Museum von Ephesos" in *Studien zur hellenistischen Keramik in Ephesos,* ed. by F. Krinzinger: 51–70. Vienna: Österreichisches Archäologisches Institut, 2001.

Hausmann, U., *Hellenistische Reliefbecher aus attischen und böotischen Werkstätten.* Untersuchungen zur Zeitstellung und Bildüberlieferung. Stuttgart 1959.

———. *Hellenistische Keramik aus Olympia.* Berlin: De Gruyter, 1996.

Hellström, P., *Pottery of Classical and Later Date, Terracotta Lamps and Glass, Labraunda II,1.* Lund: C. W. K. Gleerup, 1965.

Herbert, S.C., *Tell Anafa II,I: The Hellenistic and Roman Pottery (The Plain Wares by Andrea Berlin. The Fine Wares by Kathleen Warner Slane).* Ann Arbor: Kelsey Museum of the University of Michigan, 1997.

Hübner, G., *Die Applikenkeramik von Pergamon. Eine Bildersprache im Dienst des Herrscherkultes.* Berlin, 1993.

Karadima, Ch., "Tafika synola ellenistikes keramikes apo te Samothrake" in *A epistematikke synastisi gia ten ellenistike keramike,* 381–384. Athens 1997.

Kossatz, A.U., *Funde aus Milet V, 1, Die megarischen Becher.* Berlin 1990.

Krinzinger, F., *Studien zur hellenistischen Keramik in Ephesos.* Vienna: Österreichisches Archäologisches Institut, 2001.

Künzl, S., *Ein Komplex der Formschüsseln für Megarische Becher in Mainz. Die "Mainzer Werkstatt."* Bonn: Römisch-German. Zentralmuseum, 2002.

Laumonier, A., *La céramique hellénistique à reliefs, 1, Ateliers ioniens, Délos 31.* Paris: De Boccard, 1977.

Lévêque, P. and Morel, J.-P., *Céramiques hellénistiques et romaines*. Paris: Les Belles Lettres, 1987.

Levi, E., *Olvija I*. Kiev, 1940.

Marazov, I., *Thrace and the Ancient World, Vassil Bojkov collection*. Sofia, 2011.

Margreiter, I., *Alt-Ägina 2/3: Die Kleinfunde aus dem Apollon-Heiligtum*. Berlin: Magonza, 1988.

Massa, M., *La ceramica ellenistica con decorazione a relievo della botegha di Efestia*. Rome: Scuola Archeologica Italiana di Atene, 1990.

Metzger, I.R., *Eretria, Fouilles et recherches II: Die hellenistische Keramik in Eretria*. Basel: Francke Verlag, 1969.

Mlynarczyk, J., "Pottery from the Hellenistic cistern at Sha'ar ha-Amakim" in *Epsilon' epistemoniki synanthese gia ten ellenistiki kerameiki, Chania 1997*, 225–235. Athens 2000.

Muller, A., "Description et analyse des productions moulées, création et production dérivée" in *Le moulage en terre cuite dans l'antiquité, Actes du XVIII colloque du Centre de recherches archéologiques*, ed. by A. Muller, 437–463. Lille, 1997.

Neuru, L.L., "Megarian bowls" in *Paphos III: The Hellenistic and Roman Pottery*, ed. by J.W. Hayes, 18–22. Nicosia, 1991.

Pappa, V., "Minoa Amorgou, Ellenistiki keramike apo ten tome ton voreio tochio tou Gymnasiou" in *Epsilon' epistemoniki synanthese gia ten ellenistiki kerameiki, Chania 1997*, 105–114. Athens, 2000.

Papuci-Wladyka, E., "Hellenistic Pottery from Nea Paphos, First results of scientific analysis" in *Nieborów Pottery Workshop II 1995: Hellenistic and Roman pottery in the Eastern Mediterranean, Acts of the IInd Nieborów Pottery Workshop 1993*, ed. by H. Meyza and J. Mlynarczyk, 243–275. Warsaw, 1995.

Petrova, A., "Pontijska grupa keramika s reliefna okrasa ot elinisticheskaja epocha" in *Collegium historicum Tom 1*, ed. by M. Barakova and T. Stoyanov, 11–36. Sofia, 2011.

Pierobon, R., "La ceramica e la vita della città: Le coppe a rilievo." *Bollettino d'Arte Supplemento* 31–32 (1986): 83–99.

Pierobon R. and R. Benoit, "Coppe elenistiche a rilievo de Iassos, un bilancio" in *Delta' epistemoniki synanthese gia ten ellenistiki kerameiki, Mytilene 1994*, 371–380. Athens, 1997.

Puppo, P., *Le coppe megarese in Italia*. Naples 1995.

Rogl, Ch., "Eine Vorschau zu den reliefverzierten Trinkbechern der ephesischen Monogramm-Werkstätte" in *Studien zur hellenistischen Keramik in Ephesos*, ed. by F. Krinzinger, 99–112. Vienna: Österreichisches Archäologisches Institut, 2001.

Rosenbaum-Heginbottom, R., "Moldmade relief bowls from Tell Dor, Israel: A preliminary report" in *Nieborów Pottery Workshop II 1995: Hellenistic and Roman pottery in the Eastern Mediterranean, Acts of the IInd Nieborów Pottery Workshop 1993*, ed. by H. Meyza and J. Mlynarczyk, 365–396. Warsaw, 1995a.

———. "Imported Hellenistic and Roman pottery" in *Excavations at Dor, Final Report, IB: Areas A and C, The Finds,* ed. by E. Stern, 183–288. Jerusalem: Hebrew University of Jerusalem - Institute of Archaeology, 1995b.

Rotroff, S., *Hellenistic Pottery: Athenian and Imported Moldmade Bowls, Athenian Agora 22.* Princeton: American School of Classical Studies at Athens, 1982.

———. "Moldmade relief bowls from Sardis" in *Gamma' epistemoniki synanthese gia ten ellenistiki kerameiki, Thessaloniki 1991,* 359–366. Athens, 1994.

———. "Moldmade bowls at Samothrace" in *Samothracian Connections, Essays in Honor of J. D. McCredie,* ed. by O. Pelagia and B.D. Westcoat, 60–73. Oxford: Oxbow Books, 2010.

Schmidt, S.G., "A group of Early Hellenistic pottery from a well in Eretria" in *Epsilon' epistemoniki synanthese gia ten ellenistiki kerameiki, Chania 1997,* 361–372. Athens, 2000.

Schwabacher, W., "Hellenistische Reliefkeramik aus Kerameikos." *American Journal of Archaeology* 45 (1941): 182–228.

Semiraro, G., "Hierapolis de Phrygie: la céramique à relief hellénistique et romaine" in *Les céramiques en Anatolie des époques hellénistique et romaine,* ed. by C. Abadie-Reynal, 84–89. Istanbul: Institut Français d'Études Anatoliennes, 2003.

Siebert, G., "Bols à reliefs d'ateliers grecs dans le dépot marin de Santa Sabina en Apulie." *Ricerce e Studi Brindisi* 10 (1977): 111–150.

———. *Recherches sur les ateliers de bols à relief du Péloponnése à l'époque hellénistique.* Paris: De Boccard, 1978.

———. "Les bols à relief. Une industrie de l'art de l'époque hellénistique" in *Céramiques hellénistiques et romaines,* ed. by P. Lévêque and J.-P. Morel, 55–83. Paris: Les Belles Lettres, 1980.

Sinn, U. *Die homerischen Becher.* Berlin: Mann, Gebr., 1979.

Sirbu, V., "Bols geto-daces à decor en relief et représentations figuratives" in *Miscellanea Historica et Archeologica in Honorem Professoris Ionel Candea,* ed. by V. Sirbu and L. Cristian, 19–31. Brăila, 2009.

Smetana-Scherrer, R., "Spätklassische und hellenistische Keramik." *Alt-Ägina 2/1* ed. by H. Walter, 56–91. Mainz: Verlag Philipp von Zabern in Wissenschaftliche Buchgesellschaft, 1982.

Sokolovska, V., *Isar – Marvinci i Povardarjeto v antično vrreme.* Skopje, 1986.

Tsakos, K., "Pilines metres megarikon skyfon apo to Samo" in *Gamma' epistemoniki synanthese gia ten ellenistiki kerameiki, Thessaloniki 1991,* 294–301. Athens, 1994.

Varbanov, V., "Late Hellenistic bowls with Reliefs from Ruse District, NW Bulgaria." *Archaeologia Bulgarica* 16 (2012): 59–76.

Waagé, F.O., "Hellenistic and Roman Tableware from North Syria" in *Antioch on the Orontes IV–1: Ceramics and Islamic Coin,* ed. by F.O. Waagé, 1–60. Princeton, 1948.

Zabelina, V.S., "Importnyje "megarskyje" chashi iz Pantikapaja." *Soobshchenia Gosudarstvennogo Muzeja Istorii Izkusstva* 7 (1984): 153–172

Ziegenhaus, O. and G. De Luca, *Das Asklepieion.* Berlin, 1968.

Pre-Classical Lithic Sites in Western Rough Cilicia

Nicholas Rauh[1]

I would like to take this opportunity to express my gratitude to Charles and Marie-Henriette Gates for their tireless support through the years. My debt to them dates as far back as my graduate school days at UNC-Chapel Hill, where they both taught before relocating to Bilkent University in the late 1980s. Charles and Marie-Henriette have been instrumental in fostering my career in Anatolian archaeology. They assisted me during my tenure as a Fulbright student in İstanbul in 1984–1985, and they introduced me to scholars and ministry authorities to facilitate the development of my Rough Cilicia Archaeological Survey Project in 1995. Since that time I have not only enjoyed the opportunity to direct the survey for sixteen seasons, but I have come to develop close ties with several of the Gates' faculty colleagues at Bilkent University. I have delivered guest lectures on campus, and I sat on two MA theses defenses (Ayşe Atauz and Jason DeBlock). In 2006, I conducted my Anatolian Archaeology Field School there. None of this, and so much more, would have been possible without the guidance and support afforded me by Charles and Marie-Henriette Gates. I remain singularly indebted to them for the tutelage and friendship they have furnished me with through the years.

Abstract

Finds from three sites in the upper Bıçkıcı river canyon, and those of Günnercik Yayla on the Taşeli Plateau in the Taurus Mountains, indicate regional occupation in the highlands above Gazipaşa, Turkey from the Pre-Pottery Neolithic through the early Iron Age Periods. At the rock outcrops at Sivritaş Tepe, the Rough Cilicia Survey Team encountered high concentrations of lithic and hand-made ceramic remains, as well as scores of fragments of lithic debitage. Stone forms include flakes, blades, and two intact arrowheads. At Günnercik Yayla, team members observed a number of minimally worked lithic forms, including broken hammer stones of granite, worked adage flakes, and literally dozens of highly polished beads.

1 School of Languages and Cultures, Purdue University, 640 Oval Drive, West Lafayette, IN 47907-2039, USA.

Both sites exhibit characteristics of sustained stone knapping activities. Based on a preliminary investigation, the region was far more actively exploited by pre-Classical inhabitants than it was at any time prior to Ptolemaic occupation at the end of the fourth century BC.

Introduction

Very briefly, I have decided to share in this publication some survey data relevant to the Gates' decades-long work as Bronze and Iron Ages specialists in Greece and Anatolia. Although the orientation of my survey in Gazipaşa (Gazipaşa District; Antalya Province) is predominantly Greco-Roman in character, during the last few years of the survey, my team began to encounter lithic remains and lithic era sites in the highlands above the Mediterranean coast. Admittedly, I have no competence as a lithic specialist, and the team itself has for the most part lacked the necessary expertise. Nonetheless, it seems useful to publicize these lithic finds and site locations to make them available to the wider archaeological community. Interested scholars are welcome to apply for permission to examine the materials we collected at the Alanya Archaeological Museum, where they are stored.

In this paper I will focus on finds from four sites in two locations: those of Karaçukur (RC 0303), Sivritaş Tepe (RC 0802), and Kenetepe (RC 0304) in the upper Bıçkıcı river canyon, and those of Günnercik Yayla (RC 1101) on the Taşeli Plateau in the Taurus Mountains. The first three stand within a kilometer of one another and indicate regional occupation in the highlands from the Chalcolithic through the early Iron Age Periods. Günnercik Yayla appears to be Pre-Pottery Neolithic in character and may represent a seasonal stone knapping site of early pastoralists.

From the outset, members of the Rough Cilicia Survey Team have been concerned by the apparent lack of pre-Roman materials encountered in the coastal terrain of the survey area, either amid the built landscapes of ancient urban sites such as Selinus or Nephelion (which are presumed to have been occupied as early as the Iron Age) or in rural transects.[2] Apart from our finds of Cypriot style painted wares (decorated with concentric circles) at Alaca Dağı (RC 9717), we have encountered very little to demonstrate pre-Roman occupation at any of the sites along the coast, let alone pre-Classical settlement.[3] Precisely why lithic

2 For discussion, see Rauh *et al.* 2009.

3 The finds at Alaca Dağı were reported preliminarily in Laflı 2001; *cf.* Rauh *et al.* 2009, 268–272. A mere handful of ceramic remains, Phoenician amphora rims and Attic black slipped sherds, help to identify pre-Hellenistic or pre-Classical occupation at sites such as Iotape, Selinus, Nephelion, and Charadros. Most settlement appears to have commenced during the Ptolemaic occupation of the area after 305 BC. For the evidence of Hellenistic occupation, see Rauh *et al.* 2013.

remains have been encountered exclusively in the highlands remains uncertain. One theory holds that the immense scale of urban development during the Early Roman era (67 BC-250 AD) tends to conceal earlier levels of occupation along the coast beneath accumulated layers of artificial terracing and Roman structural remains. Most coastal settlements were minimal in size until the Roman era and developed rapidly only at that time, making it difficult to reconstruct earlier phases of occupation apart from the evidence of a few, random, pre-Roman (predominantly Hellenistic) potsherds. A second explanation posits that the region of western Rough Cilicia exhibits a truncated chronology due to significant landscape deformation. Our geomorphological research indicates that some 3 m of alluvium was deposited in the Gazipaşa lowlands (the Delice, Bıçkıcı, and Hacımusa river basins) since the end of antiquity.[4] Since pre-Classical occupation is likely to have occurred in the lowlands near the shore, the limited remains of this occupation conceivably lie buried deep beneath more recent deposition.

All I can say for now is that as the work of the project progressed into the midlands,[5] lithic remains began to surface with increasing regularity. The shallow soils and exposed limestone bedrock of the midlands and highlands, combined with more limited evidence of Roman-era construction, tend to reveal a broader range of historical occupation or no evidence of occupation at all. Again, the presence of lithic remains in the Rough Cilician midlands and Taurus Mountains highlands might seem logical to scholars with long experience in such terrain, but for members of the survey team who labored for years through dense assemblages of Early and Late Roman ceramic remains along the coast, the exposed character of pre-Roman settlement in the uplands comes as something of a surprise. Our highland survey work remains restricted for the most part to the narrow canyon of the Bıçkıcı River, just north of the modern city of Gazipaşa (Fig. 1).

Approximately 30 km in length, the Bıçkıcı River is the second longest river of the Gazipaşa basin. It also represents the narrowest, most direct route from the sea to the crest of the Taurus Mountains. The Bıçkıcı catch basin can be classified according to four distinct zones: the highland meadows and barren peaks of the Taşeli Plateau (1400–2100 m elev.), the upper basin of the Bıçkıcı at Karatepe (500–1400 m), the rapidly descending ridges of the midlands (500–300 m), and the coastal plain. Today, the Taşeli Plateau where Günnercik Yayla is located, resembles a lunar landscape. Barren rock and enclosed highland meadows extend along the triangular shaped plateau for approximately 30 km. Every enclosed *yayla* that I have visited exhibits a sinkhole at its lowest point. Some of these sinkholes present

4 See Akkemik *et al.* 2012; Rauh *et al.* 2009, 264–268.

5 By our reckoning, the ridge lines and river canyons between 500 and 1000 m in altitude represent Ptolemy the Geographer's *mesogeia*; for discussion see Rauh *et al.* 2009: 279, n. 100.

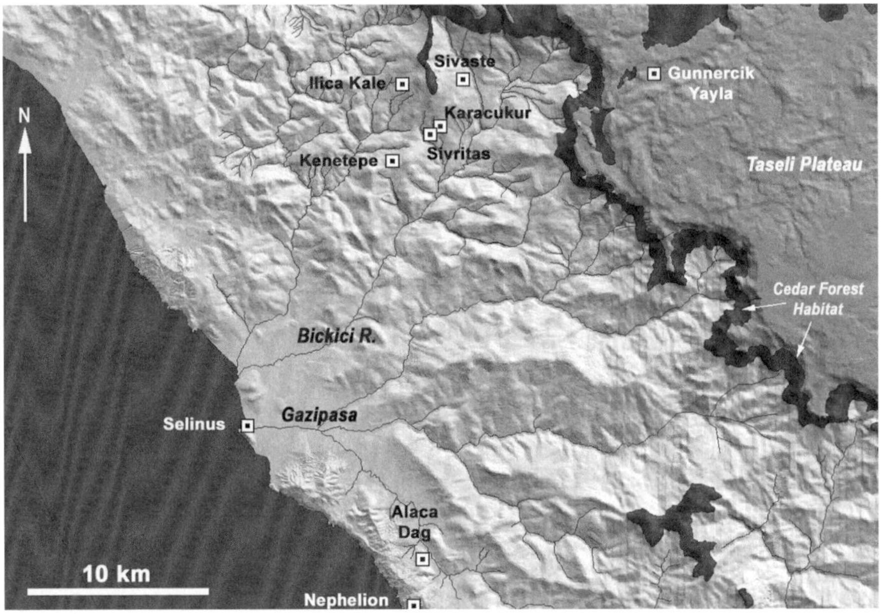

FIG. 1 Map of Western Rough Cilicia

themselves as vast cave entrances, where rain water collects to enter underground channels that feed various lines of springs in the midlands below. Günnercik Yayla, for example, is essentially enclosed by limestone bluffs on all sides. A slight rise resembling an island sits in the middle of the meadow (FIG. 2). Local residents who stay there during summer months told us that the flooded meadow forms a shallow lake in spring time. Overall, the plateau experiences as much as 3 m of snow during winter, and all but one of the roads passing through the highlands remain closed during that season.

As our assembled pollen data indicates, many of these *yaylas* stand at the elevation of the natural habitat of highland forests such as cedar and fir (1500 -1800 m). Today limited stands of relic cedars survive, invariably mixed with fir, black pine and widely scattered juniper, the last two of which represent secondary growth of invasive plants consequent to deforestation. The meadows remain as critical to modern livestock production as they did in antiquity. These top lawn or *pelouse* grasses are believed to furnish four times the nutrients that grazing animals can obtain in the lowlands. In antiquity, pastoralists would drive their herds of sheep and goats into the highlands along precipitous tracks; today, they typically truck the animals, including large cows, to the highlands.

The other region that concerns us in this paper is the broad naturally sculpted bowl of the upper Bıçkıcı basin. This landscape is 9 km wide and characterized by

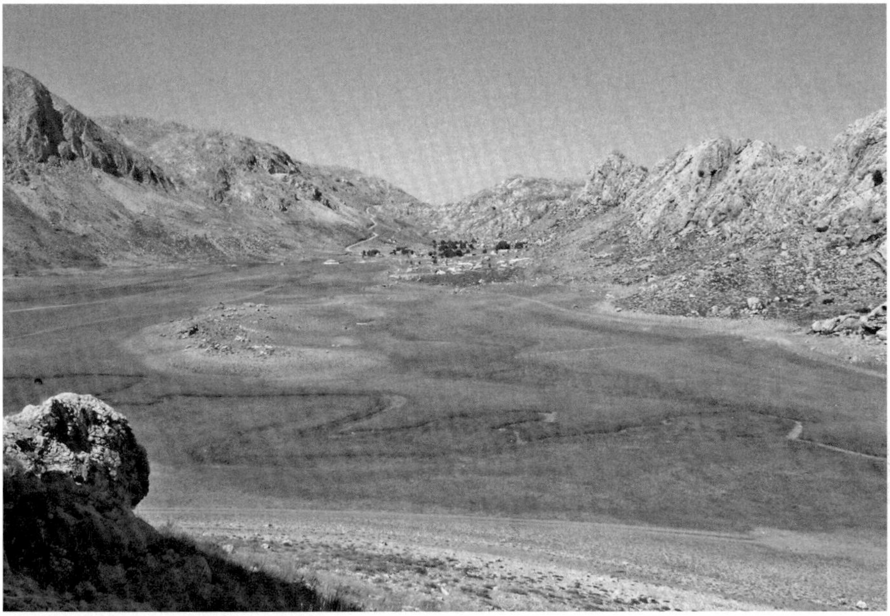

FIG. 2 View of Günnercik Yayla (RC 1101) from the north

a high altitude river terrace surrounded on three sides by steep limestone cliffs. Below the basin, the Bıçkıcı River tumbles along a narrow gorge to the lowlands below. The river terrace at the floor of the canyon has been dissected by Bıçkıcı tributaries into a V-shaped headland (500 m elevation) scarred by 180 m deep incisions to either side. At the head of the canyon the terrain rises from 500 m elevation to 1581 m at the Karaboğaz pass to the Taşeli plateau. On the west side of the canyon the mountain of Karatepe rises step-like from the river terrace through a series of benches, minor peaks and saddles until it joins with the crest of the plateau. The flanks of the northern and eastern sides of the canyon rise more precipitously as nearly vertical walls. A consistent spring line is visible between 600–900 m elevation around the entire rim of the canyon, offering perennial water to the tumbling hills and valleys below.

The scattered communities of Karatepe extend along the lower slopes of the semicircular landscape that surrounds the terrace. Small neighborhoods such as Çınarcık, Şahinler, Kaynarca, Akkaya, Çomruk, and Sugözü are nestled in sloping terrain between 400 and 900 m elevation. Along the steep slopes of the canyon between 1500–1800 m stand mixed forests of cedar and fir of very recent growth. A dense, recently planted pine forest occupies most of the terrain of the river terrace itself. Along the lower flanks, particularly on the western side of the basin which is well watered by perennial springs and exposed to abundant sunlight, farmers

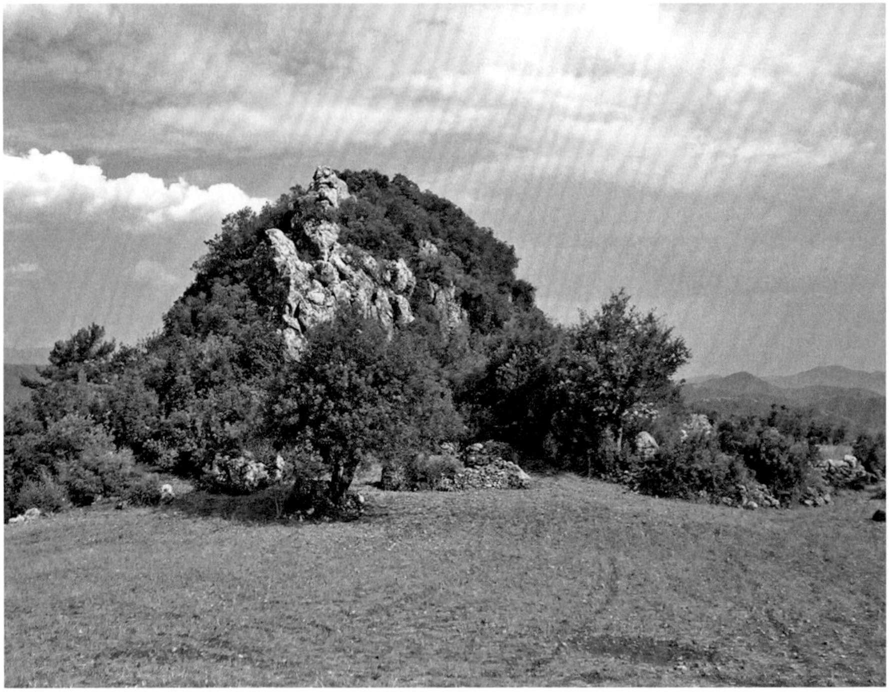

Fig. 3 View of the butte at Karaçukur (RC 0303)

have constructed complex networks of steeply ascending terraces for agricultural purposes. Some terraces harbor nut (almonds and black walnuts) and fruit trees, but most are used to raise wheat and hay.

Since 2003, the survey team has devoted considerable attention to this highland in order to obtain archaeological and geoarchaeological data capable of calibrating past human exploitation of highland resources in Rough Cilicia. Data obtained from the Turkish Forestry Service and from older inhabitants reveal that the cedar forest at the crest of the Bıçkıcı River has been continuously harvested from the late Ottoman era until 1980, when the Forestry Service prohibited all cedar timbering operations in the area.[6] The narrowness of this river basin, its lack of divergent arms, and the directness with which it descends from the crest of the Taurus to the sea all recommended it as an ideal landscape for evaluating the effects of long term deforestation.

The Rough Cilicia Archaeological Project has conducted repeated archaeological and geoarchaeological research in the Bıçkıcı Canyon area, including

6 As early as 1896, illegal timbering in the wider Alanya vicinity was punishable by fines; see Akkemik *et al.* 2012.

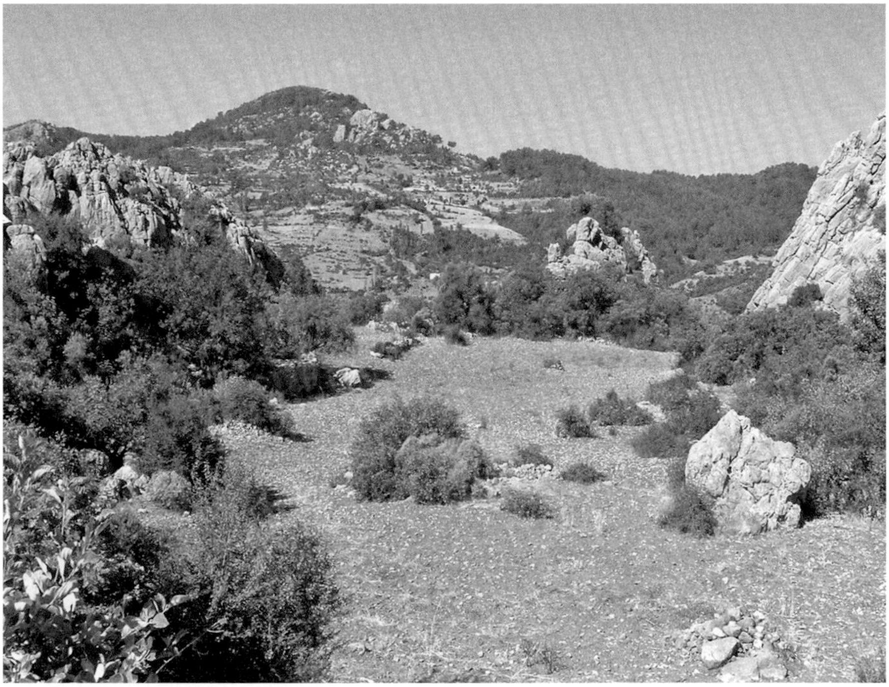

FIG. 4 View of the knapping area at Sivritaş Tepe (RC 0802)

four survey campaigns (2003, 2007, 2008, and 2011). In 2003, team members investigated a vast portion of the Bıçkıcı watershed, visiting and recording six ancient sites in the upper basin, including RC 0301 Sivaste, RC 0302 Akkaya Mah., RC 0303 Karaçukur, RC 0304 Kenetepe, RC 0308 Kilise Taş Mevki, and RC 0309 Gevinde or Ilıca Kale. At Sites RC 0301, RC 0302, RC 0303 and RC 0304, the team conducted intensive, systematic flag survey of all visible architectural elements and surface pottery. Site RC 0304 proved to be so large, however, that the director had little choice but to restrict flag survey procedures to the most exposed area of the acropolis.

Three significant urban sites displaying abundant monumental architecture (RC 0301 Sivaste, RC 0304 Kenetepe and RC 0309 Ilıca Kale) existed on the west slope of the canyon. Evidence of a network of Roman roads identified at RC 0302 (Akkaya Mahalle) that converged toward RC 0301 Sivaste indicates that these urban complexes were carefully integrated with the communities on the coast. One of the urban sites, RC 0304 Kenetepe, qualifies as an extremely large site. All three urban sites (Kenetepe, Sivaste, and Ilıca Kale) exhibit strong evidence of monumentality, inscribed literacy, and importation of transport amphoras and ceramic finewares from abroad. More significantly, pottery analysis at each site demonstrates that habitation in this region spanned the same pre-modern phases as those of the large urban sites along the coast. The team identified a significant quantity of Hellenistic fineware at RC 0304 Kenetepe and at least a minimum of the same at RC 0301 Sivaste and RC 0309 Ilıca Kale. All three sites exhibit abundant Early Roman finewares (predominantly Cypriot Sigillata, but some ESA as well), and all three exhibited significant quantities of Late Roman finewares (Cypriot Red Slip, Phocaean Ware). The team also recorded samples of Byzantine pottery (green glazed ware) at RC 0304 Kenetepe and RC 0309 Ilıca Kale (where the remains of a Late Roman complex resembling a monastery are visible). In short, the ceramic contexts for the urban sites of the Bıçkıcı watershed appear to resemble those of the coastal region, indicating that the region remained occupied and fully utilized in an unbroken sequence from the Hellenistic to Late Roman and Byzantine eras.

Precisely how early this watershed was inhabited is suggested by the lithic finds at RC 0303 Karaçukur and RC 0802 Sivritaş Tepe. The former is situated below a distinctive rock butte directly above the modern village of Karatepe; the latter is situated directly across the road from the butte, 600 meters down the sloping terrain (Fig. 3, Fig. 4). In terrace fields at the base of the butte at Karaçukur (740 m elevation), the team found wall remains constructed from rough hewn blocks. In some places the lowest courses of the wall appear to rest *in situ*. In the fields beside the walls, a good quantity of pre-Roman lithic and ceramic remains were systematically identified and recorded. Remains include one obsidian flake, several fragments of hand-turned prehistoric or Bronze Age pottery (blackened and probably cookware), several Classical era kylix rims with triangular beveled rims, and a few Hellenistic incurved rim bowls and amphora handles. The most impressive find was the largely intact remains of a piriform jug with flat base and hand-molded strainer spout (Fig. 5). Closest comparanda for the form suggest a date of the sixth century BC.[7]

Reinvestigation of the site by Richard Rothaus and Nicholas Rauh in July 2005 yielded additional lithic debitage of obsidian and flint (chert), fragments of burnished hand-turned pottery, a black-slipped kylix rim fragment, and two small bone fragments. During a preliminary visit to the same location in 2008, the team obtained a grab collection of worked fragments of red and gray flint, two pieces of worked obsidian, and two worked pieces of a soft white stone resembling onyx. One worked piece of limestone exhibited a hand-worked bore hole. Several fragments of hand-made cooking ware were identified, including two large ledge handles (one exhibiting a unique reddish exterior slip and a blackened interior surface indicating the presence of food residue), one blackened stewpot fragment

7 See Rauh and Wandsnider 2005.

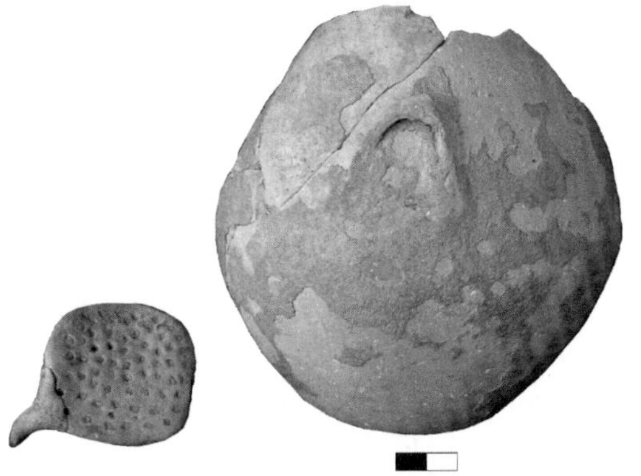

FIG. 5 Fragments of the strainer pot from Karaçukur (RC 0303)

with upright rim, and another fragment exhibiting a piriform shoulder with an upright rim. Other pre-Roman forms recovered in 2008 include a Classical kylix rim, a black slipped ring foot to a Classical fineware bowl, two black slipped Hellenistic incurved rim fragments and a ring foot to a Hellenistic coarseware bowl. Large "Roman era" coarseware fragments and a few fragments of Early Roman Cypriot Sigillata fineware were also recovered at the site. It may be significant, however, that few if any sherds at Karaçukur exhibit wheel ridging characteristic of the second to sixth centuries AD.

The combined assemblage indicates that human settlement at Karaçukur was sustained from perhaps as early as the Chalcolithic era until Early Roman times.[8] Despite this consistent pattern of finds recovered at the site, the team remained uncertain about its implications. For one thing, the location exhibits no recognizable architectural remains to support the conclusion.[9] For another, team members were informed by residents that as recently as 50 years ago, farmers in Gazipaşa commonly obtained flint blades from this location for use as teeth in wooden, animal-drawn threshing sleds. An inspection of the teeth of one such sled on display in the Baysal Hotel in Gazipaşa revealed the same red and gray flint blades as those recovered by the team at Karaçukur. In other words, despite the presence of hand-turned ceramic remains at this location, the production of worked flint stone at Karaçukur offered no certain proof of pre-Classical lithic

8 The Chalcolithic date for the handmade cookware was suggested by Soner Ateşoğulları, a prehistorian employed at the Museum of Anatolian Civilizations in Ankara, who served as our government representative in 2007. Most of the amphora sherds investigated in this area are smooth walled, and have thick, oval, upright handles, a likely indication that the site was occupied through the late Hellenistic or at the latest Early Roman era.

9 In 2003, the team recorded the terrace walls mentioned above, and in 2005 Rauh climbed to the crest of the butte itself to observe similar remains of poorly fashioned walls along its length. However, these and the terrace walls are conceivably modern.

production at this site. For this reason, the team concluded that additional investigation of the highland canyon was necessary.

A second season of pedestrian survey was conducted in the Bıçkıcı highland canyon in July 2008. The research agenda of the 2008 season consisted of off-site pedestrian survey in the terraced agricultural terrain in the village of Karatepe. The intention of the survey team was to investigate some portion of the terrain to better understand patterns of land use in this highland basin during antiquity. Off-site pedestrian survey was conducted in the vicinity of several of the sites identified in 2003 to determine the wider extent of ancient occupation. Given the difficulty of the terrain—which slopes steeply and is heavily obstructed by terraces enclosed by fences and stone walls—not to mention programmatic time constraints and the imposing size of the canyon, the team decided to restrict the survey to the rural areas neighboring the three most significant sites, Kenetepe (RC 0304), Karaçukur (RC 0303), and Sivaste (RC 0301).

In all, the 2008 RCSP pedestrian team walked 16 transects comprising 53 units of 100 m length at 3 to 5 m intervals. Three new sites, RC 0810, 0802 and 08083, were identified in this vicinity, one of which, RC 0802, Sivritaş Tepe, pertains directly to the question of pre-Classical settlement in this vicinity. In and around a cluster of upturned rock outcrops, the team encountered high concentrations of lithic and hand-made ceramic remains, as well as strong evidence of a lithic knapping area.[10] This site lies directly across the modern asphalt road and 600 m southwest of the lithic deposit that was identified beside the butte at Karaçukur. Sivritaş Tepe (RC 0802; 670 m elevation) presents itself as a natural alluvial bench framed by an irregular wall of vertical rock faces (hence the name, "Pointy Rock Hill").

The investigation of the rock outcrop of Sivritaş Tepe revealed two significant features: a large cave on the north face of the outcrop and a narrow, flat ravine at the interior of the rock formation (Fig. 4). The cave is quite large, nearly 3 m tall and 5 m wide at its entrance. It exhibits two passageways with a 2 m wide tree growing in a chute-like opening at its interior. Near its entrance team members found ceramic remains and a fragment of worked red flint. Several additional remains of worked lithics were identified in the vicinity. Several pre-Classical forms were likewise identified, including a large storage jar with upright rim and piriform shoulder, a hand-turned stewpot fragment with an upright, visibly rolled rim and additional hand-turned cookware sherds.

As stated above, the exposed outcrop of Sivritaş is extremely jagged and irregular and exhibits several deep fissures along its length. A long (200 m) narrow winding ravine is visible along its midsection. Pursuing a narrow path into

10 Rauh 2009; Rauh 2012.

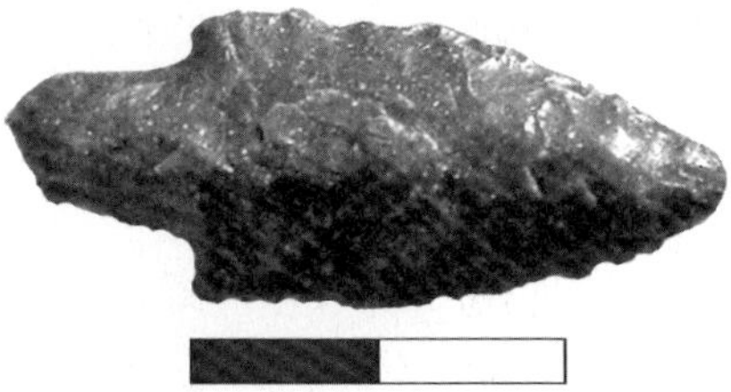

Fig. 6 Red flint arrowhead from Sivritaş Tepe (RC 0802)

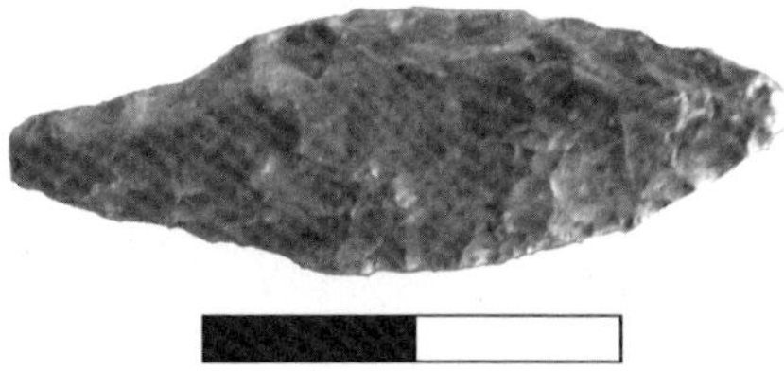

Fig. 7 Gray flint arrowhead from Sivritaş Tepe (RC 0802)

the ravine, team members encountered a small agricultural field approximately 40 x 100 m, exhibiting small areas of terracing along its margin. From this 'east ravine' a narrow brushy path leads further along the ravine to a second, smaller opening (20 x 70 m) labeled by the team as the 'west ravine'. Worked lithic remains were identified in both ravines, particularly in the terraced area on the south side of the east ravine, where literally hundreds of fragments of flint debitage identified the place as a knapping area. Handfuls of debitage, mostly gray flint, were collected. Lingering concern about the likely modernity of the knapping area was allayed by the identification of a red flint arrowhead 3.9 cm long and a broken red flint sickle blade. During a visit to the site in 2011, a similarly worked gray flint arrowhead was recovered by the team (Fig. 6, Fig. 7). Similar concentrations of debitage were found in the west ravine. Ceramics recorded in the ravine areas include several coarse ware sherds of various periods and one hand-made blackened stewpot fragment with upright rim and sloping shoulder. The team saw little evidence of structural habitation apart from the dense layer of small (hand-sized) stone blocks on the ground. Striations on the face of the rock ledge near the lithic remains were possibly hand worked. Labeled site RC 0802, the lithic remains at Sivritaş Tepe surpass those found at Karaçukur (RC 0303). The finds of two intact arrowheads combined with handmade pottery and literally scores of fragments of lithic debitage clearly marks this as a pre-Classical (possibly Chalcolithic) stone-knapping area and settlement.

Transect data obtained from terraced agricultural terrain immediately below the outcrop demonstrated that the horizon of lithic and handmade ceramic remains extended 200 m. In steeply sloping fields, numerous additional lithic remains were identified, including worked fragments of red and gray flint, possibly onyx, and several pieces of imported obsidian. Other finds include a large lump of iron ore and in particular a hand-turned cook pot or storage basin with a large ledge handle. The exterior surface of this sherd appears to be slipped or painted bright red (Fig. 8).

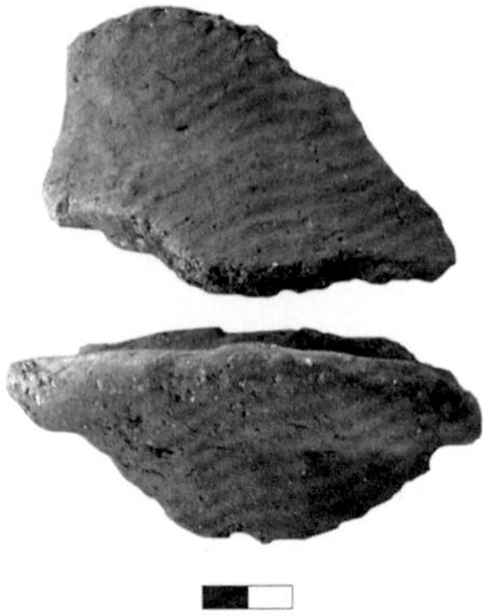

Fig. 8 Fragments of a hand-turned cook pot or storage basin with ledge handle from Sivritaş Tepe (RC 0802)

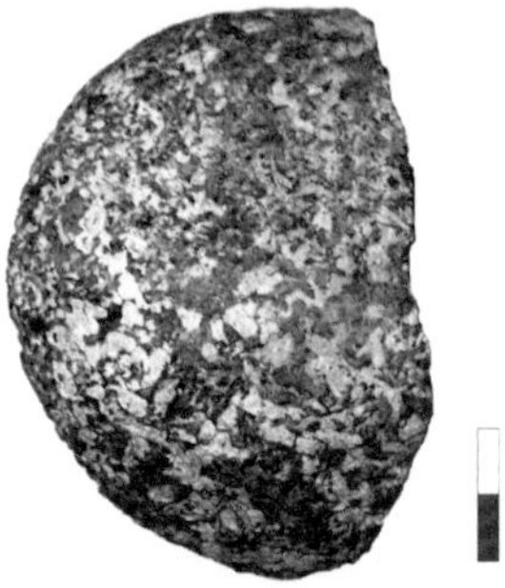

Fig. 9 Broken granite hammer stone from Günnercik Yayla (RC 1101)

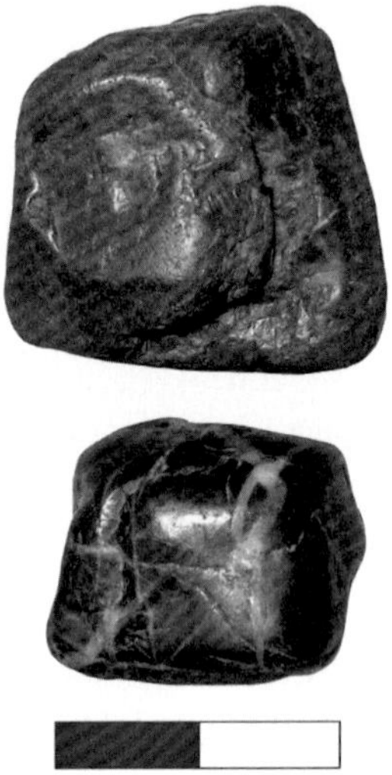

Fig. 10 Rectangular polished beads with drill hole impressions from Günnercik Yayla (RC 1101)

In addition, approximately 150 m below (south of) the cliffs, Rauh investigated several large mounds of extremely small-flake gray flint debitage; there were at least three large "slag heaps" easily 1 m tall. Unquestionably, an enormous amount of gray flint was worked in this area, but the debitage fragments were so small as to suggest that they represent the leavings of modern stone knapping, for example, residue piles resulting from the production of flint teeth for the modern plough sleds discussed above. Either way—ancient or modern—these slag heaps offer another telling detail about the stone knapping industry that occurred at the Sivritaş Tepe outcrop. No springs were visible in the vicinity, but the ravine some 200 m west bears spring water coming down from a large spring that emerges on a saddle of the ridge below Kenetepe (RC 0304).

It is worth noting that similar fragments of flint and obsidian debitage were likewise encountered amid the ruined structural remains at Kenetepe (RC 0304) in 2003. At the time they were identified as possible fragments of mosaic tesserae. However, in view of the widely dispersed lithic remains encountered along the agricultural terraces on the western slope of the Bıçkıcı highland basin, the likelihood that these remains represent pre-Classical debitage seems high. The entire landscape of tumbling benches and fields surrounding the stone-knapping area at Sivritaş Tepe appears to mark a significant Chalcolithic or pre-Classical settlement that seems to have continued in use through early Iron Age (Archaic) times.

With funding from the National Geographic Society, the Rough Cilicia Archaeological Survey Project relocated its operations in July 2011 to the highland Taşeli Plateau itself. The primary research agenda of the 2011 season was to investigate the degraded character of highland cedar forests in the plateau. Pedestrian survey remained secondary to the main task of obtaining pollen and carbon data from geomorphic excavations of selected alluvial deposits in the region. If time allowed, the team walked limited transects in the vicinity of the trenches themselves. Despite this limitation, the team identified one significant pre-ceramic lithic production site near Trench 5 at Günnercik Yayla (RC 1101; 1799 m elevation).

While excavating Trench 5 in a dry stream gulley in the plain of Günnercik Yayla, the team walked 3 transects. Extending approximately 220 m, a low rocky rise at the center of the meadow caught the attention of the team and was investigated briefly. Team members observed a number of minimally worked lithic forms, including numerous broken hammer stones of granite, worked adage flakes, fragments of parent material with evidence of percussion strikes and dozens of highly polished beads, some rectangular, some rounded (Fig. 9, Fig. 10). Drill hole impressions were observable on several of the beads. The team returned to the site a few days later to conduct a more detailed survey of the area. Team members walked at 30 m intervals from the "island" feature at the center of the *yayla* toward houses situated on higher ground at the base of the hills that enclose the western flank of the valley. Hundreds more lithic remains were observed at this time, including dozens of polished beads. Team members mapped these remains for 270 m across the meadow to the flank of the hill until they reached the yards of the houses. The density of beads and worked stone (approximately 1 per meter^2) indicate that lithic remains extend possibly along the entire northern flank of the valley. At the base of the enclosing ridge near Trench 5, the team also encountered a shallow cave with sparse ceramic and skeletal remains. Wheel-ridged ceramic remains indicate that this locus was occupied in the Late Roman era.

In short, the site exhibited an extensive pre-ceramic lithic horizon. It possibly served as a production center for polished beads of chert, adage, and limestone. Given the elevation and the high likelihood that the location was inaccessible during winter, this was probably a seasonal site. Conceivably, it was occupied during the summer season by pastoralists who drove their herds into the highlands to take advantage of the top lawn grasses. While camping there, elements of the group possibly cut timber in the surrounding forest (now denuded) and quarried the available exposed rock (adage, flint) to generate these polished beads and square-shaped ornaments. The fact that the ground on the west side of the valley lies strewn with hundreds if not thousands of these polished stone artifacts indicates that it was heavily worked over many years by visitors who otherwise left no visible sherd scatter. This suggests that the site was occupied seasonally by visitors during the Pre-Pottery Neolithic era. The absence of any visible structural remains prohibits us from classifying the site further as PPNA or PPNB. But the scale of the stone knapping and polishing that occurred here indicates that settlements of either era probably existed in the lowlands below the plateau.

The lithic site at Günnercik Yayla thus furnishes the earliest evidence for human occupation in the Gazipaşa District encountered thus far by the Rough Cilicia Survey Team. It offers a potential clue to the kind of settlements that existed in the lowlands prior to the rapid development in the Early Roman era. In this regard it is worth noting that the survey team has encountered far more substantial lithic remains at this site and in the highland bowl of Karatepe in the upper Bıçkıcı river basin than it has Classical era finewares anywhere in the Gazipaşa District. Based on the results of our investigation, the region was seemingly far more actively exploited during the prehistoric era than it was at any time prior to Ptolemaic occupation at the end of the fourth century BC. At the very least, the finds of lithic sites in the highlands of western Rough Cilicia have significantly altered the paradigm of a truncated chronology for the region.

REFERENCES

Akkemik, Ü., H. Caner, G. Conyers, N. Karlıoğlu, M. J. Dillon, N. K. Rauh and L. Theller., "The Archaeology of Deforestation in South Coastal Turkey." *International Journal of Sustainable Development and World Ecology* 1/1 (2012): 1–11

Laflı, E., "Alacadağ: Eine neue Fundstelle von späteisenzeitlicher Keramik im westlichen Rauhen Kilikien" in *La Cilicie: Espaces et Pouvoirs locaux (2e millénaire av. J.-C. - 4e siècle ap. J.C.). Actes de la Table Ronde Internationale d'Istanbul, 2–5 Novembre 1999*, ed. by E. Jean, A. M. Dinçol and S. Durugönül, 195–214. Paris: Institut Français d'Études Anatoliennes Georges Dumézil, 2001.

Rauh, N. K., "Dağlık Kilikya Yüksek Arazi Arkeoloji Araştırması: 2011 Yılı Raporu." *Araştırma Sonuçları Toplantısı* 30/2 (2012): 223–234.

———. "Sivritaş Tepesi in Gazipaşa İlçesi: The Discovery of a Prehistoric Stone-Knapping Site." *ANMED* 7 (2009): 113–116.

Rauh, N. K., M. J. Dillon and R. Rothaus., "Anchors, Amphoras and Ashlar Masonry: New Evidence for the Cilician Pirates" in *Rough Cilicia: New Historical and Archaeological Approaches*, ed. by M. Hoff and R. Townsend, 59–86. Oxford: Oxbow Books, 2013.

Rauh N., R. Townsend, M. Hoff, M. Dillon, M. Doyle, C. Ward, R. Rothaus, H. Caner, Ü. Akkemik, L. Wandsnider, S. Ozaner and C. Dore., "Life in the Truck Lane: Urban Development in Western Rough Cilicia." *JOAI (Jahreshefte des Österreichischen Archäologischen Instituts in Wien)* 78 (2009): 253–312.

Rauh N. K. and L. Wandsnider, "Dağlık Kilikya Yüzey Araştırma Projesi: 2002 ve 2003 Sezonlarının Raporu." *Araştırma Sonuçları Toplantısı* 22/1 (2005): 125–138.

The "Sacrilegious, Accursed and Tomb-breaker": Sarcophagus Re-use at Aphrodisias

Esen Öğüş[1]

Abstract

The ancient Roman site of Aphrodisias in Caria was well-known in antiquity for its marble sculpture production. Part of this production encompasses c. 600 sarcophagi from the second and third centuries CE. These are decorated in relief with the portraits of their patrons, allegorical and mythological figures. A substantial number of funerary inscriptions, either carved on sarcophagi or on separate marble blocks, were also preserved at the site. Even though these inscriptions clearly condemn the practice of sarcophagus re-use with imprecations and fines, many sarcophagi were still re-used for subsequent burials, or for entirely different purposes, such as building blocks in various monuments. This paper gathers the archaeological and epigraphic evidence from the city to demonstrate the reasons why this phenomenon persisted despite the bans and understand the secondary life of the funerary monuments. In addition, the paper presents enigmatic phenomena related to the re-use of sarcophagi. For instance, the tomb-breakers changed the names on the inscriptions, but often did not touch the portraits, which sometimes led to bizarre disjunctions of image and text.

Introduction

Aphrodisias in Caria, the city of Aphrodite, was well known in the Roman Empire for its marble quarries, sculptors and signature style that appealed to both local and external patrons. Marble sarcophagi from the city played a significant role in the overall funerary landscape of Roman Asia Minor, and it rivaled other centers of production such as Proconnesos and Dokimeion in the number of sarcophagi produced. There are about 105 fully or mostly preserved marble sarcophagus chests

1 Texas Tech University School of Art, 18th St. and Flint Ave., Lubbock, TX, 79409 USA.
I am thankful to R.R.R. Smith and New York University Excavations at Aphrodisias. 'S' numbers are excavation inventory numbers. All translations are my own unless otherwise noted. 'School' of Aphrodisias: Erim 1967; Squarciapino 1983; sculpture workshops: Van Voorhis 1998; and Aphrodisias sculptors in Italy: Squarciapino 1983; Moltesen 1990.

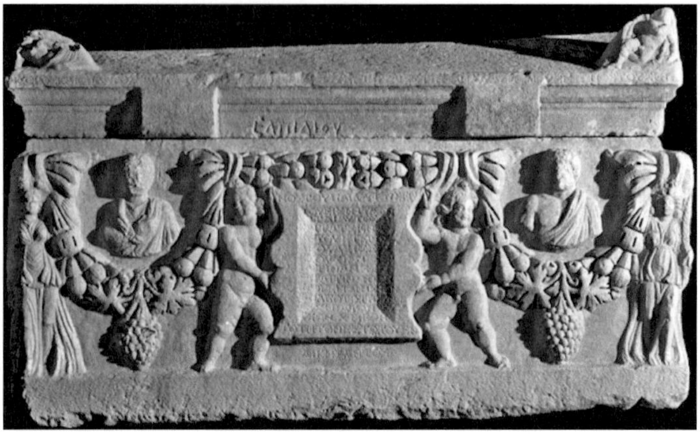

FIG. 1 Garland sarcophagus from Aphrodisias (S-709). Courtesy New York University Excavations at Aphrodisias.

and about 700 fragments of chests and lids from the city. All of these sarcophagi were produced at Aphrodisias out of local marble to satisfy local demand.

Around 12% of the sarcophagi from Aphrodisias are inscribed with the names of their owners. Though the remaining are not inscribed, they were accompanied by inscriptions on separate marble blocks that were built into the tomb monuments. As will be explained in greater detail below, these funerary inscriptions strictly prohibit re-use of the sarcophagi, announce a fine for the illegal act of reuse and name the violators as "sacrilegious, accursed and tomb-breakers." Still, the sarcophagi were occasionally re-used by other families as burial chests, or as raw building material for various structures.

This paper gathers the archaeological and epigraphic evidence for sarcophagus re-use, and sheds light on the reasons why this phenomenon persisted, despite being banned. The aim is to understand the secondary life of funerary monuments and to demonstrate the changing perception of material culture in the Roman and post-Roman periods of the city. The initial section of this paper introduces sarcophagus production at Aphrodisias; discussion then moves to the extant evidence of sarcophagus re-use, and the final section explores the reasons for this re-use and the broader implications of this practice.

Aphrodisian Sarcophagi

The vast majority of the Aphrodisian sarcophagus chests are decorated in relief. They can be categorized into types according to this decoration, and by far the two most common types are garland sarcophagi and columnar sarcophagi. There

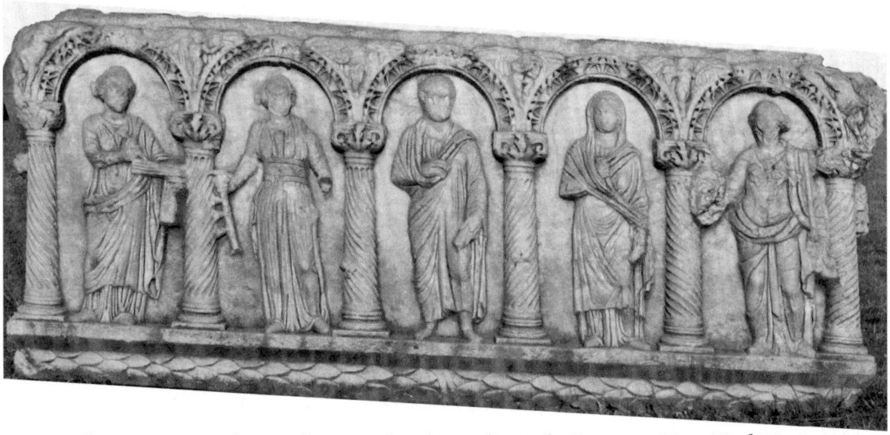

Fig. 2 Columnar sarcophagus from Aphrodisias (S-432). Courtesy New York University Excavations at Aphrodisias.

are about 350 garland sarcophagi (about 70 fully preserved chests or front panels and about 280 fragments from chests), which are decorated with two or three hanging garlands supported by Erotes or less commonly by bucrania.[2] If there are only two garlands, the space between them is usually filled with a molded *tabula*, which was either left empty or less commonly inscribed with the names of the patrons (Fig. 1).

The second most commonly produced chest form is the columnar sarcophagus, of which there exist about 215 in total (15 fully preserved chests or front panels and about 200 fragments from chests).[3] These sarcophagi feature a columnar façade supporting an arcade in relief (Fig. 2). The intercolumniations display standing portrait figures of the patrons and ideal and mythological characters, most commonly the Muses. There also exist far less common types with frieze or fluted decorations.

Chronology

There are three main data sets to consider in determining the chronology of the sarcophagi: the carving style of the chests, portrait hairstyles, and the nomenclature in the inscriptions.[4] Broad dating (in centuries) by the carving style of the chests is

2 Garland sarcophagi were published in a monograph, Işık 2007, in addition to various articles, for instance, Işık 1982; Işık 1984.

3 Öğüş Uzun 2010; Öğüş 2014a.

4 Other possibilities are *stephanephorates* (the name of the priest called *stephanephoros* to indicate the year, although this is not a viable option, as the *stephanephorates* are held in consecutive years or *post mortem*), the fines (a large as

quite straightforward at Aphrodisias, especially for the garland sarcophagi. In the first and second centuries, the garland sarcophagi were usually large and decorated with three garlands carried by bucrania or herms.[5] In the third century, however, the sarcophagi become more standardized, are relatively smaller and appear mass-produced.[6] They commonly have a tabula in the center carried by Erotes and two flanking garlands. Usually there are busts of the deceased inside the lunettes of the garlands. In rare cases, the busts were replaced by representations of Eros and Psyche or other mythological scenes, such as Ganymede being abducted by the eagle.

The columnar sarcophagi, on the other hand, were first produced at the end of the second century CE, with the majority dating to the third century CE. The difference between the earlier and later examples is less obvious, and only a few can be dated relatively securely to the second century CE.[7] On these earlier examples, the human figures are small in proportion to their architectural background. However, in the third-century examples, the dating of which is confirmed by hairstyles, the figures fill most of the space inside the aediculae.

A second and more reliable dating criterion is portrait hairstyles.[8] Male hairstyles do not necessarily follow the emperor's hairstyles, and they may be retrospective. For example, there are representations of men in the mid-third century that still have an Antonine-style beard.[9] Female hairstyles, on the other hand, tend to closely follow the fashionable contemporary styles worn by the Roman empresses. Though the faces and the details of the hair are sometimes unfinished, the intended hairstyle can often still be determined. Accordingly, the most common hairstyle represented on the sarcophagi is that worn by Julia Domna, with centrally parted bulky hair gathered at the nape of the neck. This hairstyle dates the sarcophagi to around 193–220 CE.[10] Another common hairstyle is that of Julia Mamaea, mother of Alexander Severus, with centrally parted hair tucked behind the ears and gathered at the back of the head, dating the sarcophagi to around 220–235 CE.

---

opposed to small amount might be indicative of inflation in the third century CE, but it is not possible to suggest a consistent system to determine the date), or lettering and layout (could be misleading). See Reynolds and Rouché 2007, 150–152.

5 For instance, S-12 (Işık 1982, figs. 50–52; 2007, cat. 13) or S-418 (Işık 2007, cat. 2). Generally, sarcophagi produced before the third century CE are 2.30–3 m in width, 1–1.2 m in height, and 1–1.4 m in depth. This dating is the author's observation.

6 The third century sarcophagi are usually 2 m in width and 0.70–0.80 m in height and depth.

7 S-356 and S-357.

8 Broadly discussed in Smith 2008.

9 This is a broad phenomenon in portraiture of the Empire, see Fejfer 2008, 280–281, 355–356.

10 Of course, one should not assume that these date ranges of reigns are precisely reflected in the changes in portrait hairstyles. These are only broad approximations.

A third criterion for dating is the nomenclature used in the inscriptions. Out of 120 inscribed sarcophagi, about 65 of them have preserved names. And 40 of these 65 (about 62%) belong to citizens with the *nomina* Marcus Aurelius and Aurelia, the family name of the emperor Caracalla. It is most likely that these individuals received their citizenship and new names with Caracalla's *Constitutio Antoniniana* (Antonine Constitution), which granted citizenship to all of the free inhabitants of the Empire. 212 CE, the date at which this constitution was promulgated, sets a *terminus post quem* for the sarcophagi.[11] Other than these inscriptions on sarcophagus chests, there are about 100 additional marble blocks from the city walls that belong to Marci Aurelii.

Considering all the criteria above, it is possible to say that the production of sarcophagi at Aphrodisias began in the first century CE and continued through the end of the third century CE. The majority of the production, however, dates to the early third century CE, with a particular peak in the early Severan period (193–220 CE), and a slight drop in the late Severan period (220–235 CE). The most significant drop in production, however, occurred after 250 CE, when the re-use of the existing chests became common.[12]

Archaeological context

The extant sarcophagi are mostly accidental finds that were discovered outside the city walls during agricultural work. Other fragments found inside the city had been re-used for various purposes in post-antiquity. They originally come from tomb structures located outside the city walls along roads that ran west, northwest, northeast, east, southeast, south and southwest directions out of the city.[13]

Funerary inscriptions at Aphrodisias use varied terminology for different burial types, such as: *eisōstē* (an individual burial niche, inside a sarcophagus or in another kind of monument); *platos*/ *platas*/ *platē* (a burial place or platform inside of which burial niches were placed); *mnēma* (a tomb structure with the function of a memorial); *bōmos* (an altar-shaped platform, usually with a burial niche); and *bathrikon* (a stepped base with burial niches inside). All of these terms but *eisōstē* indicate a built monument that is visible above the ground. Similar terms are found in the inscriptions of other cities in Asia Minor, for instance in Hierapolis, Termessos and Elaiussa

11 As also suggested in Smith 2008.

12 The reasons for the rise and fall of the sarcophagi have been discussed elsewhere, see Smith 2008; Öğüş 2014b.

13 The original contexts of the sarcophagi and remaining tomb structures were studied in Turnbow 2011. For the city walls and gates in these directions, see De Staebler 2007, 162–173.

Sebaste.[14] Epigraphic information also suggests that the sarcophagi were placed 'on' the tomb buildings rather than inside. Visual evidence from the nearby city of Hierapolis supports this suggestion. There, the sarcophagi were placed back to back on top of the funerary structures, whether they are altar-shaped tombs, platforms, or house-formed memorials.[15] This outdoor context of the sarcophagi suggests that their intended audience was not only the bereaved family, but also the general public.

Today, several barrel-vaulted hypogeum-type (underground) chamber tombs with *eisōstai* (burial niches) are preserved. These can be descended into via a flight of steps. However, the superstructures on which the sarcophagi were placed were torn down in the fourth century CE, and the blocks, including inscribed ones, were re-used to construct the city walls.[16] Some sarcophagi shared the same fate as the tomb blocks – cut into pieces and built into the city walls.[17] Nonetheless, a few hypogeum-type tombs recovered in rescue excavations reveal a long span of use for these structures, beginning in the Roman period and extending well into Late Antiquity.[18] This continuous use of the substructures suggests that the tombs were dismantled not because they lost their value as burial structures, but out of necessity and extenuating circumstances.

Funerary Inscriptions

The dismantling of tomb monuments and the re-use of blocks, including inscribed ones, in the city walls allowed for the preservation of a considerable number of funerary inscriptions in good condition.[19] The inscriptions are mostly formulaic texts that announce the legal owner(s) of the tomb and the sarcophagus; forbid anyone to exhume the bodies and inhume others; and in the event that the sarcophagus is violated, they accuse the "accursed" violators of the prosecutable crimes of sacrilege (*asebeia*) and tomb-breaking (*tymborychia*) and state a fine to be paid to various institutions, such as the Treasury of the Roman people (*tamieion*), the Treasury of the Emperor (*kuriakos phiskos*) or the Temple of Aphrodite.[20] The prescribed funerary fine varies between 1,500 and 12,000 denarii (inflation in the third century CE

14 Kubińska 1968, 73–93, 101–108.

15 For the tomb structures in Hierapolis, see Schneider Equini 1972. For the funerary inscriptions at Hierapolis, see Judeich 1898 and Ritti 2006.

16 On re-use of the blocks from the tombs: De Staebler 2007, 203–222.

17 For example, S-22, S-358.

18 As dated by coins and lamps, for instance, see Tulay 1991.

19 Roueché 1989, 22–23.

20 For a general discussion of funerary imprecations, see Strubbe 1997 and Cormack 2004, 126–133. For evidence from Aphrodisias, see Chaniotis 2004, nos. 23 and 26; and Reynolds and Roueché 2007.

should be taken into consideration in this rather varied range), one third of which was offered to the prosecutor as an incentive for private individuals to pursue violators. However, there is no evidence as to whether any tomb-breakers were ever prosecuted. Furthermore, judging from the numerous sarcophagi that were re-used in the Roman period, it seems that the fines alone were not deterrent enough.

Sarcophagus Re-use

Despite the imprecations of the funerary inscriptions, sarcophagi were commonly re-used, especially after the second half of the third century CE, when the rate of sarcophagus production dropped drastically. As previously mentioned, there are two principal ways in which sarcophagi were re-used: (1) as secondary or later sarcophagi and (2) as building material and utilitarian objects. This section examines the evidence for each type of re-use.

Re-use as Sarcophagi

Sarcophagi from Aphrodisias were normally not intended for a single person but rather for several individuals, and often a family group. Obviously the individuals from the same family group did not all die at the same time, but whenever one did, the lid of the sarcophagus was re-opened, and the newly deceased was inhumed alongside the other body or bodies. The inscriptions do not ban the subsequent inhumation of the bodies of authorized family members, but rather the exhumation of the existing bodies and inhumation of unauthorized ones, who were unaffiliated with the owner family. However, despite this ban, the sarcophagi were often re-used as secondary or perhaps tertiary burial chests for individuals not authorized by the initial owners. Evidence for such re-use exists in the erased and re-carved inscriptions that indicate the names of the new owners; repairs on the chests; and disjunctions between inscriptions and busts.

Modified and Added Inscriptions

On some sarcophagi, the inscriptions were modified by chiseling off the original inscription and replacing it with a new one or simply by leaving the original inscription intact and adding a new one on a blank space elsewhere on the chest or lid. A large garland sarcophagus of the third century CE provides an example of the former practice (Fig. 3).[21] The center of the chest is dominated by a tabula,

21 S-1. Published in Işık 1982, 77–83, figs. 24–26; Işık 1984, 265–266, fig. 42; Işık 2007, cat. 157; Reynolds *et al.* 2007, 13.106.

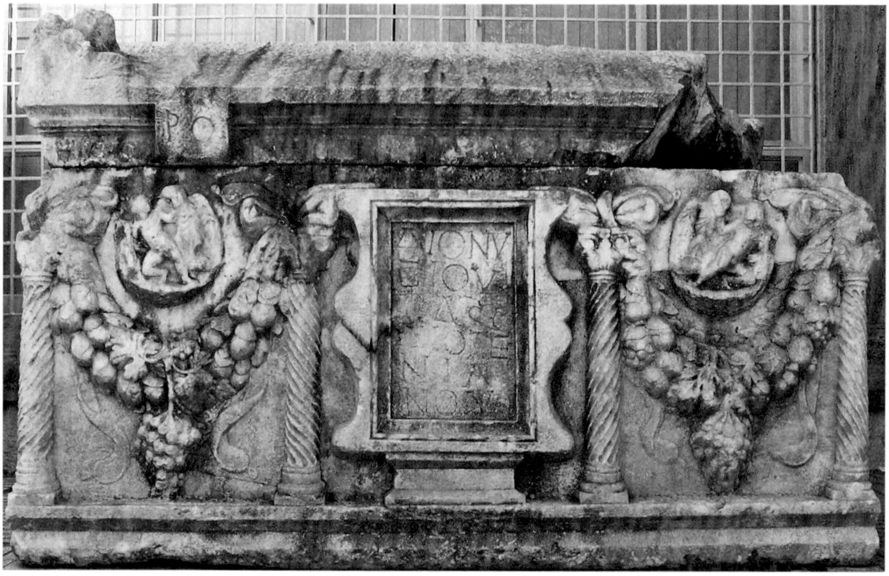

FIG. 3 Garland sarcophagus from Aphrodisias (S-1). Courtesy New York University Excavations at Aphrodisias.

on either side of which there is a garland carried by columns, in lieu of the more common Erotes. Inside the lunettes of each of the garlands, there is a circular relief that shows Ganymede abducted by the eagle. The original inscription inside the tabula was erased, as evident by the claw chisel marks, and replaced by an inscription with unusually large and irregular letters. This secondary inscription begins on the lid and continues in the tabula, and suggests that the sarcophagus and the spot on which it stands (*topos*) belonged to a Dionysios. The crude and unprofessional lettering of the inscription does not conform with the delicate styling of the garlands and mythological reliefs, which confirms that it was most likely added by the secondary owners.

Another example of the later addition of an inscription is the garland sarcophagus of the third century CE with a tabula in the center, two garlands on either side, and a male portrait inside each of the lunettes of the garlands (FIG. 1).[22] The original owners are indicated in the inscription that starts on the lid and continues in the tabula: "Marcus Aurelius Zenon and his sons." Later users, however, left the original inscription and the busts untouched (they show no signs of re-working), but inscribed a single word on the lid, in between the two lifting bosses: *Elpidiou*,

22 S-709. Unpublished sarcophagus. Translation provided in the field report of Angelos Chaniotis I 07.15 (unpublished).

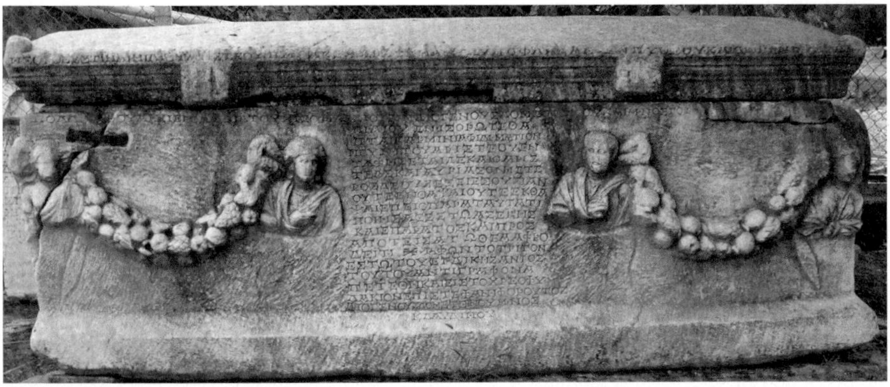

FIG. 4 Garland sarcophagus from Aphrodisias (S-11). Courtesy New York University Excavations at Aphrodisias.

"of Elpidios." This word is written in a crude and unprofessional letter form. It is clear that Elpidios, however he acquired the sarcophagus, was not at all bothered by the presence of the names and likenesses of the original owner, and was satisfied to announce his ownership simply by adding his own name to the lid.

Repairs. Traces of ancient repair on the chests are clearly visible on a few examples. Repair by itself does not prove that the sarcophagus was re-used, since it is quite possible that a newly commissioned sarcophagus may have been broken during transportation or by earthquakes. However, traces of repair combined with rudimentary inscriptions or modified relief decoration might indicate that a sarcophagus was in fact re-used.

One example of such repair and re-use is provided by a garland sarcophagus that was significantly modified from its original design (FIG. 4).[23] The whole left and back corner of the chest was broken and was re-attached with three clamps in the back and two in the front. The upper right corner of the chest was also broken and repaired with the insertion of a long rectangular piece of marble. In addition to this extensive repair scheme, the chest shows further signs of later additions and modifications. On the front of the chest, the space is divided into three, and two garlands hanging from busts flank an open area in the center. In this central space, there is a floating inscription. Immediately to the left of the inscription, there is a fully finished female bust and immediately to the right is a male bust. In the corners of the chest, there are two unfinished busts; the one on the left is female and the one on the right is male.

23 S-11. Published in Jones and Smith 1994; Işık 2007, cat. 6; Reynolds *et al.* 2007, 13.604.

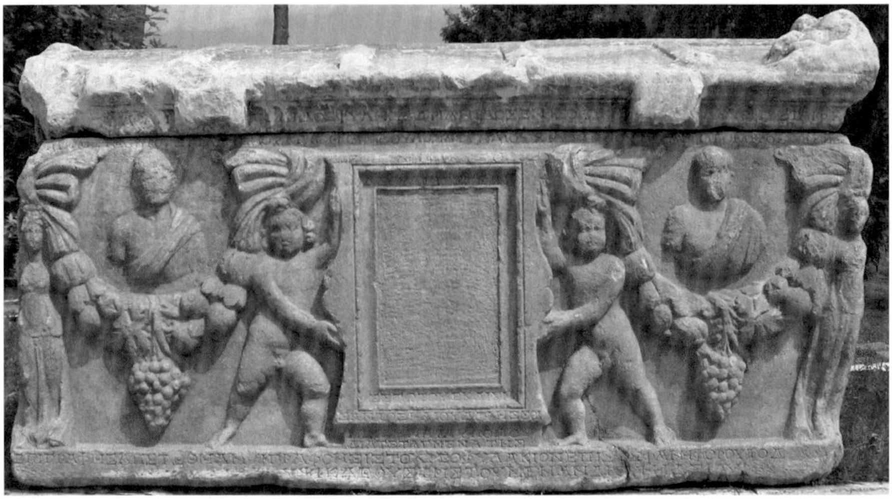

Fig. 5 Garland sarcophagus from Aphrodisias (S-478). Courtesy New York University Excavations at Aphrodisias.

The original tripartite scheme and the style of the garlands are typical for a triple-garland sarcophagus of the first or second century CE.[24] It seems that the secondary owners of the sarcophagus modified the whole chest by chiseling away the third garland in the center, replacing it with an inscription, and adding the two portrait heads on either side of the garland and in the corners. This modification is confirmed by the later dating of the busts compared to the style of the chest. The male bust has a short, cropped haircut squared on his forehead and a short groomed beard, datable broadly to the second half of the third century CE. As was suggested in a previous publication, the hairstyle of the female bust, with the braided bun reaching to the crown of the head, dates the sarcophagus more specifically to 260–290 CE.[25]

The twenty-line inscription matches the suggested dating of the portrait hairstyle, as well as further confirming the re-use of the sarcophagus. It suggests that the sarcophagus belongs to an "Aemilius Aristeas, conceded to him (*parakechorēmenē*) by Flavius Antonios Pytheas and Flavius Antonios Diogenes, sons of Apollonios the high priest..."[26] The inscription also mentions that in the sarcophagus has been buried Carminia Philemation, the wife of Aeristeas, and Aristeas himself. Furthermore, the inscription indicates that Aur(elia) Iasone would also

24 Işık 2007.

25 Jones and Smith 1994, 465–466.

26 Translation and commentary by Jones and Smith 1994, 468.

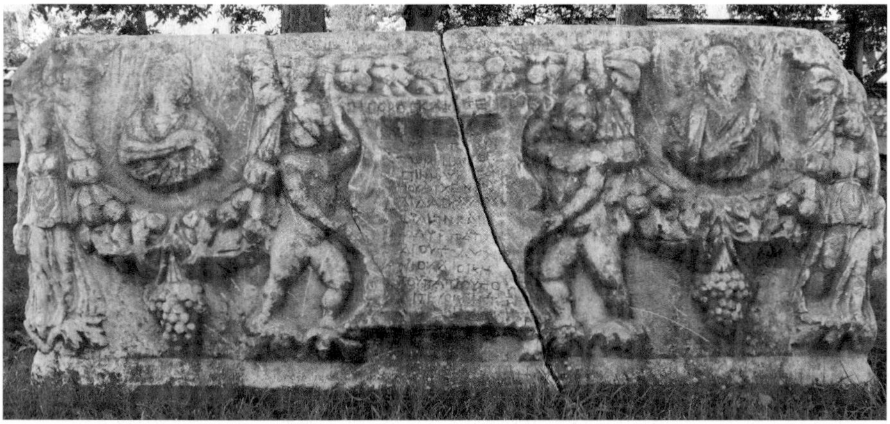

FIG. 6 Garland sarcophagus from Aphrodisias (S-39). Courtesy New York University Excavations at Aphrodisias.

be inhumed in the same sarcophagus upon her death. The concession of the sarcophagus here is a common practice for tombs in Asia Minor and implies a gift, probably made upon the death of Carminia Philemation, wife of Aristeas. In this case, it seems that the re-use was legal. The secondary owners, however, had to make a series of considerable changes to accommodate the tastes and needs of their own family.

Disjunction between Iconography and Inscription

Several sarcophagus patrons seem to have paid particular attention to ensuring that the genders of the legal owners and the busts were in agreement with each other. This is true for the aforementioned sarcophagus re-used by Elpidios, which originally belonged to Marcus Aurelius Zenon and his sons, and fittingly features two male busts. Such congruity is also evident in a garland sarcophagus owned by an ex-slave and his son, who was probably still a slave (FIG. 5).[27] The busts represent two males in what appear to be work clothes, each with one shoulder bare. Therefore, several patrons were clearly invested in the agreement and clarity of the iconography and the text.

However, there are occasional disjunctions between the names announced in the inscriptions and the genders of the portrait busts. For example, the inscription may suggest that both the owners are male, while the busts may represent a male

27 S-478. Unpublished sarcophagus. Translation provided in the field report of Angelos Chaniotis I 02.022 (unpublished).

and a female. Such a disjunction between the names and busts might indicate re-use. This is the case for the late Severan garland sarcophagus whose inscription starts on the frame of the tabula and is written in irregular letters (FIG. 6).[28] The tabula itself shows signs that the previous inscription was chiseled off, which confirms that the chest was re-used. The inscription attributes the ownership of the sarcophagus and the surrounding memorial to a Marcus Aurelius Leontius Auchenios, teacher of friends, and a M. Aurelius Papaios Polychronios, steward of Papias, *curialis*.[29] Both of these owners are obviously male, although the portrait bust on the left belongs to a female, now with a broken face.

Even though assuming a gender disjunction between the busts and the inscription as evidence for re-use might be the immediate tendency, one must refrain from hasty interpretations. An example of this kind of disjunction that does not necessarily attest to re-use is presented by an inscribed garland sarcophagus with unfinished portrait faces (FIG. 7).[30] This sarcophagus was found in a tomb context with other sarcophagi (i.e. not a stray find), and neither the inscription nor the portraits on it appear to have been changed. The inscription mentions that it belongs to Marcus Aurelius Proklos and his son, along with whomever they wish. The portraits, however, are those of one female and one male with unfinished faces. In this case, there is no evidence that the sarcophagus was re-used. On the contrary, since it was found in a funerary context, it probably remained untouched until it was discovered. It is quite possible to explain the gender disjunction by considering the personal wishes of the owner Proklos: he may have wanted to represent his son and his wife on the sarcophagus instead of himself. Or else, Proklos (and other patrons like him) perceived the busts as decorative and generic representations of the deceased, rather than attributing individual identity to them. The unfinished nature of the faces may confirm this perception of busts. Therefore, the disjunction between inscriptions and busts may not always be interpreted as evidence for re-use and must be supported by other evidence in order to be conclusive.

Re-use as Building Material and Utilitarian Objects

In building projects undertaken in the late and post-Roman periods, sarcophagus chests were treated as marble building material and were often cut into flat slabs so they could be utilized in paving or wall construction. When the city walls

28 S-39. Işık 2007, cat. 176; Reynolds *et al.* 2007, 15.345.

29 See the translation and commentary in Roueché 2004, IX.11. Also published in Reynolds and Roueché 2007, 179; Işık 2007, cat. 176.

30 S-414. Işık 2007, cat. 116; Reynolds *et al.* 2007, 13.110.

of Aphrodisias were built in the fourth century CE, the superstructures of the tombs were torn down to provide building materials for the project. The sarcophagi themselves were surely displaced in this period, and shortly thereafter many were broken into pieces and built into the walls.

Sarcophagus chests frequently found later use in renovation and building projects as in the Temple-Church conversion at Aphrodisias, or were commonly used as cover slabs in Byzantine tombs. The Temple-Church project involved major reconstruction and renovation work. The Temple was originally completed in the early first century CE as an 8 x 13 Ionic temple, and was dramatically transformed into a cathedral around 500 CE.[31] The conversion process involved the dismantling of the cella of the temple and the repositioning of columns on its east and west sides in alignment with those along its north and south flanks. In addition, an exterior wall was built around the colonnade, an apse was added on the east end of the building, as were narthexes and an atrium on the west, and the temenos enclosure was modified. The church was used in this condition for many centuries until it underwent a second renovation in the Middle Byzantine period. At that time, new floors were laid throughout the church. Many of the slabs that were used as paving stones in this second renovation are in fact pieces of sarcophagi that were cut into slabs and installed as paving stones so that the decorated surface was hidden on the underside of the stone. Sometimes, the relief decoration was also chiseled off, even though the decorated side remained hidden from view. Clearly, by the Middle Byzantine period, these sarcophagi had lost their value as a container for inhumed remains and were lying around the city in disarray.

Sarcophagus fragments were also treated as slabs of marble to cover the Middle Byzantine graves found around the Tetrapylon. One such example is a fragment of a columnar sarcophagus whose two aediculae survive (Fig. 8).[32] The aedicula on the left includes a fragmentary inscription that could have been carved later. The aedicula on the right originally represented a male figure, which was chiseled off, flattened and was provided with a large cross in relief in the middle of his torso.

In the later Islamic periods of the city, the re-use continued, and the sarcophagi were again treated as building material, sometimes even built into the walls of homes in the modern Turkish village. Several fully preserved sarcophagus chests were even re-used in the 1960s as wine vats by residents of Geyre, the village that had developed on top of the ancient settlement before the excavations began.

31 Building of the temple in Reynolds 1990; transformation of the Temple into a church: Hebert 2000, esp. 12–14.

32 S-754 (Inv. No. 83–067). Unpublished sarcophagus.

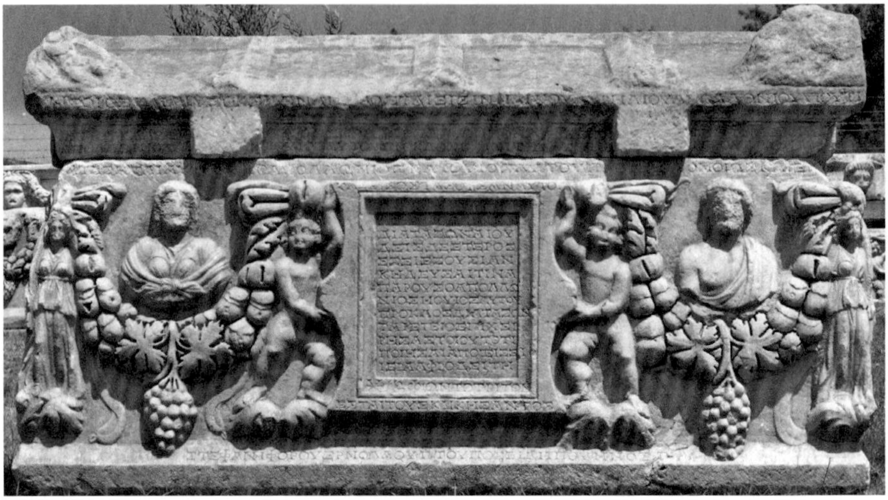

Fig. 7 Garland sarcophagus from Aphrodisias (S-414). Courtesy New York University Excavations at Aphrodisias.

Reasons and Implications of Sarcophagus Re-use

As demonstrated, despite imprecations and illegality, sarcophagi were commonly re-used. The two types of re-use examined here, namely re-use as sarcophagi versus re-use as building material, point to different issues, each deserving a separate focus.

In the Roman period, re-using the sarcophagi as secondary burial chests seems to have been quite common. Such re-use is evident from the modified or added inscriptions, the all too common repairs, and the many disjunctions of gender between the listed owners and the busts. As demonstrated, some individuals acquired these 'second-hand' sarcophagi legally. For others, there is no evidence to suggest whether or not the fine for tomb violation was ever charged by the prosecutors or paid by the violators. However, since tomb violation was clearly a quite common practice, the fine system and execution of legal sanctions was probably not functioning efficiently. It is also a possibility that the announced fines were paid by the violators without further consequences, and in practice, if not in theory, these fines acted like purchase prices. Such an act must have been especially easy if the family members had long since died out and there were no living relatives left to complain about the violation of the family tomb.

Economic decline, especially in the second half of the third century CE, might have contributed to the re-use of sarcophagus chests by others. The tightening control of the Roman government, the narrowing budgets of the councilors, and increased inflation must all have contributed to the declining economy. Mar-

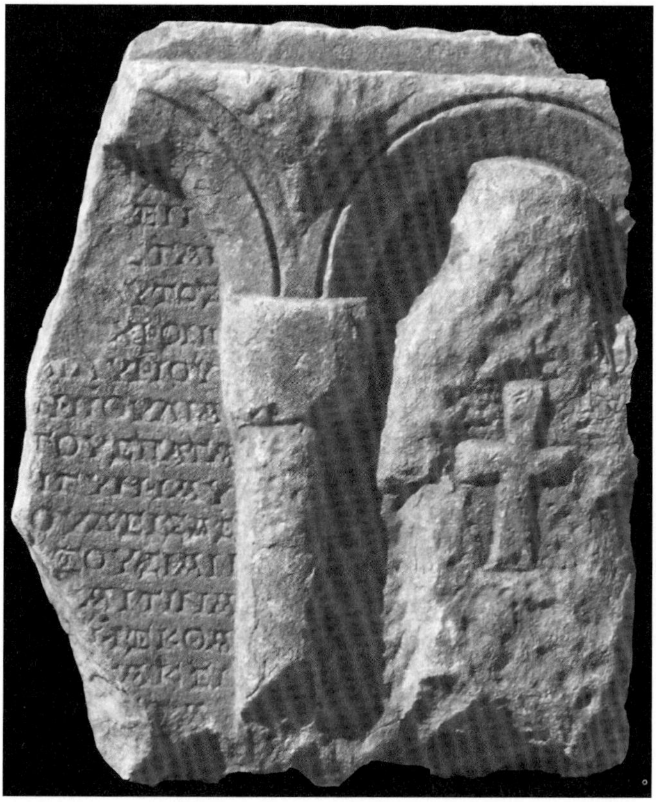

FIG. 8 Fragment of columnar sarcophagus from Aphrodisias (S-754). Courtesy New York University Excavations at Aphrodisias.

ble quarries might also have become dysfunctional in this period and may have stopped producing marble for private use or else greatly reduced their output. In fact, epigraphic evidence suggests that some major monuments of the city, for example the South Agora Gate, were left in ruins for some time, probably due to financial problems, only to be repaired in Late Antiquity.[33]

In any case, some who chose to re-use sarcophagi clearly did not pay much attention to the existing inscriptions and busts or could not afford professional letter cutters and bust carvers to modify the sarcophagi to their liking. This indifference could be due to a sense of respect for the previous owners, if not pure neglect or financial exigencies. The perception of the busts might have also determined how they were treated. Some secondary owners did not touch the portraits even when they exhibited a clear disjunction between their genders and the newly added text. Of course, it must have required a considerable amount of money to hire a sculptor to modify the bust, which the later users might not have

33 For example, an inscription honors a Dulcitius, the governor, who "stretching out his strong hand, raised me [the Agora Gate] too, who had suffered for unnumbered years." See Roueché 1989, doc. 38–40, pp. 69–73.

been easily able to afford. However, it is curious to observe that they did not simply chisel off the busts themselves, which is fairly easy to do. In that case, it is quite possible that some perceived the busts as part of the decoration of the chest and as generic busts that represented the rather broad category of the "deceased," rather than markers of ownership or a specific identity. When ownership was indicated by an added secondary inscription, there might have been no need to touch the portraits. Therefore, it may be possible to consider the inscriptions as primary and the images as a secondary means of claiming ownership of sarcophagi, rather than necessarily interdependent and inseparable agents.[34]

A funerary monument from Rome displays a similar disjunction between its inscription and relief sculpture.[35] While the relief depicts three individuals, a standing boy, a seated man and a standing girl, the inscription only refers to a man, Cornutus Doliens, and his son. The explanation for this monument has been that the portraits were devalued to the status of being mere decorative motifs.[36] Although such a judgment may be a bit overstated, still, the monument shows that the text and images did not have to be dependent upon one another, and in certain cases, it is clearly the inscription that provided the essential and primary information regarding the owners.

The second type of re-use for the sarcophagi, namely as building materials, points to extenuating circumstances and the changing burial culture under Christianity. As mentioned, the tomb buildings were dismantled in the fourth century CE, and their blocks, as well as some sarcophagi, were used to build the city walls. Even though such a major building project might be thought of as an indication of civic prosperity, many other spolia from the city center, such as statue bases, statues, and public decrees, were also used as building material, which suggests that this project was done out of insecurity rather than prosperity.

In fact, Aphrodisians may have faced serious outside threats during this period. Gothic invasions were part of the panorama of problems in mid-third century CE Anatolia.[37] Zosimus, for instance, speaks of a Gothic incursion into Asia Minor under Gallus and Volusianus that reached as far as Ephesus, Pessinus and Cappadocia.[38] Syncellus, in his list of places attacked by the Goths under Valerian and Gallienus enumerates Ionia, Galatia and Pessinus.[39] Jordanes asserts that Ephesus

34 Several studies demonstrated the interdependence and complementary nature of text and images in artworks. See for example, Koortbojian 1996.

35 *CIL* vi.16483.

36 Sanders 1970, 93.

37 The exact chronology of Gothic invasions in Asia Minor is not entirely clear. For a thorough evaluation of the sources, see Salamon 1971 and Magie 1950, 1566–1568.

38 Zos. I 26, 1–2; 27,1; 28,1.

39 Syncellus, 716.

and many other Asian cities were attacked under Gallienus (260–268 CE).[40] In fact, the Goths seem to have come as close to Aphrodisias as Hierapolis in Phrygia and perhaps also Stratonikeia in Caria, the latter of which sought a response from the oracle of Zeus Panamara as to whether or not the barbarians were going to destroy their city in the next year.[41] Similarly, the Sassanians were felt as a real threat in southeastern Anatolia and particularly in Cilicia in the mid-third century CE. Although their raids were not physically felt in western Asia Minor, Valerian, intending to lead a major force against the Sassanians beyond the Euphrates, initiated a major propaganda campaign to prepare the Greek cities of Asia Minor against possible raids by the Persians.[42]

While such external threats may have led to the re-use of tombs and sarcophagi, changing burial customs by this date may also have been a reason for this practice. It is quite possible that the house-shaped tombs with sarcophagi placed on top of them were no longer the preferred means of inhumation in Late Antiquity. Christians might have been content with simple pit graves, or underground chambers. As the torso of the male figure on the aforementioned fragment was marked out with a cross, the human figures on the sarcophagi might even have been deemed inappropriate for Christians, at least in the Middle Byzantine period. Later re-use of sarcophagi as slabs of pavement in the cathedral or as grave covers suggests that by the Middle Byzantine period, sarcophagi had completely lost their significance as sacred burial structures. Instead, they were merely valued as available pieces of stone.

Conclusion

In conclusion, the many different modes of sarcophagus re-use demonstrated here provide clues regarding the shifting perception and treatment of funerary monuments in the Roman period into post-antiquity. The elaborate chests that helped to distinguish a third-century CE citizen from his fellow citizens and sought to express a clear individual identity quickly fell out of favor in Late Antiquity. In these later periods, the chests were even reduced to the rank of building materials. The secondary life of funerary monuments not only illuminate a changing burial culture, but also demonstrate how volatile material culture and its perception can be under changing social conditions.

40 Jornades, *Getica*, 107.

41 Hierapolis: Salamon 1971, 127–128 and Loewe 1922, 254–256. Stratonicea: *CIG* II 2717; Magie 1950, 706.

42 *Res Gestae Divi Saporis*, published by Maricq 1958, lines 6–10. Also see Mitchell 1993, 237 and Magie 1950, 1568–1569.

REFERENCES

Chaniotis, A., "New Inscriptions from Aphrodisias (1995–2001)." *American Journal of Archaeology* 108 (2004): 377–416.

Cormack, S., *The Space of Death in Roman Asia Minor.* Vienna: Phoibos, 2004.

de Staebler, P.D., *The City Wall of Aphrodisias and Civic Identity in Late Antique Asia Minor.* PhD. Thesis, New York University, Institute of Fine Arts, 2007.

Erim, K.T., "The School of Aphrodisias." *Archaeology* 20 (1967): 18–26.

Fejfer, J., *Roman Portraits in Context.* Berlin: De Gruyter, 2008.

Hebert, L., *The Temple-Church at Aphrodisias.* PhD. Thesis, New York University, Institute of Fine Arts, 2000.

Işık, F., "Kleinasiatische Girlandensarkophage mit Pilaster- oder Säulenarchitektur." Jahreshefte des Österreichischen Archäologischen Institutes in Wien (ÖJh) 53 (1982): 30–146.

———. "Die Sarkophage von Aphrodisias" in *Symposium über die Antiken Sarkophage, Pisa 5.-12. September 1982: Marburger Winckelmann-Programm*, ed. by B. Andreae, 243–281. Marburg/Lahn: Verlag des Kunstgeschichtlichen Seminars, 1984.

———. *Girlanden-Sarkophage aus Aphrodisias. Mit einem Beitrag zu den Inschriften von J. M. Reynolds and C. Roueché.* Mainz am Rhein: Von Zabern, 2007.

Jones, C.P. and R.R.R. Smith, "Two Inscribed Monuments at Aphrodisias." *Archäologischer Anzeiger* (1994): 455–472.

Judeich, W., *Altertümer von Hierapolis.* Berlin: Dietrich Reimer Verlag, 1898.

Koortbojian, M., "*In Commemorationem Mortuorum*: Text and Image along the 'Streets of Tombs'" in *Art and Text in Roman Culture*, ed. by J. Elsner, 210–233. Cambridge: Cambridge University Press, 1996.

Kubińska, J., *Les Monuments Funéraires dans les Inscriptions Grecques de l'Asie Mineure.* Travaux du Centre d'archéologie méditerranéenne de l'Académie polonaise des sciences, 5. Warsaw, 1968.

Loewe, R., "Der gotische Kalender." *Zeitschrift für Deutsches Altertum und deutsche Literatur* 59 (1922): 245–290.

Magie, D., *Roman Rule in Asia Minor to the End of the Third Century after Christ.* Princeton: Princeton University Press, 1950.

Maricq, A., "Classica et Orientalia: 5. Res Gestae Divi Saporis." *Syria* 35 (1958): 295–360.

Mitchell, S., *Anatolia. Land, Men and Gods in Asia Minor,* Vol. 1. Oxford: Clarendon Press, 1993.

Moltesen, M., "The Aphrodisian Sculptures in the Ny Carlsberg Glyptotek" in *Aphrodisias Papers: Recent Work on Architecture and Sculpture*, ed. by C. Roueché and K. T. Erim, *Journal of Roman Archaeology* Suppl. 1 (1990): 133–146.

Öğüş Uzun, E., *Columnar Sarcophagi from Aphrodisias: Construction of Elite Identity in the Greek East.* PhD. Thesis, Harvard University, 2010.

Öğüş, E., "Columnar Sarcophagi from Aphrodisias: Elite Emulation in the Greek East." *American Journal of Archaeology* 118 (2014a): 1–24.

———. "Rise and Fall of Sarcophagus Production at Aphrodisias." *Phoenix* 68 (2014b): 137–156.

Reynolds, J.M., "Inscriptions and the Building of the Temple of Aphrodite" in *Aphrodisias Papers: Recent Work on Architecture and Sculpture*, ed. by C. Roueché and K. T. Erim, *Journal of Roman Archaeology* Suppl. 1 (1990): 37–40.

Reynolds, J.M. and C. Roueché, "The Inscriptions" in F. Işık, *Girlanden-Sarkophage aus Aphrodisias. Mit einem Beitrag zu den Inschriften von J. M. Reynolds and C. Roueché*, 147–185. Mainz am Rhein: Philipp von Zabern, 2007.

Reynolds, J.M, C. Roueché and G. Bodard. *Inscriptions of Aphrodisias*. Available at http://insaph.kcl.ac.uk/iaph2007 (retrieved on 13 Aug 2014), 2007.

Ritti, T., *An Epigraphic Guide to Hierapolis (Pamukkale)*. Ege Yayınları: İstanbul, 2006.

Roueché, C., *Aphrodisias in Late Antiquity*. London: Society for the Promotion of Roman Studies, 1989.

———. *Aphrodisias in Late Antiquity: The Late Roman and Byzantine Inscriptions*. Available at http://insaph.kcl.ac.uk/ala2007 (retrieved on 13 Aug 2014), 2004.

Salamon, M., "The Chronology of Gothic incursions into Asia Minor in the Third century AD." *Eos* 59 (1971): 109–139.

Sanders, G., "Les éléments figuratifs des *Carmina Latina Epigraphica*" in *Lapides Memores. Païens et chrétiens face à la mort: le témoignage de l'épigraphie funéraire latine*, ed. by A. Donati, D. Pikhaus and M. Van Uytfanghe, 87–110. Faenz: Fratelli Lega, 1970.

Schneider Equini, E. *La Necropoli di Hierapolis di Frigia*. Rome: Accademia nazionale dei Lincei, 1972.

Smith, R.R.R., "Sarcophagi and Roman Citizenship" in *Aphrodisias Papers 4. New Research on the City and its Monuments*, ed. by R.R.R. Smith and C. Ratté, *Journal of Roman Archaeology* Suppl. 70 (2008): 347–395.

Squarciapino, M.F., "La Scuola di Aphrodisias (40 Anni Dopo)." *Archeologia Classica* 35 (1983): 74–87.

Strubbe, J. Arai Epitumbioi: *Imprecations against Desecrators of the Grave in the Greek Epigraphs of Asia Minor*. Bonn: Rudolf Halbert Verlag Gmbh, 1997.

Tulay, S., "Kabalar Kurtarma Kazısı 1989." *Müze Kurtarma Kazıları Semineri 1990* (1991): 25–39.

Turnbow, H. N. *Sarcophagi and Funerary Display in Roman Aphrodisias*. PhD. Thesis, New York University, Institute of Fine Arts, 2011.

van Voorhis, J., "Apprentices' Pieces and the Training of Sculptors at Aphrodisias." *Journal of Roman Archaeology* 11 (1998): 175–192.

Miniature Cream Vessels from Tatarlı Höyük Dated to the Hellenistic Period

Hayriye Akıl[1]

Abstract

Tatarlı Höyük is located near the Tatarlı village (Yedioluk, Yedigöz), which is 5 km to the north of Mustafabeyli at the Osmaniye border and 24 km to the east of Ceyhan. The mound is situated in the eastern part of Çukurova (Cilicia) and is located in a place where two important routes, one with a south-north and the other with an east-west direction, overlap. The excavations at Tatarlı Höyük began in 2007. During these excavations, which still continue today, levels dated to the Hellenistic period, the Iron Age, the Late Bronze Age and the Middle Bronze Age have been unearthed. Six miniature baked clay vessels were found in the Hellenistic levels during the 2007 to 2013 seasons. The vessels in question, which have been discovered in small numbers during these excavations, are called miniature cream vessels.[2]

Introduction

Tatarlı Höyük[3] is located in the Ceyhan district of the Adana province of Turkey (Fig. 1). This ancient settlement, which is situated close to the Tatarlı village, entered scholarly literature after its discovery by Seton-Williams in 1951.[4] S. Lloyd and J. Mellaart indicated Tatarlı Höyük on a map showing the distribution of "volute handle/feet" type pottery dated to the Early Bronze Age IIIb,[5] and in 1991, M. H. Sayar reported a spring and some ruins around Tatarlı Village.[6] But the first comprehensive research at this *höyük* started during the "Ceyhan I" phase of the Cilician Surveys of Serdar Girginer,[7]

1 Arkeoloji Bölümü, Fen-Edebiyat Fakültesi, Çukurova Üniversitesi, 01330, Adana.

2 Işın 2002, 85.

3 Girginer, Girginer and Akıl 2010, 454.

4 Seton-Williams 1954, 128–129, 170, no. 39.

5 Lloyd and Mellaart 1962, 257, map X.

6 Sayar, Siewert and Taeuber 1993, 179.

7 Girginer 2007, 177.

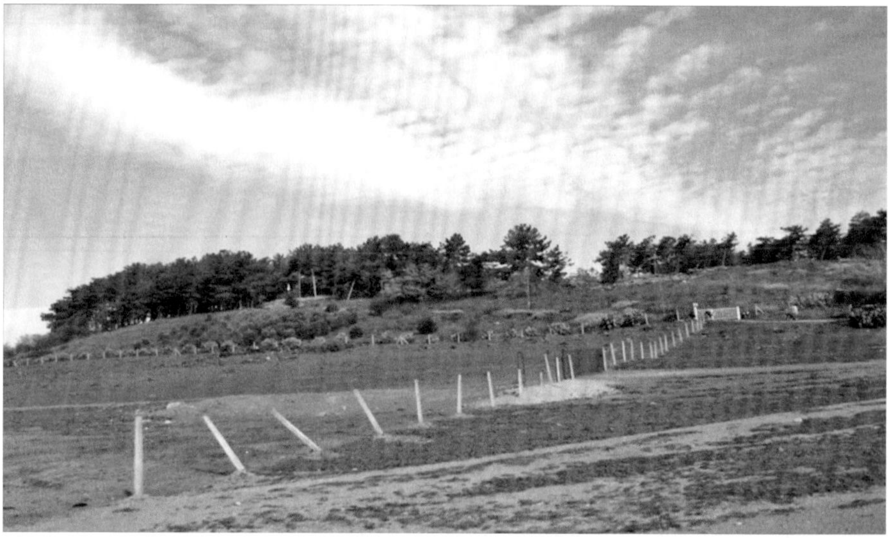

FIG. 1 Tatarlı Höyük from the south

who initiated the excavations at the site in 2007. During these excavations Hellenistic, Iron Age, Late Bronze Age and Middle Bronze Age levels were discovered (FIG. 2).

Hellenistic miniature cream vessels, of which six examples were found at Tatarlı Höyük, have their origins in third millennium BC Egypt.[8] These vessels became widespread especially in Greece and Lydia during the sixth century BC. The small number of Hellenistic-Roman cream vessels from the excavations makes it hard to make a typological analysis of the examples from Tatarlı Höyük. These vessels were not generally defined in a definite manner in the Hellenistic period, and they were referred to with various names, such as *unguentarium, kothon, aryballos, alabastron* and *lydion*.

The Functions of the Miniature Cream Vessels

The miniature cream vessels were used as oil and balm containers, so they became very popular in the ancient Greek world. Some local forms for these were developed during the fifth century BC. The Hellenistic vessels, which were used in Athens in the fifth and fourth centuries BC, are believed to be vanguards of the cream/ medial bottles and poison vessels.[9] These vessels were not used in sacred environments. The varieties of these vessels grew because of the increasing popularity of aromatic oils

8 Smith 1870, 1214.

9 Rotroff 1997, 198.

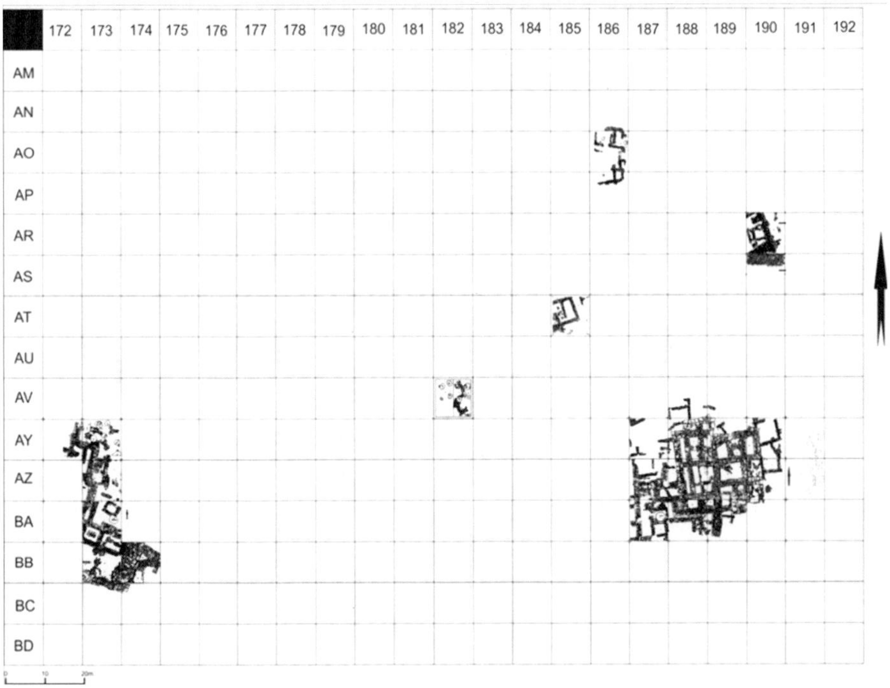

FIG. 2 Plan of the citadel (Tatarlı Höyük 2012 excavations)

and perfumes, scientific improvements, and new methods and technics of producing vessels in the Hellenistic period.

Putting labels on these vessels is another innovation for the period in question. These inscriptions included some information about the ingredients of the vessels, and the names of pharmacists were also written in some cases as a guarantee of quality.[10] The most popular medicine that appears on the inscriptions is *lykion*, which received its name from the Lycian region of southwestern Anatolia.[11] Dioscorides[12] recommended *lykion* in order to cure various diseases, such as staunching, psoriasis, itchiness, some diseases related with eyelids, ears and

10 Işın 2002, 85–87.

11 Pliny, XII, 15.

12 Jackson 1999, 72. Pedanius Dioscorides, who was born in Anazarbos in the Cilician region, is the most famous pharmacologist of the Archaic age. He lived in the first century AD, and he traveled very much. Dioscorides wrote his book, *De Materia Medica,* in which he rejected spells and superstitions, in 64 AD. The writer in question was educated in the Cilicia region, and he might have written this work as a means of recording the medical prosperity of this region from as far back as the second millennium BC.

tonsils, gingiva, lip fissures, ulcers, lyssa, coeliac and dysentery. [13] Scribonius Largus, who earned a remarkable reputation as a physician in the early first century AD, indicated that Indian *lykion* surpasses all other eye balms.

A small number of lead jars containing this valuable material has been unearthed at various sites. *Lykion* of Iasos, *Lykion* according to Moses's prescription, and *Nymphodorus Lkion* as seen on one vessel from Priene vessel dated to the third-second century BC, are examples of inscriptions on these. [14] *Lykion,* like many other medicines and cosmetic products, were actually creams and they could be applied by means of a spatula or fingers. [15] It is known that most of Pliny's medical suggestions in his *Natıral History* were made of a mixture including honey and animal fats. [16]

The Locations where the Hellenistic Miniature Cream Vessels were Unearthed

At Tell Anafa, 26 miniature vessels defined as medical containers were unearthed. [17] These artifacts are stylistically divided into four groups. Ten of these examples constitute the first group. These vessels, which have no parallels from other sites but are related to some Persian vessels, have a cylindrical body with a raised, straight base. Six miniature vessels belong to the second group. This form with a partially protruding body was from the Hellenistic 2B layer (110–100 BC). The third group includes nine miniature vessels. These vessels with a protruding body were from the Hellenistic 2A layer (125 BC). The fourth type includes only one vessel, which is called the "Galelian medical container", and it is dated to 10–20 AD.

Examples found at Samaria have a red lining on their exterior and their heights vary between 3–7 cm. [18] The functions of these could not be determined. The one example found at Tarsus-Gözlükule, which is 4.1 cm high, has a raised base and is made of light brown clay with a reddish-brown lining on its exterior and the rim. [19] The vessel is believed to be from the period between the mid-second century BC and mid-first century BC, although the date can be extended to the end of the first century BC.

During the excavations at Tralleis between 1996 and 2002, one miniature

13 Sjöqvist 1960, 81

14 Jackson 1999, 75. *Lykion* has been used in India until recent times, and it was brought to the United Kingdom in the early 19th century BC. *Lykion* is used to treat conjunctivitis.

15 Smith 1992, 163–164.

16 Pliny, XX, 10.

17 Berlin and Slane 1997, 70–72, figs. 119–129

18 Reisner, Fisher and Lyon 1924, 302.

19 Goldman 1950, 217, pl. 123, 93.

vessel, which was called a "medical bottle," was unearthed in the Hellenistic level.[20] This artifact was compared with the Morgantina type IIIB vessels, and it was dated to a period between the last quarter of the third century BC and the first quarter of the second century BC. Miniature vessels of Morgantina Type IVA were dated to the Roman period.

The miniature cream vessels from Patara were stylistically divided into three types, with the biconical type without a handle being the characteristic form, and there are little differences between them.[21] A hundred vessels, which were unearthed during the Patara excavations, were defined as cream vessels with a medical purpose. They are mostly 4–5 cm tall, and their capacities differ, ranging from 10 gr to 30 gr. These vessels were dated to the period between the third century BC and the first century BC.

The cream vessels from Ephesos are believed to form the early beginnings of the small sachets, which can be distinguished from cream vessels by their low necks, that were more appropriate to use as containers for solid materials.[22] The comparison of cream vessels from Ephesos, Delos, Morgantina and Corinth indicate that the examples from Ephesos are dated to the period between the third century BC and the first century BC.

Eight miniature vessels of this type were found at Corinth, and their heights vary from 2.6 cm to 4.2 cm.[23] Surprisingly, a few of them were discovered in sacred places. The results of the excavations have clearly shown that these were not manufactured before the third century BC.

Seventeen miniature vessels from Agora have a varying height of 2.5 to 4.2 cm.[24] The evaluation of their forms, especially when compared with similar terracotta or lead vessels, has shown that these were mostly used to contain medicine or cosmetics. Most of them are local products, except five, based on their different forms and technique of production. These vessels have raised or straight bases, wide, slightly outturned rims, and their inner and outer surfaces are mostly lined. These pear shaped vessels have no handle. The examples from Agora were divided into three groups. The vessels in the first, and probably the best represented, group have a an outturned profile and a straight base. The second type has a vertical bottom edge. This group, which is only represented by one artifact, is dated to 175 BC. The ones in the third group have a raised base, and they are dated to the third century BC or early second century BC.

20 Dinç 2012, 178, fig. 10.

21 Işın 2002, 91.

22 Mitsopoulos-Leon 1991, 148–149.

23 Edwards 1975, 99–100.

24 Rotroff 1997, 198, pl. 1309–1313.

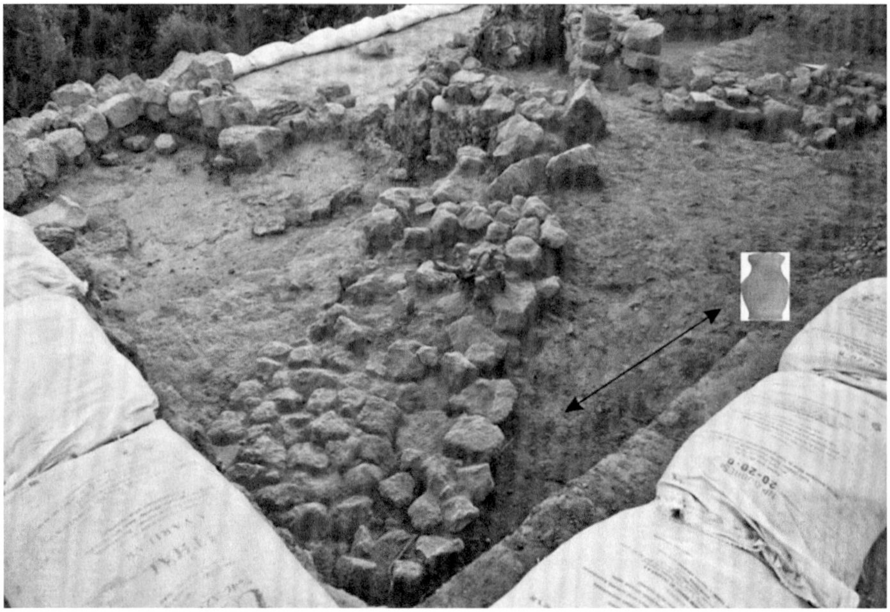

FIG. 3 AP 186 trench during the Tatarlı Höyük 2010 excavations (Location of Object 1)

Fifty four miniature vessels were unearthed at Morgantina in total.[25] These vessels were divided into four main stylistic groups, but there are also many subdivisions which are based on the little differences among them. Types 1 and 2 were discovered in residences and stores, Type 3 just around the Demeter and Kore temples and Type 4 in both sacred and unsacred places. These vessels show a heterogeneous distribution and were never found as a group at a special place. The vessels from Morgantina usually have a height of 2.5 to 5.6 cm. Some of them had *ΛYKION* inscribed on them. These light brown, grey or pink colored vessels usually have thick walls with a shiny blackish brown or red colored lining. Based on the numismatic and ceramic evidence gathered from the locations where these vessels were discovered, the miniature cream vessels from this site were dated to the third-second centuries BC.

Miniature Cream Vessels from Tatarlı Höyük

Six baked clay miniature vessels were found in the Hellenistic level of Tatarlı Höyük in between 2007 and 2013, each of which shows stylistically different characteristics.

25 Sjöqvist 1960, 79–80, pl. 19

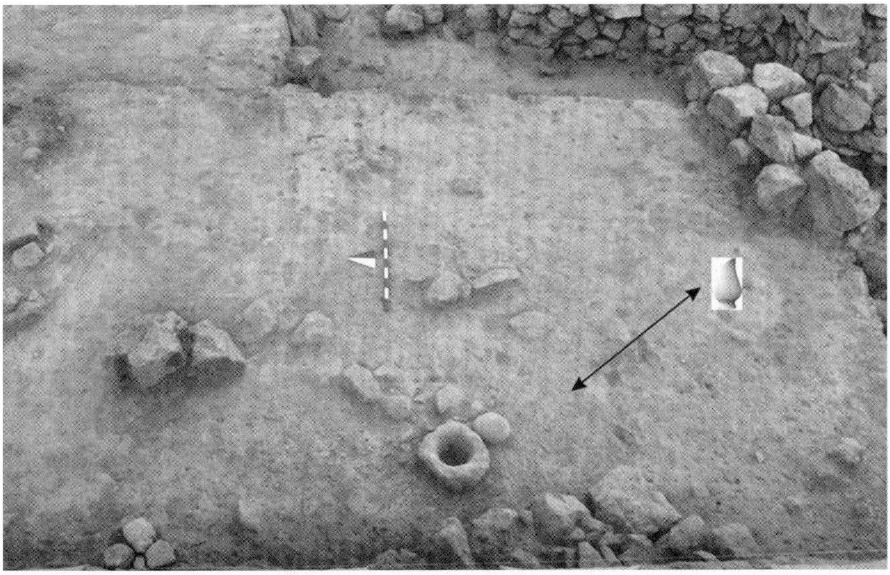

FIG. 4 AZ 187 trench during the Tatarlı Höyük 2012 excavations (Location of Object 2)

A step-trench was opened on the steep northern slope of the *höyük* in order to uncover all the stratigraphic layers of the mound. During the excavations that were carried out at the first level of this trench, a miniature vessel was unearthed in AP-186 (FIG. 3). The rim of this low vessel, which has a lightly bulging body with a low base and a straight bottom, is outturned, and it is not lined. Examples with the most similar forms were discovered at Agora,[26] Corinth[27] and Ephesos.[28] These miniature vessels were dated to third and second centuries BC, based on the dating of a lamp from the same trench.[29]

During the 2011 and 2012 seasons, some Hellenistic remains were discovered that were annexed to the northern, eastern and western walls of a building dated to the second millennium BC on the eastern side of the citadel, where three miniature vessels were unearthed. The first example (Catalogue no: 2) has an outturned rim, a tall neck, a bulged body, a low base ending with a straight bottom and a cream color lining (FIG. 4). This piece resembles type IV of Morgantina, which is dated to the second century BC, in terms of its style.

26 Rotroff 1997, 198, pl. 100, fig. 1309.

27 Edwards 1975, 99–100, pl. 58, fig. 600.

28 Mitsopoulos-Leon 1991, 148–149, pl. 215, fig. O33.

29 Bailey 1975, 235–236, pl. 102, Q509. Bailey corresponded the similar form of this lamp with the Levantine lamps, and so he dated it to the second half of the second century BC.

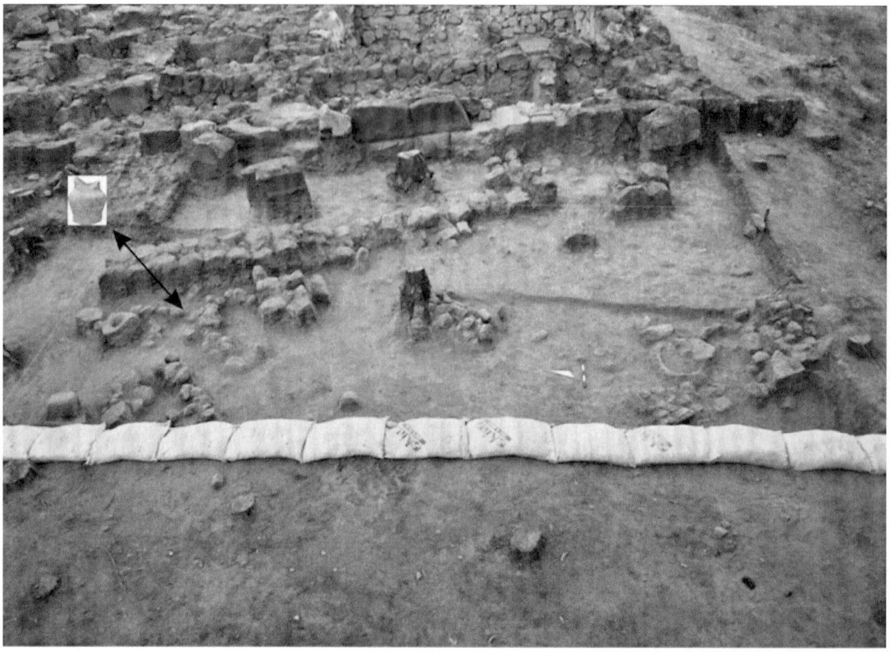

Fig. 5 AZ 187 trench during the Tatarlı Höyük 2009 excavations (Location of Object 3)

The second example (Catalogue no: 3), which is unlined, has a bulged body with a low neck and a tall base with straight bottom. Because of the raised base and the thick body wall, the capacity of this vessel is relatively low (Fig. 5). The third vessel (Catalogue no: 4) has a simple rim and is unlined. Like the second example (Catalogue no: 3), it has a relatively low capacity because of the raised base and the thick wall of the body (Fig. 6). Morgantina Type IIIA vessels are the most similar comparative examples to the second and third examples (Catalogue 3 and 4), although the bases of these vessels are lower. Examples from Morgantina are dated to the period in between the third and second centuries BC. It should be noted that the body of a vessel from Morgantina had the the impression of a seal including a representation of the head of Asclepius, which is an implication of its medical function.[30] No vessels that look similar to the first example (Catalogue no: 2) could be found.

Two miniature vessels were found in the Hellenistic levels in trenches BA-174 and BA-186, which were opened on the southern part of Tatarlı Höyük in 2013. One of them (Catalogue no: 5) has a simple rim and a body which bulges slightly at the transition point to the base; it has also a raised base. This vessel with a straight base

30 Sjöqvist 1960, 79–80, pl. 19, figs. 7, 10.

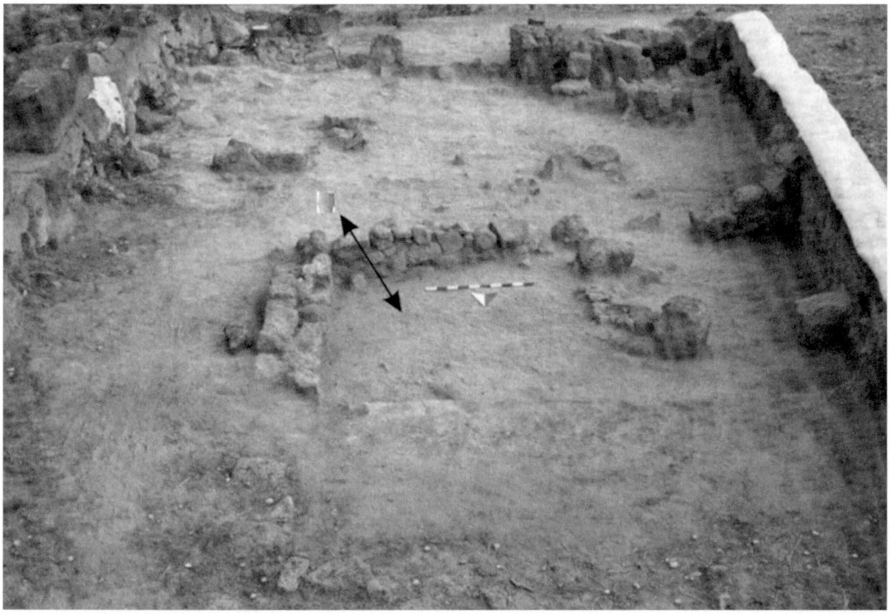

FIG. 6 AZ 187 trench during the Tatarlı Höyük 2009 excavations (Location of Object 4)

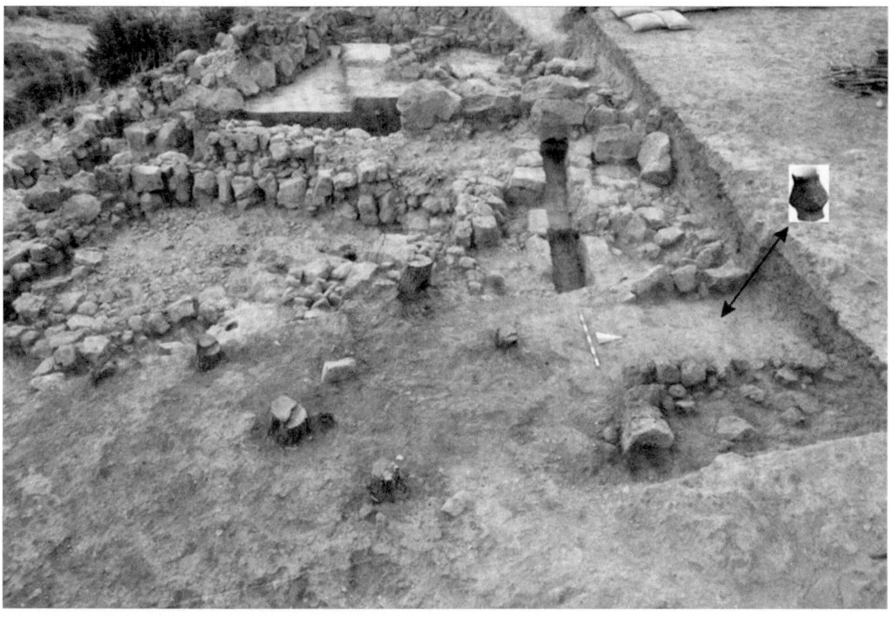

FIG. 7 BA 174 trench during the Tatarlı Höyük 2013 excavations (Location of Object 5)

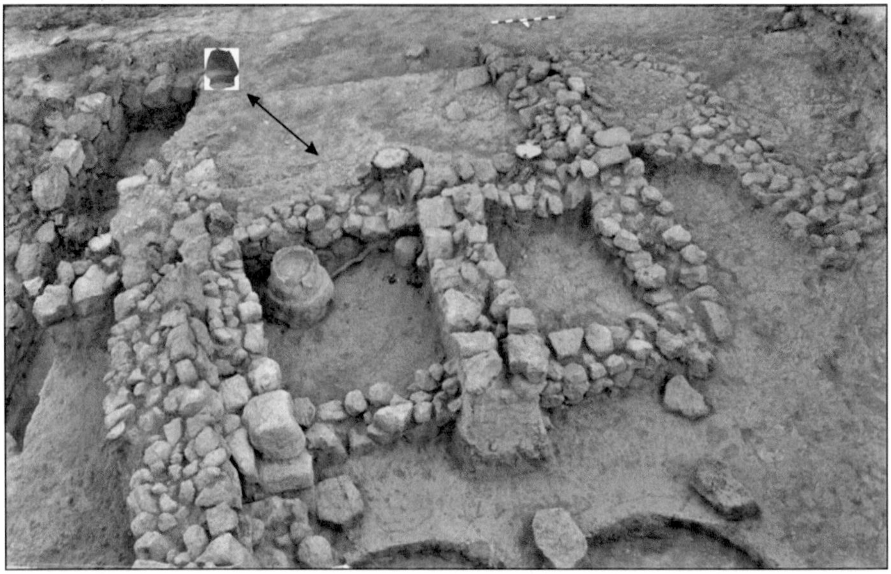

FIG. 8 BA 186 trench during the Tatarlı Höyük 2013 excavations (Location of Object 6)

has a slip on its exterior surface (FIG. 7). The vessels from Agora[31] and Corinth,[32] which are stylistically similar to this example, are dated to the third and second centuries BC. The other example (Catalogue no: 6) has a simple rim and a body which gradually bulges downwards from the mouth and then makes a concave turn to join the straight bottom. (Catalogue no: 6). Like the vessels found in trench AZ-187 (Catalogue no: 3 and 4), the capacity of this unlined vessel is relatively low because of its thick wall (FIG. 8). Similar examples were unearthed at Ephesos, and the examples from Ephesos were dated to the third-second century BC based on the comparisons made with examples from Corinth and Delos.[33]

Conclusion

Each miniature vessel that was found during the Tatarlı mound Hellenistic Period settlement excavations from the 2007 to 2013 excavation seasons has a different form and different features. Only two of the six examples were slipped (Catalogue no: 2 and 5) and the rest were self slipped. Their clay is composed of sand, mica, and limestone. Their height ranges from 2.2 cm to 2.7 cm.

31 Rotroff 1997, 198, pl. 100, fig. 1312.

32 Edwards 1975, 99–100, pl. 58, fig. 602.

33 Mitsopoulos-Leon 1991, 148–149, pl. 215, fig. O34.

Since the number of examples from Tatarlı Höyük (which share morphological similarities with the finds from Agora, Corinth, Ephesos, and Morgantina) is limited, it was not possible to classify these vessels in terms of their forms and manufacturing techniques. These miniature vessels, which seem to have been used for medical/cosmetic purposes in the ancient world, will be examined in more detail in terms of their typological characteristics and functions, and the new results will be shared with the research community when the archeological studies are completed.

CATALOGUE

Catalogue No: 1
Locus: TH.10. AP 186–3505/3
Rim Diameter: 3.1 cm
Preserved Height: 5.1 cm
Clay Colour: 5YR 6/6
Exterior Colour: 5YR 6/6 reddish yellow
Description: complete preserved. Clay, mica and lime inclusions.

Catalogue No: 2
Locus: TH.12. AZ 187–7113/1
Rim Diameter: 3.1 cm
Preserved Height: 7.8 cm
Clay Colour: 5YR 7/6 reddish yellow
Exterior Colour: 10YR 7/4 very pale brown
Description: a large part of the rim portion not preserved. Clay, mica inclusions.

Catalogue No: 3
Locus: TH.2009. AZ 187–711/2
Rim Diameter: 2.1 cm
Preserved Height: 3.8 cm
Clay Colour: 7.5YR 6/6 reddish yellow
Exterior Colour: 7.5YR 6/4 light Brown
Description: a large part of the rim portion not preserved. Clay, mica and sand inclusions.

Catalogue No: 4
Locus: TH.11. AZ 187–721/2
Rim Diameter: 2.2 cm
Preserved Height: 2.7 cm
Clay Colour: 10YR 7/6 yellow
Exterior Colour: 2.5Y 7/6 yellow
Description: complete except for small piece broken off rim. Clay, mica inclusions.

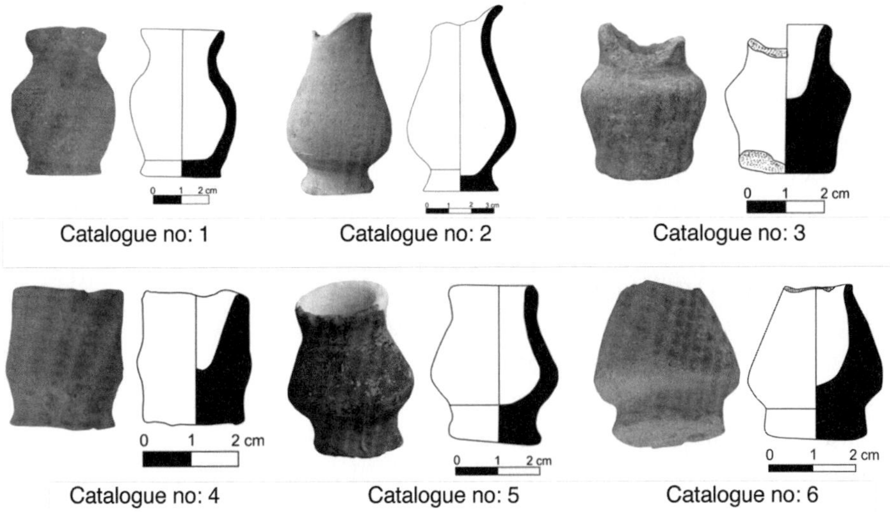

FIG. 9 Catalogue of vessels

Catalogue No: 5
Locus: TH.13. BA 174–67/1
Rim Diameter: 2.1 cm
Preserved Height: 3.5 cm
Clay Colour: 10YR 7/4 very pale brown
Exterior Colour: 10R 4/4 weak red
Description: a large part of the rim portion not preserved. The rim has been restored. Clay, mica inclusions. This vessel has a slipped outer surface.

Catalogue No: 6
Locus: TH.13. BA 186–41/2
Rim Diameter: 1.5 cm
Preserved Height: 3.3cm
Clay Colour: 10YR7/4 very pale brown
Exterior Colour: 10YR7/4 very pale brown
Description: a large part of the rim portion not preserved. Clay, mica and sand inclusions.

REFERENCES

Bailey, D.M., *A Catalogue of the Lamps in the British Museum, I. Greek, Hellenistic and Early Roman Pottery Lamps.* London: British Museum Publications, 1975.

Berlin, A. and W.K. Slane, *Tell Anafa II, The Hellenistic and Roman Pottery.* Ann Arbor: Kelsey Museum of the University of Michigan, 1997

Dinç, R., "Tralleis (1996–2002) Kazı Buluntuları Işığında Mesogis Şarapçılığı ve Sağlık" in *Stratonikeia'dan Lagina'ya Ahmet Adil Tırpan Armağanı,* ed. by B. Söğüt, 173–198. İstanbul: Ege Yayınları, 2012.

Edwards, G., *Corinthian Hellenistic Pottery, Corinth Vol.VII, Part III.* New Jersey: The American School Of Classical Studies At Athens, 1975.

Girginer, K.S., "2005 Yılı Adana (Ceyhan) ve Kayseri (Develi) Yüzey Araştırmaları." *Araştırma Sonuçları Toplantısı* 24/2(2007): 173–196.

Girginer, K.S., Ö. Girginer and H. Akıl, "Tatarlı Höyük (Ceyhan) Kazısı İlk İki Dönemi." *Kazı Sonuçları Toplantısı* 31/3 (2010): 453–476.

Goldman, H., *Excavations at Gözlü Kule,* Tarsus I. Princeton: Princeton University Press, 1950.

Işın, G. 2002., "Ointment or Medicine Vessels from Patara: An Overview of a Simple Hellenistic From in the Ancient Mediterranean World." *Archäologische Anzeiger* 2002/1 (2002): 85–96.

Jackson, R., *Roma İmparatorluğu'nda Doktorlar ve Hastalıklar,* trans. Ş. Mumcu). İstanbul: Homer Kitabevi Yayınları, 1999.

Lloyd, S. and J. Mellaart, *Beycesultan I: The Chalcolithic and Early Bronze Age Levels.* London: British Institute at Ankara Publication, 1962.

Mitsopoulos-Leon, V., *Die Basilika am Staatsmarkt in Ephesos, Kleinfunde, Forschungen in Ephesos IX 2/2.* Vienna: Österreichische Akademie der Wissenschaften, 1991.

Pliny. *Natural History,* trans. by H. Rackham, W.H.S. Jones, D.E. Eichholz, ed., W. Heinemann. London: William Heinemann Ltd. 1949–1954.

Reisner, G.A., Fisher, C.S. and D.G. Lyon, *Harvard Excavations at Samaria 1908–1910.* Cambridge, MA 1924.

Rotroff, S.I., *Hellenistic Pottery Athenian and Imported Wheelmade Table Ware and Related Material, Agora 29.* Princeton: American School of Classical Studies at Athens, 1997.

Sayar, M.H., Siewert, P. and H. Taeuber, "Doğu Kilikya'da Epigrafi ve Tarihi-Coğrafya Araştırmaları." *Araştırma Sonuçları Toplantısı* 10 (1993): 175–197.

Seton-Williams, M.V., "Cilician Survey." *Anatolian Studies* 4 (1954): 121–174.

Sjöqvist, E., "Morgantina Hellenistic Medicine Bottles." *American Journal of Archaeology* 64 (1960): 78–83.

Smith, W. *Dictionary of Greek and Roman Antiquities.* London: John Murray, 1870.

Smith, R.H., "Bloom of Youth A Labelled Syro-Palestinian Unguent Jar." *Journal of Hellenic Studies* 112 (1992): 163–167.

PART 6

Late Antique to Ottoman

Size Matters!
Scale and Demography of the Deli Halil Settlement

Füsun Tülek[1]

Abstract

Size is vital for identifying a settlement, along with layout and demography. If the power and wealth of a settlement depends on the extent of its territory and population, then size matters. A settlement is inhabited by a number of people who consume and produce artifacts in demand. To a degree, a settlement is also dependent on the production of its hinterland. It must be self-sustaining to the extent of having resources: water, and land for farming and grazing.

Three years of the Osmaniye archaeological survey recorded a Late Antique settlement on the slope of an inactive volcano. Deli Halil, named after the volcano, is an unfortified settlement that covers quite a large area close to the ancient city of Epiphaneia and its harbor, Burnaz. The present study aims to estimate the demography of the Deli Halil settlement, taking into consideration its structures and the size of the area. The significant number of residential structures and storage cellars of the Deli Halil settlement are expected to illuminate issues concerning its demography and identification.

Demographic estimation can enhance our understanding of the ancient settlement of Deli Halil. It is important to know the number of structures, size of the area covered and number of inhabitants to give us some grasp of the administrative, economic, social and political status of a settlement. The quality and density of structures and population provide an insight into the planning of a settlement, demonstrating its sociological and administrative organization. It is crucial to retrieve this information from archaeological documentation in order to understand the status of the Deli Halil settlement compared with other settlements of various sizes in its territory, in particular its relations with the region's metropolis, Epiphaneia. The present study is concerned with assessing the demography of the ancient

1 Department of Archaeology, Faculty of Sciences and Humanities, Kocaeli University, Umuttepe Campus, 41380 Kocaeli, Turkey.

settlement at Deli Halil with regard to its size and the number and density of its structures, to support further examination of the settlement. Area and population size are significant, as they are important parameters for defining the economic and social structure of its inhabitants, as well as its administrative status.

The ancient settlement of Deli Halil, situated on the south slope of a 460 m high volcano, is within the town of Toprakkale of the Osmaniye Province and has been documented by the Osmaniye Archaeological Survey (FIG. 1).[2] The geomorphological rises of the volcano, the Deli Halil basalt formation, begin at the coast, at the northeasternmost point of the Gulf of Issos, stretch eastwards to the first heights of the Amanus Mountains and delineate the southern border of East Plain Cilicia, separating it from the Issos Plain. The ancient settlement, at a height of 347 m, has a broad view of the Gulf of Issos, Burnaz, the harbor of the Epiphaneia on the southeast outskirts of the Deli Halil volcano, the southern entrance to the Kısık Pass and various other settlements of the Issos Plain.

An intensive archaeological survey of the ancient settlement included mapping of the volcanic land and the widespread remains of streets and structures of the settlement in three separate sections using geographic positioning systems. The layout of the settlement has been drawn in places where archaeological contexts remain intact, and all the rectangular and round structures of the settlement have been measured; *in situ* and scattered architectural elements have been recorded, as well as potsherds and various ornamented terracotta fragments. Archaeo-geological examination of the volcanic land and its vicinity was conducted to understand the impact of land type on the foundation and sustainability of the settlement.

The layout indicates a settlement built on terraces conforming to the topography in which streets intersect where the land is relatively level. Fortification walls and public structures are absent, other than a temple for worship. The settlement layout presents a premeditated plan laid out in one phase with structures that are similar in plan, building technique and function.

Rectangular structures are built with dry wall masonry technique without mortar, whereas round structures are built using mortar and their interiors are

2 The Deli Halil ancient settlement was first identified as such by the remains of its masonry, which presented a visible and recordable layout in 2008, by the Osmaniye Archaeological Survey Project, conducted by the present author. Preliminary reports of the Archaeological Survey of the site have been published in proceedings of the Survey Results Meeting of the Turkish Ministry of Tourism and Culture (see Tülek 2009; 2010; 2011; 2012). Archaeo-geological examination of the Deli Halil settlement has also been the subject of a project of the TÜBİTAK-SOBAG no. 109K025, which was completed in 2011. The ancient settlement of Deli Halil was mapped by cartographer H. Akan, and its drawings were accomplished by architect C. Sudaş. The present paper was prepared in the winter of 2013 with the support of the Library Research Grant given by the German Archaeology Institute to benefit library facilities of the Berlin Branch.

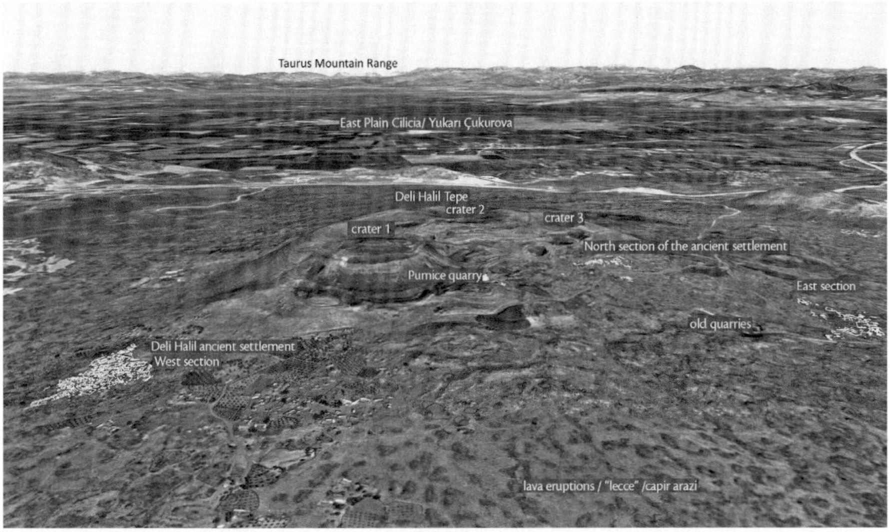

FIG. 1 Deli Halil volcano and landscape of the Ancient Settlement of Deli Halil.

covered with a thick layer of fine plaster demonstrating that the different building techniques were both known and their application was a deliberate choice. The construction material is uniformly black-brown basalt rock; both an amorphous-shaped very light type and very heavy column-type basalt have been used to build walls.

Founded on a basalt bedrock the settlement yields no former layers of culture to illuminate past foundations. The rough surface of the volcano comprises pyroclastic heaps of lava eruptions difficult to walk and live on. Dating of the settlement to the beginning of the fifth and the end of the sixth century CE is mainly based on pottery; ornamented terracotta fragments, pottery of common ware, fine ware, and transport amphorae are contemporaneous and uniformly belong to one phase. The absence of fortification walls is a feature of contemporaneous settlements in the region, such as Akören.[3]

Strategically located up on the volcano, the Deli Halil settlement controls the Burnaz harbor at the northeasternmost point of the Mediterranean Sea, watching over the main sea route and maritime trade, as well as the intersection of land routes which merge in the Issos Plain as the pilgrimage route heading to Jerusalem via Antioch. It also guards the route leading to Kısık Pass, the only access from the Issos Plain to the east Cilician Plain, taken by caravans heavily loaded with goods for the Cilician Plain.

3 Wulf-Rheidt 2003.

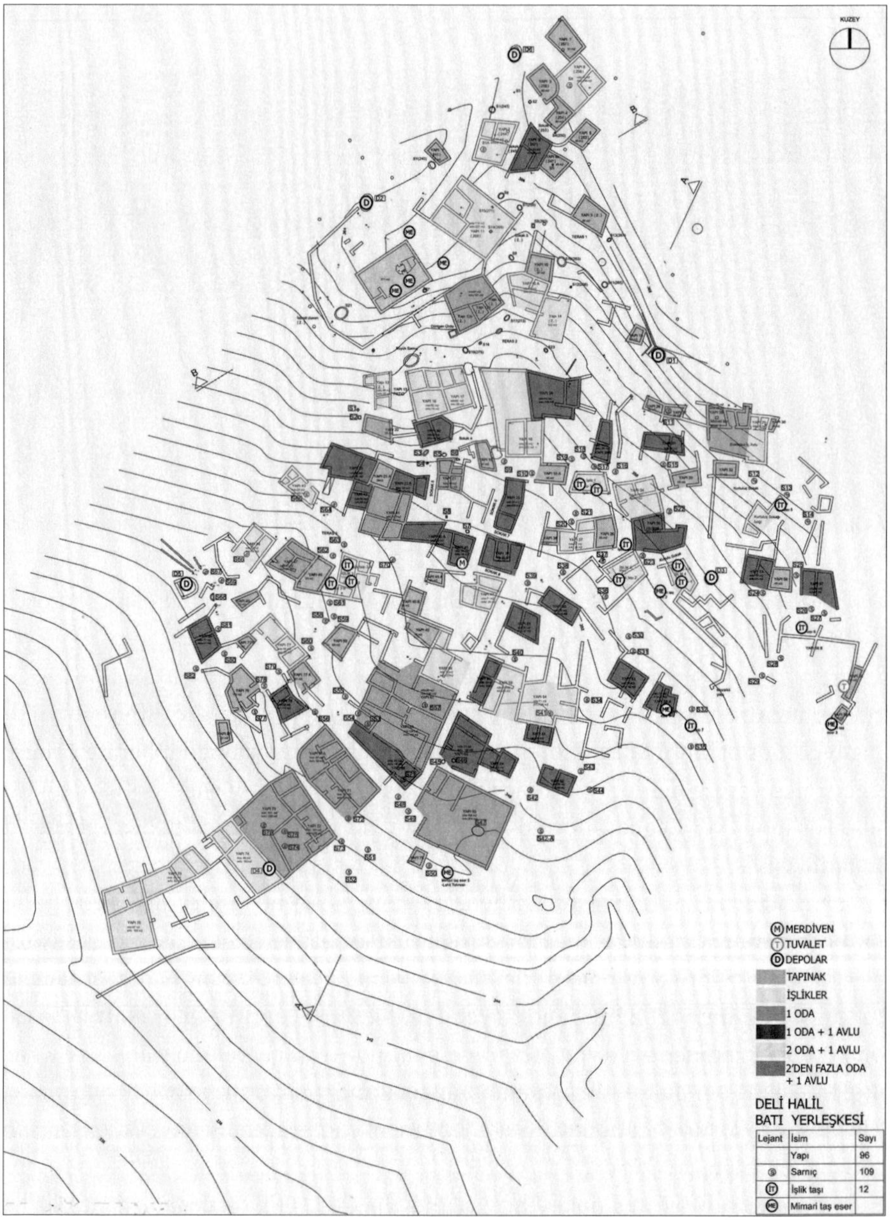

FIG. 2 Plan of the West Section of the Deli Halil settlement.

Ancient settlements are usually located where there is arable land, where fresh water for drinking, home use and irrigation is available and where main routes can be conveniently accessed. Fertile land for agricultural activities, farming, and grazing for animals is necessary for a food supply sufficient to sustain the population. Water is vital not only for human consumption and home use, but also for husbandry and farming. Population sustainability can also be achieved to some extent by producing food and goods, either with local resources or those from other sites. A convenient location with easy access to the main land and sea routes is a must for a settlement to provide raw materials for production and trade surplus goods. The Amanus region was a very well-known supplier of both timber and olive oil in the Late Antique period.

Founded on basalt bedrock, the Deli Halil ancient settlement does not have a large enough area of fertile soil to cultivate and supply food for its inhabitants. The small olive groves of the present day indicate that in the past, olives could have been cultivated. Peasants can only pasture small herds, since there is not enough land for big flocks of livestock to graze. Rainwater runs over the surface of the basalt bedrock, enabling water to be collected in cisterns. The basalt bedrock varies in thickness from 200 m in the upper parts, to just 25 m at the outskirts.[4] Cracks in the bedrock only allow water to deposit beneath the layers, however, drilling a well requires modern technologies.

A site without any water source and with insufficient arable land, as is the case with the Deli Halil settlement, could be anticipated to be a temporary settlement or a settlement for a purpose. A collection of a considerable quantity and quality of potsherds in the archaeological survey testify to the livelihood of the settlement over a period of around two hundred years, from the beginning of the fifth to the end of the sixth centuries CE. Sherds of fine tableware almost uniformly belong to Red Slip Phocaean ware, while most of the amphorae fragments bear features of North African production of the Late Antique period. The well-planned layout indicates that the settlement was not founded *ad hoc*, and that the location of the site was chosen deliberately.

Remains of the settlement stretching from east to west on the south slope of the volcano survive in three clusters named the East, North, and West Sections (Fig. 2). The distance between the East and North Sections is only 300 m, whereas the distance between the North and West Sections is roughly ±1,000 m. The archaeological survey indicates a densely built settlement on a premeditated plan, in which rectangular structures are aligned side by side along intersecting streets or horizontal terraces accessed by ramparts. The plan of the settlement displays rectangular structures, as well as remarkable round structures that functioned as both cisterns and storage cellars (Fig. 3). The surviving walls of some of the buildings rise to a height of 1.5 m, enclosing the perfectly laid out rectangular structures of houses, each preceded by a courtyard with a cistern and storage cellar (Fig. 4, Fig. 5). It is a large settlement, with olive presses and mills, and the number of storage cellars exceeds the number of residences. Parts of ruins retaining

4 Yılmaz 2011.

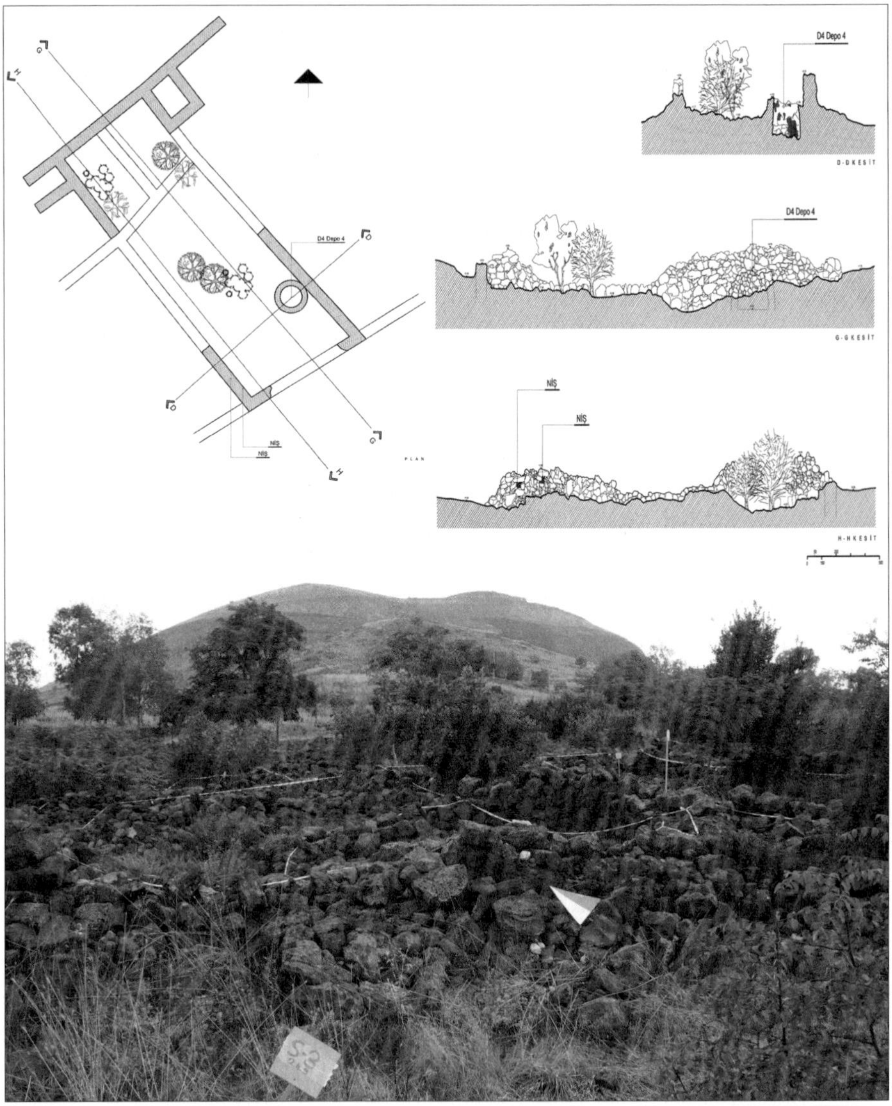

FIG. 3 Plan of House nr. 74 with storage cellar courtyard in the West Section of the Deli Halil Settlement.

their archaeological context intact and unspoiled have been documented in the archaeological survey. Archaeologically intact, preserved areas of ±2.36 ha have been measured in the North Section, ±10.36 ha in the East Section and ±13 ha in the West Section. It has been conjectured that the North and East sections were originally one body of the settlement, but today they are detached and heavily damaged due to the dirt track and gorges of the pumice quarries.

The West Section of the settlement yielded 96 rectangular structures and 115 round structures, housed in 19 insula, laid out on three terraces and 15 streets covering 13 ha, which is one third of the settlement proper. The total documented area of the North and East sections of the settlement is 40 ha, meaning that the ancient settlement was originally roughly 80 ha in size. Although the area covered by the Deli Halil ancient settlement is about one fifth that of its metropolis, Epiphaneia, it seems too large to be just an ordinary small village, a *kome*.

The fifth century CE was a period of economic boom in the Eastern Mediterranean and the Levant, as well as a time of prosperous village settlements in the Late Antique period. Archaeological studies of Late Antique settlement patterns of both North Syria and the Antioch periphery demonstrate an increase in the number of settlements and a population boom, parallel with economic improvement.[5] The increase in the number of settlements, as well as the population of the settlements, is evidenced in the villages of North Syria, the Lime Massif,[6] with populations varying from 1,000 to 5,000.[7] In Egypt in Late Antiquity, provincial metropolises were recorded as occupying 80 ha and housing 16,000 people, such as Shivta, which occupied an area of 90 ha, and Karanis, at 80 ha. A village in the countryside was estimated to house 2,000 to 2,500 people.[8]

Demographic examinations of Late Antique settlements—villages or fortified towns—in Asia Minor are still too few to determine methodologies to guide the present study or providing examples for analogy.[9] Studies demonstrate that a typical Anatolian village of the sixth century CE housed 250 to 700 people, and a big village would have 1,000 people.[10] A Late Antique settlement in the territory of Lampsacus in northwestern Anatolia, present-day Lapseki, with roughly 1,000 people, was considered a big village, *kome megale*.[11] Another sixth century CE village, Arif in Lycia, southwest Anatolia, situated at 800 m above sea level, was a fortified town measuring 100 x 250 m, covered two and a half hectares and was estimated to house some 800 people.[12] Mokissos in Central Anatolia, a sixth century CE fortified town of the emperor Justinianus, covered

5 Özgen and Gates 1992; Wilkinson *et al.* 2004; Lehmann *et al.* 2007; Ongoing Osmaniye Archaeological (2007–2013); Ongoing Archaeological Survey of the territory of Antioch by Pamir (2013).

6 Tate 1997, 74–75.

7 Laiou 2005, 38.

8 Morrison and Sodini 2002.

9 Harrison 1979; Wulf 2003; neither of the studies present a demographic examination.

10 Trombley 1985, 331.

11 Trombley 1985, 341.

12 Harrison 1979, 234.

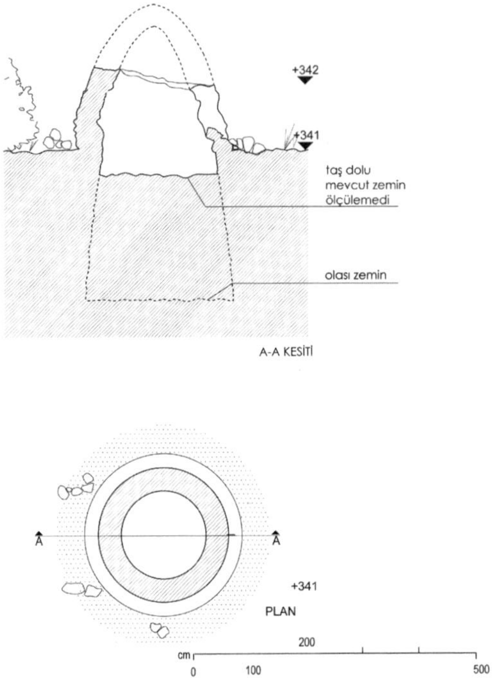

FIG. 4 Plan of the storage cellar nr. 1 in the East Section of the Deli Halil Settlement.

50 ha, and Justiniana Prima occupied around 10 ha.[13] Akören II in East Cilicia had 90 houses with roughly 700 people.[14]

Development of the countryside and the rural economy in the sixth century CE is also observed in settlements called *metrokomai*, which had no form of civic structures or public squares, but were densely built, with a population of 1,000 to 5,000.[15] Akören, an unfortified sixth century CE early Byzantine village in Cilicia in the Taurus mountain range, which is 100 km north of Adana at an altitude of 300 m similar to the Deli Halil settlement, covered an area of 300 x 150 m. The settlement of Akören yielded 90 residential structures, and archaeologists examining the site estimated 5–8 people per household and a population of 450–700 people.[16] Olive presses and millstones were recorded at the village, also similar to the Deli Halil settlement. Archaeological examination shows that the Deli Halil ancient settlement, covering around 80 ha on basalt bedrock, is also unfortified. Although the settlement covers a large area, its population may not have been very dense, considering that it is a rural settlement with no arable land.

13 Kirilov 2007, 14.

14 Wulf-Rheidt 2011, 198

15 Dagron 1979, 29.

16 Wulf-Rheidt 2003, 302.

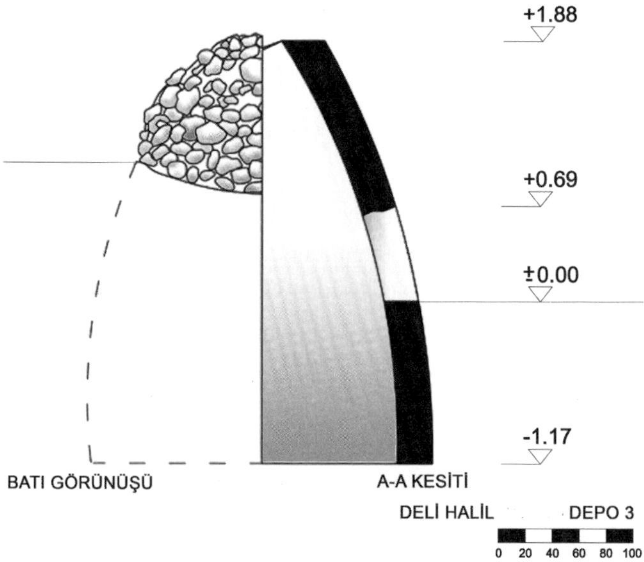

FIG. 5 Plan of the storage cellar nr. 3 in the North Section of the Deli Halil Settlement.

Demographic analysis of past populations is a topic of scholarship producing a plethora of publications.[17] The historiography of demographic studies primarily demonstrates an interest in the growth of past populations to present day values. In general, the scope of demographic studies is limited to examining the size, structure and development of human populations.[18] Scholars employ numerous methodologies to study the size of past populations, which results in the use of eclectic approaches.[19] Data available for the size of past populations is inadequate, since it is not intended for demographic purposes. For example, in the demographic estimations of Classical Period settlements, the contribution of each settlement to the Delian League is used as data that is reliable enough to calculate the population size of the participating cities.[20] In the Roman Imperial period, the first census was taken at the time of Emperor Augustus, recording people for tax collection. Data provided from such censuses are used in present day studies to estimate the demography of the Roman settlements. Similarly, records of the church synods provide insight into the size and strength of towns, since they had a hierarchical structure based on the size of the population. Accounts of the conversion of pagans to Christianity provide an estimation of the size of the Early Christian population.[21]

17 Among many studies, those of Russel 1958; Naroll 1962; Hansen 2008 and Zorn 1994 have been of benefit to this study.

18 Scheidel 2001, 1.

19 Russel 1958.

20 Hansen 2008, 280.

21 Trombley 1985, 330

However, all of these records either omit women, children, the elderly and slaves, or they record men and women as citizens but exclude the rest, since they were created for specific purposes.

In addition, scholars of historical demography and archaeologists try to make use of other forms of data, such as skeletal remains recovered at ancient sites, to estimate the size and demographic characteristics of that settlement. Present day ethnographic data also provide an analogy and an understanding of sites that retain environmental and economic conditions, as well as lifestyles that are comparable to past settlements. Thus, ethno-archaeology is frequently consulted in demographic estimates of ancient settlements.[22] Analysis of food consumption based on remains and residue that is indicative of rates of consumption is another method used by archaeologists. The space occupied by inhabitants and the number of people per household are also taken as reasonable and reliable parameters in calculating the number of people living in an ancient settlement.[23] In all of these approaches, ethnography provides supporting data for analogy, particularly when there is no evidence of a constant number of persons in one ancient household. Macro- and micro-level approaches are employed in demographic studies: the first for regional population estimations and settlement patterns, while the second is a site-specific approach more concerned with the socio-economics of a particular settlement.[24]

The micro-level approach, which is a site-specific level of estimation, should be appropriate for demographic estimation of the Deli Halil settlement, since the major concern is to identify the nature of its livelihood and the reasons for its establishment at the given location. Methods applied in the micro-level approach for estimating the demography of a site include area estimation, dwelling-based estimates and availability of natural resources.

The 'area estimation' method takes a density coefficient for an area of 1 ha and calculates the number of people according to the size of the settlement. However, in area estimation, the method of calculating the amount of floor space occupied by an individual has been elaborated further by calculating the amount of roofed space required per person in a house.[25] With regard to dwellings and households, an additional method has also been employed in estimating the number of persons that constitute a family. Estimating the number of family members in a household draws directly on ethno-archaeology, particularly where the structure of family and society has changed little.

---

22 Wulf 2003, 302. Wulf estimated the demography of Akören relying on ethno-archaeological data.

23 Zorn 1994, 32

24 Zorn 1994, 31.

25 A method developed by Naroll (1962) and later improved by Le Blanc (1971).

'Dwelling based estimation' of demography has mostly been applied at settlements where partial archaeological excavations yield one third or one tenth of the entire settlement. The number of residential structures in an excavated area of a certain size is taken as the criterion for estimating the total number of houses in the settlement.[26] The shortcoming of this method is that the residential structures may not be found in the same density and scale all across the settlement, as is the case at the Deli Halil settlement.

'Natural resource estimation' considers the capacity of farming and grazing land, as well as the availability and capacity of water sources. Natural resource estimation requires knowing the climatic conditions and annual rainfall of the area in the past, based on the present day.[27] The number and capacity of cisterns and grain stores at the Deli Halil settlement immensely facilitate the estimation of demography.

Studies taking the 'density coefficient method' as an approach either use the estimated number of people living in a certain unit of area or the number of houses at a site as a coefficient of the number of people living in a household. The approach that takes the constant of the number of people constituting a household can be adopted in estimating the population of the Deli Halil settlement.

The Deli Halil archaeological survey results give us the number of houses in one third of the area of the West Section. However, the constant of the number of people living in a household must be estimated. Studies have used different numbers for estimating household size, depending on the variable of city or rural life.[28] For the estimation of pre-modern Middle Eastern populations, the constant of 4–5.5 for a household has been taken.[29] Regarding the eastern Cilician Plain, particularly inhabitants of the modern Erzin Plain, the geographical setting of the Deli Halil settlement, a number of 5.5 people living in a household should be a valid and relevant constant.[30] The constant of 5.5 applied to the 96 houses of the West Section of the ancient settlement of Deli Halil gives 528 people, being only one third of the population; thus in total we can estimate 1,584 people living in the West Section of the settlement.

'Area estimation' can be also employed when calculating living space with regard to how many people live in 1 ha.[31] In case of the Deli Halil settlement, the

26 Zorn 1994, 33.

27 Zorn 1994, 32.

28 Russel 1958.

29 Hansen 2008, 280.

30 The author is a native of the town of Erzin town.

31 Shiloh 1980, 25; Figures provided by Finkelstein contradict the results of Shiloh (Finkelstein 1990, 50).

above approach of taking the number of households can be pursued further. If 528 people lived in 13 ha of the Deli Halil settlement, then there were 48 inhabitants in 1 ha. Indeed, the density coefficient figure of 48 inhabitants in 1 ha matches the calculations of Broshi.[32] A constant density coefficient of 48 is in line with the figure that has been calculated, and found mostly reasonable, as the basis of population data in Middle Eastern cities.[33] The West Section of the Deli Halil settlement has been measured to be around 40 ha, meaning that 1,920 people lived in this part of the settlement.

As part of area estimation, an approach taking into account the roofed and unroofed living space required per person in a dwelling was first proposed by Naroll and was developed by others.[34] The archaeological survey recording the settlement elaborated on the plans of its units; thus data of roofed and unroofed space is available. Naroll took a coefficient of 10 m^2 living space required per person in the roofed area of a house.

For demographic estimation of the Deli Halil settlement, the adoption of coefficients taken for ancient settlements of neighboring regions and culturally close societies should be effective. The coefficient of 5.31 m^2 of living space required per person in a roofed area taken for the ancient city of Nippur sounds reasonable.[35] Roofed living spaces calculated in all 96 houses of the Deli Halil ancient settlement measure around 4,800 m^2, and dividing this by 10 m^2 living space per person would give a figure of 480 people as one third of the population; that is to say, a total of 1,440 people living in the West Section of the Deli Halil ancient settlement. However, as conjectured by the traditional way of life in the region, it seems appropriate to take a constant of 5.31 m^2 to calculate the required roofed living space per person. This gives us 903 people in one third of the West Section, and a total of 2,700 inhabitants living in the West Section of the settlement.

As for the consumption of natural resources, the West Section of the Deli Halil settlement yielded 109 round structures built in the ground and six round structures, cylindrical in shape, built above the ground. The round structures built in the ground have vaulted tops, whose surface is either flat or corbelled, but always with an opening at the top covered by a stone lid. The openings of the round structures built into the ground are either rectangular or circular in shape. Some of these circular openings have a nicely burnished stone bracelet, reminiscent of the wellheads common in traditional Anatolian vernacular rural housing. The round structures of the Deli Halil settlement are roughly the same size and

---

32 Broshi 1975, 6.

33 Shiloh 1980, 26.

34 Naroll 1962; Le Blanc 1971.

35 Stone 1981.

shape: cylindrical, bottle- or pear-shaped. They generally measure 3 to 3.5 m in diameter and 5 m in height. All the interiors are thickly and very well plastered. While the general masonry in the settlement uses the dry wall technique, these round structures are built with a strong mortar including grains of pumice, lime and terracotta, evenly plastered at 2.5 cm thickness. Each house contained one round structure built in the ground in its courtyard. Some of the round structures are clustered on terraces, and they are numerous around the oil presses. Some of the round structures are thought to be cisterns, since there is no natural water source. Evidently some of the round structures, even those built in the ground, may be storage cellars for storing goods.

109 round structures built in the ground have been recorded in the archaeologically examined one third of the West Section of the Deli Halil settlement. The measurements given above show that one round structure has a capacity of roughly 19 m^3. A standard coefficient for the water consumption required by an adult in a Mediterranean country is taken as 9 liters per day.[36] Considering average precipitation in the area falls over six months, water storage capacity for six months or 183 days should be 1,647 l per person. In the above demography calculations, if we take a population of 528 and multiply it by 1,647 liters, dividing this figure by 19 m^3 results in the need for 45 cisterns for the given number of people for six months. The highest number produced above in one of the demographic estimations can be taken as a parameter for calculating the number of water reservoirs required at the settlement: that is, 903 people need 1,487,241 l of water, meaning 77 cisterns. Regardless of whether the number of cisterns required is 45 or 77, the number of round structures exceeds the required amount, meaning that either 64 or 32 are storage cellars.

In sum, the Deli Halil settlement has a surplus number of cisterns to store water for its population for six months. A figure of 528 people sounds reasonable for the population of one third of the West Section of the Deli Halil settlement. The nature of the surplus round structures can be pursued by further examination of food consumption of other sorts: for example, grain supply.

The daily nutrition of the Deli Halil people definitely consisted of grain, olives and olive oil, evident in the excessive quantity of dolia fragments found at the site, as well as garum and probably North African wine, evidenced by spatheia and amphorae fragments.[37] Studies concerning food consumption in modern rural areas of Anatolia and the Near East in general take a constant of 140 kg grain consumption per person per year.[38] In this case, 528 people would need 73,920 kg

36 Zorn 1994, 42.

37 Tülek 2012, 374.

38 Zorn 1994, 43.

grain per year at the Deli Halil settlement. Since the Deli Halil settlement does not have arable land, the grain must have been brought from somewhere else, probably from inland of the eastern Cilician Plain, namely the chora of the ancient city of Hireapolis Castabala, and kept in storage. Four round storage cellars would suffice to store a year's supply of grain for 528 people in the Deli Halil settlement. This leaves 60 round storage cellars to store around 115 tons of olive oil, or 28 round structures built in the ground with a capacity of around 54 tons of olive oil. Olive oil was a major daily necessity of Roman society; it was not only consumed as food, but also used in oil lamps for illumination, and even used as medicine.

The amount of olive oil presumably kept in the round storage containers is still more than enough for the annual consumption of a population of which one third is roughly calculated to be 528 inhabitants. Annual per capita consumption of olive oil in a Mediterranean culinary society can be estimated at 10 kg; taking into account other forms of use, such as the Romans made, of oil triples this number, to a rough total consumption of 15 tons of olive oil a year. Still, a huge storage capacity is left, possibly for olive oil, if not also for grains.

Examination of potsherds collected at the settlement yielded an excessive number of fragments of fine tableware and amphorae that could only have been acquired via maritime trade from Phocaea and North Africa. The people of the Deli Halil settlement seem not only to have produced olive oil in their own mills, they may also have traded it via the Mediterranean. Most probably they acted as merchants, collecting olive oil and grain from both the hinterland of Epiphaneia and eastern Plain Cilicia, through Burnaz, the harbor of Epiphaneia. A cobbled Roman road stretching from the coast and heading 3 km in the direction of the Deli Halil Basalts is solid evidence of direct contact between its inhabitants and the harbor.[39] Although there is no evidence of the role they played in trading the grain of the eastern Cilician Plain and the lumber of the Amanus Mountains, the settlers of Deli Halil may have well dealt in all the goods and raw materials of the region and controlled the trade.

39 Özgen and Gates 1992, 390.

REFERENCES

Broshi, M., "La populations de l'ancienne Jerusalem." *Revue Biblique* 82 (1975): 5–14.

Dagron, G., "Entre village at cite: la bourgade rurale des IVe-VIIe siècle en Orient." *Koinonia* 3 (1979): 29–52.

Finkelstein, I., "A Few Notes on Demographic Data From Recent Generations and Ethnoarchaeology." *Palestine Exploration Quarterly* 122 (1990): 47–52

Hansen, M.H., "An Update on the Shotgun Method." *Greek, Roman and Byzantine Studies* 48 (2008): 259–286

Harrison, R.M., "Nouvelle Découvertes Romaines Tardives et Paléobyzantines en Lycie." *Comptes Rendus de L'Academie des Inscriptions and Belles-Lettres.* Paris (1979): 222–239.

Kirilov, C., "The Reduction of the Fortified City Area in Late Antiquity: Some Reflections on the end of the 'Antique City' in the Lands of the Eastern Roman Empire" in *Post-Roman Towns, Trade and Settlement in Europe and Byzantium 2* , ed. by J. Henning, 3–24, Berlin: De Gruyter, 2007.

Laiou, Angeliki E., "The Byzantine Village (5th–14th Century)" in *Les Villages dans l'Empire byzantine IV-XV siècle. Réalités Byzantines 11,* ed. by J. Lefort, C. Morrisson, J-P. Sodini, 31–53. Paris: Association des Amis du Centre d'Histoire et Civilization de Byzance, 2005.

Le Blanc, S., "An Addition to Naroll's Suggested Floor Area and Settlement Population." *American Antiquity. Society for American Archaeology* 36/2 (1971): 210–211.

Lehmann, G., A.E. Killebrew and M.-H. Gates, "Summary of the 2006 Cilicia Survey (İskenderun Bay Region)." *Araştırma Sonuçları Toplantısı* 25/3 (2007): 171–188.

Morrisson, C. and J.- P. Sodini, "The Sixth Century Economy" in *The Economic History of Byzantium: From the Seventh through the Fifteenth Century,* ed. by A. E. Laiou, 171–220. Washington D.C.: Dumbarton Oaks, 2002.

Naroll, R., "Floor Area and Settlement Population." *American Antiquity. Society for American Archaeology* 27/4 (1962): 587–589.

Özgen, İ. and M.-H. Gates., "Report on the Bilkent University Archaeological Survey in Cilicia and the Northem Hatay: August 1991." *Araştırma Sonuçları Toplantısı* 10 (1992) 387–394.

Pamir, H., "Antakya ve Çevresi Yüzey Araştırması." *Araştırma Sonuçları Toplantısı* 31/2 (2013): 278–298.

Russel, J.C., "Late Ancient and Medieval Population." *Transactions of the American Philosophical Society, New Series* 48/3 (1958): 1–152.

Scheidel, W., "Progress and Problems in Roman Demography" in *Debating Roman Demography,* ed. by W. Scheidel, 1–81. Leiden: Brill, 2001.

Shiloh, Y., "The Population of Iron Age Palestine in the Light of a Sample Analysis of Urban Plans, Areas and Population Density." *Bulletin of the American Schools of Oriental Research* 239 (1980): 25–35.

Stone, E.C., "Texts, Architecture and Ethnographic Analogy: patterns of Residence in Old Babylonian Nippur." *Iraq* 43 (1981): 19–33.

Tate, G., "The Syrian Countryside during the Roman Era" in *The Early Roman Empire in the East*, ed. by S. E. Alcock, 55–71. Oxbow Monograph 95. Oxford: Oxbow Books, 1997.

Trombley, F.R., "Paganism in the Greek World at the End of Antiquity: The Case of Rural Anatolia and Greece." *Harvard Theological Review* 78/3–4 (1985): 327–523.

Tülek, F., "Osmaniye Arkeolojik Yüzey Araştırması 2008 Yılı Çalışması." *Araştırma Sonuçları Toplantısı* 27/3 (2009): 69–78.

———. "Osmaniye Arkeolojik Yüzey Araştırması 2009 Yılı Çalışması." *Araştırma Sonuçları Toplantısı* 28/1 (2010): 373–388.

———. "Osmaniye Arkeolojik Yüzey Araştırması 2010 Yılı Çalışması." *Araştırma Sonuçları Toplantısı* 29/1 (2011): 491–504.

———. "2011 Yılı Osmaniye Arkeolojisi Çalışma Raporu." *Araştırma Sonuçları Toplantısı* 30/2 (2012): 243–254.

Wilkinson, T. J., J. Ur and J. Casana, "From nucleation to dispersal: trends in settlement pattern in the northern fertile crescent" in *Side-by-Side Survey, Comparative and Regional Studies in the Mediterranean World* ed. by S. E. Alcock and J. F. Cherry, 189–205. Oxford: Oxbow Books, 2004.

Wulf, U., "Akören. Zur Stadtplannung und Wohnarchitektur zweier Siedlungen in Kilikien" in *Die spaetantike Stadt und Ihre Christianisierung: Symposion vom 14. Bis 16. February 2000 in Halle/ Saale,* 299–307. Wiesbaden: Reichert, 2003.

Wulf-Rheidt, U., "Akören: Two Late Antique Villages in Cilicia" in *Archaeology and the Cities of Asia Minor in Late Antiquity* ed. by Ortwin Dally and Christopher Ratté. Ann Arbor: Kelsey Museum of Archaeology, 2011.

Yılmaz, İ., "Geological Examination of the Deli Halil Hill" in unpublished final report of the project entitled *Doğa Olaylarının Antik Deli Halil Yerleşimi Üzerine Etkileri.* TUBİTAK-SOBAG 109K025, 83–156. İstanbul, 2011.

Zorn, J.R., "Estimating the Population Size of Ancient Settlements: Methods, Problems, Solutions and a Case Study." *Bulletin of the American Schools of Oriental Research* 295 (1994): 31–48.

Tracing the Hoof-prints of Byzantine History: Horses and Horse Breeding in the Middle Byzantine Period

Filiz Tütüncü-Çağlar[1]

This article is based on my M.A. Thesis, entitled "The Land of Beautiful Horses: Stables in Middle Byzantine Settlements of Cappadocia," which I completed at Bilkent University in 2008, under the supervision of Dr. Charles Gates. I extend him my sincerest thanks. If it were not for his enthusiasm and generous support every step of the way, neither the thesis nor this article would have come into existence.

Abstract

The horse was the most important and the most valuable animal of Byzantine society for its extensive use in daily life and in battle. Although the warhorse has received considerable attention from historians, their interest has concentrated particularly on the military aspect of the horse, at the expense of non-military subjects such as horse breeds, stables and horse management. Despite the absence of scholarly works devoted to the history of horse breeding in Byzantium, archaeological studies along with historical documents from various contexts do in fact offer rich information. Intending to serve as a departure point, the present paper combines such textual and archaeological evidence in order to investigate the nature and the significance of horse breeding in the Middle Byzantine period. Focusing on the example of Cappadocian magnates of the tenth and eleventh centuries CE, who presumably bred horses in their monumental mansions, this study ultimately intends to demonstrate how the study of horses and horse breeding can contribute to the social and economic history of the Middle Byzantine period.

Introduction

The horse was essential to the Byzantines in peace as well as war. It was the most important animal in the Byzantine army, played a prominent role in chariot races

1 Department of Art History and Visual Studies, University of Victoria, Victoria, BC, V8W 2Y2, Canada.

and was a prime vehicle for travel and transportation. Likewise, it was utilized for hunting and ceremonial purposes and served as a status symbol exchanged between rulers and aristocrats. Moreover, good horses were selected for the breeding of their own kind and of mules. Despite the fairly widespread use of horses throughout the Byzantine world, the horse has never been the subject of an extensive study, and the history of horse breeding in Byzantium is yet to be written. Being the most valuable domestic animal and thanks to its role in warfare, the horse appears in primary and secondary literature more often than other types of livestock. In particular, the warhorse has received considerable attention from historians, both medieval and contemporary, who were interested in military subjects like the organization of the cavalry, its tactics, strategy and equipment. On the other hand, non-military subjects have been entirely overlooked. As a result, secondary literature is extremely meagre on subjects such as horse breeds, stables and horse management. Although scholarly works devoted to the history of horse breeding are scarce, archaeological studies along with historical documents from various contexts (including military treatises, *hippiatric* texts, chronicles and travel accounts) do in fact provide ample information that would enhance our understanding of horse breeding in Byzantium.

With an aim to serve as a departure point, the present study combines such textual and archaeological evidence in order to investigate the nature and significance of horse breeding in the Byzantine world with a focus on the Middle Byzantine period (843–1204).[2] A critical phenomenon that had a strong impact on horse breeding at this time was the emergence of a rural aristocracy on frontier zones, who gained power and wealth through border defense. As well reflected in the epic of *Digenis Akritas*,[3] these magnates owned great estates and large private troops and held high positions both in the military and in the provincial administration.[4] When necessary, they supplied the imperial army with animals and equipment, amongst which horses had the largest share. Focusing on the example of Cappadocian magnates of the tenth and eleventh centuries, who bred horses in their monumental mansions, this study ultimately intends to demonstrate how the study of horses and horse breeding can contribute to the social and economic history of the Middle Byzantine period.

The present article is based on a survey project on the archaeology of horse breeding in Byzantine Cappadocia. As discussed in detail below, Cappadocia provides ample evidence for the neglected field of the history of horse breeding and animal husbandry thanks to its peculiar rock-cut architecture that allows the

2 All dates are CE unless otherwise stated.

3 Jeffreys 1998.

4 Vryonis 1971, 24–25; Cheynet 2006.

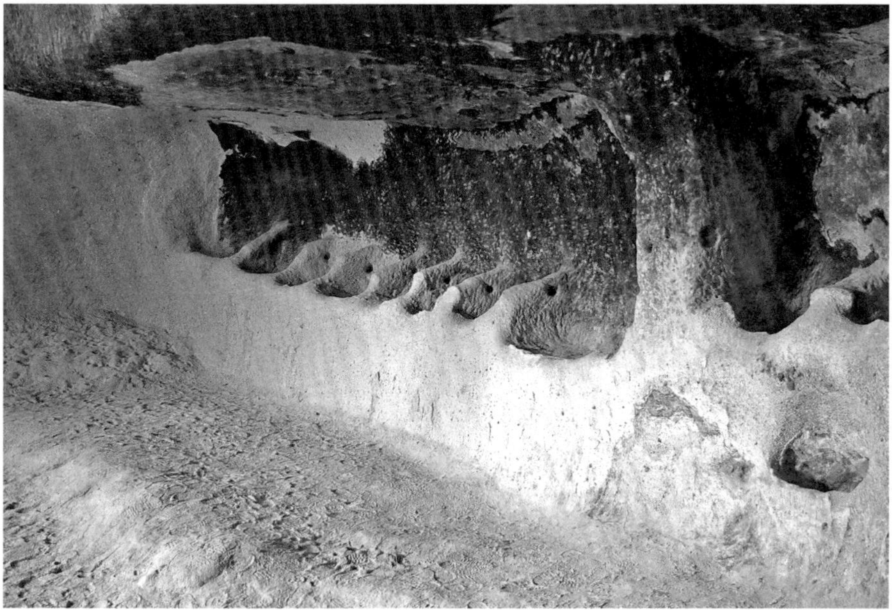

FIG. 1 Detail of mangers in the stable of Açık Saray Complex No. 2a. Photo by Mehmet Tütüncü.

exceptional preservation of features such as stables. Having remained in their original contexts with complete floor plans, elevations and in situ mangers, the stables of Cappadocia are rich sources of evidence for understanding horse breeding activities in Byzantium, as well as contributing to the interpretation of the true nature of the elite settlements that emerged in the region during the Middle Byzantine period.[5]

The article is mainly concerned with the conditions under which the Byzantines bred and used their horses, particularly during the Middle Byzantine Period. Initially it provides an overview of the difficulties posed by both the textual and the archaeological sources, which is followed by a summary of the history of horse breeding in Cappadocia. It concludes with some further insights on the subject for future research.

The Challenge of Detecting Sources

The major reason why the study of horse breeding in Byzantium has not yet received adequate scholarly attention is largely due to the difficulty in locating and

5 Tütüncü 2008.

retrieving relevant information, which is an arduous task that requires a close scrutiny of both textual and archaeological sources. It necessitates surveying the primary literature, as well as field reports of archaeological expeditions of Byzantine sites in order to collect shreds of evidence. Far from achieving such an ambitious goal, the present paper limits its scope to published primary and secondary literature with a focus on sources pertinent to horse breeding and animal husbandry directly or indirectly.

The main class of primary sources consists of military treatises dealing mainly with the warhorse. Among the most important for our purposes are the *Strategikon* that is credited to Emperor Maurice (*r.* 582–602), the *Taktika* by Leo VI (*r.* 886–912), the *Three Treatises on Imperial Military Expeditions* attributed to Constantine VII Porphyrogenitos (*r.* 913–959), the *Praecepta militaria* ("military precepts") by Nikephoros II Phokas (*r.* 963–969) and the *Taktika* of Nikephoros Ouranos (*c.* 980-*c.* 1010).[6] Focusing on the theory and practice of warfare, these texts yield extensive information regarding the organization of the cavalry and its equipment, while they are less helpful on the subjects of breeding or stabling. The most beneficial is the *Three Treatises* of Constantine VII, which describes at length how the horses were cared for by the *komēs* and *logothetēs* of the imperial stables. With a clear emphasis on horses amongst all equids, the book offers vivid details such as the type and amount of fodder required for each type of horse.[7] Likewise, the evidence in the secondary literature is rather scarce, since contemporary historians also focused on war tactics and cavalry strategies. To name a few historians of Byzantine warfare, Nicolle, Treadgold and Hyland, who have written on warhorses at length, provide sparse information on where they were bred or how they were supplied.[8]

Given the importance of horses in the army and their status in social life, it is not surprising to find a large body of literature devoted to horse medicine going back to antiquity. A rich source of information for the study of horses, *Hippiatrika*, is an encyclopedic compilation of ancient Greek texts on horse medicine compiled on orders from Constantine VII Porphyrogenitos in five Byzantine recensions in twenty-two manuscripts that range in date from the tenth to the sixteenth century.[9] There are two copies of the original manuscript, one in Berlin and the other in Paris.[10] A. McCabe has recently discussed the sources and transmission of the original text in her book, *A Byzantine Encyclopedia of Horse Medicine*. Since

6 Dennis 1984; Kazhdan 1991a, 353; Haldon 1997; 1999, 5; McGreer *et al.* 1995.

7 Constantine and Haldon 1990.

8 Nicolle 1992; Treadgold 1995; Hyland 1994.

9 *Hippiatrica* ed. E. Oder and C. Hoppe Corpus hippiatricorum Graecorum (Leipzig, 1924, repr. Stuttgart 1971).

10 Regrettably neither source was available to me at the time of writing this article.

the author has concentrated on the philological examination of the texts themselves rather than their content, the book stands more as a literary work than a source of technical information. Despite its promising title, it contains only partial translations of the original text and lists only a handful of horse diseases and their treatments, providing snippets of information on horse care.[11]

The second book relevant to horse breeding is the *Geoponika*, an encyclopedic compilation of rural life. It is a collection of writings on agriculture that was dedicated to Constantine VII, assumed to have been compiled around 944–959, though its originality is controversial.[12] Its Book XVI, dedicated to horses, is mainly concerned with horse medicine, providing remedies for various diseases, and lacks references to horse breeding, horse management or stabling.[13] The limitations resulting from the fragmentary nature of primary evidence requires referring to archaeological sources in order to fill in the gaps of texts and to contextualize the information obtained from the literary sources.

The archaeological sources are also problematic in nature due to the meagre number of studies on the subject. However, recent archaeological work at the Yenikapı excavation project in Istanbul has yielded ample zooarchaeological evidence on Byzantine horses. An exceptional find is the discovery of twenty intact horse skeletons, which is the largest number of horse skeletons ever found on a Byzantine site.[14] Having the largest animal bone inventory of the Byzantine Empire dating to a broad time span from the Early Byzantine until the Late Byzantine period, the site has produced bones belonging to fifty-four different animal species, whose skeletons had been scattered across the entire area of 58,000 m^2 under excavation. A considerable part of the total bone assemblage at Yenikapı is made up of horse bones, the largest group among all animals attested at the site.[15] The published results of pathological analyses offer invaluable insights for the study of Byzantine horse use in urban environments.[16]

---

11 A second source on medieval horse medicine is a thirteenth century Armenian book, recently translated into German by J. Dum-Tragut (2005) as *Kilikische Heilkunst für Pferde: das Vermächtnis der Armenier*. Only available in Germany, it was not possible to obtain the entire work. Although Dr. T. Zimmermann (Bilkent University) very kindly arranged a part of it to be sent from Germany, unfortunately, no conclusions could be reached based on the section I received, which made no mention of horses or horse breeding in the Byzantine world.

12 Kazhdan 1991b, 834.

13 Owen 1805.

14 Onar *et al.* 2012.

15 For 178 (0.9%) of the equid bones, it was not possible to differentiate between the horse and mule bones.

16 Onar *et al.* 2012. The morphological evaluations will also be published in the near future.

Breeding and Supply of Horses

Byzantine horses were defined and differentiated by their various contexts of use rather than their particular breeds. It is not clear from the sources whether or not there was a designation of breed in the modern sense. Military texts provide some clues about warhorses, again mostly to do with the difference in their sizes and in their uses. Yet, a thorough investigation of the equid composition of the Byzantine cavalry in the light of literary evidence necessitates more extensive research, far beyond the scope of the present study. On the other hand, the archaeological evidence, at least for now, is less helpful due to the small number of published studies and the absence of comparative material. This said, the results of ongoing morphological analyses and perhaps a taxonomical classification of the Yenikapı horse skeletons might provide some clues on Byzantine breeds in the future.

The horse in the Byzantine Empire was the animal of the rich and noble. It was expensive and considered a luxury, thus rare in peasant households.[17] It is well documented that large-scale raising of livestock, especially the breeding of horses, was undertaken in imperial ranches and aristocratic farms.[18] According to late Byzantine *praktika*, only prosperous peasants could afford horses, whereas fiscal surveys describe less affluent ones as owners of only "half-a-horse," shared between two neighbors.[19] A great landowner in the fourteenth century, John VI Kantakouzenos, complains of how he lost 1,500 mares after his property was confiscated by the state.[20] Monasteries also held fairly large numbers of equids. For instance, the Athonite Monastery of Xenophon had 100 dray horses and donkeys in the eleventh century.

The main imperial horse breeding ranches in the Middle Byzantine period were located in Malagina, Thessaly and Cappadocia.[21] Malagina was the first *aplekton*, military staging post, on the way to the eastern frontier, thus the site where the imperial army met the *strategoi* (military governors) of Thrakesion and Opsikion. In relation to horses, Malagina's name is first attested in the context of its capture by Arabs in 798, who seized the royal saddle and horses at Malagina. In successive centuries, the site continued to serve as the main imperial ranch for the breeding of horses, as widely attested in historical sources. Horse breeding activities and imperial ranches in Byzantine Thessaly are also briefly mentioned in literary sources. Unfortunately, archaeological investigations undertaken at the Byzantine fortresses and monasteries in the region has not provided any information on the subject.

17 Kazhdan 1997, 53.

18 Lefort 1993, 109.

19 Kazhdan and Nesbitt 1991b, 948.

20 Rautman 2006, 184; Kazhdan and Nesbitt 1991b, 948; 1997, 53.

21 Foss 1990b.

Renowned since antiquity as the legendary "Land of Beautiful Horses," Cappadocia has been a leading horse breeding center throughout its history. The reputation of Cappadocian horses goes back to the Iron Age, and the horse breeding tradition is frequently attested in literary sources, although no particular research has been conducted so far on the history of horse breeding in Cappadocia. One question is whether the title "Cappadocian horse" implies breed or place of origin. In the third century, a Roman didactic poet, Oppian, listed the Cappadocian horse amongst the best breeds of the ancient world. Hierokles, a *hippiatric* writer, also refers to horses of Cappadocian breeds.[22] Thus it can be hypothesized that the label "Cappadocian" was likely a horse breed rather than a place of origin, one which has lost its purity over time and become forgotten. Yet, there may be some link, however tenuous, between the famous Cappadocian breeds of the past and the so-called "local breed" or the "Anatolian breed" of modern times.[23]

Late Roman Cappadocia was one of the three provinces that had imperial stud farms, the other two being Thrace and Spain.[24] A fourth century historian, Vegetius, lists Cappadocia amongst the principal sources of horses.[25] Located in Caesarea, these imperial farms raised highly prized horses not only for chariot races but also for the army.[26] It was stipulated by law that retired Cappadocian horses from these particular stud farms were to be maintained for their remaining days on fodder from state granaries.[27] The exact location of these stud farms remains obscure, but Caesarea in the fourth century was described as a city lying in the middle of an entirely agrarian region with large numbers of imperial horse ranches.[28] A fifth century source, the *Theodosian Code*, mentions imperial herds in Cappadocia as including valuable breeds such as Hermogenian and Palmatian studs, which were the most famous breeds in the late fourth century, renowned for their speed and high quality.[29] In the sixth century, Emperor Justinian tried to reserve Cappadocia for the breeding of large cavalry mounts.[30] Apart from the imperial stud farms, horses were also bred in the large estates of local landowners; these provincial aristocrats of the Roman era are extensively discussed by Van

22 McCabe 2005, 219.

23 Tutel 1998, 131–134.

24 Drummond 1994, 88.

25 Toynbee 1973, 168.

26 Toynbee 1973; Drummond 1994, 88.

27 Jones 1964, 706.

28 Brown 2002, 39.

29 Pharr 1952, Title 6. 10. 6. 1; Hyland 1990, 9–13, 19, 213; 1994, 28; MacMullen 1962, 277–279.

30 Nicolle 1992, 7.

Dam, with special reference to the accounts of the Cappadocian fathers.[31] As previously mentioned, these were highly regarded landowners in the region who were closely familiar with horses and horse races.[32]

In contrast to the rich literary evidence on horse breeding activities in Roman Cappadocia, there are no Byzantine sources mentioning stud farms in the region after the sixth century.[33] Hyland asserts that they continued to function during the reign of Honorius (*r.* 625–638) but does not cite the source for this information.[34] The major military texts and chronicles from the Middle and Late Byzantine period, which might be expected to mention horses, such as *Maurice's Strategikon*, the *Chronicle of Theophanes*, *Strategikon of Kekaumenos*, *Praecepta Militaria*, the *Alexiad of Anna Comnena*, the *Histories of Niketas Choniates* and the *Treatises* by Constantine VII Porphyrogenitos, as well as some anonymous texts from the same time period, do not mention horse ranches in Middle Byzantine Cappadocia.[35] This does not, however, necessarily indicate the absence of stud farms, but could be explained by other reasons. First, the decline in the literary tradition in Cappadocia after Late Antiquity ought to be considered. Secondly, it is probable that by this time the importance of the imperial ranches had diminished, and they were replaced by private farms, that is, those of the elite, seeing as the burden of supplying the armies fell chiefly upon the *themata*, the main administrative divisions of the Middle Byzantine Empire.

After the pastoral territories on the central Anatolian plateau and southern Italy were lost in the eleventh century, the role of Thrace, Bulgaria, Macedonia and Serbia in stock raising and horse breeding increased. Horses were now bred in large estates in these provinces, as well as by transhumant peoples, the Vlachs of Byzantium and Serbia, who were specialized in this practice.[36] Taken from the aforesaid imperial ranches, horses were transported from one place to another by roads, along with sailing ships and galleys. A tenth century account by Leo of Synada mentions that Pylae, modern Yalova, was a port for the shipment of livestock, including horses, to the capital.[37] Horses may have been brought from imperial ranches in Malagina and Cappadocia to such ports and then shipped to further distances. Leo the Deacon describes how Nikephoros II Phokas in his invasion

31 Van Dam 2002.

32 Nicolle 1992, 7.

33 Nicolle 1992.

34 Hyland 1994, 28.

35 Dennis 1984; Haldon 1990; Theophanes, Mango 1997; McGeer 1995; Comnena and Sewter 2009; Choniates and Işıltan 1995.

36 Laiou and Morrisson 2007, 97.

37 Nesbitt and Kazhdan 1991, 1243.

of Crete in 960 used ramps for unloading horses and reports that they were run from galleys used for closing the shore and unloading horses across ramps.[38] This was also the case elsewhere in Europe during the Middle Ages. In the manner of a modern car ferry, horses were loaded onto ships, and when the destination was reached, mounted men would disembark.[39]

The treatises of Constantine VII list a great number of horses and pack animals serving the imperial train on its way to campaigns.[40] In addition to the imperial ranches, the provincial magnates, and more rarely the rural population, was required to breed and supply pack animals to the military contingents or imperial officials.[41] As the architectural evidence suggests, this might have been the case for the provincial elite in Cappadocia during the tenth and eleventh centuries, who, in their houses, had large stables used most likely for breeding horses (see below).

Various Uses of Horses in Transportation, Agriculture, Travel and Leisure

Historical sources extensively mention that the Byzantine stud farms raised horses of all types. Apart from the expensive war, or riding horses, there were also packhorses and other beasts of burden bred for the imperial baggage train that is described in treatises on imperial expeditions.[42] However, in contrast to the imperial baggage trains, horses were not commonly used in daily life for transport or cartage since they were expensive luxury animals. The main pack animals were mules and donkeys. Although not as swift as horses, they offered the great advantage of being tougher and not requiring shoeing.[43] Loads were mostly transported by beasts of burden rather than pulled in carts, which were not suitable for mountainous areas.[44] As opposed to the light chariot, the cart was a heavy and slow vehicle with four wheels. Drawn by oxen, it was used in everyday life for the transportation of burdens, harvests or even people for short distances.[45]

In travel, only well-to-do people used horses, while the majority of people traveled on foot or rode on mules or donkeys. For instance, a metropolitan, aristocratic

38 Pryor (1982) discusses Byzantine transportation of cavalry by sea, dating from as early as the eighth century, and surveys the means of horse transport and possible problems encountered during the journey, as well as the distances for which horses could be transported.

39 Rose 1999, 565–566.

40 Constantine and Haldon 1990, 118–119.

41 Nesbitt *et al.* 1991, 271.

42 Laiou and Morrisson 2007, 67–68.

43 Teall 1971, 53.

44 Nesbitt *et al.* 1991, 271.

45 Kazhdan and Nesbitt 1991a, 383–384.

and highly educated traveler, Nikolaos Mesarites, traveled from Nicaea to Constantinople in 1206 and 1208 by mule.[46] In his travel accounts, he narrates that after an exhausting day of mule riding, he finally came to an inn. He complains about the dangers and discomforts of the travel: "sitting very uncomfortably on a mule, riding on in precarious balance, being whipped by tree branches." In his account, he also relates being warned about how wrong he was to beat the mule so hard.[47]

When chariot races lost their significance after the seventh century, other equestrian sports like polo became the leisure activity of the elite.[48] Hunting was one of the most popular leisure activities, as well as a means of training for war.[49] It was a favorite activity amongst the members of the imperial family and the elite, for whom hunting was a sign of imperial qualifications, status, and power. Hunting took place on horseback, often in wild territory, either just outside Constantinople or on remote mountains. Chronicles of various emperors include many stories about their adventures in hunting. There were game parks with pavilions, landscaped and managed with care.[50] An indication for the continued popularity of horse races into the ninth century is the order of Emperor Michael III (*r.* 842–867) to dismantle the aforementioned beacon system on account of his preoccupation with a horse race at the time when the warning of the Arab raid reached the capital.[51]

It has been argued that during the ninth and tenth centuries, a new system of harnessing animals to a cart and plow was introduced.[52] It has also been suggested that transferring the force of dragging from the neck to the chest could have easily allowed replacing the ox with the horse, thereby increasing the use of horses in everyday life.[53] However, the extent to which horses were used for rural practices is unclear, as historical sources tend to suggest that horses were rarely used for agrarian purposes. For instance, the *Farmer's Law* written in the seventh-eighth centuries does not mention horses at all, while focusing on the oxen and the mules, which were major work animals and beasts of burden, as they were cheaper, stronger and more effective.[54] This absence of horse power from farms might have continued well into the later centuries.

---

46 Kazhdan and Nesbitt 1991a.

47 Galatariotou 1993, 222–228.

48 Kazhdan and Nesbitt 1991b, 948.

49 Hyland 2003.

50 Ševčenko 2002, 69–70.

51 Pattenden 1983.

52 Kazhdan and Nesbitt 1991b, 948.

53 Kazhdan and Nesbitt 1991b; Kazhdan and Nesbitt 1991a, 384.

54 Teall 1959, 129.

The Managing and Stabling of Horses

We have only scanty knowledge of where and how horses were housed in the Byzantine world. Stables almost never appear in primary accounts. The only exception is the *Three Treatises*, which provides a great deal of detail on the officers responsible for various duties in the imperial stables, both in the cities and in the provincial stables, as well as the cost of different animals, the amount of fodder needed for each type of animal, the prices of horse equipment and by whom each of these expenses were covered. While offering rich evidence also on the care and condition of different types of horses, it lists the technical terms describing different types of equids used for different purposes. The book is also remarkable for providing qualitative data for the study of horses, which is otherwise lacking in current scholarship.[55]

In the *Hippiatrika,* stables are only mentioned in a few instances as relevant to medical issues.[56] The *hippiatric* writers advise that the horse must be kept in a dry place for the health of its body, especially its hooves; the floor should be covered with wood or pebbles to harden the feet, and a bedding made of chaff should be available.[57] They also suggest the use of amulets as a means of magical protection from shrewmice, lizards and scorpions, and advise darkening the stable to cure 'horse madness.'[58] However, there is no information on how the stables were designed or maintained.

The research carried out by the author on the architecture of rock-cut stables of the Middle Byzantine settlements of Cappadocia draws attention to the stables here, which are unique examples of their kind.[59] Being amongst the few examples of horse stables surviving from the Byzantine era, they are an invaluable source of information for the history of horse breeding in the region in accordance with the legendary title of Cappadocia.[60] All of the stables accompany elite mansions situated in three rock-cut settlements within the volcanic area of the Aksaray and Nevşehir provinces: Açık Saray, Çanlı Kilise and Selime-Yaprakhisar.[61] Each set-

55 Constantine and Haldon 1990, 99–103.

56 McCabe 2006.

57 McCabe 2006, 275.

58 McCabe 2006, 252.

59 Tütüncü 2008.

60 The stables have been only briefly noted in the publications of the three settlements. Some of them have been explored and documented for the first time in my own study. The first scholar to draw attention to the stables was Veronica Kalas (2000, 137–138), who emphasized their potential value for Byzantine studies. I am grateful to Dr. Kalas for introducing me to this topic and sharing her expertise on the Cappadocian architecture with me.

61 Rodley 1985; Ousterhout 2005; Kalas 2000.

tlement contains several large stables furnished with various kinds of mangers.[62] Although it is possible to use a standard manger for all types of large domestic animals, the systematic variation in the size and height of mangers seems to be an indicator of design for different species. The majority of the mangers are higher than 80 cm, affirming their function for tall animals, such as horses. The width of mangers is approximately 50 cm, ruling out the possibility that they might have been used for camels, which would require a much wider space.

Rock-cut stables in large courtyard complexes constitute the main archaeological evidence for horse breeding activities in Middle Byzantine Cappadocia. They can be defined basically as rectangular rock-hewn rooms with barrel-vaulted or flat ceilings, sometimes with more articulated features. They are all furnished with rock-cut mangers carved into the walls as deep niches for holding fodder and pierced on the sides to form loops for the tethering of individual animals. It is argued here that different types of mangers were used for different animals; thus the function of a stable can potentially be ascertained through the analysis of its mangers. In addition to the analysis of interior features, it is also necessary to examine the stables within their broader context by comparing them with each other, as well as taking into account their relation with the complexes to which they belong. The large dimensions of the stables seem to signify the prosperity of their owners, who probably gained affluence through border defense, for which horse breeding was essential.

More information on stables might be available in the Arab sources, since Byzantine expertise on horse medicine heavily influenced the Arab world. Moreover, it has been documented that the Arabs modeled their stables and their organization on those of Byzantium.[63] Although earlier than the designated time period with which this paper is concerned, the Ghassanid sources of the sixth century convey a three-level hierarchy of personnel responsible for the stables: the *sahib al-istabl*, the stable master, was the most important officer, followed by the *sa'is*, groom, and at the lowest level was the *ghulam*, the person responsible for chore duties such as cleaning.[64] One can speculate a similar arrangement for horse management in the Byzantine world. Furthermore, although slightly later, the Mamluks have a large body of literature on horses and horse breeding, which would be worth exploring.

62 The uncertainty in the number of stables is due to the vagueness of the exact function of some rooms, which have been labeled as "stables" in the aforementioned publications.

63 Shahîd 2002, 230–231.

64 Shahîd 2002.

Caring for Horses

The Yenikapı excavations have provided interesting results on how horses were looked after in the Byzantine world. The skeletal remains at Yenikapı were classified into four categories according to their developmental stage. According to this classification, 80.5% of the horses were adults, while there were no newborn or fetus bones. Curiously, 95% of the horses were below 10 years of age, an indicator of the poor level of care conditions, while the majority were between 7–10 years. In terms of sex, the majority appear to be male, which demonstrates that they were not used for breeding purposes, at least on the excavated site itself, but most probably for riding or as pack animals.[65]

A relatively large number of the unearthed horse bones have butchery marks, especially on the hind limbs and the skulls, which is interpreted as an indication of separating the flesh or the skin from the bones. The pathological findings indicate that the horses were not treated very well, as demonstrated by the backbone deformations and damage in the jaws, which are suggested to have resulted from faulty riding practices and wrong use of the bridle. Moreover, it has been suggested that the animals had been utilized for heavy-duty purposes at early ages.[66] Examining the bones and skeletons in comparison with the diseases mentioned in the *Hippiatrica*, the researchers have found common bone issues, swelling of the hoof and degenerative vertebra disorders described by the *hippiatric* writers.[67]

The researchers explain the large number of horse skeletons found on the site as the corpses of horses that died of old age or disease and were discarded in the silt of the Lycos River. It is also suggested that the horses were bred and trained outside the Theodosian walls, which is located next to the port that has been excavated. From the butchery traces on the skeletons and bones themselves, it is thought that the horses were dumped after removing useable parts such as the skin, tail or mane, as well as long bones and the skull. From these findings, they reached the conclusion that horse meat might have been a part of the Byzantine diet, although they believe horse flesh was also used for feeding other animals.[68]

From an economic perspective, the horses were consumed entirely by humans. Their meat was used as a source of protein either for themselves or for their animals, and bones were used as raw material for making small objects.[69] Another curious point is the absence of any horse equipment or riding gear accompanying the horse skeletons, except for a single bridle discovered in the excavations. The

65 Onar 2010; Onar *et al.* 2013.

66 Onar *et al.* 2013.

67 Onar *et al.* 2013.

68 Onar *et al.* 2013.

69 Onar *et al.* 2013.

lack of equipment supports the conclusion that this was a dump area.[70] Further morphological analysis on the horse skeletons would provide more clues about the care condition of horses and perhaps would even enable defining different horse breeds.[71]

Conclusion

At the current stage of knowledge, there are more questions than answers concerning the nature and importance of horse breeding in Byzantium. What is necessary is further multi-faceted research incorporating all strands of available evidence from textual, archaeological and even art-historical sources. As a starting point, it would be meaningful to conduct a survey of the Byzantine as well as the Arabic, Turkish and Mamluk literature –as they bear a strong Byzantine influence– in order to find out more about the role of horses, how they were utilized for non-military purposes and where and how they were bred. Such a study should be illuminating in identifying the social composition of horse owners and horse breeders. Where possible, defining the number and proportion of stallions and mares in a certain ranch or stable might offer clues about the practice of horse breeding. Moreover, the proportion of horses to other equids, that is, to mules and donkeys, would provide clues about the economic status of their owners. Additionally, a study of this sort might yield quantitative evidence, which is absent in current scholarship.

Also needed are further archaeological investigations, especially in regions such as Malagina, Cappadocia and Thessaly, where the imperial ranches and stables were located. Excavations in these regions may produce material evidence corresponding to the horse breeding practices in these regions for centuries, as well as possible remains from the imperial ranches. Malagina, a place of considerable strategic importance in the Middle Byzantine period, as the major *aplekton* that contained the imperial ranches, may provide some evidence on the history of horse breeding in Byzantium. While the stables in Malagina are frequently mentioned by literary sources,[72] archaeological studies focusing on the fortifications are entirely silent about them. Furthermore, the exact location of the site has not yet been identified, although its approximate location is known to be within the boundaries of the modern Turkish province of Sakarya.[73] On the other hand, our knowledge of Byzantine Cappadocia is unfortunately still restricted to historical texts and art historical studies concentrating on the religious art and architecture

70 Onar *et al.* 2013.

71 Onar 2010.

72 Constantine and Reiske 1829.

73 Foss 1990b.

of the region, although the rock-cut settlements with their exceptional level of preservation offer rich evidence for the social and economic history of Byzantium.[74]

As regards art-historical approaches, it is significant that horses were the most commonly represented animals in Byzantine art. Therefore, it can be proposed that pictorial evidence on manuscripts, coins and wall paintings, especially the ones located within the Byzantine churches of Cappacodia, should produce interesting clues and details on the use of horses for various purposes.

In Byzantine studies, the horse has thus far been discussed primarily in relation to its role in warfare, although horses were not merely war machines, nor did Byzantine history comprise only wars. With their broad range of uses, horses were important actors in all fields of life both in cities and rural areas. Hence, their study is hoped to contribute to the social and economic history of Byzantium. Revealing the potential of the subject, this study simply intends to be "a drop in the ocean" leading to further research.

74 Kalas 2009.

REFERENCES

Ashburner, W., "The Farmer's Law." *Journal of Hellenic Studies* 30 (1910): 85–108.

Bivar, A. D. N., "Cavalry Tactics and Equipment on the Euphrates Frontier." *Dumbarton Oaks Papers* 26 (1972): 273–291.

Cheynet, J-C., *The Byzantine Aristocracy and Its Military Function*. Aldershot: Ashgate 2006.

Choniates, N. and F. Işıltan, *Historia. Ioannes ve Manuel Komnenos Devirleri*. Ankara, 1995.

Comnena, A., *The Alexiad* ed. by P. Frankopan, trans. by E.R.A. Sewter. London: Penguin Classics, 2009.

Constantine, Emperor of the East and J. J. Reiske. *Constantini Porphyrogeniti Imperatoris De ceremoniis aulae Byzantinae*. Corpus scriptorum historiae Byzantinae. Bonnae 1829.

Constantine, Emperor of the East and J. F. Haldon. *Three Treatises on Imperial Military Expeditions*. Vienna 1997.

Dennis, G.T., *Three Byzantine Military Treatises*. Washington D.C.: Dumbarton Oaks, 1985.

Drummond, S.K. and L.H. Nelson, *The Western Frontiers of Imperial Rome*. London-New York: Routledge, 1994.

Dum-Tragut, J., *Kilikische Heilkunst für Pferde: das Vermächtnis der Armenier: Kommentar – Übersetzung – Glossar*. Hildesheim: Olms, 2005.

Eichner, I., "Surveys of Early Byzantine Houses in Rough Cilicia, 2003." *Anatolia's Mediterranean Areas* 2004/2 (2004): 74–78.

Equini Schneider, E., "Classical Sites in Anatolia: 1993, Archaeological Survey in Cappadocia." *Araştırma Sonuçları Toplantısı* 12 (1994): 15–33.

Foss, C., *History and Archaeology of Byzantine Asia Minor*. Aldershot: Ashgate, 1990a.

———. "Byzantine Malagina and the Lower Sangarius." *Anatolian Studies* 40 (1990b): 161–183.

———. "Cappadocia" in *The Oxford Dictionary of Byzantium*, (v. 1) ed. by A. Kazhdan, *et al.*, 378. Oxford: Oxford University Press, 1991.

Galatariotou, C., "Travel and Perception in Byzantium." *Dumbarton Oaks Papers* 47 (1993): 221–241.

Haldon, J.F., "Military Service, Military Lands, and the Status of Soldiers: Current Problems and Interpretation." *Dumbarton Oaks Papers* 47 (1993): 1–67.

———. *Warfare, State and Society in the Byzantine World, 565–1204*. London: Routledge, 1999.

———. "Roads and Communications in the Byzantine Empire: wagons, horses and supplies" in *Logistics of Warfare in the Age of the Crusades*, ed. by J. Pryor, 131–158. Aldershot: Ashgate, 2006.

Heath, I., *Byzantine Armies, 886–1118*. Men-at-arms series. London: Osprey Publishing, 1979.

Hyland, A., *Equus, the Horse in the Roman World*. New Haven: Yale University Press, 1990.

———. *The Medieval Warhorse: From Byzantium to the Crusades*. Stroud: Sutton, 1994.

———. *The Horse in the Middle Ages*. Stroud: Sutton, 1999.

Jeffreys, E., *Digenis Akritis: the Grottaferrata and Escorial Versions,* ed. and trans. by E. Jeffreys. Cambridge: Cambridge University Press, 1998.

Jones, A.H.M., *The Later Roman Empire 284–602: A Social, Economic and Administrative Survey.* (3 vols.) Oxford: Blackwell, 1964.

Kalas, V.G., *Rock-Cut Architecture from the Peristrema Valley: Society and Settlement in Byzantine Cappadocia.* Unpublished Ph.D. Thesis, New York University, 2000.

———. "The Byzantine Kitchen in the Domestic Complexes of Cappadocia" in *Archaeology of the Countryside in Medieval Anatolia,* ed. by T. Vorderstrasse and J. Roodenberg, 109–127. Leiden: The Netherlands Institute for the Near East, 2009.

Karantabias, M., "The Crucial Development of the Heavy Cavalry under Herakleios and His Usage of Steppe Nomad Tactics." *Hirundo: The McGill Journal of Classical Studies* 4 (2005/6): 28–41.

Karpozilos, A. and A. Kazhdan, "Travel" in *The Oxford Dictionary of Byzantium* (v. 3), ed. by A. Kazhdan *et al.*, 2109. Oxford: Oxford University Press, 1991.

Kazhdan A., "Byzantium, History of" in *The Oxford Dictionary of Byzantium* (v. 2.), ed. by A. Kazhdan *et al.*, 345–362. Oxford: Oxford University Press, 1991a.

———. "Geoponika" in *The Oxford Dictionary of Byzantium* (v. 2), ed. by A. Kazhdan *et al.*, 834. Oxford: Oxford University Press, 1991b.

———. "The Peasantry" in *The Byzantines* ed. by G. Cavallo, 43–73. Chicago, 1997.

Kazhdan, A. (editor in chief), *The Oxford Dictionary of Byzantium.* (Vols 1–3.) Oxford: Oxford University Press, 1991.

Kazhdan, A. and G. Constable, *People and Power in Byzantium: An Introduction to Modern Byzantine Studies*. Washington, D.C.: Dumbarton Oaks, 1982.

Kazhdan, A. and J. W. Nesbitt, "Cart" in *The Oxford Dictionary of Byzantium* (v. 1), ed. by A. Kazhdan *et al.*, 383–384. Oxford: Oxford University Press, 1991a.

———. "Horses" in *The Oxford Dictionary of Byzantium* (v. 2), ed. by A. Kazhdan *et al.*, 948. Oxford 1991b.

Laiou, A.E. and C. Bouras, *The Economic History of Byzantium: From the Seventh Through the Fifteenth Century.* Dumbarton Oaks Studies 39, ed. by A E. Laiou and C. Bouras. Washington, D.C.: Dumbarton Oaks, 2002.

Laiou, A.E. and C. Morrison, *The Byzantine Economy.* New York 2007.

Lefort, J., "Rural Economy and Social Relations in the Countryside." *Dumbarton Oaks Papers* 47 (1993): 101–113.

MacMullen, R., "Three Notes on Imperial Estates." *The Classical Quarterly* (New Series) 12/2 (1962): 277–282.

Maurice, *Maurice's Strategikon: Handbook of Byzantine Military Strategy*. trans. by G.T. Dennis. Philadelphia: University of Pennsylvania Press, 1984.

Mavrogordato, J. *Digenes Akrites,* edited and translated by J. Mavrogordato. Oxford 1956.

McCabe, A., "Horses and Horse-doctors on the Road" in *Travel in the Byzantine World: papers from the thirty-fourth Spring Symposium of Byzantine Studies, Birmingham, April 2000* ed. by R. Macrides, 91–97. Aldershot: Ashgate, 2002.

———. *A Byzantine Encyclopaedia of Horse Medicine: The Sources, Compilation, and Transmission of the Hippiatrica.* Oxford: Oxford University Press, 2006.

McGeer, E., N. Phocas and N. Uranus, *Sowing the Dragon's Teeth: Byzantine Warfare in the Tenth Century.* Washington, D.C.: Dumbarton Oaks, 1995.

Nesbitt, J.W. *et al.*, "Beasts of Burden" in *The Oxford Dictionary of Byzantium* (v. 1), ed. by A. Kazhdan *et al.*, 274. Oxford: Oxford University Press, 1991.

Nesbitt, J. W. and A. Kazhdan, "Livestock" in *The Oxford Dictionary of Byzantium* (v. 2), ed. by A. Kazhdan *et al.*, 1242–1243. Oxford: Oxford University Press, 1991.

Nicolle, D., *Romano-Byzantine Armies 4th–9th Century.* London: Osprey Publishing, 1992.

Onar, V., "İstanbul'u anlatan kemikler." İ.Ü. *Bilim, Kültür ve Sanat Dergisi* 3 (Nisan, Mayıs, Haziran 2010): 22–29.

Onar, V., H. Alpak, G. Pazvant, A. Armutak and A. Chroszcz, "Byzantine Horse Skeletons of Theodosius Harbour: 1. Paleopathology." *Revue De Medicine Veterinaire* 163/2 (2012): 139–146.

Onar, V., H. Alpak, G. Pazvant, A. Armutak, N. Gezer İnce and Z. Kızıltan, "A Bridge from Byzantium to Modern Day Istanbul: An Overview of Animal Skeleton Remains Found During Metro and Marmaray Excavations." *The Journal of the Faculty of Veterinary Medicine* 39/1 (2013): 1–8.

Oppian, *Oppian, Colluthus, Tryphiodorus,* trans. by A. W. Mair. Loeb Classical Library. Cambridge: Harvard University Press, 1987.

Ousterhout, R.G., *A Byzantine Settlement in Cappadocia.* Washington, D.C.: Dumbarton Oaks, 2005.

Owen, T. (trans.) *Geoponika. Agricultural Pursuits.* London: J. White, 1805.

Pattenden, P., "Byzantine Early Warning System." *Byzantion* 53 (1983): 258–297.

Pharr, C. (trans.) *The Theodosian Code and Novels, and the Sirmondian Constitutions.* Princeton: Princeton University Press, 1952.

Pryor, J. H., "Transportation of Horses by Sea during the Era of the Crusades: Eighth century to 1285 A.D." *The Mariner's Mirror* 68 (1982): 103–125.

Rautman, M., *Daily Life in the Byzantine Empire.* Westport: Greenwood, 2006.

Rodley, L., *Cave Monasteries of Byzantine Cappadocia.* Cambridge: Cambridge University Press, 1985.

Rose, S., "Islam Versus Christendom: The Naval Dimensions, 1000–1600." *The Journal of Military History* 63/3 (1999): 561–578.

Ševčenko. N.P., "Wild Animals in the Byzantine Park" in *Byzantine Garden Culture* ed. by A. Littlewood, H. Maguire and J. Wolschke-Bilmahn, 69–86. Washington, D.C.: Dumbarton Oaks, 2002.

Shahîd, Irfan, *Byzantium and the Arabs in the sixth century. Volume II. Part 1, Volume II. Part 1.* Washington, D.C.: Dumbarton oaks, 2002.

Teall, J. L., "The Grain Supply of the Byzantine Empire, 330–1025." *Dumbarton Oaks Papers* 13 (1959): 87–139.

———. "The Byzantine Agricultural Tradition." *Dumbarton Oaks Papers* 25 (1971): 39–59.

Theophanes, Mango, C.A., R. Scott and G. Greatrex, *The Chronicle of Theophanes Confessor: Byzantine and Near Eastern History, AD 284–813.* Oxford: Clarendon Press, 1997.

Toynbee, J.M.C., *Animals in Roman Life and Art.* Ithaca: Cornell University Press, 1973.

Treadgold, W.T., *Byzantium and its Army, 284–1081.* Stanford: Stanford University Press, 1995.

Tutel, E., *At ve Atçılık.* İstanbul: İletişim Yayınları, 1998.

Tütüncü, F., *The Land of Beautiful Horses: Stables in Middle Byzantine Settlements of Cappadocia.* Unpublished M.A. Thesis, Bilkent University. Ankara, 2008.

Van Dam, R., *Kingdom of Snow. Roman Rule and Greek Culture in Cappadocia.* Philadelphia: University of Pennsylvania Press, 2002.

Vryonis, S., *The Decline of Medieval Hellenism in Asia Minor and the Process of Islamization.* Berkeley: Univrsity of California Press, 1971.

Getting Smashed and Ending up in the Bottom of a Pit: The Kinet Beakers and their Tragic Fate

Franca Cole[1] — *Scott Redford*[2]

We offer the following essay as a token of appreciation to Marie-Henriette and Charles Gates, their devotion to excavations at Kinet Höyük, their kindness and generosity to members of the Kinet team, and to their highly developed, but very different, senses of humour.

Hubris and historiography

With great self-assurance, the 1997 excavator of Operation K2, a 10 x 10 meter excavation unit on the east terrace just below the mound of Kinet Höyük, a harbour city on the bay of İskenderun, wrote the following on his locus sheet for Locus 56:

> This pit was not finished. It was excavated for an hour or so. It consisted of mainly murex and other shells with some evidence of burning (heavily burnt white m[ud]b[rick]). This pit is either just above M[iddle]B[ronze]A[ge] occupation in the NW quadrant, or it belongs to some other intermediate phase. *It is not medieval.* [Emphasis added.]

In his phasing of the medieval deposit, the same excavator persisted in his refusal to date this pit, which appeared at the same level as the very first medieval settlement, as medieval.[3]

The next year, excavators of the same unit, Cédric Bodet and Çağatay Karabulut, encountered the opposite problem. While searching for floor levels in the

---

1 UCL Qatar, PO Box 25256, Georgetown Building, Education City, Doha, Qatar.

2 Department of the History of Art and Archaeology, School of Oriental and African Studies, University of London, Thornhaugh Street, Russell Square, London WC1H 0XG, UK.

3 In his defence, this hour's worth of excavation in Pit 56 produced animal bone, murex shells and Hellenistic and Bronze Age pottery, but no medieval pottery.

Middle Bronze Age palace remains there, with loom weights and complete vessels popping up right and left, Bodet and Karabulut could naturally have assumed that they were finally through dealing with intrusive medieval pits. However, on page 57 of the K2 1998 notebook, in noting excavation activity on July 9th, at 9:30 am, for Locus 74, Lot 124, the excavators wrote:

> For that lot, the medieval pit 56 from 1997 seems to continue from where the shells, pebbles, and bones concentrate on its surface [this last refers to a floor the excavators were trying to trace —authors].

In an addendum to the locus sheet for Locus 74, written anonymously, but in a hand recognizable to any Kinet team member, Marie-Henriette Gates notes the presence of medieval pottery in Locus 74, Lot 124.

From the combination of these two seasons of day books and locus sheets, we understand that the medievalist excavator thought Pit 56 was pre-medieval, and the students excavating the Bronze Age thought that this pit had long since ceased to descend until, at its very bottom, it yielded up something not found elsewhere at Kinet—a discrete cache of medieval glass vessel fragments—a glass hoard. From the (revised) stratigraphy of the site, we can now date the vessels, and the pit they were found in, to the first level of the medieval occupation at Kinet, sometime in the middle of the 12th century AD.

Quantification and Evaluation

Initial evaluation of the glass hoard showed it to be composed of 354 vessel fragments, all except for eight of which were clear, with a slight greenish hue. The 'group of eight' comprised one pale pink and one blue-green bodysherd, and six sherds of de-coloured (colourless) glass.[4] As the sherds could not be differentiated further by colour, the remaining fragments were arranged by vessel part instead, revealing 111 rim sherds, 223 body sherds and 12 thick-walled base sherds. It was at this point that it became clear that the hoard was almost exclusively composed of fragments of near-identical heavy-based glass beakers with flared rims (see Fig. 1). At the same time, it was realised that this was not, as might be expected, the simple remains of a group of broken vessels which, once reconstructed, would yield similar numbers of rims and bases. Instead, the hoard fragments comprised more than 17 beaker upper bodies and only two bases (see Figs. 1–3).

While a vast majority of rim sherds were from beakers, there were also fragments from two vessels with restricted necks and everted rims (Fig. 4). Overall,

4 Bamford 1977, 79.

only ten sherds could be securely identified as coming from vessels other than beakers. Both the restricted range of vessel types represented and the uneven ratio of upper bodies to bases, indicate the hoard to be a systematic collection of glass, rather than the detritus of accidental breakage (a common problem when attempting to wash-up in the *çeşme*).

Condition and Conservation

At the time of its discovery, the hoard was loosely embedded in fine silty sediment. All sherds were coated with a fine layer of dust, but in some areas the sediment had cemented onto the surfaces. While the core of the sherds was transparent and greenish, surfaces and break-edges had deteriorated to an opaque black or pearlescent grey-white. In many cases, these deteriorated surfaces were flaking and delaminating to reveal poorly- or un-bonded iridescent layers beneath. In areas where the iridescent layers had detached, the exposed glass core beneath was greenish and transparent with a pitted and uneven surface.

Cleaning initially focused on sherd break-edges, to improve the chances of making joins. Break edges were mechanically cleaned using a scalpel and modified bamboo skewers. Surfaces of adjoining sherds were swabbed with isopropanol to remove loose sediment. Cemented sediment that could be removed mechanically, without risk of detaching the delaminating surface, were also cleaned. In some cases, the exposed cleaned surfaces were unstable and flaking. These were consolidated with a solution of 5% Paraloid B-72 in acetone. (Lower concentrations of resin were found to be ineffective in the >35°C daily temperatures and 85–100% relative humidity that are habitually enjoyed by inhabitants of modern Kinet.)

Fragments were examined individually during the cleaning process, allowing body sherds to be orientated by curvature and variation in wall thickness. (Wall thickness was variable, but in general increased with proximity to the base. Vessels had flared rims and tapered toward the base, so sherds with the broadest curvature were located closest to the rim.)

Desperation and Redemption

Reconstruction of newly-orientated fragments was a war of attrition and proceeded slowly, by a process of trial and error. (Many trials. Many errors.) Visitors to the lab frequently required fortification with ethanol-based substances, while two (of non-local origin) subsequently required hospitalization for dehydration and heat-prostration. (It has yet to be proven that their decline was beaker-related, but it does suggest care should be taken to prevent further outbreaks of beaker-trauma.) Fragments were joined, one at a time, using a solution of 25–35%

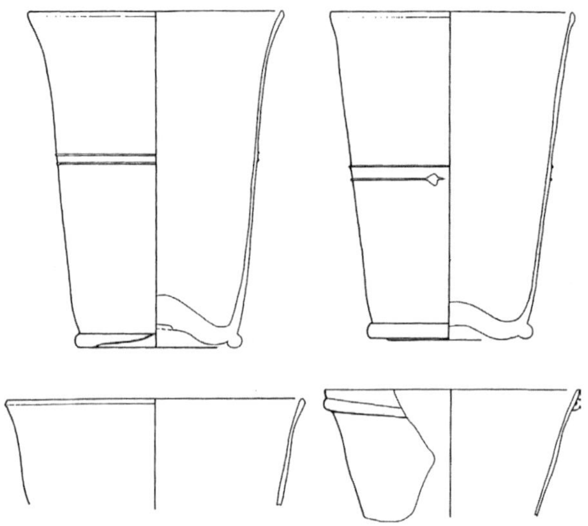

Fig 1 Complete beakers with fluting and trailed decoration. Right: KT10371 a, H 144mm, rim 120mm, base 71mm. Left: KT10371 b, H 139mm,
rim 110mm, base 73mm.

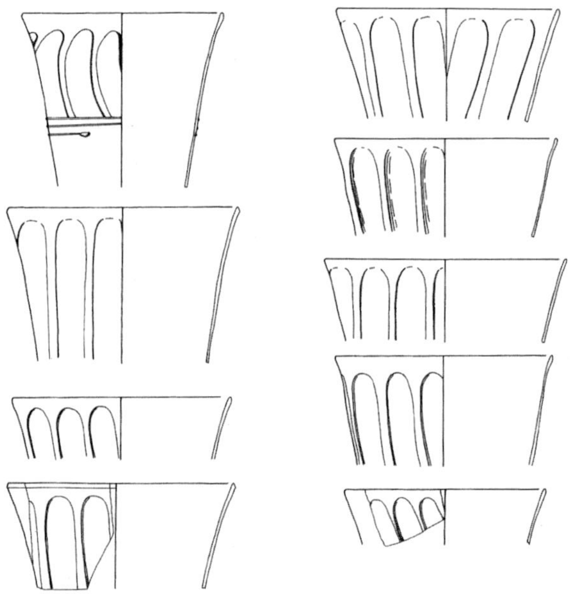

Fig 2 Beaker rims and upper bodies. Largest rim diameter 120mm, smallest 105mm.

Paraloid B-44 in acetone, applied with a fine brush. Fragments were 'pegged' into position using dots of cyanoacrylate adhesive to hold the join in place while the solvent-based adhesive cured. This exhaustive and aromatic process culminated in the construction of two complete beaker profiles, the substantially-preserved upper-bodies of 11 further vessels, and substantial fragments of another four. It was possible to join a total of 223 sherds to known vessels, leaving a further 131 sherds representing at least four further upper-bodies of vessels.

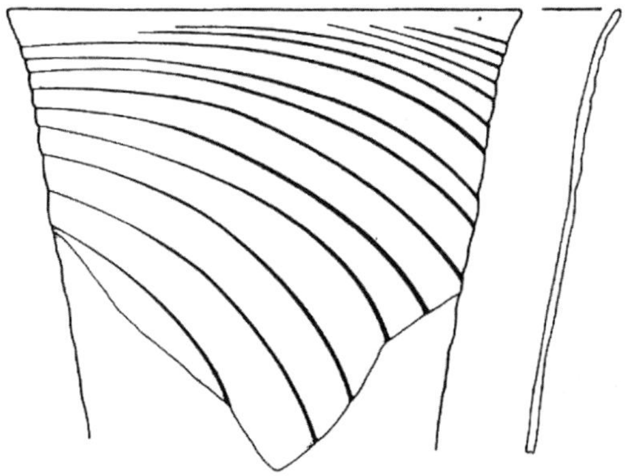

FIG 3 Vessel with twisted decoration. H 104mm, rim 105mm.

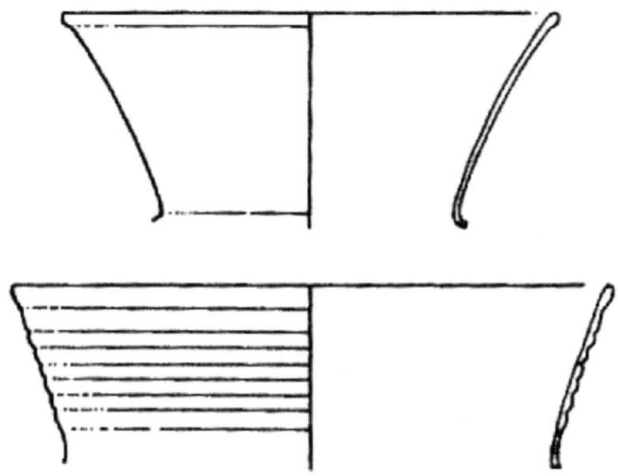

FIG 4 Restricted vessels. Upper: H 30mm, rim 74mm. Lower: H 20mm, rim 90mm.

Destruction — by Design?

Patterns of breakage visible amongst the reconstructed elements showed breakages radiating from the mid-body, as well as from the rims of the beakers, and many curved fragments exhibited midway breakage patterns that did not continue on adjacent sherds. These breakage patterns indicate that the fragmentation of the Kinet beakers was not the result of a single breakage event, such as an accident.

Research into intersecting fracture behaviour has largely been driven by forensic osteology,[5] but much of the experimental work underpinning this research was undertaken on brittle structures including glass and eggshell.[6] Following these rules, a previously unbroken glass vessel will fracture with fault-lines radiating from the point of impact. Where a vessel is already broken, fault-lines will only radiate as far as the nearest broken edge and terminate at that point, thus enabling an observer to reconstruct the order in which individual impact events occurred.

5 E.g. Dixon 1984; Madea *et al.* 1986; Madea and Staak 1988; Viel *et al.* 2009

6 Puppe 1903; Schüttrumpf 1966.

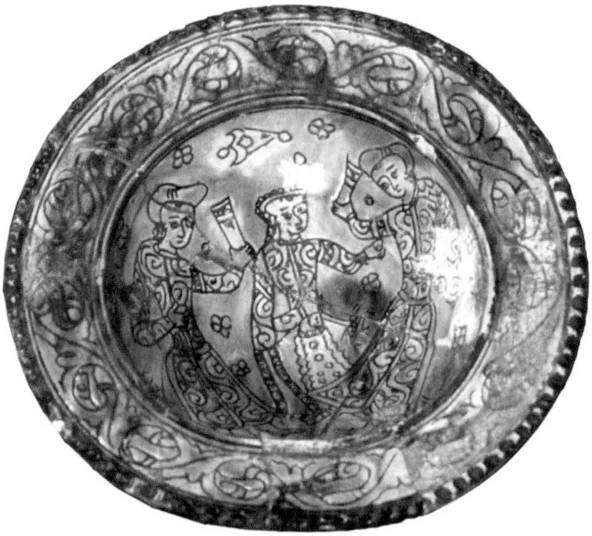

Fig 5 A 13th or early 14th century bowl from Misis

Getting Smashed and Ending up in a Pit...

Given the narrow base and flared rim of the Kinet beakers, the natural percussion point for accidental breakage would be at the rim itself. Instead, a number of the beakers exhibited breakage patterns demonstrating impact points at their mid-bodies, a place that, due to the concave curvature of the wall, would be least likely to be impacted during a fall. These patterns suggest that at least some of the Kinet vessels were deliberately broken by a blow or blows to their mid-body. Larger fragments have been broken into smaller fragments and long, curved fragments appear to have been broken in half—perhaps to make them more compact for storage. When viewed together, this pattern of breakages points to the Kinet beakers having been broken deliberately, rather than accidentally. A secondary point suggests that their breakage may relate more to a desire for compaction than for breakage alone.

Why was a fairly substantial number (17) of glass beakers seemingly deliberately smashed and deposited in the bottom of a pit, perhaps even a pit dug expressly for them? The first answer that comes to mind is an ethnographic one—a 13th or early 14th century bowl from Misis, not so far from Kinet, depicts a party or other ceremony: in it, a woman is flanked by two men hoisting glass beakers (Fig. 5). Other glazed earthenware bowls from Kinet and other sites in the region depict a cupbearer, also proffering a glass beaker (like the other beakers, presumably filled with wine) as a symbol of elite hospitality (Fig. 6). What could be more profligate than to toss the beaker one held in such a celebration of ceremony, after tossing back its contents, of course? Alas, the answer seems to lie in a more sober, commercial aspect of medieval life in this part of the world.

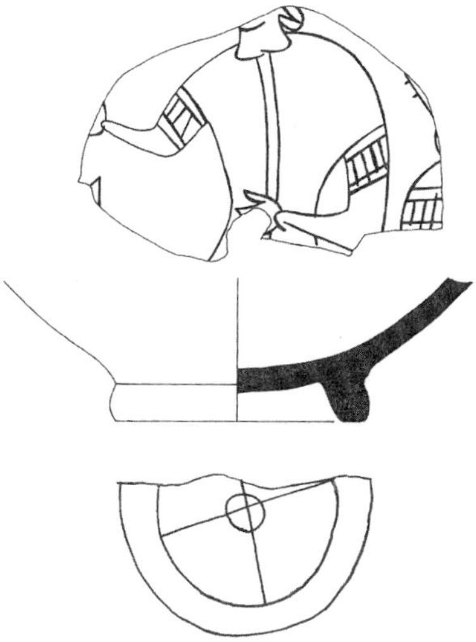

Fig 6 A glazed earthenware bowl from Kinet

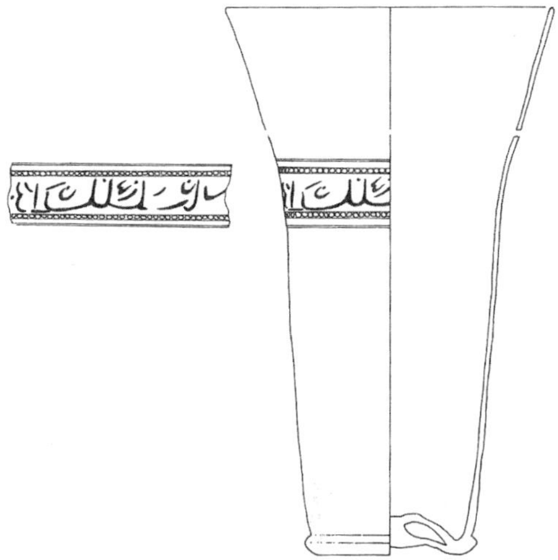

Fig 7 A 14th century enamelled beaker from Kinet. H 168mm, rim 103mm.

Kinet did not have a large number of glass finds. The one other beaker that survived in good enough condition to be reconstructed (Fig. 7) comes not, like these beakers, from the beginning of the medieval occupational sequence, but from its very end, in the early decades of the 14th century. This was a time when a range of different ceramics and other finds were making their way to the site. Finds included this enamelled beaker, originating from Islamic lands, under Mamluk control, in northern Syria.[7]

7 See similar beakers in Lane 1938, 72, fig. 13a-b; Jackson-Tal and Tal 2013, 93; Redford 1994, 91.What remained of the inscription can be read as part of a series of standardised titles of both Ayyubid and Mamluk monarchs. A similar piece of an enamelled Ayyubid or Mamluk beaker was recovered at the port of Antioch (Lane 1938, 72, and fig. 13, A-B). The Kinet beaker's inscription displays some overlap with that found on Lane's Plate 13 A: (*'Izz l-Mau)lana(?) al-Malik a(l-'Alim*): (Glory to) our Lord (?) the King…) Similar beakers with similar inscriptions were found in two elite contexts, the first Crusader, the second Islamic. The first is the citadel at Arsuf/Arsus, used by the Hospitallers there before first the city and then the citadel were taken by the Mamluks in 1265; see Jackson-Tal and Tal (2013, 93) for an enamelled beaker with an inscription. The 13th century palace at Samsat had a "glass room". Redford (1994, 91) shows one enamelled beaker with an inscription from this palace. Based on stylistic criteria, these beakers have been dated to the period of 1225–1250 (Kenesson 1998, 46). Archaeological evidence seems to cast some doubt on this dating. The author himself contradicts this dating when he labels the generic inscriptions like that on the Kinet enamelled beaker as of "Ayyubid or early Mamluk provenance."

Unlike the beakers in the cache, the Kinet enamelled beaker owes its survival to destruction—of the site—which was burned and abandoned at this time. The enamelled beaker was broken and burned, but relatively intact compared to most glass finds at Kinet. Many complete pots were found in this final level, where they had seemingly fallen from their storage places as the site burned.[8]

Profligacy versus Parsimony

The question remains: Why did the Kinet beakers end up smashed and in the pit? It is unlikely that even an elite group at a site that had just been settled, likely by the Knights Templar, would squander a whole lot of drinking vessels, no matter how joyous the occasion. Even if they had, why would these broken vessels be buried in a pit? To answer this question, we may have recourse to the rich history of medieval glass production in the Levant and the hopes of redemption for these smashed beakers in the international glass trade of the medieval eastern Mediterranean.

The presence of quartz-rich sands and potash in the region comprising present-day Syria, Lebanon, and Israel led to a flourishing glass industry here in Roman and medieval times,[9] as well as an allied industry producing artificial paste bodied ceramics. The recycling of glass became common in the Roman period. Glass was produced from its raw materials in primary workshops. These workshops supplied the secondary workshops, where glass-blowing and vessel manufacture took place and where scraps and recycled vessel fragments were re-melted along with glass from ingots or pre-prepared lumps.[10] Using prepared or recycled glass to make new glass vessels is advantageous even in regions where the raw materials are available because the fluxes present in the prepared glass lower its melting temperature, allowing for substantial savings in fuel.[11]

Our knowledge of medieval glass recycling is largely based on evidence from the Serçe Limanı shipwreck.[12] The 15-metre vessel was carrying 4 tonnes of raw glass and cullet when she sank in a southwestern Anatolian harbour in the third decade of the 11th century. Analysis of the assemblage indicates the vessel first stopped to take on cargo in Egypt, stopping again on the Levantine coast and was likely on its way to Constantinople at the time of its sinking.[13]

---

8 For a consideration of some of the ceramics found in the debris of the same room as this beaker, see Redford (2015).

9 Freestone *et al.* 2000.

10 Freestone 2006.

11 Stern 1999.

12 Bass *et al.* 2004; Bass *et al.* 2009.

13 Bass *et al.* 2004; Bass *et al.* 2009.

The eastern Mediterranean practice of glass recycling continued into the period of the Crusades. There is a well-known trade treaty, dated 1277, between Jacopo Contarini, the Doge of Venice and Prince Bohemond VII of Antioch. The treaty exempted the Venetians from duty charged on all goods exported from the port of Tripoli (in today's northern Lebanon), with the notable exception of broken glass.[14] This is a strong indication of the high commercial value attached to broken glass at this time and goes further towards explaining why people may have hoarded this material. Another hoard example is found at Al-Mina, the port of Antioch, which lies between Kinet and Tripoli.[15] British excavations in the 1930s uncovered a glass "hoard" dated by Arthur Lane to the 9–10th centuries that could also have been stored for export and recycling.[16] The Kinet hoard may have been unique within Kinet, but fits closely with regional archaeological and historical evidence for recycling and hoarding at this time.

Technology and Style

The Kinet beakers themselves fall comfortably within the parameters of what we know about 12th–13th century production of glass beakers, both in Frankish/Crusader and Islamic contexts. Discussion of glass from medieval Syria is dominated by enamelled glass, which finds such favour in histories of art and the museums of the world. Beyond this, it is important to consider what the majority of the production actually was, be it plain or decorated, and to understand what existed before enamelled glass started being produced in quantity in the 13th century in Syria. Most Kinet beakers seem to have been made of clear glass, with a slight greenish hue. This is a natural colour for glass made without the addition of a decolourizer.[17]

The pontil scars visible on the base of vessels KT 10371 and KT 10371a demonstrate them to have been blown, and their wall-facets suggest marvering on a grooved board. Their flared rims indicate that they were hot-worked to the chosen shape. Shallow, roughened spiral grooves located near the lip of the vessel interior indicate the use of tools (probably glassmakers' jacks) to 'open' the rim while the glass was still hot and, therefore, malleable.[18] Following shaping, trailed body-decoration was

14 Comments on this tax are made in Whitehouse (2009, 566) and Carboni (1998, 101–102) "...that, if the Venetians wanted to import *verrebrizé*, or *vitrum deslaboratum* (broken glass) together with the *alumen album* (the soda necessary to make glass) and beach sand, they had to pay a tax on them."

15 Lane 1938; Woolley 1953, 182–185.

16 See hoard E2 in Lane 1938, 65.

17 Bamford 1977, 79.

18 Gudenrath 1991.

added to a majority of vessels. The solid glass base-rings visible on KT10371 and KT10371a, and the hollow rim decoration on KT10371m, are also trailed additions. The surface ripple-effect seen on vessel KT10371f is most likely to have been produced by pinching the end and rotating the pontil to create a twisted ripple effect.[19]

The production sequence for the beakers with faceted decoration is more difficult to determine with certainty. Vessels KT10371e, g, i, j, k, l, o, p and q have linear facets which are visible on the outer surface only. Facets are more sharply defined in the mid and lower body, are more diffuse towards the rim and are absent from the base. These facets are likely to have been produced by rolling the partially-blown glass (on the pontil) across a grooved plate. The occasional soft facets visible on the interior surfaces seem to be a result of indirect pressure from the faceting of the outer surface, rather than the result of direct hot working of the interior. The spiral grooves on the inner vessel lips are evidence of direct hot working, and the flaring of the vessel rim was probably sufficient to cause smoothing of the external facets as the glass was stretched. This was most probably achieved with sofietta and jacks.[20] The rounding visible on all facets just beneath the rim is likely to relate to the smoothing and finishing of the rim following its separation from the blowpipe, rather than indicating the use of a deliberately rounded tool. All the faceted vessels and one of the twisted vessels had applied trailed decoration around their mid-bodies. A small bulb of glass was attached to the body and then pulled away, to produce a fine thread which was wound between 1 ¾ and 2 ¼ full turns around the body. Of the eleven vessels with trailed decoration, ten showed the attachment bulb positioned closest to the base and the vessel rotated in a clockwise direction, while only one vessel had an attachment bulb closer to the rim and anti-clockwise decoration.

Chronology and Comparanda

Comparanda from Frankish cities and, of course, Serçe Limanı show that, like ceramic traditions, traditions of glass-making were not altered by the establishment of the Frankish states on the coast of the Levant, and that a tradition of drinking from cylindrical beakers pre-dated the establishment of the Crusader states of the Outremer and continued under their rule. Although clear Islamic archaeological contexts are less common, beakers seem to have been an equally important feature of medieval Islamic glassmaking in the region.

Clear or nearly-clear glass beakers *not* decorated with enamel have been found in cities under Frankish rule like Beirut, Acre, and Arsur/Arsuf. They share many

19 See Gudenrath 1991, figs. 163–165.

20 See Gudenrath 1991, figs. 65–87.

features with the Kinet beakers. In terms of decoration, they are finished with trailed decorations of applied threads in both the same and contrasting colours of glass (Kinet examples are all single-colour), with similar hot-worked facets and forms, with thick bases and applied base-rings,[21] elsewhere described as "rolled bases with raised concave centers", and "cylindrical shapes [...] gently flaring towards the rim."[22]

While the Serçe Limanı assemblage contained a range of vessels including stacked groups of narrow-based beakers that were similar to each other, the Kinet glass hoard/cache was composed solely of beakers and, while broadly similar in style and size, these beakers differed the one from the next. One possible origin for the Kinet beakers would be Antioch. In the 12th century, Kinet lay on the northern borders of the Principality of Antioch, an area guarded by forts and castles granted to the Knights Templar. Benjamin of Tudela mentions a small Jewish glass-making community in Antioch at about this time.[23] It is also possible that the beakers were manufactured somewhere in Cilicia. While we know next-to-nothing about glass production in medieval Cilicia, excavators at the site of Yumuktepe, at the western end of the Cilician plain, found a complete beaker from a church burial in a level they date to the 11th century. With its rolled base, flared upper body and two parallel applied threads on the body, this beaker greatly resembles Kinet beakers 10371a and b.[24]

If we range further afield, we find that clear, or very lightly colored glass beakers have been found at many sites to the south of the Kinet/Cilicia/Antioch region. Sarah Jennings' publication of the Beirut glass notes that beakers were "predominantly a plain form and only three were decorated."[25] As concerns their

21 The concave base formed around the pontil scar is described as a 'kick' (Kröger 1995, 41–42; Gudenrath 1991).

22 Kitson-Mim Mack (2009,72) states "Intact beakers and the five stacks of three to five beakers were clustered in only two areas of the site, both areas representing living spaces on the ship." What the author calls "truncated cone" beakers had no out-folded or applied bases, allowing for the stacking she reports. The simpler forms and smaller sizes of beakers found in this early 11th century context (not to mention their scratch-incised designs) provide a baseline for developments in the 12th–13th centuries.

23 Benjamin of Tudela, *The Itinerary of Benjamin of Tudela* (Malibu, Calif: John Simon, 1983), p. 76. "Ten Jews dwell here, engaged in glass-making." The glass from the 1930s Antioch-on-the-Orontes excavations was never published. Some of this will be published by Tasha Vorderstrasse. We thank Asa Eger for this information.

24 See Köroğlu (2002, 520) for the dating of the church where this burial was found to the late 10th through 11th centuries, p. 523 for description of the glass found at the site, and p. 535, pl. 15 for a photograph of the beaker and see Köroğlu (2004, 129, pl. VII-9) for a drawing of this beaker.

25 Jennings 2004–2005, 229.

manufacture, she notes that "[B]ases associated with these beakers either have a fold that projects at the base edge or have a single fine trail around the basal edge. Most have high domed and often pointed bases with distinct pontil scars."[26] All these observations could be equally applied to the Kinet beakers. In addition, she notes one beaker whose decoration recalls those of Kinet beakers 10371e and g-l. This is a "beaker with raised vertical ribs unevenly spaced."[27]

Excavations in the Crusader castle of Montfort discovered one example of these beakers.[28] In addition, glass vessels were decorated with applied threads and prunts. Indeed, this article on Montfort may be the origin of ongoing attempts to associate prunted beakers with Frankish habitation, and even manufacture.[29]

Excavations at Jerusalem, while only loosely dated to the 13th–15th centuries, also recovered beakers whose form recalls those of the Kinet beakers.[30] Recent excavations in the citadel at Arsus/Arsuf, which was taken over by the Hospitallers before the capture of the city by the Mamluks in 1265, have uncovered a large cache of vessels in ceramic and glass. Appropriate to the elite setting, there are gilded and enamelled beakers, including one with an inscription referred to above. More germane to our subject, clear glass beakers without decoration were also found.[31]

The largest collection of medieval beakers from an Islamic context was recovered by the Danish excavations at Hama in the 1930s. These were only published after the Second World War, by which time much information about the find spots of the objects had been lost. These, too, are only loosely, or stylistically, dated. There are many beakers that resemble KT 10371 and 10371a, well known "types" of medieval Levantine glass production. However, those that resemble the facets or panel decoration on KT 10371e and g-l are classified, due to their technique, state of conservation, and other reasons, as being post-medieval.[32]

---

26 Jennings 2004–2005, 229. Beaker bases illustrated in fig. 10.10, 12–16.

27 Jennings 2004–2005, 230.

28 Dean 1927, fig. 56D. On page 40, the author describes this rim fragment as follows: "...in one case, (D), a radial design in bands was formed by moulding the surface of the object."

29 Dean 1927. For more prunted beakers from Monfort, see Whitehouse 2005, 191 and colour plate 42. For a recent instance of a continuation of the prunted beaker – Frankish use, or production hypothesis, see Gorin-Rosen 1997, 75–85.

30 Brosh (2005, 188), "The ten fragments of beakers found in the group have cylindrical bodies with incurving flared openings near the rim."

31 Jackson-Tal and Tal (2013, 95) mention "wide-mouthed conical beakers with pushed-in tubular bases," illustrated on p. 96, nos. 5–7.

32 Riis 1957, 49, in which these beakers are called "verre transparent côtelé."

Beyond the Pit: A Non-Enamelled Majority and the Quest for More

The Kinet cache of beakers fits comfortably within our current understandings of the history of glass making, use and disposal in the medieval Levant. While the circumstances of its deposition, and the predominance of a single type of vessel (without being matched, or of a set) remain a mystery, it seems to us as if they were deposited in order to be recovered subsequently, and that their deliberate smashing gives us a clue as to the reason for their intended recovery: selling for recycling. What it does not tell us (sadly), is the fate of the 'missing' 15 beaker bases.

In terms of shape and decoration, the beakers pertain to the general parameters of medieval glass production and the importance placed on glass drinking-vessels in high-status situations (while the rest of the population drank from wooden or ceramic vessels). The predominance of beakers decorated with hot-worked facets or panel decorations marks the Kinet beakers as unusual (or points to under-identification of these facets elsewhere). Regardless of the reason, the growing corpus of plain and hot-worked vessels increasingly points to the need to focus on the non-enamelled majority of glass beaker production. More knowledge about these would be smashing!

REFERENCES

Bamford, C.R., *Colour Generation and Control in Glass*. Oxford: Elsevier Scientific Publishing, 1977.

Bass, G., S. Matthews, J.R. Steffy and F. Jr. van Doorninck, *Serçe Limanı: An Eleventh Century Shipwreck. The Ship and its Anchorage, Crew, and Passengers*. Volume 1. College Station, 2004.

Bass, G., R. Brill, B. Lledó and S. Matthews, *Serçe Limanı: The Glass of an Eleventh Century Shipwreck*. Volume 2. College Station, 2009.

Benjamin of Tudela, *The Itinerary of Benjamin of Tudela*. Pasadena 1983.

Brosh, N., "Islamic Glass Finds of the Thirteenth to Fifteenth Century from Jerusalem-Preliminary Report" *Annales du 16è Congrés de l'Association Internationale pour l'Histoire du Verre*, 186–190. Loosdrecht: AIHV Publications, 2005.

Carboni, S., "Gregorio's Tale; or, Of Enamelled Glass Production in Venice" in *Gilded and Enamelled Glass from the Middle East*, ed. By R. Ward, 101–106. London: British Museum Press, 1998.

Carboni, S. and D. Whitehouse, *Glass of the Sultans*. New York: Metropolitan Museum of Art Publications, 2001.

Dean, B., "The Exploration of a Crusaders' Fortress (Monfort) in Palestine." *Bulletin of the Metropolitan Museum of Art* 22 (1927): 5–46.

Dixon, D.S., "Pattern of Intersecting Fractures and Direction of Fire." *Journal of Forensic Sciences* 29 (1984): 651–654.

Freestone, I.C., "Glass Production in Late Antiquity and the Early Islamic Period: A Geochemical Perspective." *Geological Society, London, Special Publications* 257 (2006): 201–216.

Freestone, I.C., Gorin-Rosen, Y. and M. Hughes, "Primary Glass from Israel and the Production of Glass in Late Antiquity and the Early Islamic Period" in *La Route du Verre. Ateliers Primaires et Secondaires du Second Millénaire av. J. C.* ed. by. M.-D. Nenna Maison de L'Orient Mediterranean 33 (2000): 65–83.

Gorin-Rosen, Y., "Excavation of the Courthouse Site at 'Akko: Medieval Glass Vessels (Area TA)." *Atiqot* 31 (1997): 75–85.

Gudenrath, "Appendix: Techniques of Glassmaking and Decoration" in *Five Thousand Years of Glass*, ed. by H. Tait, 213–241, London: British Museum Press, 1991.

Jackson-Tal, R. and O. Tal, "Crusader Glass in Context: The Destruction of Arsur (Apollonia-Arsuf, Israel), April 1265." *Journal of Glass Studies* 55 (2013): 85–100.

Jennings, S., "Vessel Glass from Beirut BEY 006, 007, and 045." *Berytus* 48–49 (Special edition 2004–2005).

Kenesson, S., "Islamic Enamelled Beakers: A New Chronology" in *Gilded and Enamelled Glass from the Middle East*, ed.by R. Ward, 45–49, London: British Museum Press, 1998.

Kitson-Mim Mack, J., "Beakers" in *Serçe Limanı: The Glass of an Eleventh Century Shipwreck*, Volume 2, ed. by. G. Bass, R. Brill, B. Lledó, S. Matthews, 41–76. Texas: Texas A&M University, 2009.

Köroğlu, G., "Yumuktepe in the Middle Ages" in *Mersin-Yumuktepe: A Reappraisal*, ed. by I. Caneva / V. Sevin, 103–134. Lecce: Congedo, 2004.

———. "Yumuktepe Höyüğü Ortaçağ Kazısından Küçük Buluntular" in *VI. Ortaçağ ve Türk Dönemi Kazı Sonuçları ve Sanat Tarihi Sempozyumu*, ed. by M. Denktaş, Y. Özbek, A. Sağıroğlu Arslan , 515–535, Kayseri, 2002.

Lane, A., "Medieval Finds at al-Mina in North Syria." *Archaeologia* 87, (1938): 19–78.

Madea, B., C. Henßge and H.B. Lockhoven, "Priorität bei mehrfachen Schußverletzungen des Schädels." *Zeitschrift für Rechtsmedizin* 97 (1986): 213–218.

Madea, B. and M. Staak, "Determination of the Sequence of Gunshot Wounds of the Skull." *Journal of the Forensic Science Society* 28 (1988): 321–328.

Puppe, G., "Traumatische Todesursachen" in *Gerichtliche Medizin, Zwölf Vortrage*, ed. by R. Kutner, 65–84. Jena: Fischer, 1903.

Redford, S., "Ayyubid Glass from Samsat, Turkey." *Journal of Glass Studies* 36 (1994): 81–91.

———. "Port Saint Symeon Ceramics and Cyprus" in *Cypriot Medieval Ceramics: Reconsiderations and New Perspectives.*, ed. by D. Bakirtzis and N. Coureas, 125–151. Nicosia: The Cyprus Research Centre & The Leventis Foundation, 2015.

Riis, P.J., "Les verreries" in *Hama Fouilles et Recherches 1931–1938*. Volume 4, Part 2, ed. by P.J. Riis / V. Poulsen, 30–116, Copenhagen, 1957.

Schüttrumpf, G., "Untersuchungen über die Priorität der Schädelbrüche." *Deutsche Zeitschrift für die Gesamte Gerichtliche Medizin* 58 (1966): 94–100.

Stern, M.E., "Roman Glassblowing in a Cultural Context." *American Journal of Archaeology* 103, (1999): 441–484.

Viel, G., A. Gehl and J.P. Sperhake, "Intersecting Fractures of the Skull and Gunshot Wounds. Case Report and Literature Review." *Forensic Science, Medicine, and Pathology* 5 (2009): 22–27.

Whitehouse, D., "Glass from the Crusader Castle at Monfort" in *Annales du 16é Congrès de l'Association Internationale pour l'Histoire du Verre* 191–193. Loosdrecht: AIHV Publications, 2005.

Woolley, C.L., *A Forgotten Kingdom*. London: Penguin, 1953.

Bronze Surgical Instruments from Tüpraş Field and the Islamic-Byzantine Medical Trade

Asa Eger[1]

Abstract

In 2011, excavations at Tüpraş Field, the Early Islamic and Middle Byzantine settlement north of Kinet Höyük, revealed a set of long thin bronze tools with a decorated center, each one slightly different than the other. Parallels for these have been found around the Early Islamic world, however scholars have diverged on how to interpret their function. They have been published either as applicators for kohl or instruments for surgery. This contribution will discuss the tools in their site context and examine similar published and unpublished ones elsewhere to determine their date and geographical distribution. From the archaeological evidence, parallels, and Islamic medical texts, this paper will argue that their function was primarily surgical. The presence of these tools and other related objects in a small frontier settlement provide evidence for a wider trade in pharmacological and medical supplies that took place across the Islamic-Byzantine frontier.

> *The yron is most excellent but that it is offensive to the eye and bringeth the patient to great sorrowe and dread of the burning and the smart.* [2]

Islamic metalwork is well-known for its intricacy, beauty and craftsmanship, manifesting in the most pragmatic and every-day objects, such as candlesticks, lamp-stands, incense burners, boxes, bowls, basins, ewers and pen boxes. These qualities have attracted scholars to study and exhibit the most highly-decorated and lavish examples, works of art that have graced the pages of both art historical publications and exhibition and auction catalogues, alike.[3] However, many of

---

1 Department of History, The University of North Carolina at Greensboro, 2135 MHRA Building, PO Box 26170, Greensboro, NC 27402–6170.

2 William Clowes to Queen Elizabeth. via Bennion 1979, 183.

3 See for example: Porter and Rosser-Owen 2012; Ziffer 1996; Allan 1986; Baer 1983; Melikian-Chirvani 1982.

the smaller objects found in excavations have escaped notice and have not been treated synthetically or categorically. Objects in archaeological contexts, when examined as an aggregate group in light of their contexts, geographical distribution and function can reveal much about not only their individual or communal value, but their role in larger movements of goods, and ideas and networks of trade.

In 2011, excavations at Tüpraş Field, the Early Islamic and Middle Byzantine settlement north of Kinet Höyük, revealed five beautiful but curious artifacts that soon caught the attention of members working at the Kinet dig house. They were long thin bronze tools with a decorated center, each one slightly different than the other. Marie-Henriette Gates, who greatly appreciated and loved all of the early medieval objects we were finding, was delighted as these presented a puzzle. What were they used for, and how did they relate to each other? Parallels for these have been found around the Early Islamic world, however, scholars have diverged on how to interpret their function. They have been published either as applicators for kohl or instruments for surgery. This contribution will discuss the tools in their site context and examine similar published (and unpublished) ones elsewhere to first determine their date and geographical distribution. From the archaeological evidence, parallels and Islamic medical texts, I will hypothesize that their function was primarily surgical. The presence of these five tools and other related objects in a small frontier settlement provide evidence for a wider trade in pharmacological and medical supplies that took place across the Islamic-Byzantine frontier.

The Objects

The five tools are polished bronze (copper alloy) with rounded tips and a central decoration on the shaft. The decoration falls into one of three styles with some sub-variations:

1) **a.** a cut faceted diamond shape flanked by discs
   b. a cut faceted diamond shape flanked by incised square collars, often resulting in a square cross-section and not protruding much past the thickness of the rest of the instrument
2) two inverted triangles creating a single hourglass flanked by two discs with a disc in the middle
3) double spheres
4) single lozenge bead flanked by two discs (seen only in parallels).

The central decoration functioned as a grip handle for the fingers and suggests that the tool was used for delicate work. The tools were probably made in a single piece lost-wax mold. There is no evidence of mold flashing on the edges, and this would have just left the tips needing polishing. Many thanks go to Dr. Franca Cole, the conservationist for these finds, whose meticulous notes and observations are included here. Measurements are in centimeters. Not all the information for all objects was recorded during the season they were recovered, as they were all (save one) taken to the Hatay Museum for registration at the end of the 2011 season.

No.	KT No.	Trench	Locus. Lot	Length object	Length shafts	Diam. handle	Diam. shaft	Date	Type
1	26755	TF 16	5.30	12.05	5.4/5.6	.55	.4 to .25/.3	7/4/11	1a
2	26884	TF 17	17.33	11.5	5.0/5.0	.4 to .5			1b
3	27021	TF 19	1.1	6.7		1.8	.5 to .35	7/18/11	2
4	27324	TF 17	12.39	11.8	4.75/4.0		.5 to .35	7/13/11	2
5	27453	TF 16	5.26	9.9	4.6/4.55	.45 to .25	.4 to .3	7/13/11	3
6	27454	TF 16?	5.26					7/13/11	
7	27280	TF 16	5.42					7/20/11	
8	26459	TF 17	6.13	6.85		.4		6/21/11	Undec.
9	27450	TF 16	24.39	10.25		.5	.45	7/18/11	Undec.

1) KT 26755 has a shaft that tapers toward the center, and one side is slightly longer than the other. The double-headed tool has blunt rounded tips and is also bent at the border of the decorated handle. The decorative area is cast with a square cross section edged by two discs. It is formed by cutting wedges from the corners of the square to produce a faceted diamond shape flanked with pairs of incised lines. This style is our type 1a, protruding past the shaft body (Fig. 1).
2) KT 26884 has a faceted cut diamond flanked by two incised squares. The decorated handle does not protrude much past the body of the shaft itself. This style is our type 1b. Both shaft ends are even in length. It is not in the Hatay Museum but in storage at Bilkent University (Fig. 2).
3) KT 27021 is half the size of the others with a decorated head and blunt rounded end. It appears as if one half of the shaft is broken, but there is no indication of a break. If it was broken, the tool has been polished smooth and refinished. The decoration is formed of two truncated cones whose narrow ends point to the center, producing an hourglass shape, and joined by a raised rounded band. The bi-cones exhibit traces of shallow incised rings, partially preserved. The tool is most similar to KT 27324 and is type 2 (Fig. 3).
4) KT 27324 features a central hourglass shape formed of truncated cones, tapered ends inwards, joined with a raised band in the middle and discs or

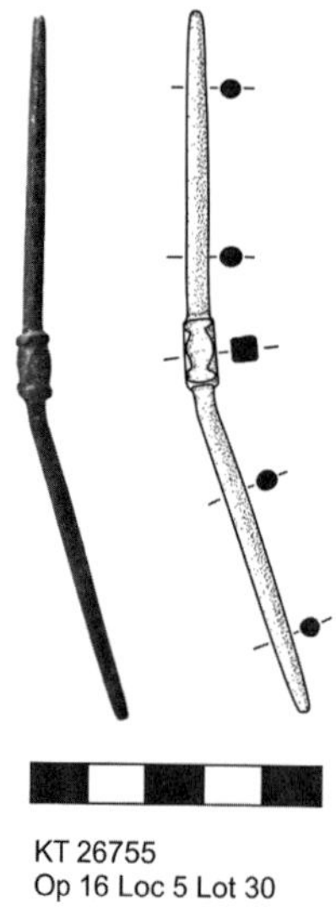

FIG 1. KT 26755 (drawing by S. Demir, photograph by M.-H. Gates)

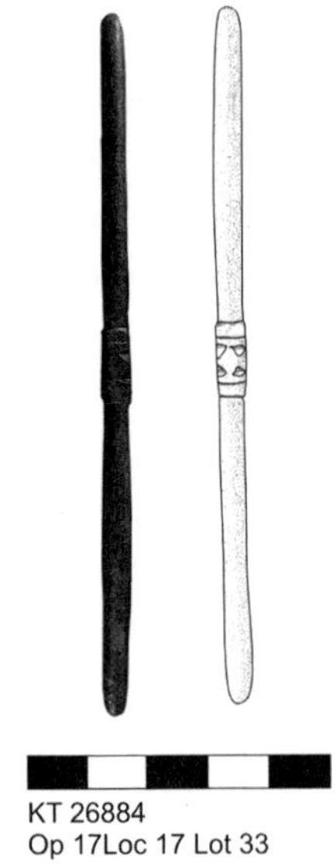

FIG 2. KT 26884 (drawing by S. Demir, photograph by M.-H. Gates)

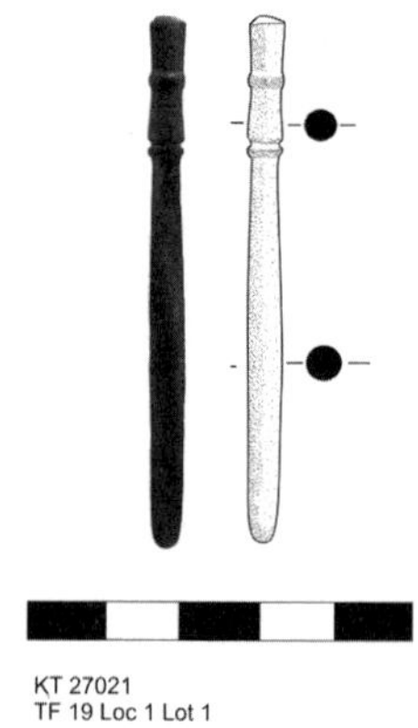

FIG 3. KT 27021 (drawing by S. Demir, photograph by M.-H. Gates)

collars at either end at the wide end of each cone. The truncated cones are decorated with a series of six parallel lines. One rounded tip appears to have been flattened, but this may be a result of damage rather than intention. It is type 2, like KT 27021 (FIG. 4).

5) KT 27453 has rounded blunt shaft ends and a central double sub-spherical beaded handle. The tool was cast as a single piece and polished. It is type 3 (FIG. 5).
6) and 7) were not studied.

Two other objects were related and can be added here, although of a different type with undecorated handles. They are included as they may have been part of the set of bronze tools described above with the same general function.

8) KT 26459 is undecorated with one rounded end and one pointed end. The shaft is bent near the center. While this may have not been original, one cannot discount the possibility of a tool with a deliberately bent half. The piece is hammered unevenly to a point, and the head was snipped with shears, partly smoothed. The cross-section is circular at all points along the body. Its function serves as a pin or needle.

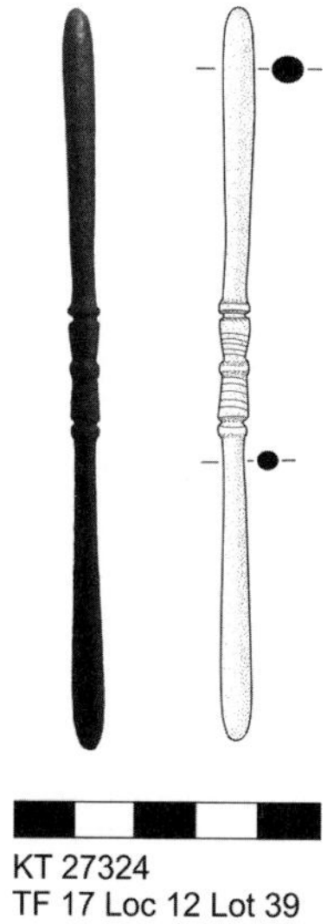

Fig 4. KT 27324 (drawing by S. Demir, photograph by M.-H. Gates)

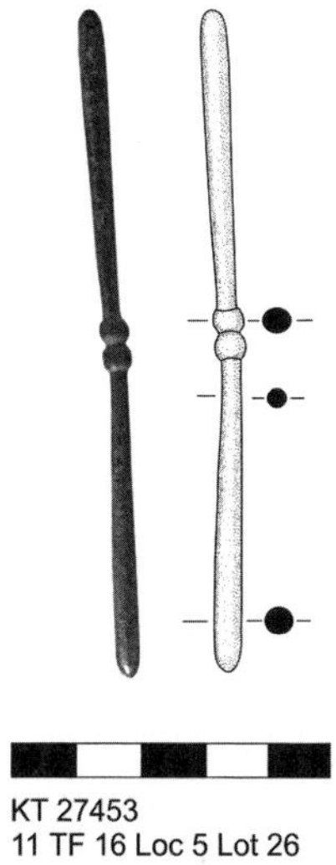

Fig 5. KT 27453 (drawing by S. Demir, photograph by M.-H. Gates)

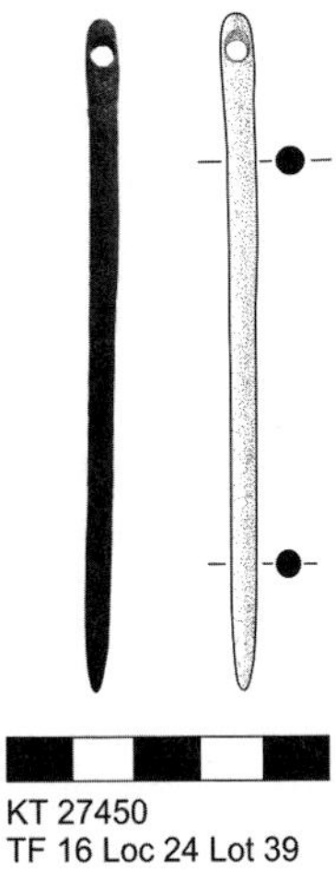

Fig 6. KT 27450 (drawing by S. Demir, photograph by M.-H. Gates)

9) KT 27450 is a long needle or awl, pierced at one end with a large hole and a pointed tip at the other. The perforated end would have been hammered flat then drilled on a diagonal. Faceting along the shaft suggests that it was re-sharpened subsequently on a stone (Fig. 6).

Context

Unfortunately, the Murphy's Laws of archaeology are unavoidable. The contexts for every one of these objects were mixed, and most were from an upper layer corresponding with the fill of the second occupation of Tüpraş Field. The second occupation, Phase II, is the re-use of the 'Abbāsid site in the Middle Byzantine period, the eleventh and twelfth centuries. Curiously, all were found only in the 2011 season when excavation focused on the eastern rooms, wall, and gate of the main fortified enclosure. Three were found in TF 16, three were found in TF 17 just north and only one was found in TF 19 located just north and outside the fortified enclosure walls. The bronze tool in TF 19 was in the upper surface layer (Fig. 7). All the ones in TF 16 were in poor mixed layers or destruction layers of the site. One was found within a robbing trench that was along the outside of the eastern exterior wall whose purpose was to remove its large ashlars. One of the three in TF 17 was in a stone collapse, a poor context. The second was in a similar mixed fill in the center of the trench just south of the rooms along the north.

The only one in a potentially good context was KT 26459, the long awl or needle that was not of the same type as the set of five with decorated handles. The object came from a trench excavated as an initial exploratory sounding in the east of TF 17. It was found within a room bound by two parallel north-south walls of rather loosely built large rubblestones outside the structure. Similar to burning and destruction evidence in the fortified enclosure, all rooms had a burnt layer, although the extramural rooms had far less burning than those rooms within the larger structure to the west. However, these rooms had only one period of occupation that could be discerned. Mid-tenth to early twelfth century material was associated with these burnt contexts, including ceramics (colorsplash sgraffiato), metal nails, blades and bone, all suggestive of domestic contexts. These may have been extramural occupational houses built against the outside fortified enclosure wall. Their exact phasing is unclear; their materials are similar to Phase II (eleventh-twelfth century Middle Byzantine) and Phase III (tenth century) with the polychrome sgraffiato. Although Phase III (eighth-tenth century) extramural structures were found, the walls in TF 17 were also quite different and poorly made, and they are at a much higher elevation.

In lieu of any good context, does this suggest that these belong to the Phase II eleventh-twelfth century phase when only the fortified enclosure was used, and some more poorly built structures outside its walls, rather than earlier, when there is substantial material culture from the eighth-tenth centuries in structures outside the walls? The earliest/latest date range is most comfortably the tenth to mid-twelfth century, after which the entire site was damaged by an earthquake, burned and abandoned. This corresponds mainly with the Faṭimid period and the period of Byzantine reconquest of the region and early Crusader rule. Several other objects relate to the Faṭimid period and are of Egyptian origin that date to this phase, such as a glass bottle (discussed below) and a fragment of Faṭimid lusterware.

Parallels

Similar bronze tools have been discovered and published elsewhere in regions and sites important throughout the Early Islamic world ranging as far east as Nīshāpūr, to the south at Fusṭāṭ and Edfu, to the west at al-Andalus and in Bilād al-Sham: in the south in Palestine and in northern Syria and the *thughūr* in nearby Anṭakīya and Ḥamā. In all cases, the parallels are nearly exact; the only difference usually being the decorated center portion and, in several cases, the tip of the tool. Most interpretations are that these tools were for surgery, however some say that their

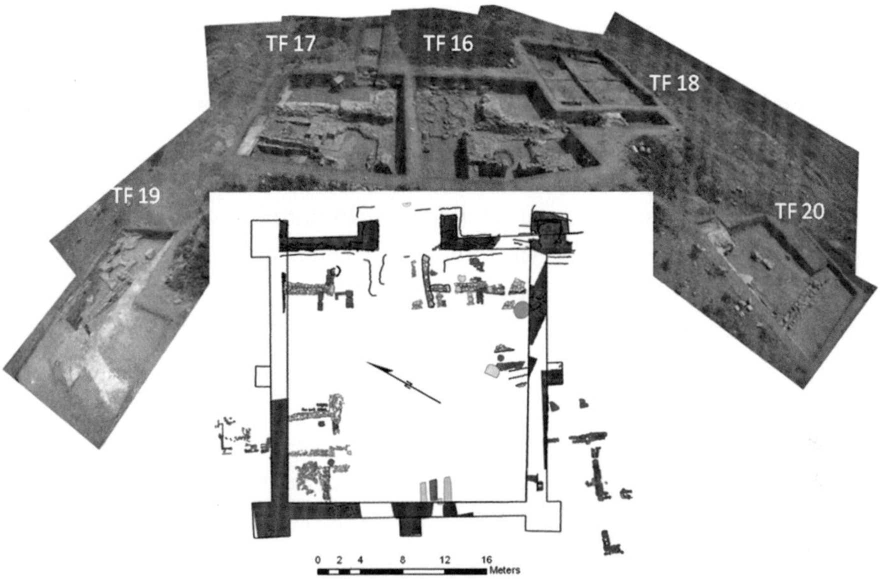

FIG 7. Tüpraş Field Excavations, 2011 Season (photograph by M. –H. Gates)

function was for the application of cosmetics, specifically kohl. In other cases, similar tools have also been considered as forks.[4] The parallels will be presented from the eastern to western Islamic world.

Nīshāpūr

In the excavations at Nīshāpūr, conducted by the Metropolitan Museum of Art, they were classified as kohl sticks although some hesitation is present in the publication.[5] Allan noted that similar tools have been known in Iran since the third or fourth century BCE and were introduced by the Greeks. They occurred in the Parthian levels of the excavations at Taxila and were thought to be toothpicks or ear cleaners.[6] However, Allan cautions against using much more ancient parallels to help determine their function in the Early Islamic period, particularly as there are no Sasanian examples. He also notes that they appeared frequently at Rayy and Sīrāf.

They consisted of two forms, published under the same function: one undecorated and the other with a decorated center grip. The published types are of our

4 Warland 2012, 372, pl. 1, 4.

5 Allan 1982, 38, 76.

6 Marshall 1951, vol. 2, 585; vol. 3, pl. 173, no. 221

Type 2b, with an angular geometric cut design. The decoration on Number 83 is too difficult to read from the photo but does not protrude past the shaft's thickness. Number 84 has a double faceted diamond motif and protrudes slightly as a rectangular handle with square cross-section which we may call a slight variation, Type 1c. Some broke in the center, an obvious weak point, and were published as halves (and perhaps still functional). Two of them (numbers 83 and 84) were 7.6 and 7.4 cm long, respectively.[7] The total length would have been between 14–15 cm. These are slightly longer than our examples.

Sāmarrā'

An undecorated bronze tool with rounded blunt points was published in the Sāmarrā' excavations conducted by the Iraqi Department of Antiquities.[8] There is no more specific information on the object or its context; however, it is likely from the mainly ninth century occupation of the site and, with the exception of a palace, from any one of a number of residences that were excavated.

Ḥamā

The excavations at Ḥamā yielded the largest number of examples that were published. Fifteen examples were found undecorated, while twenty-six were decorated in the center. The excavators also posited that they were also kohl sticks, "sondes pour maquillage des yeux et similaires."[9] The undecorated polished tools were similar in shape, length, and thickness/diameter as the decorated ones and had the same rounded tips. The thickness was equal throughout the length of the instrument. In some cases, one tip was thicker/wider or more pointed/narrower than the other, giving the tool two different ends. The length was up to 16 cm, but most examples were between 11–13 cm. Among those published was a smaller tool quite different than the others (fig. 24.4). It had a loop on one end that was hinged. No further comments were made in the publication; however, it appears that it was used for tooth extraction.

The decorated examples were all of our Type 1 and had a rounded or angular central bead-like part that was chiseled or incised and framed by two shapes, often discs. Some had a protruding decorated handle as in our Type 1a (fig. 24.5, fig. 24.8), and others were like our Type 1b with a non-protruding handle and square cross-section in many variations of design (fig. 24.6, fig. 24.7, fig. 24.9, fig. 24.11),

7 Allan 1982, 76, nos. 83–84.

8 Iraq Government Department of Antiquities 1940, pl. 142.

9 Ploug *et al.* 1969, Riis, fig. 24.

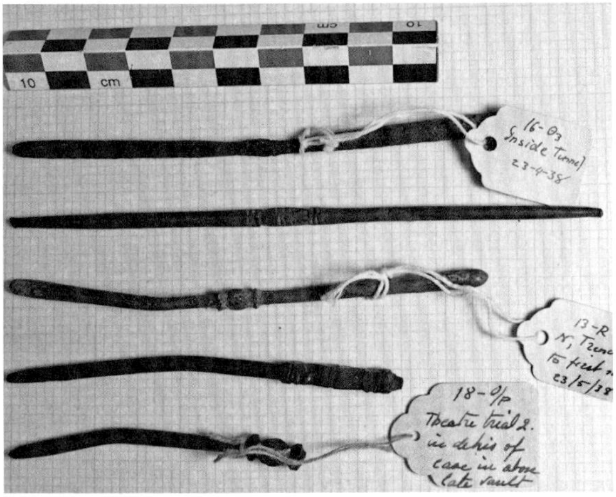

FIG 8. Bronze tools from Antioch (photograph by A. Eger, courtesy of the Princeton University Art Museum)

while the less protruding rectangular handle of Type 1c is also present (figs. 24.10, 24.12, 24.13). The tips were slightly tapered. They measured similar in length, 12–14 cm. Nearly all were cast bronze.

The publishers also included instruments with spatula or more spoon type ends and those with needle or pin tips. While all are separated into different classes, these may all be treated as similar instruments of cast bronze of similar length and thickness (spatulas: 11–12 to 16–17 cm, needles 10.9–14.6 cm, pins 8.9–13.6 cm). The spoons seem to have been for cooking and were much longer. It is difficult to see how the spatulas may have been used for cooking; their flattened shovel end would only be useful in measuring out minute quantities of a substance, or as an instrument.

Anṭākiya

Five unpublished examples were found in the Antioch (Anṭākiya) excavations by Princeton in the 1930s. They are currently housed in the Princeton University Art Museum, and I examined them in the first week of January in 2014 (FIG. 8).

Three of them have rounded tips that are not flattened like a spatula. One has a hook-like end that has been broken on one side. The fifth, which is broken just past the decorated center, has a rounded tip that is more pointed. The three complete tools range from 8.8 g to 12.1 g and 11.31 cm to 13.6 cm. The thickness is very uniform: four of the five are 0.31 cm thick between the center and tip (the fifth is 0.41), and three of the five are 0.41 cm thick in the decorated center (the other two are 0.45 and 0.52 cm.). Despite the uniformity in thickness, each have a decorated center that is completely different. Like the other excavated examples from Nīshāpūr and Ḥamā, the motifs are square, angular, rounded and disc, and usually a combination of two of these. Only three of the tools had labels, and these were found in excavated trenches around the city (13-R, 16-O, and 18-O/P). The context for the theater 18-O/P tool found in debris above a late vault mainly consisted of Early and Middle Islamic glazed ceramics.

Ṭarsūs

Nine bronze tools were found at Ṭarsūs of varying size and shape, suggesting a set of different tools. They are from the recent Boğaziçi excavations and two feature near exact parallels: a polished shaft and rounded blunt tip on either end, with a central decorated grip. Using the classification here, one is Type 1 (TGK 2014 C7 16 nr. 2532) and one is Type 3 (TGK 2012 C7 07 nr. 689). The excavators note that the concentration of these tools in one area (Goldman's excavations did not reveal any) may suggest a single location where they were used by a physician. The tools date to the Early Islamic period, likely before the eleventh century, according to the excavators.[10]

Montfort

Two bronze tools were published from the Metropolitan Museum of Art's excavations at Montfort, the Crusader castle in northern Israel. The publication in the Metropolitan's Bulletin shows at least two instruments (maybe more), one of which is a parallel to those at Tüpraş with a central decorated grip and rounded ends. The shaft tapers, however, on either side near the central grip.[11] The decorated portion is of the faceted cut diamond type (1b) that does not protrude past the shaft's thickness. The other tool has the same rounded blunt end and a spatulate opposite end with a Type 1a protruding faceted diamond flanked by discs. Both tools are published as needles or probes. Interestingly, a much smaller bronze tool with spatulate end on one side is published as a kohl-stick. The context is dated to 1226/7–1271; the site was destroyed in 1272.[12]

Syria (provenance unknown)

A set of similar tools came from Syria. They range in length from 9.2 to 17.5 cm and are in the Sabah collection in Kuwait.[13] One of these, the second from the left in the published photo, is similar, with a central decorated handle. The dec-

10 Özyar *et al.*, 2016. I am grateful to Oya Pancaroğlu for sharing this information with me.

11 Dean 1927, 39, fig. 54.C.

12 Adrian Boas, personal communication.

13 Institut du monde arabe 2005, 175.

oration is raised, but not central, and consists of a series of adjacent discs. The tools are dated broadly as a group from the eighth to twelfth centuries. However, this style is more similar to Roman examples and has no other known Islamic parallels. The ends are different than one another, and it has a thinner shaft but more spatulate end.

A set of bronze tools from the Baron Ustinov collection, which were later bought by S. Hoth, contained some closer parallels. The exact provenance is unknown, but they came from Ashqelon (ʿAsqalān), Palmyra (Tadmur), Gaza or Caesarea (Qayṣārīyah), where the Baron acquired his objects. A similar tool (pl. II.6) with a rounded blunt end and pointed opposite end had a slightly off-centered grip of three adjacent discs that are the same thickness as the shaft, which tapers a little in the center of each end. Hoth describes it as a double sound with one 'olive' end and one 'stiletto' end. Hoth dates it to the Hellenistic or Roman period and most likely from Ashqelon based on the sale statements accompanying the group when it was sold. A group of six tools (pl. III, 16–21), all virtually identical, were also described as double sounds with rounded blunt ends. Two were broken in half at the central handle. The tools have a protruding incised rectangular grip with square cross-section, Type 1c. Their length is between 7.3 and 15.8 cm. Hoth dates these to the Islamic period and not the Hellenistic or Roman on the basis that they all have central squared grips as opposed to off-centered (excentric) rounded ones. Four other tools in the collection (pl. III, 11–14) all had one spatulate end and no central handle. One had an Arabic inscription on the spatula bearing the name of the owner or maker, *atiʿakāb*, possibly a Palmyrene name, but subsequent resident of ʿAsqalān.[14] Hoth argues that these are all surgical instruments.

Egypt (provenance unknown), Edfu, and Fusṭāṭ

Petrie published some examples in his *Objects of Daily Use* catalogue of Egyptian objects from the "Graeco-Roman period." To be sure, the dating is general at best, and, I would argue, faulty, as there is no supporting evidence for dating these objects to these periods. He published the double-ended tools as kohl-sticks or unguent spoons of bronze.[15] It is likely from this publication that the attribute of kohl sticks was attached to the tool and taken up as the primary identifying function in later studies. Numbers 47–50 on Plate 23 are exact parallels in size, shape, and style to the set from Tüpraş Field. They were double-ended with rounded blunt tips. Number 47 had a Type 1b double faceted diamond and Number 48 had a single lozenge bead flanked by discs, a variation on Type 1a but a new motif.

14 Holth 1919, 10–11; Bliquez 1984, 189.

15 Petrie 1927, 28, pl. XXIII: nos. 47–50.

It can be categorized in a different class, Type 4. Number 49 was too corroded to discern the decoration, and Number 50 was undecorated.

Two similar tools, although made of iron and not bronze, were published in the catalogue *L'art du métal au début de l'ère chrétienne* from the Louvre. Their provenance is from Edfu (Atfū) from the excavations of H. Henne. The first (AF 1426) is 16 cm long and 0.6 cm thick, while the second (1427) is 14.8 cm long and 0.4 cm thick. The first tapers in near the central grip and has a cut/angular decoration producing two faceted diamond shapes and incised with parallel lines (Type 1b). The second is of the same type (1b) but does not protrude past the thickness of the shaft with parallel lines. Both have rounded tips. The publication dates these possibly to the "Coptic" period (fourth-seventh centuries) although is ultimately uncertain.[16] As nearly exact parallels, these may now be more comfortably assigned later to the Islamic periods of occupation. Edfu was occupied in the Faṭimid period from the tenth century onwards as a provincial town in Upper Egypt.[17]

The largest number, although how many is unknown for certain, was from Scanlon's excavations in Fusṭāṭ. These tools, along with many other variations, were part of the Henri Amin Awad Collection, which then gave them to the Islamic Arts Museum in Cairo. They have been studied by H. Awad, a medical doctor, and S. Hamarneh, a specialist on Islamic medical science.[18]

They interpret the tools as surgical. Several of their medically-based interpretations are very useful and combine their own knowledge with those of medical texts from the Byzantine and Islamic periods. Some of their other conclusions are without much basis. They date the tools to the eighth-early ninth centuries, or pre-Faṭimid, although there is no solid evidence to support any of this dating. Second, they associate the presence of these with a military post at Fusṭāṭ. Their exact locations are unknown. However, these have come from Scanlon's excavations, which were largely in domestic areas with extensive Faṭimid occupation but poor stratigraphy overall. The ninth-twelfth century date encompasses a greater and more comfortable range for these excavations, however it is important to keep in mind that much of the material culture from Scanlon's excavations was Faṭimid (tenth-twelfth century). One is published in color in the catalogue *La médecine au*

16 Bénazeth 1992, 278. Similar tools with rounded tips or spatulate ends of iron but no decorated central grip were found at the village Anibeh, the northern Nubian site of Karanog, in a cemetery. For example, an undecorated but similar tool (7388) was in tomb G 131 and was mentioned as an iron kohl-stick. Kohl boxes were also found in association with other items, including one example of an iron kohl stick pushed into a kohl box. The cemetery was dated from the first to fifth century CE or a Roman/Byzantine date. Wooley and Randall-MacIver 1910, 66, 71, 244.

17 Gascoigne 2005, 153–190.

18 Hamarneh and Awad 1977, 520–524, fig. 1; Hamarneh 1977, 3–14, fig. 6; Hamarneh and Awad 2002. These three articles are all largely identical. See also: Hamarneh 1961, 82–94.

temps de calife and dated to the ninth century.[19] The decoration of a single lozenge bead flanked by discs is Type 4, seen in an example by Petrie above.

Al-Andalus (Provenance Unknown), Seville

Two examples from the Museo Arqueológico Provincial de Córdoba that appear in the catalog *El Esplendor de Los Omeyas Cordobeses* were published as surgical instruments from the tenth-twelfth centuries (No. Inv 6.849 and 11.557).[20] No. 6.849 is 12 cm long and cylindrical with rounded ends, and the catalogue states that it could have been used either as a long handled spoon for mixing and application of drugs or makeup or as a probe. No. 11.557 is a close parallel, but with one end quite different. It is longer, at 16.7 cm, with a double beaded center (Type 3), and one end is a small spoon or spatula. The entry states that this is for the extraction and application of various substances, either medicine or cosmetics, or perhaps for other medical uses. This last tool presents the only variation seen on the bronze instrument with a raised central portion. J. Zozaya pubished four bronze tools that he calls, with relative certainty, surgical instruments.[21] Three are from the National Archaeological Museum in Madrid, and one is from the Ethnographic Museum "Leite de Vasconcelos" in Belem, Lisbon. The first (Inventory Number: 83/165/1) is 10.7 cm long and 3.5 mm in diameter, found in the region of Seville. It is broken on either end but has a protruding incised rectangular grip with square cross-section, Type 1c. Zozaya believes that both ends formed spoons, one larger than the other. Based on Milne's volume on surgical instruments in the Greek and Roman periods, Zozaya speculates on function. This tool resembles a probe called the *cyathiscomele*, and a variant of the *spathomele* which features a spatula end.[22] Since this piece is broken, the function is unclear. It may have also functioned to mix drugs or apply make-up. The second tool (83/165/2) is 8.2 cm long and 2.7 mm in diameter, also from the area of Seville, and broken on one side. The complete side comes to a pointed end, while the other end is speculated to have also been a small spoon. The grip is the same as the first, Type 1c. For these last two, the grips were likely not centered on the instrument. The form is a *ligula* and used for extracting unguents or ointments from jars.[23]

19 Institut du monde arabe 1996, 166, fig. 103 (third tool from the left).

20 Viguera and Castillo Castillo 2001.

21 Zozaya 1984, 255–259.

22 For a color photograph: Morales and Molina Lopez 1999, 219 where it is called a surgical instrument. These first three are also published in color: Ginés and Samsó 1992, 271. Note: the third tool is called 83/166/3 in Zozaya's article, but in the color publication *El Legado* it is: 83/165/3. They are the same.

23 For a color photograph: *El Legado*, 280, where it is called a surgical instrument.

The third tool (83/165/3), also from the region of Seville (Ishbīliyah), is the nearest parallel to the examples from Tüpraş. It is 12.2 cm long and 4.5 mm in diameter. The tool is cylindrical, but the grip is squared and centered, composed of a double faceted diamond with square collars on either end and the center with minimal protrusion, Type 1b. The ends are rounded. One half of it was bent, like KT26459. This instrument is called a double probe or *specillum,* and Zozaya states that it was the most common tool.

The fourth tool is quite different and its provenance unknown (983–274–18). It is 14.5 cm long and square in cross section in the center grip, which is similar to the other tools. One end is perforated, allowing the passage of a thread, while the other is bifurcated into two points. Zozaya states that this probe is for the extraction of nasal polyps. The tools were made with the lost-wax method. Their chronology, from more reliably dated parallels in Spanish museums (which are unfortunately not shown), is the end of the tenth/beginning of the eleventh century.

A bronze tool very similar to those from Tüpraş was published as a color photograph and also from the Museo Arqueológico de Madrid. The decoration does not protrude and is of Type 1b: two diamond carved lozenges with flanking square collars and incised with three parallel lines and a central square collar.[24]

Chronology and Distribution

Based on the examples from Tüpraş and parallels, what can be surmised about the chronology and distribution of these specific tools? Obtaining a tight date is impossible at the moment due to the fact that they occur in poor or undocumented contexts. Generally, they can be seen as Early or Middle Islamic (eighth-thirteenth centuries) and not Roman, as Petrie thought. Although Islamic tools were very similar and most likely derived from Roman examples (see below), our specific tool with its polished bronze double rounded blunt ends and central decorated handle falling under one of four types of motif has no exact Roman parallel.[25] The Tüpraş excavations, only encompassing an occupation from the eighth to twelfth century, makes this last point fairly definite. Their context at Tüpraş, although unreliable, suggests that they are from the latest phase of the site: eleventh/early twelfth century. Hamarneh and Amin's work on the Fusṭāṭ material posits that they are seventh

24 De Morales and Molina 1999, 126. Two other tools, both seemingly of bronze, dated to the twelfth to thirteenth centuries appear in the Museo Arqueológico de Alicante and are published in color. One is pierced at one end and pointed at the other, as an awl or needle, and the other has a long thin shaft with one part twisted and one end a small spoon, *Ibid*, 216, 221.

25 See the work of Bliquez 1994 who catalogs tools mainly from Pompeii.

or eighth century or definitely pre-Faṭimid; however, this is not based on any evidence. Zozaya's comparison with well-dated parallels of the tenth/eleventh century in Spain is more convincing, although he does not illustrate his publication with these parallels. Their occurrence from contexts at Montfort allows for a later date of the thirteenth century. With finely crafted objects designed for a narrow range of functions, we have to consider the likely possibility of re-use of these specially designed tools. A safe dating would be between the ninth and thirteenth centuries, and a hypothetical one, the tenth and eleventh centuries, that is, the Faṭimid period.

Distribution shows that these tools were fairly common throughout the Islamic world and appear in some of the most major urban areas, from Nīshāpūr to Sāmarrā' to Fusṭāṭ to Seville and Cordoba. They also appear in mid-range towns near the Islamic-Byzantine frontier such as Ḥamā, Anṭākiya and Ṭarsūs, and even waystations, such as Ḥiṣn al-Tīnāt, and Crusader castles like Montfort. It can be deduced that they are of Islamic origin and not Byzantine, however, where they were manufactured is unknown at present.[26] The function of these tools can be best understood through textual corroboration.

Surgical Instruments in Medical Texts

The field of medicine, including pharmacology and surgery, was certainly known and practiced throughout the Early Islamic world. It was directly influenced by Roman and Byzantine texts. Literature on the subject of *de materia medica* after Dioscorides (from Anazarbus or 'Ayn Zarba, 40–90 CE) and Galen (from Pergamon, 131–200 CE) inspired translations and also stimulated studies and practice in the broader field of medicine in the Early and Middle Islamic periods. These treatises were mainly concerned with anatomy, pathology and the drugs themselves, with descriptions of plants and provenance in what could be classed as pharmacology.

Surgery was more obscure, and while there were volumes on instructing the surgeon, many of the authors had not necessarily practiced all the techniques, but were transmitting knowledge from Byzantine Greek sources.[27] Paulus of Aegina was a surgeon from Alexandria who lived around the time of the Islamic conquest in 642 CE and wrote seven volumes on medicine and surgery, the *De re medica*

26 There are about 180 tools in the Benaki Museum, 15 of which are nearly identical to those from Tüpraş Field, and most come from Egypt; however their archaeological contexts are unknown (Mara Verykokou, forthcoming). These, coupled with those from the Fusṭāṭ excavations, raise the strong likelihood that they were being produced in Egypt during the Faṭimid period.

27 Ullmann 1978, 44–45. Physicians sometimes mentioned that no one had actually performed or seen such a procedure performed before, and the ideas were taken from older (i.e. Greek) manuals. See Pormann and Savage-Smith 2007, 62, 121.

libri septem. His work was translated into Arabic by the Christian Ḥunayn b. Isḥaq al-Ibāḍī (808/809–873 CE) and became incredibly influential for Islamic doctors. Some later Byzantine treatises survive that discuss surgery and provide lists of surgical instruments that specify types of surgical tools. The Codex Parisinus Latinus 11219 (ninth century) has Latin names adapted from Greek of 66 tools. Another list is the Laurentianus gr. LXXIV 2 of the eleventh century with 89 entries. Both were published first by H. Schoene and then L. J. Bliquez.[28] Some included tools (knives) to use for tonsils, embryos, bladder stones, uvulas, fistulas and eyelids. The *Typikon* of the Pantocrator monastery gives instructions for the "sharpener" to keep, store and sterilize all manner of surgical instruments for a variety of ailments.[29]

As knowledge on surgery and surgical tools was transmitted from the Roman and Byzantine periods, the tools themselves also were strongly influenced from earlier periods. Most tools bore a basic shape that has remained relatively unchanged from the Roman period until today, as dictated by function. They were mainly of bronze with a specific tool at either end and most commonly with an embellished and raised center handle or grip, which implies both well-crafted and highly valued instruments that were also functional. Roman tools from the first-third centuries have been extensively studied, and they show the persistence of function and style into the medieval periods.[30] The Arabic inscription on the Ustinov spatula may be the maker's mark of a specialized craftsman.

Byzantine physicians' works, like the one by Paul of Aegina, directly influenced Abū al-Qāsim Khalaf b. al-'Abbās al-Zahrawī (known by his Latinized name Albucasis, *c.* 936–1013 CE), who was a Muslim surgeon who lived in al-Andalus and was from Madināt al-Zahra', outside of Cordoba. He has been regarded by some as the father of modern surgery. His book, *Kitāb al-tasrīf li man 'ajiza 'an al-ta'alīf* (*The Arrangement of Medical Knowledge for One Who is Not Able to Compile a Book for Himself*), is an important encyclopaedic text written as an instructional

28 Schoene 1903, 280–284; Bliquez 1984, 187–204.

29 For more on Greek and Roman surgical tools, see also Parani 2003, 204–205; Meyer-Steineg 1912; Tabanelli 1956, idem, Tabanelli 1958; Künzl 1983.

30 See Bliquez 1992, 35–36, figs. 2, 4, 5. He calls the decorated center a "knotty limb" pattern. A doctor's tool kit was found at Kyzikos (modern Balıkesir, Turkey) with a variety of instruments including two long probes/hooks with decorated handle: Heres 1992, 158–159. See the tools from Corinth, classified as "ear spoons" and "unguent spoons" and other spatulate instruments, as well as surgical tools, Davidson 1952, 181–182, pls. 82–84, where many are from Byzantine contexts and ultimately from "inconclusive evidence." For more on these, see Bliquez 1984, 187–188 where he states they are mainly dated to the ninth-twelfth centuries and thus contemporary with the Tüpraş tools. See Institut du monde arabe 2005, 175, pl. 103 for a set of Islamic two headed instruments with a decorated handle, dated eighth-twelfth century from Syria in the al-Sabah collection in Kuwait.

manual that became widely used in Europe and was translated into Latin, *Liber Alsaharavi de Cirugia,* in the late twelfth century by Gerard of Cremona and also to Hebrew in 1258 by Shem-Tov ben Isaac de Tortose.

There were other surgeons, who lived, practiced and wrote in central Islamic lands in the twelfth and thirteenth centuries. Abu Nasr b. al-Ayn Zarbī (d. 1153) was an Arab physician who worked in Baghdad and Cairo under the ʿAbbāsids and Faṭimids, respectively. He was native to ʿAyn Zarba, the home of Diuscurides and part of the Islamic-Byzantine frontier, and lived there under Saljūq rule. He wrote on surgery, as well as other medical fields in *al-Kafi fī Sina'at al-Tibb* and described instruments. Another Arab physician, a Melkite from Jordan, Abū al-Faraj b. al-Quff al-Karakī (1233–1286), was based in the citadel of Damascus and published a surgical manual entitled, *al-ʿUmdah fī ṣināʿat al-jirāḥah* (*Basics in the Art of Surgery*) and described instruments as well.[31] Zahrawī's volume, which discusses nutrition, the relationship between food and disease, diagnosis, medical specialization, pharmacology, diseases and symptoms and even doctor-patient relationships devotes its last (thirtieth) chapter to surgery. The chapter is divided into three parts: 1) cautery; 2) incision, puncturing, venesection, cupping, surgery on abscesses and removal of foreign bodies; 3) and treating broken bones and bandaging. He includes diagram illustrations of the roughly two hundred instruments necessary, many of which he created, with specific purposes.[32] Nearly all the instruments comprise an elongated metal tool with various ends (much like dentist's tools). While the instrument drawings are fairly diagrammatic and stylized and vary from each manuscript and translation, it is possible to find several that are near the examples from Tüpraş and their widespread parallels. As implied by the lengthy and first section of Zahrawī's thirtieth chapter on surgical techniques, cauterization (*al-kay*) was a common and popular form of medicine in the medieval Islamic world and recommended for all sorts of ailments. Cautery by fire (*al-kay bi-nar*) was recommended for the treatment for blood flow in arteries (for which it is still used today), infections around wounds, tumors and growths, amputation and matters related to ophthalmology. As a result, there were many different types of cautery tools.[33] For these procedures, the end of the tool would be heated to cauterize tissue. Several of the tools illustrated in Zahrawī's text are most similar to those from Tüpraş. As specific cauteries, they were used for treating a range of ailments that al-Zahrawī describes, such as removing tumors, treating stomach troubles, incising fistulae,

31 Ibn al-Quff 1994.

32 Institut du monde 2005, 169–171.

33 Bennion 1979, 183–184. Cautery is still practiced in many parts of the world today. For cauterization according to Greek and Roman authors, see Jackson 1986, 154–156.

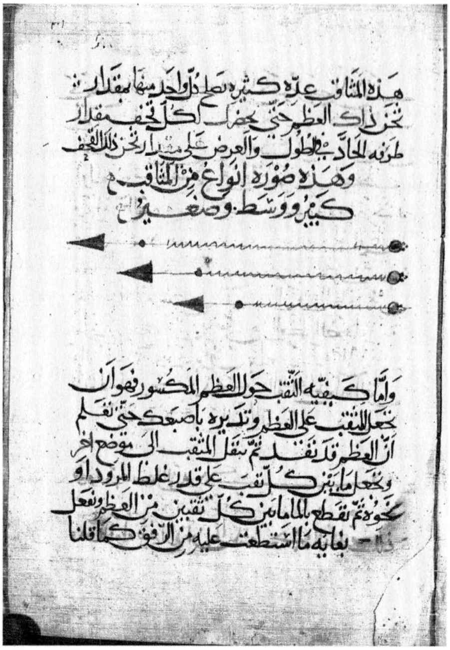

FIG 9. Page from *Kitāb al-tasrīf li man ʿajiza ʿan al-taʾalīf* by al-Zahrawī'. Khuda Bakhsh Oriental Library (India), manuscript no. 3146, (201 r.) (Courtesy of Bibliotheca Alexandrina).

treating haemorrhoids, penile warts and a variety of other orthopedic and genetic disorders. A long tool with a rounded probe on one end and diamond shaped opposite end had a central grip. It was used to treat a lachrymal fistula in the eye. Ideally, al-Zahrawī stated that the tool (called *al-makwāh* or *mismariya*) should be hollow, possibly perforated, but it could also be solid like a probe or stylet (*al-mirwad*).[34] Probe-type cauteries were used for treating liver tumors, spleen ailments, and a range of other maladies. Another tool with a central grip had pointed tips on either end. It was for the cauterization of the toothache. Al-Zahrawī gives some explanation for one purpose of the decorated central handle, stating that it should have some "thickness in the body of it so that the intensity of the fire does not reach the patient's mouth" (*wayakūn fī kharamhā bʿaḍ al-ghalṭ lʾllāl yuṣil ḥarr al-nār ilā fam al-ʿalīl*). After the physician held the cautery to the site "until the cautery gets cold" the patient filled their mouth with good butter and held it there before spitting it out.[35]

Probes, stylets, or explorers are described in the second section, where he discusses instruments for perforating or incising. The probe was also called *barīd*, *misbār*, and also *mirwad*. The *misbār* was perforated (like the awl/needle tool from Tüpraş and al-Andalus), allowing a thread to be used. Zahrawī stated these tools

34 Zahrawī 1973, 56–57.

35 Zahrawī 1973, 66–67. The treatment of butter appears to be a form of oil pulling.

should be round, polished, and smooth, like packing-needles, of Chinese copper or of white copper, or of brass, silver or iron. They were best used to treat fistulae, which are abnormal connections between organs or vessels. Probes could gauge their depth, resistance of the surrounding skin and the effect of the fistula on the bone. The *mirwad* was a small straight blunt probe used for eyelids, teeth, sinuses and inguinal hernia.[36] Spoon-probes (like those found in Ṭarsūs and al-Andalus) were given the same word or a variation, *mal'aqah al-marūd*. One example featured a small spoon at one end for applying a caustic or medicine and the other end a probe for removal of a tumor of the uvula. Hook probes (like in Anṭākiya) were for removing foreign object in the throat. Probes were derived from similar Greco-Roman tools, the Latin *specillum* or Greek *méle*. The spoon probe (like in al-Andalus, Ḥamā, Ṭarsūs) was derived from the Greek *spathoméle, cyathiscoméle, specillum auricularium* (an ear scoop).

Function

The function of the tools from Tüpraş and their parallels has been posited either as a tool for surgery or an applicator for kohl or other makeup. Based on the material and textual evidence, it seems clear that the primary function for this type of instrument was for use in medical procedures. That variations were found with more spatulate ends (al-Andalus) or hooks (Anṭākiya) suggests the existence of a range of tools, like a dentist's office, each one for a purpose. Indeed, sets have been discovered, such as the group of tools from Fusṭāṭ and a group of instruments from Syria from the eighth-twelfth century, published as surgical instruments. They range in length from 9.2 to 17.5 cm and are in the Sabah collection in Kuwait.[37] Each tool has one or two different tips, whether spatulate, 'olivary', double-pronged, or circular/spoon-like on one end and a rounded blunt tip at the other, while they are of the same family in having a decorated handle portion.

Based on material evidence, the specific tools from Tüpraş and around the Islamic world, a bronze probe with double rounded blunt ends and a central decorated grip seems the most widespread and common of these tools. It would be ideal if these tools matched one in Zahrawī's medical illustrations, however, despite the widespread distribution of our type of instrument, his treatise was written two centuries later across the Mediterranean and subjected to numerous recopies and versions of the illustrations.[38]

36 Zahrawī 1973, 348, fn. iv.

37 Institut du monde 2005, 175. Unfortunately, there is no specific provenance.

38 For example, see Hamarneh (1961), who discusses published drawings of Zahrawī and unpublished manuscripts and their variation.

Nevertheless, the general parallels for our tools appear either (or both) to be cauteries and probes.[39] Based on functions derived from the Islamic texts, this is perhaps unsurprising. The thickness of the grip would have insulated the user from the heat. A piece of fabric or leather could also have been used to insulate the user. They were made of either bronze or iron. The lack of an iron example from our parallels may be an indication of preservation or preference. Furthermore, the instrument could have been used for a wide range of medical procedures including ophthalmic and dental, most of which do not involve incision. Given the hesitation at the actual practice of surgery by Islamic physicians and the preference for procedures such as cauterization, it seems that our tool would have been easier to use and multi-purpose.[40]

The types of cauteries that Zahrawī illustrated are numerous, but the main ones are calviform (club or spade-shaped tip), olivary (olive- or spatulate-shaped end), circular (spoon end), punctuate (pierced) and lenticular. Probes carried similar designations. Those from Tüpraş and the other areas with close parallels are the double-bladed (derived from the Greek *apurenoméle, apuroméle* or Latin *specillum*) or even double-olivary variety (derived from the Greek *dipúrenos méle* or *amphísmilos*). Milne and Bliquez illustrate similar Italian examples that Greco-Roman medical authors state were used both as probes and cauteries and even for mixing medicaments.[41]

As one application of the "spoon-probe" was for applying medicine, there is no reason that it could have not been used for cleaning wounds with the help of a cloth wrapped around the instrument[42] or for the application of make-up. Indeed, Milne mentions that the probe was also used as an applicator, and the olivary-probe specifically resembled similar instruments, such as kohl-sticks, found in early Egyptian tombs with accompanying pigment boxes (such as the ones at Karanog).[43] Therefore, the function of a kohl-stick is but one use for these multi-functional instruments, which were primarily designed as surgical instruments.

39 See Milne 1976, 57.

40 Bliquez also argues, based on the popularity of cauterization and the dearth of obvious cauteries from Pompeii, that other tools also fulfilled this function, such as the small spatulate tools, or *ligulae*, in *Roman Surgical Instruments,* 1994, 45 D(f).

41 Bliquez 1994, 52, see nos. 209–212, 160–162. These are 17–18 cm long. He says that he groups numbers 221–230, which he identified as "socketed shafts" for the treatment of cataracts or used in cauterizing operations, p. 53. For the double simple probe see Milne 1976, 56, pl. 10, fig. 4 which has a raised ring and rounded tips and is 14.5 cm long, 2 mm thick. For the double-olivary probe/cautery see pl. 11, fig. 1 , 4. D, 56–58; Meyer-Steineg 1912, 22ff.

42 Many thanks to Mara Verykokou of the Benaki Museum for this suggestion.

43 Milne 1976, 55.

The Medical Trade

What were so many of the same exact surgical instruments doing in a small waystation on the Islamic-Byzantine frontier? These were not the only medically related objects found at Tüpraş Field. Several nearly complete glass vessels were recovered that were studied by C. Swan.[44] A small squat jar of light purplish glass 6 cm tall with a 3.5 cm diameter and 4.0 base diameter had a mold-blown honeycomb pattern of rounded indents and a short neck and slightly flared rim. This type of glass vessel is typically called an *albarello,* and its function has been suggested to store medicine. Parallels can be found in both Byzantine and Islamic lands that date to the eleventh-twelfth centuries.[45]

A second vessel is a small blue glass flask decorated with a series of opaque white trails in a "festoon" pattern and marvered. Although broadly dated to the eighth-thirteenth centuries, this example seems to date to the tenth-twelfth centuries. The blue variety may be Egyptian, while a purple variety is primarily Levantine. The contents may have been unguents or perfumes or kohl.[46] The third vessel is a molar flask 5–6 cm high and colorless. It dates from the ninth-eleventh centuries, and this class of vessel typically contained unguents or perfumes. The last glass vessel was a small teardrop-shaped flask of light olive green. These vessels dispensed liquid in single drops, and parallels from Fusṭāṭ were dated around 1000 CE and thought to have held drugs or perfume.

The first three vessels were most likely imported from Islamic lands bound for Byzantine lands and important for what they contained, whether medicines, perfumes, oils, or cosmetics. Imported glass from Islamic lands was present at Amorion. A fourth glass vessel was found in TF 19 (Locus 7, lot 7), which was a fill attributed to Phase III (tenth century), part of buildings built outside the walls of the fortified enclosure and a good context.It was part of a spout either from a cupping device for bloodletting or from an alembic (*al-anbīq*), a distilling device, often used in medicine.

Early Islamic evidence exists for glass vessels specifically manufactured to hold *materia medica*. From the Fusṭāṭ excavations, glass fragments from vessels were found with stamps or seals mentioning their contents, measurement and weight.[47] They are dated by identifying the officials named to the first half of the eighth century or Umayyad period. Many of the contents are foods or spices such as fava beans, hemp oil, lentils, anise, peas, sesame seeds, cumin seeds,

44 Swan 2012, Chapter 4.

45 For example, see Institut du monde arabe 1996, 147, fig. 68 from La Haye, Gemeentemuseum, OG (1) 369–54 from Iran, twelfth century.

46 For example, see Institut du monde arabe 1996, 213, fig. 155 from the National Museum of Damascus 602 A.

47 Hamarneh and Awad 2002.

aloe, and olive oil. Whether they were containers meant for shops or trade is unclear.[48]

Transportation of these substances is not often mentioned. Al-Bīrūnī mentions certain substances carried in small wooden boxes or leather bags and bottles. It is logical to assume that small glass bottles with limited volume capacity also functioned in this way. Too often, the vessel itself is regarded as a manufactured, imported, or traded item. However, glass bottles (which are preserved in the archaeological record, as opposed to wooden boxes or leather bags and bottles) were likely used to transport the precious and costly medical substances.

K. Durak argues convincingly and extensively, utilizing several medical texts and non-medical texts, for an active trade in medical substances between Byzantium and the lands of Islam.[49] While his research deals primarily with substances of pharmacology—plant, animal, and mineral—one can infer great significance to the medical trade. This trade between Byzantium and the Islamic World was a part of larger international commercial activity linking numerous networks. As Durak argues, it was so well established and significant that it continued past the Byzantine reconquest of North Syria (including the coastal strip where Tüpraş Field was located) in the late tenth century.[50] Trade of goods from Islamic lands to Byzantine lands actually appears to increase in the late tenth and eleventh centuries.[51] It is interesting to note that ʿAyn Zarba played a role in this as the home of both Dioscurides and Abu Nasr. Perhaps a medical school formed around Dioscurides in this Islamic-Byzantine frontier town?

The exchange of knowledge alongside a trade in medical implements and pharmaceutical substances contributed to an active medical trade between Islamic and Byzantine lands. Caught in the middle, the small frontier waystation and port of Tüpraş Field (Ḥiṣn al-Tīnāt) exhibited a range of glass vessels and specialized bronze tools whose primary function was medical. They likely had a number of secondary uses, among them as applicators for cosmetics. The five tools studied here, when examined alongside similar bronze tools as a group, show that they were found throughout the Islamic world from al-Andalus to Nīshāpūr between

48 Morton 1985; Miles 1985, 385.

49 Durak 2008, Chapter 2.

50 Durak 2008, 232.

51 The widespread distribution with the most frequent occurrence at Cairo, alignment of chronology and dating of other medical vessels may support other scholars who contend that the Faṭimid period witnessed an age of great growth and innovation in sciences, particularly the medical ones. This is in part due to the number of preserved texts, which mention hospitals and practitioners. Anees 1983, 61–93. The influence may have spread or risen independently in Islamic Spain during the period of the Umayyad Caliphate, as evidenced by the presence of tools there and of al-Zahrawī.

the ninth to thirteenth centuries, and hypothetically more narrowly, during the tenth and eleventh centuries. These specifically designed tools add to the existing corpus of Islamic metalwork as both objects of everyday use and finely crafted physical representations of scientific achievement in the early medieval world.

REFERENCES

Allan, J.W., *Metalwork of the Islamic World: The Aron Collection*. London: Sotheby's, 1986.

———. *Nishapur: Metalwork of the Early Islamic Period.* New York: The Metropolitan Museum of Art, 1982.

Anees, M.A., *Health Sciences in Early Islam*. Volume 1. *Collected Papers by Sami K. Hamarneh.* Blanco, ed. by M. A. Anees. Texas: Zahra Publications, 1983.

Baer, E., *Metalwork in Medieval Islamic Art.* Albany: SUNY Press, 1983.

Bénazeth, D., *L'art du metal au début de l'ère chrétienne.* Paris: RMN, 1992.

Bennion, E., *Antique Medical Instruments.* Berkeley: University of California Press, 1979.

Bliquez, L.J., "Two Lists of Greek Surgical Instruments and the State of Surgery in Byzantine Times." *Dumbarton Oaks Papers* 38 (1984): 187–204.

———. "Hercules Motif on Greco-Roman Surgical Tools" in *From Epidauros to Salerno: Symposium Held at the European University Centre for Cultural Heritage, Ravellow, April, 1990,* ed. by A. Krug, 35–50, PACT 341992.

———. *Roman Surgical Instruments and Other Minor Objects in the National Archaeological Museum of Naples.* Mainz: Von Zabern, 1994.

Davidson, G., *Corinth. Vol. XII The Minor Objects.* Princeton: American School of Classical Studies at Athens, 1952.

Dean, B., "The Exploration of a Crusader's Fortress (Montfort) in Palestine." *The Metropolitan Museum of Art Bulletin,* Part 2: "A Crusader's Fortress in Palestine: A Report of Explorations Made by the Museum 1926" 22/9 (Sept., 1927).

de Morales, C.A. and E. Molina, *La Medicina en al-Andalus*. Granada: Fundación El legado andalusí, 1999.

Durak, K., *Commerce and Networks of Exchange Between the Byzantine Empire and the Islamic Near East from the Early Ninth Century to the Arrival of the Crusaders.* Unpublished PhD Thesis. Harvard University, 2008.

Gascoigne, A., "Dislocation and continuity in early Islamic provincial urban centres; the example of Tell Edfu." *Mitteilungen des Deutschen Archäologischen Instituts, Abteilung Kairo* 61 (2005): 153–190.

Ginés, J.V. and J. Samsó, *El Legado Científico Andalusí,* April-June 1992. Madrid, 1992.

Hamarneh, S.K., "Drawings and Pharmacy in al-Zahrawi's 10th-Century Surgical Treatise." *United States National Museum Bulletin* 228 (1961): 82–94.

———. "Excavated Surgical Instruments from Old Cairo, Egypt." *Annali dell'Istituto e museo di storia della scienza di Firenze* 2 (1977): 3–14.

Hamarneh, S.K. and H.A. Awad, "Early Surgical Instruments Excavated in Old Cairo, Egypt." *International Surgery* 62/10 (1977): 520–524

———. "Medical Instruments" in *Fustat Finds: Beads, Coins, Medical Instruments, Textiles, and Other Artifacts from the Awad Collection*, ed. by J. Bacharach. Cairo: American University in Cairo Press, 2002.

———. "Glass Vessel Stamp Data for Materia Medica" in *Fustat Finds: Beads, Coins, Medical Instruments, Textiles, and Other Artifacts from the Awad Collection* ed. by J. Bacharach. Cairo: American University in Cairo Press, 2002.

Heres, H., "Ein römisches Arztkästchen aus Kyzikos" in: *From Epidauros to Salerno: Symposium Held at the European University Centre for Cultural Heritage, Ravellow, April, 1990,* ed. by A. Krug, 157–166. PACT 34 1992.

Holth, S., *Greco-Roman and Arabic Bronze Instruments and their Medico-Surgical Use.* Kristiania: Kommission Hos Jacob Dybwad, 1919.

Ibn al-Quff, Ya'qūb ibn Isḥāq, *Al-'Umdah fī ṣinā'at al-jirāḥah.* Amman: Maṭb'ah al-Jāmi'ah al-Urdunnīyah, 1994.

Institut du monde arabe. *La médecine au temps des califes:à l'ombre de l'Avicenne: exposition présentée du 18 novembre 1996 au 2 mars 1997.* Paris: Institut du monde arabe, 1996.

Institut du monde arabe. *L'Age d'or des sciences arabes: exposition présentée à l'Institut du monde arabe, Paris 25 octobre 2005–19 mars 2006*. Arles: Actes Sud; Paris: Institut du monde arabe, 2005.

Iraq Government Department of Antiquities. *Excavations at Samarra 1936–1939. Part II Objects*. Baghdad: Government Press, 1940.

Jackson, R., "A Set of Roman Medical Instruments from Italy." *Britannia* 17 (1986): 119–167.

Künzl, E., *Medizinische Instrumente aus Sepulkralfunden der römischen Kaiserzeit* Cologne: Reinland Verlag, 1983.

Marshall, J., *Taxila. 3 Volumes*. Cambridge: Cambridge University Press, 1951.

Melikian-Chiryani, A.S., *Islamic Metalwork from the Iranian World, 8th–18th Centuries.* Victoria and Albert Museum Catalogue. London: Her Majesty's Stationery Office, 1982.

Meyer-Steineg, T., *Chirugische Instrumente des Altertums: ein Beitrag zur antiken Akiurgie.* Jena: G. Fischer, 1912.

Miles, G.C., "Egyptian Glass Pharmaceutical Measures of the 8th century CE." *Journal of the History of Medicine and Allied Sciences* XV (1985): 384–389.

Milne, J.S., *Surgical Instruments in Greek and Roman Times.* Chicago: Ares Publishers, 1976.

Morton, A.H., *A Catalog of Early Glass Stamps in the British Museum.* London: British Museum Press, 1985.

Özyar, A., O. Pancaroğlu, E.Ünlü and A. Vokaer. "Tarsus-Gözlükule Kazılarında Ele Geçen Erken İslami Dönem Buluntuları Hakkında Bazı Gözlemler." *KST* 28 (2016): forthcoming.

Petrie, Sir W.M.F., *Objects of Daily Use.* Encino, CA: Joel L. Malter & Co., 1927.

Ploug, G., E. Oldenburg, E. Hammerschaimb, R. Thomsen and F. Lokkegaard, "Les petits objets médiévaux sauf les verreries et poteries" in *Hama: Fouilles et Recherches 1931–1938.* Copenhagen: Carlsbergfondet, 1969.

Pormann, P.E. and E. Savage-Smith, *Medieval Islamic Medicine.* Washington, D.C.: Georgetown University Press, 2007.

Porter, V. and M. Rosser-Owen, *Metal Work and Material Culture in the Islamic World: Art, Craft, and Text. Essays Presented to J. W. Allan.* ed. by V. Porter and M. Rosser-Owen. London: I.B. Tauris, 2012.

Schoene, H., "Zwei Listen Chirurgischer Instrumente." *Hermes* 38 (1903): 280–284.

Swan, C,. *In Flux: Glass, Technology, and the Glassmaking Industry of the Middle Byzantine and Early Islamic Eastern Mediterranean—The Archaeology and Archaeometry of a High-Temperature Craft.* Unpublished PhD Thesis. Brown University, 2012.

Tabanelli, M., *Chirurgia nell'antica Roma.* Torina: Minerva Medica, 1956.

———. *Lo strumento chirurgico e la sua storia dale epoche greca e romana al secolo decimosesto.* [Forli]: Romagna medico,1958.

Ullmann, M., *Islamic Medicine.* Edinburgh: Edinburgh University Press, 1978.

Viguera, M.J. and C. Castillo Castillo, *El Esplendor de Los Omeyas Cordobeses: La Civilización Musulmana de Europa Occidental.* Granada: Junta de Andalucía, Consejería de Cultura a través de la Fundación El Legado Andalusí, 2001.

Warland, R., "Der Gegenstand im Bild Zur Kontextualisierung von Realien in der byzantinischen Wandmalarei Kappadokiens" in *Byzantine Small Finds in Archaeological Contexts,* ed. by B. Bohlendorf-Arslan and A. Ricci. *Byzas 15.* İstanbul: Ege Yayınları, 2012.

Woolley, C.L. and D. Randall-MacIver, *Karanòg: The Romano-Nubian Cemetary.* Vol. 3. Philadelphia: University Museum, 1910.

al-Zahrawī, Abū al-Qāsim Khalaf ibn 'Abbās. [*Albucasis*] *On Surgery and Instruments: a definitive edition of the Arabic text with English translation and commentary* [*Kitāb al-tasrīf li man 'ajiza 'an al-ta'alīf*]. Trans. by M. S. Spink and G. L. Lewis. London: Wellcome Institute of the History of Medicine, 1973.

Ziffer, I., *Islamic Metalwork.* Tel Aviv: Eretz Israel Museum, 1996.

Zozaya, J., "Instrumentos quirurgicos andalusies." *Boletin de la Asociación Española de Orientalistas* 20 (1984): 255–259.

Ottoman Identity as Material Culture

Fahri Dikkaya [1]

Abstract

Historical sources place the foundation of the Ottoman state at the end of the 13th century.[2] However, it is not possible to say that the material culture in the archaeological record reflects the same phenomenon. This paper will discuss the relationship between Ottoman identity in its early stages of emergence and archaeological remains with particular focus on the identification of material culture significant to early Early Ottoman identity.

Introduction

The Ottoman state came into existence sometime around 1300 as a small principality in northwestern Anatolia, on the frontiers between the Anatolian Seljukid Sultanate and the Byzantine Empire. This small principality was founded by Osman I, and it was named after him in accordance with Turkish patrimonial tradition. This initial period of Ottoman history presents a transformation from a rather insignificant frontier principality into an empire.

The Mongol invasions reached the Near East in the 1220s, and following the Mongol victory at the Battle of Kösedağ in 1243, the Anatolian Seljukid Sultanate became a vassal state of the Ilkhanids in Iran. The immediate result of the Mongolian invasion was the westward migration of Turkmens into the mountainous regions of western Anatolia. The Turkmens rose up against the Mongols in 1277. Thus, over the period from 1260 to 1320, Turkmens founded a number of independent principalities in western Anatolia, among them the Germiyanid, the Karamanid, the Menteşe and the Aydinid. While these principalities were static, the Ottomans followed a dynamic conquest policy in the Balkans, and sometimes in Anatolia as well. The first attempt by the Ottomans to unify Anatolia was undertaken by Bayezid I, but failed after a crushing defeat at the Battle of Ankara in 1402. During the interregnum following this defeat, the Anatolian principalities reestablished themselves.

---

1 Department of History, Bilkent University, 06800 Ankara, Turkey.

2 All dates are CE unless stated otherwise.

The Ottomans recovered, and stability returned during the reigns of Mehmed I and Murad II (between 1413 and 1451), owing to the fact that durable institutions of the Ottoman state had survived in the Balkans. According to İnalcık, “after Timur’s blow to [the] first Ottoman empire under Bayezid I, the center of gravity of the state shifted to the Balkans.”[3] In other words, the Ottoman dominion was re-established by Mehmed I and Murad II in the Balkans. In Anatolia, it was Mehmed II who established Ottoman dominion. A very long process of Turkish conquest, settlement, and political unification in Anatolia, which had begun with the Battle of Manzikert in 1071, was finally achieved with the final Ottoman reunification brought about by Mehmed II in the late 15th century.[4]

Pottery

In this period, the main characteristic feature of the material culture of the Anatolian principalities was red fabric and fine glazed painted wares consisting of Slip Painted Ware, Turkish Sgraffito Ware, Glazed Monochrome Painted Ware, Impressed Ware, and Miletus Ware. The most common type is Miletus Ware, first recognized by Friedrich Sarre during excavations at Miletus in 1939.[5] The most common forms include everted rim deep bowls with a low flaring ring foot and high, concave walls; and everted flanged rimmed large dishes with low a flaring ring foot and concave walls.[6] Floral or geometric ornaments around a central motif (such a flower rosette, rosette, or sunburst) were the most common decorative patterns. The typical fabric of this pottery tradition is orange-reddish to reddish with some lime and many fine micaceous inclusions.[7] Red clay is very characteristic of this pottery tradition. The production of these wares is dated to a period between the 14th and 16th centuries. Archaeological research has shown that these painted wares were actually produced in several towns in Anatolia, such as İznik, Kütahya, Konya, Çanakkale, Ankara and Miletus.[8] They were distributed from Troy and Miletus in the west to Korucutepe in Elazığ and Samsat in the east.[9] The

3 İnalcık 2005, 13.

4 Vryonis 1971, 104.

5 Sarre 1939, 341–345.

6 Crane 1987, 53.

7 Vroom 2005a, 157.

8 For İznik, see Aslanapa 1987; Aslanapa, Yetkin and Altun 1989; Fındık 2001, 36–84. For Kütahya, see Paker 1964–1965, 157; Şahin 1979–1980, 261. For Çanakkale, see Hayes 1995, 205; Akarca 1979, 503. For Miletus, see Sarre 1935, 72.

9 Crane 1987, 53; Parman 2002, 74; Parman, Parla and Bursalı 2006, 5; Aslanapa 1987; Aslanapa, Yetkin and Altun 1989; Fındık 2001, 36–84; 2003, 106; Paker 1964–1965, 157; Şahin 1979–1980, 261; Hayes 1995, 205; Hayes 1992; Akarca 1979, 503; Sarre 1935, 72; Vroom 2005b, 24–26; Deveci 2003, 125; Ünal 1974, 27.

production centers and patterns of distribution indicate that the wares were a common element of material culture in Anatolian principalities. In fact, following the publication of Oktay Aslanapa's articles about Miletus Ware in İznik,[10] Mükerrem Paker criticized the periodization of this pottery type as "Early Ottoman," instead identifying them as "Anatolian Principalities Pottery."[11]

By the end of the 15th century, a different pottery tradition began in Anatolia, in both fine tablewares and unglazed common wares. This glazed pottery tradition was named *İznik Ware* by Aslanapa because of the location of its production.[12] The comprehensive analysis of this pottery is provided by J.W. Hayes in his published volume on the pottery from the Saraçhane excavations,[13] and İznik tiles and pottery were first given a typology by Arthur Lane.[14] In Lane's view, this pottery could be divided into three main groups according to the colors used for its decorative themes. The first group dated to 1480/90–1525/30 was termed the İznik I or "Abraham of Kütahya" type. İznik I is characterized by its blue painted decoration on a white surface. The second group, termed the İznik II or "Damascus" type, was dated to 1525–1560. İznik II has a polychrome decorative scheme, but the well-known red color of İznik ware had not yet been applied to this type. The final group, the İznik III or "Rhodian" type, was dated to 1555–1700, and is characterized by green, İznik red (or 'tomato-red') and blue, with decorative black lines painted on. In addition to this typology, there are two other types, namely the "Golden Horn" type dated to 1510- 1540, and the monochrome vessel type dated to 1550. The shapes of İznik pottery include highly decorated large dishes with a ring base and everted rim, deep bowls of different sizes with a ring base, and delicate jugs.[15] A notable difference from the previous tradition dating to the 14th and 16th centuries is that the body of vessels in these groups is composed of a hard, compact, and fine off-white clay with quartz frit. White clay is very characteristic of this pottery tradition.

Identity

Once the centralist and absolutist Ottoman system in Anatolia and the Balkans was completed by Mehmed II following the conquest of Constantinople, the city, now İstanbul and the new capital of the Ottomans, became the symbol of

10 Aslanapa 1965a; 1965b.

11 Paker 1964–1965.

12 Aslanapa *et al.* 1989.

13 Hayes 1992.

14 Lane 1957a, 45–60; Lane 1957b.

15 Atasoy and Raby 1994, 38–39.

Mehmed's ambition for a universal empire.[16] Thus, the transformation from state to "empire" created a new phenomenon based on an immense and unprecedented Ottoman identity. This phenomenon was nourished by the supposed notion of a glorious past as a disinterred historical truth created through atavistic memory. In this context, Oghuz and his son Gök Khan, the most important name in Oghuz geneology, were mentioned amongst the Ottoman dynasties' ancestors by the chroniclers. The first Ottoman chronicles –such as those of Aşıkpaşazade, Neşri, and İbn Kemal –were written during this period. These chroniclers composed a genealogical work by introducing a descent from Qayi. Thus, these chronicles record the glorious past of the early Ottomans through Oghuz mythology and their kinship with the early Seljukid sultans as a way of legitimizing their immense universal history. The policies of Mehmed II and his successor Bayezid II founded the imperial state system and the novelty of its Ottoman. Thus, the Ottoman Empire reassembled a heterogeneous Anatolia and the Balkans under an Ottoman rubric, reflecting a homogeneous and holistic Ottoman identity as a universal form in its mentality. As such, Mehmed II styled himself as a Roman emperor, the ruler of the two continents and two seas.[17]

As a reflection of this new phenomenon, material culture was transformed into a new style, entailing radical modifications. The heterogeneous and common material culture of the first pottery tradition, characterized by Miletus Ware, was a product of a disparate Anatolia and distributed throughout the Anatolian principalities. Therefore, it cannot be described as exclusively Ottoman. On the other hand, the second pottery tradition, characterized by İznik Ware by the end of the 15th century, reflects a homogeneous and imperial Ottoman identity. Therefore, this pottery tradition can be identified as one of the first examples of a truly Ottoman material culture. This applies to architectural development in the Ottoman Empire as well. According to Kuran, there are three successive stages of Ottoman architecture:[18]

> In the first stage, deviating Seljuk practice as used in a single dome in front of the mihrab or a row of triple domes for special effects, and each bay of the traditional hypostyle mosque was placed under a dome. In the second stage, a larger dome was erected at the center of the hall. In the final stage, the smaller bays surrounding the big central space were integrated under half domes on one, two, three, or four sides.[19]

16 İnalcık 2005, 17–18.

17 İnalcık 2005, 18.

18 Kuran 1968, 202.

19 *Ibid.* 1987, 18.

The first and second stages can be seen in the Anatolian principalities, but the final stage can only be described as Ottoman. According to architectural historians,[20] the Mosque of Bayezid was erected as an imperial mosque complex in Istanbul by Bayezid II in the years 1501–1506. It represents the beginning of the classical period in Ottoman architecture. Both İznik Ware and the architecture of the classical period lasted into the middle of the 17th century.

Conclusion

In conclusion, Ottoman archaeological material culture can only be identified as a distinct phenomenon from the late 15th century, although Ottoman political history actually begins at the end of the 13th century. The archaeological data between the 14th and 16th centuries possesses heterogeneous and transitional features common to all contemporary Anatolian principalities. The transformation of the Ottoman state into an "empire" by Mehmed II and his unification of Anatolia and the Balkans under Ottoman dominion were what created a uniform "Ottoman" material culture. Consequently, it is problematic to identify Miletus Ware and other similar material culture as Ottoman. The homogeneity of the material remains from this period of the initial stages of the Ottoman state's formation is questionable. To resolve this dispute, "Late Medieval Turkish Pottery" has been deemed acceptable as a general name for the Turkish pottery of this period.

20 Meriç 1958; Öz 1936; Necipoğlu-Kafadar 1986; Necipoğlu 1991; 2010.

REFERENCES

Akarca, A., "Çanakkale'de Yeni Bir Çanak Çömlek Merkezi" in *VII. Türk Tarih Kongresi, Kongreye Sunulan Tebliğler* (vol. I), 501–506. Ankara, 1979.

Aslanapa, O., "Kırmızı Hamurlu İlk Osmanlı Keramikleri." *Türk Kültürü* 3 (1965a): 35–43.

———. *Türkische Fliesen und Keramik in Anatolien.* İstanbul: Baha Matbaası, 1965.

———. "Osmanlı Devri Keramik Sanatı." *Antika* 27 (1987): 4–8.

Aslanapa, O., Ş. Yetkin and A. Altun, *The Iznik Tile Kiln Excavations.* İstanbul 1989.

Atasoy, N. and J. Raby, *Iznik: Pottery of Ottoman Turkey.* London: Thames & Hudson, 1994.

Crane, H., "Some Archaeological Notes on Turkish Sardis." *Muqarnas* 4 (1987): 43–57.

Deveci, A., "Bilecik Orhan Gazi İmareti Kazısında Bulunan Seramikler" in *Anadolu Tarikat Yapılarına Bakış (13–15. YY.). Bilecik Orhan Gazi İmareti Kazı Sonuçları,* ed. by E. Altınsapan, 125–135. Eskişehir, 2003.

Fındık, N.Ö., *İznik Roma Tiyatrosu Kazı Buluntuları (1980–1995) Arasındaki Osmanlı Seramikleri.* Ankara: T.C. Kültür ve Turizm Bakanlığı, 2001.

———. "Turkish Glazed Pottery" in *Amorium Reports II, Research Papers and Technical Reports* ed. by C.S. Lightfoot, BAR International Series, 105–118. Oxford: British Archaeological Reports, 2003.

Hayes, J.W., *Excavations at Saraçhane in Istanbul* (vol. 2). Princeton: Princeton University Press, 1992.

———. "A Late Byzantine and Early Ottoman Assemblage from the Lower City of Troia." *Studia Troica* 5 (1995): 197–210.

İnalcık, H., *An Economic and Social History of the Ottoman Empire I: 1300–1600.* Cambridge: Cambridge University Press, 2005.

Kuran, A., *The Mosque in Early Ottoman Architecture.* Chicago: University of Chicago Press, 1968.

———. *Sinan, the Grand Old Master of Ottoman Architecture.* İstanbul: Ada Press, 1987.

Lane, A., *Later Islamic Pottery: Persia, Syria, Egypt, Turkey.* London: Faber & Faber, 1957a.

———. "The Ottoman Pottery of Iznik." *Ars Orientalis* 2 (1957b): 247–281.

Meriç, R.M., *Bayezid Camii Mimarı.* Ankara 1958.

Necipoğlu, G., *Architecture, Ceremonial and Power: The Topkapı Palace in the Fifteenth and Sixteenth Centuries.* Boston: The MIT Press, 1991.

———. *The Age of Sinan: Architectural Culture in the Ottoman Empire.* London: Reaktion Books, 2010.

Necipoğlu-Kafadar, G., "Plans and Models in 15th–16th Century Ottoman Architectural Practice." *Journal of the Society of Architectural Historians* 45 (1986): 224–243.

Öz, T., "Eski Cami Planları ve Tarihi Vesikalar." *Yedigün* 172 (1936): 4.

Paker, M., "Anadolu Beylikler Devri Keramik Sanatı." *Sanat Tarihi Yıllığı* 1 (1964–1965): 155–182.

Parman, E., "Eskişehir Karacahisar'da Ortaçağ Kalesi" in *V. Hacettepe Üniversitesi Edebiyat Fakültesi Sanat Tarihi Bölümü Ortaçağ Kazı ve Araştırma Sempozyumu,* 70–75. Ankara 2002.

Parman, E., C. Parla and M. Bursalı, "Eskişehir (Merkez Karacaşehir Köyü) Karacahisar Kalesi" in *Kazı Sonuçları Toplantısı* 28/2 (2006): 1–12.

Şahin, F., "Kütahya Çini ve Keramik Sanatı ve Tarihinin Yeni Buluntular Açısından Değerlendirilmesi." *Sanat Tarihi Yıllığı* 9–10 (1979–1980): 259–273.

Sarre, F., "Die Keramik der Islamischen Zeit von Milet" in *Das Islamische Milet,* ed. by K. Wulzinger, P. Wittek and F. Sarre, 341–345. Berlin-Leipzig, 1935.

———. "Die Fayencen von Niceea und ihr Export nach dem Abendland." *Pantheon* 24 (1939): 341–345.

Ünal, İ., "Antalya Bölgesinde Çinili Eserler." *Etnografya Dergisi* 14 (1974): 15–28.

Vroom, J., *Byzantine to Modern Pottery in the Aegean: An Introduction and Field Guide.* Utrecht: Brepols, 2005a.

———. "Medieval Pottery from the Artemision in Ephesus: Imports and Locally Produced Wares" in *Spätantike und mittelalterliche Keramik aus Ephesos,* ed. by F. Krinzinger, 17–49. Vienna: Österreichische Akademie der Wissenschaften, 2005.

Vryonis, S. Jr., *The Decline of Medieaval Hellenism in Asia Minor and the Process of Islamization from Eleventh through the Fifteenth Century.* Berkeley: University of California Press, 1971.

PART 7

Archaeological Science, Heritage and Ethnoarchaeology

Synthesis of Geoarchaeological Research around Kinet Höyük, Hatay, Turkey

Timothy Beach — Sheryl Luzzadder-Beach — Jonathan M. Flood[1]

Abstract

The factors of environmental change in any region are complicated, especially so in the Mediterranean with its seismicity, geomorphic and vegetation diversity and long history of varied land uses. Here we consider three of the most important aspects of environmental history: soil erosion, sedimentation and soil and water geochemistry. Based on our own field studies and others in the Hatay province of Turkey, the most intensive erosion occurred during and at the end of the Roman period. Exemplifying this, the ancient Roman road on the alluvial plain near Kinet Höyük is buried by 1–6 m of alluvium and the Roman road through the Amanus Mountains is eroded by as much as 2 m. In contrast to the degradation, soil and agricultural systems were also being built up extensively during the Roman period, as we observed in the foothills above Kinet. Another major period of Mediterranean environmental change was the Little Ice Age period, more than a millennium later, which many sources link with landscape instability. Although our research focused on landscape instability from the middle Holocene, and especially during or after the Roman period, the Little Ice Age was another period of environmental dynamism, which would likely show up with wider research in the drainage basin. Another line of evidence that also bears witness to human use and impacts on this environment is geochemistry. We show that there are distinct geochemical signatures of human activities associated with eras and with sites. Four metals, cadmium (Cd), mercury (Hg), lead (Pb) and strontium (Sr), indicated the largest differences between archaeological and natural loci and had higher means for anthropogenic loci (streets, rooms, floors and artifacts). Mercury, cadmium and lead varied the most across eras, and all three elements peaked in the Medieval and Bronze Ages, showing medium to high levels in Hellenistic and Modern samples and lowest levels in the Iron Age sites. Elevated phosphorus (P) on the *höyük* also indicated higher human enrichment and pollution potentials. An analysis of surface water and groundwater mineral characteristics in the region indicates potential for good water quality in support of domestic and agricultural

1 Department of Geography and Environment, University of Texas at Austin, 305 E 23rd Street, CLA 3.306, A3100, Austin, TX 78712, USA.

needs, as reflected by the long-term geologic controls on water chemistry. This would be outside of anthropogenic pollution potentials from runoff from human activities such as smelting and animal herding. The groundwater analysis showed that the dissolved ion load reflects the local geology and is mainly from calcium and bicarbonate, with a noticeable contribution from sulfate, and a high electrical conductivity.

Introduction

Every sedimentary sequence tells a somewhat different story. Such sequences come from lakes, floodplains or any other long- or short-term resting place for sediment cascading downhill. Every layer indicates some aspect of the energy, timing, local environment and watershed, agents of erosion and transport and *in situ* weathering. Geoarchaeology, soil science, sedimentology and geomorphology, among others, study these sediments and their history. Indeed, one floodplain or lake often tells a very different story from an adjacent valley or even from a different floodplain within the same valley. Nonetheless, larger patterns emerge from synthesis of enough depositional sequences, though it may take many studies and years of research.

Likewise, historical geographers and historians as well as archaeologists sift through historical documents from multiple sources to show myriad human actions and responses in different environments. Over time they build local accounts into larger stories, which may reflect larger historical or environmental trends. Human interactions with the environment are as complicated as the multiple scientific lines of evidence, and several fields have grown up around these complicated interactions: geography, historical ecology, political-cultural ecology and geoarchaeology.

This chapter assesses the environmental history of Kinet Höyük and its watershed based on sedimentary, erosion and geochemical evidence and compares it with surrounding watersheds of the Hatay region to understand the big drivers of environmental change. Sediments, and their implied erosion, are a key but highly complicated proxy for understanding environmental change around the world.[2] Our studies from the Kinet area found that the Roman Period witnessed the greatest quantity of environmental change, though access limited the geographic scope of our surveys. We also must consider all environmental factors as geomorphic drivers, such as climatic variation in the change from moister to drier conditions in the sixth century CE around the "536 CE Event",[3] the Medieval

2 Beach *et al.* 2008, 301–331; 2009, 1710–1724; Luzzadder-Beach *et al.* 2011, 119–129; 2012, 3646–3651.

3 McCormick *et al.* 2012, 169–220.

Climate Anomaly (MCA) and the Little Ice Age (LIA). Sediment geochemistry provides important evidence about the patterns and impacts of human activity through space and time, and water chemistry allows a window on the geologic influences and potential limiting factors on water use in this environment.

Environmental Background

Kinet Höyük[4] lies on the alluvial plain of the northern tip of the Bay of İskenderun, in a region of great dynamic forces and multiple drivers of environmental change[5] (Fig. 1). The *höyük*, near the mouth of the Deli Çay, collects water and sediments from the coastal-alluvial plain, foothills and the Amanus (or Nur in Turkish) Mountains. The alluvial fans and plains developed here over 5 million years of coalescing deltas and fans, forming a piedmont along the sinking Amanus front.[6] The Quaternary (last 2.6 million years) deposits alone are about 10–20 m thick,[7] though one of our excavations displays 6 m of alluvium deposited in only the last 2000 years.[8]

The Amanus Mountains are composed of Paleozoic sandstone and siltstone, and quartzite and ophiolite rocks, with limestone and serpentine thrust from the bottom of ancient seas above younger rocks. This geological dynamism results from an active tectonic triple junction of plates, in which the African Plate is jammed in the middle of the Anatolian Plate on its west and Arabian Plate on its east. The mountains rose as they folded up between the Plates in a NE-SW running anticline.[9] The Amanus are still rising at about 10 cm per 1000 years, or about 5 cm since the historical sources first mentioned the range.[10] The Amanus zone also has a small strike-slip or transform motion.[11]

There have been at least four major historical earthquakes in the region, including one earthquake in 1268 CE that devastated Cilicia.[12] Three other large, nearby, historical earthquakes occurred at *c.* 500 BCE,[13] 50 CE,[14] and the great earthquake of 551 CE. Archaeoseismicity is a young field but of interest to envi-

4 Gates 2004, 405–416.

5 Woodward 2009.

6 Erol 1991, 99–102; Mülazımoğlu 1979; Ozaner and Russell 1995, 135–151.

7 Doyuran 1982, 151.

8 Beach and Luzzadder-Beach 2008, 416–428.

9 Lyberis *et al.* 1992, 1–15.

10 Bridgland *et al.* 2003, 1080–1089.

11 Yurtmen *et al.* 2002, 207–246.

12 Ganse and Nelson 1981.

13 Pirazzoli *et al.* 1991, 295–311.

14 Ozaner and Russell 1995, 135–151.

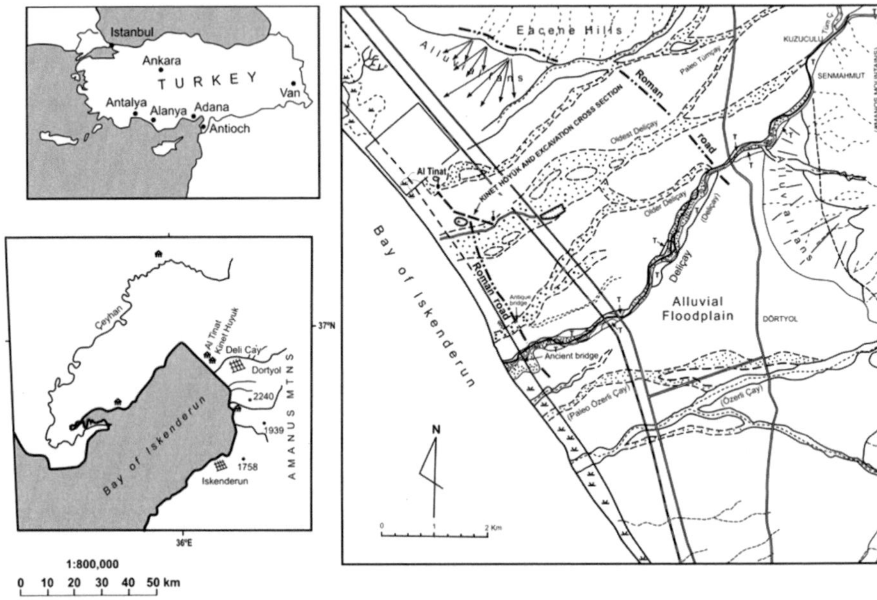

Fɪɢ. 1 Maps of the Kinet region and the Eastern Mediterranean (after Beach and Luzzadder-Beach 2008).

ronmental history since earthquakes can have major impacts on the environment, such as triggers for landslides and sedimentation.[15] For example, a series of major tectonic events in early Byzantine times, around the 551 CE event, affected the wide region momentously. Seismic events can lead to high rates of landslides, erosion, offsets of architecture, dramatic fluctuations in groundwater levels and temperature, and large scale surface changes that have major impacts on river systems and settlements.[16] Altunel *et al.* reported more than 30 historical earthquakes since 184 BCE for the northern part of the Dead Sea Fault east of the Amanus Mountains. A 6.2 magnitude earthquake occurred outside Adana in 1998 and caused major structural damage within the city and up to 150 km away from the epicenter.[17]

The Amanus region is also climatically diverse, ranging from semi-aridity caused by rainshadow east of the Taurus, Misis, and Amanus Mountains to high humidity and precipitation (rising above 2300 mm per year) produced by air currents rising and cooling as they climb up the mountain front. Near Kinet, the average temperature is 19.7°C with a range moderated by the surrounding mountains

15 Keefer 1994, 265–284.

16 Nur and Cline 2000, 43–63; Nur and Burgess 2008; Contadakis and Asteriadis 1993, 333–337.

17 Çelebi 2000, 283–288.

that block continental air masses and the sea. Precipitation is also high, with a mean of 1080 mm, but it varies highly from year to year.[18] The seasonal rainfall is more typical of Mediterranean climates with wet winters and dry summers.[19]

The Amanus has similar forests to those of the Balkans and Black Sea at elevations above 750 m but has a more typical Eastern Mediterranean ecosystem below 750 m. Tree species here are generally soil specific with limestone formed soils being dominated by Turkey oak (*Quercus cerris*) and Oriental hornbeam (*Carpinus orientalis*), while sandstone formed soils are dominated by Oriental beech (*Fagus orientalis*) and black pine (*Pinus nigra*). On lower slopes, Turkish pine (*Pinus brutia*) is dominant with an undergrowth of Holm oak (*Quercus ilex*) and hornbeam. Ravines are dominated by laurel (*Laurus nobilis*), with linden (*Tilia argentea*) and yew (*Taxus baccata*). Near the tree line, around 2200 m above sea level, black pine and Clicician Fir (*Abies cilicica*), and reportedly some Lebanon Cedar (*Cedrus libani*), give way to shrubs or herbs of the genera *Lamiaceae* and *Eremurus*.[20] Surprisingly, Kehl could not find serpentine rock ecosystems (often patchy and depauperate), despite the wide regional distribution of such rocks and the high frequency of these 'serpentine barren' associations around the world.[21]

Attempts to study paleoecology and paleoclimatology in cores from regional wetlands and lakes have been met with poorly preserved pollen and other fossil proxies, perhaps because of the region's alkaline pH, often above 8 in soils and groundwater.[22] Regional paleoecology studies are quite distant, 200 km westward in the Taurus and 100 km southeastward and in a much drier climate. These are important because they bring to bear one of the largest drivers of environmental change, namely, flooding, which in Europe and the Mediterranean is associated with cooler periods.[23] Among the most cited paleoecology studies come from the sediments of Lake Van and speleothems of Soreq Cave, some 600 km west and south of Kinet, respectively.[24] Lake Van's oxygen isotope and trace element records show that the most profound drying occurred during the Younger Dryas, *c*. 12,900–11,500 BP at the end of the Pleistocene, periodic and significant drying in the Middle and Late Bronze Age and in the Hellenistic and Roman periods at a time when land-use and human population pressures accelerated.[25] The Bar-Mat-

18 Beach and Luzzadder-Beach 2008, 416–428.

19 Erinç 1955, 363–391; Kehl 1998.

20 Kehl 1998.

21 Kehl 1998; Kazakou *et al.* 2008, 495–508.

22 Beach and Luzzadder-Beach 2008, 416–428.

23 Butzer 1969; Macklin *et al.* 2006, 145–154.

24 Wilkinson 2005, 169–192.

25 Lemcke and Sturm 1997; Wilkinson 2005, 169–192.

thews *et al.*[26] cave study uses speleothem oxygen isotope ratios and analogs of modern precipitation, which provide cross cutting lines of evidence. The Soreq cave record shows a similar pattern, but with the maximum aridity from about 5000 to 7000 BP, a jump to higher rainfall about 5000 BP, decreasing rainfall up to 2000 BP, an increase until *c.* 1500 BP, increased drought until 1300 BP, and steady conditions over the last millennium.[27] A speleothem record from southern Turkey's Kocain Cave, *c.* 500 km west of Kinet, provided more nuance for the last 2 millennia: steady moisture from 2000 BP to 1400 BP, drying from 1400 to 1300 BP, steady effective moisture until 700 BP, when another hundred year drying period occurred and instability to 400 BP, stable, moist conditions to 200 BP, and then drying conditions up to the increased moisture conditions of the last century.[28]

We still await a reliable paleoclimate study from the Hatay, which should have plenty of sites for speleothem work because of the region's numerous caves. Given that the Kinet climate is wetter and more humid than many other parts of the region, the surrounding records may be less useful for the climate influences on the historical trajectory of Kinet. Nonetheless, the main climatic drivers of landscape change are the abrupt and large changeover from the wetter Pleistocene to the very dry Younger Dryas at 12800 BP; the rapid change around 11500 BP to the wetter and warmer early Holocene through the Holocene Thermal Maximum to another abrupt drying around 4200 BP followed by a longer dry regime until around 2000 BP; steady conditions until the cooler and dryer interlude from 1500 to 1400 BP; warmer conditions in the MCA; and colder conditions in the LIA, followed by warming in the last century. Several records indicate deteriorating conditions in the sixth century CE,[29] especially in terms of cold, come from all over the world and may be connected to a large volcanic eruption.[30]

The first historical mention of the Amanus occurred in Bronze Age cuneiform documents, referring to the range as a source for Cedar (*Cedrus libani*), boxwood (*Buxuus longfolia*), and cypress (*Cupressus sempervirens*). Thus lumbering, likely together with fire, may have had the first important human impacts, since timber was probably cut high in the mountains and slid and then floated east down the Aksu into the Euphrates and west down into the Mediterranean.[31] Redford *et al.*[32] note that early Arabic sources cited al-Tīnāt (which we now think is just

26 Bar-Matthews *et al.* 1998.

27 Orland *et al.* 2009, 27–35.

28 Graham *et al.* 2011, 1217–1245.

29 Büntgen *et al.* 2011, 578–582.

30 McCormick *et al.* 2012, 169–220.

31 Rowton 1967, 261–277.

32 Redford *et al.* 2001.

meters northwest of Kinet) as a timber-exporting frontier fort during the early Arab expansion.[33] This implies timber harvesting in the Amanus and foothills and sliding and floating the trees down the Tüm Çay and Deli Çay (rivers) during high runoff in winter and spring. Nineteenth century sources report both that the Amanus Mountains had extant forests[34] but deforested conditions around one port.[35] Forest cover is still extensive today across the range.[36]

Environmental History of Erosion and Sedimentation in the Eastern Mediterranean

The history of human impact on the Mediterranean environment provides a rich context for Kinet. Human impact was probably imperceptible in the Early Holocene, even with the nearby earliest domestication of plants and animals and use of fire (though there is a lively debate about the "early Anthropocene" hypothesis that humans have influenced climate from 7,000 BP onward and ecosystems since the late Pleistocene.[37]) For the Amanus and regions eastward, Wilkinson has noted that the early to mid-Holocene cultures (Neolithic, Chalcolithic, and Bronze Age) focused their settlement on river valleys and low plains, and that only in later first millennium BCE did empires expand onto the uplands and marginal steppes.[38] Classical Greek civilization arose about this time, and many papers have recounted Classical Greek writers on erosion and land degradation, as evidence of an eroded landscape or a degraded civilization or both.[39]

Two scientists, Butzer and Vita-Finzi, are especially important for bringing the question of Mediterranean erosion into prominence by focusing on sedimentary sequences.[40] Butzer interpreted sediment stratigraphy to be multifaceted, but Vita-Finzi hypothesized two general layers: an upper and younger layer, colored gray or yellow, dating from the third century CE to the last century and a lower and older layer colored red with Paleolithic artifacts, formed from the Late Quaternary.[41] He argued the ubiquity of these layers was evidence for

33 Redford *et al.* 2001; Eger 2010, 49–76.

34 Rowton 1967, 261–277.

35 Seton-Williams 1954, 126.

36 Beach and Luzzadder-Beach 2008, 416–428.

37 Ruddiman 2003; 2013; Kennett and Beach 2013, 88–100; Braje *et al.* 2014, 26–29.

38 Wilkinson 2005.

39 Kraft *et al.* 1975, 1191–1208; Eisma 1978.

40 Butzer 1964; Vita-Finzi 1969; Van Andel 1998, 361–390, Wilkinson 2003; Cordova 2008, 443–457; Casana 2008, 429–442.

41 Butzer 1964; 1980; Vita-Finzi 1969.

a climatic change driver sometime during the Roman period. Although these general facies are common in valley fills,[42] subsequent studies have interpreted many more sediment layers, regional diversity and multiple drivers.[43] To be sure, some still interpret climate as a principal driver.[44] The World Systems sociologist Tabak[45] synthesized many sources[46] to argue for a higher incidence of "deluges" during the Little Ice Age in CE 1320, 1600, 1700, and 1810, and the 1320 event corresponds to increased flooding around Europe.[47] These bred flooding and erosion and mass wasting and the formation of coastal swamps. Tabak was looking for high magnitude and long duration impacts. This can be a controversial area today, however, because of the slippery slope toward environmental determinism. Tabak carefully navigated away from environmental determinism by following the intricate interactions of three *longue durée* drivers of change in this large and unwieldy region.[48] These were the Little Ice Age (1300–1450 and 1550–1870), the shift in the center of world-economic power to northwestern Europe (1590s-1830s) and the economic downturn known as the 17th Century Crisis (1620/1650–1730/1750). The Little Ice Age had two major effects: colder temperatures (and lower evapotranspiration) and "deluges," both of which caused increased flooding of valleys and coastal plains. This increased wetness in the lowlands vexed traditional cereal farming, and, along with the economic and demographic contractions of the 17th century, caused cereal to withdraw upslope. Two of these factors, the increased intensity of rainfall and the intensified land use on the slopes, would also have accelerated erosion and valley sedimentation. Others have attributed the building out of river deltas to Post-Glacial sea-level rise,[49] and still others have interpreted human-induced landscape alteration from farming, livestock, and deforestation.[50] Brückner and colleagues have studied many cores and geophysical data and differentiated multiple mechanisms, from tsunamis to Hellenistic and Roman accelerated erosion.[51]

42 Beach and Luzzadder-Beach 2008, 416–428; Casana 2008, 429–442.

43 E.g., Kraft *et al.* 1975, 1191–1208; Eisma 1978; Butzer 1980; Davidson 1980; Van Andel *et al.* 1990, 379–396; Van Andel 1998, 361–390; Butzer 2005, 1773–1800; Fuchs 2007, 349–356.

44 Faust *et al.* 2004, 1757–1775; Verschuren *et al.* 2000, 410–414.

45 Tabak 2008.

46 Especially Grove 2001; Grove and Rackham 2001.

47 Macklin *et al.* 2006, 145–154.

48 Tabak 2008.

49 Kayan 1999, 541–548.

50 Van Andel 1998, 361–390.

51 E.g., Brückner 2003; Brückner *et al.* 2006, 63–83.

The Amuq Valley, to the east of the Amanus from Kinet, provides a nearby and comparable record, though with half the rainfall.[52] In a series of publications, Wilkinson discerned a varied and complicated chronology of erosion and sedimentation.[53] Overall the studies demonstrated large-scale, upslope population movements, intensive slope erosion, and high sedimentation in alluvial plains and on foothills during the Roman period. Similarly, a study near Petra in southern Jordan using pollen from Syrian rock hyrax middens, suggests deforestation of Jordan's Mediterranean forests from *c.* 100–300 CE, during Roman rule of the region, transforming the area into scrubland from forest. Central Spain provides a more distant but parallel Mediterranean record, with increased deforestation and erosion and sedimentation with Roman administration of this area after 80 BCE, moister conditions from *c.* 100–400 CE, and followed by increased aridity and the complete desiccation of the lake around 715 CE.[54] Around the Mediterranean are many other local examples of deforestation, accelerated flooding, and erosion,[55] especially widespread evidence for over the last two centuries from increased human impacts and the Little Ice Age.[56] As indicated by Kaplan's meta-analysis,[57] scholarship agrees that deforestation occurred across the Mediterranean during the Roman period, and that the climate changed to greater aridity after 400 CE.

Because of the evidence for multiple drivers of environmental change in the form of soil erosion and sedimentation, more and more have argued for the coincidence of multiple factors such as climatic together with human induced land use changes.[58] The factors could be amplified and may reach tipping points for high magnitude change.

Alluvial Exposures in the Watershed around Kinet Höyük

Our lines of evidence for the environmental history around Kinet include sedimentary sequences exposed along riverbanks and within excavations and erosion scars in uplands. Essentially, we divided this landscape into three parts—mountains, foothills, and the coastal plain—but there are other parts we assume play smaller roles, and each part we recognize has multiple subdivisions that play roles in the cascade of sediment. Security concerns have limited our access to the

52 Wilkinson 1999, 555–571; Wilkinson 2003; Casana 2008, 429–442.

53 Wilkinson 1999; 2003; 2005; 2010.

54 Curras 2012, 31–53.

55 Rosen 1997, 396–416; Van Andel 1990, 379–396.

56 McNeill 1992.

57 Kaplan *et al.* 2009.

58 Bintliff 2002, 417–435; Butzer 2005, 1773–1800.

mountain and foothill regions and to high resolution maps and air photos. Hence, we focused on the plain around Kinet, which is an aggrading and sinking alluvial plain about 10 km west of the Amanus Mountains. The plain has been built by streams that have left their steep mountain canyons carrying high sediment loads by meandering and avulsing (rapidly changing) their courses. The main channel has been the Deli Çay to the south of Kinet, but a northern stream, the Dikilitaş, through an arm called the Tüm Çay has also flowed spasmodically back and forth across this plain. Indeed, the Tüm Çay was once an independent stream, but the Deli Çay has pirated it through channel migration.[59] Ozaner provided the main, earlier geomorphologic research around Kinet, formulating a history of changing river channels based on historical aerial photography and field studies.[60] Overall, since Kinet Höyük's Neolithic founding, the alluvial plain built out (prograded) by *c.* 500 m into the Bay of İskenderun, assuming the *höyük*'s early settlement was indeed coastal, though we should note that coastal sites are prone to the brunt of the sea and its many whims. The plains around nearby Kara Höyük and Muttalip Höyük prograded similarly,[61] as did other parts of the Turkish coast such as Ephesus and Miletus.[62] The channel also shifted periodically, with an early baseline, Mid-Holocene channel passing north of Kinet Höyük. Subsequently, into the Hellenistic period, the river ran to a harbor and port to the south of the mound. Later in the Hellenistic to Roman era, when Kinet Höyük was abandoned until the 13th century, the river migrated 2 km farther southward. In the last few hundred years, the stream moved another 500 m south to its current channel.[63] So much abstraction of the stream's flow has probably limited further migration to extreme events that overwhelm the modern water diversion infrastructure. Otherwise, a wilder Deli Çay may reoccupy some of the other channels that we suppose are older, though they may still act as distributary channels for large and rare events.

Stream channels are both meandering and braiding over the plain, which has created a plain of coarse channel sediments and fine overbank deposits when stream leave their channels during high magnitude floods. Current streams have incised into their channels, creating shallow canyons with steep alluvial cutbanks ranging from 4 m near the coasts to 12 m high near the foothills. Based on numerous cutbank exposures, the alluvial plain has 2 to 3 buried surfaces that indicate some periods of regional stability and instability. The current topsoils are

59 Ozaner and Russell 1995, 135–151.

60 Ozaner 1995, 513–527.

61 Ozaner 1995, 513–527.

62 Beach and Luzzadder-Beach 2008, 416–428; Brückner 2003; Brückner *et al.* 2006, 63–83; Stock *et al.* 2013, 57–69.

63 Ozaner and Russell 1995, 135–151.

moderately developed soils formed in 85 to 150 cm deep loams and sandy loams with gravel, cobble, and boulder layers. The 20–30 cm deep, dark brown topsoils have formed in sediments that lie above a moderately developed paleosol (earlier topsoil surface). This upper paleosol in the profile is common at about 1–1.5 m deep and is dominated by Roman or Hellenistic artifacts and building foundations that along with radiocarbon evidence argues for a date from 2300 to 1700 cal. BP.[64]

A second paleosol occurs buried at 2.5 m, 1 to 1.5 m below the Roman/Hellenistic soil. This moderately developed clay loam soil had associated Bronze Age and unidentifiable, eroded ceramics and a radiocarbon sample in the soil dates to 3975–3705 cal. BP. This later Bronze Age paleosol was built on 1 to 2.5 m of loamy sediments with ceramics throughout, which reach down to a third paleosol, found beneath these sediments buried by 4 to 5.2 m of sediment. This paleosol is distinct in the Deli Çay cutbanks, but converges with the overlying paleosol on the Tüm Çay and Özerli Çay. Like paleosol 2, paleosol 3 is a clay loam soil, and above it are associated Bronze Age ceramics, and one radiocarbon date is Chalcolithic at 5925 to 5710 cal. BP. Paleosol 3 formed in low energy, fine alluvium, with stronger red hues, and it lies above a high energy cobble and gravel layer that has been cemented by calcium carbonate. Red hues may have come from long periods of soil formation or from erosion from more weathered, older Red Mediterranean soils such as terra rosas.[65] They are probably a combination of both, with the older weathered soils lying below red sediments deposited from the earliest erosion of the upland red, weathered soils. In the Deli Çay channel, the high energy cobble and gravel are now cemented to form a calcrete conglomerate. It is clear this occurred in some portions of the Bronze and Iron Ages as well, because buildings at Kinet used these as building stones. Paleosols 2 and 3 have evidence of significant human use in more sherd and tile scatters and a longer period of soil formation than the modern and Roman/Hellenistic soils, including more clayey textures, greater weathering in the B horizons and evidence of clay translocation. The Roman topsoils had the highest levels of phosphorous and artifacts, probably indicating the most intensive human inputs.[66]

The second striking aspect of regional geomorphology is that sometime between the Chalcolithic and Early Bronze, the river had high competence, i.e., boulder-sized serpentine exposed in its present channel about 4 m lower in the landscape. The evidence for this is the present channel has cut through a cemented boulder and gravel bed sandwiched by two paleosols with artifacts and charcoal dated to 5925–5710 and 3975–3705 cal. BP at depths of 5.15 and 3.4 m.

64 All radiocarbon dates at the 95% probability.

65 Atalay 1997, 247–260.

66 Beach and Luzzadder-Beach 2008, 416–428.

The second lowest paleosol (paleosol 3) occurs in many exposures across the region from the foothills to near the coastline and is significantly different from the other alluvial soils. It is buried by 5 to 7 m in the alluvial plain and deeper in some parts of the bajada that rings the Amanus front. The paleosol lies below the calcrete conglomerate in each exposure from the foothills into the alluvial plain. This soil shows the most intensive pedogenesis: it is the only clay textured soil in the alluvial plain, with 48% clay (39% fine clay), dark red colors, great depths (more than 1 m in a Tüm Çay exposure) and is the only paleosol with highly weathered gravels. We found no evidence for artifacts in this paleosol in alluvial contexts, though similar soils form the modern surface in older foothill and high terrace landscapes. Since it lies at least 1 to 3 m below high energy sediments and the mid Holocene paleosol, it probably represents a surface from the late Quaternary. All of these lines of evidence point to an older stable surface with high rates or a long period of weathering and much lower rates of erosion and deposition. The boulder calcrete in many exposures indicates the low energy environment of the underlying paleosol gave way to high energy deposition at some period, perhaps due to base level changes, river channel changes, or Pleistocene high energy runoff.

About 500 m inland from the coast and parallel with Kinet, at and below modern sea level, the oldest paleosol merges with a layer that may represent the ancient coastline. These sediments are a series of sands and sandy clays deposited at shoreline—beach and low energy estuarine swamp deposition, respectively. The coastline inundated up to 500 m inland in the past but not at a higher elevation. Sea levels reached near present levels about 5,000 to 6,000 BP, and in many parts of the Mediterranean and the world, these earliest high stands reached far inland before receding as streams have prograded with high sediment loads accelerated in many places by human impacts.[67]

Taken together, the aggradation evidence, thus far based on radiocarbon dates and many artifacts, suggests a long-term rate of *c.* 1 m per millennium. Aggradation proceeded in three waves, starting with the filling of sediments on top of Late Quaternary terra rosa and other paleosols, soil formation in this fill, aggradation during the Bronze Age, pedogenesis of the Bronze Age fill, aggradation during and after the Hellenistic and Roman periods, and then spotty instability in Medieval times. Stream channel dredging and stream divergence in the last three decades has greatly altered stream channels and the sediment supplies for coasts all over the Mediterranean.

67 Brückner 1998.

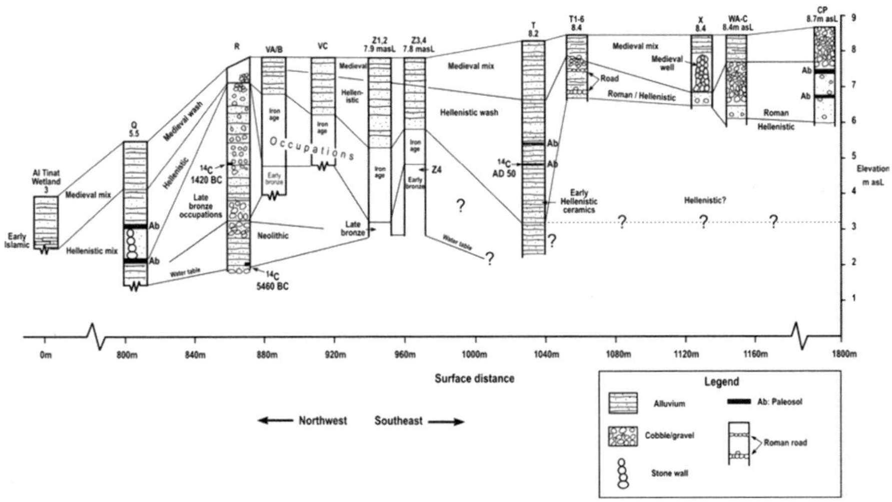

FIG. 2 Excavations and Eras of Deposition around Kinet Höyük (after Beach and Luzzadder-Beach 2008).

Excavations around Kinet Höyük

Beach and Luzzadder-Beach reported findings from 15 excavation units along a 1000 m transect northwest to southeast adjacent to Kinet Höyük (FIG. 2).[68] This excavation transect reached to depths of 7 m and pointed to a complicated history of sediment burial and alluvial plain formation (FIG. 2). The whole region has a 1–2 m cover of Hellenistic and Medieval sediments as dated by artifacts and ceramics, though some areas have much deeper post-Hellenistic aggradation. One area of the coastal plain covering about 100 m of the transect was an off-mound tell of Early Bronze to Iron Age date, which had been built up through the eras by collapses, middens, floods, and reoccupations. What is left of this smaller occupation is *c.* 3–4 m higher than the surrounding plain sediments through the Iron Age, and the remains of a small Bronze Age occupation is about 3–4 m above the plain as well. Both of these indicate the wider expanse of Bronze and Iron Age settlement beyond the *höyük*.

One larger area became buried in a surrounding glut of Hellenistic to Late Roman alluvium of up to 6 m depth in one excavation. High energy cobbles and gravels through this zone and finer silts indicate that channel flows and overbank floods were occurring through this period as the channel was filling and migrating southward. This zone of excavations, the Ts, also uncovered a segment of the Roman Road that provides both insight into the region's Roman past and

68 Beach and Luzzader Beach 2008.

evidence for the floods that buried it. Exposed in four excavations over a 50 m span were a lower Roman Road, more than 10 m wide in places, at 1.6 m deep from before the fourth century CE, and an upper, narrower Roman Road, buried by another 1 m of flood sands and gravels. By the Roman period, Kinet Höyük's 20 m high mound had been abandoned for the migrating river's banks at Roman Issos, 2 km south, where a Roman bridge, connected to the buried Roman roads, stands testament today above the buried channel and abreast the Issos settlement. The upper Roman road was probably still near the surface during Medieval times, because a well-worn surface associated with the upper road dated to CE 1180 to 1280, and Early Islamic ceramics occurred at this level. Moreover, this road ran in the direction of the fort along the elevated fault scarp that parallels the coastline. The upper Roman road at Kinet had been buried again by later Medieval flooding, which may be associated with Little Ice Age floods that many scholars such as Tabak[69] recount.

These lines of data indicate that 3–4 m of the *c.* 6 m of Hellenistic to Roman sedimentation around this landscape had occurred before the lower Roman road. Hence Hellenistic through Late Roman environmental change was rapid, and given how much of the human landscape was buried, another, lower, buried road may be present, though for preservation purposes, we could not excavate below the lower road. Still, despite the river's 2.5 km post-13th century flooding, much of the landscape was buried again, probably as large scale floods periodically filled older, subsidiary channels.

Excavations around Hisn al-Tīnāt

More insight into the region's environmental history came from excavations around the eighth-tenth centuries Tüpraş Field site, 800 m northwest of Kinet and which we now identify with the Early Islamic *thaghr* Hisn al-Tīnāt.[70] If the multiple lines of evidence for drying from the fifth to seventh centuries CE are a guide for this region, by the time of Hisn al-Tīnāt the climate was becoming wetter (or we should also note that geomorphic events such as stream capture or seismicity may have reactivated flow in the paleo Tüm Çay) and thus more conducive to floating logs out of the Amanus.[71] Most of the excavations occurred on the local summit of a broad, low rise, above the plain. These parallel the excavations at Kinet in that the top 1 m is largely Medieval, but unlike Kinet this has an Early Islamic level.

69 Tabak 2008.

70 Eger 2010, 49–76.

71 Orland *et al.* 2009, 27–35.

The al-Tīnāt excavations revealed the fort was mostly buried by collapsed mud brick and flood, aeolian silts and fine sands. One excavation downhill and seaward revealed an early Islamic wetland and paleosol level buried by 120 cm of high energy gravels and river worn ceramics and glass. The buried level had an extraordinarily rich sequence of well preserved ceramics and bone adjacent to large, parallel-lying wood logs. We have interpreted this level as a midden along the edge of a harbor or port, perhaps where the paleo Tüm Çay met the sea. The map of paleo stream channels (FIG. 1) indicates the Tüm Çay and/or Deli Çay coursed to the south of al-Tīnāt in what must have been a deep enough channel to transport lumber. These were then buried by deep layers of medieval alluvium after site abandonment.[72]

Results of Erosion around Roman Road in Foothills

An underlying impulse for this research from the start has been the long and ongoing debate about the cause of Mediterranean erosion. Around the region are numerous landscapes that are eroded, and many studies for decades have attempted to answer when and what caused this landscape degradation over this broad region.[73] These questions are keys to the fundamental problems of landscape formation and human-environmental sustainability. The next line of evidence in this paper derives from field surveys into the eroded foothills of the Amanus Mountains. These surveys indicated that the Roman period had by far the most intensive investment in rural infrastructure or *landesque capital,* including another Roman road through the Amanus, Roman-Byzantine farmsteads, extant Roman terrace systems and a buried Roman dam. This expanded Roman settlement footprint is also evident in the neighboring Amuq watershed.[74]

The Roman road through the Amanus zigzagged over the steep hillslopes and created bare expanses, where runoff could concentrate and erode the landscape. Indeed, after less than 2 millennia, the deep channels have dissected the road up to 2 m deep and as much 1 m into serpentine bedrock. Abandoned and unmaintained roads are notorious locales of sediment production in landscapes[75] because they allow the direct impacts of raindrops, little infiltration, concentrated turbulent flows into ruts, piping below the road construction and waterfalls where the road turns for a switchback.[76] Indeed, because of concentrated runoff cascading off switchbacks, erosion away from a road is often more extensive than on the road.

72 Eger 2010, 49–76.

73 Butzer 2005, 1773–1800; Butzer 2012, 3632–3639.

74 Gerritsen 2008, 241–314.

75 Wilkinson 1993, 548–562; Wilkinson 2003, 31; Bekker-Nielsen 2004.

76 Luce and Wemple 2001, 111–232.

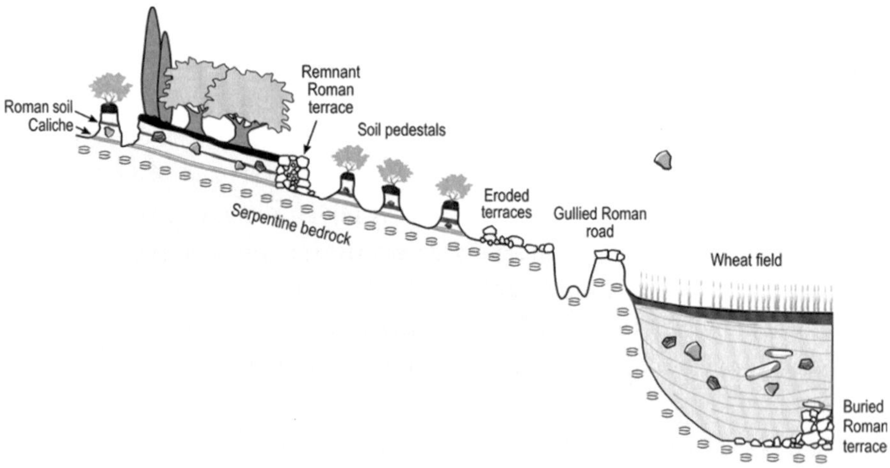

FIG. 3 Landscape diagram from the Amanus Lower Slopes

No evidence was available to date road gullying, but a Roman villa and farmstead near the route of the Roman road provide some insight into Roman landscape erosion connected to sedimentation (FIG. 3). The site has the remains of the foundations of villas with columns, mosaics, abundant ceramics and masonry. Around it are gullies that have incised into the soil surface by 1–3 m in depth through the soil and into serpentine bedrock, leaving a field of pedestal soil remnants capped by Holm oaks (*Quercus ilex*) that lead upslope into an extant Roman agricultural terrace that has been breached in places by the gullies (FIG. 3). The gullies thus have sliced into soils, providing extensive exposures of stratigraphy. These soils have a consistent profile of 50–100 cm, which reveal a thin buried soil filled with Roman artifacts about 30–50 cm below the surface, sitting unconformably atop a 20 cm thick layered caliche, or K horizon, built on weathered serpentine bedrock. The caliche horizons form from CaCO3 precipitating beneath a soil profile from long periods of CaCO3 leaching from the overlying soils.[77] This sequence is complicated, but the half of the exposed soil profiles with the Ab horizons are young soils, formed only since Roman times, because abundant Roman artifacts occur through the layers to the caliche layer. These soils are rich in phosphorous, calcium and magnesium, indicative of a short period of leaching in an environment with high potential for leaching. Thus, these are soils largely formed behind Roman terraces *c.* 2000 years ago. The thick caliche, however, indicates more leaching from deeper soil profiles and longer time periods, and hence, the Roman terraces

77 Birkland 1999, 127.

signify that much of the landscape was eroded when the terraces were built, perhaps as attempts to curb and compensate for earlier erosion.

But dating soil erosion from a surface is notoriously difficult on the relatively short timescales involved; we can only conclude the soils eroded after some baseline and stopped centuries ago for topsoils to form. We know the soils existed since the Roman period because of the remnant soil pedestals that correspond to the Roman terrace and building foundations. To get at the question of when erosion occurred, we studied deposition at several sites, including downslope from the Roman terraced upland, where there are Roman field terraces that are buried by stream channel and floodplain sediments. One 4 m deep exposure here revealed a Roman or Hellenistic terrace from *c.* 2000 years ago that is buried by 4 m of alluvium, and another blown-out terrace from *c.* 1400 years ago is buried by 2 m. Hence, 2 m of sediment deposited in this floodplain in 600 years old, and another 2 m has been deposited since that time. Another nearby slope exposure revealed a buried level at 1.75 m that dated to *c.* 1360 years ago and one at 0.55 m that dated to 1300 years ago. Moreover, deeper sediments in depositional sequences are more red in color, indicative of erosion from iron oxide-rich, older and more weathered red soils that formed over millennia, whereas shallower soils are more green in color, indicative of freshly eroded serpentine bedrock leftover after the red soils were exhausted.

These dates and measurements represent only one part of the Kinet watershed where authorities permitted research, but they give an indication of soil erosion and deposition in Roman and Late Roman times, as well as the rich *landesque capital*, the terraces and other rural infrastructure, invested in the landscape at this time.

Elemental Chemistry around Kinet

Another line of information for environmental history of a region is the elemental chemistry record in surface samples on habitations and rural sites. Beach and Luzzadder-Beach found very high levels of phosphorous on the *höyük*, especially through dense occupations, and some paleosols near the main *höyük* settlement.[78] This indicates significant human enrichment, possibly to the extent of water pollution. But the rest of this section synthesizes and expands on research we presented in more detail in Luzzadder-Beach *et al.*[79]

We collected soil samples systematically by age, archaeological setting, and natural situation. The archaeological age divisions were Bronze and Iron Ages,

78 Beach and Luzzadder-Beach 2008.

79 Luzzadder-Beach *et al.* 2011.

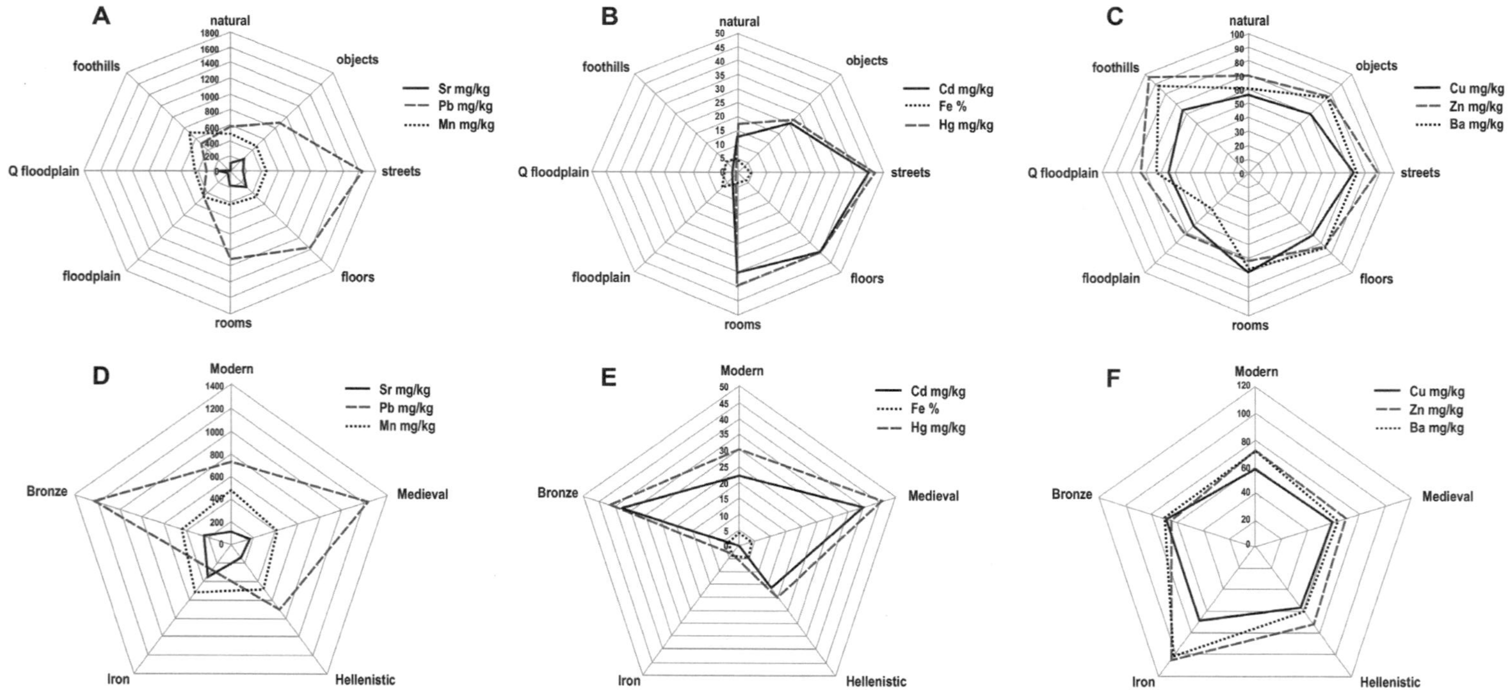

FIG. 4 Radar Diagrams of Kinet, Turkey ICP-NP Trace Element Analysis mean concentrations by site types (A-C) and ages (D-F). Samples digested in nitric and perchloric acid. Concentrations determined by ICP-AES, n=51 (from Luzzadder-Beach, Beach *et al.* 2011).

Hellenistic, Roman, Medieval and Modern eras. Natural (geomorphic) settings include such landscape positions as floodplains, hill-slopes, terraces, soil horizons, and bedrock. We compared samples by locus (4A-C) and by era (4D-F), and their mean elemental chemistry values (Fig. 4). The line lengths of each spoke of the radar charts in Fig. 4 indicate the mean concentration of the elements, and each spoke on the radar chart indicates a different sample locus or a different era.

Site and Typology Analysis

Using ICP-AES with a total acid digestion (nitric-perchloric acid[80]), we determined the concentrations of nine metal elements for 51 samples. We classified these samples according to mean concentration by site and by the archaeological ages of each deposit (see Table 1a & Table 1b).[81]

Elemental Comparisons by Locus

For each locus, we compared heavy metal means for archaeological (anthropogenic) settings with means for natural settings. We also compared these measurements to crustal averages for the region.[82] As reported by Luzzadder-Beach *et al.*[83] the four metals that indicated the largest differences between archaeological and natural loci and had higher means for anthropogenic loci (streets, rooms, floors and artifacts) were cadmium (Cd), mercury (Hg), lead (Pb) and strontium (Sr) (Fig. 4). Cadmium and lead levels for the anthropogenic settings of streets, floors and rooms exceeded both natural and crustal means; in fact, the natural settings also exceeded crustal averages.[84] Mean lead (Pb) concentrations (896 to 1643 mg/kg) for anthropogenic settings also exceeded natural (290–586 mg/kg) and crustal (16 mg/kg) averages for the region. Luzzadder-Beach *et al.*, and Chiarucci and Baker[85] point out that the geology of Kinet includes elevated levels of metals in its serpentine rocks, which may explain why both sets of means exceed broader regional crustal averages. Strontium (Sr) is associated with ocean sediments and the shells of organisms, and the crustal average for the region is 300 mg/kg.[86] Floor deposits and artifacts exhibited higher Sr means than for natural sites, yet lower

80 Luzzadder-Beach *et al.* 2011, 119–129.

81 See also Luzzadder-Beach *et al.* 2011 for more tables of detailed individual results.

82 See Herz and Garrison 1998, 196; Chiarucci and Baker 2007, 1–2.

83 Luzzadder-Beach *et al.* 2011.

84 Luzzadder-Beach *et al.* 2011, 119–129.

85 Luzzadder-Beach *et al.* 2011; Chiarucci and Baker 2007.

86 Luzzadder-Beach *et al.* 2011, 119–129.

TABLE 1A. Kinet Elemental Analysis means by site (a) and age (b), n=51 (from Luzzadder-Beach *et al.* 2011).

	NATURAL	OBJECTS	STREETS	FLOORS
CHEMISTRY				
Ba mg/kg	60.4	76.4	74.5	75.1
Cd mg/kg	12.8	25.6	45	39.8
Cu mg/kg	55.7	59.9	71.9	62.1
Fe %	5.1	3.5	4.4	4
Hg mg/kg	17.6	26.8	47.2	39.2
Mn mg/kg	500.8	457.6	457.9	462.7
Pb mg/kg	585.6	896	1642.7	1367.3
Sr mg/kg	106.4	226.1	159.3	282.7
Zn mg/kg	69.8	77.1	88.5	73.4
	ROOMS	FLOODPLAIN	Q FLOODPLAIN	FOOTHILLS
CHEMISTRY				
Ba mg/kg	68.4	36.7	63.4	88.2
Cd mg/kg	35.5	2.4	1.9	2.1
Cu mg/kg	70.2	53.3	55	64
Fe %	3.7	7.3	4.7	5.7
Hg mg/kg	40.1	0.9	3.2	0.7
Mn mg/kg	428	452.1	439.8	712.3
Pb mg/kg	1120.6	464.5	290.4	501.5
Sr mg/kg	186.6	41.9	136.8	0
Zn mg/kg	62.8	61.6	73.8	96.4

than the crustal average. In this setting, Sr likely indicates human enrichment through use of marine resources such as fish bones and murex shells for dye. Other geologies that are limestone dominated may exhibit a higher Sr background, so these interpretations vary by geology and geography. Sr is also highly elevated in the Hellenistic House Site Q, where there was a distinctive shell horizon. Prior to its burial by floodplain and coastal deposition, Site Q was once closer to the sea and subject to marine inputs.[87]

87 Beach and Luzzadder-Beach 2008, 416–428; Luzzadder-Beach *et al.* 2011, 119–129.

TABLE 1B. Kinet, Turkey AGES and mean values.

	MODERN	MEDIEVAL	HELLENISTIC	IRON	BRONZE
CHEMISTRY					
Ba mg/kg	73.40	64.00	60.90	101.90	70.10
Cd mg/kg	22.20	39.90	16.40	1.60	37.70
Cu mg/kg	58.50	60.00	57.30	69.70	68.40
Fe %	4.10	4.00	4.60	3.60	3.90
Hg mg/kg	30.00	45.90	19.90	3.30	41.40
Mn mg/kg	473.80	415.00	481.60	526.00	445.10
Pb mg/kg	731.90	1228.50	699.60	258.40	1231.30
Sr mg/kg	107.60	161.70	139.00	342.30	245.30
Zn mg/kg	73.30	69.60	72.40	105.60	65.00

TABLE 2. Kinet, Turkey, Pearson's Coefficient table, matrix comparing elements, NP (n=51). High correlations are shown in bold. (from Luzzadder-Beach *et al.* 2011, 123).

	BA	CD	CU	FE	HG	MN	PB	SR	ZN
BA	1								
CD	0.12	1							
CU	0.253	0.208	1						
FE	–0.219	–0.273	0.041	1					
HG	0.128	0.942	0.138	–0.251	1				
MN	0.283	–0.292	0.076	0.472	–0.164	1			
PB	0.166	0.944	0.342	–0.117	0.828	–0.207	1		
SR	0.498	0.234	0.135	–0.54	0.126	–0.289	0.241	1	
ZN	0.698	–0.189	0.175	0.111	–0.17	0.403	–0.084	0.304	1

We conducted a parallel study using a different ICP AES method (with DTPA and total digestion[88]) to focus on the lead and cadmium results and to compare our results with regional work done by Karanlık *et al.*[89] Our parallel study in Kinet

88 See Luzzadder-Beach *et al.* 2011, 119–129.

89 Karanlık *et al.* 2011.

TABLE 3. Descriptive statistics, Turkey ICP-NP (TYNP, n=51) elemental analyses (from Luzzadder-Beach *et al.* 2011, 123).

		BA	CD	CU	FE	HG	MN	PB	SR	ZN
TYNP	Mean	67.14	25.70	61.36	4.41	28.97	470.00	928.61	172.77	70.97
TYNP	Median	63.44	41.15	56.73	4.09	39.41	446.91	1174.95	152.59	69.48
TYNP	Std Dev	20.37	20.94	26.90	1.27	24.89	84.20	560.10	123.01	17.42
TYNP	CV	30.33	81.49	43.84	28.90	85.94	17.92	60.32	71.20	24.54

TABLE 4. Water quality in Kinet Region
4A. Field measurements 1999 and 2000

SITE	DATE	ELECTRICAL CONDUCTIVITY	TOTAL DISOLVED SOLIDS	SALINITY
(Location)	(mm/dd/yyyy)	(µS)	(mg/L)	(ppt)
Spring near Kullu	06/28/2000	361	174	0.2
Deli Çay at super highway	06/29/2000	443	215	0.2
Özerli Çay	06/30/2000	386	185	0.2
Well at Kinet Dig House, inside	07/03/2000	606	289	0.3
Well at Kinet Dig House, spigot	07/05/1999	651	314	0.3
Farm well NW of *höyük*, nr 'Q'	06/28/1999	778	371	0.4
Delta Petrol Well, E of *höyük*	07/04/1999	629	299	0.3

4B. Laboratory analysis of Delta Petrol Well, 03/13/1991, provided by owner 06/28/1999

EC	NA	CA	CATION	BICARB	CL	SO_4	ANION	SODIUM	SAR	pH
(µS)	(epm)	(epm)	(Sum)	(epm)	(epm)	(epm)	(sum)	(%)	(index)	(paper)
540	0.2	5.2	5.4	3.7	0.6	1.1	5.4	3.85	0.15	7.5

also demonstrated higher levels of Pb and Cd than those of Karanlık and especially levels in anthropogenic loci near Kinet Höyük. Again, these results point towards concentrated human inputs and geological source material (e.g., serpentine rocks) differences within the watershed.

Elemental Era Analysis

We divided the samples by archaeological era in the next step of the analysis, comparing elemental means by Bronze Age, Hellenistic, Medieval, and Modern samples (Table 1b & Fig. 4d–f). Ages of deposits showed broad variation in elemental means, and these did not correlate with increasing time (not simply accumulating through the years), and they did not systematically decrease with erosion and weathering.[90] Mercury (Hg), Cadmium (Cd) and Lead (Pb) all showed the greatest variability across the ages. These three were the most highly correlated elements among the nine, and each had very consistent and comparable magnitudes of variation, shown by an analysis of coefficient of variation and standard deviation for the elements reported in Luzzadder-Beach *et al.*[91] All three elements peaked in the Medieval and Bronze Ages, showing medium to high levels in Hellenistic and Modern samples and lowest levels in the Iron Age sites (Table 1b, Fig. 4d–f).

Discussion

Potential sources of concentration of cadmium and mercury in ancient Turkey are pottery glazing and metalworking.[92] The individual locations showing the highest levels of lead and cadmium were streets, floors, hearths and a buried soil. Copper (Cu) also was elevated in this group. Mercury (Hg) was found at its highest level in two Middle Bronze Age loci, a hearth and a destruction layer; Hg could indicate the presence of cinnabar (HgS) used for pigments since the Neolithic.[93]

Strontium (Sr) was more positively correlated with age, ranging from Iron Age concentrations of 342 mg/kg, to Modern concentrations around 107.6 mg/kg.[94] A possible explanation is that in these earlier time periods the site was closer to the coast than today, and strontium correlates strongly with coastal resources and large shell deposits, including many *Murex* and other marine shells, associate with Bronze and Middle Bronze Age sites and grinding stone sediments. Two Iron Age activity sites had among the highest levels of strontium (Sr) as well (the other six elements did not have significant levels associated with archaeological loci).[95]

Human activities leave distinguishable patterns of elemental chemistry in the archaeological landscape. These patterns can be distinguished from natural geomorphic settings and from background geology. Although our work and

90 Luzzadder-Beach *et al.* 2011, 119–129.

91 Luzzadder-Beach *et al.* 2011, Tables 2 and 3.

92 Luzzadder-Beach *et al.* 2011, 119–129.

93 Lambert 1997, 78; Luzzadder-Beach *et al.* 2011, 119–129.

94 Luzzadder-Beach *et al.* 2011, 119–129.

95 Luzzadder-Beach *et al.* 2011, 119–129.

others' have shown that this can vary broadly by geology and with geography,[96] site specific analyses may reveal significant clues to human industrial activities ranging from cooking to pottery glazing to metallurgy. This was the case in Kinet Höyük, where the chemical signatures of activity sites were strikingly different from natural background settings, and where chemical signatures of archaeological eras varied widely from one another. Some of these differences were orders of magnitude higher over natural background or crustal averages for some elements. Other elements, such as Fe, were only slightly elevated in natural settings, such as weathered red soils. Both ICP-AES NP and ICP-AES DTPA analytical methods and treatments were useful for making these distinctions. Luzzadder-Beach *et al.*[97] also discuss the relative advantages and limitations of these methods.

Water Quality

To complete our environmental geochemical analysis, we sampled waters of the basin surrounding Kinet, including two sites in 1999 and four sites in 2000. Table 4 includes results of field water testing of spring water, surface water, and groundwater in the region (Table 4a), including water chemistry data (Table 4b) for the water well east of and nearest to Kinet Höyük, provided by the owner, Delta Petrol Headquarters. We know local people used groundwater in earlier periods, judging by at least one Medieval well we discovered in excavation unit X (Fig. 2) northeast of the *höyük* in 2000. In general, the electrical conductivity (EC, µS) and total dissolved solids measurements (TDS, mg/l) indicated low to medium amounts of dissolved ions in the upper watershed springs and surface waters of the region. Salinity was moderate to low at 0.2 ppt in all surface sources. The EC ranged from 386–443 µS, and the TDS ranged from 174–215 mg/l in the region's surface waters. The ground water wells produce water with approximately twice the dissolved ion load. Groundwater EC in the three sources sampled ranged from 606–778 µS, the TDS ranged from 289–371 mg/l and salinity ranged from 0.3 to 0.4 ppt. These findings are underscored by the chemical analysis of the well at Delta Petrol, whose water table was reported at 22 m in 1999, and the well depth was drilled to 40 m. The analysis showed that the dissolved ion load is mainly from calcium and bicarbonate, with a noticeable, but lesser contribution from sulfate, and a high EC. This is not surprising and reflects the local geology. This last part links to the archaeology of the site by indicating water quality in the past was probably very likely similar, except in the early occupations of the site when the sea was closer and salt water more of a problem for use. We can also say that

96 Luzzadder-Beach *et al.* 2011, 119–129.

97 Luzzadder-Beach *et al.* 2011.

water quality is generally excellent and should have produced no limitations on agriculture and human health, except where runoff occurred from human pollution or heavy metals from smelting.

Conclusions

The factors of environmental change in any region are complicated, especially so in regions like the Mediterranean that are seismically active, mountainous, have complicated climate change evidence and have long histories of human use. This article focused on three important aspects of environmental history: geochemical enrichment, soil erosion, and aggradation. We demonstrated that human activities such as cooking, smelting and pottery glazing made distinct inputs to the geochemistry of sediments in and around the site, distinguished both by era and locus, and distinct from the surrounding geology. The most significant indicators of these activities by site were cadmium, lead, mercury and strontium. Water chemistry studies showed a potentially good water quality for domestic and agricultural uses, based on the calcium carbonate geologic character of the local springs, surface water and groundwater. Nonetheless, runoff pollution from mining and smelting and human and agricultural waste could have undermined natural water quality, hinted at by high levels of phosphorous and some heavy metals in the sediments.

For the Kinet watershed, the balance of evidence from depositional and upland sites points to the Roman period as the most erosive. Symbolic of this conclusion, the Roman road on the alluvial plain is buried by 1–2 m of alluvium, and the Roman road through the Amanus Mountains is the eroded by 1–2 m in gullies. This evidence parallels evidence from the closest studied sites near Antioch in the Amuq Plain and numerous other sites around Turkey and the Mediterranean. One of the debates about this erosion was whether it occurred before, during, or after (the abandonment) of Roman *landesque capital*. Different studies cite evidence for all three, but more and more evidence supports the most intensive erosion during and at the end of the Roman period, though the current study and others confirm that soils were also being built up by terracing during this period. These lines of evidence correlate with both the intensive nature and abandonment of Roman terraces and other *landesque capital,* but it also correlates with the broader change of wetter to more arid conditions in the Late Roman period.

Much of the wider research focused on the Little Ice Age (LIA) period demonstrated from numerous archival and scientific sources that landscape instability during this time was an important factor to human land use and activities. This paper also offers evidence for landscape instability after the Roman period, and we hope further research will more precisely identify if the periods like the LIA may indeed correlate with environmental instability as did the Roman period before. We will need more contribution of scientific and broad syntheses to bring together multiple lines of archival and environmental sources to make more localized studies aware of other big drivers and periods of change that might be comfortably overlooked.

REFERENCES

Altunel, E., M. Meghraoui, V. Karabacak, H.S. Akyüz, M. Ferry, Ç. Yalçıner and M. Munschy, "Archaeological Sites (Tell and Road) Offset by the Dead Sea Fault in the Amik Basin, Southern Turkey." *Geophysical Journal International* 179 (2009): 1313–1329.

Atalay, I., "Red Mediterranean Soils in Some Karstic Regions of the Taurus Mountains, Turkey." *Catena* 28 (1997): 247–260.

Beach, T., S. Luzzadder-Beach, N. Dunning and D. Cook, "Human and Natural Impacts on Fluvial and Karst Depressions of the Maya Lowlands." *Geomorphology* 101/1–2 (2008): 301–331.

Beach, T., S. Luzzadder-Beach, N. Dunning, J. Jones, J. Lohse, T. Guderjan, S. Bozarth, S. Millspaugh and T. Bhattacharya, "A Review of Human and Natural Changes in Maya Lowlands Wetlands over the Holocene." *Quaternary Science Reviews* 28 (2009): 1710–1724.

Beach, T. and S. Luzzadder-Beach, "Aggradation Around Kinet Höyük, an Archaeological Mound in the Eastern Mediterranean, Turkey." *Geomorphology* 101/3 (2008): 416–428.

Bekker-Nielsen, T., *The Roads of Ancient Cyprus*. Copenhagen: Museum Tusculanum Press, 2004.

Bintliff, J., "Time Process and Catastrophism in the Study of Mediterranean Alluvial History: A Review." *World Archaeology* 33/3 (2002): 417–435.

Birkland, P., *Soils and Geomorphology*. Oxford: Oxford University Press, 1999.

Braje,T.J., J.M. Erlandson, C.M. Aikens, T. Beach, S. Fitzpatrick, S. Gonzalez, D.J. Kennett, P.V. Kirch, G.A. Lee, K.G. Lightfoot, S.B. McClure, L.M. Panich, T.C. Rick, A.C. Roosevelt, T.D. Schneider, B. Smith and M.A. Zeder, "An Anthropocene Without Archaeology-Should We Care?" *The Society for American Archaeology Archaeological Record* 14/1 (2014): 26–29.

Bridgland, D., G. Philip, R. Westaway and M. White, "A Long Quaternary Terrace Sequence in the Orontes River Valley, Syria: A Record of Uplift and of Human Occupation." *Current Science* 84/8 (2003): 1080–1089.

Brückner, H., "Coastal Research and Geoarchaeology in the Mediterranean Region" in the *German Geographical Coastal Research: The Last Decade. Institute for Scientific Co-operation, Tübingen and Committee of the Federal Republic of Germany for the International Geographical Union, 253–258.* Tübingen: Institute for Scientific Co-operation, 1998.

———. "Delta Evolution and Culture – Aspects of Geoarchaeological Research in Miletos and Priene" in *Troia and the Troad: Scientific Approaches*, ed. by G.A. Wagner, E. Pernicka, and H. P. Uerpmann, 121–144. Berlin: Springer Verlag, 2003.

Brückner, H., M. Müllenhoff, R. Gehrels, A. Herda, M. Knipping and A. Vött, "From *Archipelago to Floodplain – Geographical and Ecological Changes in Miletus and its Environs During the Past Six Millennia (Western Anatolia, Turkey)." Zeitschrift für Geomorphologie, Supplementband* 142 (2006): 63–83.

Büntgen, U., W. Tegel, K. Nicolussi, M. McCormick, D. Frank, V. Trouet, J. Kaplan, F. Herzig, K. Heussner, H. Wanner, J. Luterbacher and J. Esper, "2500 Years of European Climate Variability and Human Susceptibility." *Science* 331 (2011): 578–582.

Butzer, K., *Environment and Archaeology. An Introduction to Pleistocene Geography.* Chicago: Aldine Publishing Company, 1964.

———. "Holocene Alluvial Sequences: Problems of Dating and Correlation" in *Timescales in Geomorphology*, ed. by R. A. Cullingford, D. A. Davidson and J. Lewin, 333–354. New York: Wiley, 1980.

———. "Environmental History in the Mediterranean World: Cross-disciplinary Investigation of Cause-and Effect for Degradation and Soil Erosion." *Journal of Archaeological Science* 32/12 (2005): 1773–1800.

———. "Collapse, Environment, and Society." *Proceedings of the National Academy of Sciences* 109 (2012): 3632–3639.

Casana, J., "Mediterranean Valleys Revisited: Linking Soil Erosion, Land Use and Climate Variability in the Northern Levant." *Geomorphology* 101/3 (2008): 429–442.

Çelebi, M., "Revelations from a Single Strong-motion Record Retrieved during the 27 June 1998 Adana (Turkey) Earthquake." *Soil Dynamics and Earthquake Engineering* 20 5 (2000): 283–288.

Chiarucci, A. and A. Baker, "Advances in the Ecology of Serpentine Soils." *Plant Soil* 293 (2007): 1–2.

Contadakis, M.E. and G. Asteriadis, "Variations on the Shallow Underground Water Level and Temperature Related to the Seismic Activity" in *Proceedings of the XXIII General Assembly of the European Seismological Commission, Prague Czechoslovakia 1992, Vol.II*, 333–337. Prague, 1993.

Cordova, C.E., "Floodplain Degradation and Settlement History in Wadi al-Wala and Wadi ash-Shallalah, Jordan." *Geomorphology* 101 (2008): 443–457.

Curras, A., L. Zamora, J.M. Reed, E. Garcia-Soto, S. Ferrero, F. Armengol, F. Mezquita-Joanes, M.A. Marques, S. Riera and R. Julia, "Climate Change and Human Impact in Central Spain During Roman Times: High-resolution Multi-proxy Analysis of a Tufa Lake Record (Somolinos, 1280 m asl)." *Catena* 89/1 (2012): 31–53.

Davidson, D., "Erosion in Greece During the First and Second Millennium BC" in *Timescales in Geomorphology*, ed. by R.A. Cullingford, D.A. Davidson and J. Lewin, 142–158. New York: Wiley, 1980.

Doyuran, V., "Erzin ve Dörtyol Ovalarının Jeolojik ve Hidrolojik Özellikleri." *Türkiye Jeoloji Kurumu Bülteni* 25 (1982): 151–160.

Eger, A., "Hisn al-Tinat on the Islamic-Byzantine Frontier: Synthesis and the 2005–2008 Survey and Excavation on the Cilician Plain (Turkey)." *Bulletin of the American Schools of Oriental Research* 357 (2010): 49–76.

Eisma, D., "Stream Deposition and Erosion by the Eastern Shore of the Aegean" in *The Environmental History of the Near and Middle East Since the Last Ice Age,* ed. by W. Brice, 67–81. London: Academic Press, 1978.

Erol, O., "Geomorphological Evolution of the Taurus Mountains,Turkey." *Zeitschrift für Geomorphologie, Supplementband* 82 (1991): 99–102.

Erinç, S., "Climatic Types and the Variation of Moisture Regions in Turkey." *Annals of the Association of American Geographers* 44 (1955): 363–391.

Faust, D., C. Zielhofer, R. Baena Escudero and F. Diaz del Olmo, "High-resolution Fluvial Record of Late Holocene Geomorphic Change in Northern Tunisia: Climatic or Human Impact?" *Quaternary Science Reviews* 23 (2004): 1757–1775.

Fuchs, M., "An Assessment of Human Versus Climatic Impacts on Holocene Soil Erosion in NE Peloponnese, Greece." *Quaternary Research* 67 (2007): 349–356.

Ganse, R. and J. Nelson, *Catalog of Significant Earthquakes: 2000 BC – 1979, Including Quantitative Casualties and Damage. Report SE-27, National Oceanic and Atmospheric Administration, Environmental Data and Information Service.* Washington 1981.

Gates, M.H., "2002 Season at Kinet Höyük (Yeşil-Dörtyol, Hatay)." *Kazı Sonuçları Toplantısı* 25/1 (2004): 405–416.

Gerritsen, F., A De Giorgi, A. Eger, R. Özbal and T. Vorderstrasse, "Settlement and Landscape Transformations in the Amuq Valley, Hatay: A long-term Perspective." *Anatolica* 34 (2008): 241–314.

Graham, N. E., C.M. Ammann, D. Fleitmann, K.M. Cobb and J. Luterbacher, "Support for Global Climate Reorganization During the Medieval Climate Anomaly." *Climate Dynamics* 37 (2011): 1217–1245.

Grove, A., "The 'Little Ice Age' and its Geomorphological Consequences in Mediterranean Europe." *Climatic Change* 48/1 (2001): 121–136.

Grove, A. and O. Rackham, *The Nature of Mediterranean Europe: An Ecological History.* New Haven: Yale University Press, 2001.

Herz, N. and E.G. Garrison, *Geological Methods for Archaeology.* Oxford: Oxford University Press, 1998.

Kaplan, J. O., K.M. Krumhardt and N. Zimmermann, "The Prehistoric and Preindustrial Deforestation of Europe." *Quaternary Science Reviews* 28/27–28 (2009): 3016–3034.

Karanlık, S., A. Necat and Y. Mehmet, "Spatial Distribution of Heavy Metals Content in Soils of Amik Plain (Hatay, Turkey)." *Environmental Monitoring and Assessment* 73 (2011): 181–191.

Kayan, I., "Holocene Stratigraphy and Geomorphological Evolution of the Aegean Coastal Plains of Anatolia." *Quaternary Science Reviews* 18 (1999): 541–548.

Kazakou, E., P. Dimitrakopoulos, R. Reeves, A. Baker and A. Troumbis, "Hypotheses, Mechanisms, and Trade-offs of Tolerance and Adaptation to Serpentine Soils: From Species to Ecosystem Level." *Biological Reviews* 83 (2008): 495–508.

Keefer, D., "The Importance of Earthquake-induced Landslides to Long-term Slope erosion and Slope-failure Hazards in Seismically Active Regions." *Geomorphology* 10/1–4 (1994): 265–284.

Kehl, H., *Lokat: Eine Landschaftsokologische Komplexanalyse im Amanus der Sudost-Turkei*. Berlin, 1998.

Kennett, D. and T. Beach, "Archaeological and Environmental Lessons for the Anthropocene from the Classic Maya Collapse." *The Anthropocene* 4 (2013): 88–100.

Kraft, J., Jr. G. Rapp and S. Aschenbrenner, "Late Holocene Paleogeography of the Coastal Plain of Messenia, Greece and its Relationships to Archaeological Settings and to Coastal Change." *Bulletin of the Geological Society of America* 86 (1975): 1191–1208.

Lambert, J.B., *Traces of the Past: Unraveling the Secrets of Archaeology through Chemistry*. New York: Basic Books, 1997.

Lemcke, G. and M. Sturm, "δ18O and Trace Element Measurements as Proxy for the Reconstruction of Climate Changes at Lake Van (Turkey): Preliminary Results" in *Third Millennium BC Climate Change and Old World Collapse*, ed. by N. Dalfes, G. Kukla and H. Weiss, 653–678. Berlin: Springer Verlag, 1997.

Luce, C. and B. Wemple, "Hydrologic and Geomorphic Effects of Forest Roads (Special Issue)." *Earth Surface Processes and Landforms* 26/2 (2001): 111–232.

Luzzadder-Beach, S.L., T.P. Beach, R.E. Terry and K.Z. Doctor, "Elemental Prospecting and Geoarchaeology in Turkey and Mexico." *Catena* 85/2 (2011): 119–129.

Luzzadder-Beach, S., T. Beach and N. Dunning, "Maya Models and Distant Mirrors: Wetland Fields, Drought and the Maya Abandonment." *Proceedings of the National Academy of Science* 109 (2012): 3646–3651.

Lyberis, N., E. Kasapoglu, T. Yurur and N. Gundogdu, "The East Anatolian Fault: An Oblique Collisional Belt." *Tectonophysics* 204 (1992): 1–15.

Macklin, M.G., G. Benito, K.J. Gregory, E. Johnstone, J. Lewin, D.J. Michczyńska, R. Soja, L. Starkel and V. Thorndycraft, "Past Hydrological Events Reflected in the Holocene Hydrological Record of Europe." *Catena* 66/1–2 (2006): 145–154.

McCormick, M., U. Büntgen, M.A. Cane, E.R. Cook, K. Harper, P. Huybers, T. Litt, S.W. Manning, P.A. Mayewski, A.F. More, K. Nicolussi and W. Tegel, "Climate Change During and After the Roman Empire: Reconstructing the Past from Scientific and Historical Evidence." *Journal of Interdisciplinary History* 43/2 (2012): 169–220.

McNeill, J., *The Mountains of the Mediterranean World: An Environmental History*. Cambridge: Cambridge University Press, 1992.

Mülazımoğlu, N.S., *İskenderun Körfezi Tabanı, Kıyıları ve Çevresinin Kuvarterner Jeolojisi ve Jeomorfolojisi*. Unpublished PhD Thesis submitted to Institute of Geography, Istanbul University, 1979.

Nur, A. and E. Cline, "Poseidon's Horses: Plate Tectonics and Earthquake Storms in the Late Bronze Age Aegean and Eastern Mediterranean." *Journal of Archaeological Sciences* 27 (2000): 43–63.

Nur, A. and D. Burgess, *Apocalypse: Earthquakes, Archaeology, and the Wrath of God.* Princeton: Princeton University Press, 2008.

Orland, I., M. Bar-Matthews, N. Kita, A. Ayalon, A. Matthews and J. Valley, "Climate Deterioration in the Eastern Mediterranean as Revealed by Ion Microprobe Analysis of a Speleothem that Grew from 2.2 to 0.9 ka in Soreq Cave, Israel." *Quaternary Research* 71 (2009): 27–35.

Ozaner, F. and J. Russell, "Diachronic Study of Coastal Changes at Anemurium: Geomorphological and Archaeological Applications." *Arkeometri Sonuçları Toplantısı* 10 (1995): 135–151.

Ozaner, F., "Dörtyol-Payas (Issos) Ovası'nda (Antakya) Tarihi Çağlardan Günümüze Süregelen Jeomorfolojik Değişikliklerin Kinet Höyük Üzerindeki Etkileri." *Araştırma Sonuçları Toplantısı* 12 (1995): 513–527.

Pirazzoli, P. A., J. Laborel, J.F. Saliege, O. Erol, I. Kayan and A. Person, "Holocene Raised Shorelines on the Hatay Coasts (Turkey): Palaeoecological and Tectonic Implications." *Marine Geology* 96 (1991): 295–311.

Redford, S., S. Ikram, E. Parr and T. Beach, "Excavations at Medieval Kinet, Turkey: a Preliminary Report." *Ancient Near Eastern Studies* 38 (2001): 58–138.

Rosen, A., "The Geoarchaeology of Holocene Environments and Land Use at Kazane Höyük, Southeast Turkey." *Geoarchaeology* 12/4 (1997): 396–416.

Rowton, M.B., "The Woodlands of Ancient Western Asia." *Journal of Near Eastern Studies* 26 (1967): 261–277.

Ruddiman, W.F., "The Anthropogenic Greenhouse Era Began Thousands of Years Ago." *Climatic Change*, No. 61/3(2003): 261–293.

———. *Earth Transformed* (1st ed.). New York: W. H. Freeman, 2013.

Seton-Williams, M.V., "Cilician Survey." *Anatolian Studies* 4 (1954): 121–171.

Stock, F., Pint, A., Horejs, B., Ladstätter, S. and H. Brückner, "In Search of the Harbours: New Evidence of Late Roman and Byzantine Harbours of Ephesus." *Quaternary International* 312 (2013): 57–69.

Tabak, F., *The Waning of the Mediterranean 1550–1870: A Geohistorical Approach.* Baltimore: Johns Hopkins University Press, 2008.

Van Andel, T., "Paleosols, Red Sediments, and the Old Stone Age in Greece." *Geoarchaeology* 13 (1998): 361–390.

Van Andel, T., E. Zanger and A. Demitrack, "Land Use and Soil Erosion in Prehistoric and Historical Greece." *Journal of Field Archaeology* 17 (1990): 379–396.

Verschuren, D., K. Laird and B. Cumming, "Rainfall and Drought in Equatorial East Africa During the Past 1,100 years." *Nature* 403 (2000): 410–414.

Vita-Finzi, C., *The Mediterranean Valleys: Geological Changes in Historical Times.* Cambridge: Cambridge University Press, 1969.

Wilkinson, T., "Linear Hollows in the Jazira, Upper Mesopotamia." *Antiquity* 67 (1993): 548–562.

———. “Holocene Valley Fills of Southern Turkey and Northwestern Syria: Recent Geoarchaeological Contributions.” *Quaternary Science Reviews* 18 (1999): 555–571.

———. *Archaeological Landscapes of the Near East*. Tucson: University of Arizona Press, 2003.

———. “Soil Erosion and Valley Fills in the Yemen Highlands and Southern Turkey: Integrating Settlement, Geoarchaeology, and Climate Change.” *Geoarchaeology* 20/2 (2005), 169–192.

———. “Empire and Environment in the Northern Fertile Crescent” in *Landscapes and Societies-Selected Cases*, ed. By I. P. Martini and W. Chesworth, 135–151. Dordrecht: Springer Verlag, 2010.

Woodward, J., *The Physical Geography of the Mediterranean*. Oxford: Oxford University Press, 2009.

Yurtmen S., H. Guillou, R. Westaway, G. Rowbotham and O. Tatar, “Rate of Strike-slip Motion on the Amanos Fault (Karasu Valley, Southern Turkey) Constrained by K-Ar Dating and Geochemical Analysis of Quaternary Basalts.” *Tectonophysics* 344 (2002): 207–246.

Regional and Long-Distance Movements of Animals and Animal Parts in Ancient Turkey: the Zooarchaeological Evidence

Canan Çakırlar[1]

I dedicate this paper to Marie-Henriette and Charles Gates, devoted teachers and scholars of ancient Anatolian cultures and their connectivity with surrounding lands.

I arrived at the Kinet dig house in 1999 on an (of course) hot and humid night in July from a trip to Syria, Jordan and eastern Turkey –a trip that was inspired by Bayan Gates's legendary Archaeology of Syria and Palestine course. I had no idea at the time that this was only the first of many trips to be not only inspired but skillfully encouraged by the Gateses, including a two-year (!) 'trip' to Beirut, and an incredible ongoing journey through the magical world of zooarchaeology. Yes, like many other archaeology students, I can easily claim that I owe my career to the directors of the excavation where I grew up. But the reason why I feel tremendously grateful to them is not only because they provided the best possible training in a professional setting, but because they made me feel protected and cherished throughout my twenties, no matter how far I was from home.

We have been, we are, very lucky to have them by our side.

Abstract

This paper presents a survey of the zooarchaeological (taxonomic, metric and molecular) evidence for movements of animal and animal parts in ancient Turkey from the Epipalaeolithic to the Byzantine Period. The survey shows that the transportation of animal parts over long distances up to 200 km began in the Epipalaeolithic, became an intensive and large scale activity during the Bronze Age and ultimately evolved into a commonplace

1 Groningen University, Institute of Archaeology, Poststraat 6, 9712ER, Groningen-Netherlands.

method to astound and impress both citizens and foreigners during the Byzantine Era. Recent developments show that molecular (isotopic, aDNA) research and surveys of gray literature have great potential to contribute to building up evidence for this over-looked aspect of cultural contact and exchange in ancient Anatolia.

Introduction

Describing subsistence economies and reconstructing local environments are perhaps the best known uses of zooarchaeology. Animal bone assemblages are assumed to reflect the available fauna in the immediate vicinity of the settlements in which they originate, and based on this assumption they are used to infer how people raised domestic animals, which cohorts of the wild populations they took from their immediate environment, if stratigraphic sequences are long enough and how environmental conditions changed over time. In Turkey too, the majority of zooarchaeological research aims at reconstructing subsistence and environment.

One often overlooked aspect of zooarchaeological assemblages is their potential to provide evidence for human-mediated regional and long-distance movements of animals and animal parts, which contribute to the understanding of the nature of human mobility and cultural contact over long distances. Remains of taxa found outside of their natural distribution range make up the bulk of the evidence in this respect. These remains may end up outside their natural range as commodities, as curiosities brought from exotic lands, as booty or as herded livestock. Since the social mechanisms through which animals and animal parts were carried away from their birth place must have been very diverse and must have varied from one period to the other, I will be using the word 'movement' instead of 'trade', 'exchange,' etc. throughout the paper. In Turkey, while such evidence from taxonomic identifications is fairly abundant, evidence from re-invested and relatively new methods of analysis, such as isotopic and palaeogenetic analyses, is limited. Although Anatolia is a particularly interesting region to put zooarchaeological evidence in the service of research agendas focusing on ancient cultural networks, its potential has hardly been realized.

In this paper, I survey the taxonomic, metric and molecular evidence for long-distance movements of animals and animal parts in ancient Turkey, from the Epipalaeolithic to the Byzantine Period.[2] The survey of zooarchaeological evidence shows that activities involving movements of animals and animal parts had formal beginnings in the Epipalaeolithic and were conducted to serve purpos-

2 The time period I cover is aligned with the time scope of the majority of the excavations conducted in Turkey. To ensure accessibility, I use common names for taxa throughout the body of the paper unless absolutely necessary, and take advantage of footnotes to provide scientific names.

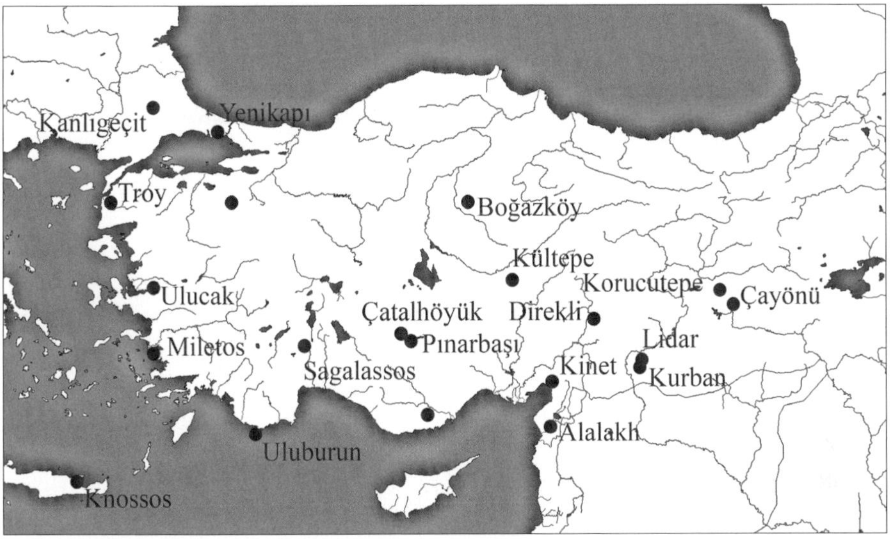

FIG. 1 Sites mentioned in the text.

es other than subsistence; these activities saw remarkable changes in scale and intensity during the following Neolithic and Bronze Ages, becoming on the one hand an essential part of the everyday lives of farmers and pastoralists, and on the other hand, fueling recently formed but rapidly growing demands of elite and/or ruling classes of society turning definitively into an ultimate political vehicle to astound citizens and showcase international wealth and power in the Byzantine Period. The groundbreaking results of recent zooarchaeological research in Turkey indicate that the picture drawn by this survey is far from complete, showing just the tip of the iceberg.

Inland Foragers and Marine Shells

The earliest evidence for faunal exchange over some distance consists of shells of marine origin and comes from inland Epipaleolithic sites such as Öküzini in the western Taurus, Pınarbaşı on the Konya Plain and Direkli Cave in Maraş (TABLE 1, FIG. 1). While the *ca.* 30 km distance shells travelled from the Mediterranean coast can be considered to fall within the catchment area of cave-dwelling foragers of the western Taurus,[3] Mediterranean shells found in a forager camp in southern central Turkey, which must have travelled up to 215 km before their final deposition, should be regarded as remnants of trips to the coast, trips by

3 Storch *et al.* 1992.

TABLE 1. Summary of evidence for regional and long-distance movements of animals and animal parts in ancient Turkey.

PERIOD	ANIMAL PART	SPECIES	SITE/LOCATION	ESTIMATED WALKING DISTANCE BETWEEN SITE AND ORIGIN
Epipaleolithic	Shell	*Nassarius, Columbella*	Direkli Cave	174 km
Epipaleolithic	Shell	*Dentalium* sp., *Collumbella rustica, Arcularia gibbosula*	Öküzini, Karain	30 km to the Mediterranean coast
Epipalaeolithic	Shell	*Dentalium* sp., *Nassarius* sp.	Pınarbaşı	215 km to the Mediterranean coast
Neolithic	Shell (also fossil)	Various	Çatalhöyük	215 km to the Mediterranean coast
Aceramic Neolithic	Shell	*Columbella rustica, Nassarius* sp.	Ulucak VI	11 km to the Aegean coast
Neolithic	Shell	Red Sea shells	Kurban Höyük	>1000 km to the Gulf of Aqaba
Pottery Neolithic	Shell, shellfish	Lagoon cockles, various	Ulucak V-IV	11 km to the Aegean coast
Neolithic	Domestic herds	Sheep, goat	Into western Anatolia	From Central Anatolia and/or Southwest Asia
Neolithic	Domestic herds	Pig	Into Europe	From western Anatolia
Early Bronze Age	Domestic herds	(Woolly) Sheep	Korucutepe, Boğazköy, Demircihöyük	1000 to 2000 km
Middle Bronze Age	Population overturn	European Pig	Lidar Höyük	1800 km
Late Bronze Age	Wild, exotic herds, hippo and elephant ivory	Asian Elephant	Sites in Hatay, Adana, Gaziantep, and Kahramanmaraş	4000 km (for elephant)
Iron Age	Live domestic animals, preserved fish, hide	Bactrian and dromedary camel, Nile perch and catfish, gazelle	Various sites all over Anatolia	1000 to 2000 km
Hellenistic, Roman and Byzantine Periods	Preserved exotic fish, live menagerie animals	Nile perch and catfish, elephants, ostriches, gazelles	Sagalassos, Yenikapı	3000–4000 km

coastal dwellers to remote inland locations or trips undertaken by middle-men who facilitated the exchange.[4]

What is noteworthy about this evidence, other than its early date and forager context, is its uniform character and probable continuity from the Upper Paleolithic, perhaps even from 8000 years ago,[5] as well as its similarity with the evidence from the Levant. The mollusk species preferred for 'export' are identical or similar across the eastern Mediterranean during the Epipaleolithic and they are commonly naturally or artificially perforated.[6] Choices for a limited amount of taxa, especially those with small-sized, smooth-surfaced and roundish shells, persist from the earlier Paleolithic periods of Africa and the Levant.[7] Furthermore, the same taxa are preferred in the Paleolithic and Mesolithic of Europe.[8] All these point at a nearly global pattern of raw material procurement serving to fulfill a common symbolic behavior. Anatolia, including its inland areas, did not remain out of the loop.

Early Farmers

The agricultural transition, or Neolithization, may have involved arguably one of the most remarkable of the human-induced faunal movements Anatolia has witnessed until modern times. With new palaeogenetic, zooarchaeological and archaeological evidence from central and western Turkey, it is becoming increasingly clear that Neolithic lifestyles were transmitted through communities who moved together with—at least—sheep and goat herds.[9] According to our present knowledge, the natural distribution area of the ancestral forms of domestic sheep and goat does not reach western Anatolia.[10] Although this knowledge is based more on a lack of data rather than a thorough pre-Neolithic zooarchaeological record in the regions west of central Anatolia and east of the Aegean Sea, palaeogenetic and zooarchaeological evidence strongly supports the hypothesis that sheep and goat were initially domesticated in Southwest Asia, including the Upper Euphrates Basin and Cappadocia, were transported to western Anatolia and then further into southeastern Europe by early farmers.[11] One of the most likely places for the

4 Baysal 2013a; Erek 2008.

5 Here I refer to the Middle Stone Age of Africa, i.e. anatomically modern humans, not the Neanderthals of the Levant or Europe.

6 Bar-Yosef 2005; 2008.

7 Kuhn *et al.* 2001; D'errico 2005.

8 Alvarez 2011.

9 Çakırlar 2012.

10 Uerpmann 1987.

11 Arbuckle *et al.* 2014; Scheu *et al.* 2012.

origin of domestic sheep, goat and cattle transported to Aceramic Knossos at the beginning of the seventh millennium BC [12] is the submerged coasts of southwestern Anatolia. Palaeogenetic evidence clearly shows that the first domestic pigs of Europe originated from a local western Anatolian lineage, not directly from pigs domesticated in Southwest Asia. [13]

In addition to moving domestic livestock, the early farming communities of Anatolia also transported wild animal populations. The most obvious and better-researched of these is the fallow deer, [14] a deer species which is endemic to Anatolia. The Anatolian subspecies of fallow deer was transported to the island of Rhodes in the mid-seventh millennium BC, most probably from the southwestern Anatolian mainland, which is located less than 11 nautical miles away. [15] In view of the fact that the Persian subspecies of fallow deer was brought to Cyprus from the Levant along with other wild and domestic animals prior to the seventh millennium BC, [16] this situation is hardly surprising. The species is common in the Neolithic and Chalcolithic contexts of western Anatolia and was spread rapidly into southeastern Europe through humans. [17] Whether the Anatolian fallow deer were ranched or simply captured alive, transported, and subsequently released in the wild is subject to current research. [18]

Exchange of marine shells to inland areas continued during the Neolithic and afterwards. The interest in taxa which were already popular in the Epipalaeolithic survived supra-regionally well into the Pottery Neolithic. For example, small marine snails like *Nassarius* and *Columbella* with suspension (?) holes are the most common elements of early Neolithic worked shell assemblages both in the İzmir and the Konya regions. [19] Some shells, such as certain species of cowrie shells, originated from the Red Sea. [20] They must have been transported over more than 1000 km, directly or indirectly, from the Gulf of Aqaba, or else further, in the Red Sea. Fossil shells were also transported long distances during the pottery Neolithic. [21]

---

12 Isaakidou 2008.

13 Ottoni *et al.* 2013.

14 *Dama dama dama,* also called the European or Anatolian fallow deer, is a subspecies of *Dama dama.* The other subspecies, *Dama dama mesopotamica* was distributed in the Levant and Mesopotamia.

15 Masseti *et al.* 2006.

16 Vigne *et al.* 2011.

17 Çakırlar and Atıcı forthcoming.

18 Sykes 2014.

19 Baysal 2013b; Bar-Yosef 2013; Çakırlar 2015.

20 Reese 1990.

21 Bar-Yosef *et al.* 2010.

By the mid-seventh millennium BC, fresh or preserved shellfish had begun to be transported to settlements that were near but not right on the coast.[22] Accumulations of complete (i.e. both valves present), well preserved lagoonal bivalves in the Pottery Neolithic and Chalcolithic layers of the inland site of Ulucak, which was located 5 to 10 km from the coastline at the time, are ample evidence for short distance transportation of low calorie food resources.[23] Small amounts of marine fish in Neolithic Ulucak provide further support to the view that transport of marine food took place between inland and the coast over a distance that could be covered in about six hours because the trip included a steep uphill walk.[24] The mechanisms involved in the transportation of low calorie marine foods between coastal and inland regions are difficult to determine: were marine foods items of exchange between inland and coastal dwellers? Were they gifts from the coastal dwellers? Or were they procured during day excursions to the sea coast?

Transportation of marine animals and animal parts into inland regions and the spread of herding further west and north continued throughout the Neolithic and the Early Chalcolithic (until *ca.* 5500 BC). All types of archaeological evidence dating to the Middle and Late Chalcolithic (5500–3000 BC) are scarce in Anatolia, especially in the western regions.[25] With the Ubaid influence and the Uruk expansion in the southeast and intensified interactions with southeast Europe in the west, we must expect large scale movement of herds, as well as the exchange of other faunal elements between migrants and locals in the late fifth and fourth millennia BC, but we currently have no concrete zooarchaeological evidence to confirm this expectation.

The Bronze Age

The Bronze Age witnessed substantial additions to the faunal spectrum of ancient Turkey; as much as our present knowledge allows, most of these, if not all, are introductions from other regions. The donkey, for example, originates from northeastern Africa and is found as far west as Troy already in the Early Bronze Age.[26] The earliest domestic horses in the southern Balkans were uncovered in Kırklareli-Kanlıgeçit, located in modern Turkey.[27] Based on bone measurements, Benecke argued that the Kanlıgeçit horses are more likely to have originated from

22 Çakırlar 2015.

23 Çakırlar 2009, 100–102, 121.

24 Çakırlar 2012.

25 Düring 2011, 200–256.

26 Uerpmann 2003.

27 Benecke 2009.

Anatolia rather than Eastern Europe, but this argument was recently questioned by Bendrey, who contested the methodology Benecke used to compare bone measurements.[28] While the question of whether Benecke's methodology is applicable to hypothesize the geographical origin of domestic horse populations does not fall into the scope of this paper, the problem remains that there is not enough data to sufficiently describe the morphological characteristics of early domestic horses in Anatolia.[29]

The ancestral form of domestic sheep is not a woolly animal. Wool in sheep is a phenotypic trait which evolved through the course of domestication. When and how the production of wool from sheep began is much debated, because wool production is difficult to assess archaeologically.[30] Southwest Asia is usually considered to be the earliest region of wool of production.[31] In the 1970s, German zooarchaeologists interpreted the significant size change in archaeological sheep of Early Bronze Age Anatolia as an indication of the introduction of woolly sheep from Southwest Asia.[32] Although this hypothesis was commonly accepted for a long time, probably because it fit well into Sherratt's Secondary Products Revolution model,[33] the issue of wool is currently being re-investigated.[34] For the moment, concrete evidence for exchange in raw wool in Anatolia is confined to textual evidence, most notably from Middle Bronze Age Kültepe, texts from which mention imported wool from Assyria.[35]

While texts attest to the long-distance movement of livestock after the Middle Bronze Age,[36] because it is difficult, if not impossible to pinpoint introduced individuals of domestic animals with macroscopic methods, zooarchaeological evidence is largely lacking in this regard. Two recent studies at the molecular level, however, are promising.

The first one is a pilot study of isotopic ratios of sheep teeth from Alalakh, the Late Bronze Age capital of the lower Orontes Valley.[37] The ratios of two different

---

28 Bendrey 2012.

29 Also see Arbuckle 2009, for a discussion of the possible earlier appearance of domestic horses in central Anatolia in the Late Chalcolithic. Arbuckle suggests that further research may identify central Anatolia as an independent center of horse domestication.

30 Greenfield 2010.

31 Helmer *et al.* 2007.

32 Rauh 1981, 44.

33 Sherratt 1983.

34 http://www.topoi.org/project/a-4–1/ (accessed 8–1-2015).

35 Atıcı 2014.

36 Collins 2007.

37 Meiggs 2010.

strontium isotopes incorporated into an individual's skeletal tissue through water and food intake are determined by the ratio of strontium isotopes in that individual's geological environment. Differences and changes in the ratios of the strontium extracted from the hard tissue of organisms represent patterns of mobility across different geologic areas. Strontium isotopic values of enamel layers of sheep teeth in Middle and Late Bronze Age Alalakh suggest that at least one individual sheep may have been raised further south in the Orontes Valley.[38] This individual might represent trade in livestock among the Bronze Age cities located along the Orontes.

More concrete evidence for the movement of domestic livestock in the Bronze Age comes from pig palaeogenetics. According to the results of a large series of ancient DNA analyses of pig bones from a vast region, domestic pigs originating from western Anatolia interbred with wild boar in Europe.[39] Within a short period of time, the female[40] wild boar in Europe became integrated into the domestic livestock. By the Middle Bronze Age, these 'Europeanized' domestic pigs began to appear in the archaeological record of Turkey, as a result of continuous human contact between Europe and Anatolia.

One of the most archaeologically visible drives behind the remarkable increase in the transportation of wild animal parts during the Bronze Age was the international demand for ivory and ivory products.[41] Finds of finished and unfinished elephant and hippopotamus ivory from the Uluburun shipwreck are perfect examples of the lively trade that supplied the demand for ivory.[42] In direct or indirect relation to the ivory exchange in the Bronze Age, live individuals of elephants were also transported to Turkey during the Late Bronze Age, from India via northern Mesopotamia.[43] Zooarchaeological finds of elephant bones in Turkey are distributed at sites in the provinces of Hatay and Maraş.[44] The fact that a considerable amount of the elephant bones found in sites in Turkey, Syria, Lebanon and Iraq belongs to the postcranial body (i.e., neither the head nor the teeth), along with 'natural' deposits of elephant skeletal remains in Turkey, strongly suggest that herds of Indian elephants lived in the region between roughly 1500 and 700 BC.[45] There is no evidence to suggest that the human-mediated movements of individuals or herds of Indian elephants took place prior to the Late Bronze Age.

---

38 *Ibid.*

39 Ottoni *et al.* 2013.

40 There is no information about males.

41 Potts 1997, 260–262, among others.

42 Pulak 1998.

43 Caubet and Poplin 2010.

44 Lister *et al.* 2013.

45 Çakırlar and Ikram 2014.

While the transplanted Indian elephant herds most likely died out completely by the seventh century BC, texts indicate that live elephants continued to be transported to Turkey, mainly as war elephants and sometimes as items of curiosity in the subsequent millennia.[46]

The Iron Age

The amount of zooarchaeological data available for Iron Age Anatolia is much more limited than it is for the Neolithic and the Bronze Ages. We have no 'hard' zooarchaeological evidence among domestic animals for the consequences of historically well-known population movements, such as the enigmatic phenomenon of the 'Sea Peoples', the Ionian migration, the Greek colonization or the Persian invasion. Such possibly large-scale human movements can be expected to have accelerated the wholesale establishment of imported breeds in new regions and interbreeding between local and imported breeds, giving rise to new breeds.

Nevertheless, the little zooarchaeological data there is indicates that intensified cultural contacts led to significant changes in the availability of faunal resources in Anatolia. Most notable of these is the introduction of camels. At least five sites produced camel remains dating to the Iron Age in Turkey. The sites are widely distributed from the western coast of Anatolia (e.g., Kalabaktepe-Miletos) to the southeastern coast (e.g., Kinet).[47] The Bactrian is thought to have been domesticated in the third millennium BC and the Dromedary in the second millennium BC.[48] Which of the species arrived in Anatolia first, whether they arrived simultaneously and whether hybrids were also already produced in the first millennium BC in Turkey or elsewhere are issues that require further research.[49]

Another important domesticate that makes its clear appearance in the Anatolian kitchen during the Iron Age is the chicken. The chicken was domesticated in Southeast Asia probably sometime in the third millennium BC, and although a few individuals seem to have made their way into Southwest Asia—most likely as curiosities—during the second millennium BC, the wholesale spread of domestic chicken populations in the Eastern Mediterranean took another eight or nine hundred years.[50] The earliest record of domestic chicken in Anatolia involves a small number of finds from the Late Bronze Age layers of Korucutepe.[51] The

46 Kistler 2005.

47 Çakırlar and Berthon 2014.

48 Zeder 2012.

49 Çakırlar and Berthon 2014.

50 Peters 2014.

51 Boessneck and von den Driesch 1975.

scarce evidence from Iron Age Anatolia suggests that chickens became much more common during this period. For example, chickens are the most common birds in seventh-sixth century BC Kinet Höyük.[52]

The Late Iron Age witnesses the first long-distance fish imports into Anatolia from the Levant or the Nile. Nile perch (*Lates niloticus*) and the Nile catfish bones (*Clarias*) found at Kilisetepe in Rough Cilicia indicate trade or exchange in processed non-local fish, in the case of Nile perch definitely from the Nile (see below for the discussion of *Clarias*).[53]

The only other zooarchaeological evidence for long-distance movements of animals and animal parts in first millennium BC Turkey,[54] which I am aware of, consists of a single gazelle bone found in Kabalaktepe, the Iron Age settlement of Miletos.[55] This is a horn core, which according to the faunal analyst, Zimmermann, represents a Dorcas gazelle,[56] a species whose ancient distribution did not include Turkey.[57] The horn may have been transported to Miletos as an isolated piece, attached to a trophy (?) skull or on a live animal.

Hellenistic, Roman and Byzantine Periods

Zooarchaeological data for the Hellenistic, Roman and Byzantine periods in Turkey are, like the Iron Age, not abundant. Nevertheless, studies carried out in a handful of Hellenistic and post-Hellenistic sites bring a colorful faunal world into light. Among these, Sagalassos in Burdur and Yenikapı in Istanbul stand out with fascinating results.

Thanks to a systematic sieving program, a large and rich fish assemblage has been recovered at Roman Sagalassos, an inland city located at an elevation of 1400–1700 m. In addition to locally available taxa, the fish assemblage included various species of Mediterranean fish, which were imported from at least a distance of *ca.* 110 km,[58] and four taxa of exotic freshwater fish.[59] The latter group consists of three taxa which are endemic to the Nile (*Lates niloticus*, the Nile perch, *Bagrus*, a genus of the catfish, and *Clarias gariepinus,* the Nile catfish), and one taxon which

52 Çakırlar and Bosman, in prep.

53 Van Neer and Waelkens 2007.

54 Excluding marine mollusk shells found in inland locations.

55 Zimmermann 1993.

56 *Ibid* 52.

57 Uerpmann 1987.

58 De Cupere 2001; Van Neer *et al.* 2000; 2008. The nearest coast to Sagalassos is the Antalya Bay.

59 Arndt *et al.* 2003; De Cupere 2001.

is endemic to the African continent (*Tilapia*, also commonly known as Tilapia). The natural distribution ranges of the Nile catfish and Tilapia, however, extend well beyond Africa. The distribution of the Nile catfish extends all the way northeast up to the Seyhan-Ceyhan River basin in Adana and the natural distribution of Tilapia extends up to the Litany River basin in Lebanon.[60] While it is clear that Nile perch and *Bagrus* were material products of trade relations with Egypt, the large distribution ranges of the Nile catfish and Tilapia hampered the possibility of pinpointing their origins based on taxonomic identifications alone. In order to determine a more exact geographic origin of the Nile catfish found in Sagalassos, zooarchaeologists working at the site teamed up with a team of geneticists, who could cluster the mitochondrial DNA of ancient and modern individuals of Nile catfish into phylogenetic lineages from different regions. The analyses designated the lower Nile as the source of the Nile catfish bones in Sagalassos.[61]

Zooarchaeological remains found in the recently excavated Theodosian harbor of Constantinople (Yenikapı) open a whole new window to the lively cosmopolitan lifestyle of the capital of the Byzantine Empire. The gradually silted sediments in the harbor, which were uncovered as part of a development project, were packed with pottery, especially amphorae, shipwrecks and animal bones. Among these, in addition to the bones of common domestic and wild animals, a large range of exotic species was identified, including elephants, ostriches, gazelles and even macaques.[62] The mixed context of the remains does not allow inferences as to whether these exotic animals belonged to the royal menageries or other elite households or if they (or at least some) were the remains of luxury foods. The involvement of Medieval İstanbul in the processed fish trade was well-known from historical sources,[63] but the discovery of a shipwreck containing amphorae filled with preserved fish[64] represents a unique opportunity to investigate a frozen moment in this lively trade. The zooarchaeological study of these fish remains awaits undertaking.

Conclusion

Human-mediated long-distance movements of animals and animal parts have taken place at least since the Palaeolithic, starting with the transportation of marine shells to inland locations. People were already willing to transport fresh

60 Arndt *et al.* 2003.

61 Arndt *et al.* 2003.

62 Onar *et al.* 2013.

63 Dalby 2003, 67–68.

64 Kocabaş 2008.

or preserved animal-based food stuffs over considerable distances starting in the seventh millennium BC at the latest, even though these foodstuffs had very little nutritional value. Also in the seventh millennium BC, people were transporting not only domestic livestock but also untamed captives, such as the fallow deer, over land and sea. Evidence for the long-distance movements of animals and animal parts in the Bronze and Iron Ages demonstrate how interwoven the demand for imported items (e.g., precious and rare metals) and the demand for trading vehicles (e.g., camels) have become throughout time. Exotic animals attested in the Byzantine capital show how transported live animals have doubtlessly become objects to inspire, awe and to impress (status symbols, in other words) in urbanized Medieval contexts.

Evidence indicating the transport of dead animals, animal parts, livestock and wild animal populations can greatly enhance discussions about connectivity, mobility and long-distance contact in Anatolian prehistory in particular, and the prehistory of the Eastern Mediterranean in general. The majority of the examples I gave come from macroscopic studies (e.g., conventional zooarchaeology), and few come from research looking at the molecular constituents and biometric properties of animal remains. The latter kind of research is becoming more common and more advanced in archaeological sciences, which makes it increasingly potent to recover hidden evidence in bones and reveal patterns of the regional and long-distance mobility of animals. Hopefully, we will be seeing intensified efforts towards this direction in the archaeology of Turkey, not only covering its prehistory, but all time periods. Bridging the obvious divide between the so-called material culture studies in archaeology, the domain which normally studies regional and long-distance relationships among ancient communities, and environmental archaeology, which is usually assigned to focus on reconstructing subsistence, diet and environment, will certainly make a contribution towards better understanding of the mechanisms that were devised to expand long-distance relations.

REFERENCES

Alvarez, E., "Personal Ornaments Made from Mollusc Shells in Europe During the Upper Paleolithic and Mesolithic: News and Views" in *Archaeomalacology Revisited. Non-Dietary Use of Molluscs in Archaeological Settings,* ed. by C. Çakırlar. 1–8. Oxford: Oxbow Books, 2011.

Arbuckle, B.S., "Chalcolithic Caprines, Dark Age Dairy, and Byzantine Beef." *Anatolica* 35 (2009): 179–224.

Arbuckle, B.S., S.W. Kansa, E. Kansa, D. Orton, C. Çakirlar, L. Gourichon, L. Atıcı, A. Galik, A. Marciniak, J. Mulville, H. Buitenhuis, D. Carruthers, B. De Cupere, A. Demirergi, S. Frame, D. Helmer, L. Martin, J. Peters, N. Pöllath, K. Pawłowska, N. Russell, K. Twiss and D. Würtenberger, "Data Sharing Reveals Complexity in the Westward Spread of Domestic Animals across Neolithic Turkey." *PLOS ONE* 9/6 (2014): e99845.

Arndt, A., W. van Neer, B. Hellemans, J. Robben, F. Volckaert and M. Waelkens, "Roman Trade Relationships at Sagalassos (Turkey) Elucidated by Ancient DNA of Fish Remains." *Journal of Archaeological Science* 30 (2003): 1095–1105.

Atıcı, L., "The Secondary Products Revolution in Light of Textual Evidence from Kültepe-Kanesh, Central Turkey" in *Animal Secondary Products: Domestic Animal Exploitation in Prehistoric Europe, the Near East and the Far East,* ed. by H. Greenfield, 233–252. Oxford: Oxbow Books, 2014.

Bar-Yosef, D., B.A. Gümüş and Y. İslamoğlu, "Fossil Hunting in the Neolithic: Shells from the Taurus Mountains at Çatalhöyük, Turkey." *Geoarchaeology* 25 (2010): 375–392.

Bar-Yosef, D., "Dentalium Shells Used by Hunter-gatherers and Pastoralists in the Levant. *Archaeofauna* 17 (2008):103–110.

Bar-Yosef, D., "Mollusc Exploitation at Çatalhöyük" in *Humans and Landscapes of Çatalhöyük: Reports From the 2000–2008 Seasons,* ed. by I. Hodder 329–338. London: Oxbow Books, 2013.

Bar-Yosef, D., "The Exploitation of Shells as Beads in the Palaeolithic and Neolithic of the Levant." *Paléorient* 31 (2005): 176–185.

Baysal, E., "A Tale of Two Assemblages: Early Neolithic Manufacture and Use of Beads in the Konya Plain." *Anatolian Studies* 63 (2013b): 1–15.

Baysal, E., "Epipalaeolithic Marine Shell Beads at Pınarbaşı. Central Anatolia from an Eastern Mediterranean Perspective." *Anatolica* 39 (2013a): 261–276.

Bendrey, R., "From wild Horses to Domestic horses: A European Perspective." *World Archaeology* 44 (2012): 135–157.

Benecke, N., "On the Beginning of Horse Husbandry in the Southern Balkan Peninsula – The Horses from Kırklareli-Kanlıgeçit (Turkish Thrace)." *Tuba-Ar-Turkish Academy of Science Journal of Archaeology* 12 (2009): 13–24.

Boessneck, J. and A. von den Driesch, *Tierknochenfunde vom Korucutepe bei Elaziğ in Ostanatolien.* Fundmaterial der Grabungen 1968 und 1969, in *Korucutepe 1.* ed. by van Loon, M. Amsterdam and New York: North-Holland and Elsevier, 1975.

Çakırlar, C., "Adaptation, Identity, and Innovation in Neolithic and Chalcolithic Western Anatolia (6800–3000 cal. BC): the Evidence from Mollusk Shells." Quaternary International 390; 117–125.

———. *Mollusk Shells in Troia, Yenibademli, and Ulucak: An Archaeomalacological Approach to the Environment and Economy of the Aegean*. Oxford: British Archaeological Reports, International Series, 2009.

———. "The Evolution of Animal Husbandry in Neolithic Central-west Anatolia: the Zooarchaeological Record from Ulucak Höyük (*c.* 7040–5660 cal. BC, Izmir, Turkey)." *Anatolian Studies* 62 (2012): 1–33.

Çakırlar, C. and R. Berthon, "Caravans, Camel Wrestling and Cowrie Shells: Towards a Social Zooarchaeology of Camel Hybridization in Anatolia and Adjacent Regions." *Anthropozoologica* 49 (2014): 237–252.

Çakırlar, C. and S. Ikram, "Ivory, Elephant Bones, and the Relationship between the two in Syria and Beyond." Paper presented at the *International Congress of the Archaeology of the Ancient Near East*. 2014.

Çakırlar, C. and L. Atıcı, "Patterns of Animal Exploitation in Western Turkey: from Palaeolithic Molluscs to Byzantine Elephants" in *Oxford Handbook of Zooarchaeology,* ed. by U. Albarella, H. Russ, K. Vickers and S. Viner-Daniels. Oxford: Oxford University Press, forthcoming.

Caubet, A. and F. Poplin, "Réflexions sur la question de l'éléphant syrien" in *Dur-Katlimmu 2008 and Beyond, Studia Chaburensia I,* ed. by H. Kühne, 1–9. Wiesbaden: Harrassowitz Verlag, 2010.

Collins, B.J., *The Hittites and Their World.* Atlanta: Society of Biblical Literature, 2007.

Dalby, A., *Flavours of Byzantium*. London: Prospect Books, 2003.

De Cupere, B., *Animals at Ancient Sagalassos: Evidence of the Faunal Remains.* Leuven: Brepols, 2001.

d'Errico, F., C. Henshilwood, M. Vanhaeren and K. van Niekerk, "Nassarius Kraussianus Shell Beads from Blombos Cave: Evidence for Symbolic Behaviour in the Middle Stone Age." *Journal of Human Evolution* 48 (2005): 3–24.

Düring, B.S., *The Prehistory of Asia Minor: from Complex Hunter-Gatherers to Early Urban Societies*. Cambridge: Cambridge University Press, 2011.

Erek, M.C., "2007 yılı Direkli Mağarası Kazıları." *Kazı Sonuçları Toplantısı* 30 (2008): 323–346.

Greenfield, H. J., "The Secondary Products Revolution: the Past, the Present and the Future." *World Archaeology* 42 (2010): 29–54.

Helmer, D., Gourichon L. and E. Vila, "The Development of the Exploitation of Products from Capra and Ovis (Meat, Milk and Fleece) from the PPNB to the Early Bronze in the Northern Near East (8700 to 2000 BC cal.)." *Anthropozoologica* 42 (2007): 41–69.

Isaakidou, V., "The Fauna and Economy of Neolithic Knossos' Revisited" in *Escaping the Labyrinth. The Cretan Neolithic in Context. Sheffield Studies in Aegean Archaeology.* ed. by V. Isaakidou and P. Tomkins. 95–112. Oxford: Oxbow Books, 2008.

Kistler, M., *War Elephants*. Nebraska: University of Nebraska Press, Bison Books, 2005.

Kocabaş, U., *The 'Old Ships' of the 'New Gate'*. İstanbul: Ege Yayınları, 2008.

Kuhn, S., M.C. Stiner, D.S. Reese and E. Güleç, "Ornaments of the Earliest Upper Paleolithic: New Insights from the Levant." *Proceedings of the National Academy of Sciences* 98 (2001): 7641–7646.

Lister, A.M., W. Dirks, A. Assaf, M. Chazan, P. Goldberg, Y.H. Applbaum, N. Greenbaum and L.K. Horwitz, "New Fossil Remains of *Elephas* from the Southern Levant: Implications for the Evolutionary History of the Asian Elephant." *Palaeogeography, Palaeoclimatology, Palaeoecology* 386 (2013): 119–130.

Marciniak, A., "The Secondary Products Revolution: Empirical Evidence and its Current Zooarchaeological Critique." *Journal of World Prehistory* 24 (2011): 117–130.

Masseti, M., A. Cavallaro, E. Pecchioli and C. Vernesi, "Artificial Occurrence of the Fallow Deer, Dama Dama Dama (L., 1758), on the Island of Rhodes (Greece): Insight from mtDNA Analysis." *Human Evolution* 21 (2006): 167–175.

Meiggs, D., "Herding Practices, Urban Provisioning, and Human Mobility at tell Atchana (Alalakh): 2009 Strontium Isotope (87Sr/86Sr) Results." *Arkeometri Sonuçları Toplantısı* 26 (2010): 51–68.

Onar, V., H. Alpak, G. Pazvant, A. Armutak, N. Gezer İnce and Z. Kızıltan, "A bridge from Byzantium to Modern Day Istanbul: An Overview of Animal Skeleton Remains Found During Metro and Marmaray Excavations." *Journal of the Faculty of Veterinary Medicine, Istanbul University* 39 (2013): 1–8.

Ottoni, C., L.G. Flink, A. Evin, C. Geörg, B. de Cupere, W. van Neer, L. Bartosiewicz, A. Linderholm, R. Barnett, J. Peters, R. Decorte, M. Waelkens, N. Vanderheyden, F.-X. Ricaut, C. Çakirlar, Ö. Çevik, R. Hoelzel, M. Mashkour, A. Mohaseb Karimlu, S. Sheikhi Seno, J. Daujat, F. Brock, R. Pinhasi, H. Hongo, M. Perez-Enciso, M. Rasmussen, L. Frants, H.-J. Megens, R. Crooijmans, M. Groenen, B. Arbuckle, N. Benecke, U. Starnd Vidarsdóttir, J. Burger, T. Cucchi, K. Dobney and G. Larson, "Pig Domestication and Human Mediated Dispersal in Western Eurasia Through Ancient DNA and Geometric Morphometrics." *Molecular Biology and Evolution* 30 (2013): 823–832.

Peters, J., "Chicken: Domestication" in *Encyclopedia of Global Archaeology*. 1382–1384. New York: Springer, 2014.

Potts, D., *Mesopatamian Civilization. The Material Foundations*. Ithaca: Cornell University Press, 1997.

Pulak, C., "The Uluburun Shipwreck: An Overview." *International Journal of Nautical Archaeology* 27 (1998): 188–224.

Rauh, H., *Knochenfunde von Säugetieren aus dem Demircihüyük* (*Nordwestanatolien*). *Dissertation submitted to the Institut für Paläoanatomie, Domestikationsforschung und Geschichte der Tiermedizin* der Universität München, 1981.

Reese, D.S., "Marine and Worked Shells" in *Town and Country in Southeastern Anatolia*, Vol. 2, *The Stratigraphic Sequence at Kurban Höyük* ed. by G. Algaze. 410–416. Chicago: University of Chicago Press, 1990.

Scheu, A., C. Geörg, A. Schulz, J. Burger and N. Benecke, "The Arrival of Domesticated Animals in South-Eastern Europe as Seen from Ancient DNA." *Population Dynamics in Prehistory and Early History: New Approaches Using Stable Isotopes and Genetics* 5 (2012): 45–54.

Sherratt, A., "The Secondary Exploitation of Animals in the Old World." *World Archaeology* 15 (1983): 90–104.

Storch, G., W. Schoch, W. Rähle, J. Moser, D. Burger, H. Berke, B. Albrecht, G. Albrecht and H.-P. Uerpmann, "Late Pleistocene and Early Holocene finds from Öküzini: A Contribution to the Settlement History of the Bay of Antalya, Turkey." *Paléorient* 18 (1992): 123–141.

Sykes, N., "Hunting and Hunting Landscapes" in *Encyclopedia of Global Archaeology*. 3592–3611. New York: Springer, 2014.

Uerpmann, H.-P., "Environmental Aspects of Economic Changes in Troia" in *Troia and the Troad: Scientific Approaches*, ed. by G. A. Wagner, E. Pernicka and H.-P. Uerpmann. 251–262. Berlin: Springer, 2003.

———. *The Ancient Distribution of Ungulate Mammals in the Middle East: Fauna and Archaeological Sites in Southwest Asia and Northeast Africa*. Wiesbaden: Reichert Verlag, 1987.

Van Neer, W. and M. Waelkens, "Fish Remains from Bronze Age to Byzantine Levels" in *Excavations at Kilise Tepe, 1994–98,* ed. by J. Postgate and D. Thomas. 607–612. Ankara 2007.

Van Neer, W., R.H. Wildekamp, F. Küçük and M. Ünlüsayın, "The 1997–1999 Surveys of the Anatolian Fish Fauna and their Relevance to the Interpretation of Trade at Sagalassos." *Geo-and Bio-Archeology at Sagalassos and in its Territory,* 299–323. Leuven: Leuven University Press, 2008.

Vigne, J.D., I. Carrere, F. Briois and J. Guilaine, "The Early Process of Mammal Domestication in the Near East." *Current Anthropology* 52 (2011): 255–271.

Zeder, M.A., "Pathways to Animal Domestication" in *Biodiversity in Agriculture: Domestication, Evolution, and Sustainability,* ed. by P. Gepts, T.R. Famula, R.L. Bettinger, *B. Brush, D. Damania*, E. McGuire and O. Qualset, 227–229. Cambridge: Cambridge University Press, 2012.

Zimmermann, E., *Die Tierreste aus dem archaischen Milet/Westtürkei* (*7. bis 5. jh. v. Chr.*). Dissertation submitted to the University of Munich, 1993.

Dove Cots and Dove Towers in the Kayseri Region

Ben Claasz Coockson [1]

Abstract

This article is about the concentrations of stone tower-like structures found in the valleys northeast of Kayseri. These 'towers' are the above ground parts of dove cots used by the Armenian population over a long period that ended in the First World War. There are two main types of towers and some variations, while the subterranean rock-cut cots show no standardized design or dimensions. The cots could house up to *ca.* 800 birds, which were used to produce guano. Some cots are made in rock-cut churches and dwellings belonging to the Byzantine period. The expansion the town of Kayseri endangers the existence of these structures.

Introduction

Since Neolithic times humans have always kept large numbers of animals for various purposes. All will be familiar with the traditional domesticated farm-animals, such as cattle, horses, sheep, goats and various types of poultry, all of which required housing of some form or another. There is, however, one class of domesticated animal that required a very specialized form of housing, namely those two principal representative of Columbidae, stout-bodied birds with short necks that we generally refer to as dove or pigeon. [2] These birds were kept partly for their meat, but more especially for their droppings, known as guano. This guano was used as fertilizer for the fields, but most especially for vineyards, and was preferred for this use above all other types of animal-derived fertilizer thanks to its high levels of phosphorus and nitrogen. However, since these birds are rather small compared with, for example a cow or a horse, their droppings are also very small, even if they are delivered on a more frequent basis!

---

1 Midas Han, Çukurca Köyü Yolu, Çukurca, Seyitgazi, Eskişehir, Turkey.

2 Although the terms "dove" and "pigeon" are often used interchangeably, the expression "dove" tends to be used for smaller species and "pigeon" for larger ones of the same general family. Note, for example, how in the local vernacular speech the same type of structure might be referred by one person as a 'Dove Cot' while another will call it a 'Pigeon Hole'.

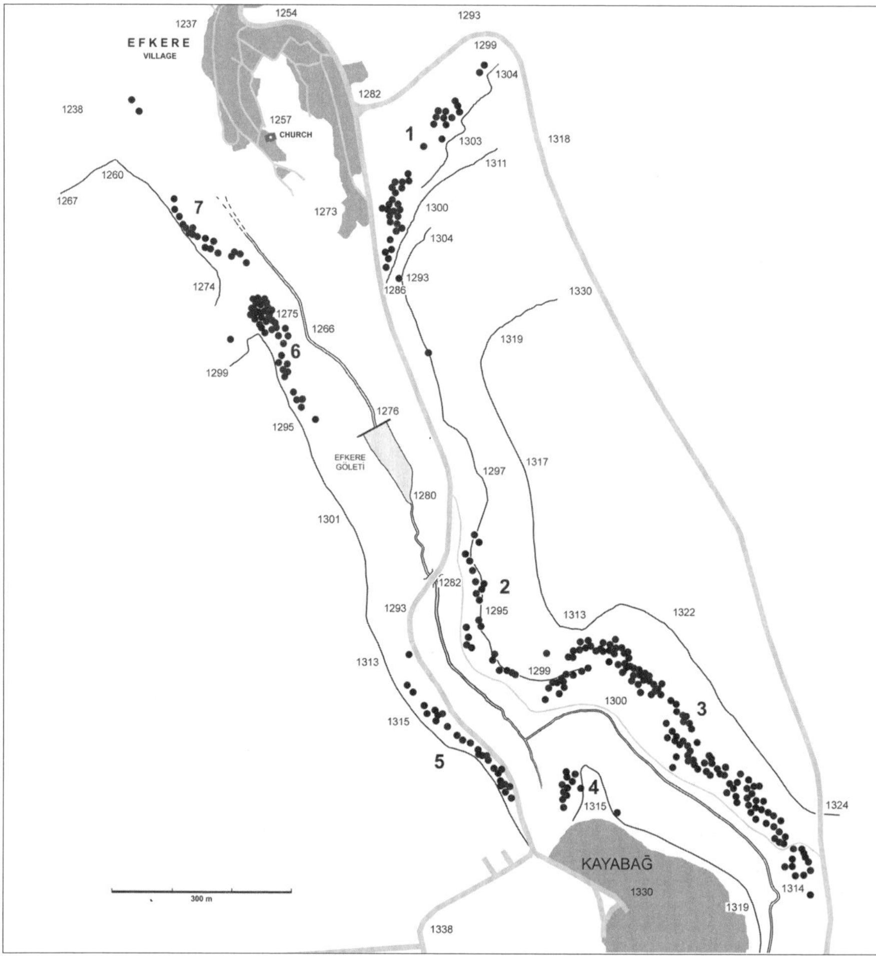

FIG. 1 Map of the Efkere valley

The point being that to get workable amounts of guano, large numbers of birds had to be kept clustered in a small area to concentrate this end product which could then be collected for use as fertilizer. To help in this concentration process, the birds were housed in masonry tower-like buildings that are generally referred to as 'dove-cots' or 'dove-towers'. Examples of these dove cots—which can often contain between 600–800 birds—can be found in many parts of Turkey, although the best, no longer used for their original purpose, exist in the Kayseri Region, a region once famous for its vineyards.[3] In this area many examples of dove cots

3 The key study of these is "A Fantasy in Central Anatolian Architectural Heritage: Dove Cots and Towers in Kayseri," İmamoğlu *et al.* 2005.

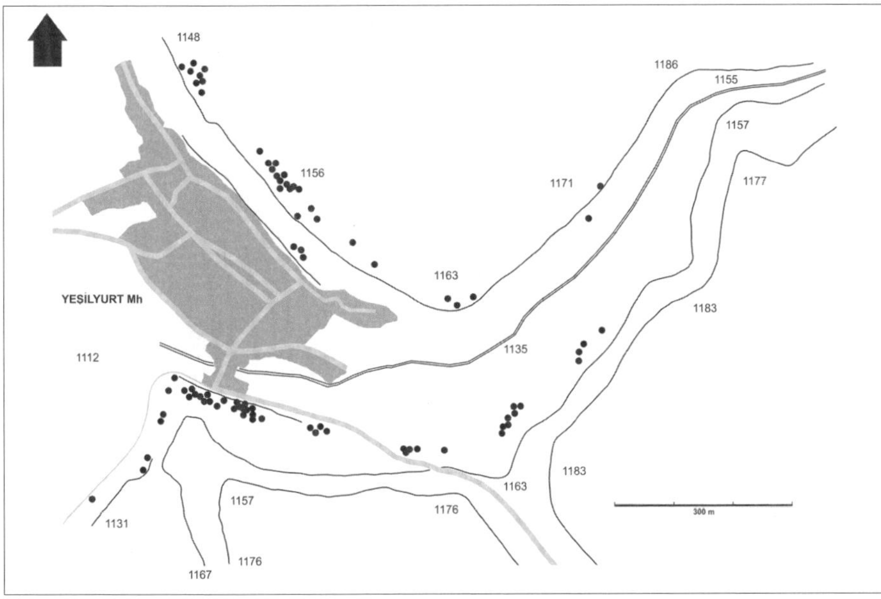

FIG. 2 Map of the Yeşilyurt area

can still be seen on the hill slopes above villages that originally had a majority or total Armenian population, as is evidenced by the domestic architecture and the now-abandoned churches.[4] The point being that with the expulsion of the Armenian population in 1915, the vineyards fell out of use, and so also the need for the dovecots. And while it might be thought that the guano produced in them would still have been of value to the remaining Turkish population in this area, the fact is that they simply felt no need of this product for the fertilization of the areas they farmed. Added to which, during the latter part of the 20th century, the density of population in the villages of central Anatolia plummeted to such an extent that even less farmland needed to be fertilized. Then, with the widespread introduction of artificial fertilizers, even less of the natural product was required, apart from which this product meant that those people who did remain in the area showed an increasing reluctance to do the dirty job of clearing out the accumulated mass of guano left by some 600–800 doves.[5]

It would be as well to stress here that dove cots and dove towers are not exclusive to the Kayseri region or even to Turkey. They exist in large parts of Europe, the Middle East and North Africa. Moreover, there are many variations in their

4 Note, however, that in some cases the dovecots are built over the remains of what are apparently settlements of Byzantine date.

5 Maybe one day someone may pick up this guano production in the organic farming trend.

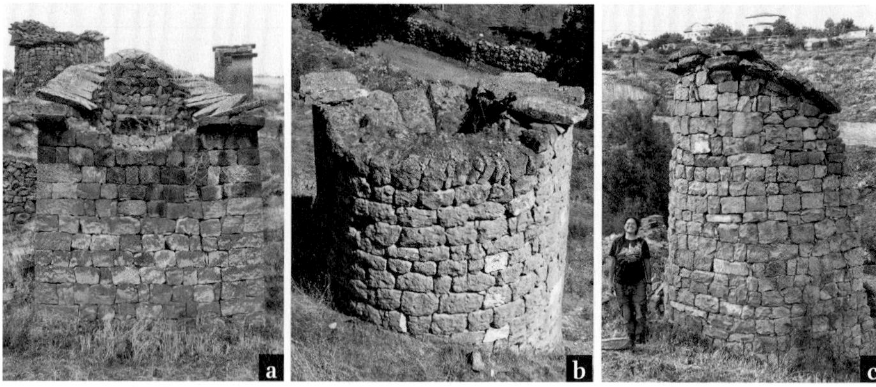

FIG. 3 Horseshoe shaped towers (type 1):

a. The 'Closed Horseshoe' type of tower, with a wide border on top used by the birds to sit on. The slot in the bottom left houses the top of the narrow hole used to feed the birds in winter. The stones are squared blocks of irregular sizes [Group 3]. Efkere Vadi, 2013.

b. An example of a smaller 'Closed horseshoe' shaped tower, the round side is on the high ground. On the wall are still some flat stones *in situ* that provide a sitting place for the doves/ pigeons and protect them from predators by the overhang preventing climbing onto the top of the wall. Özluca, 2012.

c. The height of this tower is ca. 4 m. The 'scale' is 1.6 m tall [Group 2]. Efkere Vadi, 2012.

shape and appearance. In many cases, for example, the towers house the nest-boxes themselves, and there are no underground rooms for the accumulation of the guano.

Elsewhere—and even in the Kayseri region—there are rock cut dove cots cut into the volcanic tuff, although the best examples of these are to be seen in the area now known as Cappadocia. Here, rooms were cut with the pigeon boxes covering the whole walls. But it is with the tower-like dove cots of the Kayseri region that we are concerned here, and we begin this essay with a summary of earlier research and continue with a report on more recent fieldwork by the author.

The Kayseri Dovecots: A Summary of Recent Research

These are only to be found in a small area *ca.* 18 km east of the old town centre of Kayseri, among the foothills of a group of mountains overshadowed by the volcano called Erciyes Dağı with an altitude of 3893 m. This group of mountains consists of the Turna Dağ, the Kuramaz Dağ and the Sallıhöyük Tepe; all with their peaks at around 2000 m. On their north side are the foothills with three

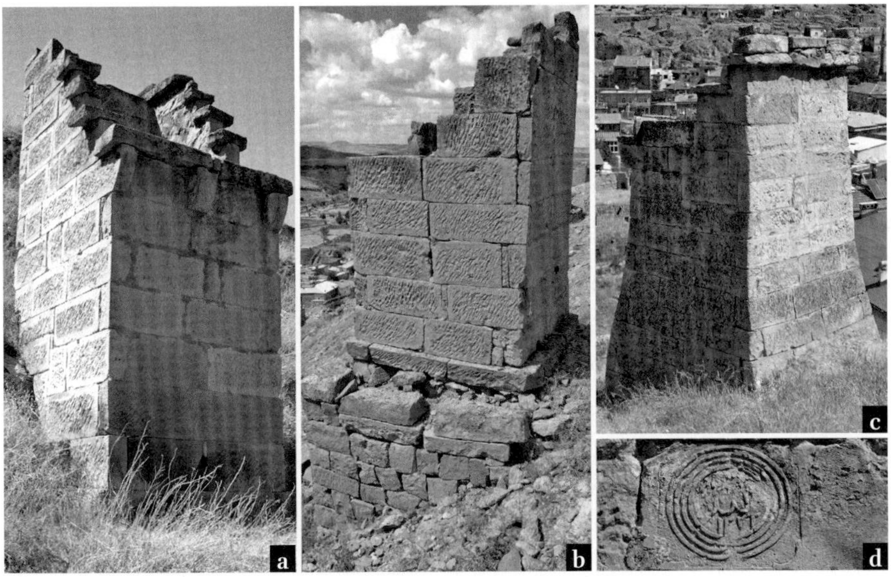

FIG. 4 Square towers (type 3):

a. A square tower. Near the bottom behind the grass in this photo a hole is visible; this was used to feed the birds in winter when there was nothing to find for them outside. Özluca, 2012.

b. A square tower built on a 'Closed Horseshoe' shaped tower. Güzelyurt, 2013.

c. A square tower with a widened base. This is the only one recorded so far. Güzelyurt, 2013.

d. Ottoman inscription on the back of a tower; nicely centred at eye-height. The date is AH 1232 = 1816/1817. Güzelyurt, 2013.

deep stream valleys, and this is where the dovecot towers are located. The towers stand usually on the higher ground of the valleys' steep sloping sides, although the tops of the towers do not rise above the valley crest. The ground level slopes so the wall at the highest side is also higher than the wall at the lower side of the slope. The rear of the tower has to be higher than the front, otherwise there is not enough height between the ground and the top to protect the entrance. The top of the tower is open to the sky, and the low front-wall side faces always towards the valley; however some small variations in orientation are possible.

These dove cot installations are divided into a subterranean part and an above surface part. Below the ground is a carved-out space measuring several meters across and high, but these are never made according to some form of standard dimensions—this space can be round, square, rectangular and everything in between, and some of these spaces have little side rooms and corridors. In the high side walls are small carved out box like holes; the nest boxes, generally called 'pigeon-holes', the total number of which can run up to 300 or 400. In each such pigeon-hole a dove family nested. These nest boxes are usually of triangular shape or with a rounded top shape.

It has been reported that each of these structures has a central dip in the floor, and which has been usually explained as a basin to collect rainwater and snow that falls through the open top of the upper structure.[6] The author of this article, on the other hand, has not observed any of these basins in the dove cots that he has personally investigated, so they might not be such a common feature as has been suggested. Moreover, however, any such water saved in these basins would almost certainly get polluted by the birds' own droppings.

In the cave's ceiling is a hole or shaft of more than a meter wide that leads straight up to the surface. Such holes would invite all kind of predators to enter and to butcher many of the birds. To prevent this from happening, the large stone towers are built on the surface and surround the holes. These towers form the 'above-ground' part of the construction.

The dove cot proper, with its nesting boxes, can be entered by humans through a *dromos*-like entrance, a very narrow trench that ends in a short tunnel. This is closed by a stone wall with a small wooden door and originally a wooden lock. This is to keep snakes and other predators locked outside. When in use, humans would not enter the dove cot very often, since it would make the birds uneasy and they might fly away in panic. The cot-room is only entered to remove the harvest of the guano. This cannot be done with large bags, since they cannot pass through the narrow doorway.

The birds used the towers all year round, and in winter when there is nothing for them to find as food, the owner had to feed the birds. For this purpose, an extra feature is added to the structure. This is a tube like hole in which grain was thrown. These tubes can be located in one of the walls or in the ground in front of the tower. The first is to allow the grain to fall into the round entrance, the second goes through the thick ceiling and ends inside the cot-room.

As expected in such small communities, the ownership of the towers was well known and undisputed. For this reason there seem to be no property markers on them, like inscriptions or graffiti. Indeed, only one of the *ca.* 400 visited towers had a decorative element (see Fig. 4d), although one other had stones reused on which a stone cutter had tried some decorative motifs. The only decorative elements are the 3 often rounded supports of the lowest stone shelf of the square towers.

The Kayseri Dove Towers can be divided into three main types:

---

6 See İmamoğlu *et al.* 2005.

Type 1: The 'Closed Horseshoe' Shaped Tower
The 'Closed Horseshoe' tower would appear to be the older type. They are larger and much heavier in construction, although there are different sizes and dimensions in this model. This type is made of small squared stones that form a neat wall-face on the exterior. The interior can be less regularly built. Between the two outer layers is a fill of stone rubble and soil, probably once a kind of clay mortar. On top there are large stone slabs that form a slanting surface on the walls; this protects the walls from rainwater penetrating into the wall construction. At the same time it forms a wide platform on which the birds can sit. In the rounded side stone 'shelves' are often added for the birds to rest on, on their way up or down the entrance shaft. The rounded side is always at the highest side, while the flat front always faces the valley's bottom.

Type 2: The Round Tower
This is very similar in construction to the type 1 tower, but the ground-plan is circular or more or less round. However as the survey shows, this type is not frequently found.

Type 3: The Square Tower
Type 3 'square' towers are much smaller in length and width and are made of thin large hewn and cut rectangular blocks that are placed and stuck together with mortar. One example in Group 1 near Efkere (tower 1–027) is 2 m wide and 2.2 m long on the exterior. Their walls are only one stone block thick, meaning that the inner space of the towers is more or less equal to the inner space of the smaller examples of types 1 and 2 towers, but with much less wall volume. The top of these type 3 towers is not slanting but stepped in the same way that the courses of the stone blocks are placed. On top of the exposed ends of the steps, horizontal stones are placed that cover the wall stones and at the same time are a platform for the birds to sit on. Also, long protruding platforms are made at the lowest sides; these are long stones over the whole width and are carried by tree supports on the exterior. These supports in the side walls are extended wall stones. Inside the tower, wooden beams can be place where the birds could rest while going in or out. On the other hand, the nice large rectangular blocks make them easy targets for people who need building material, and so many have been badly robbed.

Towers of Various Types

A significant number of the Kayseri towers occur as single examples of their type or in such low numbers that it is not worth designating them as specific types; and these are discussed in what follows.

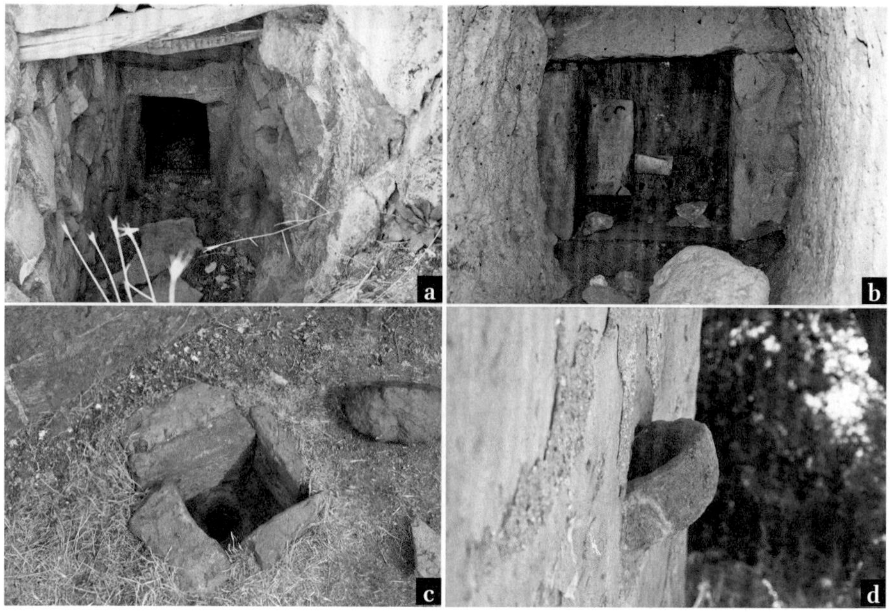

FIG. 5

a. Entrance tunnel on the valley side of the tower. Efkere Vadi, 2013.

b. Wooden door at the end of the tunnel. This lock can be opened with a large wooden key that slides from the side into the lock-block and releases the wooden 'tong' seen in the photo [Group 3]. Efkere Vadi, 2012.

c. Hole of a tube to enter food, located next to the tower [Group 1]. Efkere Vadi, 2013.

d. Stone tray that enables easy feeding [Group 4]. Efkere Vadi, 2013.

Square Towers with Widened Bases[7] and Square Towers on 'Closed Horseshoe Shaped' Tower Bases

This combination of two types is common on the North Slope above the village of Güzelyurt, and their relationship strengthens the suggestion that the square towers are a later development in tower architecture. However, the 'Closed Horseshoe' towers used as a base for these towers are in general smaller than examples of this type elsewhere. So the adduced building-type chronology that would place all of the 'Closed Horseshoe' towers as earlier than all of the square versions might not be as straightforward as it seems.

The towers are placed near the top of the steep hillslope that runs along the valley. Since the towers always stand on such steep slopes, it is easy to dig horizontally or slightly down into the hill and have enough rock ahead to carve the

7 See FIG. 4C.

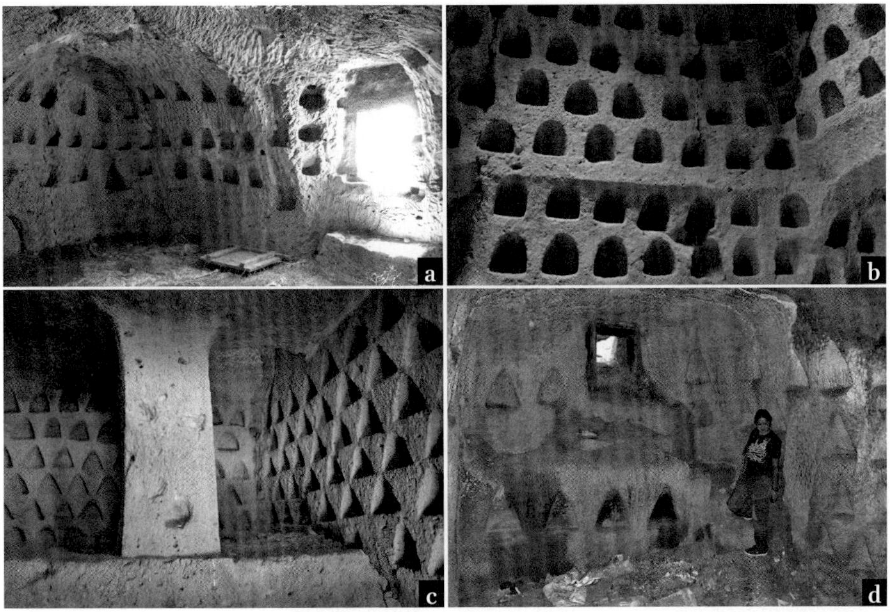

FIG. 6

a. A rectangular cut room with many pigeon-holes in the wall. The central column has to carry the roof, so the entrance hole leading into the tower is located in the corner. Özluca, 2012.

b. Reused dwelling [Group 3] with boxes cut into the walls. In the top is a blocked hole that originally might have been the chimney of the house. Efkere Vadi, 2013.

c. A rectangular cut room with many pigeon-holes in the wall. The central column has to carry the roof, so the entrance hole leading into the tower is located in the corner. Özluca, 2012.

d. This dove cot [Group 1] has a staircase inside and rather large pigeon-holes. The room has the dimensions of ca. 6 m long, 3.6 m wide and 2.6 m high. Bahçeli Köy, 2012.

required underground room, the shape of which bears no relation to the shape of the tower above the ground. The entrance tunnel for this is usually placed directly in front of the tower a few meters lower and away from the tower's base, but there are examples where the entrance is located towards one of the sides. The reason why these are a few meters lower and away from the base of the dove cot is that the ceiling of the underground room must be strong enough to carry the weight of the tower above, so usually such a ceiling will be about 1–2 m thick. In front or next to some entrances, a soil dump is often seen, where the spoil of the carving operation was discarded.

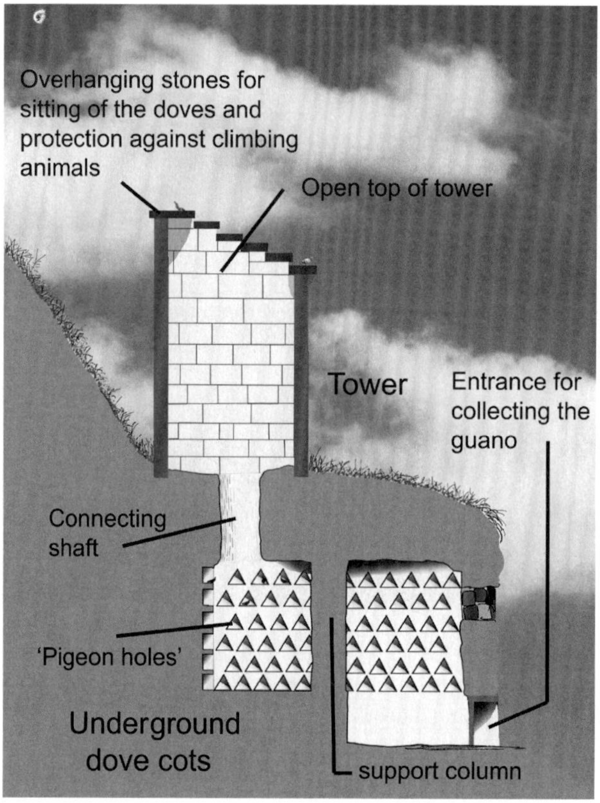

FIG. 7 Diagram of the situation in the photo of Fig. 5c. Here, there is no basin, and the guano does not fall at the same level. In the middle of the room is a supporting column left standing.

The towers are found at both sides of the valleys, more or less facing each other; wind or climate seem not to be important factors. The towers often occur in clusters above the old villages and stretch a few hundred meters to both sides if the geography allows it. In the distribution pattern, it can be observed that groups or clusters of five or six towers stand together, often separated by many meters of empty ground. This indicates probably ownership of dove cots or land, or family relations.

In general, previous work on these towers has only been concerned with the 'newly' made dove cots, those ones that have been specifically rock-cut for this function. These rooms have a single small entrance (see FIG. 5A & FIG. 5B). In front of the doorway is often a hewn platform with a few steps down to the bottom of the room. However, there are many towers that have rooms of different and earlier origin below them, in some cases even a rock-cut Byzantine church, although usually this earlier rock-cut space represents an older rock-cut dwelling. In some disused Byzantine churches, for example, a shaft was cut straight up through the ceiling or through the imitation dome of the church and a tower was constructed around this hole on the surface. If an old church or house was reused, these build-

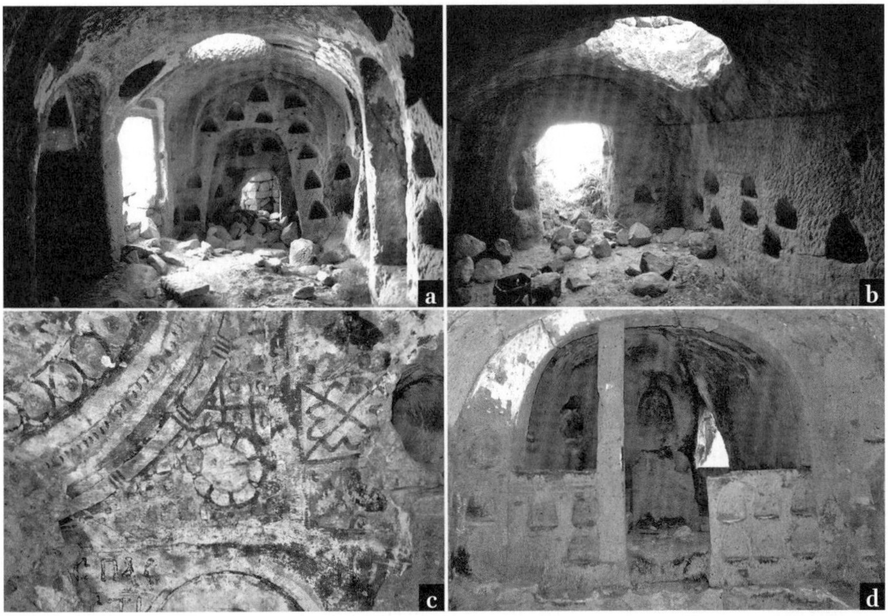

FIG. 8

a. Church reused as dove cot. The next boxes have been cut into the walls with frescos. [Group 3] Efkere Vadi, 2012.

b. A small church with the hole and the tower clearly in place, but with very few pigeon-holes. The few holes in the walls are irregularly placed and roughly cut. Bağpınar, 2012.

c. Detail of a fresco on the ceiling of a church [Group 3]. Efkere Vadi, 2012.

d. Entrance to the apse of a rock-cut church, with additional pigeon holes. Efkere Vadi, 2013.

ings usually had large doorways. These then were blocked with stones leaving only a very small square doorway, and an artificial tunnel was constructed in front of it. However, in those dove cot-churches that were visited by this writer, there was not always that many rock cut 'pigeon-holes' for the nesting birds. There were a number of these cut into the walls, but far less than what might have been expected in such a large space (see FIG. 8B). However, churches always have an apse in the east end and some side 'chapel-like' niches, and so it is possible that in these niches wooden racks were placed that formed the nesting boxes. If so, nothing remains of these putative wooden constructions. That aside, doves and their droppings were not very good occupants for the churches and their frescoes, and consequently, not many frescoes have survived to any great extent in these churches; only some patches have been preserved.

The Kayseri Dove Cots: the Results of the Field Investigation

Stimulated by the work of Vacit İmamoğlu, Mustafa Kurumaz and Çağrı İmamoğlu, the writer of this article decided to investigate the Kayseri dove cots with the aim of recording them and identifying any location pattern behind their situation. The work began with a study of Google Earth to detect towers in the landscape. This is easy when large clusters of towers occur, but difficult for single or badly preserved ones. Field investigation involved locating each tower on the ground and establishing its precise coordinate with a Garmin Etrex Summit device, this point usually being taken at the rear or the highest side of the tower, although in a few cases this was not possible, and so the coordinate was taken in front or at the lowest side. The EPE (Expected Position Error) using this device is usually between 4–6 m. Since it is extremely difficult to remember which towers had been recorded while moving around in clusters of the same type of towers that all stand close to each other, the method of study involved starting high up the hillslope and repeatedly going down and up again to move forward in what could be described as a closed front survey to record all standing towers and the remains of ruined ones. In a few instances, this method was not practical, and so the tower positions had to be established using Google Earth.

Each tower was recorded with a small Samsung camera with a sound function by which the GPS waypoint number of the site could be verbally given. Photos were taken with a Konica Minolta A2 Dimage and an Olympus e-420. To find the towers was not a problem, but to find the overgrown shafts on the hillside was difficult and not without danger. Each tower was recorded with at least one photograph that clearly showed the type and its general condition, with more photographs taken of such details as feeding tubes, or more general views showing the entrance tunnel. The state of the remains was recorded as: 1: perfect condition, 2: damaged, 3: ruined, 4: only the shaft can be seen, 5: only the collapsed underground cot-room remains (the presence of the entrance tunnel or its condition was not taken in account, since they all had one), 6: re-use of a pre-existing Byzantine rock-cut church, and 7: re-use of a pre-existing Byzantine rock-cut dwelling. [8]

Two valleys were completely covered in this field survey; these are the Güzelyurt Valley (*ca.* 1.5 km long) and the Efkere Valley (*ca.* 2 km long). Both valleys have dove cots and towers on both sides of the valley.

The Güzelyurt Valley

Eighty-one dove cots were recorded in this valley; 48 on the south side and 33 on the steep north slope. Of this total of 33, there is one rock-cut room which

8 These details are not provided here, on account of space limitations, but will be given in a final report to be published elsewhere.

is located high in the steep rock side and it was not possible to visit it to see if a tower ever existed there.

The 48 locations on the south side are divided in: four, were a hole or depression shows the former location of a cot and or a tower, one roundish tower, 17 'Closed Horseshoe' shaped towers, one square tower with a widened base and 25 square towers. Most of the square towers stand directly above the village, while most of the 'Closed Horseshoe' shaped towers stand further away in the valley, often in clusters of four.

The towers on the north side show combined designs, for example, square towers that stand on a "Closed Horseshoe' shaped base or on top of older towers. The north side shows two clusters with many towers and a few far spread-out towers. Three square towers stand on a ledge much lower just behind the village houses.

The Efkere Valley

At the north end is the old village of Efkere that before the first Wold War was inhabited by majority Armenian population as the large now abandoned and ruined Surp Stepanos church in the former center of the village shows. The remains of houses run all the way up to just below the dove towers of Group 7 at the west slope next to the village. The present village is much smaller and has been renamed Bahçeli Mahallı.

At the south end of the valley is the village of Karabağ on the west slope of the valley and opposite on the east slope is Nize now renamed as Güzelköy. In this village stands a large ruined Armenian church.

This valley is about two kilometres long and runs roughly from north to south. Along its bottom runs the Darsiakh Suyu. Dove towers occupy both sides of the valley. However there are clear clusters to be observed that can be directly associated with a nearby settlement. For example, Groups 1, 6 and 7 are evidently associated with Efkere village, while Groups 2, 3, 4 and 5 are concentrated around Karabağ. The towers of Group 2 and the north section of Group 3 are built over the remains of an earlier settlement, presumably of Byzantine date that has rock-cut churches and dwellings, graves and a water-channel.

Group 1

This group's center is located *ca.* 250 m east of the Efkere Church and forms a 390 m long line facing towards the northwest. The group has the remains of 40 dove cots and dove towers; there are two 'Closed Horseshoe' towers, four square towers, where the open top is oriented towards the southwest, 29 square towers oriented towards the northwest and five round holes that give access to the cots but without a remaining tower. The most southern tower stands about 150 m away from its nearest neighbour.

Group 2

The group's center is located about 800 m northwest of the mosque in Karabağ. It follows the rounded edge of the mountain slope and is about 250 m long and consists of 24 dove cots and dove towers. The orientation is towards the west. The cots here are frequently cut into the walls of rock-cut Byzantine dwellings and churches, located next to a long and 30 cm wide rock-cut water channel. The group contains one round or roundish tower, 17 'Closed Horseshoe' towers, two square towers and two round holes that give access to the cots but without a remaining tower.

Group 3

The group's center is located *ca.* 500 m north of the mosque in Karabağ, and is located on the north bank of the stream, with a bend near its northwest end. The group extends over some 650 m and consists of 128 dove cots and dove towers. The northwest part is built over what would appear to be the cemetery of the same Byzantine settlement. The group has one 'Closed Horseshoe' tower made of two combined towers, two oval towers made of two combined towers, seven round or roundish towers, 87 'Closed Horseshoe' towers, 31 square towers and six round holes that give access to the cots but without a remaining tower.

Group 4

The group's center is located roughly 500 m northwest of the mosque in Karabağ. The group extends for 150 m with the remains of 13 dove cots and dove towers. Twelve of these are orientated towards the west, while a single, slightly separated tower is orientated towards the north. The group has two 'Closed Horseshoe' towers, nine square towers, one round hole that gives access to the cots but without a remaining tower, and one collapsed dove cot.

Group 5

The group's center is located *ca.* 700 m northwest of the mosque in Karabağ. As it now exists, the group extends over 300 m, but it might have been longer, as it ends at a place where substantial road-widening has recently taken place, the same road having cut through a few dove cots visible on the high side of the road. The group is orientated towards the northeast. There are 24 in all, with 12 'Closed Horseshoe' towers, six square towers, five round holes that give access to the cots but without a remaining tower and one collapsed dove cot.

Group 6

This group's center is located *ca.* 400 m south of the Efkere Church, and it extends in a 200 m long line facing towards the east. There is a concentration on a steep round sloop at the north end of the group. Fifty dove cots or their remains were recorded here, 14 'Closed Horseshoe' towers, 33 square towers and two round holes that give access to the cots but without a remaining tower.

Group 7

This group's center is located *ca.* 200 m southwest of the Efkere Church and forms a 325 m long line facing east. The towers stand at the edge of the former village, and in some places there are house ruins between the towers. Of the 20 examples located here, 11 are 'Closed Horseshoe' towers, six square towers, one a round hole that gave access to the cots but without a remaining tower and two collapsed dove cots.

Conclusion

The two valleys that have been surveyed show that there still remain large numbers of dove cots and towers, although their general preservation is not very good: many are damaged to a greater or lesser extent, while others are almost completely at the point of collapse. The great danger for the future survival of these towers is the fast growing town of Kayseri, for the flat areas above the valleys are increasingly being used for construction of whole neighbourhoods that come to the edges of the valleys. There seem to be no preservation programmes for these remains, and so we end this article on the sad note that this will probably become yet one more part of the lost vernacular architecture of Ottoman Turkey.

REFERENCES

İmamoğlu, V., M. Kurumaz and Ç. İmamoğlu, "A Fantasy in Central Anatolian Architectural Heritage: Dove Cotes and Towers in Kayseri." *Middle East Technical University Journal of the Faculty of Architecture* 22/2 (2005): 79–90.

Art or Artifact?

How Museum Presentation Influences Definitions

Erica Hughes[1]

Charles and Marie-Henriette Gates each have a special place reserved in my heart. During my time at Bilkent I studied under, and developed a personal relationship with, both of these warm and engaging persons. I have fond memories of Marie-Henriette Hanım on the way to practice with her ud, or warning undergraduates not to write about the alleged "mysteries" of Egypt. Charles Bey, always approachable, even celebrated the first Hat Day[2] *with us in a fabulous peacock mask. Their attention and joy made the halls of Bilkent a wonderful place for learning. Marie-Henriette Hanım agreed to supervise first an independent study and then my Master's Thesis, the first true archaeological inquiry I ever undertook. Thus, in some small way, everything I do in archaeology will always be dedicated to her. It is to Charles Bey, then, that I specifically dedicate this paper, both in the memory of time served as his personal assistant, and in honor of his noble reaction to my infamous outburst in his History of Art seminar. May you always have students to challenge, and be challenged by.*

Abstract

This paper focuses on the many definitions of art and aesthetic value, as well as the methodologies behind their creation in order to reach conclusions about the context of museum objects and the differences between art and artifact. The treatment of this topic will be separated into three sections: I will begin by describing the ways in which our conceptions of artworks are modified through definitions, and place these definitions within the discursive space of archaeological artifacts displayed in museums. In the

1 zarathustraspeaks@msn.com. This article was written during a postdoctoral fellowship at Koç University, İstanbul.

2 Editor's note: "Hat Day" refers to March 10th, the author's birthday. In 2006, the author began asking friends and colleagues to join her in celebration by wearing a hat on that day.

second section, I will underline the special conditions of museum display. Finally, I will describe the interplay between museum context, the definition of an artwork and the role of the curator. The fundamental question then, as once I asked in class, is: "What do we mean when we discuss Art?" This is but one of a constellation of questions relevant to all archaeologists, art historians, curators, artists and philosophers of art.

Defining Artworks

To begin with, a definition is a tally of the attributed meanings to a cluster of letters or sounds created so that an outsider to a certain concept yet *still an insider linguistically* may understand that cluster and implement it in language. The definitions of many similar clusters are interrelated, such as *art* and *artist* and *artwork*, and while authors may not attempt to define any one of these terms, it is clear that they have chosen a definition when these clusters are deployed. In other words, when a theorist uses the words *art* and *artist* and *artwork*, they already have a specific definition in mind, rather than the full range of tallied possibilities. There are many different approaches to defining terms, and the type of definition chosen for deployment affects the necessary conditions and social parameters of usage for any given term.

The concept of art, until very recently, has been divorced from a physical artwork since the introduction of Platonic forms. Heidegger and Schopenhauer, with reference to these forms, both described works of art in terms of their function (to "unconceal" and to "facilitate knowledge" of these forms, respectively).[3] This focus on the relation between artworks and their effects or uses as the defining essence of art follows the paradigm of a functional approach, i.e. *What makes x an x is its serving the point of the concept of x.*[4] The point of a concept can be understood as the reason why that particular concept exists, in relation to human wants or needs. Davies provides the example of the idea of food to explain the point of a concept.[5] Food exists because we do not wish to die or be hungry. A common example of a concept that is defined functionally is that of poison, as the only thing common to poisons is their functional efficacy producing death. Beardsley, a classical functionalist, defines an artwork as "an arrangement of conditions intended to be capable of affording an experience of marked aesthetic character."[6] Yet, to this seemingly intentionalist definition, he characterizes aesthetic experience in

3 Heidegger 1975 (trans. Hofstadter); Schopenhauer 1844.

4 Davies 1991, 26.

5 Davies 1991, 26.

6 Beardsley 1981, xix.

terms of its valuable effects on the individual contemplating the artwork.[7] In his discussion of *bad art*,[8] Beardsley admits that he does not consider those artworks intended to serve the point of art, but which fail to do so, as artworks. The point of the concept of an artwork, to Beardsley, is to provide an experience valuable due to its "marked aesthetic character."[9] This does not preclude an artwork from having multiple functions, as suggested by Nietzsche in "Expeditions of an Untimely Man."[10]

If we are to view objects recovered from archaeological excavations and displayed in museums as artworks in accordance with the functional definition, we must first consider the point of the concept of any artwork. The lack of consensus as to the essence of art is largely seen as the main problem with functional definitions of artworks; in order to describe how something serves the point of art, we must know the point of art. Is a Roman *strigil* art because it achieves the function of art—whether that function is to allow the viewer to become the subject of will-less knowing,[11] or the elevation of the soul?[12] Is this function to provide pleasure brought about by the free play of understanding and imagination?[13] Simply because some object may be used *as though it were* an artwork does not necessarily make it an artwork. Let us consider this objection in more depth. Milk (placed in a mislabelled jar) can be used as if it were a poison and secreted into the food of an intended victim. Barring extreme lactose intolerance, milk is not functionally efficacious in bringing about death (the essence of a poison). Are the objects in an archaeological museum being displayed *qua* artworks? Or as objects for another, non-aesthetic, kind of reflection? In fact, a fair few publications have focused on the didactic function of artworks[14] as their true essence.

Arthur C. Danto, who rejects the idea of the "essence" of art, originally defined an artwork as the product of an "artworld" or "atmosphere of art theory,"[15] which comprises all members of the institution of art: critics, artists, gallery co-ordinators and educated consumers of art. Davies subsumes Danto's Institutional theory of art under the rubric of procedural approaches.[16] Any proponent of a

7 Beardsley 1958, 573–576.

8 Beardsley 1969.

9 Beardsley 1982, 229.

10 Nietzsche 1889.

11 Schopenhauer 1844.

12 Poe 1846.

13 Kant 2001.

14 E.g. *Art and Its Messages*. Ed. by S. Davies 1997.

15 Danto 1964.

16 Davies 2007, 44.

procedural definition would claim that art is defined by a set of rules, procedures or widely-known social conditions. An example provided by Davies of when it is appropriate to define something procedurally is the concept of knighthood, which is now bestowed for reasons other than valor in battle, thus departing from its original *function* as an official political or militaristic reward.[17] It is the process, the bestowing, that is the essence of knighthood. Where once this concept was defined in relation to merit, it is no longer used to reward service to the crown or exemplary display in tournaments, but is defined by the procedure through which the title is conferred. One becomes a knight through the procedure of bending the knee before the sovereign with a sword. More pertinent to archaeology, some objects recovered from excavation are defined procedurally, such as ground stone or chipped stone tools.

Dickie's robust institutionalism, though disagreeing with some of the "overly formal"[18] terminology of Danto, defines art as an artifact "[...] which has conferred upon it the status of candidate for appreciation by some person or persons acting on behalf of a certain social institution (the artworld)."[19] A consequence of this procedural approach to the definition of artworks is that museum display necessarily reflects the past action of status conferral. Deductively, anything that is displayed in a museum or hung on the walls of a gallery (aside from practical information such as the location of toilets and exits, or labels) becomes an artwork. Procedural definitions eschew the need for universal meaning, as *how* the artwork came to be considered *qua* artwork is the defining act. This simple approach does not privilege the intention of the artist over that of the "art world." In fact, the only necessary condition for conferral of art status is the acceptance of a pre-existing group of artists or aesthetically-minded persons. This, like any procedural approach, yields an unlimiting definition of art, as "bad art" is still art, and a person who has never attempted to create can be an artist simply by virtue of having the title conferred.

Privileging the procedure by which something acquires status over whether or how status is merited entirely divorces classificatory from evaluative issues. Other disagreements that stem from this divide include the identification of the authoritative group and the possibility of many, or elite, institutions. In the case of museum display, the authority is transparent: the curator. Yet must this authority have recourse to the historical context of an object? Margolis[20] argues that artworks are situated within a historical and cultural context, and it is only with

17 Davies 1991, 34–35.

18 Dickie 1984, 87.

19 Dickie 1974, 34.

20 Margolis 1974.

sensitivity to these factors that a piece may be considered as art.[21] An obsidian biface on display may be appreciated for its material and formal qualities such as gleam, hue and craftsmanship, and yet we have no evidence that this piece was considered worthy of aesthetic appreciation during its creation and use. According to Margolis (and other strict historicists), this tool does not become an artwork simply through modern appreciation, as it must be considered in terms of the conditions that obtained during its infancy, as well as its situation within the history of art of the culture that produced it.

Yet another approach to the definition of artworks focuses on the intention of the artist as a necessary condition.[22] In other words, if an artist did not intend for their work to be appreciated as an artwork, then it cannot be considered as an artwork. Historicist approaches to the definition of artworks consider the intention of the artist as part of the context of the creation. Even some theorists holding to proceduralist or functionalist approaches have insisted on the inclusion of intent as a necessary condition.[23] This raises the question of the autonomy of intent. Is intent alone sufficient for the determination of an object as an artwork, or can the artist's intent be subsumed as a necessary condition under functionalist or institutional approaches? There is an interesting combination of historical and intentional definitions of artworks offered by Levinson: "What makes something an artwork is an intention that it be viewed as art has properly been viewed in the past."[24] In this case, Levinson insists that intent is both a necessary and a sufficient condition for considering an object as an artwork. According to this view, any poorly-crafted, incomprehensible and generally reviled pile of matter is to be considered an artwork so long as the artist intended it to fit into a past rubric of artworks. If we presume that *only* the intention of the artist determines an object's status as an artwork, then we remain in a state of limbo in considering prehistoric objects. This renders both historical and intentional approaches to the definition of artworks an absurd exercise for the obsidian biface.

There are two other necessary conditions for artworks that are not specific to any approach, but must be discussed in terms of museum presentation: performance and artifactuality.

Performance or presentation is related to the artist's intention, as an object may have been intended to be displayed or, instead, presented in defiance of intention. Is the presentation condition necessary or sufficient for a piece to be an artwork? Those who claim that the intention to display is sufficient cause for

21 Margolis 1980

22 E.g. Hirsch 1967; Walton 1970; Levinson 2002.

23 Danto 1982, 46; Beardsley 1981.

24 Levinson 1978 as paraphrased in Davies 1991, 117.

becoming an artwork must hold that the bucrania at Çatalhöyük, which were intended to be seen, are artworks. A purely historical approach would allow for this condition, but what about objects which are both on display and in hidden contexts? An example that springs to mind from the same site are the jaws and talons buried in plaster lumps on the walls of buildings.[25] The lumps are themselves quite visible, though the bone is not. Are the bones on display? Another question raised by the performance condition is: when does an object become an artwork? When it is intended to be displayed, or when it actually is displayed? Let us again consider a Roman *strigil* as an example of an object that had not been displayed during its use-life. Does its presentation in a museum make it art? It seems then, that an understanding of the temporal context of intended presentation is important for the consideration of performance as a necessary condition for artworks.

The other important condition is that of artifactuality. It may seem unnecessary to insist that an artwork be an object, but the inclusion of musical and theatrical pieces within the set of artworks forces a reconsideration of artifactuality which, luckily, does not directly pertain to archaeologically-recovered objects in museums. The definition of artifact given in most entry-level archaeology courses depends on the human intervention in the original properties of an object.[26] A stone must be scratched, a bone pierced, a shell brought to the site through human action before it can be called an artifact. The displacement of an object's attributes need not be intentional, as a burnt stone may be the result of an uncontrolled cookfire, yet is still almost always considered an artifact. As an interesting contrast, in aesthetic theory, the words object and artifact are used interchangeably, but, as in archaeological definitions, the transformative agent that allows an object/artifact to become an artwork is human intervention. It is the type of human intervention that differs, and I would argue that one kind of intervention is necessarily physical, while the other is necessarily not.

Before I outline this argument, we must consider the relation of the object to the artwork. *Laocoön and His Sons* is both a piece of marble and a sculpture, yet we must not succumb to simple hylomorphism, as the relations between object and artwork are more complex than those of form and matter. All properties of the object are not necessarily those of the artwork. At the time of discovery, the right arm of Laocoön had been lost, so the object was disfigured. However, this did not detract from its properties *qua* artwork. Similarly, were the statue to be laid upon its side, this would not change the properties of the artwork, as orientation is a property of the object. This raises the interesting question as to the separability of the artwork from the artifact, as some properties necessarily overlap. How far can

25 Last 1998.

26 E.g. Darvill 2008.

one deform the properties of the object without affecting the artwork? Another way to ask this question is: is art status ever revoked? Or can art status exist beyond the physical object? Although the Hanging Gardens of Babylon have ceased to exist, historians still describe this wonder as a great work of art.[27]

The interpretation of objects, barring great leaps in neuroscience, is not a physical process. Judgments about style, taste and appreciation are all aspects of aesthetic interpretation. Danto,[28] among others, has claimed that the ascription of art status to an object makes a conceptual difference, that the object is transformed through interpretation. This non-physical transformation of an object into an artwork is an individual process, and the agent need not be conscious of their aesthetic appreciation. Any object that gives pleasure *qua* art to a person becomes an artwork for that person. The individual's interpretation of an object as artwork privileges the intention of the audience over that of the artist. Though Danto would have all interpretation constrained by the artist's experience,[29] clearly this is not always possible. The viewer decides that this is art..."TO ME."

Special Attributes of the Contexts of Museum Display

The crucial distinction between an artifact that is found *in situ* and an artifact displayed in a museum is that the latter is not in its original context. Many considerations arise from this basic difference. Objects have the power to transform the space around them in terms of both cultural appropriateness and object-potential. An example given by Susan Feagin is that of altar paintings, which "transform the space, and place, where they are, into one where certain ritual observances are appropriate."[30] These paintings cannot transform space in the same way when they are hung on the walls of a gallery or museum. Imagine a priest singing *Kyrie, eleison* before a triptych in an art gallery! Objects in a museum context not only appear differently apart from their original surroundings, but also function differently.[31] Paintings that once were intended to convey the sacred become vehicles for producing aesthetic pleasure (or awe at the efficacy of imperial collecting). Similarly, the altar-piece in a church suffers from a "defect of distance"[32] in that absent saints are made present through their substitute images. Once the painting is placed in a museum, this defect of distance ceases to exist, as the painting's

27 E.g. Dalley 2013, 162.

28 Danto 1982.

29 Danto 1982, 55, 56.

30 Feagin 1991, 22.

31 Feagin 1991, 23.

32 Summers 1991.

"[...] own physical presence is the object of attention."[33] While defect of distance can be a problem with representational art, museum display changes the way we would have approached an object in its original context. Three-dimensional objects are understood by the entire body through the potential for interaction. Even if we do not accept the functional definition of artworks, we can see that the object-potential of an artifact is sharply decreased by its imprisonment in a glass case. We cannot grasp a knife, don a garment, or taste a hackberry. Bodily comprehension is limited by potential. Sometimes the use-potential of an object is obscure; we cannot imagine how to grasp it, or in what way it should be used. Without some kind of bodily interaction—actual or imagined—the object remains alien to comprehension.

Another special condition of museum display is the ability to place labels near the object of attention. Labels serve to direct the visitor's attention to formal characteristics or important ideas raised by an object, and to simultaneously answer obvious questions while facilitating the generation of further ones. In this respect, the presence of labels can impose a framework for appreciation, assuming that the visitor chooses to direct some of their limited and selective capacity of attention towards the label.[34] The presentation of the historic or cultural context of a displayed artifact allows the audience to begin to place the object within the discursive space of its original deployment. While a visitor may appreciate the color or shape of Egyptian faience without a label, the information provided can promote the appreciation of vitrification craftsmanship or the uses and meanings associated with the technique in antiquity. While the artifact, rather than the content of its representations, becomes the subject, there is a new defect of distance, namely that of use-potential rather than substitution. The visitor may not be able to handle an object, but a label gives enough information to set the context. The presence of a label is unimportant for a proceduralist, yet crucial for a historicist.

The ability to control the arrangement and association of objects in museums also affects the ways in which we interact with material artifacts. Though attention is more likely directed towards objects set apart from others, the creation of a scenario of related objects helps promote a bodily understanding of context. Most museum visitors will be familiar with the shape of a sword, and so the creation of a fantasy wherein the visitor is wielding the sword is easy to imagine. A visitor may be less sympathetic to the uses of less familiar objects. A grinding stone is much harder to imagine oneself using, so a situational reconstruction with mannequins using this potentially unfamiliar tool; illustrations of use; or setting a scene with a combination of related artifacts wherein the visitor more easily can understand the

33 Feagin 1991, 23.

34 Bitgood 2000.

use-potential of this artifact can be created to facilitate contextual information. In this way, the context of museum presentation allows for appreciation of past experiences, not simply aesthetic pleasure. Similarly, archaeological artifacts can improve knowledge, as well as provide an aesthetic experience.

Conclusions

Without labels or scenarios, the audience is invited to search their reactions to displayed archaeological artifacts as mere artworks or as mere objects. However, there are other ways in which the curator may be able to take advantage of the special conditions of museum context.

To begin with, the visitor assumes that any object in a museum is worthy of attention according to some authority, that the display of each object serves a purpose. This authority, the one who makes these determinations, is the curator. However, visitors might not care about the purpose of any given exhibit; they may be too tired, in a hurry, or only interested in the extraordinary. For example, an exhibit of the seriation of protogeometric jugs could easily be passed by as just another case full of nearly-identical pots. Placement, orientation and the relations between objects can be tweaked to pique interest, to instruct, or to force an aesthetic interpretation. Setting a piece apart from the others, in isolation on a pedestal or in its own case is a conscious attribution of higher value. Without a label, a common assumption is that the isolated piece is an artwork and should be appreciated as such. A visitor is then more likely to approach the object and attempt a bodily understanding. The orientation of an object can also influence the perceptions of visitors. For instance, a carved ivory spatula may be laid on its side among a jumble of other tools, as though it were in use or, instead, upended for greatest visibility. If the practical functions are emphasized, then the visitor is invited to see the object as an example of historical grooming. If the spatula is upended, the visitor is invited to consider the intricate representations carved into the artifact. The curator's choice to place objects together also affects the type of definition afforded by the visitor, as each object can be seen as part of a constellation of past actions or as a work of art worthy of appreciation on its own merits. Disparate items that are placed together challenge the visitor to divine their relationship, as in the instance of a bronze ladle which could be displayed with other items of worked bronze, or associated with implements made from other materials in a kitchen context.

The decision to include more or less information with each exhibit affects both the probability that a bronze ladle will be seen as a representative of bronze workmanship or as part of a set of culinary tools; or as belonging to both groups. The location and size of an informative label in relation to the object or scenario it describes affect the visitor's approach to an exhibit. A curator may decide to label less spectacular items, in the assumption that they are less likely to be appreciated *qua* artworks, or label fabulous examples of craftsmanship in hopes that the physical properties of an object can entice a visitor to learn about its technical properties and historical context. The special conditions of museum presentation allow for the creation of a definition through the properties of the information provided with an object or set of objects.

The interplay between museum context, the definition of an artwork, and the role of the curator in taking advantage of the museum conditions to direct attention towards certain properties of an exhibit create a liminal situation in which an object is neither wholly an artwork, nor wholly a teaching aid. The display of an artifact recovered through archaeological excavation in a museum then has a twofold goal: to improve knowledge and to provide aesthetic experience. The curator guides the conscious appreciation of museum exhibits through the creation and use of the special contexts of display. The attributes of both object and artwork are subsumed within archaeological artifacts, and the tension between these properties engages the visitor and encourages them to define what they view. Thus, an object's categorization as art or artifact by the visitor depends on the physical, relational and informative contexts provided by the curator.

REFERENCES

Beardsley, M., *Aesthetics: Problems in the Philosophy of Criticism*. 2nd ed. Indianapolis: Hackett Publishing Company, Inc., 1981.

———. *Aesthetics: Problems in the Philosophy of Criticism*. New York: Harcourt Brace and World, 1958.

Bitgood, S., "The Role of Attention in Designing Effective Interpretive Labels." *Journal of Interpretation Research* 5.2 (2000): 31–45.

Dalley, S., *The Mystery of the Hanging Garden of Babylon: An elusive world wonder traced*, Oxford: Oxford University Press, 2013.

Danto, A., "The Artworld." *Journal of Philosophy* LXI(1964): 571–584.

———. *Transfiguration of the Commonplace: A Philosophy of Art*. Cambridge: Harvard University Press, 1982.

Darvill, T., "Artefact" in *The Concise Oxford Dictionary of Archaeology*. Oxford: Oxford University Press, 2008.

Davies, S., *Definitions of Art*. Ithaca: Cornell University Press, 1991.

———. (ed) *Art and its Messages: Meaning, Morality and Society*. University Part: Pennsylvania State University Press, 1997.

———. *Philosophical Perspectives on Art*. Oxford: Oxford University Press, 2007.

Dickie, G., *Art and the Aesthetic: An Institutional Analysis*. Ithaca: Cornell University Press, 1974.

———. *The Art Circle: A Theory of Art*. New York: Haven, 1984.

Feagin, S., "Paintings and Their Places." *Australasian Journal of Philosophy* Pp. 260–268. Reprinted in *Art and Its Messages: Meaning, Morality, and Society*, ed. by S. Davies, 17–25 Pennsylvania State University Press, 1994.

Heidegger, M., *Poetry, Language, Thought* trans. by A. Hofstadter. New York: Harper and Row, 1975.

Hirsch, Jr, E., *Validity in Interpretation*. New Haven: Yale University Press, 1967.

Kant, I., *Critique of the Power of Judgment* trans. by P. Guyer and E. Matthews. Cambridge: Cambridge University Press, 2001.

Last, J., "A Design for Life: Interpreting the Art of Çatalhöyük." *Journal of Material Culture* 3.3 (1998): 355–378.

Levinson, J., "Defining Art Historically." *British Journal of Aesthetics* 19.3 (1979): 232–250.

———. "Hypothetical Intentionalism: Statements, Objectives and Replies" in *Is There a Single Interpretation*? ed. by M. Krausz, University Park: Pennsylvania State University Press, 2002.

Margolis, J., "Works of Art as Physically Embodied and Culturally Emergent Entities." *British Journal of Aesthetics* 14.3 (1974): 187–196.

———. *Art and Philosophy*. Atlantic Highlands: Humanities Press, 1980.

Nietzsche, F., "Expeditions of an Untimely Man" in *Twilight of the Idols* trans. by D. Large. Oxford: Oxford University Press, 1998.

Poe, E.A., "The Philosophy of Composition." *Graham's Magazine* XXVIII.4 (1846): 163–167.

Schopenhauer, A., *The World as Will and Representation,* trans. by E.F.J. Payne, 1958. Colorado: The Falcon's Wing, 1844.

Summers, D., "Real Metaphor" in *Visual Theory: Painting and Interpretation*, ed. by N. Bryson, M. Holly and K. Moxey, 231–259. New York: Harper Collins, 1991.

Walton, K., "Categories of Art." *The Philosophical Review* 79 (1970): 334–367.

A New Interpretation of Beads in their Archaeological and Cultural Context

Sinan Kılıç[1]

Abstract

Beads are known to have been used as early as the Palaeolithic period and have been an essential aspect of human life ever since. Even though they are usually used for decorative purposes today, evil-eye beads are also used for protection. This helps us understand different functions of beads in the past as well. Folk legends from Eastern Turkey inform us about the non-decorative functions of beads depending on their colour, shape and size. Therefore, beads in archaeological contexts should be analysed not only typologically but culturally as well. Such analyses are possible through interdisciplinary studies including anthropology, ethnology, and folklore.

Introduction

Beads found in archaeological sites indicate their significance in human history. Regardless of their common use as ornaments today, beads probably had multiple functions in the past depending on their colour, shape and size. Evil-eye beads and prayer beads are good examples of their multi-functional use today, as mentioned in a number of folk legends from Eastern Turkey.

Some argue that ornaments could be used for interpersonal communication;[2] therefore, studying the use patterns of ornaments would help us understand early human behaviour.[3] They would also shed light on cultural behaviour of Neanderthals and even earlier hominids.[4]

Ornamentation always impresses others by displaying power and glory. It also expresses cultural identity, sexuality or personal preferences.[5] A ring on a finger

---

1 Arkeoloji Bölümü, Edebiyat Fakültesi, Yüzüncü Yıl Üniversitesi, Kampüs, Van, Turkey.

2 Nobel and Davidson 1996; Mithen 1996; Klein 2009.

3 Mc Brearty and Brooks 2000; Marshack 1990; Clark and Lindly 1989.

4 Hayden 1993.

5 Kuhn *et al.* 2001.

indicates marital status, the value of a necklace displays the level of wealth and different types of amulets could be used as expressions of faith or ideologies or for protection from the evil eye. For example, based on an ethnographic study in Turkey, a toddler with a speech delay can be 'cured' by carrying a string of blue beads.[6]

Based on the use of beads for multiple functions today, the same inference can be made about the past. A variety of ornaments found in burial sites may indicate the beliefs of people in using them in the afterlife. Anatolian Turkmen women are still buried fully adorned with their ornaments today.[7]

Semi-precious stones used for bead production have special meanings in different cultures. For example, different rocks are believed to have gender identities based on their form, colour and brightness. In ancient Mesopotamia, rocks with vivid colours were assumed to be masculine, whereas others with faded colours were assumed to be feminine.[8] Such valuable information should be used in the interpretation of beads recovered from archaeological sites.

Evidence of the Earliest Beads

The early use of beads in past human cultures has been confirmed through archaeological research.[9] In the Skhul Cave located on the east coast of the Mediterranean Sea, a perforated seashell ornament was found and dated to 135,000–100,000 years ago.[10] In the same region, a perforated seashell painted with redochre was discovered in the Quafzeh Cave that is approximately 92,000 years old.[11] In the Pigeon Rock Shelter in Morocco, a worked seashell was found in the Middle Palaeolithic layer and dated to approximately 82,000 B.P.[12] In the 1990s, numerous perforated seashells identified as beads were discovered in the Blombos Cave located on the east coast of South Africa and dated to approximately 75,000 B.P.[13]

Some experts are sceptical about the use of beads as ornaments prior to the early stages of the Upper Palaeolithic Period.[14] Some believe that the use of bead ornaments spread from Africa to Europe and Asia based on the evidence from the

6 Örnek 1995, fig. 39.

7 Tansuğ 2004.

8 Tanyu 1968; Eliade 2003.

9 Dubin 1987, 2009.

10 Vanhaeren *et al.* 2006.

11 Bar-Yosef Mayer *et al.* 2009.

12 Bouzouggar *et al.* 2007.

13 Henshilwood *et al.* 2004; d'Errico *et al.* 2005.

14 Chase and Dibble 1987; Mellars 1996, 372–375; Mc Brearty and Brooks 2000; Dubin 2009.

Early Upper Palaeolithic sites of Üçağızlı Cave in Turkey and Ksar 'Akil Rock Shelter in Lebanon, where large numbers of perforated seashells were documented.[15] A seashell with two holes was also found in Kostenki IVb in Russia dated to the same time period.[16] Perforated bear and fox teeth were recovered from the 11th level of Bacho Kiro Cave in Bulgaria dated to 38,000–35,000 B.P.[17] A perforated cattle tooth and other decorated bones with incisions are also known from Kara Bom in Russia in the Altai region,[18] also dated to the same time period. A number of worked ostrich eggshells from Enkapune Ya Muto Cave in Kenya may indicate the presence of a bead manufacturing area.[19] In Abri Castanet in France, a number of semi-finished beads exhibiting different stages of production and a number of "basket-formed" bone-beads were recovered from the early Upper Palaeolithic layers.[20]

Bead Legends from Eastern Turkey

Traditional beliefs on bead use in the Ağrı and Kars regions of Eastern Turkey are very remarkable. Beads in this area are believed to have magical powers, such as protecting one from the evil eye or having the ability to heal illness depending on their colour and shape. For example, a mother wears white beads to produce plenty of milk for her baby. Cows are decorated with larger white beads, also for the same reason (Fig. 1a). Reddish beads represent the colour of blood and are believed to heal various diseases (Fig. 1b–c). A heart-shaped bead is believed to heal heart problems (Fig. 1b). Interestingly, the supernatural powers of beads are also mentioned in folk legends such as "living beads" or beads that help women to get pregnant. In addition, sacred meanings may also be ascribed to some beads.

Four folk legends regarding bead use are documented from the Ağrı-Doğubeyazıt and Kars-Kağızman regions:[21]

Legend 1: Legend of Beads with Evil Powers from Ağrı-Doğubayazıt

An old woman used to carry an evil bead that might hurt children. One day she visited her neighbour, and as soon as she stepped in the door, the neighbour's young son started crying, and he suddenly became ill. The old

15 Kuhn *et al.* 2001; Stiner *et al.* 2013.

16 Anikovich *et al.* 2007.

17 Fernández and Jöris 2007.

18 Derevianko and Rybin 2003.

19 Ambrose 1998.

20 White 2007.

21 These legends were compiled by Ruşen Aksoy, member of the Archaeology Club of Yüzüncü Yıl University.

woman realised that this was the doing of the bead, so she put the bead in a bowl of water. In order to heal, the boy needed to drink this water. However, his condition worsened in the following days. After realising that the bead itself was the reason for his illness, the boy's family came to the conclusion that the bead was alive and needed to be killed. They burned the bead in a fire, and, as a result, the boy was cured.

Legend 2: Legend of the "Child Bead" from Ağrı-Doğubayazıt
One day, a woman who could not get pregnant found a long, oval, greyish-coloured bead in a creek. After some time, she got pregnant. Therefore, it was believed that the bead helped the woman get pregnant. So, they called it a "child bead". It was believed that it was actually a bird's egg that fell from the sky. However, this bead was also believed to possess evil powers. If it was mistakenly brought into a house with a pregnant woman or a child, the woman might have a miscarriage or the child might die. The bead must be put in water and that water in turn should be used to make bread. Eating that bread would heal the woman or the child.

Legend 3: Legend about a Bead from Akça Village near Kars-Kağızman
One day, while a man was herding his goats on the mountains, it started raining, and the rain gradually turned into hail. The man took shelter under a tree. Suddenly, a bead with white, grey, and pink colours, with a picture of the moon on one side and the sun on the other, fell from the sky. The man took the bead and believed it possessed healing powers. When a barren woman puts the bead into a bowl of water and drinks it, it is believed that she can get pregnant.

Legend 4: A Folk Belief from Kağızman-Kars
Mothers of infants who lack milk wear white beads to produce milk. It is believed that this bead comes from the Kaaba in Mecca.

Conclusion

Folk tales and beliefs provide us with plenty of material to be used in the interpretation of archaeological data. Philologist, historian and folklorist Abdülkadir İnan (1889–1980) writes: "Intangible aspects of cultures such as legends, stories and folk tales enlighten us about the unknowns of non-material culture, just as potteries and weapons recovered from archaeological sites teach us various stages of the material culture of the past."[22] These words emphasize the importance of our knowledge of

22 İnan 1938, 71.

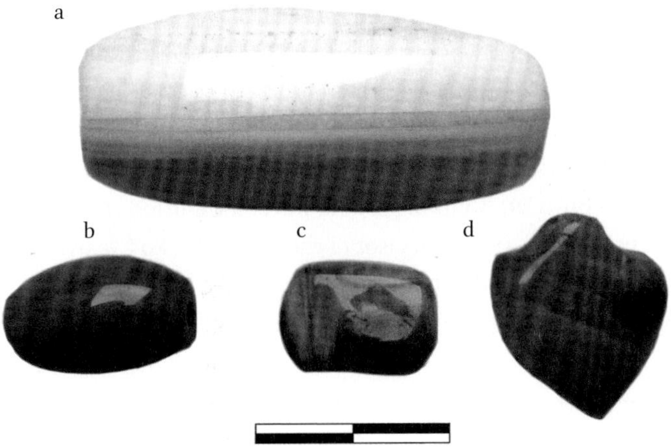

FIG. 1 Healing beads from the Ağrı region of Eastern Turkey.

beliefs and traditions accumulated through thousands of years. Products of non-material culture would help us understand the origins of traditions and beliefs. In addition, we would be able to interpret the cultural material in a better way by using the elements of non-material culture such as "ancient myths, folktales, wild spirits, and pagan traditions", instead of simply studying their production techniques.[23]

Beads recovered from archaeological sites are usually described for their visible traits or manufacturing techniques.[24] While a complex system of bead classification includes a vast variety of raw materials and production techniques, there are only a few studies that mention, for instance, the concept of the "evil eye" in the analysis of beads.[25] Due to their common use, evil-eye beads are often subject to ethnographic and folkloric research.[26] For example, in Turkey, the evil-eye beads are widely used in nearly every house, workplace or vehicle for protection from evil powers.

Evil-eye beads and shells of *monetaria moneta* used today are clearly reflections of ancient traditions in the Near East. With the help of folk beliefs, we can explore new ways in interpreting cultural material such as beads recovered at archaeological sites. Therefore, we should ask questions like how and why a specific bead was used in its cultural context. Thus, the study of archaeological findings should involve the methods of anthropology, ethnology and folklore.

23 Anhtony 1996.

24 Kenoyer 1991; Gündoğdu 2004.

25 Örnek 1995; Akpınarlı 1996.

26 Acıpayamlı 1962.

Acknowledgement

An earlier version of this paper was presented on September 7th, 2005 at the International Symposium on Mount Ararat and Noah's Ark at Doğubayazıt. The paper was revised for the Festschrift in honour of Marie-Henriette and Charles Gates. Many thanks go to the editors of this book for the interest they have shown. Also sincere thanks go to Prof. Dr. İlhan Başgöz for his contributions and suggestions, and to Mrs. Begüm Başoğlu, the supervisor of the Vitali Hakko Creative Industries Library at Nakkaştepe-İstanbul, for helping me with the library research. Special thanks go to Ayşe Taşkıran who helped me edit this paper.

REFERENCES

Acıpayamlı, O., "Anadolu'da Nazarla İlgili Bazı Âdet ve İnanmalar." *Ankara Üniversitesi Dil ve Tarih Coğrafya Dergisi* 20 (1962): 1–20.

Akpınarlı, F., "Anadolu'da Nazar ve Nazarlıklar." *I. Türk Halk Kültürü Araştırma Sonuçları Sempozyum Bildirileri*, 158–164. Ankara 1996.

Ambrose, S.H., "Chronology of the Later Stone Age and Food Production in East Africa." *Journal of Archaeological Science* 25 (1998): 377–392.

Anikovich, M.V., A.A. Sinitsyn, J.F. Hoffecker, V.T. Holliday, V.V. Popov, S.N. Lisitsyn, S.L. Forman, G.M. Levkovskaya, G.A. Pospelova, I.E. Kuz'mina, N.D. Burova, P. Goldberg, R.I. Macphail, B. Giaccio and N.D. Praslov, "Early Upper Paleolithic in Eastern Europe and Implications for the Dispersal of Modern Humans." *Science* 315 (2007): 223–225.

Anthony, D.W., "Nazi and Eco-feminist Prehistories: Ideology and Empiricism in Indo-European archaeology" in *Nationalism, Politics and Practice of Archaeology*, ed. by P. L. Kohl, 82–96. Cambridge: Cambridge University Press, 1996.

Bar-Yosef Mayer, D., B. Vandermeersch and O. Bar-Yosef, "Shells and Ochre in Middle Paleolithic Qafzeh Cave, Israel: Indications for Modern Behaviour." *Journal of Human Evolution* 56 (2009): 307–314.

Bouzouggar, A., N. Barton, M. Vanhaeren, F. d'Errico, S. Collcutt, T. Higham, E. Hodge, S. Parfitt, E. Rhodes, J.L. Schwenninger, C. Stringer, E. Turner, S. Ward, A. Moutmir and A. Stambouli, "82,000-year-old Shells Beads from North Africa and Implications for the Origins of Modern Human Behaviour." *Proceedings of the National Academy of Sciences of the United States of America* 104/24 (2007): 9964–9969.

Chase, P. and H. Dibble, "Middle Paleolithic Symbolism: A Review of Current Evidence and Interpretation." *Journal of Anthropological Archaeology* 6 (1987): 263–296.

Clark, G.A. and J. Lindly, "Modern Human Origins in the Levant and Western Asia: The Fossil and Archaeological Evidence." *American Anthropology* 91 (1989): 962–986.

Derevianko, A.P. and E.P. Rybin, "The Earliest Representations of Symbolic Behaviour by Palaeolithic Humans in the Altai Mountains." *Archaeology, Ethnology & Anthropology of Eurasia* 3/15 (2003): 27–50.

Eliade, M., *Demirciler ve Simyacılar* trans. by Mehmet Emin Özcan. İstanbul: Kabalcı Yayınları, 2003.

d'Errico, F., C. Henshilwood, M. Vanhaeren and K. van Niekerk, "Nassarius Kraussianus Shell Beads from Blombos Cave: Evidence for Symbolic Behaviour in the Middle Stone Age." *Journal of Human Evolution* 48 (2005): 3–24.

Fernández, E.Á. and O. Jöris, "Personal Ornaments in the Early Upper Paleolithic of Western Eurasia: An Evalution of the Record." *Eurasian Prehistory* 5/2 (2007): 31–44.

Gündoğdu, H., "Patterns of Black Amber Bead Making Northeast Anatolia" in *Ethnoarchaeological Investigations in Rular Anatolia*, ed. by T. Takaoğlu, 115–126. İstanbul: Ege Yayınları, 2004.

Hayden, B., "The Cultural Capacities of Neandertals: A Review and Re-evaluation." *Journal of Human Evolution* 24 (1993): 113–146.

Henshilwood, C.S., F. d'Errico, M. Vanhaeren, K. van Niekerk and Z. Jacobs, "Middle Stone Age Shell Beads from South Africa." *Science* 304 (2004): 404.

İnan, A., "Epope ve Hurafe Motiflerinin Tarih Bakımından Önemi." *Çığır*, Kasım (1938): 71–72.

Kenoyer, J.M., "Lapis Lazuli bead making in Khambat, India." *World Archaeology* 23 (1991): 44–65.

Klein, R.G., *The Human Career.* Chicago: University of Chicago Press, 2009.

Kuhn, S.L., M.C. Stiner, D.S. Reese and E. Güleç, "Ornaments of the Earliest Upper Paleolithic: New Insights from the Levant." *Proceedings of the National Academy of sciences of the U.S.A.* 98/13 (2001): 7641–7646.

Marshack, A., "Early Human Symbol and Evolution of the Human Capacity" in *The Emergence of Modern Humans: An Archaeological Perspective*, ed. by P. Mellars, 457–499. Ithaca: Cornell University Press, 1990.

Mc Brearty, S. and A. Brooks, "The Revolution that Wasn't: A New Interpretation of the Origin of Modern Human Behaviour." *Journal of Human Evolution* 39 (2000): 456–463.

Mellars, P., *The Neanderthal Legacy: An Archaeological Perspective from Western Europe.* Princeton: Princeton University Press, 1996.

Mithen, S., *The Prehistory of the Mind: A Search for the Origins of Art, Religion and Science.* London: Thames & Hudson, 1996.

Nobel, W. and I. Davidson, *Human Evolution, Language and Mind.* Cambridge: Cambridge University Press, 1996.

Örnek, S.V., *Türk Halk Bilimi.* Ankara, 1995.

Stiner, M.C., Kuhn, S.L. and E. Güleç, "Early Paleolithic shell beads at Üçağızlı Cave I (Turkey): Technology and the socioeconomic context of ornament life-histories." *Journal of Human Evolution* 64 (2013): 380–398.

Tansuğ, S., "Anadolu Takıları." *Skylife*, Eylül (2004): 96–104.

Tanyu, H. *Türklerde Taşla İlgili İnançlar.* Ankara, 1968.

Vanhaeren, M., F. d'Errico, C. Stringer, S.L. James, J.A. Todd and H.K. Mienis, "Middle Paleolithic Shell Beads in Israel and Algeria." *Science* 312 (2006): 1785–1788.

White, R., "Systems of Personal Ornamentation in the Upper Paleolithic: Methodological Challenges and New Observations" in *Rethinking the Human Revolution: New Behavioural and Biological Perspectives on the Origin and Dispersal of Modern Humans*, ed. by P. Mellars, K. Boyle, O. Bar-Yosef and C. Stringer, 287–302. Cambridge: McDonald Institute for Archaeological Research, 2007.

Index

Historical Names

Geographical and Topographical Names

E

F

G

H

Divine and Mythological Names

D-E

G-H

I-M

N

P-S

Z